THE NEUROSCIENCE OF
AUTISM SPECTRUM DISORDERS

THE NEUROSCIENCE OF AUTISM SPECTRUM DISORDERS

JOSEPH D. BUXBAUM
Seaver Autism Center for Research and Treatment
Departments of Psychiatry, Neuroscience, and Genetics and Genomic Sciences
Friedman Brain Institute
Mount Sinai School of Medicine
New York, NY, USA

PATRICK R. HOF
Fishberg Department of Neuroscience
Friedman Brain Institute
Mount Sinai School of Medicine
New York, NY, USA

AMSTERDAM • BOSTON • HEIDELBERG • LONDON
NEW YORK • OXFORD • PARIS • SAN DIEGO
SAN FRANCISCO • SINGAPORE • SYDNEY • TOKYO
Academic Press is an Imprint of Elsevier

Academic Press is an imprint of Elsevier

The Boulevard, Langford Lane, Kidlington, Oxford OX5 1GB, UK
225 Wyman Street, Waltham, MA 02451, USA

First edition 2013

Notice
No responsibility is assumed by the publisher for any injury and/or damage to persons or property as a matter of products liability, negligence or otherwise, or from any use or operation of any methods, products, instructions or ideas contained in the material herein. Because of rapid advances in the medical sciences, in particular, independent verification of diagnoses and drug dosages should be made

British Library Cataloguing in Publication Data
A catalogue record for this book is available from the British Library

Library of Congress Cataloging-in-Publication Data
A catalog record for this book is availabe from the Library of Congress

ISBN: 978-0-12-391924-3

For information on all Academic Press publications
visit our web site at books.elsevier.com

Working together to grow
libraries in developing countries
www.elsevier.com | www.bookaid.org | www.sabre.org

ELSEVIER   BOOK AID International   Sabre Foundation

Contents

Contributors

Sarrita Adams Department of Biochemistry, University of Cambridge, Cambridge, UK; Medical Microbiology and Immunology, Genome Center, MIND Institute, University of California, Davis, CA, USA

David G. Amaral Department of Psychiatry and Behavioral Sciences, and Center for Neuroscience, California National Primate Research Center, MIND Institute, University of California at Davis, CA, USA

Evdokia Anagnostou Bloorview Research Institute, University of Toronto, Toronto, Ontario, Canada

Richard J.L. Anney Department of Psychiatry and Neuropsychiatric Genetics Research Group, Trinity College Dublin, Dublin, Ireland

Bonnie Auyeung Autism Research Centre, Department of Psychiatry, University of Cambridge, Cambridge, UK

Simon Baron-Cohen Autism Research Centre, Department of Psychiatry, University of Cambridge, Cambridge, UK

Marianne L. Barton Department of Psychology, The University of Connecticut, Storrs, CT, USA

Margaret L. Bauman Harvard Medical School, Boston, MA, USA; Departments of Anatomy and Neurobiology, Boston University School of Medicine, Boston, MA, USA

Melissa D. Bauman Department of Psychiatry and Behavioral Sciences, and Center for Neuroscience, California National Primate Research Center, MIND Institute, University of California at Davis, CA, USA

Jeffrey Berman Department of Radiology, Children's Hospital of Philadelphia, University of Pennsylvania, Philadelphia, PA, USA

Armando Bertone School of Applied Child Psychology, Department of Educational and Counseling Psychology, McGill University; Director, Perceptual Neuroscience Lab (PNLab) for Autism and Development, Montreal, Canada

Catalina Betancur INSERM U952, CNRS UMR 7224 and Pierre and Marie Curie University, Paris, France

Gene J. Blatt Department of Anatomy and Neurobiology, Boston University School of Medicine, Boston MA, USA

W. Ted Brown Department of Human Genetics, New York State Institute for Basic Research in Developmental Disabilities, Staten Island, NY, USA

Joseph D. Buxbaum Seaver Autism Center for Research and Treatment, Departments of Psychiatry, Neuroscience, and Genetics and Genomic Sciences, Friedman Brain Institute, Mount Sinai School of Medicine, New York, NY, USA

Guiqing Cai Seaver Autism Center for Research and Treatment, Laboratory of Molecular Neuropsychiatry, Department of Psychiatry, Friedman Brain Institute, Mount Sinai School of Medicine, New York, NY, USA

Laura A. Carpenter Department of Pediatrics, Medical University of South Carolina, Charleston, SC, USA

Manuel F. Casanova Department of Psychiatry, University of Louisville, Louisville, KY, USA

Ira L. Cohen New York State Institute for Basic Research in Developmental Disabilities, Staten Island, NY, USA

Mary Coleman Foundation for Autism Research, Sarasota, FL, USA

Edwin H. Cook Department of Psychiatry, Departments of Neurology, Pathology, and Psychiatry, NYU Langone Medical Center, New York, NY, USA

Majannie Eloi Akintude University of California, Davis, CA, USA

Jin Fan Department of Psychology, Queens College, The City University of New York, Flushing; Departments of Psychiatry and Neuroscience, and Seaver Autism Center for Research and Treatment, Mount Sinai School of Medicine, New York, NY, USA

Deborah A. Fein Department of Psychology, The University of Connecticut, Storrs, CT, USA

Eric Fombonne Department of Psychiatry, McGill University, The Montreal Children's Hospital, Montreal, Canada

Lisa R. French Autism and ADHD Research Clinics, The Montreal Children's Hospital Research Institute, McGill University Health Centre, Montreal, Canada

Keita Fukumoto Graduate School of Biomedical Sciences, Hiroshima University, Minami, Hiroshima, Japan

Ozlem Bozdagi Günal Seaver Autism Center for Research and Treatment, Department of Psychiatry, Mount Sinai School of Medicine, New York, NY, USA

Hala Harony Seaver Autism Center for Research and Treatment, Department of Psychiatry, Mount Sinai School of Medicine, New York, NY, USA

Irva Hertz-Picciotto Department of Public Health Sciences, The MIND Institute, University of California, Davis, CA, USA

Luke Heuer University of California, Davis, CA, USA

Patrick R. Hof Fishberg Department of Neuroscience, Friedman Brain Institute, Mount Sinai School of Medicine, New York, NY, USA

Christina M. Hultman Department of Medical Epidemiology and Biostatistics, Karolinska Institutet, Stockholm, Sweden

Krista L. Hyde   Faculty of Medicine, McGill University and The Montreal Children's Hospital Research Institute; International Laboratory for Brain Music and Sound, University of Montreal and McGill University, Montreal, Canada

Humi Imaki   Department of Developmental Neurobiology, New York State Institute for Basic Research in Developmental Disabilities, Staten Island, NY, USA

Yong-hui Jiang   Departments of Pediatrics and Neurobiology, Duke University Medical Center, Durham, NC, USA

Thomas L. Kemper   Departments of Anatomy and Neurobiology, Boston University School of Medicine, Boston, MA, USA

So Hyun (Sophy) Kim   Autism Program, Yale Child Study Center, Yale University, School of Medicine, CT, USA

Alexander Kolevzon   Seaver Autism Center for Research and Treatment, Department of Psychiatry, Mount Sinai School of Medicine, New York, NY, USA

Izabela Kuchna   Department of Developmental Neurobiology, New York State Institute for Basic Research in Developmental Disabilities, Staten Island, NY, USA

Azadeh Kushki   Bloorview Research Institute, University of Toronto, Toronto, Ontario, Canada

Showming Kwok   Simons Center for the Social Brain, Picower Institute for Learning and Memory, Department of Brain and Cognitive Sciences, Massachusetts Institute of Technology, Cambridge, MA, USA

Janine M. LaSalle   Medical Microbiology and Immunology, Genome Center, MIND Institute, University of California, Davis, CA, USA

Stephen Z. Levine   Department of Community Mental Health, Faculty of Social Welfare and Health Sciences, University of Haifa, Israel

Anath C. Lionel   The Centre for Applied Genomics, The Hospital for Sick Children, and McLaughlin Center and Department of Molecular Genetics, University of Toronto, Ontario, Canada; Program in Genetics and Genome Biology, The Hospital for Sick Children, Ontario, Canada

Eric London   Department of Psychology, New York State Institute for Basic Research in Developmental Disabilities, Staten Island, NY, USA

Catherine Lord   Center for Autism and the Developing Brain, Weill Cornell Medical College, NY, USA

Kristen Lyall   MIND Institute, University of California, Davis, Sacramento, CA, USA

Shuang Yong Ma   Department of Developmental Neurobiology, New York State Institute for Basic Research in Developmental Disabilities, Staten Island, NY, USA

Christian R. Marshall   The Centre for Applied Genomics, The Hospital for Sick Children, and McLaughlin Center and Department of Molecular Genetics, University of Toronto, Ontario, Canada

Christopher J. McDougle   Department of Psychiatry, Harvard Medical School, Boston, MA, USA

Caitlyn McKeever   Department of Psychiatry, University of Toronto, Toronto, Ontario, Canada

James C. McPartland   Yale Child Study Center, New Haven, CT, USA

Nikolaos Mellios   Simons Center for the Social Brain Picower Institute for Learning and Memory, Department of Brain and Cognitive Sciences, Massachusetts Institute of Technology, Cambridge, MA, USA

John T. Morgan   MIND Institute, Department of Psychiatry and Behavioral Sciences, UC Davis, CA, USA

Sheryl S. Moy   Carolina Institute for Developmental Disabilities and Department of Psychiatry, University of North Carolina at Chapel Hill, Chapel Hill, NC, USA

Alysson Renato Muotri   University of California San Diego, School of Medicine, Department of Pediatrics/Rady Children's Hospital San Diego, Department of Cellular and Molecular Medicine, Stem Cell Program, La Jolla, CA, USA

Robert K. Naviaux   The Mitochondrial and Metabolic Disease Center, Departments of Medicine, Pediatrics, and Pathology, University of California, San Diego School of Medicine, San Diego, CA, USA

Jun Nomura   Graduate School of Biomedical Sciences, Hiroshima University, Minami, Hiroshima, Japan

Christine Wu Nordahl   MIND Institute, Department of Psychiatry and Behavioral Sciences, UC Davis, CA, USA

Krzysztof Nowicki   Department of Developmental Neurobiology, New York State Institute for Basic Research in Developmental Disabilities, Staten Island, NY, USA

Alyssa Orinstein   Department of Psychology, The University of Connecticut, Storrs, CT, USA

Abraham Reichenberg   Department of Psychosis Studies, Institute of Psychiatry, King's College London, London, UK; Department of Psychiatry, Mount Sinai School of Medicine, New York, NY, USA

Timothy P.L. Roberts   Department of Radiology, Children's Hospital of Philadelphia, University of Pennsylvania, Philadelphia, PA, USA

Sven Sandin   Department of Psychosis Studies, Institute of Psychiatry, King's College London, London, UK; Department of Medical Epidemiology and Biostatistics, Karolinska Institutet, Stockholm, Sweden

N. Carolyn Schanen   Nemours Biomedical Research, duPont Hospital for Children, Wilmington, DE, USA

Stephen W. Scherer   The Center for Applied Genomics, The Hospital for Sick Children, and McLaughlin Center and Department of Molecular Genetics, University of Toronto, Ontario, Canada

Rebecca Schmidt   Department of Public Health Sciences, The MIND Institute, University of California, Davis, CA, USA

Cynthia M. Schumann MIND Institute, Department of Psychiatry and Behavioral Sciences, UC Davis, CA, USA

Latha V. Soorya Department of Psychiatry, Rush University Medical Center, Chicago, IL, USA; Mount Sinai School of Medicine, New York, NY, USA

Kimberly A. Stigler Department of Psychiatry, Indiana University School of Medicine, Indianapolis, IN, USA

Mriganka Sur Simons Center for the Social Brain Picower Institute for Learning and Memory, Department of Brain and Cognitive Sciences, Massachusetts Institute of Technology, Cambridge, MA, USA

Toru Takumi Graduate School of Biomedical Sciences, Hiroshima University, Minami, Hiroshima, Japan; Japan Science and Technology Agency (JST), CREST, Chiyoda, Tokyo, Japan

Eva Troyb Department of Psychology, The University of Connecticut, Storrs, CT, USA

Neha Uppal Seaver Autism Center for Research and Treatment, Fishberg Department of Neuroscience, and Friedman Brain Institute, Mount Sinai School of Medicine, New York, NY, USA

Judy Van de Water Department of Internationl Medicine and the UC Davis MIND Institute, Davis, CA, USA

Ragini Verma University of Pennsylvania, Philadelphia, PA, USA

Fred R. Volkmar Yale Child Study Center, New Haven, CT, USA

Zachary Warren Department of Pediatrics and Psychiatry; Vanderbilt University, Nashville, TN, USA

Jarek Wegiel Department of Developmental Neurobiology, New York State Institute for Basic Research in Developmental Disabilities, Staten Island, NY, USA

Jerzy Wegiel Department of Developmental Neurobiology, New York State Institute for Basic Research in Developmental Disabilities, Staten Island, NY, USA

William C. Wetsel Departments of Psychiatry and Behavioral Sciences, Cell Biology, and Neurobiology, Duke University Medical Center, Durham, NC, USA

Thomas Wisniewski Departments of Neurology, Pathology, and Psychiatry, NYU Langone Medical Center, New York, NY, USA

Introduction

We are experiencing a remarkable time in the study and understanding of neurodevelopmental disorders, and chiefly among them, autism spectrum disorders (ASD). ASD and associated conditions have long represented a major clinical and scientific challenge. There have been few reliable leads that provided neurobiologists with traction for the study of their underlying pathophysiology. Recently, however, genetic and genomic approaches have led to fundamental molecular discoveries that now reliably provide the basis for further studies. These molecular discoveries resisted prior approaches because of the profound complexities in the genetic and genomic landscape of ASD noted below.

We have witnessed several crucial steps and discoveries in the field. First, many studies have shown that ASD have a significant genetic component. This is important because methods of gene discovery for genetic disorders continue to accelerate at a breathtaking pace and useful because genes are natural targets for therapeutics and represent baseline units of study for neuroscientists. Second, a staggering degree of heterogeneity in the genetic and genomic underpinnings in ASD has been uncovered, with current estimates of 500 or more genes and a similar number of CNV loci, many of latter representing contiguous gene syndromes. Third, we are seeing extremes in expressivity of gene mutations that defy diagnostic classification such that overlapping genes have been reliably identified in ASD, intellectual disability, epilepsy, and even schizophrenia, representing an additional challenge. Fourth, the genes being identified are diverse and do not fit into any single molecular pathway, cellular compartment, or even organ. However, many and even most are expressed in the brain, and a significant proportion of them are involved in nerve and synaptic function. And finally, of much interest to molecular and evolutionary biologists, an under appreciated role for *de novo* mutation in ASD is clearly emerging.

With all of these complexities, one may ask whether there are any reasons for optimism. The answer, in our view, is definitely yes. The move from a protracted period of molecular uncertainty to a period of reliable findings is enormously exciting and already leading to important findings. While it is true that most, and possibly all, of the common variant association studies are false positives, we do know of about 100 genes that are implicated in ASD through rare genetic variation of major effect, representing perhaps 20 percent of all ASD genes. Moreover, we are very likely to double this number within 2 or 3 years as the methods of next-generation sequencing are applied to existing samples. Furthermore, an important outcome from these discoveries is that neurobiological models that are being developed around these genes have construct validity. This means that as, for example, a cell or animal model is developed with a disruption in a gene associated with high-risk for ASD, the neurobiological study of that model will reveal molecular, cellular, and systems-level insights into the pathogenesis and pathobiology of ASD. Similarly, such model systems, because they have such strong construct validity, have the potential to lead to novel therapeutics, and novel clinical trials are already being tried as a result, deriving from insights from the disruption of genes such as FMR1 (fragile X syndrome), TSC1/2 (tuberous sclerosis), and SHANK3 (22q13 deletion syndrome).

Finally, we now have a much better understanding of patient-based ASD research. The clinical heterogeneity of ASD has long been under appreciated, and it has hence been difficult to draw many strong conclusions from phenotyping, neuroimaging, or neuropathological studies. With etiological heterogeneity being better appreciated, together with improvements in our clinical abilities to detect and diagnose ASD and define subgroups, as well as improved brain imaging approaches and increasingly refined postmortem brain analyses techniques, all contribute considerably to forming a more cohesive view of ASD. One important direction in this domain is genotype-driven analysis, in which subjects with similar genetic liabilities are grouped for neuropsychological, neuroimaging or other analyses. The power of such approaches is evident and will bring increased knowledge of ASD pathophysiology in the same way that the genetic basis of ASD has become much clearer.

It is in this context that we have written this book. This exciting and transformative time in ASD genetics and genomics represents an unparalleled opportunity for neurobiological discoveries in ASD. At the same time the multifaceted complexity of ASD will demand analyses at many levels, from molecular to behavioral neuroscience, as well as very creative and novel approaches. For someone considering research in ASD, or seeking to expand their research in the field, having an authoritative textbook that presents many of the key aspects of ASD will provide the necessary current knowledge of the field. Through the four sections of the book we benefitted from the highest caliber experts reporting on medical and behavioral aspects of ASD, etiological studies in ASD, neuroimaging and neuropathology in ASD, and model systems and pathways of ASD, providing the reader with the strongest, current foundation in the neurobiology of these conditions. We look forward to these next few years for decisive progress on the relationships between molecular changes and changes in human behaviors at the highest levels that present as ASD.

This book emerged in conversations with Mica Haley, a Senior Neuroscience Editor at Elsevier, in the wake of a highly successful meeting on ASD organized by the Editors that took place in November 2010 in San Diego. We are indebted to Tom Stone, Kristi Anderson, and Pauline Wilkinson at Elsevier for their help and efforts during the entire production of this book. We are especially thankful to Jessica Brownfeld whose indefatigable enthusiasm and support have been essential throughout the elaboration of this book.

J.D.B.
P.R.H.

SECTION 1

AUTISM SPECTRUM DISORDERS

Alex Kolevzon, Joseph D. Buxbaum

The first four chapters in this section discuss the autism spectrum disorders (ASD) in terms of clinical manifestations and prevalence rate. Epidemiological studies provide a prevalence estimate for ASD of about 1%, with a much higher rate in males (French, Bertone, Hyde, Fombonne). There is great interest in the increased *prevalence* of ASD observed over the past decades, which is accounted for in whole or in part by broader diagnostic criteria, better identification of individuals with ASD, and reliable diagnosis at younger ages. Whether there is an increase in the *incidence* of ASD is controversial and an area of active investigation.

One important foundation for ASD research has been the careful definition of ASD and the reliable recording of signs and symptoms associated with them (Kim and Lord). This is especially important as ASD are behaviorally defined and have no reliable biomarkers. One critical finding is that ASD manifest early in childhood development, which provides both an opportunity for earlier diagnosis and intervention, and a neurodevelopmental context for the emergence of symptoms (Barton, Orinstein, Troyb, and Fein). Within the ASD spectrum, Asperger's syndrome stands as an autism spectrum condition with preserved cognitive and verbal functioning (McPartland and Volkmar).

The second set of chapters in this section discusses interventions in ASD. Behavioral interventions remain the first line of treatment and are clearly effective (Soorya, Carpenter, and Warren). Because evidence is accumulating that early and intensive interventions are associated with the best outcomes, the early diagnosis of ASD is critical. To date, pharmacological treatments for ASD focus on symptoms observed in individuals with ASD that may be apart from the unique, core symptom domains of social and language deficits (Kolevzon). With the advent of both a better understanding of typical and atypical brain function, and with better model systems, we are seeing an emergence of novel therapeutics for ASD, which provide a basis for great optimism (Anagnostou, McKeever, and Kushki).

One note around terminology in this book. Almost all chapters use the term autism spectrum disorders (ASD) to refer to disorders manifesting as autistic disorder, Asperger's syndrome, and related pervasive developmental disorders. There is an active discussion in the field around replacing the current diagnostic categories with a single category of autism spectrum disorder (ASD). For this reason, the chapters most commonly use ASD throughout, rather than separately using ASD or ASDs in different contexts. Finally, in many chapters, autism is used as a synonym for ASD. These conventions are common in the ASD literature.

Epidemiology of Autism Spectrum Disorders

Lisa R. French*, Armando Bertone†, Krista L. Hyde**, Eric Fombonne‡
*Autism and ADHD Research Clinics, The Montreal Children's Hospital Research Institute, McGill University Health Center, Montreal, Canada †School of Applied Child Psychology, Department of Educational and Counselling Psychology, McGill University; Director Perceptual Neuroscience Lab (PNLab) for Autism and Development, Montreal, Canada **Departments of Psychiatry, and Neurology and Neurosurgery, McGill University and The Montreal Children's Hospital Research Institute, McGill ‡Department of Psychiatry, McGill University, Montreal Children's Hospital, The Montreal, Canada

INTRODUCTION

In this chapter, we provide a comprehensive review of the findings and methodological features of published epidemiological surveys concerned with the prevalence of autism spectrum disorders (ASD[1]). This chapter builds upon previous reviews (Fombonne, 2003a; 2009a; 2011; Williams et al., 2006) and includes the results of pertinent studies since published. The specific questions addressed in this chapter are as follows:

1. What is the range of prevalence estimates for autism and related pervasive developmental disorders (PDDs)?
2. What are the correlates of ASD in epidemiological surveys?

[1]Autism spectrum disorders (ASD) is the modern term that replaces the former 'pervasive developmental delay' (PDD). Throughout this paper, the term PDD will only be used in direct quotations and when referring to diagnostic nosologies; otherwise, 'ASD' will be used.

3. How should the time trends observed in the current prevalence rates of ASD be interpreted?

SELECTION OF STUDIES

The studies selected for inclusion in this analysis were identified through systematic searches using the major scientific literature databases (MEDLINE, PSYCINFO, EMBASE, PUBMED), and from previous reviews published by our group and others (Fombonne, 2003a, b; 2009a; Fombonne et al., 2011; Williams et al., 2006). *A priori*, we established a population minimum of 5,000 for the current review; studies involving smaller populations were excluded. Emerging evidence from smaller studies around the world is largely consistent with the findings discussed below; the interested reader is encouraged to review studies conducted in Brazil (Paula et al., 2011), in Sweden (Arvidsson et al., 1997; Gillberg, 1987; Gillberg et al., 1995; Kadesjo et al., 1999), in the UK (Tebruegge et al. 2004), and elsewhere for more information. Only studies published in English were included, but several studies published in other languages (e.g., from China) are available for consideration. Finally, surveys that relied on a questionnaire-based approach for behavioral phenotyping (or diagnosis) (e.g., Ghanizadeh, 2008) were excluded.

Overall, 66 studies published between 1966 and 2011 met our criteria and were selected. Of these, 49 studies provided information on rates specific to autistic disorder, 13 studies on Asperger disorder (later referred to as Asperger syndrome; AS), and 12 studies on childhood disintegrative disorder (CDD). A total of 34 studies provided estimates on ASD combined, of which 18 also provided rates for specific ASD subtypes.

The surveys used were conducted in 21 different countries, including the UK (16 studies), the United States (13 studies), and Japan (7 studies). The results of over half of the studies (n = 40) were published after 2001, with most studies relying on school-aged samples. Finally, a very large variation in the size of the population surveyed was evidenced (range: 5120 to 4.9 million; mean: 291,944; median: 56,946), with some recent studies conducted by the US Centers for Disease Control (CDC, 2007b; 2009) relying on samples of several hundreds of thousands of individuals.

STUDY DESIGNS

In designing a prevalence study, two major features are critical for the planning and logistics of the study, as well as for the interpretation of its results: case definition, and case ascertainment (or case identification methods) (Fombonne, 2007).

Case Definition

Over time, the definition of autism has changed, as illustrated by the numerous diagnostic criteria that were used in both epidemiological and clinical settings (see Table 1.1.1). Starting with the narrowly defined Kanner's autism (Kanner, 1943), definitions progressively broadened in their criteria, from that proposed by Rutter (1970), and subsequently ICD-9 (1977), APA, (1980) and APA, (1987), including the two more recent major nosographies used worldwide: ICD-10 (1992) and DSM-IV (APA, 1994). The early diagnostic criteria reflected the more qualitatively severe forms of autism's behavioral phenotype, usually associated with severe delays in language and cognitive skills. In the 1980s, less severe forms of autism were recognized, either as a qualifier for autism occurring without mental retardation (i.e., 'high-functioning' autism), or as separate diagnostic categories (pervasive developmental disorders not-otherwise-specified – PDD-NOS, or autism spectrum disorders – ASD) within a broader class of autism spectrum disorders (ASD) denominated 'pervasive developmental disorders' (PDD, an equivalent to ASD) in current nosographies.

While it had been described by Asperger in 1944 (Asperger, 1944), Asperger disorder only appeared in official nosographies in the 1990s, with unclear validity, particularly with respect to its differentiation from 'high-functioning' autism. Other ASD subtypes that were described in DSM-III subsequently disappeared (i.e., autism-residual state). While there is generally high interrater reliability and commonality of concepts across experts regarding ASD diagnosis, some differences still persist concerning the operationalized criteria of ASD. For example, DSM-IV (APA, 1994) has a broad category of PDD-NOS, sometimes referred to loosely as 'atypical autism', whereas ICD-10 (1992) has several corresponding diagnoses for clinical presentations that do not allow an autistic disorder diagnosis and include: atypical autism (F84.1, a diagnostic category that existed already in ICD-9), other PDD (F84.8), and PDD-, unspecified (F84.9). As a result, studies that refer to 'atypical autism' must be carefully interpreted, and equivalence with the DSM-IV concept of PDD-NOS should not be assumed. As no diagnostic criteria are available for these milder forms of the autism phenotype, the resulting boundaries with the spectrum of ASD are left uncertain. Whether or not this plays a role in more recent epidemiological studies is difficult to ascertain, but the possibility should be considered in assessing results for subsequent epidemiological surveys.

TABLE 1.1.1 Prevalence Surveys of Autistic Disorder

Year of publication	Authors	Country	Area	Size of target population	Age	Number of subjects with autism	Diagnostic criteria	% with normal IQ	Gender ratio (M/F)	Prevalence rate/10,000	95% CI
1966	Lotter	UK	Middlesex	78,000	8–10	32	Rating scale	15.6	2.6 (23/9)	4.1	2.7; 5.5
1970	Brask	Denmark	Aarhus County	46,500	2–14	20	Clinical	–	1.4 (12/7)	4.3	2.4; 6.2
1970	Treffert	USA	Wisconsin	899,750	3–12	69	Kanner	–	3.06 (52/17)	0.7	0.6; 0.9
1976	Wing et al.	UK	Camberwell	25,000	5–14	17[1]	24 items rating scale of Lotter	30	16 (16/1)	4.8[2]	2.1; 7.5
1982	Hoshino et al.	Japan	Fukushima-Ken	609,848	0–18	142	Kanner's criteria	–	9.9 (129/13)	2.33	1.9; 2.7
1983	Bohman et al.	Sweden	County of Västerbotten	69,000	0–20	39	Rutter criteria	20.5	1.6 (24/15)	5.6	3.9; 7.4
1984	McCarthy et al.	Ireland	East	65,000	8–10	28	Kanner	–	1.33 (16/12)	4.3	2.7; 5.9
1986	Steinhausen et al.	Germany	West Berlin	279,616	0–14	52	Rutter	55.8	2.25 (36/16)	1.9	1.4; 2.4
1987	Burd et al.	USA	North Dakota	180,986	2–18	59	DSM–III	–	2.7 (43/16)	3.26	2.4; 4.1
1987	Matsuishi et al.	Japan	Kurume City	32,834	4–12	51	DSM-III	–	4.7 (42/9)	15.5	11.3; 19.8
1988	Tanoue et al.	Japan	Southern Ibaraki	95,394	7	132	DSM-III	–	4.07 (106/26)	13.8	11.5; 16.2
1988	Bryson et al.	Canada	Part of Nova-Scotia	20,800	6–14	21	New RDC	23.8	2.5 (15/6)	10.1	5.8; 14.4
1989	Sugiyama & Abe	Japan	Nagoya	12,263	3	16	DSM-III	–	–	13.0	6.7; 19.4
1989	Cialdella & Mamelle	France	1 département (Rhône)	135,180	3–9	61	DSM-III like	–	2.3	4.5	3.4; 5.6
1989	Ritvo et al.	USA	Utah	769,620	3–27	241	DSM-III	34	3.73 (190/51)	2.47	2.1; 2.8
1991	Gillberg et al.	Sweden	Southwest Gothenburg + Bohuslän County	78,106[4]	4–13	74	DSM-III-R	18	2.7 (54/20)	9.5	7.3; 11.6
1992	Fombonne & du Mazaubrun	France	4 régions 14 départements	274,816	9 & 13	154	Clinical-ICD-10 like	13.3	2.1 (105/49)	4.9	4.1; 5.7
1992	Wignyosumarto et al.	Indonesia	Yogyakarita (SE of Jakarta)	5,120	4–7	6	CARS	0	2.0 (4/2)	11.7	2.3; 21.1
1996	Honda et al.	Japan	Yokohama	8,537	5	18	ICD-10	50.0	2.6 (13.5)	21.08	11.4; 30.8

(Continued)

TABLE 1.1.1 Prevalence Surveys of Autistic Disorder – cont'd

Year of publication	Authors	Country	Area	Size of target population	Age	Number of subjects with autism	Diagnostic criteria	% with normal IQ	Gender ratio (M/F)	Prevalence rate/10,000	95% CI
1997	Fombonne et al.	France	3 départements	325,347	8–16	174	Clinical ICD-10-like	12.1	1.81 (112/62)	5.35	4.6; 6.1
1997	Webb et al.	UK	South Glamorgan, Wales	73,301	3–15	53	DSM-III-R	–	6.57 (46/7)	7.2	5.3; 9.3
1998	Sponheim & Skjeldal	Norway	Akershus County	65,688	3–14	34	ICD-10	47.1[3]	2.09 (23/11)	5.2	3.4; 6.9
1999	Taylor et al.	UK	North Thames	490,000	0–16	427	ICD-10	–	–	8.7	7.9; 9.5
2000	Baird et al.	UK	Southeast Thames	16,235	7	50	ICD-10	60	15.7 (47/3)	30.8	22.9; 40.6
2000	Powell et al.	UK	West Midlands	25,377	1–5	62	Clinical/ICD10/DSM-IV	–	–	7.8	5.8; 10.5
2000	Kielinen et al.	Finland	North (Oulu and Lapland)	27,572	5–7	57	DSM-IV	49.8[7]	4.12[7] (156/50)	20.7	15.3; 26.0
2001	Bertrand et al.	USA	Brick Township, New Jersey	8,896	3–10	36	DSM-IV	36.7	2.2 (25/11)	40.5	28.0; 56.0
2001	Fombonne et al.	UK	England and Wales	10,438	5–15	27	DSM-IV/ICD-10	55.5	8.0 (24/3)	26.1	16.2; 36.0
2001	Magnússon & Saemundsen	Iceland	Whole island	43,153	5–14	57	Mostly ICD-10	15.8	4.2 (46/11)	13.2	9.8; 16.6
2001	Chakrabarti & Fombonne	UK (Midlands)	Staffordshire	15,500	2.5–6.5	26	ICD10/DSM-IV	29.2	3.3 (20/6)	16.8	10.3; 23.2
2001	Davidovitch et al.	Israel	Haiffa	26,160	7–11	26	DSM-III-R/DSM-IV	–	4.2 (21/5)	10.0	6.6;14.4
2002	Croen et al.	USA	California DDS	4,950,333	5–12	5,038	CDER 'Full syndrome'	62.8[5]	4.47 (4116/921)	11.0	10.7;11.3
2002	Madsen et al.	Denmark	National Register	63,859	8	46	ICD-10	–	–	7.2	5.0–10.0
2005	Chakrabarti & Fombonne	UK (Midlands)	Staffordshire	10,903	4–7	24	ICD-10/DSM-IV	33.3	3.8 (19/5)	22.0	14.4; 32.2
2005	Barbaresi et al.	USA, Minnesota	Olmstead County	37,726	0–21	112	DSM-IV	–	–	29.7	24.0; 36.0
2005	Honda et al.[6]	Japan	Yokohama	32,791	5	123	ICD-10	25.3	2.5 (70/27)	37.5	31.0; 45.0
2006	Fombonne et al.	Canada (Quebec)	Montreal	27,749	5–17	60	DSM-IV	–	5.7 (51/9)	21.6	16.5; 27.8

Gillberg et al.	Sweden	Göteborg	2006	32,568	7–12	115	Gillberg's criteria	–	35.3	3.6 (90/25)	29.2; 42.2
Baird et al.	UK	South Thames, London	2006	56,946	9–10	81	ICD-10	47	38.9	8.3 (≈ 72/9)	29.9; 47.8
Ellefsen et al.	Denmark	Faroe Islands	2007	7,689	8–17	12	ICD-10 Gillberg criteria for AS	–	16.0	3.0 (9/3)	7.0; 25.0
Oliveira et al.	Portugal	Mainland and Azores	2007	67,795	6–9	115	DSM-IV	17	16.7	2.9	14.0; 20.0
Latif & Williams	UK	Wales	2007	39,220	0–17	50	Kanner	–	12.7	–	9.0;17.0
Williams et al.	UK	Southwest (Avon)	2008	14,062	11	30	ICD-10	86.7	21.6	5.0 (25/5)	13.9; 29.3
van Balkom et al.	Netherlands	Aruba (Caribbean)	2009	13,109	0–13	25	DSM-IV	36.0	19.1	7.3 (22/3)	12.3; 28.1
Lazoff et al.	Canada	Montreal	2010	23,635	5–17	60	DSM-IV	–	25.4	5.0 (50/10)	19.0; 31.8
Kim et al.	S. Korea	Goyang City	2011	55,226	7–12	27	DSM-IV	55.6	94	4.4	
Leonard et al.	Australia	Western Australia	2011	393,329	0–21	826	DSM-III, IV & TR	–	30	–	
Parner et al.	Denmark	National Register	2011	404,816	0–10	767	ICD-10	–	21.8	–	
Parner et al.	Australia	Western Australia	2011	152,060	0–10	516	DSM-IV & TR	–	39.3	–	

[1] This number corresponds to the sample described in Wing & Gould (1979).
[2] This rate corresponds to the first published paper on this survey and is based on 12 subjects among children aged 5 to 14 years.
[3] In this study, mild mental retardation was combined with normal IQ, whereas moderate and severe mental retardation were grouped together.
[4] For the Göteborg surveys by Gillberg et al. (Gillberg, 1984; Gillberg et al., 1991; Steffenburg & Gillberg, 1986) a detailed examination showed that there was overlap between the samples included in the three surveys; consequently only the last survey has been included in this table.
[5] This proportion is likely to be overestimated and to reflect an underreporting of mental retardation in the CDER evaluations.
[6] This figure was calculated by the author and refers to prevalence data (not cumulative incidence) presented in the paper (the M:F ratio is based on a subsample).
[7] These figures apply to the whole study sample of 206 subjects with an ASD.

Case Identification

When an area or population has been identified for a survey, different strategies have been employed to find individuals matching the case definition retained for the study. Some studies have relied solely on existing service providers databases (Croen et al., 2002), on special educational databases (Fombonne et al., 2006; Gurney et al., 2003; Lazoff et al., 2010), or on national registers (Madsen et al., 2002) for case identification. These studies have the common limitation of relying on a population group that was readily accessible to the service provider or agencies, rather than sampling from the population at large. As a result, individuals with the disorder who are not in contact with these services are not included as cases, leading to an underestimation of the prevalence proportion. Recent studies that have systematically surveyed the general population and have included children without known developmental/behavioral difficulty and no contact with existing services have identified a large undetected prevalence pool (Kim et al., 2011).

Other investigations have relied on a multistage approach to identify cases in underlying populations (e.g., CDC, 2009; Kim et al., 2011). The aim of the first screening stage of these studies is to cast a wide net in order to identify subjects possibly affected with an ASD, with the final diagnostic status being determined at subsequent stages. This process often consists of sending letters or brief screening scales requesting school and health professionals, and/or other data sources, to identify possible cases of autism. Few of these investigations rely on systematic sampling techniques that would ensure a near-complete coverage of the target population. Moreover, such investigations differ in several key aspects with regards to this screening stage. First, the thoroughness of the coverage of all relevant data sources varied enormously from one study to another. In addition, the surveyed areas were not comparable in terms of service development, reflecting the specific educational or health care systems of each country and of the period of investigation. Second, the type of inclusion information sent out to professionals invited to identify children varied from a few clinical descriptors of autism-related symptoms (or diagnostic checklists) to more systematic screening strategy based on questionnaires or rating scales of known reliability and validity. Third, variable participation rates in the first screening stages provide another source of variation in the screening efficiency of surveys, although refusal rates tended, on average, to be very low.

Few studies provided an estimate of the reliability of the screening procedure. The sensitivity of the screening methodology is also difficult to gauge in autism surveys, as the proportion of children truly affected with the disorder but not identified in the screening stage (the 'false negatives') remains generally unmeasured. The usual approach, which consists of sampling at random screened negative subjects in order to estimate the proportion of false negatives and adjusting the estimate accordingly, has not been used in these surveys. The main reason is that, due to the relatively low frequency of the disorder, it would be both imprecise and very costly to undertake such estimations. As a consequence, prevalence estimates must be understood as underestimates of 'true' prevalence rates, with the magnitude of this underestimation unknown in each survey.

When the screening phase is completed, subjects identified as positive go through the next step, involving a more in-depth diagnostic evaluation to confirm their case status. Similar considerations regarding the methodological variability across studies apply to these more intensive assessment phases. In the studies reviewed, participation rates in second-stage assessments were generally high (over 80%). The source of information used to determine diagnosis usually involved a combination of data from different informants (parents, teachers, pediatricians, other health professionals, etc.) and data sources (medical records, educational sources), with an in-person assessment of the person with autism being offered in some but not all studies. Obviously, surveys of very large populations, such as those conducted in the United States by the CDC (2007a, b; 2009) or in national registers (Madsen et al., 2002), did not include a direct diagnostic assessment of all subjects by the research team. However, these investigators could generally confirm the accuracy of their final determination by undertaking, on a randomly selected subsample, a more complete diagnostic workup. The CDC surveys have established a methodology for surveys of large populations that relies on screening of a population using multiple data sources, a systematic review and scoring system for the data gathered in the screening phase combined with, in the less obvious cases, input from experienced clinicians with known reliability and validity. This methodology is adequate for large samples, and is likely to be used in the future for surveillance efforts.

When subjects were directly examined, the assessments were conducted using various diagnostic instruments, ranging from a typical unstructured examination by a clinical expert (but without demonstrated psychometric properties), to the use of batteries of standardized measures by trained research staff. The Autism Diagnostic Interview (Le Couteur et al., 1989) and/or the Autism Diagnostic Observational Schedule (Lord et al., 2000) have been increasingly used in the most recent surveys.

PREVALENCE ESTIMATIONS

Autistic Disorder

Prevalence estimates for autistic disorder are summarized in Table 1.1.1. There were 49 studies (including 12 in the UK, 6 in the United States, and 6 in Japan), with over half of them published since 2000. The sample size varied from 5,120 to 4.95 million, with a median of 46,500 (mean: 228,528) subjects in the surveyed populations. Age ranged from 0 to 27 years, with a median age of 8.5 years. The number of subjects identified with autistic disorder ranged from 6 to 5,038 (median: 53). Males consistently outnumbered females in 40 studies where gender differences were reported, with a male/female ratio ranging from 1.33:1 to 16.0:1 in 39 studies (1 small study had no girls at all), leading to an average male/female ratio of 4.4:1. Prevalence rates varied from 0.7/10,000 to 94/10,000 with a median value of 13/10,000. Prevalence rates were negatively correlated with sample size (Spearman's r: -0.5; $p < 0.001$), with small-scale studies reporting higher prevalence rates.

The correlation between prevalence rate and year of publication was significant (Spearman's r: 0.77; $p < 0.001$), indicative of higher rates in more recent surveys. Therefore, a current estimate for the prevalence of autistic disorder must be derived from more recent surveys with an adequate sample size. In 26 studies published since 2000, the median rate was 21.6/10,000 (mean rate: 25.3/10,000). After exclusion of the 2 studies with the smallest and largest sample sizes, the results were very similar (mean rate: 26.2/10,000). Thus, the best current estimate for autistic disorder is 26/10,000. In 24 studies where the proportion of subjects with IQ within the normal range was reported, the median value was 32% (interquartile range: 17.3–54%). In these surveys, there was a significant correlation between a higher proportion of normal IQ subjects and a higher male/female ratio (Spearman's r: 0.54; $p = 0.007$), a result consistent with the known association between gender and IQ in autism. Over time, there were minor associations between the year of publication of the survey and the sample male/female ratio (Spearman's r: 0.36; $p = 0.02$) and the proportion of subjects without mental retardation (Spearman's r: 0.38; $p = 0.07$). Taken in conjunction with the much stronger increase over time in prevalence rates, these results suggest that the increase in prevalence rates is not entirely accounted for by the inclusion of milder forms (i.e., less cognitively impaired) of autistic disorder, albeit this might have contributed to it to some degree.

Asperger Syndrome

Epidemiological studies of Asperger syndrome (AS) are sparse, due to the fact that it was acknowledged as a separate diagnostic category in both ICD-10 and DSM-IV only in the early 1990s. Two epidemiological surveys (not featured in the current analysis due to relatively small population sizes) have been conducted which *specifically* investigated AS prevalence (Ehlers & Gillberg, 1993; Kadesjo et al., 1999). However, only a handful of cases (N < 5) were identified in these surveys, with the resulting estimates varying greatly. In addition, since there was no separate report for children meeting criteria for autistic disorder, it remains unclear whether these subjects would have also met criteria for autistic disorder and how prevalence rates would be affected if hierarchical rules were followed to diagnose both disorders. A recent survey of high-functioning ASD in Welsh mainstream primary schools has yielded a relatively high (uncorrected) prevalence estimate of 14.5/10,000, but no rate was available specifically for AS (Webb et al., 2003).

Other recent surveys have examined samples with respect to the presence of both autistic disorder and Asperger syndrome. Thirteen studies (already listed in Table 1.1.1) published since 1998 provided usable data (Table 1.1.2). The median population size was 23,635, and the median age 8.5 years. Numbers of children with AS varied from 21 to 826, with a median sample size of 45. There was a six-fold variation in estimated rates of AS (range: 4.9 to 28/10,000). The median value was 21.3/10,000. With the exception of one study (Latif & Williams, 2007), the number of children with autistic disorder was consistently higher than that of children with AS. The prevalence ratio (Table 1.1.2, right-hand column) exceeded 1, with a median value of 2.4, indicating that the rate of AS was consistently *lower* than that for autism (Table 1.1.2). The unusually high rate of AS relative to autistic disorder obtained in Latif and Williams's (2007) study appeared to be inflated due to the inclusion of high-functioning autism in the AS definition. The epidemiological data on AS are therefore of dubious quality, reflecting the difficult nosological issues that have surrounded the inclusion of AS in recent nosographies as well as the lack of proper measurement strategies that ensure a reliable difference between AS and autistic disorder.

Childhood Disintegrative Disorder

Twelve surveys provided data on childhood disintegrative disorder (CDD) (Table 1.1.3). In 5 of these, only 1 case was reported; no case of CDD was identified in 4 other studies. Prevalence estimates ranged from 0 to 9.2/100,000, with a median rate of 1.8/100,000. The pooled estimate, based on 11 identified cases and a surveyed population of about 560,000 children, was 1.9/100,000. Gender was reported in 10 of the 11 studies, and males appear to be overrepresented, with

TABLE 1.1.2 Asperger Syndrome (AS) in Recent Autism Surveys

Study	Size of population	Age group	Informants	Assessment Instruments	Diagnostic criteria	Autism N	Autism Rate/10,000	Asperger Syndrome N	Asperger Syndrome Rate/10,000	Autism/ AS ratio
Sponheim & Skjeldal, 1998	65,688	3–14	Parent Child	Parental interview + direct observation, CARS, ABC	ICD-10	32	4.9	2	0.3	16.0
Taylor et al., 1999	490,000	0–16	Records	Rating of all data available in child record	ICD-10	427	8.7	71	1.4	6.0
Powell et al., 2000	25,377	1–4.9	Records	ADI-R Available data	DSM-III-R DSM-IV ICD-10	54	–	16	–	3.4
Baird et al., 2000	16,235	7	Parents Child Other data	ADI-R Psychometry	ICD-10 DSM-IV	45	27.7	5	3.1	9.0
Chakrabarti & Fombonne, 2001	15,500	2.5–6.5	Child Parent Professional	ADI-R, 2 wks multidisciplinary assessment, Merrill-Palmer, WPPSI	ICD-10 DSM-IV	26	16.8	13	8.4	2.0
Chakrabarti & Fombonne, 2005	10,903	2.5–6.5	Child Parent Professional	ADI-R, 2 wks multidisciplinary assessment, Merrill-Palmer, WPPSI	ICD-10 DSM-IV	24	22.0	12	11.0	2.0
Fombonne et al., 2006	27,749	5–17	School registry	Clinical	DSM-IV	60	21.6	28	10.1	2.1
Ellefsen et al., 2007	7,689	8–17	Parent Child Professional	DISCO, WISC-R, ASSQ	ICD-10 Gillberg AS criteria	21	28.0	20	26.0	1.1
Latif & Williams, 2007	39,220	0–17	?	Clinical	Kanner, Gillberg AS criteria	50	12.7	139	35.4	0.36
Williams et al., 2008	14,062	11	Medical records and educational registry	Clinical	ICD-10	30	21.6	23	16.6	1.3
van Balkom et al., 2009	13,109	0–13	Clinic series	Review of medical records	DSM-IV	25	19.1	2	1.5	12.5
Lazoff et al., 2010	23,635	5–17	School registry	Review of educational records	DSM-IV	60	25.4	23	9.7	2.6
Leonard et al., 2011	393,329	0–12	Records	Available data	DSM-IV & TR	826	21.0	64	1.6	12.9

TABLE 1.1.3 Surveys of Childhood Disintegrative Disorder (CDD)

Study	Country (Region/State)	Size of target population	Age group	Assessment	N	M/F	Prevalence estimate (/100,000)	95% CI (/100,000)
Burd et al., 1987	USA (North Dakota)	180,986	2–18	Structured parental interview and review of all data available-DSM-III criteria	2	2/–	1.11	0.13–3.4
Sponheim & Skjeldal, 1998	Norway (Akershus County)	65,688	3–14	Parental interview and direct observation (CARS, ABC)	1	?	1.52	0.04–8.5
Magnússon & Saemundsen, 2001	Iceland (whole island)	85,556	5–14	ADI-R, CARS and psychological tests—mostly ICD-10	2	2/–	2.34	0.3–8.4
Chakrabarti & Fombonne, 2001	UK (Staffordshire, Midlands)	15,500	2.5–6.5	ADI-R, two weeks multidisciplinary assessment, Merrill-Palmer, WPPSI-ICD-10/DSM-IV	1	1/–	6.45	0.16–35.9
Chakrabarti & Fombonne, 2005	UK (Staffordshire, Midlands)	10,903	2.5–6.5	ADI-R, two weeks multidisciplinary assessment, Merrill-Palmer, WPPSI-ICD-10/DSM-IV	1	1/–	9.17	0–58.6
Fombonne et al., 2006	Canada (Montreal)	27,749	5–17	DSM-IV, special needs school survey	1	1/–	3.60	0–20.0
Gillberg et al., 2006	Sweden (Götenborg)	102,485	7–24	DSM-IV, review of medical records of local diagnostic center	2	1/1	2.0	0.2–7.1
Ellefsen et al., 2007	Denmark (Faroe Islands)	7,689	8–17	DISCO, Vineland, WISC-R, ICD-10/DSM-IV	0	–	0	–
Kawamura et al., 2008	Japan (Toyota)	12,589	5–8	DSM-IV, population based screening at 18 and 36 mths	0	–	0	–
Williams et al., 2008	UK (Avon)	14,062	11	ICD-10, educational and medical record review	0	–	0	–
van Balkom et al., 2009	Netherlands (Aruba)	13,109	0–13	Clinic medical record review	0	–	0	–
Lazoff et al., 2010	Canada (Montreal)	23,635	5–17	DSM-IV, special needs school survey	1	1/0	4.23	0.0–24.0
Pooled Estimates		559,951			11	9/1	1.96	1.1–3.4

a male/female ratio of 9:1. The upperbound limit of confidence interval associated to the pooled prevalence estimate (3.4/100,000) indicates that CDD is a rare condition, with about 1 case occurring for every 112 cases of autistic disorder.

Prevalence for Combined ASD

A new objective of more recent epidemiological surveys was to estimate the prevalence of all disorders falling onto the autism spectrum, thereby prompting important changes in the conceptualization and design of surveys. However, before reviewing the findings of these studies (mostly conducted since 2000), we examine to what the extent findings from the first generation of epidemiological surveys of a narrow definition of autism also informed our understanding of the modern concept of autism spectrum disorders.

Unspecified Autism Spectrum Disorders in Earlier Surveys

In previous reviews, we documented that several studies performed in the 1960s and 1970s had provided useful information on rates of syndromes similar to autism but not meeting the strict diagnostic criteria for autistic disorder then in use (Fombonne, 2003a, b; 2005). At the time, different labels were used by authors to characterize these clinical pictures, such as the 'triad of impairments' involving deficits in reciprocal social interaction, communication, and imagination (Wing & Gould, 1979), autistic mental retardation (Hoshino et al., 1982), borderline childhood psychoses (Brask, 1970) or 'autistic-like' syndromes (Burd et al., 1987). These syndromes would fall within our currently defined autistic spectrum, probably with diagnostic labels such as atypical autism and/or PDD-NOS.

In 8 of 12 surveys providing separate estimates of the prevalence of these developmental disorders, higher rates for the atypical forms were actually found compared to those for the more narrowly defined autistic disorder (see Fombonne, 2003a). However, this atypical group received little attention in previous epidemiological studies, and these subjects were not defined as 'cases' and therefore were not included in the numerators of prevalence calculations, thereby underestimating systematically the prevalence of what would be defined today as the spectrum of autistic disorders. For example, in the first survey by Lotter (1966), the prevalence would rise from 4.1 to 7.8/10,000 if these atypical forms of autism had been included in the case definition. Similarly, in Wing et al.'s study (1976), the prevalence was 4.9/10,000 for autistic disorder, but the prevalence for the whole ASD spectrum was in fact 21.1/10,000 after the figure of 16.3/10,000 (Wing & Gould, 1979), corresponding to the triad of impairments, was added. The progressive recognition of the importance and relevance of these less typical clinical presentations has led to changes in the design of more recent epidemiological surveys (see below), that now use case definitions that incorporate a priori these milder phenotypes.

Newer Surveys of ASD

The results of surveys that estimated the prevalence of the whole spectrum of ASD are summarized in Table 1.1.4. Of the 34 studies listed, 18 also provided separate estimates for autistic disorder and other ASD subtypes; the other 16 studies provided only an estimate for the combined ASD rate. All these surveys were published since 2000, with the majority (71%) published after 2006; the studies were performed in 12 different countries (including 10 in the UK and 8 in the United States). Sample sizes ranged from 7,333 to 4,247,206 (median: 50,863; mean: 282,827). One recent study was specifically conducted on adults and provided the only estimate (9.8/1,000) thus far available for adults (Brugha et al., 2011). In the remaining studies, the average age of samples ranged from 5.0 to 12.5, with 8 years being the mean, modal and median age. When specified, the diagnostic criteria used in the 32 studies reflected the reliance on modern diagnostic schemes (8 studies used ICD-10, 20 the DSM-III, DSM-IV or DSM-IV-TR; both schemes being used simultaneously in 2 studies). In 20 studies where IQ data were reported, the proportion of subjects within the normal IQ range varied from 30% to 100% (median: 54.4%; mean: 53.4%), a proportion that is higher than that for autistic disorder and reflects the lesser degree of association, or lack thereof, between intellectual impairment and milder forms of ASD. Overrepresentation of males was the rule, with male/female ratio ranging from 2.7:1 to 15.7:1 (mean: 5.2; median: 4.5). There was a 42-fold variation in prevalence proportions that ranged from a low of 6.26/10,000, to a high of 264/10,000. However, some degree of consistency is found in the center of this distribution, with a median rate of 62/10,000 and a mean rate of 74/10,000 (interquartile range: 49.3–82.7/10,000). This mean rate is close to the rate reported recently for ASD in 14 sites (CDC, 2007b); the CDC value represents, however, an average, and that study conducted at 14 different sites utilizing the same methodology found a three-fold variation of rate by state. Across individual states, Alabama had the lowest rate of 3.3/1,000 whereas New Jersey had the highest value with 10.6/1,000 (CDC, 2007b). As expected, a new CDC report on 307,000 US children aged 8 and born 4 years later than children from the previous survey reported an average prevalence of

TABLE 1.1.4 Newer Epidemiological Surveys of Pervasive Developmental Disorders

References	Country	Area	Size	Age	N	Diagnostic criteria	% with normal IQ	Gender ratio (M:F)	Prevalence/ 10,000	95% CI
Baird et al., 2000	UK	Southeast Thames	16,235	7	94	ICD-10	60%	15.7 (83:11)	57.9	46.8–70.9
Bertrand et al., 2001	USA	New Jersey	8,896	3–10	60	DSM-IV	51%	2.7 (44:16)	67.4	51.5–86.7
Chakrabarti & Fombonne, 2001	UK	Stafford	15,500	4–7	96	ICD-10	74.2%	3.8 (77:20)	61.9	50.2–75.6
Madsen et al., 2002	Denmark	National Register	–	8	738	ICD-10	–	–	30.0	–
Scott et al., 2002	UK	Cambridge	33,598	5–11	196	ICD-10	–	4.0 (–)	58.3[1]	50 / 67[1]
Yeargin-Allsopp et al., 2003	USA	Atlanta	289,456	3–10	987	DSM-IV	31.8%	4.0 (787:197)	34.0	32–36
Gurney et al., 2003	USA	Minnesota	–	8–10	–	–	–	–	52.0[5] 66.0	– –
Icasiano et al., 2004	Australia	Barwon	≈ 54,000	2–17	177	DSM-IV	53.4%	8.3 (158:19)	39.2	–
Chakrabarti & Fombonne, 2005	UK	Stafford	10,903	4–6	64	ICD-10	70.2%	6.1 (55:9)	58.7	45.2–74.9
Baird et al., 2006	UK	South Thames	56,946	9–10	158	ICD-10	45%	3.3 (121:37)	116.1	90.4–141.8
Fombonne et al., 2006	Canada	Montreal	27,749	5–17	180	DSM-IV	–	4.8 (149:31)	64.9	55.8–75.0
Harrison et al., 2006	UK	Scotland	134,661	0–15	443[4]	ICD-10, DSMIV	–	7.0 (369:53)	44.2[4]	39.5–48.9
Gillberg et al., 2006	Sweden	Göteborg	32,568	7 12	262	DSM-IV	–	3.6 (205:57)	80.4	71.3–90.3
CDC, 2007a	USA	6 states	187,761	8	1,252	DSM-IV-TR	38% to 60%[2]	2.8 to 5.5	67.0	–[2]
CDC, 2007b	USA	14 states	407,578	8	2,685	DSM-IV-TR	55.4%[3]	3.4 to 6.5	66.0	63–68
Ellefsen et al., 2007	Denmark	Faroe Islands	7,689	8–17	41	DSM-IV, Gillberg's criteria	68.3%	5.8 (35:6)	53.3	36–70
Latif & Williams, 2007	UK	South Wales	39,220	0–17	240	ICD-10, DSM-IV, Kanner's & Gillberg's criteria	–	6.8 –	61.2	54–69[1]
Wong and Hui, 2008	China	Hong Kong	4,247,206	0–14	682	DSM-IV	30	6.6 (592:90)	16.1 (1986–2005) 30.0 (2005)	– –
Nicholas et al., 2008	USA	South Carolina[6]	47,726	8	295	DSM-IV-TR	39.6%	3.1 (224:71)	62.0	56–70
Kawamura et al., 2008	Japan	Toyota	12,589	5–8	228	DSM-IV	66.4%	2.8 (168:60)	181.1	158.5–205.9

(Continued)

TABLE 1.1.4   Newer Epidemiological Surveys of Pervasive Developmental Disorders – cont'd

References	Country	Area	Size	Age	N	Diagnostic criteria	% with normal IQ	Gender ratio (M:F)	Prevalence/ 10,000	95% CI
Williams et al., 2008	UK	Avon	14,062	11	86	ICD-10	85.3%	6.8 (75:11)	61.9	48.8–74.9
Baron-Cohen et al., 2009	UK	Cambridgeshire	8,824	5–9	83	ICD-10	–	–	94[7]	75 – 116
Kogan et al., 2009	USA	Nationwide	77,911	3–17	913	–	–	4.5 (746:167)	110	94 – 128
Van Balkom et al., 2009	Netherlands	Aruba	13,109	0–13	69	DSM-IV	58.8	6.7 (60:9)	52.6	41.0–66.6
CDC, 2009	USA	11 states	307,790	8	2,757	DSM-IV	59	4.5 (–)	89.6	86 – 93
Lazoff et al., 2010	Canada	Montreal	23,635	5–17	187	DSM-IV	–	5.4 (158:29)	79.1	67.8–90.4
Barnevik-Olsson et al., 2010	Sweden	Stockholm	113,391	6–10	250	DSM-IV	0	–	22	–
Al-Farsi et al., 2011	Oman	National Register	528,335	5–14[8]	98	DSM-IV- TR	–	2.9	190	150–230
Brugha et al., 2011	UK	England	7,333	16–98	72	ADOS	100	3.8	98	30–165
Kim et al., 2011	S. Korea	Goyang City	55,266	7–12	201	DSM-IV	31.5	3.8	264	191–337
Leonard et al., 2011	Australia	Western Australia	393,329	0–21	1179	DSM-III, IV, & TR	38.5	5.55	30	–
Parner et al., 2011	Australia	Western Australia	152,060	0–10	678	DSM-IV & TR	–	–	51	47–55.3
Parner et al., 2011	Denmark	National Register	404,816	0–10	2002	ICD-10	–	–	68.5	65–721
Samadi et al., 2011	Iran	National Register	1,320,334	5	826	ADI-R	–	4.3	6.26	5.84–6.70

[1] This was calculated by the author.

[2] Specific values for % with normal IQ and confidence intervals are available for each state's prevalence.

[3] This is the average across seven states.

[4] This was estimated using a capture–recapture analysis; the number of cases used to calculate prevalence was estimated to be 596.

[5] These are the highest prevalences reported in this study of time trends. The prevalence in 10-year-olds is for the 1991 birth cohort, and that for 8-year-olds is for the 1993 birth cohort. Both prevalences were calculated in the 2001–2002 school year.

[6] This refers to children aged 8, born either in 2000 and 2002, and included in the two CDC multisite reports.

[7] This was rate based on a Special Education Needs register. A figure of 99/10,000 is provided from a parental and diagnostic survey. Other estimates in this study vary from 47 to 165/10,000 deriving from various assumptions made by the authors.

[8] Al-Farsi et al. (2011) provided a breakdown of age groups; for methodological reasons (i.e., ASD is not typically diagnosed in the age group 0–4), we used only available prevalence rates for age groups 5–9 and 10–14.

89.6/10,000 (CDC, 2009). Again, substantial variation across states was reported, as prevalence ranged from 4.2/1,000 in Florida to 12.1/1,000 in Arizona and Missouri. One factor associated with the prevalence increase in the CDC monitoring survey was the improved quality and quantity of information available through records, indicative of greater awareness about ASD among community professionals. As surveillance efforts continue, it is likely that awareness and services will develop in states that were lagging behind, resulting in a predictable increase in the average rate for the United States as time elapses. These CDC findings apply to other countries as well, and prevalence estimates from any study should always be regarded in the context of the imperfect sensitivity of case ascertainment that results in downward biases in prevalence proportions in most surveys.

As an illustration, the four surveys in Table 1.1.4 with the lowest rates probably underestimated the true population rates. In a Danish investigation (Madsen et al., 2002), case finding depended on notification to a national registry, a method which is usually associated with lower sensitivity for case finding. The Hong Kong survey (Wong and Hui, 2008) and an Australian (Icasiano et al., 2004) survey have relied on less systematic ascertainment techniques. The Atlanta survey by the CDC (Yeargin-Allsopp et al., 2003) was based on a very large population and included younger age groups than subsequent CDC surveys, and age-specific rates were in fact in the 40–45/10,000 range in some birth cohorts (Fombonne, 2003a, b). Case-finding techniques employed in the other surveys were more proactive, relying on multiple and repeated screening phases, involving both different informants at each phase and surveying the same cohorts at different ages, which certainly enhanced the sensitivity of case identification (Baird et al., 2006; Chakrabarti & Fombonne, 2005). Assessments were often performed with standardized diagnostic measures (i.e., ADI-R and ADOS) which match well the more dimensional approach retained for case definition.

Overall, results of recent surveys agree that an average figure of (74/10,000) can be used as the current estimate for the spectrum of ASD. The convergence of estimates around 70–90 per 10,000 for all ASD combined, conducted in different regions and countries by different teams, is striking especially when derived from studies with improved methodology. This is now the best estimate for the prevalence of ASD currently available. However, it represents an average and conservative figure, and it is important to recognize the substantial variability that exists between studies, and within studies, across sites or areas. The prevalence figure of 80/10,000 (equivalent to 8/1,000 or 0.80%) translates into 1 child out of 125 with an ASD diagnosis.

TIME TRENDS IN PREVALENCE AND THEIR INTERPRETATION

The debate on the hypothesis of a secular increase in rates of autism has been obscured by a lack of clarity in the measures of disease occurrence used by investigators, or in the interpretation of their meaning. In particular, it is crucial to differentiate prevalence from incidence. Whereas prevalence is useful to estimate needs and plan services, only incidence rates can be used for causal research. Both prevalence and incidence estimates will increase when case definition is broadened and case ascertainment is improved. Time trends in rates can therefore only be gauged in investigations that hold these parameters under strict control over time. These methodological requirements must be borne in mind while reviewing the evidence for a secular increase in rates of ASD, or testing for the 'epidemic' hypothesis. The 'epidemic' hypothesis emerged in the 1990s when, in most countries, increasing numbers were diagnosed with ASD. This lead to an upward trend in children registered in service providers' databases that was paralleled by higher prevalence rates in epidemiological surveys. These trends were interpreted as evidence that the actual population incidence of ASD was increasing (what the term 'epidemic' means). However, alternative explanations to explain the rise in numbers of children diagnosed with ASD had to be ruled out before supporting this conclusion, and include those covered in the following sections.

Use of Referral Statistics

Increasing numbers of children referred to specialist services or known to special education registers have been taken as evidence for an increased incidence of ASD. Upward trends in national registries, medical, and educational databases have been seen in many different countries (Gurney et al., 2003; Madsen et al., 2002; Shattuck, 2006; Taylor et al., 1999), all occurring in the late 1980s and early 1990s. However, trends over time in *referred* samples are confounded by many factors such as referral patterns, availability of services, heightened public awareness, decreasing age at diagnosis (see Shattuck et al., 2009), and changes over time in diagnostic concepts and practices.

Failure to control for these confounding factors was obvious in previous reports (Fombonne, 2001), such as the widely quoted reports from California Developmental Database Services (CDDS, 1999; 2003). First, these reports applied to numbers rather than rates, and failure to relate these numbers to meaningful denominators left the interpretation of an upward trend vulnerable to changes in the composition of the underlying population. For example, the population of California was 19,971,000 in 1970 and increased to 35,116,000 as of July 1, 2002, a change of +75.8%. Second, the focus on the year-to-year changes in absolute numbers of subjects known to California State-funded services detracts from more meaningful comparisons. For example, as of December 2007, the total number of subjects with an ASD diagnosis was 31,332 in the 3–21-year-old age group (including all CDER autism codes) (CDDS, 2007). The population of 3–21-year-olds in California was 9,976,768 on July 1, 2007 (Census Bureau for the US, 2009). If one applies the 2007 average US rate of 67/10,000 deriving from the CDC (2007b), one would expect to have 66,844 subjects with an ASD, within this age group, living in California. The expected number is twice as high as the number of subjects actually recorded in the public service at the same time.

The discrepancy would be more pronounced if the latest CDC figures of 9/1,000 (Table 1.1.4; CDC, 2009) were used to estimate the expected number of Californian residents with an ASD. Certainly, these calculations do not support the 'epidemic' interpretation of the California DDS data, and confirm the selective nature of the referred sample. The upward trends in the DDS database simply suggest that children identified in the California DDS database were only a subset of the population prevalence pool, and that the increasing numbers reflect merely an increasing proportion of children receiving services. Third, with one exception (see below), no attempt was made to adjust the trends for changes in diagnostic concepts and definitions. However, major nosographical modifications were introduced during the corresponding years with a general tendency in most classifications to broaden the concept of autism (as embodied in the terms 'autism spectrum' or 'pervasive developmental disorder'). Fourth, the age characteristics of the subjects recorded in official statistics were portrayed in a misleading manner, where the preponderance of young subjects was presented as evidence of increasing rates in successive birth cohorts (Fombonne, 2001). The problems associated with disentangling age from period and cohort effects in such observational data are well known in the epidemiological literature and deserve better statistical handling. Fifth, the decreasing age at diagnosis results in itself to increasing numbers of young children being identified in official statistics (Wazana et al., 2007) or referred to specialist medical and educational services. Earlier identification of children from the prevalence pool may therefore result in increased service activity that may lead to a misperception by professionals of an 'epidemic'. However, it is important to note that an increase in referrals does not necessarily mean increased *incidence*.

A more refined analysis of the effect of a younger age at diagnosis using cumulative incidence data by age 5 years showed that 12% of the increase in incidence from the 1990 to the 1996 birth cohort could be explained by this factor, and up to 24% with an extrapolation to the 2002 cohort (Hertz-Picciotto & Delwiche, 2009). Although younger age at diagnosis can explain only a small proportion of the increase in diagnoses in this analysis, it does play a role in several published reports, though its effect would attenuate as the cohort becomes older. Hertz-Picciotto and Delwiche's (2009) analysis of the California DDS data is also limited by their reliance on the DDS database that reflected changes in regional referral patterns, especially during that period.

Another study of this dataset was subsequently launched to demonstrate the validity of the 'epidemic' hypothesis (MIND, 2002). The authors relied on DDS data and aimed at ruling out changes in diagnostic practices and immigration into California as factors explaining the increased numbers. While immigration was reasonably ruled out, the study comparing diagnoses of autism and mental retardation over time was impossible to interpret in light of the extremely low (< 20%) response rates. Furthermore, a study based solely on cases registered for services cannot rule out the possibility that the proportion of cases within the general population who registered with services has changed over time. For example, assuming a constant incidence and prevalence at two different time points (i.e., hypothesizing no epidemic), the number of cases known to a public agency delivering services could well increase by 200% if the proportion of cases from the community referred to services rises from 25% to 75% in the same interval. In order to eliminate this plausible (see above) explanation, data over time are needed *both* on referred subjects *and* on non-referred (or referred to other services) subjects. Failure to address this phenomenon precludes any inference to be drawn from a study of the California DDS database population to the California population (Fombonne, 2003a). The conclusions of this report were therefore simply unfounded.

The Role of Diagnostic Substitution

One possible explanation for increased numbers of a diagnostic category is that children presenting with the same developmental disability may receive one particular diagnosis at one time, and another diagnosis at a subsequent time. Such diagnostic substitution (or switching) may occur when diagnostic categories become increasingly familiar to health professionals and/or when access to better services is ensured by using a new diagnostic category. The strongest evidence of 'diagnostic switching' contributing to the prevalence increase was produced in all US states in a complex analysis of Department of Education data in 50 US states (Shattuck, 2006), indicating that a relatively high proportion of children previously diagnosed as having mental retardation were subsequently identified as having an ASD diagnosis. Shattuck showed that the odds of being classified in an autism category increased by 1.21 during 1994–2003. Concurrently, the odds of being classified in the learning disability (LD) (odds ratio: OR = 0.98) and the mental retardation (MR) categories (OR = 0.97) decreased significantly. Shattuck (2006) further demonstrated that the growing prevalence of autism was directly associated with decreasing prevalence of LD and MR within states, and that a significant downward deflection in the historical trajectories of LD and MR occurred when autism became reported in the United States as an independent category in 1993–94. Finally, Shattuck (2006) showed that, from 1994 to 2003, the mean increase for the combined category of *Autism + Other Health Impairments + Trauma Brain Injury + Developmental Delay* was 12/1000, whereas the mean decrease for MR and LD was 11/1000 during the same period. One exception to these ratios was California, for which previous authors had debated the presence of diagnostic substitution between MR and autism (Croen et al., 2002; Eagle, 2004). The previous investigations have largely relied on ecological, aggregated data that have known limitations. Using individual-level data, a new study has re-examined the hypothesis of diagnostic substitution in the California DDS dataset (King & Bearman, 2009) and has shown that 24% of the increase in caseload was attributable to such diagnostic substitution (from the mental retardation to the autism category). It is important to keep in mind that other types of diagnostic substitution are likely to have occurred as well for milder forms of the ASD phenotype, from various psychiatric disorders (including childhood schizoid 'personality' disorders; Wolff & Barlow, 1979) that have not been studied yet (Fombonne, 2009b). For example, children currently diagnosed with Asperger disorder were previously diagnosed with other psychiatric conditions (i.e., obsessive-compulsive disorder, school 'phobia', social anxiety, etc.) in clinical settings, before the developmental nature of their condition was fully recognized.

Evidence of diagnostic substitution within the class of developmental disorders has also been provided in UK-based studies. Using the General Practitioner Research Database, Jick et al. (2003) demonstrated that the incidence of specific developmental disorders (including language disorders) decreased by about the same amount that the incidence of diagnoses of autism increased in boys born from 1990 to 1997. A more recent UK study (Bishop et al., 2008) showed that up to 66% of adults previously diagnosed as children with developmental language disorders would meet diagnostic criteria for a broad definition of ASD. This change was observed for children diagnosed with specific language impairments, but was even more apparent for those diagnosed with a pragmatic language impairment.

Comparison of Cross-Sectional Epidemiological Surveys

Epidemiological surveys of autism each possess unique design features that could account almost entirely for between-studies variation in rates. Therefore, time trends in rates of autism are difficult to gauge from published prevalence rates. The significant aforementioned correlation between prevalence rate and year of publication for autistic disorder could merely reflect increased efficiency over time in case identification methods used in surveys as well as changes in diagnostic concepts and practices (Bishop et al., 2008; Kielinen et al., 2000; Magnússon and Saemundsen, 2001; Shattuck, 2006; Webb et al., 1997). In studies using capture-recapture methods, it is apparent that up to a third of prevalent cases may be missed by an ascertainment source, even in recently conducted studies (Harrison et al., 2006). Evidence that method factors could account for most of the variability in published prevalence estimates comes from a direct comparison of eight recent surveys conducted in the UK and the United States (Fombonne, 2005). In each country, four surveys were conducted around the same year and with similar age groups. As there is no reason to expect large variations in between-area differences in rates, prevalence estimates should be comparable within each country. However, there was a 6-fold variation in rates for UK surveys, and a 14-fold variation in US rates. In each set of studies, high rates were derived from surveys where intensive population-based screening techniques were employed, whereas lower rates were obtained from studies relying on passive administrative methods for case finding. Since no passage of time was involved, the magnitude of these gradients in rates can only be attributed to differences in case identification methods across surveys.

Even more convincing evidence comes from the large survey by the CDC on 408,000 US children aged 8 and born in 1994 (CDC, 2007b) where an average prevalence of 66/10,000 was reported for 14 US states. One striking finding of this report is that there was more than a three-fold variation in state-specific rates that ranged from a low of 33/10,000 for Alabama to a high of 106/10,000 in New Jersey. It would be surprising if there were truly this much variance in the number of children with autism in different states in the United States. These substantial differences most certainly reflected ascertainment variability across sites in a study that was otherwise performed with the same methods and at the same time. In the more recent CDC 11 across-state study (CDC, 2009), the same variability is reported again. Prevalence was significantly lower (7.5/1,000) in states that had access to health sources only compared to that (10.2/1,000) of states where educational data was also available. The authors also reported that the quality and quantity of information available in abstracted records (the main method for case ascertainment) had increased between 2002 and 2006. Together with a reported average decrease of 5 months for the age at diagnosis and a larger increase in the non-mentally retarded population, these factors suggest that improved sensitivity in case ascertainment in the CDC monitoring network has contributed substantially to the increase in prevalence. Thus, no inference on trends in the incidence of ASD can be derived from a simple comparison of prevalence rates over time, since studies conducted at different periods are likely to differ even more with respect to their methodologies.

Repeat Surveys in Defined Geographical Areas

Repeated surveys, using the same methodology and conducted in the same geographical area at different points in time, can potentially yield useful information on time trends provided that methods are kept relatively constant. The Göteborg studies (Gillberg, 1984; Gillberg et al., 1991) provided three prevalence estimates that increased over a short period of time from 4.0 (1980) to 6.6 (1984) and 9.5/10,000 (1988), the gradient being even steeper if rates for the urban area alone are considered (4.0, 7.5, and 11.6/10,000, respectively) (Gillberg et al., 1991). However, comparison of these rates is not straightforward, as different age groups were included in each survey. Secondly, the increased prevalence in the second survey was explained by improved detection among those with intellectual delays, and that of the third survey by cases born to immigrant parents. That the majority of the latter group was born abroad suggests that migration into the area could be a key explanation. Taken in conjunction with a change in local services and a progressive broadening of the definition of autism over time that was acknowledged by the authors (Gillberg et al., 1991), these findings do not provide evidence for an increased incidence in the rate of autism. Similarly, studies conducted in Japan at different points in time in Toyota (Kawamura et al., 2008) and Yokohama (Honda et al., 1996 and 2005) showed rises in prevalence rates that their authors interpreted as reflecting the effect of both improved population screening of preschoolers and of a broadening of diagnostic concepts and criteria.

Two separate surveys of children born between 1992–1995 and 1996–1998 in Staffordshire, UK (Chakrabarti & Fombonne, 2001; 2005), were performed with rigorously identical methods for case definition and case identification. The prevalence for combined ASD was comparable and not statistically different in the two surveys (Chakrabarti & Fombonne, 2005), suggesting no upward trend in overall rates of ASD, at least during the short time interval between studies. In two recent CDC surveys (2007a, b), the prevalence at six sites included in the 2000 and 2002 surveys remained constant at four sites, and increased in two states (Georgia and West Virginia), with the reported increase most likely due to improved quality of survey methods at these sites. In the 2009 CDC report, an average increase of 57% in prevalence was reported in 10 sites with 2002 and 2006 data, with a smaller increase in Colorado. Increases of different magnitudes and directions were reported in all subgroups, making it difficult to detect a particular explanation. The CDC researchers identified a number of factors associated with the change in prevalence but could not conclude on the hypothesis of a real change in the risk of ASD in the population.

Successive Birth Cohorts

In large surveys encompassing a wide age range, increasing prevalence rates among most recent birth cohorts could be interpreted as indicating a secular increase in the incidence of ASD, provided that alternative explanations can confidently be eliminated. This analysis was used in two large French surveys (Fombonne & du Mazaubrun, 1992; Fombonne et al., 1997). The surveys included birth cohorts from 1972 to 1985 (735,000 children, 389 of whom had autism), and when pooling the data of both surveys, age-specific rates showed no upward trend (Fombonne et al., 1997).

An analysis of special educational data from Minnesota showed a 16-fold increase in the number of children identified with an ASD from 1991–1992 to 2001–2002 (Gurney et al., 2003). The increase was not specific to autism since, during the same period, an increase of 50% was observed for all disability categories (except severe intellectual deficiency) especially for the category including attention deficit hyperactivity disorder (ADHD). The large sample size allowed the authors to assess age, period, and cohort effects. Prevalence increased regularly in successive birth cohorts; for example, among 7-year-olds, the prevalence rose from 18/10,000 in those born in 1989, to 29/10,000 in those born in 1991 and to 55/10,000 in those born in 1993, suggestive of birth cohort effects. Within the *same* birth cohorts, age effects were also apparent, since for children born in 1989 the prevalence rose with age from 13/10,000 at age 6, to 21/10,000 at age 9, and 33/10,000 at age 11. As argued by Gurney et al. (2003), this pattern is not consistent with that expected from a chronic nonfatal condition diagnosed during the first years of life. Their analysis also showed a marked period effect that identified the early 1990s as the period where rates started to increase in all ages and birth cohorts.

Gurney et al. (2003) further argued that this phenomenon coincided closely with the inclusion of ASD in the federal Individuals with Disabilities Education Act (IDEA) funding and reporting mechanism in the United States. A similar interpretation of upward trends had been put forward by Croen et al. (2002) in their analysis of the California DDS data, and by Shattuck (2006) in his well-executed analysis of trends in the Department of Education data in all US states.

Conclusion on Time Trends

As it now stands, the recent upward trend in rates of *prevalence* cannot be directly attributed to an increase in the *incidence* of the disorder, or to an 'epidemic' of autism. There is good evidence that changes in diagnostic criteria, diagnostic substitution, the policies for special education, and the increasing availability of services are responsible for the higher prevalence figures. It is also noteworthy that the rise in the number of children diagnosed occurred at the same time in many countries (in the early 1990s), when radical shifts occurred in the ideas, diagnostic approaches, and services for children with ASD. Alternatively, this might, of course, reflect the effect of environmental influences operating simultaneously in different parts of the world. However, there has been no proposed and legitimate environmental risk mechanism to account for this worldwide effect. Moreover, due to the relatively low frequency of autism and ASD, power is a significant limitation in most investigations, and variations of small magnitude in the incidence of the disorder are very likely to go undetected. Equally, the possibility that a true increase in the incidence of ASD has also partially contributed to the upward trend in prevalence rates cannot, and should not, be eliminated based on available data.

OTHER CORRELATES: RACE, IMMIGRANT, AND SOCIOECONOMIC STATUS

Some investigators have mentioned the possibility that rates of autism might be higher among immigrants (Barnevik-Olsson et al., 2010; Gillberg, 1987; Gillberg et al., 1991; 1995; Wing, 1980). A total of 5 of the 17 children with autism identified in a Camberwell, UK, study were of Caribbean origin (Wing et al., 1976; see also Wing, 1980) and the estimated rate of autism was 6.3/10,000 for this group as compared to 4.4/10,000 for the rest of the population (Wing, 1993). However, the large

confidence intervals associated with rates from this study (Table 1.1.1) indicate no statistically significant difference. In addition, this area of London had received a large proportion of immigrants from the Caribbean region in the 1960s and, under circumstances where migration flux in and out of an area are occurring, estimation of population rates should be viewed with greater caution. Findings from a 1999–2003 census report in Stockholm, Sweden (Barnevik-Olsson et al., 2010), revealed that the prevalence rate of autism (autism and 'PDD-NOS/autistic-like condition') with learning disability was 0.98% in the Somali group and 0.21% in the group of non-Somali children. Moreover, 18 out of 250 children registered in the Autism Center for Schoolchildren were of Somali origin (7.2% compared to 1.6% among the total child population during 1999–2003; $p < 0.001$); Barnevik-Olsson et al. (2010) hypothesized that lower levels of vitamin D in immigrant Somali mothers, compared to Swedish-born mothers, may have affected fetal brain development, and possibly led to autism and other concerning behavioral characteristics. After adjusting for socioeconomic and healthcare factors, an epidemiological study in Texas revealed that Hispanic schoolchildren were *less* likely to suffer from an ASD than their Caucasian counterparts (Palmer et al., 2010), probably reflecting lower access to services by this population.

Moreover, the research on immigrant parents and ASD shows variable results. In the Icelandic survey (Magnússon & Saemundsen, 2001), 2.5% of the autism parents were from non-European origin compared to a 0.5% corresponding rate in the whole population, but it was unclear whether this represented a significant difference. In the study by Sponheim and Skjeldal (1998), the proportion of children with autism and a non-European origin was marginally, but not significantly, higher than the population rate of immigrants (8% versus 2.3%); it is notable that this was based on a very small sample (two children of non-European origin). A relatively recent UK survey found comparable rates in areas contrasting for their ethnic composition (Powell et al., 2000). Taken together, the combined results of these reports should be interpreted with caution. Given context-specific methodologies in each study, it may be difficult or unwarranted to generalize more broadly about 'overall' findings. All studies had low numbers of identified cases, and in particular, small numbers of autistic children born from immigrant parents, and many authors in these studies relied upon broadened definitions of autism. Statistical testing was not always rigorously conducted and doubts could be raised in several studies about the appropriateness of the comparison data that were used. Thus, the overall proportion of immigrants in the population is an inappropriate figure to which to compare observed rates of children from immigrant parents amongst autistic series; fertility rates of immigrant families are likely to be different from those in the host populations and call for strictly age-adjusted comparisons of individuals at risk of the disorder. The proportion of immigrants in the entire population might seriously underestimate that of younger age groups, and, in turn, this could have given rise to false positive results.

Finally, studies were generally poor in their definition of immigrant status, with some unclear amalgamation of information on country of origin, citizenship, immigrant status, race, and ethnicity. In the Utah study, where a clear breakdown by race was achieved (Ritvo et al., 1989), the autism parents showed no deviation from the racial distribution of this state; the proportion of non-whites in this study and in the state was, however, noticeably low, providing little power to detect departures from the null hypothesis. Unfortunately, other studies have not systematically reported the proportion of immigrant groups in the areas surveyed. However, in four studies where the proportions of immigrant groups were low (Bryson et al., 1988; Honda et al., 1996; Tanoue et al., 1988; Webb et al., 1997), rates of autism were in the upper rate range. Conversely, in other populations where immigrants contributed substantially to the denominators (Cialdella & Mamelle, 1989; Fombonne & du Mazaubrun, 1992; Fombonne et al., 1997), rates were in the 'rather low' band.

It is unclear what common mechanism could explain the putative association between immigrant status and autism, since the origins of the immigrant parents (especially in Gillberg et al., 1991; see also Gillberg & Gillberg, 1996) were very diverse and represented, in fact, all continents. With this heterogeneity in mind, what common biological features might be shared by these immigrant families and what would be a plausible mechanism explaining the putative association between autism and immigrant status? The possibility of an increased vulnerability to intrauterine infections in non-immunized immigrant mothers was raised but not supported in a detailed analysis of 15 autistic children from immigrant parents (Gillberg & Gillberg, 1996). These authors instead posited that parents, and in particular fathers, affected with autistic traits would be inclined to travel abroad in order to find female partners more naïve to their social difficulties. This speculation was based, however, on three observations only, and assessment of the autistic traits in two parents was clearly not independently obtained.

The hypothesis of an association between immigrant status or race and autism, therefore, remains largely unsupported by the empirical results. Most of the claims about these possible correlates of autism derived from *posthoc* observations of very small samples and were not subjected to rigorous statistical testing.

With regard to social class, 14 studies provided such information on the families of autistic children. Of these, 6 studies (Brask, 1970; Durkin et al., 2010; Hoshino et al., 1982; Leonard et al., 2011; Lotter, 1966; Treffert, 1970) suggested an association between autism and social class or parental education. The year of data collection for 4 investigations was before 1980 (Table 1.1.1), but some studies conducted thereafter (e.g., Leonard et al., 2011) provided evidence for the association. Using CDC data, Durkin et al. (2010) noted significantly higher prevalence of ASD in high SES children with a previous diagnosis of ASD (versus no diagnosis); they concluded that this supposed 'higher prevalence' was merely a reflection of diagnostic bias and likely SES disparity in access to services to children with autism. Leonard et al. (2011) remain open to other explanations, but also acknowledge the likelihood of access to services being what results in 'higher' prevalence rates of autism in higher socioeconomic groups. Thus, the epidemiological results suggest that the earlier findings were probably due to artifacts in the availability of services and in the case finding methods (see also Wing, 1980).

> While existing estimates are variable, the evidence reviewed does not support differences in ASD prevalence by geographic region nor of a strong impact of ethnic/cultural or socio-economic factors. However, power to detect such effects is seriously limited in [most] existing datasets, particularly in low-income countries. *Elsabbagh et al., in press*

CONCLUSION

Epidemiological surveys of autism and ASD have now been conducted in many countries. Methodological differences regarding case definition and finding procedures make comparisons between surveys difficult to perform. However, from recent studies, a best estimate of (74/10,000) (equivalences = 7.4/1,000, or 0.74%, or 1 child in about 70–90 children) can be confidently derived for the prevalence of ASD. Current evidence does not strongly support the hypothesis of a secular increase in the incidence of autism, but power to detect time trends is seriously limited in existing datasets. While it is clear that prevalence estimates have increased over time, this increase most likely represents changes in the concepts, definitions, service availability, and awareness of autistic-spectrum disorders in both the lay and professional public. To assess whether or not the incidence has increased, methodological factors that account for an important proportion of the variability in rates must be stringently controlled for. New survey methods have been developed for use in multinational comparisons; ongoing surveillance programs are currently under way and will soon provide more meaningful data to evaluate this hypothesis. The possibility that a true change in the underlying incidence has contributed to higher prevalence figures remains to be adequately tested. Meanwhile, the available prevalence figures carry straightforward implications for current and future needs in services and early educational intervention programs.

CHALLENGES AND FUTURE DIRECTIONS

- The phenotypic boundaries differentiating the spectrum of ASD from both severe developmental and neurogenetic disorders, and mild forms of atypical development remain uncertain and unreliable. Measures of impairment will need to be added to symptom and developmental assessments in order to refine case definitions for epidemiological studies and other research endeavors.
- Future epidemiological surveys should estimate the proportion of 'false negatives' in order to estimate the sensitivity of case ascertainment methods and obtain more accurate rates. Current prevalence rates underestimate the 'true' rates as they are not adjusted to compensate for missed cases.
- The monitoring of prevalence and incidence trends is needed. It will require methods that allow meaningful comparisons over time of cases defined and ascertained with stable approaches.

Suggested Reading

Centers for Disease Control, 2009. Prevalence of autism spectrum disorders – autism and developmental disabilities monitoring network, United States, 2006. Morbidity and Mortality Weekly Report Surveillance Summary 58, 1–14.

Chakrabarti, S., Fombonne, E., 2001. Pervasive developmental disorders in preschool children. Journal of the American Medical Association 285, 3093–3099.

Fombonne, E., 2007. Epidemiology. In: Martin, A., Volkmar, F. (Eds.), Lewis's Child and Adolescent Psychiatry: A Comprehensive Textbook, fourth ed. Lippincott, Williams, and Wilkins, pp. 150–171.

Shattuck, P.T., 2006. The contribution of diagnostic substitution to the growing administrative prevalence of autism in US special education. Pediatrics 117, 1028–1037.

References

Al-Farsi, Y.M., Al-Sharbati, M.M., Al-Farsi, O.A., Al-Shafaee, M.S., Brooks, D.R., Waly, M.I., 2011. Brief Report: Prevalence of Autistic Spectrum Disorders in the Sultanate of Oman. Journal of Autism and Developmental Disorders 41, 821–825.

American Psychiatric Association (APA), 1980. Diagnostic and Statistical Manual of Mental Disorders, third ed. American Psychiatric Association, Washington, DC.

American Psychiatric Association (APA), 1987. Diagnostic and Statistical Manual of Mental Disorders, third ed., rev. American Psychiatric Association, Washington, DC.

American Psychiatric Association (APA), 1994. Diagnostic and statistical manual of mental disorders. DSM-IV, fourth ed. American Psychiatric Association, Washington, DC.

Arvidsson, T., Danielsson, B., Forsberg, P., Gillberg, C., Johansson, M., Kjellgren, G., 1997. Autism in 3–6 year-olds in a suburb of Goteborg, Sweden. Autism 2, 163–173.

Asperger, H., 1944. Die 'autistischen psychopathen' im kindesalter (autistic psychopathology of childhood). Archiv für Psychiatrie und Nervenkrankheiten 177, 76–136.

Baird, G., Charman, T., Baron-Cohen, S., Cox, A., Swettenham, J., Wheelwright, S., et al., 2000. A screening instrument for autism at 18 months of age: A 6-year follow-up study. Journal of the American Academy of Child and Adolescent Psychiatry 39, 694–702.

Baird, G., Simonoff, E., Pickles, A., Chandler, S., Loucas, T., Meldrum, D., et al., 2006. Prevalence of disorders of the autism spectrum in a population cohort of children in South Thames: The special needs and autism project (SNAP). Lancet 368, 210–215.

Barbaresi, W.J., Katusic, S.K., Colligan, R.C., Weaver, A.L., Jacobsen, S.J., 2005. The incidence of autism in Olmsted County, Minnesota, 1976–1997: Results from a population-based study. Archives of Pediatrics & Adolescent Medicine 159, 37–44.

Barnevik-Olsson, M., Gillberg, C., Fernell, E., 2010. Clinical Letter: Prevalence of autism in children of Somali origin living in Stockholm: Brief report of an at-risk population. Developmental Medicine and Child Neurology 52, 1167–1168.

Baron-Cohen, S., Scott, F.J., Allison, C., Williams, J., Bolton, P., Matthews, F.E., et al., 2009. Prevalence of autism-spectrum conditions: UK school-based population study. British Journal of Psychiatry 194, 500–509.

Bertrand, J., Mars, A., Boyle, C., Bove, F., Yeargin-Allsopp, M., Decoufle, P., 2001. Prevalence of autism in a United States population: The Brick Township, New Jersey, investigation. Pediatrics 108, 1155–1161.

Bishop, D.V., Whitehouse, A.J., Watt, H.J., Line, E.A., 2008. Autism and diagnostic substitution: Evidence from a study of adults with a history of developmental language disorder. Developmental Medicine and Child Neurology 50, 341–345.

Bohman, M., Bohman, I., Bjorck, P., Sjoholm, E., 1983. Childhood psychosis in a northern Swedish county: Some preliminary findings from an epidemiological survey. In: Schmidt, M., Remschmidt, H. (Eds.), Epidemiological Approaches in Child Psychiatry. Georg Thieme Verlag, Stuttgart, pp. 164–173.

Brask, B., 1970. A prevalence investigation of childhood psychoses. Paper presented at the Nordic Symposium on the Care of Psychotic Children, Oslo.

Brugha, T.S., McManus, S., Bankart, J., Scott, F., Purdon, S., Smith, J., et al., 2011. Epidemiology of Autism Spectrum Disorders in adults in the community in England. Archives of General Psychiatry 68, 459–466.

Bryson, S.E., Clark, B.S., Smith, I.M., 1988. First report of a Canadian epidemiological study of autistic syndromes. Journal of Child Psychology and Psychiatry and Allied Disciplines 29, 433–445.

Burd, L., Fisher, W., Kerbeshan, J., 1987. A prevalance study of pervasive developmental disorders in North Dakota. Journal of the American Academy of Child and Adolescent Psychiatry 26, 700–703.

California Department of Developmental Services (CDDS), 1999, March 1. Changes in the population of persons with autism and pervasive developmental disorders in California's Developmental Services System: 1987 through 1998. Report to the Legislature March 1, 1999, 19 pages. Available at. <http://www.dds.ca.gov> (accessed 14.05.12.).

California Department of Developmental Services (CDDS), 2003, April. Autism Spectrum Disorders: Changes in the California Caseload – An Update 1999 Through 2002 Available at. <http://iier.isciii.es/autismo/pdf/aut_ar03.pdf> (accessed 18.05.12.).

California Department of Developmental Services (CDDS), 2007, December. Table 34 Available at: <http://www.dds.ca.gov/FactsStats/docs/Dec07_QRTTBLS.pdf> (accessed 28.01.09.).

Census Bureau for the US. Available at. <http://www.census.gov/> (accessed 18.05.12.).

Centers for Disease Control (CDC), 2007. Prevalence of autism spectrum disorders—Autism and developmental disabilities monitoring network, six sites, United States, 2000. Morbidity and Mortality Weekly Report Surveillance Summary 56, 1–11.

Centers for Disease Control (CDC), 2007. Prevalence of autism spectrum disorders—Autism and developmental disabilities monitoring network, 14 sites, United States, 2002. Morbidity and Mortality Weekly Report Surveillance Summary 56, 12–28.

Centers for Disease Control (CDC), 2009. Prevalence of autism spectrum disorders—Autism and developmental disabilities monitoring network, United States, 2006. Morbidity and Mortality Weekly Report Surveillance Summary 58, 1–14.

Chakrabarti, S., Fombonne, E., 2001. Pervasive developmental disorders in preschool children. Journal of the American Medical Association 285, 3093–3099.

Chakrabarti, S., Fombonne, E., 2005. Pervasive developmental disorders in preschool children: Confirmation of high prevalence. American Journal of Psychiatry 162, 1133–1141.

Cialdella, P., Mamelle, N., 1989. An epidemiological study of infantile autism in a French department (Rhone): A research note. Journal of Child Psychology and Psychiatry and Allied Disciplines 30, 165–175.

Croen, L.A., Grether, J.K., Hoogstrate, J., Selvin, S., 2002. The changing prevalence of autism in California. Journal of Autism and Developmental Disorders 32, 207–215.

Davidovitch, M., Holtzman, G., Tirosh, E., 2001, March. Autism in the Haifa area: An epidemiological perspective. Israeli Medical Association Journal 3, 188–189.

Durkin, M.S., Maenner, M.J., Meaney, F.J., Levy, S.E., DiGuiseppi, C., Nicholas, J.S., et al., 2010. Socioecnomic inequality in the prevalence of Autism Spectrum Disorder: Evidence from a U.S. cross-sectional study. PLoS ONE 5, e11551.

Eagle, R.S., 2004. Commentary: Further commentary on the debate regarding increase in autism in California. Journal of Autism and Developmental Disorders 34, 87–88.

Ehlers, S., Gillberg, C., 1993. The epidemiology of Asperger syndrome: A total population study. Journal of Child Psychology and Psychiatry and Allied Disciplines 34, 1327–1350.

Ellefsen, A., Kampmann, H., Billstedt, E., Gillberg, I.C., Gillberg, C., 2007. Autism in the Faroe islands: An epidemiological study. Journal of Autism and Developmental Disorders 37, 437–444.

Elsabbagh, M., Divan, G., Koh, Y.-J., Kim, Y.S., Kauchali, S., Marcin, C., et al., 2012. Global Prevalence of Autism and other Pervasive Developmental Disorders. Autism Research. John Wiley & Sons.

Fombonne, E., 2001. Is there an epidemic of autism? Pediatrics 107, 411–413.

Fombonne, E., 2003. Epidemiological surveys of autism and other pervasive developmental disorders: An update. Journal of Autism and Developmental Disorders 33, 365–382.

Fombonne, E., 2003. The prevalence of autism. Journal of the American Medical Association 289, 1–3.

Fombonne, E., 2005. Epidemiology of autistic disorder and other pervasive developmental disorders. Journal of Clinical Psychiatry 66, 3–8.

Fombonne, E., 2007. Epidemiology. In: Martin, A., Volkmar, F. (Eds.), Lewis's child and adolescent psychiatry: A comprehensive textbook, fourth ed. Lippincott, Williams, and Wilkins, Philadelphia, pp. 150–171.

Fombonne, E., 2009. Epidemiology of Pervasive Developmental Disorders. Pediatric Research 65, 591–598.

Fombonne, E., 2009. Commentary: On King and Bearman. International Journal of Epidemiology 38, 1241–1242.

Fombonne, E., du Mazaubrun, C., 1992. Prevalence of infantile autism in four French regions. Social Psychiatry and Psychiatric Epidemiology 27, 203–210.

Fombonne, E., du Mazaubrun, C., Cans, C., Grandjean, H., 1997. Autism and associated medical disorders in a French epidemiological survey. Journal of the American Academy of Child and Adolescent Psychiatry 36, 1561–1569.

Fombonne, E., Quirke, S., Hagen, A., 2011. Epidemiology of pervasive developmental disorders. In: Amaral, D.G., Dawson, G., Geschwind, D.H. (Eds.), Autism Spectrum Disorders. Oxford University Press.

Fombonne, E., Simmons, H., Ford, T., Meltzer, H., Goodman, R., 2001. Prevalence of pervasive developmental disorders in the British nationwide survey of child mental health. Journal of the American Academy of Child and Adolescent Psychiatry 40, 820–827.

Fombonne, E., Zakarian, R., Bennett, A., Meng, L., McLean-Heywood, D., 2006. Pervasive developmental disorders in Montreal, Quebec, Canada: Prevalence and links with immunizations. Pediatrics 118, e139–150.

Ghanizadeh, A., 2008. A preliminary study on screening prevalence of pervasive developmental disorder in school children in Iran. Journal of Autism and Developmental Disorders 38, 759–763.

Gillberg, C., 1984. Infantile autism and other childhood psychoses in a Swedish urban region: Epidemiological aspects. Journal of Child Psychology and Psychiatry and Allied Disciplines 25, 35–43.

Gillberg, C., 1987. Infantile autism in children of immigrant parents. A population-based study from Goteborg, Sweden. British Journal of Psychiatry 150, 856–858.

Gillberg, I.C., Gillberg, C., 1996. Autism in immigrants: A population-based study from Swedish rural and urban areas. Journal of Intellectual Disability Research 40, 24–31.

Gillberg, C., Cederlund, M., Lamberg, K., Zeijlon, L., 2006. Brief report: The autism epidemic. The registered prevalence of autism in a Swedish urban area. Journal of Autism and Developmental Disorders 36, 429–435.

Gillberg, C., Schaumann, H., Gillberg, I.C., 1995. Autism in immigrants: Children born in Sweden to mothers born in Uganda. Journal of Intellectual Disability Research 39, 141–144.

Gillberg, C., Steffenburg, S., Schaumann, H., 1991. Is autism more common now than ten years ago? British Journal of Psychiatry 158, 403–409.

Gurney, J.G., Fritz, M.S., Ness, K.K., Sievers, P., Newschaffer, C.J., Shapiro, E.G., 2003. Analysis of prevalence trends of autism spectrum disorder in Minnesota. Archives of Pediatrics and Adolescent Medicine 157, 622–627.

Harrison, M.J., O'Hare, A.E., Campbell, H., Adamson, A., McNeillage, J., 2006. Prevalence of autistic spectrum disorders in Lothian, Scotland: An estimate using the "capture-recapture" technique. Archives of Disease in Childhood 91, 16–19.

Hertz-Picciotto, I., Delwiche, L., 2009. The rise in autism and the role of age at diagnosis. Epidemiology 38, 84–90.

Honda, H., Shimizu, Y., Misumi, K., Niimi, M., Ohashi, Y., 1996. Cumulative incidence and prevalence of childhood autism in children in Japan. British Journal of Psychiatry 169, 228–235.

Honda, H., Shimizu, Y., Rutter, M., 2005. No effect of MMR withdrawal on the incidence of autism: A total population study. Journal of Child Psychology and Psychiatry and Allied Disciplines 46, 572–579.

Hoshino, Y., Kumashiro, H., Yashima, Y., Tachibana, R., Watanabe, M., 1982. The epidemiological study of autism in Fukushima-Ken. Folia Psychiatrica et Neurologica Japonica 36, 115–124.

Icasiano, F., Hewson, P., Machet, P., Cooper, C., Marshall, A., 2004. Childhood autism spectrum disorder in the Barwon region: A community based study. Journal of Paediatrics and Child Health 40, 696–701.

Jick, H., Kaye, J.A., Black, C., 2003. Epidemiology and possible causes of autism changes in risk of autism in the UK for birth cohorts 1990–1998. Pharmacotherapy 23, 1524–1530.

Kadesjo, B., Gillberg, C., Hagberg, B., 1999. Brief report: Autism and Asperger syndrome in seven-year-old children: A total population study. Journal of Autism and Developmental Disorders 29, 327–331.

Kanner, L., 1943. Autistic disturbances of affective contact. The Nervous Child 2, 217–250.

Kawamura, Y., Takahashi, O., Ishii, T., 2008. Reevaluating the incidence of pervasive developmental disorders: Impact of elevated rates of detection through implementation of an integrated system of screening in Toyota, Japan. Psychiatry and Clinical Neurosciences 62, 152–159.

Kielinen, M., Linna, S.-L., Moilanen, I., 2000. Autism in northern Finland. European Child and Adolescent Psychiatry 9, 162–167.

Kim, Y.S., Leventhal, B.L., Koh, Y.J., Fombonne, E., Laska, E., Lim, E.C., et al., 2011. Prevalence of Autism Spectrum Disorders in a total population sample. American Journal of Psychiatry [Epub ahead of print].

King, M., Bearman, P., 2009. Diagnostic change and the increase in prevalence of autism. International Journal of Epidemiology 38, 1224–1234.

Kogan, M.D., Blumberg, S.J., Schieve, L.A., Boyle, C.A., Perrin, J.M., Ghandour, R.M., et al., 2009. Prevalence of parent-reported diagnosis of autism spectrum disorder among children in the US, 2007. Pediatrics 124, 1395–1403.

Latif, A.H., Williams, W.R., 2007. Diagnostic trends in autistic spectrum disorders in the South Wales valleys. Autism 11, 479–487.

Lazoff, T., Zhong, L., Piperni, T., Fombonne, E., 2010. Prevalence rates of PDD among children in a Montreal School Board. The Canadian Journal of Child Psychiatry 55, 715–720.

Le Couteur, A., Rutter, M., Lord, C., Rios, P., Robertson, S., Holdgrafer, M., et al., 1989. Autism diagnostic interview: A standardized investigator-based instrument. Journal of Autism and Developmental Disorders 19, 363–387.

Leonard, H., Glasson, E., Nassar, N., Whitehouse, A., Bebbington, A., Bourke, J., et al., 2011. Autism and intellectual disability are differentially related to sociodemographic background at birth. PLoS ONE 6, e17875.

Lord, C., Risi, S., Lambrecht, L., Cook Jr., E.H., Leventhal, B.L., DiLavore, P.C., et al., 2000. The Autism Diagnostic Observation Schedule-Generic: A standard measure of social and communication deficits associated with the spectrum of autism. Journal of Autism and Developmental Disorders 30, 205–223.

Lotter, V., 1966. Epidemiology of autistic conditions in young children: I. Prevalence. Social Psychiatry 1, 124–137.

Madsen, K.M., Hviid, A., Vestergaard, M., Schendel, D., Wohlfahrt, J., Thorsen, P., et al., 2002. A population-based study of measles, mumps, and rubella vaccination and autism. New England Journal of Medicine 347, 1477–1482.

Magnússon, P., Saemundsen, E., 2001. Prevalence of autism in Iceland. Journal of Autism and Developmental Disorders 31, 153–163.

Matsuishi, T., Shiotsuki, M., Yoshimura, K., Shoji, H., Imuta, F., Yamashita, F., 1987. High prevalence of infantile autism in Kurume city, Japan. Journal of Child Neurology 2, 268–271.

McCarthy, P., Fitzgerald, M., Smith, M., 1984. Prevalence of childhood autism in Ireland. Irish Medical Journal 77, 129–130.

MIND Institute, 2002, October 17. Report to the Legislature on the Principal Findings From the Epidemiology of Autism in California. A Comprehensive Pilot Study. University of California, Davis.

Nicholas, J.S., Charles, J.M., Carpenter, L.A., King, L.B., Jenner, W., Spratt, E.G., 2008. Prevalence and characteristics of children with autism-spectrum disorders. Annals of Epidemiology 18, 130–136.

Oliveira, G., Ataide, A., Marques, C., Miguel, T.S., Coutinho, A.M., Mota-Vieira, L., et al., 2007. Epidemiology of autism spectrum disorder in Portugal: Prevalence, clinical characterization, and medical conditions. Developmental Medicine and Child Neurology 49, 726–733.

Palmer, R.F., Walker, T., Mandell, D., Bayles, B., Miller, C.S., 2010. Explaining low rates of autism among Hispanic schoolchildren in Texas. American Journal of Public Health 100, 270–272.

Parner, E.T., Thorsen, P., Dixon, G., de Klerk, N., Leonard, H., Nassar, N., et al., 2011. A comparison of autism prevalence trends in Denmark and Western Australia. Journal of Autism and Developmental Disorders 41, 1601–1608.

Paula, C.S., Ribeiro, S., Fombonne, E., Mercadante, M.T., 2011. Brief report: Prevalence of pervasive developmental disorder in Brazil: A pilot study. Journal of Autism and Developmental Disorders 41, 1738–1742.

Powell, J., Edwards, A., Edwards, M., Pandit, B., Sungum-Paliwal, S., Whitehouse, W., 2000. Changes in the incidence of childhood autism and other autistic spectrum disorders in preschool children from two areas of the West Midlands, UK. Developmental Medicine and Child Neurology 42, 624–628.

Ritvo, E., Freeman, B., Pingree, C., Mason-Brothers, A., Jorde, L., Jenson, W.R., et al., 1989. The UCLA-University of Utah epidemiologic survey of autism: Prevalence. American Journal of Psychiatry 146, 194–199.

Rutter, M., 1970. Autistic children: Infancy to adulthood. Seminars in Psychiatry 2, 435–450.

Samadi, S.A., Mahmoodizadeh, A., McConkey, R., 2011. A national study of the prevalence of autism among five-year-old children in Iran. Sage Publications and The National Autistic Society, 1–13.

Scott, F.J., Baron-Cohen, S., Bolton, P., Brayne, C., 2002. Brief report: Prevalence of autism spectrum conditions in children aged 5–11 years in Cambridgeshire, UK. Autism 6, 231–237.

Shattuck, P.T., 2006. The contribution of diagnostic substitution to the growing administrative prevalence of autism in US special education. Pediatrics 117, 1028–1037.

Shattuck, P.T., Durkin, M., Maenner, M., Newschaffer, C., Mandell, D.S., Wiggins, L., et al., 2009. Timing of identification among children with an autism spectrum disorder: Findings from a population-based surveillance study. Journal of the American Academy of Child and Adolescent Psychiatry 48, 474–483.

Sponheim, E., Skjeldal, O., 1998. Autism and related disorders: Epidemiological findings in a Norwegian study using icd-10 diagnostic criteria. Journal of Autism and Developmental Disorders 28, 217–227.

Steffenburg, S., Gillberg, C., 1986. Autism and autistic-like conditions in Swedish rural and urban areas: a population study. The British Journal of Psychiatry 149, 81–87.

Steinhausen, H.-C., Gobel, D., Breinlinger, M., Wohlloben, B., 1986. A community survey of infantile autism. Journal of the American Academy of Child Psychiatry 25, 186–189.

Sugiyama, T., Abe, T., 1989. The prevalence of autism in Nagoya, Japan: A total population study. Journal of Autism and Developmental Disorders 19, 87–96.

Tanoue, Y., Oda, S., Asano, F., Kawashima, K., 1988. Epidemiology of infantile autism in southern Ibaraki, Japan: Differences in prevalence in birth cohorts. Journal of Autism and Developmental Disorders 18, 155–166.

Taylor, B., Miller, E., Farrington, C., Petropoulos, M.-C., Favot-Mayaud, I., Li, J., et al., 1999, June 12. Autism and measles, mumps, and rubella vaccine: No epidemiological evidence for a causal association. Lancet 353, 2026–2029.

Tebruegge, M., Nandini, V., Ritchie, J., 2004. Does routine child health surveillance contribute to the early detection of children with pervasive developmental disorders? An epidemiological study in Kent, UK. BMC Pediatrics 4, 4.

Treffert, D.A., 1970. Epidemiology of infantile autism. Archives of General Psychiatry 22, 431–438.

van Balkom, I.D.C., Bresnahan, M., Vogtländer, M.F., van Hoeken, D., Minderaa, R., Susser, E., et al., 2009. Prevalence of treated autism spectrum disorders in Aruba. Journal of Neurodevelopmental Disorders 1, 197–204.

Wazana, A., Bresnahan, M., Kline, J., 2007. The autism epidemic: Fact or artifact? Journal of the American Academy of Child and Adolescent Psychiatry 46, 721–730.

Webb, E., Lobo, S., Hervas, A., Scourfield, J., Fraser, W., 1997. The changing prevalence of autistic disorder in a Welsh health district. Developmental Medicine and Child Neurology 39, 150–152.

Webb, E., Morey, J., Thompsen, W., Butler, C., Barber, M., Fraser, W.I., 2003. Prevalence of autistic spectrum disorder in children attending mainstream schools in a Welsh education authority. Developmental Medicine and Child Neurology 45, 377–384.

Wignyosumarto, S., Mukhlas, M., Shirataki, S., 1992. Epidemiological and clinical study of autistic children in Yogyakarta, Indonesia. Kobe Journal of Medical Sciences 38, 1–19.

Williams, J.G., Brayne, C.E., Higgins, J.P., 2006. Systematic review of prevalence studies of autism spectrum disorders. Archives of Disease in Childhood 91, 8–15.

Williams, E., Thomas, K., Sidebotham, H., Emond, A., 2008. Prevalence and characteristics of autistic spectrum disorders in the ALSPAC cohort. Developmental Medicine and Child Neurology 50, 672–677.

Wing, L., 1980. Childhood autism and social class: A question of selection? British Journal of Psychiatry 137, 410–417.

Wing, L., 1993. The definition and prevalence of autism: A review. European Child and Adolescent Psychiatry 2, 61–74.

Wing, L., Gould, J., 1979. Severe impairments of social interaction and associated abnormalities in children: Epidemiology and classification. Journal of Autism and Developmental Disorders 9, 11–29.

Wing, L., Yeates, S., Brierly, L., Gould, J., 1976. The prevalence of early childhood autism: Comparison of administrative and epidemiological studies. Psychological Medicine 6, 89–100.

Wolff, S., Barlow, A., 1979. Schizoid personality in childhood: A comparative study of schizoid, autistic and normal children. Journal of Child Psychology and Psychiatry 20, 29–46.

Wong, V.C., Hui, S.L., 2008. Epidemiological study of autism spectrum disorder in China. Journal of Child Neurology 23, 67–72.

ICD-10, 1977. The ICD-9 Classification of Mental and Behavioural Disorders: Clinical Descriptions and Diagnostic Guidelines. World Health Organization, Geneva.

ICD-10, 1992. The ICD-10 Classification of Mental and Behavioural Disorders: Clinical Descriptions and Diagnostic Guidelines. World Health Organization, Geneva.

Yeargin-Allsopp, M., Rice, C., Karapurkar, T., Doernberg, N., Boyle, C., Murphy, C., 2003. Prevalence of autism in a US metropolitan area [comment]. Journal of the American Medical Association 289 49–55.

The Behavioral Manifestations of Autism Spectrum Disorders

So Hyun Kim*, Catherine Lord†

*Autism Program, Yale Child Study Center, Yale University, School of Medicine, CT, USA †Center for Autism and the Developing Brain, Weill Cornell Medical College, NY, USA

HISTORICAL PERSPECTIVES ON ASD BEHAVIORAL MANIFESTATIONS

The first documentations of autism spectrum disorders (ASD) as a syndrome were made in the early 1940s, in parallel by a psychiatrist and a pediatrician in different countries. Leo Kanner (1943) described 11 children with social aloofness, insistence on sameness, and language delays or oddities. At about the same time, Hans Asperger (1944) described 4 children whom he called 'little professors' who showed social awkwardness and circumscribed interests, with intact abilities in vocabulary and syntactic aspects of language. Later, Frith (1989) compared these different descriptions of ASD, which have formed the base for conceptualizations of ASD until now.

Due to the influence of psychodynamic theories in the 1960s, many believed that autism, also known as a childhood form of schizophrenia, was caused by social

deprivation and/or poor parenting (Bettelheim, 1967). However, even in the 1940s, both Kanner and Asperger recognized familial, and presumably genetic, qualities that they observed in children with ASD in the parents of their child-patients. These broader phenotypes, believed to run in families, are being studied currently but it was not until the late 1960s that a number of clinical researchers began to question the psychodynamic approach, and suggested that ASD was a neurologically based disorder. In fact, researchers have found associations between autism and seizures, intellectual disability, language, and cognitive deficits arising from attentional difficulties and sensory and vestibular systems (Hermelin and O'Connor, 1970; Rimland, 1964; Rutter and Schopler, 1978). In addition, Folstein and Rutter's (1978) twin study found much greater concordance for autism in monozygotic than dizygotic twins. However, identical twins with autism-related symptoms were NOT *identical* in ASD symptoms, providing important evidence for

The Neuroscience of Autism Spectrum Disorders.
http://dx.doi.org/10.1016/B978-0-12-391924-3.00002-8

another feature of ASD – heterogeneity – which was found even within the restricted range of identical genotypes in identical twins.

Shortly thereafter, another group of researchers carried out an epidemiological study of children in London, and described a triad of impairments in social reciprocity, language comprehension, and play (Wing and Gould, 1978). This led to a broader definition of autism, and the term 'pervasive developmental disorders' (PDD) was used in the Diagnostic and Statistical Manual of the American Psychiatric Association (DSM-IV) and the International Classification of Diseases code (ICD-10), which determine current diagnostic categorizations (APA, 1994; WHO, 1990). In the past few years, professional and parent advocacy groups have strongly argued for its replacement by *autism spectrum disorders* (ASD), a more straightforward term. It has been suggested that the term ASD reflects *autism* as the best-characterized core syndrome, within a *spectrum* of the disorder, distinguished from autism by several factors as well as severity within those factors, thus constituting a spectrum.

CORE FEATURES OF ASD

Social and Communication Deficits

In the past 20 years, our understanding of social and communication deficits in individuals with ASD has become increasingly refined. In the DSM-IV (APA, 1994) and the ICD-10 (WHO, 1990), social and communication impairments in autism are conceptualized as separate entities. Existing criteria distinguish the communication deficits in autism, such as severe delays in expressive language level, as a separate symptom domain from social impairments. However, research on the behavioral manifestation of ASD highlights that several communication impairments in ASD, such as limited engagement in social chat, difficulties in reciprocal conversation, and limited gestures, are both social factors and communication (Snow et al., 2009). Moreover, several recent studies have also shown that it is more valid and parsimonious to think of the social and communication symptom domains as a single factor rather than being separate (Gotham et al., 2007; Kim and Lord, 2011a).

There are several aspects of the communication impairments in ASD which go beyond speech/language delays. Language delays in individuals with ASD are not compensated by other modes of communications, such as eye contact, gestures, and facial expressions, as one would expect to see in other populations. Problems with speech quality have been noted in individuals with ASD (e.g., unusual prosody, rhythm) as well as a tendency towards using repetitive speech patterns such as stereotyped speech or delayed echolalia (e.g., repeating lines from a Disney movie).

Children with ASD show delays or failures to achieve various social communication milestones during the first year or two of life. As infants, children later diagnosed with ASD often show difficulties such as following another person's shift in gaze, smiling at someone who smiles or vocalizes at them, and vocalizing 'back' to someone who is talking to them (Baranek, 1999). As they become older and more verbally fluent, children and adolescents with ASD show impairments in reciprocity while conversing with others, such as building on what the other person says or listening to how someone else feels about a particular experience. Other conversational deficits include difficulties initiating and maintaining meaningful conversation (e.g., not responding to others' leads or questions).

Other social and communication deficits occur in different developmental milestones such as complex imaginative play, cooperative play in a group, and gestures (APA, 2000). Many individuals with ASD whose verbal abilities are intact still tend to use limited gestures that are not well integrated with other modes of communication (e.g., eye contact, vocalizations). All of these deficits and delays may negatively affect the development of meaningful social relationships with peers and others.

Restricted and Repetitive Behaviors and Interests

Another hallmark of ASD is restricted and repetitive behaviors and interests (RRBs). Based on the proposed DSM-5 criteria of ASD (APA, 2010), RRBs include a very broad category of behaviors such as intense preoccupations and interests (e.g., having very specific knowledge about vacuum cleaners); adherence to specific, nonfunctional routines (e.g., insisting on taking a certain route to school); repetitive motor manners (e.g., hand flapping); and preoccupation with parts of objects (e.g., peering at the wheels of toy cars while spinning them).

Many examples of RRBs represent deviance because the presence of most of these behaviors is generally considered abnormal at any age. However, during infancy and toddlerhood, some of the behaviors conceptualized as examples of RRBs have been found to be also present in typically developing children and children with other non-ASD developmental disorders (Charman and Baird, 2002; Kim and Lord, 2010; Ventola et al., 2006). For example, some children with other developmental disorders such as intellectual disabilities without autism have been found to show some types of RRBs such as unusual sensory interests and complex mannerisms. These kinds of RRBs have been usually conceptualized as 'lower-order' RRBs that are associated with lower intellectual functioning (Turner, 1999). However, even though RRBs have been observed in very young children without autism, they have been found to be significantly more prevalent and/or severe in children and adolescents with ASD aged 1 to 20 years than those with other developmental disorders, or in typically developing children and adolescents (Kim and Lord, 2010; Richler et al., 2007; South et al., 2005).

Previous studies have examined heterogeneity in RRBs using factor analyses and found support for two different RRB factors: repetitive sensory-motor behaviors (RSMB; e.g., hand/finger mannerisms, unusual sensory interests, repetitive use of objects, complex mannerisms) and insistence on sameness (IS; e.g., difficulties with change in routine, compulsions/rituals, unusual attachment to objects; Bishop et al., 2006; Szatmari et al., 2006). These different types of RRB vary in their associations with NVIQ and age. For example, studies have found that RSMB, including sensory interests, hand and finger mannerisms, and complex mannerisms, were negatively associated with NVIQ and stable over time (Kim and Lord, 2010; Richler et al., 2010). While RSMB was frequently associated with lower cognitive and adaptive functioning, IS had been shown to be relatively independent of other phenotypic features (Richler et al., 2010). These different types of RRB also varied in their trajectories over time (see below). Some of these behaviors overlap with symptoms of other disorders, including obsessive-compulsive disorder (OCD; Leyfer et al., 2006).

In addition to the RSMB and IS factors, Lam and colleagues (2008) recently reported a third factor, circumscribed interests (CI), which included behaviors such as intense, focused hobbies; strong preoccupations with particular topics (e.g., Egyptian history, sewer systems); and unusually strong attachment to certain objects. In this study, CI was found to be independent of participant characteristics such as gender, age, and IQ, as well as presence of language loss/regression and autism symptoms. These results suggested that CI might be more specific to autism than RSMB and IS, as the latter two are found among other non-ASD developmental disorders. It was also argued that there have been no other psychiatric and developmental disorders that include CI as a manifestation of RRBs. In addition, Lam et al. (2008) suggested that the CI and IS factors may be of use in genetic investigation since both factors showed significant familial associations. Research has been limited in this area and the results from different studies have varied by sample and analytical methods, thus replication is needed.

HETEROGENEITY IN BEHAVIORAL MANIFESTATIONS OF ASD

Behavioral manifestations of ASD vary widely from one individual to another. This heterogeneity is impacted by variability in different factors, such as developmental trajectories, level of language, cognitive ability, gender, adaptive behaviors, and sensory and motor impairments. Given the extreme heterogeneity in behavioral manifestations of ASD, it is not clear whether the same etiological factors can explain different phenotypes (e.g., a nonverbal child with severe intellectual disability and verbally fluent child with advanced intellectual functioning; Lord and Corsello, 2005). These groups of children would also differ in their response to interventions. Thus, it is important to review past literature to examine how heterogeneity in behavioral manifestations of ASD is affected by variability in other factors.

Patterns of Onset and Regression

Some children with ASD start to show symptoms that are specific to ASD as early as 8 months (Watson et al., 2007). Patterns of onset of ASD have been examined, particularly in children who exhibit a loss of language and/or social skills in the first few years of life. Regression is highly specific to ASD. Some children who show loss in the domain of language then regain skills close to typical development prior to disruption, but others do not (Pickles et al., 2009). However, Lord et al. (2004b) also argued that, for many children with language loss, development prior to loss was rarely reported as entirely normal. In addition, a sample of multiplex families in which both affected family members had a history of regression showed an evidence of linkage on chromosome 7q and 21q, including regions containing genes expressed in fetal brain (Molloy et al., 2005). On the other hand, several studies found that children with a history of regression, by later childhood, do not show differences in autism symptom severity, intellectual functioning, adaptive behaviors, seizures, and gastrointestinal difficulties compared to children without a history of regression. Many of these studies have relied on retrospective parent-reporting of regression, which may not capture the more subtle losses observed in prospective studies (Ozonoff et al., 2011).

Developmental Trajectories

Past studies generally report overall gains in abilities for children with ASD over time, with considerable variability in outcomes (e.g., Mawhood et al., 2000; Sigman and Ruskin, 1999). Even though the diagnosis of autism has been found to be reasonably stable from the second or third year of life to early childhood and adolescence, different symptom domains or abilities show different trajectories (Lord et al., 2006; Moore and Goodson, 2003). Using a sample of 26 children with ASD, Charman et al. (2005) found that the heterogeneity in the severity of symptoms, language levels, and nonverbal IQ scores increased over time from 2 to 7 years of age. In addition, communication skills have been found to show variability in trajectory from large gains to decreases in verbal skills over time relative to age norms (e.g., Anderson et al., 2007; Charman et al., 2005; Sigman and McGovern, 2005). RRBs have also shown variability in trajectories, showing both increases and stability over time depending on different samples and age groups (Charman et al., 2005; Piven et al., 1996; Starr et al., 2003).

Many studies have reported improvements in ASD symptoms over time. For example, improvements in adaptive behavior and social responsiveness have been reported from early childhood to late adolescence (McGovern and Sigman, 2005). In this study, parents of individuals with ASD reported fewer symptoms in the areas of socialization and RRBs when their children were in adolescence than in early childhood.

Even though some improvements have been observed from early childhood into teen years, adolescents with ASD continue to experience significant degrees of autism symptoms and dependency despite a small subgroup with more favorable adult outcomes (Seltzer et al., 2004). Although autism symptoms and maladaptive behaviors in adolescents and young adults with ASD showed improvements during the secondary school years, improvement may slow after high school exit for internalizing behavior problems and most autism symptoms (Taylor and Seltzer, 2010). Thus, developmental trajectories and prognoses of ASD are quite variable, and are linked to factors such as the severity of autism-specific difficulties in social and communication functioning and repetitive behaviors, and the general level of functioning, including adaptive behaviors and intellectual functioning.

Intellectual Impairments

Cognitive abilities observed in ASD range from severe intellectual disability to scores in the superior range on tests of intellectual functioning. In the past, it was believed that more than 50% of individuals with ASD had nonverbal IQ scores below 70 (e.g., mild to severe intellectual disability). However, recent studies have suggested that the proportion of children with ASD with nonverbal IQ scores below 70 is somewhere between 20 and 50% (Charman et al., 2011). In addition,

nonverbal IQ scores in most children with ASD are found to be stable over time from age 2 to later school age.

Research has also focused on examining the differences in cognitive functioning between Asperger syndrome (AS) and those referred to as 'high functioning autism' (HFA). In the DSM-IV, AS is differentiated from autism by the absence of a history of language delay. Individuals with HFA generally include those who have IQs in the average to above average range. Studies examining the differences in cognitive functioning between these two groups have provided mixed results. For instance, the results of some studies have suggested that individuals with AS have higher verbal and/or nonverbal IQs than those with HFA (e.g., Klin et al., 1995). In contrast, results from other studies have indicated that there is no difference between these groups (e.g., Ozonoff et al., 2000).

Individuals with ASD have also varied in their IQ profiles, specifically in the discrepancy between verbal IQ (VIQ) and performance IQ (PIQs). Earlier, it was suggested that children with ASD had relative strengths in PIQs compared to VIQs (e.g., Lockyer and Rutter, 1970). However, more recent studies have shown that, as IQs approach the average range or higher, a few individuals, though not all, have significantly higher VIQs than PIQs (Klin et al., 1995), though the most common profile was similar PIQs and VIQs (Charman et al., 2011). Individuals with discrepant cognitive profiles (VIQs < PIQs) were shown to have increased gray matter volume (Joseph, 2011).

Language Level and Verbal IQ

Language abilities in ASD vary from individuals who do not develop functional speech to those who are verbally fluent. In the past, it was believed that 50% of the ASD population did not acquire any functional language (Lord et al., 2004a). Overall, it has been shown that about 30% of preschoolers with ASD have no functional use of language across different diagnostic subtypes (Chakrabarti and Fombonne, 2001).

Given the tremendous variability in language levels, the presence of distinct ASD subgroups based on language profiles has been suggested. For instance, Tager-Flusberg and colleagues (2011) highlighted three language subgroups within ASD:

1. Individuals who are verbally fluent and do not have difficulties with structural aspects of language (e.g., vocabulary, syntax, phonology);
2. Individuals who acquire varying degrees of functional language, though acquisition may be delayed, development may be slowed, and they may

have ongoing difficulties in different areas of language;

3. Individuals who remain nonverbal (i.e., do not develop the ability to speak).

Past longitudinal studies of young children with ASD have indicated that the emergence of spoken language is one of the most important variables predicting better outcomes in later childhood and adulthood (Howlin et al., 2004; Venter et al., 1992). Children who have not developed language by age 5 are more impaired on early measures of social, communication, joint attention, and imitation skills (Thurm et al., 2007). Improvements in spoken language and communication skills have become one of the main goals in early treatments of ASD (Kasari et al., 2010). A handful of past studies examined the potential factors associated with development of verbal skills in ASD. One of the most widely studied factors related to development of language skills in ASD is joint attention, which includes 'behaviors used to follow or direct the attention of another person to an event or object to share an interest in that event or object' (Siller and Sigman, 2002). A child's ability to initiate or attend to bids for joint attention (e.g., pointing, showing, and alternating gaze) is a strong predictor of verbal abilities, based on multiple studies with preschoolers, older children, adolescents, and/or adults with ASD (Dawson et al., 2004; Mundy and Neal, 2001; Sigman and McGovern, 2005).

In addition to joint attention skills, the severity of autism symptoms has been also examined as one of the predictors of verbal abilities in ASD. Poor language outcomes at age 7 were associated with impairment at age 3 in the areas of restricted and repetitive behaviors and socialization (Charman et al., 2005). Compared to children with receptive language disorder only, a verbally able autism group was more impaired on language and verbal IQ measures at age 7.5 years (Mawhood et al., 2000). Moreover, preschoolers with a diagnosis of autism, compared to those with a broader diagnosis of PDD-NOS, showed poorer language outcome 2–3 years later (Charman et al., 2003), even after accounting for initial nonverbal and language scores (Thurm et al., 2007). Finally, several studies showed a relatively high concordance rate for verbal/nonverbal status in sibling and twin pairs (e.g., Spiker et al., 2001) though results were not consistent. As of now, little is known about the biological mechanisms underlying the failure to acquire spoken language (Tager-Flusberg et al., 2011).

Gender

Gender is also one of the most important factors associated with heterogeneity in ASD. ASD is approximately 3–4 times more prevalent in boys than girls (CDC, 2007). In the past, early studies reported that females with ASD were more impaired than males in both cognitive and adaptive functioning, (Lord et al., 1982; Tsai et al., 1981). Recent studies have shown more complex relationships between gender and cognitive ability. Volkmar and colleagues (1993) suggested that autism is 'rare' in females with average cognitive ability. Furthermore, it has been argued that the association between gender and cognitive ability might differ by simplex (families with one affected child and one or more unaffected siblings) versus multiplex status (families with more than one child affected) based on the finding that cognitive ability was less variable across genders in multiplex samples but not in simplex samples (Spiker et al., 2001). Similarly, Banach and colleagues (2008) found no significant gender differences in NVIQ for multiplex samples, but found a gender difference in NVIQ in simplex cases of autism.

Gender differences were also examined in autism symptom severity. Some past studies have shown that females demonstrate milder impairments due to less severe RRBs and more intact imitation and play skills. For example, Lord et al. (1982) found that boys demonstrated more unusual visual interests and poorer play behavior than girls, based on 384 boys and 91 girls aged 3 to 8 years. Similarly, Hartley and Sikora (2009) found that preschool-age boys showed more RRBs compared to girls. However, a specific subtype of RRB, 'insistence on sameness', was found to be independent of gender in past studies based on young children, adolescents, and adults with ASD (Hus et al., 2007; Richler et al., 2010).

The findings with respect to the relationship between gender and social and communication deficits are less clear than those on RRBs. For samples of school-age children, no gender differences were found on clinical ratings of social relatedness and interest (Lord et al., 1982), while more recent work on toddlers with ASD suggested that boys demonstrated significantly better adaptive communication and less clinical impairment than girls in pragmatic and nonverbal forms of communication (Carter et al., 2007; Hartley and Sikora, 2009). On the other hand, McLennan et al. (1993) reported that male children under 5 years of age with autism showed significantly greater impairments in communication and social interaction, while after age 10, females in adolescence and adulthood demonstrated poorer current social functioning, as assessed by a distal outcome, accounted for by a lower likelihood of friendships (McLennan et al., 1993). Although the results from the previous studies are inconsistent, these studies point to the possibility of greater symptom expression in males. Future studies, however, should further examine the nature of gender differences in social and communication functioning.

Various theoretical explanations have been suggested for the gender differences manifested in ASD. One prominent theory is that some gender differences in autism are a reflection of the sexual dimorphism in the normative population with respect to nonverbal and verbal functioning (Wing, 1981). It has been also suggested that females have less brain lateralization (and therefore require greater brain damage to be affected with autism), which may be associated with lower NVIQ scores in females than those of males (Baron-Cohen et al., 2005; Lord et al., 1982; Wisniewski, 1998). Thus, it is possible that the relationship between gender and the phenotypic expression of autism may be an interaction between changes in brain function necessary for autism impairment to occur and the greater lateralization of brain functioning in the normative male population.

Genetic studies have also provided inconsistent findings on gender differences. Specific linkage associations with male-only families and families including females have been found in some genetic studies (Lamb et al., 2005; Stone et al., 2004). Moreover, the proportion of individuals carrying *de novo* copy number mutations is lower (1.8:1 male:female) than the overall ratio of affected males:females in the population (Sebat et al., 2007). Even though results have not been always consistent, most evidence points to the possibility that the gender differences in autism symptom manifestations have strong neurogenetic components.

Sensory and Motor Impairments

Even though sensory and motor impairments are not currently part of diagnostic criteria, parents of children with ASD often report abnormal sensory behaviors and deficits in motor skills. Both increased and decreased responsiveness to sensory stimuli have been observed in children with ASD (Rogers et al., 2003). For instance, some individuals with ASD may visually inspect others by peering out of the corners of their eyes or examining things at very close range. Others may show extreme disturbances associated with certain tactile sensations such as brushing, washing, or cutting hair and strong resistance to wearing socks or shoes. Other common complaints include severe behavioral reactions to loud or unusual noises or sometimes even common sounds such as singing or coughing. One caveat is that sensory-seeking behaviors and strong disturbances are not unique to autism, but are also prevalent in children with general intellectual disabilities. However, the severity and frequency of sensory impairments have been found to differentiate children with

ASD from those with other non-ASD disorders (Kim and Lord, 2010).

Motor impairments have been also reported to be prevalent in individuals with ASD. Up to 33% of cases of individuals with ASD show delays in motor milestones (Mayes and Calhoun, 2003). Some children with ASD, though not all, show problems with coordination and balance (Ghaziuddin and Butler, 1998), gait disturbances such as tiptoeing (Kielinen et al., 2004), and significant postural abnormalities (Minshew et al., 2004).

Adaptive Behaviors

Individuals with ASD, including more able adolescents and young adults with ASD, have significant impairments in adaptive behaviors (Howlin, 2004). Most children with early diagnoses of autism will not be completely independent as adults; many will need support in employment and residential living (Howlin, 2000). The standard scores of adaptive behaviors in individuals with ASD are seen to decline over time (Fisch et al., 2004). However, a significant minority of individuals with ASD, especially those with milder symptoms and fluent language skills by age 5, will be able to take responsibility for activities in daily living and complete higher education (Szatmari et al., 2003).

A typical profile of adaptive skills in ASD, as measured by the Vineland Adaptive Behavior Scales (Sparrow et al. 1984), is marked by greatest delays in socialization with lesser delays in communication and relative strengths in daily living skills (Bolte and Poustka, 2002). However, cognitive functioning, as one of the most important predictors of daily living skills in children with ASD, will be likely to affect this profile of adaptive behaviors in ASD. Specifically, individuals with lower intellectual functioning show more impairment in adaptive behaviors (Schatz and Hamdan-Allen, 1995). Thus, variability in adaptive functioning may be mediated by cognitive levels to a certain extent. Nevertheless, impairments in adaptive behaviors were found even in very able children with autism who showed a notable gap between IQ and adaptive skills, which widened with increasing age (Klin et al., 2007). This implies that individuals with ASD are failing to acquire skills that are expected based on their chronological and cognitive development.

Results of studies examining relations between adaptive skills and autism symptoms have been inconsistent. Some studies have found a weak relation between autism symptoms and adaptive behavior measured using the Autism Diagnostic Observation Schedule (ADOS) and the Vineland respectively (Kanne et al., 2010; Klin et al., 2007). Others have found a moderate to strong association between adaptive behaviors and autism severity (Perry et al., 2009). It is not yet clear whether intact cognitive skills or milder autism symptoms are necessarily protective factors in adaptive behaviors in individuals with ASD.

In addition, studies found that a significant minority of individuals with ASD showed relatively optimal outcomes (e.g., average or above average IQ, intact verbal skills, and age appropriate adaptive skills), who have been referred to as 'more able' children with ASD (Howlin, 2000). For example, Szatmari et al. (1989) studied a group of 26 individuals with ASD of normal IQ from 11 to 27 years. Educationally, half the group had received special schooling but the other half had attended college or university, with 44% obtaining a degree. Among these individuals, 75% had fairly intact adaptive behaviors. However, these individuals still had clear social impairments such as limited eye contact, gestures, and facial expressions. About one-third of these individuals also showed problems in initiating and maintaining conversations and two-thirds had overly formal speech. Despite these social and communication difficulties, a quarter of these individuals had dated regularly or had long-term relationships. Among 26 individuals, two people were unemployed and four were in sheltered workshop schemes; three were still studying; one worked in the family business; and six were in regular, full time employment. Five individuals lived independently and, although ten were still at home, three of these were reported to be completely independent, five required some minimal supervision, one required moderate care and one needed constant supervision. These results show that there is a significant minority of individuals with ASD who show optimal outcomes, especially those whose intellectual, verbal and adaptive abilities are fairly intact.

Comorbidity

Individuals with ASD have been found to have symptoms of many other psychiatric disorders such as attention deficits, hyperactivity, anxiety, obsessive-compulsive behaviors, depression, and even psychosis. Not all individuals with ASD show symptoms of other psychiatric disorders, but a significant proportion have been diagnosed with psychiatric disorders other than ASD. Although differentiating symptoms as either a comorbid psychiatric disorder or a manifestation of autism is challenging, the phenomenon of comorbidity is of interest to researchers because it may indicate important neurochemical, neuroanatomical, or genetic overlaps between ASD and these other disorders.

As mentioned above, intellectual disability (ID) is one of the most commonly diagnosed disorders in individuals with ASD, and it has been suggested that the proportion of children with ASD with nonverbal IQ scores below 70 is somewhere between 20 and 50% (Charman et al., 2011). Besides ID, the most commonly recognized co-occurring symptoms in individuals with ASD are attention deficits and hyperactivity and/or anxiety disorder (Goldstein and Schwebach, 2004; Kanne et al., 2009). By definition according to the DSM-IV, an ASD is an exclusionary criterion for making an attention-deficit/hyperactivity disorder (ADHD) diagnosis. However, about one third of individuals with ASD show attention deficits and hyperactivity symptoms which would qualify for a diagnosis of ADHD (Goldstein and Schwebach, 2004). A recent population-based study based on a sample of 112 10 - 14-year old children with ASD found that about 28% met the DSM criteria of ADHD and another 28% for oppositional defiant disorders (Simonoff et al., 2008). Thus, in the next edition of the DSM, it is likely that individuals with ASD will be able to receive the diagnosis of ADHD if their symptoms meet the criteria for the disorder (APA, 2010).

Past studies have also shown that more able individuals with ASD experience higher levels of internalizing symptoms such as anxiety and depression than typically developing individuals (Gillott et al., 2001; Kanne et al., 2009). Leyfer et al. (2006) found that high proportions of individuals met the criteria for different anxiety disorders among a sample of 109 children and adolescents with ASD. In their study, about 44% of the sample with ASD met the DSM criteria for specific phobia, 37% for obsessive compulsive disorder, and 12% for separation anxiety. In addition, about 10% of the sample had a history of major depressive disorder. A recent population-based study by Simonoff and colleagues (2008) also found anxiety disorders to be one of the most common comorbid diagnoses in individuals with ASD. In this study, about 29% of children from 12 to 14 years of age met the DSM criteria for social anxiety. Mazurek and Kanne (2010) also reported significantly elevated symptoms of anxiety and depression in a sample of 1,202 children between ages of 4 and 17, especially those with higher IQ scores. In addition, depression symptoms have been also prevalent in individuals with ASD, especially for those with Asperger syndrome or high functioning ASD, with comorbidity rates as high as 30% (Ghaziuddin et al., 2002; Wing, 1981).

It is not yet clear whether the behavioral and emotional problems that are found in individuals with ASD are truly comorbid or secondary to the core ASD symptoms. For example, Georgiades et al. (2010) found, using a principal component analysis (PCA) with items in the Autism Diagnostic Interview-Revised (ADI-R; Lord et al., 1994) and the Child Behavioral Checklist (CBCL; Achenbach and Rescorla, 2000) that the emotional and behavioral problems in ASD loaded highly on components associated with autism symptoms. It is possible that symptoms such as anxiety may stem from an awareness of social and other core deficits of ASD (Bellini, 2004; Chamberlain et al., 2007). It is also known that higher IQ scores can be associated with greater anxiety (Sukhodolsky et al. 2008), which might suggest that individuals with ASD with more insight and self awareness may experience higher levels of anxiety symptoms (Mazurek and Kanne, 2010). Further research is warranted to examine the relationship between the symptoms of ASD and behavioral and emotional problems.

DIAGNOSIS AND CLASSIFICATION OF ASD

Standardized Diagnoses

A diagnosis of ASD is a diagnosis made purely on the basis of behavior because there is not yet a reliable biological marker for the disorder. Given the extraordinary heterogeneity in genetics and other neurobiological research, it seems likely that behavioral diagnoses will be an important part of understanding and treating these disorders for many years. Generally, the syndrome of *autism* is considered the most clearly defined of all the ASD and also one of the most reliably defined psychiatric disorders emerging in childhood (Volkmar et al., 1997). An experienced clinician, using standardized methods, can reliably diagnose autism in children aged 2, and sometimes even younger. Standardized diagnostic instruments based on criteria in the Diagnostic and Statistical Manual on Mental Disorders, 4th edition (DSM-IV; APA, 1994) and in the World Health Organization's International Statistical Classification of Diseases and Related Health Problems, 10th Revision (ICD-10; WHO, 1990) have created uniform standards for a diagnosis of ASD. However, diagnoses of autism versus PDD-NOS are relatively unstable, in contrast to overall diagnoses of ASD versus other non-ASD developmental disorders, which are consistent over time (Kleinman et al., 2008; Lord et al., 2011; Turner and Stone, 2007). For this reason, recently developed diagnostic instruments and criteria for toddlers and young preschoolers include classifications of ASD vs. non-ASD rather than autism, ASD, vs. non-ASD (Kim and Lord, 2011a; Luyster et al., 2009).

The diagnosis of ASD is made based on a comprehensive assessment of developmental history, cognitive and communicative functioning, and observation of autism symptoms using multiple diagnostic and cognitive instruments. Providing a comprehensive review of ASD diagnostic instruments is beyond the scope of this chapter. For this purpose, see Lord and Corsello

(2005) or Worley and Matson (2011). Here, we will focus on two widely used instruments in clinical and research practice; the Autism Diagnostic Interview-Revised (ADI-R; Lord et al., 1994) and the Autism Diagnostic Observation Schedule (ADOS; Lord et al., 2000).

The ADI-R is a standardized, semi-structured, investigator-based interview for caregivers of individuals referred for a possible diagnosis of ASD. It is administered by a trained clinician with expertise in interviewing skills and knowledge of ASD. Information collected during the interview contributes to diagnostic algorithms, which provide classifications of 'autism' or 'nonspectrum'. Recently, in research, an ASD cut-off was proposed to allow inclusion of children in the broader autism spectrum (Lainhart et al., 2006; Risi et al., 2006). Additionally, new algorithms have been developed for the classifications of children from 12 to 47 months of age with a nonverbal mental age of at least 10 months (Kim and Lord, 2011a).

The ADOS is a standardized, semi-structured, clinician observation for children and adults referred for a diagnosis of ASD. Like the ADI-R algorithms, the ADOS algorithms were developed based on DSM-IV diagnostic criteria. It includes activities that require 35–45 minutes to administer, and provides the clinician with the opportunity to observe the social, communication, and restricted behaviors related to ASD. Five different modules, based on the level of language and age of the child, comprise the instrument. Children with mental ages under 15 months often meet ADOS cut-off criteria for ASD, regardless of clinical diagnosis. To address this issue, a toddler version of the ADOS (ADOS-T; Luyster et al., 2009), appropriate for children aged 12-30 months with no language or use of single words, was originally developed for research use and recently became available to clinicians.

In recent studies, it has been found that use of information from both the ADI-R and ADOS together better reflect clinical best-estimate diagnoses of ASD than when either single instrument was used alone. This is the case for toddlers and preschoolers, as well as older children and adolescents (Kim and Lord, 2011b; Risi et al., 2006). The ADI-R includes a developmental history and a detailed description of an individual's functioning in a variety of social contexts, as well as caregivers' perceptions of the level of impairment and/or frequency of different behaviors. The ADOS provides a summary of an experienced clinician's standardized observations of an individual's behaviors within contexts that elicit social initiations and responses as well as communication interchanges. These instruments make independent, additive contributions to more accurate diagnostic decisions for clinicians evaluating toddlers and young preschoolers with ASD. Combinations of alternative instruments such as the

Szatmari, P., Bryson, S.E., Boyle, M.H., Streiner, D.L., Duku, E., 2003. Predictors of outcome among high functioning children with autism and Asperger syndrome. Journal of Child Psychology and Psychiatry 44, 520–528.

Szatmari, P., Georgiades, S., Bryson, S., Zwaigenbaum, L., Roberts, W., Mahoney, W., et al., 2006. Investigating the structure of the restricted, repetitive behaviours and interests domain of autism. Journal of Child Psychology and Psychiatry 47, 582–590.

Szatmari, P., MacLean, J.E., Jones, M.B., Bryson, S.E., Zwaigenbaum, L., Bartolucci, G., et al., 2000. The familial aggregation of the lesser variant in biological and nonbiolgocial relatives of PDD propbands: A family history study. Journal of Child Psychology and Psychiatry 41, 579–586.

Tager-Flusberg, H., Edelson, L., Luyster, R., 2011. Language and Communication in Autism Spectrum Disorders. In: Amaral, D., Dawson, G. (Eds.), Autism Spectrum Disorders, first ed. Oxford University Press, USA, pp. 172–185.

Taylor, J.L., Seltzer, M.M., 2010. Changes in the autism behavioral phenotype during the transition to adulthood. Journal of Autism and Developmental Disorders 40, 1431–1446.

Thurm, A., Lord, C., Lee, L., Newschaffer, C., 2007. Predictors of language acquisition in preschool children with autism spectrum disorders. Journal of Autism and Developmental Disorders 37, 1721–1734.

Tsai, L.Y., Stewart, M.A., August, G., 1981. Implication of sex differences in the familial transmission of infantile autism. Journal of Autism and Developmental Disorders 11, 165–173.

Turner, M., 1999. Annotation: Repetitive behavior in autism: A review of psychological research. Journal of Child Psychology and Psychiatry 40, 839–849.

Turner, L., Stone, W., 2007. Variability in outcome for children with an ASD diagnosis at age 2. Journal of Child Psychology and Psychiatry and Allied Disciplines 48, 793–802.

Venter, A., Lord, C., Schopler, E., 1992. A follow-up of high-functioning autistic children. Journal of Child Psychology and Psychiatry 33, 489–507.

Ventola, P.E., Kleinman, J., Pandey, J., Barton, M., Allen, S., Green, J., et al., 2006. Agreement among four diagnostic instruments for autism spectrum disorders in toddlers. Journal of Autism and Developmental Disorders 36, 839–847.

Volkmar, F.R., Rutter, M., 1995. Childhood disintegrative disorder: Results of the DSM-IV autism field trial. Journal of the American Academy of Child and Adolescent Psychiatry 34, 1092–1095.

Volkmar, F.R., Carter, A., Sparrow, S.S., Cicchetti, D., 1993. Quantifying social development in autism. Journal of the American Academy of Child and Adolescent Psychiatry 32, 627–632.

Volkmar, F.R., Klin, A., Cohen, D.J., 1997. Diagnosis and classification of autism and related conditions: Consensus and issues. In: Cohen, D.J., Volkmar, F.R. (Eds.), Handbook of autism and pervasive developmental disorders, second ed. Wiley, New York, pp. 5–40.

Watson, L.R., Baranek, G.T., Crais, E.J., Reznick, J.S., Dykstra, J., Perryman, T., 2007. The first year inventory: Retrospective parent responses to a questionnaire designed to identify one-year-olds at risk for autism. Journal of Autism and Developmental Disorders 37, 49–61.

Wing, L., 1981. Asperger's syndrome: A clinical account. Psychological Medicine 11, 115–119.

Wing, L., Gould, J., 1979. Severe impairments of social interaction and associated abnormalities in children: Epidemiology and classification. Journal of Autism and Developmental Disorders 9, 11–29.

Wisniewski, A.B., 1998. Sexually-dimorphic patterns of cortical asymmetry, and the role for sex steroid hormones in determining cortical patterns of lateralization. Psychoneuroendocrinology 23, 519–547.

World Health Organization (WHO), 1990. International Classification of Diseases (10th revision). World Health Organization, Geneva.

Worley, J.A., Matson, J.L., 2011. Diagnostic Instruments for the core features of autism. In: Matson, J.L. (Ed.), International Handbook of Autism and Pervasive Developmental Disorders. Springer, New York, pp. 215–231.

1.3

Early Manifestations of Autism Spectrum Disorders

Marianne L. Barton, Alyssa Orinstein, Eva Troyb, Deborah A. Fein

Department of Psychology, The University of Connecticut, Storrs, CT, USA

Autism or autism spectrum disorders (ASD) are neurobiological disorders, defined by impairments in social interaction and social communication, and restricted interests and activities. ASD was first identified by Leo Kanner in 1943, who proposed that it was a biological condition characterized by 'extreme aloneness from the beginning of life' (Kanner, 1943, p. 248). While evidence in support of the biological and genetic roots of the disorder is now incontrovertible (Section 2), current data suggest that signs of the disorder are not present in the earliest months of life, but instead emerge during or after the second half of the first year (Rogers, 2009; Tager-Flusberg, 2010). Symptoms of the disorder, especially very early manifestations, seem to vary across individuals and emerge at different developmental stages, a pattern which reflects both the variability and plasticity of early development, and the heterogeneous nature of the disorder itself.

The search for the earliest manifestations of ASD is rooted in awareness of the significant theoretical and practical benefits that accrue from understanding its origins. On a theoretical level, identification of the earliest signs of ASD may advance our understanding of the nature of the disorder and the neurodevelopmental processes that underlie it. Identification of the earliest signs of disorder permits the careful study of developmental processes before those processes can be affected by an atypical developmental trajectory. Examination of early signs of ASD might also provide insights into the biological mechanisms that support typical social development. On a practical level, identification of early markers of ASD may facilitate earlier and more effective screening for the disorder, earlier identification of affected children, and earlier intervention for those children. Multiple studies have now demonstrated that intensive early intervention is associated with more positive outcomes for children with ASD, (Ben-Itzchak et al., 2008; Dawson, et al., 2009; McGovern and Sigman, 2005; Rogers and Vismara, 2008), and may be associated with extremely positive outcomes in a subset of children (Helt et al., 2008).

Often, intervention services cannot be provided until children obtain a diagnosis of an ASD. While parents may report concerns with their child's social or communicative development as early as 12–18 months (Stone, et al., 1994), several studies suggest that children may not receive an ASD diagnosis until they are 4 years of age or later (Autism and Developmental Disabilities Monitoring Network Surveillance Year 2002 Principal Investigators, 2007; Shattuck et al., 2009; Yeargin-Allsopp et al., 2003). Children from socio economically disadvantaged groups may be identified even later than children from the general population (Begeer et al., 2009; Dancel et al., 2008; Liptak et al., 2008; Mandell, et al 2002). Systematic screening for ASD, based on early manifestations of the disorder, lowers the age at which children are referred for intervention, increases intervention rates to be more consistent with prevalence rates (Earls and Hay, 2006; Pinto-Martin et al., 2005), and reduces disparities in the age of diagnosis between racial and ethnic groups (Sices et al., 2003). Some authors (e.g., Dawson, 2008) have posited that early identification of children with ASD may permit intervention to alter atypical developmental trajectories that may *prevent* the development of the full autism syndrome.

This chapter will begin with a review of the literature regarding the earliest manifestations of ASD, including biological markers and early behavioral presentations. We will then consider the implications of those data for models of the disorder. We close the chapter with thoughts about the clinical applications of an emerging understanding of early risk processes.

EARLY BIOLOGICAL MARKERS

Head Circumference and Other Growth Parameters

Given its simplicity and non-invasive nature, head circumference has been used as a proxy of brain size in many studies of young children with ASD (see Chapter 3.1). Most head circumference studies have been retrospective, and have examined the early medical records of children with ASD. Head circumference at birth for infants later diagnosed with ASD is generally normal (Dawson et al., 2007; Dementieva et al., 2005; Fukumoto et al., 2008; 2011; Hazlett et al., 2005; Muratori et al., 2012; Torrey et al., 2004; van Daalen et al., 2007; Webb et al., 2007; Whitehouse et al., 2011) or smaller than normative samples of typically developing controls (Courchesne et al., 2003; Mraz et al., 2007; Rommelse et al., 2011). Most studies have found accelerated postnatal head growth in children later diagnosed with ASD (Courchesne, et al., 2003; Dawson, et al., 2007; Dementieva, et al., 2005; Dissanayake et al., 2006; Elder et al., 2008; Fukumoto, et al., 2008; Mraz et al., 2007; 2009; Muratori, et al., 2012; van Daalen, et al., 2007; Webb, et al., 2007), resulting in a larger head

circumference sometime within the first three years of life (Courchesne et al., 2003; Davidovitch et al., 2011; Dawson et al., 2007; Fukumoto et al., 2011; Gillberg & de Souza, 2002; Mraz et al., 2007; 2009; Muratori et al., 2012; Webb et al., 2007). However, the timing of head growth acceleration is still debated. Many studies found that accelerated head circumference growth occurred within the first six months after birth (Dementieva et al., 2005; Fukumoto et al., 2008; Muratori et al., 2012; van Daalen et al., 2007), others found increased growth through the first year (Courchesne et al., 2003; Dawson et al., 2007; Elder et al., 2008; Mraz et al., 2007; Webb et al., 2007), and others still found rapid growth between the first and third years of life (Dissanayake et al., 2006; Hazlett et al., 2005). Nonetheless, increased head growth early in life appears to be an indicator for later diagnosis of ASD.

There has also been some association between early postnatal head circumference and later ASD symptoms. Infants who had a larger head circumference at 12 months, combined with deceleration of head circumference growth in the second year of life, were more likely to receive an ASD diagnosis in early childhood (Elder et al., 2008). Additionally, smaller head circumference at birth, larger head circumference between ages 1 and 2, and/or greater head circumference increase were associated with more severe autism symptoms (Mraz et al., 2007). Specifically, Courchesne et al. (2003) found that smaller head circumference at birth was associated with poorer verbal skills in early childhood, and greater increase in head circumference was associated with more repetitive behaviors.

In addition to head circumference, other growth parameters, such as height and weight, have been examined for the first three years of life in children with ASD. While not universal (Muratori et al., 2012; Webb et al., 2007), most studies have shown that children with ASD are significantly longer (Dissanayake et al., 2006; Fukumoto et al., 2008; Mraz et al., 2007; Torrey et al., 2004; van Daalen et al., 2007) and/or heavier (Dissanayake et al., 2006; Fukumoto et al., 2008; 2011; Mraz et al., 2007; 2009; Torrey et al., 2004) than their typically developing peers. Despite the abnormalities in length and weight, accelerated head circumference growth was often still present even after controlling for the other size variables (Courchesne et al., 2003; Dawson et al., 2007; Fukumoto et al., 2011). These length and weight findings, combined with the head circumference results, may suggest an early dysregulation of factors related to overall growth processes in children later diagnosed with ASD.

The rate of macrocephaly, or head circumference greater than two standard deviations above the mean, is 3% in the general population. Retrospective studies have found incidence of macrocephaly to be significantly higher in infants and toddlers later diagnosed with ASD, with rates between 11 and 25% (Dementieva et al., 2005; Gillberg & de Souza, 2002; Lainhart et al., 1997; Muratori et al., 2012; Torrey et al., 2004; van Daalen et al., 2007; Webb et al., 2007). However, not all studies have found an elevated rate of macrocephaly in young children with ASD (Barnard-Brak et al., 2011; Davidovitch et al., 2011; Rommelse et al., 2011), and macrocephaly is not found in all children with ASD. One study found a much higher rate of macrocephaly in children with Asperger disorder (25%) compared to those with autistic disorder (10%), suggesting a possible difference in underlying etiology with different behavioral phenotypes of ASD (Gillberg & de Souza, 2002).

Early Brain Abnormalities

Over the past decade, researchers have begun to examine brain abnormalities in young children with ASD (see Section 3). Studies have noted increased whole brain volume (Courchesne et al., 2001; Hazlett et al., 2005; Schumann et al., 2010), and enlarged cerebral white (Courchesne et al., 2001; Hazlett et al., 2005; 2011; Schumann et al., 2010) and gray matter (Courchesne et al., 2001; Hazlett et al., 2005; Schumann et al., 2010) in infants with ASD. Within the cerebral cortex, the frontal lobes of very young children with ASD showed the greatest increase in both white and gray matter (Carper et al., 2002). Furthermore, cerebral white and gray matter displayed abnormal growth patterns across the early postnatal years (Schumann et al., 2010). The limited findings for cerebellar volume in toddlers with ASD have been mixed, perhaps speaking to the heterogeneity of the endophenotypes of ASD. The amygdala of very young children with ASD were also found to be enlarged (Schumann et al., 2009).

Several authors have begun to investigate electrical activity, using event-related potentials (ERP) in the brains of infants at high risk of autism (typically the siblings of children diagnosed with the disorder) in response to human faces. Elsabbagh et al. (2009) report that while the neural mechanisms that support face processing appear to be intact in high risk infants, these infants show a longer latency to direct gaze and their brains may have altered patterns of connectivity. McCleery and colleagues (2009) also investigated face processing in high-risk infants at 10 months. They report that these infants showed faster responses to objects, but did not differ from typically developing children in their latency of response to faces. They also report that high-risk infants showed reduced hemispheric asymmetry in ERP responses. Other investigators have reported similarly reduced hemispheric asymmetry in language

processing in high-risk infants (Seery et al., 2010), suggesting that there may be diminished lateralization of brain function in high-risk infants during the first year of life. As Tager-Flusberg (2010) points out, these findings of differences in brain connectivity and organization emerge in the same period as the patterns of accelerated head growth described earlier.

Taken together, these neurological findings may suggest the presence of atypical brain development in very young children with ASD, which likely relates to their symptoms and functional difficulties. At the same time, the available data suggest that none of these biological markers are sufficiently reliable, sensitive or consistent across children to be used in the identification of young children with suspected ASD. As a result, most studies of early manifestations of ASD have relied upon assessment of behavioral symptoms.

BEHAVIORAL MANIFESTATIONS IN RETROSPECTIVE REPORTS

Research examining the early manifestations of ASD originally relied on retrospective studies using parent report of early symptoms, as well as early home videos of children who are later diagnosed with an ASD. These studies allow researchers to investigate participants with known diagnoses at one assessment point, reducing the length of data collection and cost of the studies. Generally, these studies identify symptoms evident as early as the first year of life within the domains of communication, socialization, and sensory reactivity, as well as motor behaviors. Additionally, retrospective studies have examined early symptoms evident among children who demonstrate symptoms of ASD following a marked loss of skills.

Delayed Communication

Retrospective studies have identified several aspects of communicative behavior that appear to differentiate infants with ASD from their typically developing peers. During the first year of life, parents' recall of early symptoms indicated that infants who were later diagnosed with ASD were less likely to respond to their parents' voices (De Giacomo & Fombonne, 1998). Additionally, the extent of expressive communication, including the frequency of simple and complex babbling, as well as delays in sound production, were found to distinguish 12-month-old infants later diagnosed with ASD from typically developing peers (Watson et al., 2007; Werner & Dawson, 2005; Wetherby & Prizant, 1998). However, delayed expressive communication is not a specific symptom of ASD and is often present among

12-month-old infants with other developmental delays (Watson et al., 2007).

Studies using home videos recorded during the first year of life to examine early gesture use among infants who later go on to receive an ASD diagnosis have yielded mixed results (Adrien et al., 1993; Clifford & Dissanayake, 2008; Colgan et al., 2006; Osterling & Dawson, 1994; Osterling et al., 2002). Some studies have shown that infants who are later diagnosed with ASD use fewer spontaneous gestures than controls, with many of these studies specifically examining the frequency of pointing (Clifford & Dissanayake, 2008; Osterling & Dawson, 1994; Osterling et al., 2002; Werner & Dawson, 2005). In fact, the frequency of declarative pointing at 12 months distinguished children who were later diagnosed with ASD from typically developing peers (Osterling & Dawson, 1994; Werner & Dawson, 2005). However, the frequency of gesture use at 12 months does not appear to distinguish infants who are later diagnosed with ASD from infants later diagnosed with other developmental disorders (Colgan et al., 2006; Osterling et al., 2002). One study has suggested that the variety of gestures used at 12 months rather than the frequency may distinguish infants who go on to develop ASD from those later diagnosed with intellectual disability, with the ASD group exhibiting a restricted range of gestures (Colgan et al., 2006).

Symptoms of ASD within the communication domain become more evident during the second year of life (Chawarska & Volkmar, 2005). Most notably, delays in communicative abilities are usually observed by parents of children who go on to receive an ASD diagnosis around the age of 2 years (Young et al., 2003). According to parental reports, by the age of 24 months, comprehension of phrases is significantly weaker among children who are later diagnosed with ASD than among children later diagnosed with developmental delays and typically developing children (Luyster et al., 2005). Furthermore, studies examining symptoms present around the child's second birthday reveal that the vocalizations of children who are later diagnosed with ASD contain significantly less complex babble, single words, and phrases (Werner & Dawson, 2005; Wimpory et al., 2000).

Lack of Social Responsiveness

During the first two years of life, aspects of social relatedness also appear to differentiate infants later diagnosed with ASD from infants diagnosed with developmental delays and from typically developing peers (Werner et al., 2005; Young et al., 2003). According to parental reports, infants who were later diagnosed with ASD tended to show less interest in peers, and were less likely to direct caregivers' attention, share their

enjoyment with caregivers, greet others appropriately, and initiate or respond to joint attention (Ozonoff et al., 2005; Werner et al., 2005). Additionally, parents reported that during the first two years of life, infants later diagnosed with ASD were less likely to imitate caregivers' actions than typically developing peers. However, imitation did not reliably differentiate infants with ASD from infants with other developmental delays (Charman et al., 1997; Maestro et al., 2001; Watson et al., 2007).

When aspects of social engagement were examined using early home videos of infants with ASD around their first birthday, the results indicated that this group was less likely to maintain appropriate eye contact, respond appropriately to a smile, look at the faces of others, orient to their name or bring objects to show to their caregivers (Adrien et al., 1993; Clifford & Dissanayake, 2008; Clifford et al., 2007; Mars et al., 1998; Osterling & Dawson, 1994; Osterling et al., 2002; Werner et al., 2000). Furthermore, analyses of home videos revealed that significant decreases in eye contact and social smiling were evident as early as 6 months of age. Decreases in responsiveness to name were consistently identified in infants as early as 8 months of age (Baranek, 1999; Clifford & Dissanayake, 2008; Werner et al., 2000). Additionally, studies using home videos revealed significant differences in initiation and response to joint attention during the second year of life between infants later diagnosed with an ASD and typically developing peers (Clifford & Disanayake, 2008). Finally, as was the case with the communication domain, abnormalities in social reciprocity became more notable during the second year of life (Clifford & Dissanayake, 2008).

Repetitive Behaviors and Other Motor Abnormalities

Retrospective studies of repetitive behaviors in infants later diagnosed with ASD revealed that, during the first year of life, infants with ASD are more likely to display unusual and repetitive hand and finger mannerisms and engage in appropriate play less frequently than do typically developing infants (Dahlgren & Gillberg, 1989; Lord, 1995; Maestro et al., 2001; Osterling et al., 2002). However, the presence of repetitive behaviors during the first year of life is not useful in differentiating between infants who will receive an ASD diagnosis and those who will be diagnosed with a developmental delay (Baranek, 1999; Osterling et al., 2002; Watson et al., 2007; Werner & Dawson, 2005, Werner et al., 2005). Nevertheless, as they age, repetitive behaviors become more reliable in differentiating children with ASD. During the second and third years of life, repetitive hand and finger mannerisms become more pronounced among children with ASD and less pronounced among children with other developmental delays and children who are developing typically (Chawarska & Volkmar, 2005; Evans et al., 1997; Moore & Goodson, 2003; Werner et al., 2005).

Other motor abnormalities identified by retrospective studies include lower levels of symmetry in the first months of life (Esposito et al., 2009), as well as low muscle tone and hypoactivity in the first year of life (Adrien et al., 1993; Maestro et al., 2005). Additionally, several studies suggest that infants and toddlers who are later diagnosed with ASD experience general delays in the development of motor skills (Landa & Garett-Mayer, 2006; Ozonoff et al., 2008c). However, infants who are later diagnosed with ASD do not appear to be more delayed within the motor domain than similarly aged infants with developmental delays. This suggests that early motor delays may result from developmental disorders generally, rather than ASD specifically (Ozonoff et al., 2008c; Rogers et al., 2003).

Sensory Reactivity

Retrospective studies of sensory reactions in infants with ASD suggest that during the first two years of life, the presence of unusual sensory behaviors distinguishes infants later diagnosed with ASD from typically developing peers (Baranek, 1999; Baranek et al., 2006; Lord, 1995; Watson et al., 2007). Most commonly, atypical sensory behaviors observed during the first and second year of life in infants later diagnosed with ASD included unusual visual inspection of stimuli, aversion to social touch, and excessive mouthing (Baranek, 1999; Chawarska & Volkmar, 2005). Abnormalities in sensory reactivity are also commonly described among children with developmental delays (Osterling et al., 2002), suggesting that the presence of this behavior may not be a specific early marker for ASD.

Temperament and Regulatory Difficulties

When asked about the first year of their child's life, parents of children with ASD often recalled that, as infants, their children exhibited extreme temperaments, describing behaviors indicative of emotional flatness, as well as irritability (Clifford & Dissanayake, 2007; Werner & Dawson, 2005). Additionally, parents of infants with ASD recalled more regulatory difficulties, including eating and sleeping difficulties, than did parents of typically developing infants. This difference in regulatory behaviors between the ASD group and the typically developing group was identified in infants as young as 3 months of age (Werner et al., 2005). However,

a significant difference in regulatory abnormalities was not detected between infants later diagnosed with ASD and infants later diagnosed with developmental delays until the children were close to 2 years of age (Werner et al., 2005). This finding suggests that the presence of regulatory difficulties in infancy is not a specific indicator of ASD.

Regression

According to their parents, between 20 and 47 percent of children with ASD exhibit few symptoms until they experience a notable loss of social interest, words or communicative intent, imitative gestures, and at times cognitive abilities (Bernabei et al., 2006; Davidovitch et al., 2000; Lord et al., 2004; Ozonoff et al., 2005; Werner & Dawson, 2005). The prevalence of the regressive onset of ASD varies considerably across studies, and depends largely on the definition of the construct that is used by the study (Bernabei et al., 2006; Ozonoff et al., 2008a). Additionally, the nature and degree of the skill loss varies considerably across cases. For example, the most common loss is of language, and may involve a loss of some words or a loss of language altogether (Lord et al., 2004; Ozonoff et al., 2005; Werner & Dawson, 2005). Most commonly, regression begins when the child is between 15 and 24 months of age, after a period of typical or delayed development (Bernabei et al., 2006; Davidovitch et al., 2000; Lord et al., 2004; Ozonoff et al., 2005; Werner & Dawson, 2005).

Several studies of regression in ASD have explored the progress of development prior to the onset of the loss of skills. These studies suggest that in many cases some degree of developmental anomaly is evident during the first year of life, prior to the onset of the regression (Lord et al., 2004; Ozonoff et al., 2005; Richler et al., 2006; Stefanatos, 2008; Werner & Dawson, 2005). Most commonly, these anomalies consisted of social delays. Additionally, regulatory difficulties have been identified before the onset of regression in ASD, including frequent difficulty sleeping and hypersensitivity to sensory stimulation (Werner & Dawson, 2005; Werner et al., 2005).

Benefits and Limitations of Retrospective Research

Studies using parent report to examine early symptoms of ASD generally depend upon questionnaires and interviews that ask parents of children with ASD to recall their child's development during infancy and toddlerhood. These studies provide considerable data from motivated observers who likely have access to the child in a variety of settings. However, the use of parental reports is complicated by the parents' inaccurate memory of events, biased recall, and limited access to an appropriate comparison group, all of which hinder a parent's ability to report accurately on the timing and development of their child's behavior (Lord et al., 2004; Reznick et al., 2007; Stone et al., 1994). Parental recall may be especially problematic when it is collected after an ASD diagnosis has been made, as parents may be unknowingly altering their reports to be more consistent with the diagnosis (Ozonoff et al., 2008a; Wimpory et al., 2000; Zwaigenbaum et al., 2007).

With the wide availability of moderately priced hand-held camcorders, retrospective studies began to rely on home videos of children later diagnosed with ASD in order to address some limitations of parental report studies. This approach has allowed access to rich behavioral samples of early childhood development, often in a natural environment, and minimized the bias introduced by parental recall of early symptoms. However, this line of research also has its limitations. The content of these videos varies considerably across studies, with some including involvement in typical family routines (e.g., bathing, eating, etc.), while others include special occasions such as birthday parties or holiday celebrations (Baranek, 1999; Werner & Dawson, 2005). This variability introduces possible differences between the content of videotapes in studies that compare children with ASD to controls that are inherent to the groups being studied (Baranek, 1999; Volkmar et al., 2007). Additionally, researchers had no control over the quality of the videotapes, the situations in which the tapes were recorded, the behaviors recorded or the impact aspects of the environment not captured on the video may have had on the behaviors of the child (e.g., prompting by a parent off camera; Colgan et al., 2006). Given these limitations, researchers increasingly recognized the need for prospective studies of children with autism from infancy through childhood.

PROSPECTIVE STUDIES

Prospective studies of any relatively rare disorder are prohibitively expensive and time consuming, and often lead researchers to look for high-risk samples where the chance of developing the disorder may be greater than in the general population. Studies have suggested that the siblings of children with ASD have a 3–8% risk of developing autism (e.g., Micali et al., 2004), making them an ideal candidate for studies of high-risk individuals.

Several studies have examined and followed the infant siblings of children diagnosed with ASD (ASD-Sibs) and siblings of typically developing children (TD-Sibs) in order to ascertain differences between the two groups very early in development. Bryson and colleagues (2008) developed the Autism Observation Scale for Infants (AOSI) to identify early signs of ASD in high-risk infants. Using this measure, their team found that there were no significant behavioral differences at 6 months of age (Zwaigenbaum et al., 2005). However, at 12 months, the presence of multiple risk factors on the AOSI predicted ASD classification at 2 years of age (Zwaigenbaum et al., 2005). Specific risk factors from the AOSI included atypical eye contact, visual tracking, disengagement of visual attention, response to name, imitation, social smiling, interest in social interaction, and sensory abnormalities (Zwaigenbaum et al., 2005).

In terms of developmental level, at 4 months, ASD-Sibs had lower mental scores on the Bayley Scales of Infant Development compared to siblings of typically developing children (TD-Sibs) (Gamliel et al., 2007). However, other studies at 6 months utilizing the Mullen Scales of Early Learning found no differences between TD-Sibs and ASD-Sibs on any domain, including Fine Motor, Visual Reception, Expressive Language, and Receptive Language (Landa & Garrett-Mayer, 2006; Ozonoff et al., 2010). By 14 months, differences were more pronounced, with consistent impairments on the Bayley Scales of Infant Development and the Mullen Scales of Early Learning for ASD-Sibs (Gamliel et al., 2007; Landa & Garrett-Mayer, 2006; Ozonoff et al., 2010). Language abilities were deficient on the scales of the Mullen Scales of Early Learning and other language measures by the end of the first year (Gamliel et al., 2007; Landa & Garrett-Mayer, 2006; Ozonoff et al., 2010; Yirmiya et al., 2006; Zwaigenbaum et al., 2005). ASD-Sibs and TD-Sibs had similar rates of directed vocalizations at 6 months; however, by 12 months, the rate of directed vocalization by ASD-Sibs was less than that of TD-Sibs (Ozonoff et al., 2010).

Social behaviors have been extensively examined in infant ASD-Sibs. ASD-Sibs as young as 4 months showed less synchrony in self-directed social interactions with their parents than TD-Sibs (Yirmiya et al., 2006) but these differences are subtle and difficult to detect. At 6 months, there was no difference between ASD-Sibs and TD-Sibs in response to name, gaze to faces, or social smiles (Nadig et al., 2007; Ozonoff et al., 2010). By 12 months, ASD-Sibs were less likely to respond to their name and displayed fewer gazes to faces (Nadig et al., 2007; Ozonoff et al., 2010). At this age, ASD-Sibs initiated fewer low-level (making eye contact to request or reaching for the toy) (Cassel et al., 2007; Rozga et al., 2011; Yirmiya et al., 2006) and high-level (pointing or giving the toy to the examiner) behavioral requests (Cassel et al., 2007). At one year of age, ASD-Sibs also were less likely to initiate or respond to acts of joint attention than TD-Sibs (Rozga et al., 2011).

The still-face paradigm (Tronick et al., 1978) has been used to assess social relatedness and emotional reactivity in ASD-Sibs. During this task, after an initial baseline play period, there is a period in which the parent is socially unrelated ('still face'), followed by a reunion play period. Studies using observation of gaze as well as more sophisticated eye tracking methodologies have found that during the still-face paradigm, 6-month-old ASD-Sibs looked at their parent's face at least as often as TD-Sibs (Ibanez et al, 2008; Merin et al., 2007; Rozga et al., 2011; Yirmiya et al., 2006), although more subtle gaze differences have been identified. Ibanez et al. (2008) noted that infant ASD-Sibs less frequently shifted their gaze to and from their parent's face and gazed away from their parent's face for longer durations at a time. Furthermore, while Merin et al. (2007) found no group differences for gaze to face versus non-face or for specific face regions, they identified a subgroup of infant ASD-Sibs who displayed reduced gaze to their parent's eye and increased gaze to their parent's mouth.

Emotional reactivity indicators from the still-face paradigm showed that infant ASD-Sibs sometimes smiled less (Cassel et al., 2007), were upset less (Yirmiya et al., 2006), and displayed more neutral affect (Yirmiya et al., 2006) than their peers.

Temperament differences have also been found in infant ASD-Sibs. At 6 months of age, ASD-Sibs who were classified as having an ASD at 24 months had a lower activity level than TD-Sibs at 6 months (Zwaigenbaum et al., 2005). Later, at 12 months of age, compared to TD-Sibs, ASD-Sibs who received an ASD diagnosis at 24 months had more severe reactions to distress and tended to fixate on objects for longer periods of time (Zwaigenbaum et al., 2005).

Studies have also tracked visual attention and eye gaze in infant ASD-Sibs. ASD-Sibs spent less time looking at their caregivers and more time looking at nonsocial objects at 6 months old compared to TD-Sibs (Bhat et al., 2010). At 6 months of age, ASD-Sibs displayed no deficits on a visual orienting task (Zwaigenbaum et al., 2005). However, by 12 months, as a group, the infant ASD-Sibs performed worse on this task than TD-Sibs. Furthermore, all of the infants who showed increased disengagement received an ASD diagnosis at age 2 (Zwaigenbaum et al., 2005). Another study of 10-month-old infants showed that ASD-Sibs had prolonged latencies to disengage their attention and reduced facilitation by an attentional priming cue (Elsabbagh et al., 2009).

Taken together, these infant sibling studies suggest that there are few very early behavioral markers implicated in later diagnosis of ASD. Atypical attention and gaze seems to be one of the earliest indicators, and subtle differences in these behaviors may be evident, at least in a subgroup of children with ASD, as early as 6 months. However, as other investigators have noted, the majority of infants at risk who will later be diagnosed with ASD, have no discernible signs at 6 months (Rogers, 2009; Tager-Flusberg, 2010). By 12 to 14 months, numerous behavioral markers emerge, including atypical social development, delayed communication development, and temperamental differences.

Studies of 12- to 24-Month-Olds with ASD

Given clinicians' increasing ability to diagnose autism in toddlers (Chawarska et al., 2007), there is increasing data available about the earliest signs of the disorder in children who meet criteria for the diagnosis. Participants in these studies comprise a broader range of children than those in studies of high-risk siblings, since they include children who may not have any increased genetic vulnerability to the disorder. To the extent that these studies include children identified after 1994, when diagnostic standards were expanded, they include an even more heterogeneous group. The following review includes prospective studies of high-risk siblings, prospective studies from the general population, and cross-sectional designs.

During the second year of life, children with ASD display deficits in the frequency of vocalization directed to others and demonstrate a significantly lower rate of communication than typical peers (Chawarska et al., 2007; Shumway & Wetherby, 2009; Wetherby et al., 2007). When infants with ASD did vocalize, their prosody was often atypical (Wetherby et al., 2004). At 12 months, children with ASD understood fewer words and phrases than controls; these deficits persisted at 18 months, when children with ASD also produced fewer words (Mitchell et al., 2006). Between ages 1 and 2, children with ASD were impaired in their use of pointing and other communicative gestures (Chawarska et al., 2007; Shumway & Wetherby, 2009; Wetherby et al., 2007). Imitation of gestures and actions was also poorer in young toddlers with ASD compared to controls (Charman et al., 1997; 1998; Young et al., 2011).

Within the social domain, between 12 and 24 months, children later diagnosed with ASD were less likely than their typical peers to orient to their name (Brian et al., 2008; Chawarska et al., 2007; Wetherby et al., 2004), make appropriate eye contact (Brian et al., 2008; Chawarska et al., 2007; Wetherby et al., 2004), engage in reciprocal social smiling (Brian et al., 2008; Chawarska et al., 2007), or show social interest and affect (Brian et al., 2008; Chawarska et al., 2007; Wetherby et al., 2004). Toddlers with ASD were also less likely to direct facial expressions to others (Chawarska et al., 2007; Wetherby et al., 2004), integrate gaze with vocalizations (Chawarska et al., 2007; Wetherby et al., 2004), or request, give, or show (Chawarska et al., 2007; Wetherby et al., 2004). Very young children with ASD often had impaired initiation of joint attention (Chawarska et al., 2007) and, less frequently, impaired response to joint attention (Charman et al., 1997; 1998; Chawarska et al., 2007; Shumway & Wetherby, 2009; Sullivan et al., 2007; Wetherby et al., 2007) in the second year of life. Toddlers aged 12–24 months with ASD paid less attention to and expressed limited concern for another person's distress compared to typically developing peers (Charman et al., 1997; 1998; Hutman et al., 2010). Between 1 and 2 years of age, infants with ASD spent less time looking at people, more time looking at objects, and less frequently shifted their attention between social and nonsocial stimuli (Swettenham et al., 1998). In one of several studies to use eye tracking methods in young children, Jones, Carr, and Klin (2008) reported that 2-year-old children with autism spent less time looking at the eyes of approaching adults, and more time looking at their mouths than either typically developing children or children with non-autistic developmental delays. In addition, children in their sample who spent less time looking at adults' eyes exhibited greater levels of social disability. In a second study, Klin et al. (2009) found that 2-year-olds with autism attend more readily to physical contingencies than to biological motion. Jones and Klin (2009) suggest that failure to attend to the eyes and to human motion may suggest that children with autism learn in a manner dominated by physical rather than social information, and that pattern may have important consequences for social development. These authors also suggest that tracking eye gaze in young children may provide an early biomarker for ASD.

During the second year of life, children with ASD demonstrated greater frequency and duration of repetitive and stereotyped behaviors with objects (Morgan et al., 2008; Watt et al., 2008; Wetherby et al., 2004) and body (Watt et al., 2008), as well as more sensory behaviors (Watt et al., 2008) compared with typically developing and developmentally delayed controls. Twelve-month-olds with ASD were more likely than developmentally delayed and typical controls to rotate and spin objects, and engage in unusual visual exploration (Ozonoff et al., 2008b). Toddlers aged 12–24 months with ASD demonstrated abnormal motor behaviors, unusual repetitive behaviors, or atypical sensory interests (Brian et al., 2008; Chawarska et al., 2007; Wetherby et al., 2004). At 12 months, children with ASD more frequently waved their arms, and at 18 months, children with ASD waved their arms and put their hands to their ears more frequently than controls (Loh et al., 2007).

Young toddlers with ASD were also more likely to be more reactive and have difficulty with transitions (Brian et al., 2008). The functional and symbolic play of young children with ASD was often impaired or abnormal (Charman et al., 1997; 1998; Chawarska et al., 2007).

These findings suggest that during the second year of life, children later diagnosed with ASD are already exhibiting impairments in communication and socialization, and may have repetitive behaviors and temperamental differences.

Studies of 24- to 36-Month-Olds

Manifestations of ASD change little between the second and third years of life. While overall language level improved and frequency of vocalizations increased between the second and third birthdays in children with ASD, abnormal qualities of communication also emerged, including atypical intonation, echolalia, and use of stereotyped language (Chawarska et al., 2007). Compared to children with other developmental delays, 24- to 36-month-old children with ASD engaged in fewer communicative acts (Stone et al., 1997). Specifically, children with ASD were more likely to communicate by making requests as opposed to making comments. Additionally, children with ASD used fewer communicative gestures than developmentally delayed children, including pointing and showing (Stone et al., 1997). Conversely, children with ASD had a higher proportion of communicative acts that involved using the examiner's hand as a tool (Stone et al., 1997). Children aged 2–3 years with ASD were less likely than their peers to integrate gestures, eye gaze, and vocalization (Stone et al., 1997). By 36 months, children with ASD continued to struggle with motor imitation compared to typically developing and developmentally delayed children (Rogers et al., 2003; Stone et al., 1997), although imitation skills improved in children with ASD between ages 2 and 3 (Stone et al., 1997). Deficits in imitation were not associated with fine motor, gross motor, or praxis difficulties (Rogers et al., 2003). Imitation skills were correlated with autism severity and joint attention skills for toddlers with ASD (Rogers et al., 2003).

Socialization skills remain consistently impaired in children with ASD between 24 and 36 months, except for improvement in response to joint attention (Chawarska et al., 2007; Goldberg et al., 2005). However, initiation of joint attention remains impaired (Chawarska et al., 2007; Goldberg et al., 2005). Furthermore, in the third year of life, young children with ASD continued to make less frequent eye contact and engage in less turn-taking behaviors than their typical peers (Goldberg et al., 2005).

Differences in affect and behavioral regulation have been noted between young children with ASD and typical peers. At age 2, children later diagnosed with ASD had less positive affect, more negative affect, and greater difficulty controlling attention and behavior than typically developing children (Garon et al., 2009). Children later diagnosed with ASD also were less likely to find social cues rewarding (Garon et al., 2009). During the third year of life, compared with typically developing children and children with developmental delays, children with ASD were more likely to use objects repetitively, engage in complex mannerisms with their bodies or hand and finger mannerisms, have difficulty with changes in routine, or have unusual attachments to objects (Richler et al., 2007). Additionally, compared with typically developing children, children with ASD had more unusual sensory interests, unusual preoccupations, and abnormal or idiosyncratic responses to sensory stimuli (Richler et al., 2007). Another study found that higher-level repetitive behaviors, such as verbal rituals, unusual preoccupations, compulsions, and difficulty with change, were more common in children diagnosed with ASD than children who are developmentally delayed without ASD, even after controlling for severity of delay, age, and adaptive functioning (Mooney et al., 2006). Conversely, lower-level repetitive behaviors, such as repetitive use of objects, hand and finger mannerisms, complex mannerisms, and self-injury, were equally common in ASD and other developmental delays, and were found more often in the third rather than fourth year of life (Mooney et al., 2006). Additionally, functional and imaginative play improved in children with ASD between 2 and 3 years of age, but still remained atypical (Chawarska et al., 2007). Symptoms of ASD in the third year of life remain fairly consistent, although atypical communicative behaviors and stereotyped interests begin to emerge at this time.

Taken together, these data provide support for the hypothesis that the earliest manifestations of ASD are evident in the domains of attention and social motivation in the latter half of the first year of life but not before. Infants at greater risk for ASD experience a decrease in the frequency of social behaviors, perhaps especially self-initiated social overtures (Bhat et al. 2010), and in ability to shift attention flexibly, beginning between 6 and 12 months. By 12 months, infants at greater risk for ASD exhibit decreased verbal and nonverbal communicative overtures (Lander and Garrett-Mayer, 2006; Yoder et al., 2009), diminished responsiveness to name (Nadig et al., 2007), atypical object exploration, and increased repetitive behaviors (Ozonoff et al., 2008a). These behaviors may be the earliest manifestations of an atypical developmental trajectory that becomes increasingly apparent as social and communication expectations increase through the preschool years.

While studies of high-risk infant siblings have been enormously helpful in describing the early behavioral patterns that predate and may predict the development of ASD, such studies have their own limitations. First, there is considerable variability in data from sibling studies based on the age at which children are enrolled, the age to which they are followed and other variables, and these differences may affect data in unspecified ways. For example, studies which enroll children at age 12 months or later may enroll more parents who already have concerns about their child's development (Rogers, 2009). Similarly, the experience of growing up in a home with a sibling with autism, and the stresses that may impose on families may also affect development. Finally, it may be the case that children with a greater genetic loading for the disorder differ from children without such a loading. For example, while there is increasing evidence that high-risk sibs who later develop ASD may present repetitive behaviors in the second year of life, there is evidence that in population samples of toddlers diagnosed with ASD, repetitive behaviors may not appear until the third or fourth year. Those divergent findings likely reflect the increased heterogeneity in population samples and suggest caution in the generalization of results from studies of children with high genetic loading for ASD. There are also methodological issues that render the interpretation of data inconclusive at times. The use of more experimental tools such as eye tracking and evoked potential in the next generation of studies of high-risk infants may help clarify some of the inconsistent findings in the existing literature.

THEORETICAL CONSIDERATIONS

What do the data regarding the earliest manifestations of ASD suggest about the nature of the disorder? At present, opinions vary. Review of the available literature suggests that very early social and communicative deficits define ASD and that the deficits in social functioning appear prior to deficits in communicative skills (Fein et al., 2011). Some researchers argue that evidence of early deficits in social responsiveness (e.g., deficits in joint attention, response to name) support the view that autism disrupts *motivation for social engagement*, and the absence of such motivation derails typical developmental trajectories and results in the multiple impairments seen in older children with autism (Dawson, 2008; Fein et al., 2011). As early as 6 months, diminished social motivation may direct children's attention away from human faces and toward inanimate objects. That disengagement may imperil developing abilities to read social communication and to share experience. It may also undermine the ability to shift attention flexibly, both of which would have negative effects on cognitive development downstream. The establishment of atypical developmental trajectories may reduce opportunities for experience-dependent brain development, leading both to behavioral patterns characteristic of the disorder and to atypical brain development. Dawson (2008) argues that this may be best understood as a set of genetically mediated risk processes that leave children unable to access and benefit from exposure to environmental interactions. Early identification of such risk processes might permit the interruption of those negative cascades at both the neurological and the behavioral level, and permit the development of compensatory processes or the restoration of more typical trajectories. Such a model, while speculative, has the potential to account for much of the variability in the presentation of ASD, and for the variable effect of intensive intervention on developmental processes. While intervention is almost uniformly helpful, it is clearly of greater help to some children than to others (see Helt et al., 2008 for review), and much of the variability in outcome appears to be related to characteristics of the child. Greater understanding of those characteristics would permit the more careful specification of interventions tailored to the needs of individual children.

Other researchers take the opposite view, and argue that the rapid deceleration in developmental progress seen in children at risk of autism between the ages of 6 and 12 months includes a variety of skills not related to social function, and sometimes regarded as secondary to the diagnosis. Rogers (2009) and Tager-Flusberg (2010) argue that emerging evidence suggests that high-risk children who later receive a diagnosis of an ASD present a variety of atypical behaviors beginning at approximately 12 months. These include increased irritability, sensory reactivity, increased activity, and possibly motor delays, although the data in support of each of these changes is much less robust than the data cited earlier in support of changes in social responsiveness. Rogers interprets the onset of broader symptoms as suggesting that autism disrupts multiple aspects of development simultaneously, and can no longer be regarded as a primarily a social communication disorder (Rogers, 2009). Rather she regards it as a disorder that affects multiple domains of function and alters the course of development across multiple areas.

Similarly, Tager-Flusberg (2010) suggests that ASD is a complex syndrome that develops gradually and reflects alterations in expected developmental pathways in multiple domains. There is no single domain of function or behavioral manifestation that predicts the development of ASD symptoms or the prognosis for an affected child. In some developmental domains, the onset of ASD is characterized by slowed development or a plateau of progress; in other domains, including social functioning, there may be a loss of previously acquired skills. Tager-Flusberg posits that the widely held belief that regression characterizes the presentation of a subset of children with ASD may be in error; rather she argues that regression, specifically in the area of social communication skills may be characteristic of *all* children with ASD and may be a consequence of a broader developmental anomaly. Both Rogers and Tager-Flusberg suggest that data from studies of high-risk siblings have suggested a significant refinement in our understanding of the nature of ASD, and especially in the role accorded to social-communicative functioning, but they acknowledge that there is much we do not yet know. Among the remaining questions they note the following: What neural mechanisms underlie the atypical developmental trajectory exhibited by young children with ASD? What precipitates the divergence of their developmental trajectory from the more typical course? Is ASD driven by a loss of interest in the social world or an exaggerated interest in the world of objects, or an inability to shift attention flexibly? These and many other questions await more careful examination of early signs of the disorder, including more data from experimental paradigms such as eye tracking and ERP.

CLINICAL IMPLICATIONS

Understanding of the early manifestations of ASD has already resulted in an improved ability to screen children for early signs of the disorder, with the resulting recommendation that all children be screened as part of routine pediatric care at age 18 and 24 months (Council on Children with Disabilities, 2006). Several groups of researchers have developed successful screening tools for toddlers based on early signs of social-communicative impairment (e.g., The Modified Checklist for Autism in Toddlers (M-CHAT) (Robins et al., 2001), or the Infant–Toddler Checklist (ITC) (Wetherby et al., 2008). These measures have been recently reviewed (Barton et al., 2011) and will not be considered in detail here. Both the M-CHAT (Chlebowski, 2011; Kleinman et al., 2008; Robins et al., 2001) and the ITC (Wetherby, 2010; Wetherby et al., 2008) consistently identify children at risk of ASD, and both require the use of follow-up measures to reduce their false positive rate. Other researchers have attempted to extend early screening to children younger than 16 months. Dietz et al. (2006) screened 31,724 14–15-month-olds and reported limited sensitivity in this age group. Pierce et al. (2011) used the ITC to screen 10,479 infants aged 12 months. Both groups of investigators report a significant false positive rate as well as difficulty differentiating children with ASD from those with other developmental concerns. Both Dietz et al. (2006) and Pierce et al. (2011) also note that many parents refused follow-up evaluations due to their low index of concern. Rogers (2009) notes that the enormous variability in the earliest signs of ASD has important implications for screening. She argues that autism screenings will have to be administered repeatedly, perhaps through age 36 months in order to identify all affected toddlers, and they should be designed to identify toddlers with less severe signs as well as those with clear-cut symptoms of ASD.

Awareness of early signs of ASD has also influenced the prevailing standards for the diagnostic evaluation of young children. The development of the Autism Diagnostic Observation Schedule (Lord et al., 2000) provided a reliable and valid tool for the assessment of reciprocal social interaction and social communication; refinements to the scoring algorithm now include increased attention to restricted interests and repetitive behaviors (Gotham et al., 2007). While diagnosis of children younger than 2 is increasingly common, the variability in early presentation of ASD symptoms as well as the rapidity of developmental change in young children warrants special diagnostic considerations. Many of the behaviors that mark early social development must be assessed relative to a child's developmental age. Children of any age whose developmental functioning is typical of children aged 10–12 months or younger cannot be expected to exhibit the social behaviors (e.g., pointing, gaze shifting) which characterize normative development, and the absence of those behaviors cannot always be interpreted as indicative of disorder. Nor are there reliable behavioral markers which might indicate an atypical trajectory in those children.

Recently proposed practice parameters recommend that the diagnostic process include standardized assessment of communication, and cognitive and adaptive skills as well as the structured observation of social, communicative, and play skills, and repetitive interests and behaviors. Data must be obtained both from detailed interviews with caregivers, and from systematic and structured observation of the child in settings designed to encourage social engagement. Finally data must be interpreted in a developmental framework by clinicians with expertise with infants and toddlers with ASD (Zwaigenbaum et al., 2009).

Most recently, data regarding the earliest manifestations of ASD have influenced changes to the standards used to define the disorder. In the proposed revision to DSM-IV, the multiple diagnoses now subsumed under the category of Pervasive Developmental Disorders will be eliminated, in large measure because it has proven difficult to make reliable distinctions between them. Instead they will now be viewed as a continuum without specific subcategories. The disorder will be defined by two sets of symptoms. The first reflects the overlap between symptoms of social engagement and intentional communication, and focuses on deficits in both social communication and interaction. This change appears related to the increased recognition of the complex relationship between early social engagement and the development of communication strategies, and the recognition that impairments in social motivation derail development in multiple areas. The second factor includes restricted and repetitive patterns of behavior and requires at least two of four specific behaviors (http://www.dsm5.org).

While this change may reflect data from studies of high-risk siblings which supports the presence of repetitive behaviors in young children, there is concern that the requirement that such behaviors be observed in all children in order to qualify for a diagnosis on the autism spectrum may result in the exclusion of children with milder forms of the disorder, or the delayed identification of children whose symptoms, especially in the area of repetitive behaviors, develop later in childhood. Those issues are currently under discussion and await further empirical data. These and other critical questions regarding diagnosis, the potential identification of subtypes of ASD, and the development of effective treatments have clearly been informed by the research efforts reviewed here and await further study of the youngest children affected by ASD.

References

Adrien, J.L., Lenoir, P., Martineau, J., Perrot, A., Hameury, L., Larmande, C., et al., 1993. Blind ratings of early symptoms of autism based upon family home movies. Journal of the American Academy of Child & Adolescent Psychiatry 33, 617–625.

Autism and Developmental Disabilities Monitoring Network Surveillance Year 2002. Principal Investigators, 2007. Prevalence of autism spectrum disorders: Autism and developmental disabilities monitoring network, 14 sites, Morbidity and Mortality Weekly Report. Surveillance Summary 56, 12–28.

Baranek, G.T., 1999. Autism during infancy: A retrospective video analysis of sensory motor and social behaviours at 9–12 months of age. Journal of Autism and Developmental Disorders 29, 213–224.

Baranek, G.T., David, F.J., Poe, M.D., Stone, W.L., Watson, L.R., 2006. Sensory Experiences Questionnaire: Discriminating sensory features in young children with autism, developmental delays, and typical development. Journal of Child Psychology and Psychiatry and Allied Disciplines 47, 591–601.

Barnard-Brak, L., Sulak, T., Hatz, J.K., 2011. Macrocephaly in children with autism spectrum disorders. Pediatric Neurology 44, 97–100.

Barton, M., Dumont-Mathieu, T., Fein, D., 2011. Screening for Autism Spectrum Disorders in primary practice. Journal of Autism and Developmental Disorders Online (accessed 13.08.11.).

Begeer, S., El Bouk, S., Boussaid, W., Terwogt, M., Koot, H., 2009. Underdiagnosis and referral bias of autism in ethnic minorities. Journal of Autism and Developmental Disorders 39, 142–148.

Ben-Itzchak, E., Lahat, E., Burgin, R., Zachor, A., 2008. Cognitive, behavioral and intervention outcome in young children with autism. Research in Developmental Disabilities 29, 447–458.

Bernabei, P., Cerquiglini, A., Cortesi, F., D'Ardia, C., 2006. Regression versus no regression in the autistic disorder: Developmental trajectories. Journal of Autism and Developmental Disorders 37, 580–588.

Bhat, A.N., Galloway, J.C., Landa, R.J., 2010. Social and non-social visual attention patterns and associative learning in infants at risk for autism. Journal of Child Psychology and Psychiatry, and Allied Disciplines 51, 989–997.

Brian, J., Bryson, S.E., Garon, N., Roberts, W., Smith, I.M., Szatmari, P., et al., 2008. Clinical assessment of autism in high-risk 18-month-olds. Autism: The International Journal of Research and Practice 12, 433–456.

Bryson, S.E., Zwaigenbaum, L., McDermott, C., Rombough, V., Brian, J., 2008. The Autism Observation Scale for Infants: Scale development and reliability data. Journal of Autism and Developmental Disorders 38, 731–738.

Carper, R.A., Moses, P., Tigue, Z.D., Courchesne, E., 2002. Cerebral lobes in autism: Early hyperplasia and abnormal age effects. NeuroImage 16, 1038–1051.

Cassel, T.D., Messinger, D.S., Ibanez, L.V., Haltigan, J.D., Acosta, S.I., Buchman, A.C., 2007. Early social and emotional communication in the infant siblings of children with autism spectrum disorders: An examination of the broad phenotype. Journal of Autism and Developmental Disorders 37, 122–132.

Charman, T., Swettenham, J., Baron-Cohen, S., Cox, A., Baird, G., Drew, A., 1997. Infants with autism: An investigation of empathy, pretend play, joint attention, and imitation. Developmental Psychology 33, 781–789.

Charman, T., Swettenham, J., Baron-Cohen, S., Cox, A., Baird, G., Drew, A., 1998. An experimental investigation of social-cognitive abilities in infants with autism: Clinical implications. Infant Mental Health Journal 19, 260–275.

Chawarska, K., Klin, A., Paul, R., Volkmar, F., 2007. Autism spectrum disorder in the second year: stability and change in syndrome expression. Journal of Child Psychology and Psychiatry, and Allied Disciplines 48, 128–138.

Chawarska, K., Volkmar, F.R., 2005. Autism in infancy and early childhood. In: Volkmar, F.R., Paul, R., Klin, A., Cohen, D. (Eds.), Handbook of autism and pervasive developmental disorders, vol. 1. Diagnosis, development, neurobiology, and behavior, third ed. Wiley, Hoboken, NJ, pp. 223–246.

Chlebowski, C., 2011. The Modified Checklist for Autism in Toddlers: A Follow Up Study Investigating the Early Detection of Autism Spectrum Disorders in a Low Risk Sample. Unpublished Doctoral Dissertation. The University of Connecticut.

Clifford, S.M., Dissanayake, C., 2008. The early development of joint attention in infants with autistic disorder using home video observations and parental interview. Journal of Autism and Developmental Disorders 38, 791–805.

Clifford, S., Young, R., Williamson, P., 2007. Assessing the early characteristics of autistic disorder using video analysis. Journal of Autism and Developmental Disorders 37, 301–313.

Colgan, S.E., Lanter, E., McComish, C., Watson, L.R., Crais, E.R., Baranek, G.T., 2006. Analysis of social interaction gestures in infants with autism. Child Neuropsychology 12, 307–319.

Council on Children With DisabilitiesSection on Developmental Behavioral PediatricsBright Futures Steering Committee and Medical Home Initiatives for Children With Special Needs Project Advisory Committee, 2006. Identifying infants and young children with developmental disorders: An algorithm for developmental surveillance and screening. Pediatrics 118, 405–420.

Courchesne, E., Carper, R., Akshoomoff, N., 2003. Evidence of brain overgrowth in the first year of life in autism. Journal of the American Medical Association 290, 337–344.

Courchesne, E., Karns, C.M., Davis, H.R., Ziccardi, R., Carper, R.A., Tigue, Z.D., et al., 2001. Unusual brain growth patterns in early life in patients with autistic disorder: An MRI study. Neurology 57, 245–254.

Dahlgren, S.O., Gillberg, C., 1989. Symptoms in the first two years of life. European Archives of Psychiatry and Neurological Science 238, 169–174.

Dancel, G., Wilson, L., Troyb, E., Verbalis, A., Fein, D., 2008. Ethnic and Linguistic Differences on the M-CHAT. Paper presented at the Meetings of the International Neuropsychological Society, Waikoloa, HI.

Davidovitch, M., Glick, L., Holtzman, G., Tirosh, E., Sarif, M.P., 2000. Developmental regression in autism: Maternal perception. Journal of Autism and Developmental Disorders 30, 113–119.

Davidovitch, M., Golan, D., Vardi, O., Lev, D., Lerman-Sagie, T., 2011. Israeli children with autism spectrum disorder are not macrocephalic. Journal of Child Neurology 26, 580–585.

Dawson, G., 2008. Early behavioral intervention, brain plasticity and the prevention of autism spectrum disorder. Development and Psychopathology 20, 775–803.

Dawson, G., Munson, J., Webb, S.J., Nalty, T., Abbott, R., Toth, K., 2007. Rate of head growth decelerates and symptoms worsen in the second year of life in autism. Biological Psychiatry 61, 458–464.

Dawson, G., Rogers, S., Munson, J., Smith, M., Winter, J., Greenson, J., et al., 2009. Randomized, controlled trial of an intervention for toddlers with autism: The Eart Start Denver Model. Pediatrics 25, 17–23.

De Giacomo, A.D., Fombonne, E., 1998. Parental recognition of developmental abnormalities in autism. European Child & Adolescent Psychiatry 7, 131–136.

Dementieva, Y.A., Vance, D.D., Donnelly, S.L., Elston, L.A., Wolpert, C.M., Ravan, S.A., et al., 2005. Accelerated head growth in early development of individuals with autism. Pediatric Neurology 32, 102–108.

Dietz, C., Swinkels, S., van Daalen, E., van Engeland, H., Buitelaar, J., 2006. Screening for autistic spectrum disorder in children aged 14-15 months: Population screening with the Early Screening of Autistic Traits Questionnaire (ESAT). Design and general findings. Journal of Autism and Developmental Disorders 36, 713–722.

Dissanayake, C., Bui, Q.M., Huggins, R., Loesch, D.Z., 2006. Growth in stature and head circumference in high-functioning autism and Asperger disorder during the first 3 years of life. Development and Psychopathology 18, 381–393.

Earls, M., Hay, S., 2006. Setting the stage for success, Implementation of developmental and behavioral screening and surveillance in primary care practice-the North Carolina assuring better child health and development (ABCD) project. Pediatrics 118, 183–188.

Elder, L.M., Dawson, G., Toth, K., Fein, D., Munson, J., 2008. Head circumference as an early predictor of autism symptoms in younger siblings of children with autism spectrum disorder. Journal of Autism and Developmental Disorders 38, 1104–1111.

Elsabbagh, M., Volein, A., Holmboe, K., Tucker, L., Csibra, G., Baron-Cohen, S., et al., 2009. Visual orienting in the early broader autism phenotype: Disengagement and facilitation. Journal of Child Psychology and Psychiatry 50, 637–642.

Esposito, G., Venuti, P., Maestro, S., Muratori, F., 2009. An exploration of symmetry in early autism spectrum disorders: Analysis of lying. Brain and Development 31, 131–138.

Evans, D.W., Leckman, J.F., Carter, A., Reznick, J.S., Henshaw, D., King, R.A., et al., 1997. Ritual, habit, and perfectionism: The prevalence and development of compulsive-like behavior in normal young children. Child Development 68, 58–68.

Fein, D., Chawarska, S., Rapin, I., 2011. In: Fein, D. (Ed.), The Neuropsychology of Autism. Oxford University Press, Oxford.

Fukumoto, A., Hashimoto, T., Ito, H., Nishimura, M., Tsuda, Y., Miyazaki, M., et al., 2008. Growth of head circumference in autistic infants during the first year of life. Journal of Autism and Developmental Disorders 38, 411–418.

Fukumoto, A., Hashimoto, T., Mori, K., Tsuda, Y., Arisawa, K., Kagami, S., 2011. Head circumference and body growth in autism spectrum disorders. Brain & Development 33, 569–575.

Gamliel, I., Yirmiya, N., Sigman, M., 2007. The development of young siblings of children with autism from 4 to 54 months. Journal of Autism and Developmental Disorders 37, 171–183.

Garon, N., Bryson, S.E., Zwaigenbaum, L., Smith, I.M., Brian, J., Roberts, W., et al., 2009. Temperament and its relationship to autistic symptoms in a high-risk infant sib cohort. Journal of Abnormal Child Psychology 37, 59–78.

Gillberg, C., de Souza, L., 2002. Head circumference in autism, Asperger syndrome, and ADHD: A comparative study. Developmental Medicine and Child Neurology 44, 296–300.

Goldberg, W.A., Jarvis, K.L., Osann, K., Laulhere, T.M., Straub, C., Thomas, E., et al., 2005. Brief report: Early social communication behaviors in the younger siblings of children with autism. Journal of Autism and Developmental Disorders 35, 657–664.

Gotham, K., Risi, S., Pickles, A., Lord, C., 2007. The Autism Diagnostic Observation Schedule: Revised algorithms for improved diagnostic validity. Journal of Autism and Developmental Disorders 37, 613–627.

Hazlett, H.C., Poe, M., Gerig, G., Smith, R.G., Provenzale, J., Ross, A., et al., 2005. Magnetic resonance imaging and head circumference study of brain size in autism: Birth through age 2 years. Archives of General Psychiatry 62, 1366–1376.

Hazlett, H.C., Poe, M.D., Gerig, G., Styner, M., Chappell, C., Smith, R.G., et al., 2011. Early brain overgrowth in autism associated with an increase in cortical surface area before age 2 years. Archives of General Psychiatry 68, 467–476.

Helt, M., Kelley, E., Kinsbourne, M., Pandey, J., Boorstein, H., Hebert, M., et al., 2008. Can children with autism recover? If so, how? Neuropsychological Review 18, 339–366.

Hutman, T., Rozga, A., DeLaurentis, A.D., Barnwell, J.M., Sugar, C.A., Sigman, M., 2010. Response to distress in infants at risk for autism: A prospective longitudinal study. Journal of Child Psychology and Psychiatry, and Allied Disciplines 51, 1010–1020.

Ibanez, L.V., Messinger, D.S., Newell, L., Lambert, B., Sheskin, M., 2008. Visual disengagement in the infant siblings of children with an autism spectrum disorder (ASD). Autism: The International Journal of Research and Practice 12, 473–485.

Jones, W., Carr, K., Klin, A., 2008. Absence of preferential looking to the eyes of approaching adults predicts level of social disability in 2 year old toddlers with autism spectrum disorder. Archives of General Psychiatry 65, 946–954.

Jones, W., Klin, A., 2009. Heterogeneity and homogeneity across the autism spectrum: The role of development. Journal of the American Academy of Child and Adolescent Psychiatry 48, 1–3.

Kanner, L., 1943. Autistic disturbances of affective contact. Nervous Child 2, 217–250.

Kleinman, J., Robins, D., Ventola, P., Pandey, J., Boorstein, H., Esser, E., et al., 2008. The Modified Checklist for Autism in Toddlers, A follow-up study investigating the early detection of autism spectrum disorders. Journal of Autism and Developmental Disorders 38, 827–839.

Klin, A., Lin, D., Gorrindo, P., Ramsay, G., Jones, W., 2009. Two-year-olds with autism orient to nonsocial contingencies rather than biological motion. Nature 459, 257–261.

Lainhart, J.E., Piven, J., Wzorek, M., Landa, R., Santangelo, S.L., Coon, H., et al., 1997. Macrocephaly in children and adults with autism. Journal of the American Academy of Child and Adolescent Psychiatry 36, 282–290.

Landa, R., Garrett-Mayer, E., 2006. Development in infants with autism spectrum disorders: A prospective study. Journal of Child Psychology and Psychiatry, and Allied Disciplines 47, 629–638.

Liptak, G., Benzoni, L., Mruzek, D., Nolan, K., Thingvoll, M., Wade, C., et al., 2008. Disparities in diagnosis and access to heath care for children with autism: Data from the National Survey of Children's Health. Journal of Developmental and Behavioral Pediatrics 29, 152–160.

Loh, A., Soman, T., Brian, J., Bryson, S.E., Roberts, W., Szatmari, P., et al., 2007. Stereotyped motor behaviors associated with autism in high-risk infants: A pilot videotape analysis of a sibling sample. Journal of Autism and Developmental Disorders 37, 25–36.

Lord, C., 1995. Follow-up of two-year-olds referred for possible autism. Journal of Child Psychology and Psychiatry 36, 1365–1382.

Lord, C., Risi, S., Lambrecht, L., Cook, E., Levental, B., DiLavore, P., et al., 2000. The Autism Diagnostic Observation Schedule – Generic: A standard measure of social and communication deficits associated with autism spectrum disorders. Journal of Autism and Developmental Disorders 30, 205–223.

Lord, C., Shulman, C., Dilavore, P., 2004. Regression and word loss in autistic spectrum disorders. Journal of Child Psychology & Psychiatry 45, 936–955.

Luyster, R., Richler, J., Risi, S., Hsu, W.L., Dawson, G., Bernier, R., et al., 2005. Early regression in social communication in autism spectrum disorders: A CPEA study. Developmental Neuropsychology 27, 311–336.

Maestro, S., Muratori, F., Barbieri, F., Casella, C., Cattaneo, V., Cavallaro, M.C., et al., 2001. Early behavioral development in autistic children: The first 2 years of life through home movies. Psychopathology 34, 147–152.

Maestro, S., Muratori, F., Cesari, A., Cavallary, M.C., Paziente, A., Pecini, C., et al., 2005. Course of autism signs in the first year of life. Psychopathology 38, 26–31.

Mandell, D.S., Listerud, J., Levy, S., Pinto-Martin, J., 2002. Race differences in the age at diagnosis among Medicaid eligible children with autism. Journal of the American Academy of Child and Adolescent Psychiatry 41, 1447–1453.

Mars, A.E., Mauk, J.E., Dowrick, P.W., 1998. Symptoms of pervasive developmental disorders as observed in pre-diagnostic home videos of infants and toddlers. Journal of Pediatrics 132, 500–504.

McCleery, J., Akshoomoff, N., Dobkins, K., Carver, L., 2009. Atypical face versus object processing and hemispheric asymmetries in 10 month old infants at risk for autism. Biological Psychiatry 66, 950–957.

McGovern, C.W., Sigman, M., 2005. Continuity and change from early childhood to adolescence in autism. Journal of Child Psychology & Psychiatry 46, 401–408.

Merin, N., Young, G.S., Ozonoff, S., Rogers, S.J., 2007. Visual fixation patterns during reciprocal social interaction distinguish a subgroup of 6-month-old infants at-risk for autism from comparison infants. Journal of Autism and Developmental Disorders 37, 108–121.

Micali, N., Chakrabarti, S., Fombonne, E., 2004. The broad autism phenotype: Findings from an epidemiological survey. Autism 8, 21–37.

Mitchell, S., Brian, J., Zwaigenbaum, L., Roberts, W., Szatmari, P., Smith, I., et al., 2006. Early language and communication development of infants later diagnosed with autism spectrum disorder. Journal of Developmental and Behavioral Pediatrics 27, S69–78.

Mooney, E.L., Gray, K.M., Tonge, B.J., 2006. Early features of autism: Repetitive behaviors in young children. European Child & Adolescent Psychiatry 15, 12–18.

Moore, V., Goodson, S., 2003. How well does early diagnosis of autism stand the test of time? Follow-up study of children assessed for autism at age 2 and development of an early diagnostic service. Autism 7, 47–63.

Morgan, L., Wetherby, A.M., Barber, A., 2008. Repetitive and stereotyped movements in children with autism spectrum disorders late in the second year of life. Journal of Child Psychology and Psychiatry, and Allied Disciplines 49, 826–837.

Mraz, K.D., Dixon, J., Dumont-Mathieu, T., Fein, D., 2009. Accelerated head and body growth in infants later diagnosed with autism spectrum disorders: A comparative study of optimal outcome children. Journal of Child Neurology 24, 833–845.

Mraz, K.D., Green, J., Dumont-Mathieu, T., Makin, S., Fein, D., 2007. Correlates of head circumference growth in infants later diagnosed with autism spectrum disorders. Journal of Child Neurology 22, 700–713.

Muratori, F., Calderoni, S., Apicella, F., Filippi, T., Santocchi, E., Calugi, S., et al., 2012. Tracing back to the onset of abnormal head circumference growth in Italian children with autism spectrum disorder. Research in Autism Spectrum Disorder 6, 442–449.

Nadig, A.S., Ozonoff, S., Young, G.S., Rozga, A., Sigman, M., Rogers, S.J., 2007. A prospective study of response to name in infants at risk for autism. Archives of Pediatrics & Adolescent Medicine 161, 378–383.

Osterling, J., Dawson, G., 1994. Early recognition of children with autism: A study of first birthday home videotapes. Journal of Autism and Developmental Disorders 24, 247–258.

Osterling, J., Dawson, G., Munson, J., 2002. Early recognition of one-year old infants with autism spectrum disorder versus mental retardation: A study of first birthday party home videotapes. Development and Psychopathology 14, 239–251.

Ozonoff, S., Heung, K., Byrd, R., Hansen, R., Hertz-Picciotto, I., 2008. The onset of autism: Patterns of symptom emergence in the first years of life. Autism Research 1, 320–328.

Ozonoff, S., Iosif, A.M., Baguio, F., Cook, I.C., Hill, M.M., Hutman, T., et al., 2010. A prospective study of the emergence of early behavioral signs of autism. Journal of the American Academy of Child and Adolescent Psychiatry 49, 256–266.

Ozonoff, S., Macari, S., Young, G.S., Goldring, S., Thompson, M., Rogers, S.J., 2008. Atypical object exploration at 12 months of age is associated with autism in a prospective sample. Autism: The International Journal of Research and Practice 12, 457–472.

Ozonoff, S., Williams, B.J., Landa, R., 2005. Parental report of the early development of children with regressive autism: The delays-plus-regression phenotype. Autism 9, 461–486.

Ozonoff, S., Young, G., Goldring, S., Greiss-Hess, L., Herrera, A., Steele, J., et al., 2008. Gross motor development, movement abnormalities, and early identification of autism. Journal of Autism and Developmental Disorders 38, 644–656.

Pierce, K., Carter, C., Weinfeld, M., Desmond, J., Hazen, R., Bjork, R., et al., 2011. Detecting, studying and treating autism early: The one year well baby checkup approach. Pediatrics Online (accessed 29.04.11.).

Pinto-Martin, J.A., Dunkle, M., Earls, M., Fliedner, D., Landes, C., 2005. Developmental stages of developmental screening: Steps to implementation of a successful program. American Journal of Public Health 95, 1928–1932.

Reznick, J.S., Baranek, G.T., Reavis, S., Watson, L.R., Crais, E.R., 2007. A parent-report instrument for identifying one-year-olds at risk for an eventual diagnosis of autism: The First Year Inventory. Journal of Autism and Developmental Disorders 37, 1691–1710.

Richler, J., Bishop, S.L., Kleinke, J.R., Lord, C., 2007. Restricted and repetitive behaviors in young children with autism spectrum disorders. Journal of Autism and Developmental Disorders 37, 73–85.

Richler, J., Luyster, R., Risi, S., Hsu, W.L., Dawson, G., Bernier, R., et al., 2006. Is there a 'regressive phenotype' of autism spectrum

disorder associated with the measles-mumps-rubella vaccine? A CPEA study. Journal of Autism and Developmental Disorders 36, 299–316.

Robins, D.L., Fein, D., Barton, M.L., Green, J., 2001. The Modified Checklist for Autism in Toddlers: An initial study investigating the early detection of autism and pervasive developmental disorders. Journal of Autism and Developmental Disorders 31, 131–144.

Rogers, S., 2009. What are infant siblings teaching us about autism in infancy? Autism Research 2, 125–137.

Rogers, S., Vismara, L., 2008. Evidence-based comprehensive treatment of early autism. Journal of Clinical Child and Adolescent Psychology 37, 8–38.

Rogers, S.J., Hepburn, S.L., Stackhouse, T., Wehner, E., 2003. Imitation performance in toddlers with autism and those with other developmental disorders. Journal of Child Psychology and Psychiatry, and Allied Disciplines 44, 763–781.

Rommelse, N.N., Peters, C.T., Oosterling, I.J., Visser, J.C., Bons, D., van Steijn, D.J., et al., 2011. A pilot study of abnormal growth in autism spectrum disorders and other childhood psychiatric disorders. Journal of Autism and Developmental Disorders 41, 44–54.

Rozga, A., Hutman, T., Young, G.S., Rogers, S.J., Ozonoff, S., Dapretto, M., et al., 2011. Behavioral profiles of affected and unaffected siblings of children with autism: Contribution of measures of mother-infant interaction and nonverbal communication. Journal of Autism and Developmental Disorders 41, 287–301.

Schumann, C.M., Barnes, C.C., Lord, C., Courchesne, E., 2009. Amygdala enlargement in toddlers with autism related to severity of social and communication impairments. Biological Psychiatry 66, 942–949.

Schumann, C.M., Bloss, C.S., Barnes, C.C., Wideman, G.M., Carper, R.A., Akshoomoff, N., et al., 2010. Longitudinal magnetic resonance imaging study of cortical development through early childhood in autism. The Journal of Neuroscience: The Official Journal of the Society for Neuroscience 30, 4419–4427.

Seery, A., Vogel-Farley, V., Augenstein, T., Casner, L., Kasparian, L., Tager-Flusberg, H., et al., 2010. Atypical Electrophysiological Response and Lateralization to Speech Stimuli in Infants at Risk for Autism Spectrum Disorder. Paper presented at the International Meetings for Autism Research, Philadelphia, PA.

Shattuck, P., Durkin, M., Maenner, M., Newschaffer, C., Mandell, D., Wiggins, L., et al., 2009. Timing of identification among children with an autism spectrum disorder: Findings from a population-based surveillance study. Journal of the American Academy of Child and Adolescent Psychiatry 5, 463–464.

Shumway, S., Wetherby, A.M., 2009. Communicative acts of children with autism spectrum disorders in the second year of life. Journal of Speech, Language, and Hearing Research 52, 1139–1156.

Sices, L., Feudtner, C., McLaughlin, J., Drotar, D., Williams, M., 2003. How do primary care physicians manage children with possible developmental delays? A national survey with an experimental design. Pediatrics 113, 274–282.

Stefanatos, G.A., 2008. Regression in autistic spectrum disorders. Neuropsychology Reviews 18, 305–319.

Stone, W.L., Hoffman, E.L., Lewis, S.L., Ousley, O.Y., 1994. Early recognition of autism: Parental report vs. clinical observation. American Journal of Diseases of Children 148, 174–179.

Stone, W.L., Ousley, O.Y., Littleford, C.D., 1997. Motor imitation in young children with autism: what's the object? Journal of Abnormal Child Psychology 25, 475–485.

Stone, W.L., Ousley, O.Y., Yoder, P.J., Hogan, K.L., Hepburn, S.L., 1997. Nonverbal communication in two- and three-year-old children with autism. Journal of Autism and Developmental Disorders 27, 677–696.

Sullivan, M., Finelli, J., Marvin, A., Garrett-Mayer, E., Bauman, M., Landa, R., 2007. Response to joint attention in toddlers at risk for autism spectrum disorder: A prospective study. Journal of Autism and Developmental Disorders 37, 37–48.

Swettenham, J., Baron-Cohen, S., Charman, T., Cox, A., Baird, G., Drew, A., et al., 1998. The frequency and distribution of spontaneous attention shifts between social and nonsocial stimuli in autistic, typically developing, and nonautistic developmentally delayed infants. Journal of Child Psychology and Psychiatry, and Allied Disciplines 39, 747–753.

Tager-Flusberg, H., 2010. The origins of social impairments in autism spectrum disorders: Studies of infants at risk. Neural Networks 23, 1072–1076.

Torrey, E.F., Dhavale, D., Lawlor, J.P., Yolken, R.H., 2004. Autism and head circumference in the first year of life. Biological Psychiatry 56, 892–894.

Tronick, E., Als, H., Adamson, L., Wise, S., Brazelton, T.B., 1978. The infant's response to entrapment between contradictory messages in face-to-face interaction. Journal of the American Academy of Child Psychiatry 17, 1–13.

van Daalen, E., Swinkels, S.H., Dietz, C., van Engeland, H., Buitelaar, J.K., 2007. Body length and head growth in the first year of life in autism. Pediatric Neurology 37, 324–330.

Volkmar, F., Chawarska, K., Carter, A., Lord, C., 2007. Diagnosis of autism and related disorders in infants and very young children: Setting a research agenda for DSM-V. In: Narrow, W.E., First, M.B., Sirovatka, P.J., Regier, D.A. (Eds.), Age and gender considerations in psychiatric diagnosis: A research agenda for DSM-V. American Psychiatric Publishing, Arlington, VA, pp. 259–270.

Watson, L.R., Baranek, G.T., Crais, E.R., Reznick, J.S., Dykstra, J., Perryman, T., 2007. The First Year Inventory: Retrospective parent responses to a questionnaire designed to identify one-year-olds at risk for autism. Journal of Autism and Developmental Disorders 37, 49–61.

Watt, N., Wetherby, A.M., Barber, A., Morgan, L., 2008. Repetitive and stereotyped behaviors in children with autism spectrum disorders in the second year of life. Journal of Autism and Developmental Disorders 38, 1518–1533.

Webb, S.J., Nalty, T., Munson, J., Brock, C., Abbott, R., Dawson, G., 2007. Rate of head circumference growth as a function of autism diagnosis and history of autistic regression. Journal of Child Neurology 22, 1182–1190.

Werner, E., Dawson, G., 2005. Validation of the phenomenon of autistic disorder regression using home videotapes. Archives of General Psychiatry 62, 889–895. Available at: http://dx.doi.org/10.1001/archpsyc.62.8.889.

Werner, E., Dawson, G., Munson, J., Osterling, J., 2005. Variation in early developmental course in autism and its relation with behavioral outcome at 3-4 years of age. Journal of Autism and Developmental Disorders 35, 337–350.

Werner, E., Dawson, G., Osterling, J., Dinno, N., 2000. Brief report: Recognition of autism spectrum disorder before one year of age – a retrospective study based on home videotapes. Journal of Autism and Developmental Disorders 30, 157–162. Available at: http://dx.doi.org/10.1023/A:1005463707029.

Wetherby, A., 2010. Identifying Children with Autism Spectrum Disorder Through General Population Screening. Paper Presented at the 9th Annual International Meeting for Autism Research, Philadelphia, PA.

Wetherby, A., Brosnan-Maddox, S., Peace, V., Newton, L., 2008. Validation of the Infant-Toddler Checklist as a broadband screener for autism spectrum disorders from 9–24 months of age. Autism 12, 487–511.

Wetherby, A.M., Prizant, B.M., 1998. Infant/Toddler Checklist for Communication and Language Development. Applied Symbolix, Chicago, IL.

Wetherby, A.M., Watt, N., Morgan, L., Shumway, S., 2007. Social communication profiles of children with autism spectrum disorders late in the second year of life. Journal of Autism and Developmental Disorders 37, 960–975.

Wetherby, A.M., Woods, J., Allen, L., Cleary, J., Dickinson, H., Lord, C., 2004. Early indicators of autism spectrum disorders in the second year of life. Journal of Autism and Developmental Disorders 34, 473–493.

Whitehouse, A.J.O., Hickey, M., Stanley, F.J., Newnham, J.P., Pennell, C.E., 2011. A preliminary study of fetal head circumference growth in Autism Spectrum Disorder. Journal of Autism and Developmental Disorders 41, 122–129.

Wimpory, D.C., Hobson, R.P., Williams, J.M.G., Nash, S., 2000. Are infants with autism socially engaged? A study of recent retrospective parental reports. Journal of Autism and Developmental Disorders 30, 525–536.

Yeargin-Allsopp, M., Rice, C., Karapurkar, T., Doernberg, N., Boyle, C., Murphy, C., 2003. Prevalence of autism in a US metropolitan area. Journal of the American Medical Association 289, 49–55.

Yirmiya, N., Gamliel, I., Pilowsky, T., Feldman, R., Baron-Cohen, S., Sigman, M., 2006. The development of siblings of children with autism at 4 and 14 months: Social engagement, communication, and cognition. Journal of Child Psychology and Psychiatry, and Allied Disciplines 47, 511–523.

Yoder, P., Stone, W.L., Walden, T., Malesa, E., 2009. Predicting social impairment and ASD diagnosis in younger siblings of children with autism spectrum disorder. Journal of Autism and Developmental Disorders 39, 1381–1391.

Young, G.S., Rogers, S.J., Hutman, T., Rozga, A., Sigman, M., Ozonoff, S., 2011. Imitation from 12 to 24 months in autism and typical development: A longitudinal Rasch analysis. Developmental Psychology 47, 1565–1578.

Young, R., Brewer, N., Pattison, C., 2003. Parental identification of early behavioural abnormalities in children with autistic disorder. Autism 7, 125–143.

Zwaigenbaum, L., Bryson, S., Lord, C., Rogers, S., Carter, A., Carver, L., et al., 2009. Clinical assessment and management of toddlers with suspected autism spectrum disorder: Insights from studies of high risk infants. Pediatrics 123, 1383–1391.

Zwaigenbaum, L., Bryson, S., Rogers, T., Roberts, W., Brian, J., Szatmari, P., 2005. Behavioral manifestations of autism in the first year of life. International Journal of Developmental Neuroscience 23, 143–152.

Zwaigenbaum, L., Thurm, A., Stone, W., Baranek, G., Bryson, S., Iverson, S., et al., 2007. Studying the emergence of autism spectrum disorders in high-risk Infants: Methodological and practical issues. Journal of Autism and Developmental Disorders 37, 466–480.

Asperger Syndrome and its Relationships to Autism

James C. McPartland*, Fred R. Volkmar†

*Yale Child Study Center, New Haven, CT, USA †Yale University School of Medicine,
Yale New Haven Hospital, New Haven, CT USA

DIAGNOSTIC CONCEPT

History

In 1944, a medical student in Vienna, working on his medical school thesis, described four boys with marked social problems and poor motor skills, but highly developed verbal language, and unusual, highly idiosyncratic and circumscribed special interests (Asperger, 1944). This student, Hans Asperger, also observed that the condition seemed familial, and he used the word 'autism' in his original description of the condition as 'Autistic Psychopathy'. Asperger made the important point that the special interests exhibited by these boys were maladaptive both because they interfered with learning in other areas and because they could come to dominate the family's life. Because of the international academic impasse caused by World War II, he was not familiar with Leo Kanner's report, published the preceding year (1943), describing the condition of early infantile autism. At that time, the current emphasis on phenomenological, research-based definitions had not yet evolved (Spitzer et al. 1978), and Asperger continued to publish on the topic until the time of his death (Asperger, 1979). Because he published in German journals, his work received relatively little attention in the English language literature at the time.

Very few English language publications on Asperger syndrome (AS) appeared for several decades after Asperger's work. Initial publications included discussion of AS as a type of personality trait/disorder (i.e., rather than a developmental disorder; Van Krevelen, 1971), as well as redescription of some Asperger's cases (Robinson

& Viatlae, 1954), though the significance and relationship to autism was not recognized at the time. Several events in the 1980s increased awareness of AS. First, the American Psychiatric Association (APA) Diagnostic and Statistical Manual (DSM-III) recognized infantile autism as an official diagnostic concept (APA, 1980). The following year, a British psychiatrist, Lorna Wing, published a highly influential review of Hans Asperger and his work (Wing, 1981). Wing's review summarized Asperger's account and provided a series of short case reports. She suggested that some aspects of his original description should be modified, for example, the presence in girls, individuals with delayed language, and individuals with intellectual disability. Wing highlighted the diagnostic concept but also greatly emphasized her impression that AS was a condition on the autism spectrum, closely related to autism, if not a variant of it. She proposed the use of the eponymous label 'Asperger syndrome' to avoid confusion with the frequent English translation of Asperger's German term, 'Autistic Psychopathy'. Although Asperger used 'psychopathy' to refer to a personality disorder, in English this term typically describes antisocial personality, a distinct diagnostic entity. Wing's report, and her ambivalence about the validity of the category, has continued to color much subsequent work on the topic.

In the ensuing years, interest in AS expanded, along with the more general interest in autism spectrum disorders. Interest was fostered by the possibility of a strong genetic condition (given observations of similar symptoms in fathers of children with AS) and because some individuals viewed it as a possible transitional disorder between autism and schizophrenia (Klin et al., 2005a). Investigators struggled to develop more concrete operational diagnostic approaches that would improve upon the descriptive classification provided by Asperger and Wing. Simultaneously, with AS having been publicized among English-speaking scientists, efforts to validate the diagnostic construct and to establish its distinct clinical meaning and utility apart from autism were undertaken.

As part of the revision process for DSM-IV (APA, 1994) a large field trial (approximating 1,000 cases) was conducted in conjunction with ICD-10 (the World Health Organization's International Classification of Diseases; Volkmar et al., 1994). As part of the field trial, clinicians were provided with potential criteria relevant to AS and also were asked to provide a best-estimate clinical diagnosis. Nearly 50 cases were assigned a clinical diagnosis of AS in the field trial. When compared to both higher functioning autism (IQ in normal range) and pervasive developmental disorder not otherwise specified (PDD-NOS; also called 'sub threshold autism' or 'atypical autism cases'), several differences emerged among these populations. These included different patterns of verbal-performance IQ in AS compared to autism (AS having elevated verbal scores), a greater frequency of circumscribed interests, and greater social symptom severity when compared to the PDD-NOS cases. Based on the results of the field trial, AS was included as a distinct diagnostic subcategory (within the pervasive developmental disorders) in DSM-IV and ICD-10 (WHO, 1994). The publication of the DSM-IV-Text Revision (DSM-IV-TR; APA, 2000) wrought significant changes to descriptive text accompanying the diagnostic criteria for AS, but no changes were made in the diagnostic algorithm.

Diagnostic Criteria

Current definitions maintain some continuity with Asperger's original description of the disorder but also differ in several ways (Woodbury-Smith et al., 2005). Current diagnostic criteria in the DSM-IV-TR distinguish AS from autism primarily by adding exclusionary criteria (APA, 2000). Children with social deficits and restricted interests who do not meet criteria for autism, did not evidence frank language delay, and possess preserved cognitive ability and daily living skills qualify for AS. Specific diagnostic criteria include two areas of impairment from among the following social behaviors:

1. Inability to use multiple nonverbal behaviors, such as eye-to-eye gaze, facial expression, body postures, and gestures to regulate social interaction;
2. Failure to develop peer relationships appropriate to developmental level;
3. Lack of spontaneous seeking to share enjoyment, interests, or achievements with other people (e.g., by a lack of showing, bringing, or pointing out objects of interest to other people);
4. Lack of social or emotional reciprocity.

These social impairments must co-occur with at least one area of impairment in terms of the following categories of restricted, repetitive, and stereotyped patterns of behavior, interests, and activities:

1. Encompassing preoccupation with one or more stereotyped and restricted patterns of interest that is abnormal either in intensity or focus;
2. Apparently inflexible adherence to specific, nonfunctional routines or rituals;
3. Stereotyped and repetitive motor mannerisms (e.g., hand or finger flapping or twisting, or complex whole-body movements);
4. Persistent preoccupation with parts of objects.

Additional diagnostic criteria specify that these symptoms cause clinically significant impairment in social, occupational, or other areas of functioning without a clinically significant general delay in language (e.g., single words used by age 2 years, communicative phrases used by age 3 years) or in the development of

functioning autism (HFA; 17% vs. 5%). Nevertheless, the preponderance of research suggests shared genetic mechanisms common to all ASD (Frith, 2004). Some studies have reported specific genetic abnormalities in case studies of patients with AS: translocations, balanced translocations, and *de novo* translocations (chromosomes 1, 5, 11, 13, 14, 15, 17; Anneren et al., 1995; Cederlund & Gillberg, 2004; Tentler et al., 2001; 2003), autosomal fragile site (Saliba & Griffiths, 1990), fragile X syndrome (Bartolucci & Szatmari, 1987), fragile Y, and 21p+ (Cederlund & Gillberg, 2004; and see Chapter 2.1). Though numerous environmental factors have been postulated to interact with genes to play an etiological role in ASD, research has not shown consistent correlations (Wing & Potter, 2002).

Psychological Factors

Several studies suggest a distinct neuropsychological profile in AS (Lincoln et al., 1998). Klin and colleagues (1995) compared individuals with AS to those with other high-functioning autism spectrum disorders on a variety of neuropsychological measures, and determined that individuals with AS exhibited deficits in fine and gross motor skills, visual motor integration, visual–spatial perception, nonverbal concept formation, and visual memory with preserved articulation, verbal output, auditory perception, vocabulary, and verbal memory. Individuals with AS have been reported to exhibit stronger verbal abilities relative to performance abilities, with particular weakness in visual–spatial organization and graphomotor skills (Ehlers et al., 1997; Ghaziuddin & Mountain-Kimchi, 2004; Rourke, 1989). Overall, individuals with AS tend to demonstrate higher scores on measures of verbal functioning relative to individuals with autism (Reitzel & Szatmari, 2003). However, this study also found that individuals with AS did not consistently demonstrate nonverbal weaknesses or increased spatial or motor problems relative to individuals with HFA. Concordant with this finding, some researchers have argued that individuals with AS evidence overall greater cognitive ability than individuals with HFA, irrespective of verbal versus nonverbal ability (Miller & Ozonoff, 2000). Resolution of this issue is complicated by the employment of heterogeneous diagnostic schemes, which have been shown to directly influence IQ differential (Klin et al., 2005b).

ASSESSMENT

Diagnostic Assessment

Diagnostic assessment of AS is made according to clinical observation of the symptoms represented in ICD-10 or DSM-IV-TR criteria. Children thought to be at risk for AS should be referred for a multidisciplinary assessment by a team with specific experience in the assessment of ASD (Klin et al., 2005c). This practice ensures that complementary disciplines are employed to differentiate ASD from disorders with overlapping symptoms, such as expressive language disorder. Interdisciplinary assessment should entail thorough developmental and health history and include the disciplines of psychology, speech, and medicine. Depending on the age of the patient and presenting concerns, specialists in the areas of motor function (e.g., occupational or physical therapists), behavior modification, neurology, psychopharmacology, academic preparation, or vocational training should be consulted in the context of the evaluation.

Rigorous assessment for AS entails parent interview, direct observation of the individual, and psychological and speech and language assessment. Parent interview should inquire about social and communicative functioning, especially in the context of peer and romantic relationships, interests and hobbies, recreational activities, insight into the perspectives of others (including the impact of one's own behavior on others), comprehension of figurative language, insight into the nature of social relationships and emotional experiences, and presence of repetitive and stereotyped behaviors and interests. Because individuals with AS may under-report or misperceive the status of social relationships, accounts should be verified independently by parents, educators, or individuals familiar with daily functioning. Given high comorbidity of anxiety and depression, mood symptoms should also be evaluated, as well as mental health status, including integrity of thought processes. The interview should include a thorough developmental history, emphasizing early social development to confirm stability of symptoms from early childhood forward.

Observation should directly assess social and communicative behavior through play- or interview-based methods, also monitoring atypical behaviors (e.g., motor mannerisms, sensory behaviors) or rigid or repetitive interests or behavioral routines. It is helpful to observe a person in both structured and unstructured contexts, as individuals with AS often display more normative behavior in highly structured or routine interactions. Social difficulties are most evident when predictability is reduced and scaffolding is not provided.

Psychological assessment should assess cognitive (or developmental) function, motor control, and adaptive functioning (Klin et al., 2007). Psychological assessment of cognitive or developmental function provides a context within which to gauge social-communicative function and to facilitate differential diagnosis, for example, learning disabilities versus AS. Speech and language assessment should measure language production, language comprehension, nonverbal communication and gesture (including gaze and joint attention in young children), pragmatic and figurative language, prosody, rhythm, volume, and content of speech (Paul, 2005).

In addition to these discipline-specific assessments, formal diagnostic evaluation should also be included using standardized diagnostic assessments. Standardized self-report, parent/teacher report, and direct observation measures have been developed to screen for and diagnose AS and the other ASD. Though many are effective for this purpose, none to date reliably distinguish among individual ASD, such as discriminating Asperger syndrome from autistic disorder (Campbell, 2005; Lord & Corsello, 2005). The current 'gold standard' diagnostic protocol for ASD consists of a parent interview, the Autism Diagnostic Interview-Revised (Lord et al., 1994), and a semi-structured conversation/play-based interview, the Autism Diagnostic Observation Schedule (Lord et al., 2000). Both instruments require specific training to administer and score reliably. Differential diagnosis among ASD continues to rely on the judgment of experienced clinicians.

Additional Assessments

Genetic screening for various inherited metabolic disturbances is best practice, given increasing evidence for links between ASD and genetic syndromes with potential medical sequelae or for the relevance of genetic counseling. Genetic testing should assess for conditions known to cause ASD, such as fragile X syndrome, or inherited disorders that may have broader impact on physical health, such as phenylketonuria. Audiological evaluation is indicated to rule out contribution of auditory dysfunction to social and language impairments; brain stem auditory evoked response can be applied for individuals unable to comply with other methods of audiological assessment. Neurological consultation is appropriate if seizure activity is suspected, if late onset is observed, or if other indications of gross neurological dysfunction or soft signs are observed. Electroencephalograms (EEGs) and brain imaging, such as sMRI, are not recommended in all cases as they are neither diagnostic nor prescriptive; they may, however, be appropriate when concurrent non-ASD brain dysfunction is suspected (Minshew et al., 2005).

TREATMENT, INTERVENTIONS, AND OUTCOME

Treatment Objectives

Treatment for AS focuses on the development of age-appropriate social and communicative abilities, and

aims to teach skills that are not naturally acquired during development by explicit instruction. Aside from considerations relevant to linguistic capability, verbal strengths, or nonverbal vulnerabilities, comparable treatment guidelines apply to AS and other high-functioning ASD (Mesibov, 1992). Limited data exist to support efficacy of particular interventions, although some progress has been made in this area (Klin & Volkmar, 2003). Recommended interventions focus on: (a) devising strategies to capitalize upon strengths (e.g., cognitive or memory skills) to compensate for areas of difficulty and (b) modifying environments to provide optimal support for learning and socialization. Intervention programs should be tailored to the individual needs of the child, based on a thorough multidisciplinary assessment as described above. Nearly all intervention programs will include acquisition of basic social and communication skills (especially pragmatic communication), adaptive functioning, and, depending on what is developmentally appropriate, academic or vocational skills (Attwood, 2000; Howlin, 1999; Myles & Simpson, 1997; Ozonoff et al., 2002).

When challenging behaviors, such as aggression, are present in individuals with AS, it is important to address the communicative intent of the behavior through functional behavior analysis and to develop a behavioral program to reduce its frequency. For older children and adults with AS, vocational training is important to teach appropriate etiquette for job interviews and workplace behavior. Explicit teaching and rote learning using a parts-to-whole approach is recommended (Klin et al., 2005c). Motor difficulties also require support and can be addressed with occupational therapies focusing on integration of learning in areas of weakness such as visual–spatial organization and body awareness. Intervention must also incorporate techniques to encourage generalization of acquired skills beyond the context of instruction.

Psycho-Educational Interventions

Many interventions capitalize upon strong language skills and a concrete cognitive style by establishing straightforward rules to guide behavior and teaching explicit verbal scripts to apply in social settings. These rules can be memorized and then practiced, first in therapeutic settings and then in more naturalistic settings. The focus on generalization has been repeatedly emphasized (Lee & Park, 2007) given the frequent tendency of individuals to be rigid and overly focused. Adopting explicit problem-solving strategies such as rules, scripts and 'self-talk' can be helpful. Assistive technology, such as organization software and personal data assistants, is a useful tool for supporting organization and work and life management in individuals with AS (Ozonoff, 1998). Similarly, specialists in communication can help to foster pragmatic language abilities in areas like self-monitory, topic management, turn taking, conversational rules, speech volume, and prosody (Paul et al., 2009).

A recommended treatment modality for children with AS is social skills groups, as they provide a forum in which children can learn skills, practice them, and be coached and reinforced *in vivo*. Social skills groups can foster social skills and offer explicit teaching of conversational rules and interactional strategies (Kaland et al., 2011; Rubin & Lennon, 2004; Saulnier & Klin, 2007). Such settings facilitate targeting of both social motivation for peer connection and improve verbal and rote memory abilities (Beaumont & Sofronoff, 2008; Macintosh & Dissanayake, 2006; Muller, 2010; Patrick, 2008). Psychotherapy using a more problem-oriented 'life-coaching' approach can also be productive (Mero, 2002; Munro, 2010; Volkmar, 2011), and increasing evidence supports the effectiveness of cognitive behavioral therapies for AS (Cardaciotto and Herbert, 2004; Weiss & Lunsky, 2010).

Pharmacological Interventions

Drug treatments that specifically target the core social vulnerability of AS have not yet been established. However, pharmacological interventions have an important place in the treatment of the frequent co-morbid conditions, particularly inattention in younger children and anxiety and/or depression in adolescents and adults (Gutkovich et al., 2007; Tsai, 2007; Volkmar & Wiesner, 2009). As is the case for psychological and educational interventions, most available literature comes from case reports or open clinical trails rather than rigorously controlled studies. It is not uncommon for younger children with AS to be given trials of stimulant medications, often prior to receiving an accurate AS diagnosis (Ehlers et al., 1997).

DEVELOPMENTAL COURSE AND OUTCOME

Direct comparisons to other ASD are intrinsically complex, given the preserved language skills in AS (Gilchrist et al., 2001; Howlin, 2003; 2005; Szatmari, 2000). Asperger's observation of similar problems in parents suggested a more positive long-term outcome in that these individuals had maintained gainful employment and raised families. Research on long-term outcomes in AS, as in other areas, is complicated by differences in overall diagnostic approach but, in general, the data suggest that relative to both classical autism (Gillberg, 1991) and more narrowly defined high-functioning autism (Gillberg, 1998), the outcome is more positive overall. However, research using divergent definitional approaches yields mixed results (Szatmari et al., 1989). Several factors may contribute to better outcome, including the impact of overall cognitive abilities and particularly good verbal abilities, as well as associated capacities for developing coping strategies and finding suitable employment. Many individuals with AS continue to have significant needs and some remain at home with few occupational opportunities (Gillberg, 1998; Howlin, 2004; 2005; Tantam, 1991). Even when overall cognitive abilities are greater, adaptive skills deficits may present a major challenge for personal independence and self-sufficiency (Saulnier & Klin, 2007). Acquisition of adaptive skills is a critical factor in predicting longer-term outcome (Szatmari et al., 2003).

FUTURE DIRECTIONS

Though excellent progress has been made since Wing (1981) brought AS to the world's attention, the disorder remains incompletely understood in several important regards. Additional nosological study is needed to validate the diagnostic construct as distinct from other autism spectrum disorders and to increase reliability in diagnosis of AS among raters (Lord et al., 2011). This could support development of standardized diagnostic tools sufficiently sensitive to reliably discriminate. Along these lines, it remains to be clarified to what extent distinct educational and social/behavioral approaches are most appropriate for AS versus other ASD. Though pharmacotherapy is a promising treatment approach, additional work must be done to develop recommendations for specific medications to treat specific symptoms with an eye towards long-term efficacy and potential side effects. Ongoing work in neuroscience and genetics, and the integration of these fields, may provide evidence for biologically based screening instruments and biologically informed medical treatments. Despite the progress made in understanding AS and its place in the broader autism spectrum, the future of AS as a psychiatric diagnosis is unclear. The release of the DSM-5, anticipated in 2013, proposes diagnostic criteria to collapse AS, as well as the autistic disorder and PDD-NOS, into a single broad category of ASD. Relative to other psychiatric disorders, AS has been intensively studied for a short period of time; nevertheless, it may soon cease to exist.

References

American Psychiatric Association (APA), 1980. Diagnostic and Statistical Manual of Mental Disorders: DSM-III. American Psychiatric Association, Washington, DC.

American Psychiatric Association (APA), 1994. Diagnostic and Statistical Manual of Mental Disorders: DSM-IV. American Psychiatric Association, Washington, DC.

American Psychiatric Association (APA), 2000. Diagnostic and Statistical Manual of Mental Disorders: DSM-IV-TR. American Psychiatric Association, Washington, DC.

Anderson, G., Hoshino, Y., 2005. Neurochemical studies of autism. In: Volkmar, F., Rhea, P., Paul, R., Klin, A., Cohen, D. (Eds.),Handbook of autism and Pervasive Developmental Disorders, third ed., Vol. 1. John Wiley & Sons, Hoboken, NJ, pp. 453–472.

Anneren, G., Dahl, N., Uddenfeldt, U., Janols, L., 1995. Asperger syndrome in a boy with a balanced de novo translocation. American Journal of Medical Genetics 56, 330–331.

Asperger, H., 1944. Die "autistichen Psychopathen" im Kindersalter. Archive für Psychiatrie und Nervenkrankheiten 117, 76–136.

Asperger, H., 1979. Problems of infantile autism. Communication 13, 45–52.

Attwood, T., 2000. Strategies for improving the social integration of children with Asperger syndrome. Autism 4, 85–100.

Autism and Developmental Disabilities Monitoring Network Surveillance Year 2002 Principal Investigators, 2007. Prevalence of autism spectrum disorders: Autism and developmental disabilities monitoring network, 14 sites, United States, 2002. Morbidity and Mortality Weekly Report Surveillance Summaries 56, 12–28.

Autism and Developmental Disabilities Monitoring Network Surveillance Year 2006 Principal Investigators, 2009. Prevalence of autism spectrum disorders: Autism and developmental disabilities monitoring network, United States, 2006. Morbidity and Mortality Weekly Report Surveillance Summaries 58, 1–20.

Baron-Cohen, S., Scott, F., Wheelwright, S., Johnson, M., Bisarya, D., Desai, A., et al., 2006. Can Asperger syndrome be diagnosed at 26 months old? A genetic high-risk single-case study. Journal of Child Neurology 21, 351–356.

Bartolucci, G., Szatmari, P., 1987. Possible similarities between the fragile X and Asperger's syndromes. American Journal of Diseases of Children 141, 601–602.

Beaumont, R., Sofronoff, K., 2008. A multi-component social skills intervention for children with Asperger syndrome: The Junior Detective Training Program. [Erratum appears in Journal of Child Psychology Psychiatry. 2008, 49:895]. Journal of Child Psychology & Psychiatry & Allied Disciplines 49, 743–753.

Berthier, M.L., Starkstein, S.E., Leiguarda, R., 1990. Developmental cortical anomalies in Asperger's syndrome: Neuroradiological findings in two patients. Journal of Neuropsychiatry & Clinical Neurosciences 2, 197–201.

Bowman, E.P., 1988. Asperger's syndrome and autism: The case for a connection. British Journal of Psychiatry 152, 377–382.

Campbell, J.M., 2005. Diagnostic assessment of Asperger's disorder: A review of five third-party rating scales. Journal of Autism & Developmental Disorders 35, 25–35.

Cardaciotto, L., Herbert, J.D., 2004. Cognitive behavior therapy for social anxiety disorder in the context of Asperger's syndrome: A single-subject report. Cognitive and Behavioral Practice 11, 75–81.

Cederlund, M., Gillberg, C., 2004. One hundred males with Asperger syndrome: A clinical study of background and associated factors. Developmental Medicine & Child Neurology 46, 652–660.

Chakrabarti, S., Fombonne, E., 2005. Pervasive developmental disorders in preschool children: Confirmation of high prevalence. American Journal of Psychiatry 162, 1133–1141.

Dawson, G., Webb, S.J., McPartland, J., 2005. Understanding the nature of face processing impairment in autism: Insights from behavioral and electrophysiological studies. Developmental Neuropsychology 27, 403–424. Available at: http://dx.doi.org/10.1207/s15326942dn2703_6.

DeLong, G., Dwyer, J., 1988. Correlation of family history with specific autistic subgroups: Asperger's syndrome and bipolar affective disease. Journal of Autism & Developmental Disorders 18, 593–600.

Ehlers, S., Gillberg, C., 1993. The epidemiology of Asperger syndrome. A total population study. Journal of Child Psychology & Psychiatry 34, 1327–1350.

Ehlers, S., Nydén, A., Gillberg, C., Dahlgren Sandberg, A., Dahlgren, S.-O., Hjelmquist, E., et al., 1997. Asperger syndrome, autism and attention disorders: A comparative study of the cognitive profiles of 120 children. Journal of Child Psychology & Psychiatry & Allied Disciplines 38, 207–217.

Eisenmajer, R., Prior, M., Leekam, S., Wing, L., Gould, J., Welham, M., et al., 1996. Comparison of clinical symptoms in autism and Asperger's disorder. Journal of the American Academy of Child & Adolescent Psychiatry 35, 1523–1531.

Ellis, H.D., Ellis, D.M., Fraser, W., Deb, S., 1994. A preliminary study of right hemisphere cognitive deficits and impaired social judgments among young people with Asperger syndrome. European Child & Adolescent Psychiatry 3, 255–266.

Fombonne, E., 2005. Epidemiology of autistic disorder and other pervasive developmental disorders. Journal of Clinical Psychiatry 10, 3–8.

Fombonne, E., Tidmarsh, L., 2003. Epidemiologic data on Asperger disorder. Child & Adolescent Psychiatric. Clinics of North America 12, 15–21.

Frith, U., 2004. Emanuel Miller Lecture: Confusions and controversies about Asperger syndrome. Journal of Child Psychology & Psychiatry 45, 672–686.

Fujikawa, H., Kobayashi, R., Koga, Y., Murata, T., 1987. A case of Asperger's syndrome in a nineteen-year-old who showed psychotic breakdown with depressive state and attempted suicide after entering university. Japanese Journal of Child & Adolescent Psychiatry 28, 217–225.

Ghaziuddin, M., 2005. A family history study of Asperger syndrome. Journal of Autism & Developmental Disorders 35, 177–182.

Ghaziuddin, M., Ghaziuddin, N., Greden, J., 2002. Depression in persons with autism: Implications for research and clinical care. Journal of Autism & Developmental Disorders 32, 299–306.

Ghaziuddin, N., Metler, L., Ghaziuddin, M., Tsai, L., Giordani, B., 1993. Three siblings with Asperger syndrome: A family case study. European Child & Adolescent Psychiatry 2, 44–49.

Ghaziuddin, M., Mountain-Kimchi, K., 2004. Defining the intellectual profile of Asperger syndrome: Comparison with high-functioning autism. Journal of Autism & Developmental Disorders 34, 279–284.

Ghaziuddin, M., Weidmer-Mikhail, E., Ghaziuddin, N., 1998. Comorbidity of Asperger syndrome: A preliminary report. Journal of Intellectual Disability Research 42, 279–283.

Gilchrist, A., Green, J., Cox, A., Burton, D., Rutter, M., Le Couteur, A., 2001. Development and current functioning in adolescents with Asperger syndrome: A comparative study. Journal of Child Psychology & Psychiatry 42, 227–240.

Gillberg, C., 1985. Asperger's syndrome and recurrent psychosis-a case study. Journal of Autism & Developmental Disorders 15, 389–397.

Gillberg, C., 1989. Asperger syndrome in 23 Swedish children. Developmental Medicine and Child Neurology 31, 520–531.

Gillberg, C., 1991. Clinical and neurobiological aspects of Asperger syndrome in six family studies. In: Frith, U. (Ed.), Autism and Asperger syndrome, pp. 122–146.

Gillberg, C., 1998. Asperger syndrome and high-functioning autism. British Journal of Psychiatry 172, 200–209.

Gillberg, C., Cederlund, M., 2005. Asperger syndrome: Familial and pre- and perinatal factors. Journal of Autism & Developmental Disorders 35, 159–166.

Gillberg, I., Gillberg, C., 1989. Asperger syndrome: Some epidemiological considerations – A research note. Journal of Child Psychology & Psychiatry & Allied Disciplines 30, 631–638.

Gillberg, C., Gillberg, I., Steffenburg, S., 1992. Siblings and parents of children with autism: A controlled population-based study. Developmental Medicine & Child Neurology 34, 389–398.

Green, J., Gilchrist, A., Burton, D., Cox, A., 2000. Social and psychiatric functioning in adolescents with Asperger syndrome compared with conduct disorder. Journal of Autism & Developmental Disorders 30, 279–293.

Greenway, C., 2000. Autism and Asperger Syndrome: Strategies to promote prosocial behaviours. Educational Psychology in Practice 16, 469–486.

Gutkovich, Z.A., Carlson, G.A., Carlson, H.E., Coffey, B., Wieland, N., 2007. Advanced pediatric psychopharmacology: Asperger's disorder and co-morbid bipolar disorder: Diagnostic and treatment challenges. Journal of Child & Adolescent Psychopharmacology 17, 247–255.

Howlin, P., 1999. Children with Autism and Asperger Syndrome: A Guide for Practitioners and Carers. John Wiley and Sons, New York.

Howlin, P., 2003. Outcome in high-functioning adults with autism with and without early language delays: Implications for the differentiation between autism and Asperger syndrome. Journal of Autism & Developmental Disorders 33, 3–13.

Howlin, P., 2004. Interventions for individuals with Asperger syndrome. Transition to adulthood. Journal of Cognitive and Behavioral Psychotherapies 4, 223–231.

Howlin, P., 2005. Outcomes in Autism Spectrum Disorders. In: Volkmar, F.R., Rhea, P., Klin, Cohen, D. (Eds.),Handbook of Autism and Pervasive Developmental Disorders, third ed., Vol. 1. Wiley, Hoboken, NJ, pp. 201–222.

Howlin, P., Asgharian, A., 1999. The diagnosis of autism and Asperger syndrome: Findings from a survey of 770 families. Developmental Medicine & Child Neurology 41, 834–839.

Howlin, P., Goode, S., 1998. Outcome in adult life for people with autism and Asperger's syndrome. In: Volkmar, F.R. (Ed.), Autism and pervasive developmental disorders. Cambridge monographs in child and adolescent psychiatry. Cambridge University Press, New York, NY, pp. 209–241.

Jones, P.B., Kerwin, R.W., 1990. Left temporal lobe damage in Asperger's syndrome. British Journal of Psychiatry 156, 570–572.

Just, M.A., Cherkassky, V.L., Keller, T.A., Minshew, N.J., 2004. Cortical activation and synchronization during sentence comprehension in high-functioning autism: Evidence of underconnectivity. Brain 127, 1811–1821.

Kaland, N., Mortensen, E., Smith, L., 2011. Social communication impairments in children and adolescents with Asperger syndrome: Slow response time and the impact of prompting. Research in Autism Spectrum Disorders 5, 1129–1137.

Kanner, L., 1943. Autistic disturbances of affective contact. Nervous Child 2, 217–250.

Kerbeshian, J., Burd, L., 1986. Asperger's syndrome and Tourette syndrome: The case of the pinball wizard. British Journal of Psychiatry 148, 731–736.

Kim, J.A., Szatmari, P., Bryson, S.E., Streiner, D.L., Wilson, F.J., 2000. The prevalence of anxiety and mood problems among children with autism and Asperger syndrome. Autism 4, 117–132.

King, M., Bearman, P., 2009. Diagnostic change and the increased prevalence of autism. International Journal of Epidemiology 38, 1224–1234. Available at. http://dx.doi.org//dyp261 [pii].

Klin, A., Jones, W., Schultz, R., Volkmar, F., Cohen, D., 2002. Visual fixation patterns during viewing of naturalistic social situations as predictors of social competence in individuals with autism. Archives of General Psychiatry 59, 809–816.

Klin, A., McPartland, J., Volkmar, F.R., 2005. Asperger syndrome. In: Volkmar, R., Rhea, P., Cohen, D. (Eds.), Handbook of Autism and Pervasive Developmental Disorders, third ed., Vol. 1, Wiley, Hoboken, NJ, pp. 88–125.

Klin, A., Pauls, D., Schultz, R., Volkmar, F., 2005. Three diagnostic approaches to Asperger syndrome: Implications for research. Journal of Autism & Developmental Disorders 35, 221–234.

Klin, A., Saulnier, C.A., Sparrow, S.S., Cicchetti, D.V., Volkmar, F.R., Lord, C., 2007. Social and communication abilities and disabilities in higher functioning individuals with autism spectrum disorders: The vineland and the ados. Journal of Autism & Developmental Disorders 37, 748–759.

Klin, A., Saulnier, C., Tsatsanis, K., Volkmar, F., 2005. Clinical evaluation in autism spectrum disorders: Psychological assessment within a transdisciplinary framework. In: Volkmar, F.R., Rhea, P., Klin, A., Cohen, D. (Eds.),Handbook of Autism and Pervasive Developmental Disorders, third ed., Vol. 2. John Wiley & Sons, Hoboken, NJ, pp. 772–798.

Klin, A., Volkmar, F.R., 2003. Asperger syndrome. Child & Adolescent Psychiatric Clinics of North America 12, xiii–xvi.

Klin, A., Volkmar, F.R., Sparrow, S.S., Cicchetti, D.V., Rourke, B.P., 1995. Validity and neuropsychological characterization of Asperger syndrome: Convergence with nonverbal learning disabilities syndrome. Journal of Child Psychology & Psychiatry 36, 1127–1140.

Kwon, H., Ow, A.W., Pedatella, K.E., Lotspeich, L.J., Reiss, A.L., 2004. Voxel-based morphometry elucidates structural neuroanatomy of high-functioning autism and Asperger syndrome. Developmental Medicine & Child Neurology 46, 760–764.

Lee, H.J., Park, H.R., 2007. An integrated literature review on the adaptive behavior of individuals with Asperger syndrome. Remedial and Special Education 28, 132–139.

Leekam, S., Libby, S., Wing, L., Gould, J., Gillberg, C., 2000. Comparison of ICD-10 and Gillberg's criteria for Asperger syndrome. Autism 4, 11–28.

Lincoln, A.J., Courchesne, E., Allen, M., Hanson, E., Ene, M., 1998. Neurobiology of Asperger syndrome: Seven case studies and quantitative magnetic resonance imaging findings. In: Schopler, E., Mesibov, G.B., Kunce, L.J. (Eds.), Asperger Syndrome or High-functioning Autism? Current issues in autism, pp. 145–163. xviii, 409.

Littlejohns, C.S., Clarke, D.J., Corbett, J.A., 1990. Tourette-like disorder in Asperger's syndrome. British Journal of Psychiatry 156, 430–433.

Lord, C., Corsello, C., 2005. Diagnostic instruments in autism spectrum disorders. In: Volkmar, F., Rhea, P., Klin, A., Cohen, D.J. (Eds.), Handbook of Autism and Pervasive Developmental Disorders, third ed., Vol. 1. Wiley, Hoboken, NJ, pp. 730–771.

Lord, C., Petkova, E., Hus, V., Gan, W., Lu, F., Martin, D.M., et al., 2011. A multisite study of the clinical diagnosis of different autism spectrum disorders. Archives of General Psychiatry. Available at: http://dx.doi.org/10.1001/archgenpsychiatry.2011.148.

Lord, C., Risi, S., Lambrecht, L., Cook Jr., E.H., Leventhal, B.L., DiLavore, P.C., et al., 2000. The autism diagnostic observation schedule-generic: A standard measure of social and communication deficits associated with the spectrum of autism. Journal of Autism & Developmental Disorders 30, 205–223.

Lord, C., Rutter, M., Le Couteur, A., 1994. Autism diagnostic interview-revised: A revised version of a diagnostic interview for caregivers of individuals with possible pervasive developmental disorders. Journal of Autism & Developmental Disorders 24, 659–685.

Macintosh, K., Dissanayake, C., 2006. Social skills and problem behaviours in school aged children with high-functioning autism and Asperger's Disorder. Journal of Autism & Developmental Disorders 36, 1065–1076.

Marriage, K.J., Miles, T., Stokes, D., Davey, M., 1993. Clinical and research implications of the co-occurrence of Asperger's and Tourette syndromes. Australian & New Zealand Journal of Psychiatry 27, 666–672.

Mayes, S., Calhoun, S., Crites, D., 2001. Does DSM-IV Asperger's disorder exist? Journal of Abnormal Child Psychology 29, 263–271.

McAlonan, G.M., Daly, E., Kumari, V., Critchley, H.D., van Amelsvoort, T., Suckling, J., et al., 2002. Brain anatomy and sensorimotor gating in Asperger's syndrome. Brain 125, 1594–1606.

McConachie, H., Le Couteur, A., Honey, E., 2005. Can a diagnosis of Asperger syndrome be made in very young children with suspected autism spectrum disorder? Journal of Autism & Developmental Disorders 35, 167–176.

McCormick, J., 2001. The effect of Asperger's syndrome on the humor perception and production of teenage boys. [Dissertation]. Dissertation Abstracts International: Section B: The Sciences and Engineering 62, 2068.

McKelvey, J.R., Lambert, R., Mottron, L., Shevell, M.I., 1995. Right-hemisphere dysfunction in Asperger's syndrome. Journal of Child Neurology 10, 310–314.

Mero, M., 2002. Asperger syndrome with comorbid emotional disorder – treatment with psychoanalytic psychotherapy. International Journal of Circumpolar Health 61, 80–89.

Mesibov, G., 1992. Treatment issues with high-functioning adolescents and adults with autism. In: Schopler, E., Mesibov, G. (Eds.), High-functioning individuals with autism. Plenum Press, New York, NY, pp. 143–156.

Miles, S.W., Capelle, P., 1987. Asperger's syndrome and aminoaciduria: A case example. British Journal of Psychiatry 150, 397–400.

Miller, J.N., Ozonoff, S., 1997. Did Asperger's cases have Asperger disorder? A research note. Journal of Child Psychology & Psychiatry 38, 247–251.

Miller, J.N., Ozonoff, S., 2000. The external validity of Asperger disorder: Lack of evidence from the domain of neuropsychology. Journal of Abnormal Psychology 109, 227–238.

Minshew, N., Sweeney, J., Bauman, M., Webb, S., 2005. Neurologic aspects of autism. In: Volkmar, F., Rhea, P., Klin, A., Cohen, D. (Eds.), Handbook of Autism and Pervasive Developmental Disorders, third ed., Vol. 1. John Wiley & Sons, Hoboken, NJ, pp. 473–514.

Mitchel, K., Regehr, K., Reaume, J., Feldman, M., 2010. Group social skills training for adolescents with Asperger Syndrome or high functioning autism. Journal of Developmental Disabilities 16, 52–63.

Muller, R., 2010. Will you play with me? Improving social skills for children with Asperger syndrome. International Journal of Disability, Development and Education 57, 331–334.

Munro, J., 2010. An integrated model of psychotherapy for teens and adults with Asperger syndrome. Journal of Systemic Therapies 29, 82–96.

Myles, B.S., Simpson, R., 1997. Asperger Syndrome: A Guide for Educators and Parents. Pro-Ed, Austin, TX.

O'Connor, K., Hamm, J.P., Kirk, I.J., 2005. The neurophysiological correlates of face processing in adults and children with Asperger's syndrome. Brain and Cognition 59, 82–95.

Ozbayrak, K.R., Kapucu, O., Erdem, E., Aras, T., 1991. Left occipital hypoperfusion in a case with the Asperger syndrome [published erratum appears in Brain and Development 1992, 14:197]. Brain and Development 13, 454–456.

Ozonoff, S., 1998. Assessment and remediation of executive dysfunction in autism and Asperger syndrome. In: Schopler, E., Mesibov, G., Kunce, L.J. (Eds.), Asperger syndrome or high functioning autism? Plenum, New York, NY, pp. 263–292.

Ozonoff, S., Dawson, G., McPartland, J., 2002. A Parent's Guide to Asperger Syndrome and High-Functioning Autism: How to Meet the Challenges and Help your Child Thrive. Guilford Press, New York, NY.

Patrick, N., 2008. Social Skills for Teenagers and Adults with Asperger Syndrome: A Practical Guide to Day-To-Day Life. Jessica Kingsley, London, England.

Paul, R., 2005. Assessing communication in autism spectrum disorders. In: Volkmar, F., Klin, A., Rhea, P., Cohen, D.J. (Eds.), Handbook of autism and pervasive developmental disorders, third ed., Vol. 2. Wiley, New York, NY, pp. 799–816.

Paul, R., Orlovski, S., Marcinko, H., Volkmar, F., 2009. Conversational behaviors in youth with high-functioning ASD and Asperger syndrome. Journal of Autism & Developmental Disorders 39, 115–125.

Pina-Camacho, L., Villero, S., Fraguas, D., Boada, L., Janssen, J., Navas-Sanchez, F.J., et al., 2011. Autism spectrum disorder: Does neuroimaging support the dsm-5 proposal for a symptom dyad? A systematic review of functional magnetic resonance imaging and diffusion tensor imaging studies. Journal of Autism & Developmental Disorders. Available at: http://dx.doi.org/10.1007/s10803-011-1360-4.

Reitzel, J., Szatmari, P., 2003. Cognitive and academic problems. In: Prior, M. (Ed.), Learning and Behavior Problems in Asperger syndrome. Guilford Press, New York, NY, pp. 35–54.

Robinson, J.F., Viatlae, L.J., 1954. Children with circumscribed interest patterns. American Journal of Orthopsychiatry 24, 755–767.

Rourke, B.P., 1989. Nonverbal Learning Disabilities: The Syndrome and the Model. Guilford, New York, NY.

Rourke, B., Tsatsanis, K., 2000. Nonverbal learning disabilities and Asperger syndrome. In: Klin, Ami, Volkmar, Fred, R. (Eds.), Asperger syndrome. Guilford Press, New York, NY, pp. 231–253.

Rubin, E., Lennon, L., 2004. Challenges in social communication in Asperger syndrome and high-functioning autism. Topics in Language Disorders 24, 271–285.

Rutter, M., 2000. Genetic studies of autism: From the 1970s into the millennium. Journal of Abnormal Child Psychology 28, 3–14.

Rutter, M., Bailey, A., Bolton, P., Le Couter, A., 1994. Autism and known medical conditions: Myth and substance. Journal of Child Psychology & Psychiatry & Allied Disciplines 35, 311–322.

Saliba, J.R., Griffiths, M., 1990. Brief report: Autism of the Asperger type associated with an autosomal fragile site. Journal of Autism & Developmental Disorders 20, 569–575.

Samson, A., Huber, O., Ruch, W., 2011. Teasing, ridiculing and the relation to the fear of being laughed at in individuals with Asperger's syndrome. Journal of Autism & Developmental Disorders 41, 475–483.

Saulnier, C., Klin, A., 2007. Brief report: Social and communication abilities and disabilities in higher functioning individuals with autism and Asperger syndrome. Journal of Autism & Developmental Disorders 37, 788–793.

Schatz, A.M., Weimer, A.K., Trauner, D.A., 2002. Brief report: Attention differences in Asperger syndrome. Journal of Autism & Developmental Disorders 32, 333–336.

Schultz, R.T., 2005. Developmental deficits in social perception in autism: The role of the amygdala and fusiform face area. International Journal of Developmental Neuroscience 23, 125–141.

Schultz, R., Robins, D., 2005. Functional neuroimaging studies of autism spectrum disorders. In: Volkmar, F., Rhea, P., Klin, A., Cohen, D. (Eds.), Handbook of Autism and Pervasive Developmental Disorders, third ed., Vol. 1. John Wiley & Sons, Hoboken, NJ, pp. 515–533.

Sofronoff, K., Dark, E., Stone, V., 2011. Social vulnerability and bullying in children with asperger syndrome. Autism 15, 355–372.

Spitzer, R., Endicott, J., Robbins, Eli, 1978. Resarch diagnostic criteria. Archives of General Psychiatry 35, 773–782.

Stein, M., Klin, A., Miller, K., 2004. When Asperger's syndrome and a nonverbal learning disability look alike. Journal of Developmental & Behavioral Pediatrics 25, S59–S64.

Sweeney, J.A., Takarae, Y., Macmillan, C., Luna, B., Minshew, N.J., 2004. Eye movements in neurodevelopmental disorders. Current Opinion in Neurology 17, 37–42.

Szatmari, P., 2000. Perspectives on the classification of Asperger syndrome. In: Klin, Ami, Volkmar, Fred, R. (Eds.), Asperger syndrome. Guilford Press, New York, NY, pp. 403–417.

Szatmari, P., Archer, L., Fisman, S., Streiner, D., Wilson, F., 1995. Asperger's syndrome and autism: Differences in behavior, cognition, and adaptive functioning. Journal of the American Academy of Child & Adolescent Psychiatry 34, 1662–1671.

Szatmari, P., Bartolucci, G., Bremner, R., 1989. Asperger's syndrome and autism: Comparison of early history and outcome. Developmental Medicine & Child Neurology 31, 709–720.

Szatmari, P., Bryson, S., Boyle, M., Streiner, D., Duku, E., 2003. Predictors of outcome among high functioning children with autism and asperger syndrome. Journal of Child Psychology & Psychiatry 44, 520–528.

Tantam, D., 1988. Asperger's syndrome. Journal of Child Psychology & Psychiatry 29, 245–255.

Tantam, D., 1991. Asperger Syndrome in Adulthood Autism and Asperger Syndrome. Cambridge University Press, New York, NY, pp. 147–183.

Tantam, D., Evered, C., Hersov, L., 1990. Asperger's syndrome and ligamentous laxity. Journal of the American Academy of Child & Adolescent Psychiatry 29, 892–896.

Tentler, D., Brandberg, G., Betancur, C., Gillberg, C., Anneren, G., Orsmark, C., et al., 2001. A balanced reciprocal translocation t(5;7)(q14;q32) associated with autistic disorder: Molecular analysis of the chromosome 7 breakpoint. American Journal of Medical Genetics 105, 729–736.

Tentler, D., Johannesson, T., Johansson, M., Rastam, M., Gillberg, C., Orsmark, C., et al., 2003. A candidate region for Asperger syndrome defined by two 17p breakpoints. European Journal of Human Genetics 11, 189–195.

Thomsen, P., 1994. Obsessive-compulsive disorder in children and adolescents: A 6–22-year follow-up study: Clinical descriptions of the course and continuity of obsessive-compulsive symptomatology. European Child & Adolescent Psychiatry 3, 82–96.

Tsai, L., 2007. Asperger syndrome and medication treatment. Focus on Autism and Other Developmental Disabilities 22, 138–148.

Tuchman, R., Rapin, I., 2002. Epilepsy in autism. Lancet Neurology 1, 352–358.

Van Krevelen, D., 1971. Early infantile autism and autistic psychopathy. Journal of Autism & Childhood Schizophrenia. 1, 82–86.

Volkmar, F., 2011. Asperger's disorder: Implications for psychoanalysis. Psychoanalytic Inquiry 31, 334–344. Available at: http://dx.doi.org/10.1080/07351690.2010.513664.

Volkmar, F., Wiesner, L., 2009. A. Practical Guide to Autism. John Wiley, Hoboken, NJ.

Volkmar, F.R., Klin, A., Schultz, R., Bronen, R., Marans, W.D., Sparrow, S., et al., 1996. Asperger's syndrome [clinical conference]. Journal of the American Academy of Child & Adolescent Psychiatry 35, 118–123.

Volkmar, F.R., Klin, A., Siegel, B., Szatmari, P., Lord, C., Campbell, M., et al., 1994. Field trial for autistic disorder in DSM-IV. Journal of American Psychiatry 151, 1361–1367.

Weiss, J., Lunsky, Y., 2010. Group cognitive behaviour therapy for adults with Asperger syndrome and anxiety or mood disorder: A case series. [Case Reports Review]. Clinical Psychology & Psychotherapy 17, 438–446.

Welchew, D.E., Ashwin, C., Berkouk, K., Salvador, R., Suckling, J., Baron-Cohen, S., et al., 2005. Functional disconnectivity of the medial temporal lobe in Asperger's syndrome. Biological Psychiatry 57, 991–998.

Williams, J.G., Higgins, J.P., Brayne, C.E., 2006. Systematic review of prevalence studies of autism spectrum disorders. Archives of Disease in Childhood 91, 8–15.

Wing, L., 1981. Asperger's syndrome: A clinical account. Psychological Medicine 11, 115–129.

Wing, L., Potter, D., 2002. The epidemiology of autistic spectrum disorders: Is the prevalence rising? Mental Retardation & Developmental Disabilities Research Reviews 8, 151–161.

Wolff, S., McGuire, R.J., 1995. Schizoid personality in girls: A follow-up study – what are the links with Asperger's syndrome? Journal of Child Psychology & Psychiatry & Allied Disciplines 36, 793–817.

Woodbury-Smith, M., Klin, A., Volkmar, F., 2005. Asperger's syndrome: A comparison of clinical diagnoses and those made according to the ICD-10 and DSM-IV. Journal of Autism & Developmental Disorders 35, 235–240.

World Health Organization (WHO), 1993. The Icd-10 Classification of Mental and Behavioural Disorders: Diagnostic Criteria for Research. World Health Organization, Geneva.

World Health Organization (WHO), 1994. International Classification of Disease: Diagnostic Criteria for Research, tenth ed., World Health Organization, Geneva.

Yeargin-Allsopp, M., Rice, C., Karapurkar, T., Doernberg, N., Boyle, C., Murphy, C., 2003. Prevalence of autism in a us metropolitan area. Journal of the American Medical Association 289, 49–55.

Behavioral and Psychosocial Interventions for Individuals with ASD

Latha V. Soorya*,†, *Laura A. Carpenter*‡, *Zachary Warren***

*Department of Psychiatry, Rush University Medical Center, Chicago, IL, USA †Mount Sinai School of Medicine, New York, NY, USA ‡Department of Pediatrics, Medical University of South Carolina, Charleston, SC, USA **Department of Pediatrics and Psychiatry; Vanderbilt University, Nashville, TN, USA

Behavioral and psychosocial treatments designed for individuals with autism spectrum disorders (ASD) have experienced a tremendous growth since the publication of Ivar Lovaas's seminal study of applied behavioral analytic (ABA) model of treatment for children with autism in 1987. To date, behaviorally based strategies are considered the first line of intervention for these individuals. The growth in the science of behavioral treatments is reflected in the recent publication of several systematic, comprehensive reviews on behavioral and psychosocial interventions in ASD (National Standards Project, 2009; Seida et al., 2009; Reichow & Wolery, 2009; Warren et al., 2011).

The availability of comprehensive reviews elsewhere sets the foundation for the overview of major treatment approaches outlined here. This chapter focuses on the approaches with the most empirical support, as well as widely used approaches in community settings. *Comprehensive programs* will be reviewed first, given the strength of the evidence and their wide use in clinical practice. Comprehensive programs are those designed to target improvements across several domains (e.g., social, language, emotional/behavioral) and may include clinic-based or educational models such as one of the first ASD-specific educational models, TEACCH (Treatment and Education

The Neuroscience of Autism Spectrum Disorders.
http://dx.doi.org/10.1016/B978-0-12-391924-3.00005-3

of Autistic and related Communication-handicapped Children). Then, reviews of the literature on interventions designed to target isolated core symptom domains will be reviewed. These primarily skill-building interventions include commonly used models such as social skills training groups and picture exchange communication systems (PECS).

In addition, interventions targeting reductions in problem behaviors both core to ASD, such as repetitive behaviors (e.g., motor mannerisms), and associated symptoms such as irritability, aggression, and anxiety management will be reviewed. Commonly used behavioral reduction treatments will be described, such as positive behavioral support. Finally, complementary and alternative treatment (CAM) approaches are reviewed, with a specific focus on the strength of the evidence for these CAM treatments.

EARLY INTENSIVE BEHAVIORAL INTERVENTION

Early intensive behavioral treatment approaches for ASD aim to intervene early in the course of the disorder (typically prior to age 5) using high-intensity therapeutic intervention. The goal of these comprehensive treatment approaches is to change the trajectory of the child's atypical development to a more typical course of development. The programs outlined below represent a class of interventions that have been instrumental in changing treatment and educational perspectives for young children with ASD.

UCLA/Lovaas Model

The most well researched of these comprehensive treatment approaches is ABA (Lovaas, 1987). ABA uses the basic principles of learning and behavior to systematically teach new skills and reduce problematic behaviors in children with ASD. The approach relies on the implementation of well-established learning procedures such as classical conditioning, operant conditioning, and observational learning. There is an extensive body of evidence supporting the use of individual behavioral treatment approaches with children with ASD (e.g., shaping, chaining, modeling). One of the core teaching strategies of traditional ABA therapy is the use of 'discrete trials,' in which a target behavior is broken into small components and then drilled to high level of accuracy through repeated teaching presentations. Intensive ABA has typically been implemented in young children (under 5 years old) for a period of 1–3 years at an intensity of 25 to 40 hours per week of mostly one-on-one intervention.

Dr Lovaas' seminal 1987 study reported on 49 children under age 4 with autism who were treated with either:

1. 40 hours per week of ABA therapy;
2. Less than 10 hours per week of ABA therapy; or
3. Treatment-as-usual in the community (Lovaas, 1987).

Therapy was delivered for 2–3 years. Results indicated that 47% of children receiving 40 hours per week of ABA achieved normal functioning by first grade, as defined by mainstream classroom placement and achievement of average cognitive skills. Conversely, only 2% of children who received less than 10 hours per week of ABA treatment or more general community treatment achieved this outcome. The publication of this study was pivotal in shifting many people's perspective from viewing autism as an untreatable mental disorder, to viewing it as a developmental disorder that could be successfully remediated. Since Dr Lovaa's initial success, eight replication studies have been conducted (Reichow & Wolery, 2009). A meta-analysis conducted by Reichow and Wolery concluded that ABA was effective for children with ASD, and that the greatest benefits are seen when the study followed the UCLA training model, when treatment duration was long, and when the total number of therapy hours was high (Reichow & Wolery, 2009). Similarly, in a meta-analysis conducted by Ospina and colleagues, ABA was found to be superior to special education on a broad range of outcome measures including adaptive behavior, socialization, and intellectual functioning (Ospina, et al., 2008).

Despite their success in research trials, discrete trial training procedures have been criticized for failing to focus on spontaneous and naturalistic use of language, a problem that some contemporary ABA procedures have attempted to address (see below). In addition, early forms of ABA (including the treatment package used in the original 1987 Lovaas trial) included aversive procedures such as thigh slaps, which are now considered to be unethical. Some advocates also feel that the procedures are coercive and do not respect the desires of the individual with ASD. Finally, ABA has also been criticized for being extremely expensive. The treatment often involves 25–40 hours per week of one-on-one intervention for 1–3 years. However, cost-benefit models suggest that the treatment may be cost-saving in the long run, as children who benefit from treatment may require fewer educational and social services across their lifetimes, and may eventually become wage-earners (Jacobson et al., 1998).

Naturalistic Behavior Therapies

The majority of research on ABA has been completed using procedures related to Discrete Trial Training, the model first evaluated by Lovaas in 1987. However, other comprehensive treatment models that use ABA principles have also been developed, many in response to the criticisms of traditional discrete trial training programs outlined above. These comprehensive programs include Applied Verbal Behavior Model, Pivotal Response Therapy, Nova Scotia Early Intensive Behavioral Intervention Model, and the Early Start Denver Model. Of these approaches, only the ESDM has demonstrated efficacy as a package intervention through a randomized controlled trial.

The Applied Verbal Behavior Model focuses on using ABA principles to teach spontaneous, functional communication. Based on the writings of famous behaviorist and philosopher B. F. Skinner, the model approaches language as a type of behavior that is controlled by antecedents and consequences (Sautter & LeBlanc, 2006). Using this approach, communication is broken down into functions such as mands (requests) and tacts (labels). While no controlled studies have been conducted evaluating the Applied Verbal Behavior Model as a comprehensive treatment program, there is an emerging body of literature supporting the effects of specific teaching strategies, such as mand training (Jennett et al., 2008).

Pivotal Response Therapy (PRT) aims to use behavioral principles to teach critical ('pivotal') skills for normal social development, such as child motivation and spontaneous initiation. The intervention uses child-directed teaching sessions (sometimes called naturalistic teaching) to teach these skills, and often involves extensive parent training. The model has also been applied to school-age children to improve motivation for academia (Koegel et al., 2010) and has been evaluated specifically as a parent-training program (Baker-Ericzén et al., 2007). While no large-scale controlled study has been conducted to demonstrate the efficacy of PRT as a comprehensive intervention program, studies have demonstrated its efficacy in improving individual skills such as play (Stahmer, 1995). The Nova Scotia Early Intensive Behavioral Intervention Model builds upon the PRT model by combining parent training and behavioral intervention. No controlled studies have evaluated the Nova Scotia model, but a naturalistic study published in 2010 demonstrated gains in language and decreases in behavior problems after one year of intervention (Smith, et al., 2010). The same study demonstrated improvement in symptoms of autism in children with IQ > 50.

The Early Start Denver Model (ESDM) was developed by Drs Sally Rogers and Geraldine Dawson to include naturalistic ABA procedures with a focus on social, emotional, and relationship development. The treatment targets very young children (often under the age of 3), and parents often take an active role in treatment and provide around one quarter of the intervention sessions. In a recent study of ESDM, 48 children under 3 years of age were randomly assigned to receive two years of ESDM treatment or community-as-usual treatment (Dawson, et al., 2010). The treatment was delivered for approximately 30 hours per week (half in a clinical setting with a therapist, and half with the parent). Those receiving ESDM treatment demonstrated greater improvements in ASD symptoms, cognitive functioning, and adaptive skills than those receiving community-based treatment.

SCHOOL-BASED TREATMENT APPROACHES

Many of the comprehensive treatment approaches described in the previous section can be implemented in the home, in a clinic setting, or in a school-based setting. However, some treatments for ASD have specifically been developed for use in an educational setting. These include TEACCH, SCERTS, and LEAP.

TEACCH (Treatment and Education of Autistic and related Communication-handicapped Children; also known as 'structured teaching') is a comprehensive treatment model that emerged in North Carolina in the early 1970s. TEACCH is often delivered within special education classroom settings. The program is structured to address common strengths and weaknesses in individuals with ASD. For example, TEACCH aims to capitalize on strengths that individuals with ASD often have in visual learning by physically arranging the classroom, the schedule, and the learning materials to support appropriate behavior. Many of the visual support procedures (picture schedules, written instructions, etc.) that are used in other teaching methods were first pioneered in TEACCH classrooms. There is a strong body of literature supporting the various component teaching strategies of TEACCH (Mesibov & Shea, 2010). While some studies have evaluated TEACCH methods in a parent-training or home-programming format, larger controlled trials of TEACCH as an educational treatment package are still required.

The SCERTS (Social Communication Emotion Regulation Transactional Support) model was designed to incorporate strategies from many leading treatment approaches including ABA, TEACCH, PRT, and others within an educational framework (Prizant, et al., 2006). The model is intended for use with individuals of all ages, including young children and adults. Although the model includes components that have been empirically supported, the model itself is relatively new and has not yet been evaluated as a package treatment. Two federally funded studies are currently underway to evaluate SCERTS in young children and in school-age children.

The LEAP (Learning Experiences: Alternative Programs for Preschoolers and Parents) program aims to use ABA principles to implement naturalistic teaching strategies in a preschool classroom. LEAP classrooms usually include children with ASD as well as typically developing children. In a recently published randomized controlled trial, children that received two years of closely monitored LEAP programming showed larger gains in all domains of cognition, language, and social skills than children that participated in classrooms that were only provided with the LEAP manual. The children receiving the closely monitored LEAP programming also showed decreases in problem behavior and symptoms of autism relative to children in the control classrooms (Strain & Bovey, 2011).

Summary of Comprehensive and Educational Treatment Models

The comprehensive and educational treatment models developed over the past 30 years have led to an important cultural shift regarding the need for intensive, wrap-around treatment programs addressing the unique needs of people with ASD. While the translation of these clinic- or university-based programs into community settings has not been tested rigorously, a focus on the 'implementation science' of autism treatments is clearly understood as a future direction for the field (Hume & Odem, 2011). In addition, the vast majority of comprehensive and educational models have yielded the strongest outcomes in altering symptoms such as IQ scores and associated symptoms. Rigorous evaluation of treatment effects on core social communication impairments is also needed. While the need to intervene early in development is clear, the limited availability of treatments or educational models for adolescents and adults with ASD is also a significant limitation in the existing research. In some cases, the functional impact of persistent impairments is striking, with long-term outcome studies suggesting the most able of the population of people with ASD continue to struggle with employment, social relationships, and mental health conditions into adulthood (Howlin et al., 2000).

INTERVENTIONS ADDRESSING SOCIALIZATION IMPAIRMENTS

Difficulty with social engagement has been reported since the earliest descriptions of ASD (Kanner, 1943) and is considered by many the unique and essential aspect that distinguishes ASD from other developmental disorders (APA, 2000; Rutter, 1978). The social impairment seen in ASD takes many forms and can vary greatly from one child to the next. Vulnerabilities related to social engagement are thought to have far-reaching implications from early childhood through adulthood.

Interventions focused on enhancing social behavior and competence in children with ASD often vary and shift targets with respect to the child's age, developmental level, and peer group (White et al., 2006). Interventions for very young children may focus on teaching parents how to engage their child and encourage back-and-forth play. Most of these interventions target impairments in early social behaviors such as imitation, shared attention, and creative play. At preschool and early childhood levels, interventions may focus on playing with peers, understanding emotions, and learning the basics of turn-taking and initiating and responding to social interactions. In the later elementary years and into adolescence, interventions may focus more on teaching perspective-taking, social problem-solving, and understanding peer-group as well as social norms. In adolescence and young adulthood, social skills interventions may increasingly focus on building skills related to occupational and functional outcomes. Despite their popularity, many social skills programs are not well researched and do not yet have an established evidence base (see Warren et al., 2011; White et al., 2006).

Behavioral Skills Training

Several approaches to addressing social impairments in young children with ASD focus on the use of behavioral strategies to improve early core skills such as joint attention, symbolic play, and imitation, either through interactions with interventionists or their parents. Such intervention approaches hypothesize that underlying skills are fundamental, or pivotal, social communication building blocks that are central to the etiology of the disorder itself (Dawson, 2008; Mundy et al., 2007; Poon et al., 2011). At a basic level, joint attention refers to a triadic exchange in which a child coordinates attention between a social partner and an aspect of the environment. Such exchanges enable young children to socially coordinate their attention with other people and their environment, to more effectively learn from others (Yoder & McDuffie, 2006). Symbolic play involves the representational use of objects, such as pretending one object is another or pretending a doll is performing an action (Kasari et al., 2008). Fundamental differences in early joint attention skills and symbolic play activities are theorized to potentially underlie the deleterious neurodevelopmental cascade of effects associated with the disorder itself, including language and social outcomes across the ASD spectrum (Kasari et al., 2008; 2010; Mundy and Neal, 2000; Poon et al., 2011). Interventions that aim to bolster these skills and facilitate effective learning with social partners in a more efficacious manner may translate into improvements in other key aspects of development over time. The accumulated sum of the joint attention and symbolic play intervention literature to date suggests that early intervention can systematically improve joint attention and play skills, and specific improvements in joint attention partially mediate improvements in other areas (Kasari et al., 2008; 2010; Poon et al., 2011). Across interventions, which vary widely in terms of scope and approach, integrated approaches that attempt to combine the advantages of developmental and discrete trial approaches via intensive graduated systems of prompts in game-like, interactional frameworks hold substantial promise for improving these core skills. This literature also suggests that these approaches are most effective when children show sustained engagement with a variety of objects, when they can be utilized within intrinsically motivating settings, and when careful adaptation to small gains and shifts can be incorporated and utilized over longer intervals of time (Kasari et al., 2008; 2010; Yoder & McDuffie, 2006).

Some intervention programs have focused on imitation, as it is theorized to be a nonverbal social-communication skill that emerges early in life and plays a crucial role in the development of other cognitive and social skills over time (Ingersoll 2008; 2010; McDuffie et al., 2007; Rogers et al., 2003). Early attempts to teach imitation often relied on very structured discrete trial training procedures and reinforcement strategies, and as such have often been criticized for the challenges these procedures hold for generalization of skills (Ingersoll 2008; 2010). Recently, interventionists have been utilizing novel methodologies for use of imitation (Ingersoll, 2010; McDuffie et al., 2007), including Reciprocal Imitation Training (RIT). RIT is a naturalistic imitation intervention that emphasizes the social role of imitation and has the ultimate goal of having children imitate a majority of actions of another rather than producing specific actions based on specified models (Ingersoll & Schreibman, 2006). As such, the intervention involves targeting multiple actions concurrently within child play. Interventionists contingently imitate nonverbal and verbal behavior, describe child actions in developmentally appropriate language, and model actions involving sensorimotor, functional, and symbolic play themes. Existing research suggests that focused imitation interventions such as RIT can significantly improve some targeted social-communication skills in the short-term (Ingersoll, 2008; 2010; McDuffie et al., 2007), with limited existing research examining long-term effects and generalization of skills across domains of social impairment.

Social Skills Groups

Social skills groups are probably the most commonly utilized method for teaching social skills for children with ASD, from the elementary- through the middle- and often high-school years. Social skills groups vary widely in terms of structure and scope. Some groups utilize time-delimited instructional models, manualized protocols, and formal curricula to teach certain core skills over a period of weeks to months (see DeRosier et al., 2011; Laugeson et al., 2011; White et al., 2006). Other groups may run continuously and involve less structured curricula, or potentially focus on providing social experiences and support versus specific instruction. Groups may be limited to children with ASD-related difficulties or can include blended programs with typically developing peer models and co-learners. Often social skills groups are embedded within educational settings or facilitated by outside agencies and professionals. Within specific skill instruction groups, adult facilitators are involved in instruction in a particular skill that is either preselected or identified via group process. Facilitators in turn engage the group in instruction via active group problem solving and discussion, role playing, practice, and rehearsal, as well as homework exercises related to skills learned. Social skills groups often target skills related to pragmatic communication and language use (e.g., socially appropriate use of language, conversation, narration), nonverbal communication (e.g., reading and utilizing gestures, facial expressions, physical proximity) as well as social cognition (e.g., theory of mind, perspective taking), the latter being a critical component for children with ASD. Instruction in these skills often involves making these abstract skills somewhat concrete and explicit. In some circumstances, parallel groups for caregivers are run in conjunction with social skills groups, which can provide linked instruction in how group skills can be reinforced in other environments.

Although recent and fairly well controlled studies of manualized curricula for social skills improvements have suggested short-term improvements in core areas of social functioning (Laugeson et al., 2011), several meta-analytic and systematic reviews have suggested that there is limited evidence for the effectiveness of group social skills intervention (Bellini et al., 2007; Matson et al. 2007; Rao et al., 2008; Warren et al., 2011; White et al., 2006). In addition to methodological challenges related to manualizing curricula and adequately assessing social outcomes for this population, these reviews have highlighted specific concerns regarding generalization and maintenance of skills from group process to other settings over time. Further research is clearly needed to examine the potential efficacy and functional impact of social skill group interventions for individuals with ASD.

Relationship Development Intervention

A somewhat different approach to improving and developing social skills is Relationship Development Intervention (RDI; Gutstein, 2001; 2009). RDI was developed by Dr Steven Gutstein and Dr Rachelle Sheely as a parent-directed intervention for fostering the social, emotional, and cognitive development of children with ASD through scaffolded learning opportunities. Within this model, parents are directed to work with training consultants to address hypothesized information-processing challenges related to ASD-associated impairments. Specifically, parents are instructed to provide challenging social learning experiences that are slightly above their children's current abilities across naturalistic settings. By graduated implementation of the program (i.e., guided participation) across daily activities, the parent provides opportunities for their child to become more flexible, adaptable, and competent (i.e., develop dynamic intelligence) across a range of activities including social interactions. The program postulates eight specific goals that are thought to be critical toward individual development: collaboration, deliberation, flexibility, fluency, friendship, initiative, responsibility, and self-management. Parents work with their specific RDI consultants to find and scaffold proximal targets across these areas (Gutstein, 2001; 2009). There is at present a fairly limited amount of supporting research regarding RDI (Gutstein 2009; Gutstein et al., 2007; Warren et al., 2011), although the authors of this work suggest that participating children are more likely to participate in typical classroom environments and show less ASD-specific impairment.

Peer-Mediated Interventions

Peer-mediated interventions utilize peers, most often classmates, to act as intervention facilitators with children with ASD. Specifically, such intervention involves training typically developing peers to be responsive social partners, capable of implementing instructional programs and techniques, as well as facilitating social interactions across a variety of settings (Garrison-Harrell et al., 1997; Laushey & Heflin, 2000). Within peer-mediated models, both identified peers and children with ASD are provided with explicit instruction in targeted skills within structured settings, as well as support and instruction as to how these techniques and skills can be employed across typical school social contexts (e.g., classroom, recess, lunch, etc.). Such instruction often involves training peer networks (e.g., several students within the school environment) that can supply intervention in daily activities across a variety of settings. The focus of intervention involves working toward increased reciprocal communication with peers, greater friendships, and decreases in negative encounters. Given the fact that such interactions may be embedded across settings and person, it is hypothesized that such interventions may have a greater chance of improving skills with better generalization across settings and maintenance over time. A growing number of studies have demonstrated positive outcomes for school-age children with ASD as well as peer interventionists, but there is at present a fairly limited evidence-base of adequately controlled research regarding efficacy (see Chan et al., 2009). More evidence regarding treatment fidelity (i.e., what aspects of peer-mediated intervention are being implemented), as well as more evidence supporting implementation of peer training in natural school environments for older students, is needed (Reichow & Volkmar, 2010).

Cognitive Behavioral Therapy

While cognitive behavioral therapy (CBT) has frequently been utilized as a treatment of comorbid symptoms in individuals with ASD (described in later section), CBT as a potential direct treatment for the social deficits associated with ASD is much less well understood (Sze & Wood, 2009; Wood et al., 2009). As contrasted with social skills training that often utilizes instruction and learned scripts, CBT utilizes a cognitive-science-informed model of psychological changes, that aims to promote active selection of memories of adaptive social responses over memories of previously learned maladaptive responses in real-world settings (see Brewin, 2006; Sze & Wood, 2009; Wood et al., 2009). Targeted CBT for ASD involves cognitive, behavioral, developmental, and emotive strategies (e.g., modeling, role playing, reinforcement, and self evaluation), which are believed to promote deep semantic processing of novel skills and, in turn, facilitate generalization across settings. Such emphasis is hypothesized to promote the retrieval of skills within applied settings over avoidant and other maladaptive strategies as contrasted with simpler skill-learning approaches.

While CBT has demonstrated clinically significant outcomes in other childhood disorders (see Seligman & Ollendick, 2011) and preliminary studies have suggested social impairments related to ASD may be positively influenced (Wood et al., 2009), potent impact on core symptoms has not yet been adequately demonstrated.

Theory-of-Mind Interventions

There is considerable evidence suggesting that many individuals with ASD display impairments related to 'theory of mind,' defined as the ability to attribute representational mental states to others and oneself in order to explain and predict behavior (see Baron-Cohen, 2000). The attribution of mental states is the process of how we interpret intentions of others based on current behavior, and is theorized to be a fairly natural way in which we understand the social world. As such, among the existing cognitive models of ASD, the hypothesis of a primary deficit in theory of mind has influenced specific intervention strategies (Happe & Fisher, 2005). In this framework, an impaired ability to understand other people's minds relates to core ASD symptoms, with inefficient 'mind-reading' affecting the development of social, communication, emotional, and imitation skills. Many interventions incorporate principles related to teaching theory-of-mind-related skills. Such interventions often provide explicit instruction on strategies for solving problems related to perspective taking and false-belief tasks. Studies have demonstrated that individuals with ASD can be taught to pass basic theory-of-mind tasks via a variety of methods from computer-administered feedback to one-on-one instruction, as well as group programs delivered in both low- and high-intensity settings (Fisher & Happe, 2005; Hadwin et al., 1996; McGregor, 1998; Ozonoff and Miller, 1995; Swettenham, 1996). However, there remain significant questions of whether such training generalizes, either to other non-learned tasks or to real-world environments (Wellman et al., 2001). Further, it is also debatable whether theory-of-mind deficits are primary deficits in ASD or simply consequences of other core deficits in terms of early social attention and orienting processes (Dawson, 2008).

Social Stories™

Social Stories™ is a popular clinical intervention that capitalizes on the relative strength in visual processing seen in many individuals with ASD. A Social Story™ provides a written description of social situations primarily using descriptive statements about the social context, and one or two directive statements regarding appropriate behavior expected from a child in a given situation (Gray, 1994). Although widely utilized, Social Stories™ have not yet been subject to rigorous investigation. The vast majority of studies on Social Stories™ were conducted using single-subject experimental designs, with limited evaluation of generalizibility (Reynhout and Carter, 2006). However, a more recent review by Karkhaneh et al. (2010) focused on six RCTs and other controlled group design research, including four dissertations. While some methodological flaws were described in the group of studies (e.g., limited use of blinded outcome evaluations, limited assessment of skill maintenance past one week of intervention), short-term outcomes were promising in improving emotion recognition skills, game-playing skills, and externalizing behavior problems. As a whole, the review also highlighted that several studies suggested the intervention was most effective in 'high-functioning' children with ASD, with stronger verbal abilities, lower autism severity, and higher IQ scores predicting response in three out of the six studies.

COMMUNICATION INTERVENTIONS

Problems with communication skills range greatly across the autism spectrum, with some children demonstrating subtle deficits in pragmatic use of language, and other children presenting as functionally non-verbal. Children with more subtle communication problems may have difficulty with conversational skills. They may produce monologue-type speech without pausing for the listener, or may fail to respond to conversational bids by others. They may have difficulty staying on topic during a conversation, and may perseverate in talking about a specific area of interest. They may have difficulty with non-literal aspects of language such as implication and irony. They may also have difficulty integrating non-verbal communication (eye contact, facial expressions, gestures) with verbal language. For these children, treatment is often provided by a 'speech language pathologist', who is trained to diagnose and treat speech and communication problems.

Children with ASD may also have more severe language impairments, including some children who fail to develop speech entirely, and others who are very delayed in speech acquisition. Communication intervention, again, is often provided by a speech language pathologist. In some cases, communication interventions for developing oral-motor functioning to promote speech are used. For example, in the PROMPT procedure (Prompts for Restructuring Oral Muscular Phonetic Targets), the speech therapist uses modeling and physical manipulation of the lips, tongue, and jaw to help the child learn to form speech sounds in the context of a motivating play session (Rogers et al., 2006). There is currently little research devoted to assessment of these types of intervention.

Communication interventions for very young children sometimes focus on training parents to use strategies to promote language. For example, Hanen's More Than Words program has been used to teach the parents of very young children (under the age of 3) to teach communication in the context of play, to respond to child to communication, to reward communication attempts, and to use play and books to elicit communication (Carter et al., 2011). Research on this intervention is limited, but suggests that it may be more effective for children who initially had more limited toy play at baseline (Carter et al., 2011).

For non-verbal or minimally verbal children, alternative forms of communication are often utilized to provide the child with a way to communicate their needs and to teach the more general concept of communication. Commonly used alternative communication strategies include sign language, augmentative communication devices, and picture-based communication systems. Simple signs are often taught to young children who have not yet developed speech, or who have very little spontaneous speech. Signs are often adapted from traditional American Sign Language (ASL) so that they are easier for children with motor-planning problems to perform. While signs can help to bridge the gap between a child's cognitive development and his or her spoken communication, it is rare for a child with ASD who cannot speak to become fully fluent in sign language.

Some children with ASD benefit from the use of an augmentative communication device, such as an electronic device with a digital voice output. For example, the child might touch a picture of a desired object (e.g., a cookie), and the computer might provide the verbal request (e.g., 'Cookie, please!'). Devices can be very simple (e.g., a single large button), or quite complex. Some devices allow the user to construct full sentences by scanning though multiple screens of pictures, and more recently applications for tablet computers such as the iPad have become popular communication training tools (Shane et al., 2011). Tablet computers and other portable electronic devices have the advantage of being more flexible, more portable, more socially acceptable and often less expensive than traditional devices. Although the majority of communication devices for ASD utilize pictures, there are also rare cases in which non-verbal individuals with ASD have been able to communicate with a traditional keyboard using text-to-speech programming. However, research is needed to better understand which interventions are effective for which individuals. In a recent meta-analysis of single-subject design

studies of augmentative communication devices, Ganz and colleagues found that interventions using such devices are effective in improving communication skills, and to a lesser extent in improving social skills and behaviors (Ganz et al., 2012b).

Picture-based communication typically involves teaching a child to point to, or hand over, a picture of a desired object or activity. The most well known picture-based communication program is the Picture Exchange Communication System (PECS). In a PECS program, children are taught to hand pictures to an adult to make requests. The initial stages of the program typically involve two teachers, one to prompt the child and one to serve as the communication partner. As the program progresses, the child is taught to seek a desired picture from a selection in a communication book, and to bring that picture to an adult. Some children eventually progress to constructing full sentences with picture symbols, which they place onto sentence strips that are also given to the adult. Two recent meta-analyses analyzed data from 13 group design studies (Bowsher et al., 2006; Ganz et al., 2012a) and 24 single-subject design studies (Allison et al., 2007 Ganz et al., 2012b) and determined that PECS improved communication skills, and had smaller but positive effects on other behaviors.

Some parents worry that teaching alternative forms of communication may delay or inhibit the development of spoken language. However, there is not good evidence to support this concern, and there is some evidence to suggest that teaching alternative forms of communication may actually promote language acquisition (Schlosser & Wendt, 2008). Teaching alternative communication strategies can also help to decrease frustration and resulting behavioral problems for minimally verbal children.

TREATMENTS FOR BEHAVIORAL AND PSYCHIATRIC PROBLEMS

Associated symptoms such as irritability, aggression, hyperactivity, and anxiety impact family life and can often create significant obstacles to the integration of individuals with ASD into social settings. Lecavalier (2006) conducted a survey with parents and teachers to evaluate problem behaviors in children with ASD. Approximately 50% of the sample of children with autism was rated as having clinically significant levels of behavioral and psychiatric disturbance. Problem behaviors were clustered into the following categories (in descending order of prevalence): ritualistic and hyperactive, hyperactive with conduct problems, anxious, and undifferentiated behavior disturbance. Similar rates of behavior problems were reported by

Skokauskas & Gallagher (2012) using the Child Behavior Checklist. Results suggested that children with ASD exhibited more internalizing (64% of ASD sample) than externalizing problems (31%). Additional analyses suggested that the most common comorbid DSM-IV (Diagnostic and Statistical Manual of the American Psychiatric Association) diagnoses in children with ASD were attention deficit/hyperactivity disorder (ADHD) and anxiety disorders (44.78% and 46.2% respectively).

The treatment approach for behavioral and psychiatric problems in individuals with ASD is dependent on several factors including the nature of the behavior (e.g., externalizing, internalizing), age/cognitive level of the child, and setting for the interventions. We will review the major approaches for treating externalizing behaviors such as impulsivity, noncompliance, and aggression as well as treatments for managing internalizing symptoms such as anxiety and rigidity/compulsiveness.

Functional Behavioral Assessment and Positive Behavioral Support

The dominant philosophy guiding behavioral interventions for problem behaviors emphasizes both compensatory and preventative approaches, generally classified as positive behavioral support (PBS) strategies. PBS represents the application of ABA principles to understanding the environmental causes of behavioral problems. The approach emphasizes the use of systematic observations and analysis known as *functional behavioral assessments* (FBAs). Interventions build upon FBAs to identify ways to prevent the need for an individual to engage in that behavior through manipulating the environment or to teach appropriate, 'replacement' behaviors.

The functional analytic approach to managing aberrant behaviors in ASD is based on the assumption that behaviors are determined by one or several motivational and contextual variables. The goal of FBAs is to develop hypotheses about the motivational and environmental causes of behaviors, and systematically test these hypotheses. A behavioral approach assumes that *behaviors* may be predicted by *setting events* (e.g., distal variables influencing behaviors such as sleep, diet) and *antecedents* (e.g., immediate predictors), and are maintained by *consequences* for the behaviors (e.g., escape from demands, obtaining desired objects). FBAs may utilize a variety of methods to test hypotheses ranging in sophistication from detailed manipulation of hypothesized causes of behavior (known as functional analyses), to observations in natural environment, and/or parent/teacher rating tools.

Results from FBAs form the basis of treatment plans, which typically incorporate various behavioral strategies. As mentioned, positive behavioral support strategies (PBS) are among the most well studied and widely used, and emphasize an approach focused on managing antecedents over consequences (i.e., prevention-based strategies). Commonly used strategies include stimulus control/environmental modifications, response interruption, extinction, and differential reinforcement of alternative, other, or incompatible behaviors (DRA/DRO/DRI) (Hume & Odem, 2011). While a review of each positive behavioral support strategy is beyond the scope of this chapter, these strategies have their basis in the experimental analysis of behavior and have been validated in both basic and human research (Sturmey, 2002).

Functional communication training (FCT) is a well-studied, widely used positive behavior support strategy that provides a good example of the integration of assessment with intervention used in PBS approaches. In general, FCT describes a set of differential reinforcement procedures in which appropriate communication (e.g., asking for help, using a picture card to request) is taught, to replace maladaptive communication strategies (e.g., screaming, hitting). FCT may be considered alone or in combination with other approaches such as extinction of undesirable behavior and/or punishment. Empirical support for FCT has been established by a series of single-case experimental design studies in children with intellectual disabilities (ID), including autism. A recent review of research on FCT identified 28 studies with over 80 participants, and utilized the American Psychological Association's (APA) criteria for empirically supported treatments. Results of the review suggest that FCT can be considered a well-established intervention for both individuals with ID and individuals with autism (Kurtz et al., 2011).

Behavioral Interventions for Restricted and Repetitive Behaviors

Restricted and repetitive behaviors (RRBs) are a core feature of autism, and have been found to be among the earliest and most persistent diagnostic markers in the condition (Bishop et al., 2010). RRBs may be conceptualized as consisting of subtypes including repetitive motor behaviors, insistence on sameness, and circumscribed interests (Lam et al., 2008). Behavioral treatments for RRBs have largely focused on improving repetitive motor behaviors (RMBs) and use FBA and behavioral strategies. Reviews of the literature suggest that strategies such as differential reinforcement of alternative behaviors, extinction, and response interruption were most effective in treating repetitive self-injury, stereotypy, and repetitive object play (Patterson et al., 2010). However, interventions for problems related to insistence on sameness or circumscribed interests are less well studied. There is some suggestion that improving engagement in a range of activities (e.g., through using picture activity schedules) and independence can improve rigidity and intense preoccupations but this remains an area requiring further investigation (Leekam et al., 2011).

Parent Management Training

Parent management training (PMT) is a well-validated program for children with disruptive behavior disorders such as attention deficit hyperactivity disorder, and meta-analytic studies suggest a large effect size for the intervention in this population (Chronis et al., 2006). PMT has been applied to managing disruptive behavior disorders in children with autism but has not been studied to the degree seen in other populations. Because PMT approaches are based in principles of operant conditioning, the interventions and strategies are similar in practice to the FBA and positive behavioral support strategies described above. PMT is differentiated by its focus on teaching parents to use established behavior management strategies in the home. In practice, intervention and comprehensive programs often incorporate behavior management strategies into the parent-training components of their treatments (see Smith et al., 2010).

Studies of PMT packages in autism are limited, but include three randomized controlled trials which suggest promise for the efficacy of PMT approaches in managing problem behaviors in individuals with ASD (Aman et al., 2009; Sofronoff et al., 2004; Whittingham et al., 2009). Sofronoff, Leslie, and Brown (2004) randomized parents of children with Asperger to PMT workshops, individual PMT, or wait-list control groups. Parents enrolled in both PMT groups reported their children as exhibiting fewer and less intense problem behaviors as measured by the Eyberg Child Behavior Inventory. No differences were seen between the treatment groups. The Research Units on Pediatric Psychopharmacology Autism Network (RUPP) conducted a multi-site study evaluating the impact of PMT alone, PMT with medication (i.e., combined therapy), or medication alone, on managing the behavioral problems in children with pervasive developmental disorders (PDDs), with the majority presenting with intellectual disabilities (Aman et al., 2009). Findings favored the combination treatment group, which demonstrated greater improvements after six months of treatment on a measure of problem behaviors at home, and on the Aberrant Behavior Checklist, a widely used measure of associated and core symptoms in autism clinical trials.

PMT treatments vary widely in the composition of their treatment packages. Traditional PMT treatments for disruptive behavior disorders often teach parents to implement reinforcement systems (e.g., token economies), provide high levels of reinforcement (e.g., catching the child being good), and to use effective consequence strategies such as time-outs. Sofronoff and colleagues integrated social skills methods such as comic strip conversations and Social Stories™ with the traditional behavior management techniques described above. In contrast, the RUPP trial utilized an individual therapy format and incorporated skill-building strategies such as visual schedules, functional communication training, and adaptive skills training. Nevertheless, the results of these well-controlled studies suggest promise for use of various forms of PMT across a wide range of individuals with ASD.

ANXIETY-MANAGEMENT INTERVENTIONS

Parsing out the core behavioral manifestations of ASD, particularly repetitive habits and rigidity, from true comorbid anxiety disorders presents several diagnostic challenges. However, the presence of debilitating anxiety symptoms in the presentation of autism is undeniable. Rates of anxiety disorders range widely, with some studies estimating upwards of 84% of individuals with ASD meet criteria for at least one DSM-IV anxiety disorder (Muris et al., 1998). Leyfer et al. (2006) found high rates of comorbid psychiatric disorders in a large (n = 109), broad sample of children with ASD aged 5–17. The most common lifetime diagnosis was specific phobia (44%), followed by obsessive-compulsive disorder (OCD) (37%), ADHD (31%), and major depression (10%).

Treatments for anxiety symptoms in autism to date represent adaptations of CBT treatments for anxiety used with typically developing individuals with anxiety disorders. Adaptations typically involve incorporation of social skills training (e.g., emotion recognition, Social Stories™) and use of visual supports into traditional CBT strategies such as exposure and response prevention, cognitive restructuring, and *in vivo* skill practice. Wood et al. (2009) evaluated a 16-week, individually delivered, version of the Building Confidence CBT program modified for children with ASD (n = 17) in a RCT with a wait-list control group (n = 23). Results of the study suggested positive improvements on blinded evaluator ratings on a commonly used clinician rating of global improvement (i.e., Clinical Global Impression-Improvement scale), as well as improvements in social functioning and autism severity as measured by the Social Responsiveness Scale. Treatment gains were maintained at a three-month follow-up. Similar findings were found by Sofronoff et al. (2005) in a comparative trial evaluating two group CBT interventions (child-only and child + parent training groups) for anxious children with autism compared to wait-list control groups. Results suggested significant improvement in the treatment groups compared to wait-list controls on anxiety symptoms.

The existing literature on interventions for behavioral and psychiatric symptoms associated with ASD suggests adaptations of empirically supported interventions developed for other disorders have been largely effective in reducing problem behaviors. Positive behavioral support strategies and parent management training may be more easily adapted, given their strong foundation in universal principles of operant conditions, and individualized treatment plans. Adapting treatments for anxiety disorders to ASD populations may be more challenging, given the overlap between behavioral manifestations of autism (e.g., rigidity, repetitive behaviors) and anxiety disorders such as OCD and generalized anxiety disorder (GAD). However, the existing research suggests promise for adapting traditional CBT approaches to high-functioning populations of people with ASD and warrants further investigation.

AUXILIARY AND COMPLEMENTARY/ALTERNATIVE TREATMENT APPROACHES

Many families of children with ASD pursue therapies outside of typical behavioral, educational, and pharmacological intervention paradigms. Recent clinic surveys have indicated that up to 30–70% of families pursue such 'complementary' and 'alternative' therapies (Hanson et al., 2007; Levy et al., 2003). Many such treatments involve dietary (e.g., gluten- and casein-free diets) and medical (e.g., hyperbaric oxygen treatment, chelation, vitamin and supplement use) approaches, which are outside the scope of this chapter. A variety of other therapeutic approaches, including sensory integration, auditory integration/training, animal therapies, and music therapy, have been developed for treating core areas of impairment or specific sensory and motor sensitivities, responses, and dysfunction that are often frequent challenges for children with ASD (Rogers & Ozonoff, 2005).

Sensory Integration

Although sensory challenges have not historically been part of the nosology of ASD (APA, 2000), sensory and motor issues have been demonstrated to seriously affect the functioning of individuals on the spectrum and their families (Bagby et al., 2012), and have been proposed for inclusion as a core feature of ASD in a future diagnostic system (DSM-5). Sensory challenges seen in ASD may include over- or under-sensitivity to sensory experiences such as touch, sound, light, pain, or movement. Sensory integration is specialized therapy, often delivered within the context of occupational therapy, with the specific intent of intervention of assisting the individual in receiving, processing, correctly interpreting, and integrating sensory information as a foundation for improving functional participation in life's tasks (Ayres, 1972; 1979; Bundy et al., 2002). Typically this therapy involves one-on-one, child-directed treatment with a trained occupational therapist, wherein the child is presented with tactile, vestibular, and proprioceptive opportunities to support the development of self-regulation, sensory awareness, and/or movement in space. Activities related to challenging postural, whole-body, ocular-motor, oral, and bilateral control are often included. Such treatment often involves numerous motor activities and physical stimulation such as swinging, massage, joint compression, weighted vests, and brushing. The intervention may also include a 'sensory diet' designed to provide the child with a range of materials addressing sensory needs. Data supporting the efficacy of sensory integration is not very strong (May-Benson & Koomar, 2010; Vargas & Camilli, 1999; Warren et al., 2011). However, many theorize that utilizing sensory activities that attract the interest of children and help them deal with difficult sensory aspects of their environment may be helpful if included within the context of broader intervention programs.

Music Therapy

Music therapy is at times employed with children with ASD, hinging on speculation that heightened engagement during musical exposure and production may translate into enhanced social communication exchanges within the therapeutic setting and beyond. This treatment method is often improvisational and unstructured, and practitioners purport that it can improve core skills often involved in shared musical process (i.e., social reciprocity, turn-taking, joint attention, eye contact). Music therapy uses musical activities such as singing, playing instruments, and music listening, either individually or in groups, to promote interaction between the therapist and the patient. Music therapy methods may involve either active music making or approaches where the patient listens to music during specified activities (Edgerton, 1994). There are only a few controlled studies of improvisational music therapy for children with ASD (Gold et al., 2006). Individual studies of music therapy have reported improvements in communication, social motivation, and social engagement via the mechanisms of imitation, repetition, cueing, and nonverbal exchanges involving rhythm and music (Edgerton, 1994; Kim et al., 2008). A recent Cochrane review of music therapy indicated that while a small number of studies have documented improvements in nonverbal and verbal communication skills, it is not clear that such improvements generalize to functional use (Gold et al., 2006).

Auditory Integration

Auditory integration training (AIT) relates specifically to auditory perception. The intervention technique attempts to improve the way individuals with ASD recognize and respond to sound and to reduce other behaviors associated with ASD. The primary hypothesis behind this treatment suggests that abnormal sensitivities to certain frequencies of sound are associated with specific communication and learning challenges. As such, training sessions with electronically altered sounds and music will improve auditory processing, lessen auditory hypersensitivities, and increase concentration (see American Speech-Language-Hearing Association, 2003). The specific physiological underpinnings of such changes remain unclear. While some early studies have reported positive outcomes associated with auditory integration training, more recent rigorously controlled trials of AIT (Corbett et al., 2008; Mudford et al., 2000) and systematic reviews (Sinha et al., 2004; Warren et al., 2011) have not indicated clear utility of AIT treatment. Currently, several professional organizations (including the American Speech-Language-Hearing Association (1993), the American Academy of Audiology (1993), the Educational Audiology Association, and the American Academy of Pediatrics (1998)) indicate that AIT should be considered an experimental rather than an evidenced-based treatment due to the lack of scientific data supporting its benefits.

Animal-Assisted Intervention

Given that science has suggested the value of pets and animals in promoting human well-being in general (Morrison, 2007), intervention approaches for individuals with ASD have also suggested a therapeutic role for animals. Animal-assisted therapy, defined as using animals within a goal-oriented setting to implement treatment, has been suggested as a possible strategy for addressing core vulnerabilities associated with ASD (Fine, 2006). Therapeutic horseback riding, a subtype of animal-assisted activities, has been used to treat populations with physical and mental disabilities and has recently been applied to individuals with ASD. Therapeutic horseback riding is defined as using horseback riding treatment to improve posture, balance, and mobility while developing a therapeutic bond between the patient and horse (All et al., 1999; Fine, 2006). Very limited systematic research regarding therapeutic horseback riding has been conducted to date, but there have been findings which suggest the potential for stimulation across multiple domains of functioning (Bass et al., 2009; Bizub et al., 2003; Macauley & Guiterrez, 2004).

Other programs have attempted to use dogs or pets as therapeutic agents and catalysts for social interaction across settings. Although beneficial effects have been suggested (Burrows et al., 2008; Viau, et al., 2010), not all children are noted to have positive reactions when interacting with animals and pets. More research is needed to better define animal-assisted intervention programs and their therapeutic benefit.

FUTURE DIRECTIONS FOR BEHAVIORAL AND PSYCHOSOCIAL INTERVENTIONS IN ASD

While there has been tremendous growth in treatments utilized to address core impairments and associated vulnerabilities of autism, there remain several critical gaps in the literature concerning optimal treatment. One gap relates to the science of early detection research, which has been critical in improving our understanding of risk factors associated with autism. Fortunately, the field has quickly heeded the call for the development of interventions targeting infants and toddlers exhibiting risk factors. Several collaborative networks including the Toddler Treatment Network funded by Autism Speaks are anticipated to provide valuable clinical and empirical data to guide treatment for this vulnerable population.

In contrast, research addressing the needs of adolescents and adults with ASD is insufficient. Behavioral interventions have improved the trajectories of individuals with ASD, but the persistence of deficits in older individuals with ASD is striking (see Howlin et al., 2004). We have a poor understanding of the behavioral manifestations of core and associated domains in adolescence and adulthood, which is a necessary first step in identifying treatment targets and developing effective interventions. It is also unclear whether adaptations of childhood interventions are sufficient for the lingering impairments in adolescents/adults with ASD, or whether more novel, targeted approaches are

CHAPTER

1.6

Current Trends in the Pharmacological Treatment of Autism Spectrum Disorders

Alexander Kolevzon

Seaver Autism Center for Research and Treatment, Department of Psychiatry, Mount Sinai School of Medicine, New York, NY, USA

OUTLINE

INTRODUCTION

There has been a significant amount of research into pharmacological treatments in autism spectrum disorders (ASD) over the past several decades. Until recently, however, the development of treatments has relied mainly on strategies only loosely related to what is known about the neurobiology of the disorders, using etiologically heterogeneous samples, and delivering intervention broadly with mixed success (King et al., 2009; McCracken et al., 2002; Research Units on Pediatric Psychopharmacology (RUPP), 2005). Based on what is known about associated psychiatric features, such as

aggression, attention deficit and hyperactivity, and anxiety, the field would attempt to 'borrow' from the existing evidence-base in other psychiatric disorders to explore potential treatment effects in ASD. Known as a 'targeted symptom domain approach,' this strategy was fruitful and led to US Food and Drug Administration (FDA) indications for associated symptoms, including 'irritability associated with autism' in the cases of risperidone and aripiprazole. Concurrently, neurobiological evidence is being aggressively pursued to support this symptom domain approach and a significant amount of literature has accumulated to describe various biochemical irregularities in ASD. The following chapter will review the current state of the evidence based on this 'top-down' approach and sections will be divided into symptom domains to facilitate clinical use.

Because these treatments are by definition symptom-driven as opposed to disease-modifying, and because few, if any, target the core symptoms of ASD (e.g., social and language impairment), polypharmacy is often required. A cross-sectional Medicaid study in 2001 in 60,641 children with ASD found that 56% used at least one psychotropic medication and 20% were prescribed three medications concurrently. Use was also common in very young children, aged 0 to 2 (18%) and 3 to 5 years (32%). Antipsychotic drugs were the most commonly prescribed (31%), followed by antidepressants (25%), and then stimulants (22%) (Mandell et al., 2008), and this study was performed *prior* to the FDA approvals of risperidone (2005) and aripiprazole (2009) in ASD.

The aim of this chapter is to describe a rational approach to symptomatic treatment in ASD and to outline the current state of evidence, in order to arm clinicians with a foundation for making informed treatment decisions. It is important to note that recent genetic discoveries and the development of animal model systems have elucidated the neurobiology of several genetic subtypes of ASD, including Rett syndrome and fragile X syndrome. These discoveries have in turn led to important opportunities for developing novel, disease-modifying therapeutics. In the following chapter, on novel therapeutics, Dr Evdokia Anagnostou will review this approach and several of the potential treatments in development.

AGGRESSION

Aggression and self-injury are associated symptoms of ASD that can result in significant harm to affected individuals and marked distress for families; they are among the symptoms most likely to trigger a psychopharmacological consultation or emergent psychiatric referral. Although the relationship between aggression or self-injurious behavior (SIB) and ASD remains unclear, these symptoms are treated with a broad range of pharmacological approaches. Various mechanisms have been proposed to underlie the presence of these symptoms in autism, and numerous targets for pharmacological intervention have been suggested. These targets include the dopaminergic, serotonergic, adrenergic, and opioid systems, among others. Reviewing controlled trials to specifically target aggression using a primary outcome measure, several medications have produced significant improvement as compared to placebo, including tianeptine, methylphenidate, risperidone, aripiprazole, clonidine, and naltrexone. However,

only risperidone, aripiprazole, and methylphenidate demonstrate results that have been replicated across at least two well-controlled studies. A summary of trials of medication for aggression is shown in Table 1.6.1.

Neuroleptics

Risperidone

Several studies support an association between the dopaminergic system and aggression (Ferrari et al., 2003; Hoglund et al., 2005; Retz et al., 2003) and most animal models of self-injury suggest dysregulation of dopamine activity (Rothenberger, 1993). Dopamine dysregulation has also been implicated in self-injurious patients with autism (Shea et al., 2004). Antipsychotic medications act as dopaminergic antagonists and can prevent the onset and maintenance of aggression and SIB (King, 2000). Many randomized controlled trials support the efficacy of risperidone, a combined dopamine and serotonin antagonist, in children with autism (McDougle et al., 2005; Nagaraj et al., 2006; Pandina et al., 2007; RUPP, 2002; 2005; Troost et al., 2005). In 2002, the Research Units on Pediatric Psychopharmacology (RUPP) Autism Network first published results from a large, multi-center trial (RUPP, 2002). This first phase of the study began as a double-blind, placebo-controlled, parallel-group trial in 101 children and adolescents with autism over eight weeks. Subjects ranged in age from 5 to 17 years and risperidone was administered for eight weeks at a final mean dose of 1.8 mg/day. The Aberrant Behavior Checklist – Irritability (ABC-I) subscale was the primary outcome measure of aggression and self-injury. Risperidone demonstrated significantly greater reductions in mean ABC-I subscore as compared to placebo (56.9% vs. 14.1%). Risperidone was also significantly more likely to produce a positive response (69%) compared to placebo (12%) on a scale of Clinical Global Impression (CGI). As part of the initial eight-week phase of the RUPP trial, parents were asked to identify one or two chief complaints of their child's behavior and reported that self-injury (effect size = 2.11) and aggression (effect size = 1.66) showed the greatest improvement with risperidone (Arnold et al., 2003).

In terms of side effects, predictably, patients on risperidone were significantly more likely to gain weight, with a mean increase of 2.7 kg as compared to 0.8 kg with placebo. Subjects receiving risperidone were also significantly more likely to experience mild (49%) or moderate (24%) increases in appetite, fatigue (59%), drowsiness (49%), drooling (27%), and dizziness (16%). Extrapyramidal symptoms, such as muscle rigidity and dyskinesias, occurred with greater frequency in patients receiving risperidone, but differences in occurrence rates as compared to placebo were not significant.

TABLE 1.6.1 Selected Controlled Trials of Medications for Aggression in Children and Adolescents with ASD

Medication	Authors	Design	Sample	Measures	Outcome
Risperidone	RUPP, 2002	Placebo parallel	101 children and adolescents	ABC-I	Positive
Risperidone	RUPP, 2005	Placebo discontinuation	38 children and adolescents	ABC-I CGI-I	Positive
Risperidone	Troost et al., 2005	Placebo discontinuation	24 children and adolescents	ABC-I CGI-SOSC	Positive
Risperidone	Shea et al., 2004	Placebo parallel	80 children	ABC-I, N-CBRF	Positive
Aripiprazole	Owen et al., 2009	Placebo parallel	98 children and adolescents	AB-I	Positive
Aripiprazole	Marcus et al., 2009	Placebo parallel	218 children and adolescents	ABC-I	Positive
Haloperidol	Remington et al., 2001	Placebo crossover	36 children and adults	ABC-I	Negative
Clomipramine				ABC-I	Negative
Methylphenidate	Quintana et al., 1995	Placebo crossover	10 children	ABC-I	Positive
Methylphenidate	Handen et al., 2000	Placebo crossover	13 children	ABC-I IOWA	Positive
Tianeptine	Niederhofer et al., 2003	Placebo crossover	12 male children and adolescents	ABC-I	Positive
Clonidine	Jaselskis et al., 1992	Placebo crossover	8 male children and adolescents	ABC-I	Positive
Naltrexone	Campbell et al., 1993	Placebo parallel	41 children	ARS	Negative
Naltrexone	Willemsen-Swinkels et al., 1996	Placebo crossover	20 children	ABC-I	Positive per teacher, negative per parent
Valproate	Hellings et al., 2005	Placebo parallel	30 children and adolescents	ABC-I OAS	Negative
Valproate	Hollander et al., 2010	Placebo parallel	27 children and adolescents	ABC-I CGI-I	Positive
Lamotrigine	Belsito et al., 2001	Placebo parallel	35 children	ABC-I	Negative
Levetiracetam	Wasserman et al., 2006	Placebo parallel	20 children and adolescents	ABC-I	Negative

ABC-I = Aberrant Behavior Checklist – Irritabilty subscale; IOWA = IOWA Conners Teacher Rating Scale; CGI-I = Clinical Global Impression – Improvement Scale; CGI-SOSC = Clinical Global Impressions – Scale of Symptom Change; N-CBRF = Nisonger – Child Behavior Rating Form; ARS = Aggression Rating Scale; OAS = Overt Aggression Scale.

Tremor was significantly more common in the risperidone group (RUPP, 2002). Results from serum analysis of lipid profile and glucose levels were not reported, but more recent studies have suggested an increased risk of elevated triglycerides with risperidone in children and adolescents (Correll et al., 2009).

Several follow-up replication studies have since been performed (McDougle et al., 2005; Pandina et al., 2007; Shea et al., 2004) and convincingly supported the initial RUPP results. Effective doses in children that have been studied range from a mean of 1.17 mg/day to 1.81 mg/day. Clinically, the principle of starting with the lowest possible dose (0.125–0.25 mg/day), depending on weight, and titrating slowly is always encouraged. There is a significant body of anecdotal evidence that supports efficacy at doses as low as 0.5 mg/day and side effects may be age- and dose-dependent. Weight gain, for example, has been associated with younger age and higher doses (Hoekstra et al., 2010).

Aripiprazole

There have been two randomized controlled trials of aripiprazole in children with ASD, and both were sponsored by the manufacturer (Marcus et al., 2009; Owen et al., 2009). Both studies were eight-week, placebo-controlled trials and both found significant improvement for aripiprazole over placebo using the ABC-I subscale and the CGI. The first study (Owen et al., 2009) began with doses of aripiprazole at 2 mg/day and titrated up to 15 mg/day based on clinical response; the mean daily dose at the end of treatment was 8.6 mg/day. The second study (Marcus et al., 2009) also started at a dose of 2 mg/day and then titrated to compare three fixed doses: 5, 10, and 15 mg/day. All three doses of aripiprazole were associated with significant improvement on the ABC-I subscale as compared to placebo.

Side effects with aripiprazole are significant and include sedation, tremor, increased appetite, drooling, and weight gain (Marcus et al., 2009; Owen et al., 2009). In one study, mean weight reportedly increased by approximately 2 kg among patients receiving aripiprazole (Owen et al., 2009). In the study by Marcus and colleagues (2009), treatment-emergent extrapyramidal side effects were reported in 22 to 23% of patients, depending on the dose, as compared to 11.8% of the placebo group. In the study by Owen and colleagues, 14.9% of subjects on aripiprazole experienced an EPS event as compared to 8% of patients on placebo. Subjects receiving aripiprazole may also be more likely to have elevated fasting lipid profiles and serum glucose values (Marcus et al., 2009). There were no differences in serum prolactin levels and no patients had clinically significant electrocardiogram (ECG) abnormalities or vital sign changes in either study with aripiprazole.

Other neuroleptics have also been studied in ASD, although not as much evidence exists to support their use as with risperidone and aripiprazole. Several studies with haloperidol (Anderson et al., 1984; Cohen et al., 1980), have demonstrated its benefit in targeting a range of maladaptive behaviors in ASD. However, the most recent controlled trial of haloperidol failed to show significant improvement as compared to clomipramine and placebo, possibly due to patient discontinuation from the study for reasons of tolerability or worsening behavioral symptoms (Remington et al., 2001). The use of haloperidol appears limited by its side effect profile, including acute dystonia and dyskinesias (Campbell et al., 1997). In addition, a recent controlled trial comparing the efficacy of haloperidol to risperidone in 30 children and adolescents with ASD found that patients receiving risperidone had significantly greater improvement in total ABC score as compared to haloperidol (Miral et al., 2007). Small open-label and retrospective studies of clozapine (Chen et al., 2001; Gobbi and Pulvirenti, 2001; Zuddas et al., 1996), quetiapine (Corson et al., 2004; Findling et al., 2004; Hardan et al., 2005; Martin et al., 1999), ziprasidone (Cohen et al., 2004; Malone et al., 2007; McDougle et al., 2002),

olanzapine (Kemner et al., 2002; Malone et al., 2001; Potenza et al., 1999), and one controlled trial with olanzapine (Hollander et al., 2006) also provide additional, albeit preliminary, evidence to support the use of these medications to treat behavioral symptoms of ASD.

Psychostimulants

Methylphenidate

Psychostimulant medications are potent dopaminergic agonists and have also been examined in the treatment of aggressive children with autism. Stimulant medications may work to reduce aggression by improving inhibitory control. They increase the availability of dopamine in the striatum and enhance prefrontal cortical function though striatal-frontal pathways (Berridge et al., 2006). Methylphenidate has been studied extensively in ASD. Historically, there was considerable reservation about the use of psychostimulants in ASD for fear they would exacerbate motor stereotypies. While benefit is modest in most patients and cannot be fairly compared to the robust effects seen in typically developing children with attention deficit/hyperactivity disorder (ADHD), the field has significant experience with methylphenidate and its safety profile is well known. Methlyphenidate has the added benefit of rapid response where response can be found. Two small, short-term, randomized controlled trials have examined the effect of methylphenidate specifically on aggression. Quintana and colleagues (1995) conducted the first in 10 subjects with autism over four weeks using a double-blind, placebo-controlled, crossover design in subjects from 7 to 11 years old and the ABC – Irritability subscale was the primary outcome measure of aggression. Methylphenidate produced significant improvements in ABC – Irritability subscore as compared to placebo and there were no significant differences in the rates of side effects between groups.

Handen and colleagues (2000) studied 13 children with ASD over seven days, also using a double-blind, placebo-controlled, crossover design. Primary outcome measures of aggression were the ABC – Irritability subscale and the aggression subscale of the IOWA Conners Teacher Rating Scale. Significant improvement was seen on both measures compared to placebo. Of 12 subjects, 5 experienced side effects while receiving methylphenidate, including social withdrawal, dullness, sadness, irritability, and skin picking.

Serotonergic Medications

Central nervous system regulation of serotonin has also been implicated in aggressive behavior and several studies have established an association between serotonin depletion and aggression in both human (Halperin et al., 2006) and animal models (Johansson et al., 1999; Vergnes et al., 1988). Worsening of ASD symptoms has also been demonstrated following acute depletion of dietary tryptophan (McDougle et al., 1996a). Serotonergic medications may affect the hypothesized serotonergic dysregulation in ASD and ameliorate associated symptoms such as aggression and self-injury.

At least two randomized controlled trials have used standardized outcome measures of aggression in examining the use of serotonergic medications as a treatment for children and adolescents with ASD. The first was by Remington and colleagues (2001) and compared clomipramine, haloperidol, and placebo in 36 subjects over seven weeks using a double-blind, placebo-controlled, crossover design with one-week washout periods in between each treatment. The ABC – Irritability subscale was the primary outcome measure of aggression and no significant differences were found between clomipramine and placebo (or between haloperidol and placebo). Tolerability was also a major confound as 20 subjects discontinued clomipramine (13 subjects discontinued haloperidol), and 12 cited side effects as the reason. The remaining 8 subjects discontinued due to lack of efficacy and worsening behavioral problems.

Tianeptine is a medication that increases serotonin reuptake (Sweetman, 2004) but is not currently available in the US. It was studied by Niederhofer et al. (2003) in 12 children with autism over 12 weeks using a double-blind, placebo-controlled, crossover design. The ABC was completed by parents and teachers and the Irritability subscale improved significantly with tianeptine as compared to placebo. However, clinician ratings did not show any difference between active medication and placebo. Drowsiness and decreased activity were significantly increased in patients receiving tianeptine.

Alpha Agonists

The adrenergic system has also been proposed to play an etiological role in aggression. Individuals with autism may experience hyperarousal in response to the environment (Toichi and Kamio, 2003), and aggression or self-injury may serve to reduce environmental stimulation (King, 2000). Adrenergic antagonists block sympathetic discharge, reduce the hyperaroused state, and have been suggested as candidate pharmacotherapy to lower levels of catecholamines (Brede et al., 2003; Ihalainen and Tanila, 2004). Clonidine has therefore been suggested as a treatment option for aggression and other associated symptoms of autism. One controlled trial with clonidine has used a standardized outcome measure of aggression in eight male children with autism over six weeks (Jaselskis et al., 1992). Teacher

ratings of the ABC – Irritability subscale improved significantly with clonidine but clinician ratings did not show improvement. Clonidine was also significantly more likely to cause drowsiness and decreased activity. Hypotension required dose reduction in three children during the study.

Naltrexone

Several studies have demonstrated elevated plasma levels of beta-endorphin in some children and adolescents with autism (Bouvard et al., 1995; Cazzullo et al., 1999; Ernst et al., 1993; Leboyer et al., 1999; Sandman, 1988) and some have proposed a relationship between the endogenous opioid system and self-injury in autism (Sandman, 1988; Sandman et al., 2000). This theoretical evidence has led to several trials with naltrexone in ASD because naltrexone is an opiate antagonist which may decrease plasma beta-endorphin levels (Bouvard et al., 1995; Cazzullo et al., 1999).

There have been at least three controlled trials with naltrexone that measured its effect on aggression but results are mixed. Campbell et al. (1993) studied 41 children with autism using a double-blind, placebo-controlled, parallel-group design over four weeks but did not find significant improvement in the severity of self-injury or aggression. In a placebo-controlled, single-dose study, Willemsen-Swinkels et al. (1995) reported significant reductions in the ABC – Irritability subscore as compared to placebo. A follow-up treatment study over eight weeks also found some improvement, but only on teacher ratings of the ABC-I, and not on parent ratings. No serious adverse effects were reported (Willemsen-Swinkels et al., 1996).

Anticonvulsant Medications

The high incidence of epilepsy in autism has led to studies of anticonvulsants in ASD, and evidence of glutamatergic dysregulation in ASD further supports these endeavors. The role of anticonvulsants is hypothesized to occur by various mechanisms, including the treatment of subclinical epilepsy and affecting intracellular processes involved in kindling-like models (Soderpalm, 2002). Valproate, lamotrigine, and levetiracetam have all been studied to reduce aggressive behavior in ASD.

Valproate

Valproate is an anticonvulsant, and one proposed mechanism of action is its effect on γ-aminobutyric acid (GABA) function (Czapinski et al., 2005). There is also evidence of anti-aggressive properties of valproate in animal and human models (Gobbi et al., 2006; Hollander et al., 2003; 2005b; Molina et al., 1986; Sival et al., 2004). Two controlled studies have examined the efficacy of valproate in ASD to reduce aggression. Hellings et al. (2005) studied 30 subjects, 6 to 20 years old, using a double-blind, placebo-controlled, parallel-group design over eight weeks. No significant improvement was found in comparison to placebo on either the ABC-I subscale or the Overt Aggression Scale (OAS). Only increased appetite was significantly more likely to be reported among patients taking valproate as compared to placebo. It should be noted, however, that the study duration may not have been sufficient to detect treatment effects, given that adequate doses were only maintained for approximately four weeks. In addition, the mean valproate blood level was 77.7 μg/dl at the end of the study, which may not have been high enough to achieve benefit.

A second study, conducted by Hollander and colleagues (2010), used a 12-week, double-blind, placebo-controlled parallel group design in 27 children and adolescents with ASD. The primary outcome measure was the ABC – Irritability subscale, plus the CGI-Improvement which also focused on irritability. Subjects receiving valproate improved significantly on the ABC – Irritability subscale as compared to placebo and 62.5% were considered responders on the CGI. Sleep-deprived electroencephalograms (EEGs) were obtained in 19 of the 27 children enrolled in this study and preliminary, exploratory results suggested that subjects with abnormal and epileptiform EEGs may be more likely to respond to valproate than subjects with normal EEG recordings. Subjects with therapeutic valproate levels between 87 and 110 μg/dl were also more likely to respond than subjects with levels below 87 or above 110 μg/dl. Side effects with valproate included insomnia, weight gain, headache, rash, polyuria, and agitation.

Lamotrigine

Lamotrigine is also an anticonvulsant and Belsito and colleagues (2001) performed the only controlled trial to use a standardized assessment of aggression and self-injury in ASD. Thirty-five children were given lamotrigine using a double-blind, placebo-controlled, parallel-group design over 18 weeks (mean final dose of 5 mg/kg/day). No significant differences were found on ABC - Irritability subscores between lamotrigine and placebo, although subjects were only maintained on therapeutic doses for 4 weeks after the required titration period. Rates of side effects also did not differ significantly between groups.

Levetiracetam

Levetiracetam is a novel anticonvulsant medication that is indicated as adjunctive therapy in the treatment of partial onset seizures and primary generalized tonic-clonic seizures in adults and children. One controlled trial has utilized a standardized outcome measure of aggression to examine the efficacy of levetiracetam in children with autism. Wasserman and colleagues (2006) studied 20 children with ASD using a double-blind, placebo-controlled, parallel-group design over 10 weeks. Participants ranged in age from 5 to 17 years and levetiracetam was titrated to a mean dose of 862.50 mg/day. No significant differences were found between parent ratings of the ABC-I subscale in subjects receiving levetiracetam and those on placebo. Teacher ratings suggested that patients who received levetiracetam increased in irritability, whereas the placebo group became less irritable. Side effects included agitation, aggression, hyperactivity, impulsivity, loss of appetite, self-injurious behavior, weight gain, and weight loss.

Summary – Aggression

Among the many studies to examine the efficacy of medication in controlling aggression in ASD using randomized controlled designs, only three medications have evidence from more than one trial to support their use. These medications are risperidone, aripiprazole, and methylphenidate. Risperidone has the most evidence to support its use for aggression in ASD, and results are consistent across several studies. Risperidone received an indication by the FDA for aggression towards others and deliberate self-injurious behavior in autism (FDA, 2006). Although sedation is a significant side effect, symptom improvement appears to be independent of somnolence according to at least one *post hoc* analysis (Shea et al., 2004). The risks of risperidone include significant weight gain and it may increase vulnerability to diabetes and cardiovascular disease later in life (Correll et al., 2009). Nutritional counseling and a physical activity regimen should therefore be included for all treated patients. Hyperprolactinemia is another safety concern with the use of risperidone (Anderson et al., 2007; Hellings et al., 2005), but prolactin release may diminish over long-term use and hyperprolactinemia may not be associated with any interference in growth or sexual maturation (Anderson et al., 2007; Malone et al., 2002; Patel et al., 2005). The utility of monitoring prolactin levels in patients treated with risperidone in the absence of clinical symptoms remains an area of debate. More studies are needed to clarify the impact of risperidone treatment in children and adolescents with autism over time. Results from long-term post-marketing trials may soon become available and contribute to this knowledge-base. They may also clarify the differential effect of dosing on the risk of metabolic and endocrine changes.

Aripiprazole should also be considered an evidence-based treatment for aggression and irritability associated with ASD. Two controlled trials support its use and one suggests that doses of 5, 10, and 15 mg/day are all associated with improvement compared to placebo. As with risperidone, risks of weight gain and metabolic disturbance persist, although levels of serum prolactin do not appear to increase with use of aripiprazole. In 2009, The FDA approved aripiprazole for the treatment of irritability associated with ASD in children aged 6 to 17 years.

Two controlled trials have found methylphenidate effective for symptoms of aggression and self-injury in ASD. Several studies have demonstrated that methylphenidate effectively targets symptoms of hyperactivity, attention deficit, and impulsivity in autism (Birmaher et al., 1988; Hoshino et al., 1977; RUPP, 2005; Strayhorn et al., 1988). It is important to note that results on symptoms of aggression are less consistent, however, and that the largest study of methylphenidate in ASD to date did not find significant differences on the ABC-I, a secondary outcome in that study, as compared to placebo (RUPP, 2005). Paradoxical effects of psychostimulants are also documented, and may confer a risk of increased irritability in some patients with developmental disability and ASD (Handen et al., 1991; RUPP, 2005).

ATTENTION DEFICIT AND HYPERACTIVITY

Symptoms of attention deficit, hyperactivity, and impulsivity are common in ASD, with estimates ranging from 50% (Lecavalier, 2006) to 75% (Sturm et al., 2004). The following section will focus on results from randomized controlled studies that utilized at least one outcome measure that included an assessment of inattention and/or hyperactivity. Retrospective and open-label studies are also reviewed when relevant to controlled trials. Results of trials of medication for attention deficit and hyperactivity are shown in Table 1.6.2.

Methylphenidate

Several randomized placebo-controlled trials have explored the use of methylphenidate in ASD (Handen et al., 2000; Quintana et al., 1995; RUPP, 2005), all with positive results. The largest controlled trial was done by the RUPP Autism Network using a crossover design in 72 children and adolescents with ASD. Methylphenidate was superior to placebo on measures of inattention and hyperactivity and 49% of subjects were classified as responders. Side effects were significantly more likely to occur in patients on methylphenidate, including decreased appetite, difficulty falling asleep, irritability, and emotional outbursts. A total of 18% of

subjects withdrew from the study due to adverse events and the most common reason for discontinuation was irritability.

A follow-up of the RUPP methylphenidate study by Posey and colleagues (2007) found that hyperactivity and impulsivity were more likely to improve than inattention. Higher doses (0.25–0.5 mg/kg) were also more consistently effective than low doses (0.125 mg/kg). Smaller studies by Quintana and colleagues (1995) and by Handen and colleagues (2000) likewise support the use of methylphenidate for hyperactivity in ASD. In one study, no significant differences in side effects were noted between groups (Quintana et al., 1995), but in the other, 38% of children experienced significant side effects as compared to placebo, including social withdrawal, dullness, sadness, and irritability (Handen et al., 2000).

Atomoxetine

Atomoxetine is a selective norepinephrine reuptake inhibitor which increases dopaminergic release in the frontal cortex because norepinephrine receptors are also sensitive to dopamine. Retrospective (Jou et al., 2005) and open-label studies (Posey et al., 2006) of atomoxetine for ADHD symptoms in children and adolescents with ASD report significant improvement on measures of hyperactivity and inattention. One small placebo-controlled, crossover study to measure ADHD symptoms in 16 children and adolescents with ASD (Arnold et al., 2006), found that atomoxetine improved symptoms of hyperactivity and impulsivity, but only approached significance on measures of inattention. Side effects with atomoxetine were significantly more common, and included gastrointestinal distress, fatigue, and racing heart. Decreased appetite and irritability were also reported, but rates did not differ significantly from placebo.

Clonidine

Clonidine is an alpha agonist that improves inattention, hyperactivity, and impulsivity in typically developing children with ADHD (Connor et al., 1999; Hazell and Stuart, 2003; Steingard et al., 1993) and more recently an extended release formulation (kapvay) was FDA- approved for ADHD. In patients with ASD, clonidine has been examined in at least two controlled, albeit small, studies with a total of 15 males. The first study (Fankhauser et al., 1992) did not show improvement in hyperactivity, but parents and clinicians reported improvement on global ratings of change. The second study (Jaselskis et al., 1992) found improvement on parent and teacher ratings of hyperactivity, irritability, and oppositional behavior, but not on clinician ratings. Predictably, side effects included sedation and hypotension and the authors suggested that

TABLE 1.6.2   Selected Controlled Trials of Medications for Attention Deficit and Hyperactivity in ASD

Medication	Authors	Design	Sample	Measures	Outcome
Methylphenidate	Quintana et al., 1995	Placebo crossover	10 children	ABC-H	↓ hyperactivity
Methylphenidate	Handen et al., 2000	Placebo crossover	13 children	Conners	↓ hyperactivity
Methylphenidate	RUPP, 2005	Placebo crossover	72 children and adolescents	ABC-H	↓ hyperactivity
Atomoxetine	Arnold et al., 2006	Placebo crossover	16 children and adolescents	ABC-H	↓ hyperactivity
Haloperidol	Campbell et al., 1978	Placebo parallel	40 children	CPRS	Negative
Haloperidol	Anderson et al., 1984	Placebo parallel	40 children	CPRS CASQ	↓ hyperactivity CASQ: negative
Haloperidol	Anderson et al., 1989	Placebo crossover	45 children	CPRS CASQ	↓ hyperactivity CASQ: ↓
Risperidone	RUPP, 2002	Placebo parallel	101 children and adolescents	ABC-H	↓ hyperactivity
Risperidone	Shea et al., 2004	Placebo	80 children	ABC-H, N-CBRF	↓ hyperactivity N-CBRF: ↓ hyperactivity (parent)
Clonidine	Fankhauser et al., 1992	Placebo crossover	7 children, adolescents, and adults	CASQ	CASQ: negative
Clonidine	Jaselskis et al., 1992	Placebo crossover	8 children and adolescents	ABC-H, ACTeRs	↓ hyperactivity (parent/teacher) ACTeRs: negative (teacher) CPRS: negative (clinician)
Amantadine	King et al., 2001	Placebo run-in	43 children and adolescents	ABC-H	↓ hyperactivity (clinician) negative (parent)
Naltrexone	Campbell et al., 1993	Placebo parallel	41 children	Conners	↓ hyperactivity (parent/teacher)
Naltrexone	Kolmen et al., 1995	Placebo crossover	13 children	Conners	↓ hyperactivity (parent) negative (teacher)
Naltrexone	Bouvard et al., 1995	Placebo crossover	10 children	Conners	Negative (teacher/parent)
Naltrexone	Willemsen-Swinkels et al., 1996	Placebo crossover	20 children	ABC-H	↓ hyperactivity (teacher) Negative (parent)
Naltrexone	Kolmen et al., 1997	Placebo crossover	11 children	Conners	Negative (parent/teacher)

ABC-H = Aberrant Behavior Checklist – Hyperactivity subscale; Conners = Conners Parent and Teacher Rating Scale; CPRS = childhood psychiatric rating scale; CASQ = Conners Abbreviated Symptoms Questionnaire; N-CBRF = Nisonger Child Behavior Rating Form; ACTeRs = Attention deficit with hyperactivity Comprehensive Teachers Rating Scale.

hyperactivity may have improved due to initial sedation; the benefit of clonidine was not sustained in some cases after six to eight weeks (Jaselskis et al., 1992).

Guanfacine

Guanfacine is another alpha agonist, but has only been studied in open-label or retrospective studies thus far in ASD. Controlled trials are under way, however, including with the newer extended release formulation (intuniv), which has been FDA-approved in ADHD. Results from published literature suggest modest benefit; one retrospective review of 80 children and adolescents with ASD and ADHD (Posey et al., 2004) found that 27% of patients showed improvement in hyperactivity and 21% showed improvement in inattention. Only 24% of patients were considered responders based on global improvement scores but there was a small, statistically significant improvement on global severity ratings. Scahill and colleagues (2006) conducted a prospective open-label trial of guanfacine in 25 children with ASD and hyperactivity and 48% of children responded; parent and teacher ratings of inattention and hyperactivity showed significant improvement for both symptoms. Although not a controlled study, reported side effects included sedation, irritability, increased aggression and self-injury, decreased appetite, sleep disturbance, constipation, headache, and nocturnal enuresis. Electrocardiogram and vital sign changes were not considered clinically significant in either of the studies with guanfacine.

Neuroleptics

Many clinical trials with neuroleptics in developmentally disabled populations have studied the effect on hyperactivity and impulsivity. In a review by Aman and Langworthy (2000), 11 clinical trials were identified that evaluated antipsychotic medications for hyperactivity in children with ASD. Four of these were controlled trials with haloperidol (Anderson et al., 1989; Campbell et al., 1978; 1984; Locascio et al., 1991), which appears to improve hyperactivity in ASD. Results were not always consistent, however, and depend on the outcome measure utilized. Results from open-label studies with risperidone (Fisman and Steele, 1996; Horrigan and Barnhill, 1997; McDougle et al., 1997; Nicolson et al., 1998; Perry et al., 1997) and olanzapine (Potenza et al., 1999) were also mostly positive and risperidone appears to significantly reduce hyperactivity in ASD. The RUPP Autism Network placebo-controlled trial of risperidone used the ABC – Irritability subscale as the primary outcome measure, but the Hyperactivity subscale was also used (2002). Risperidone significantly improved hyperactivity as compared to placebo (effect size = 1).

Amantadine

Amantadine is a noncompetitive *N*-methyl-D-aspartate (NMDA) antagonist indicated for the treatment of Parkinson's disease. King and colleagues (2001) did a placebo-controlled study of amantadine in 43 children and adolescents with ASD to assess its impact on behavioral symptoms and found significant improvement on clinician-rated measures of

hyperactivity. Parent-rated measures did not improve, however. A total of 53% of patients were considered responders on measures of global improvement although this was not significant as compared to the 25% of subjects receiving placebo who were also considered responders. The most common side effects in patients taking amantadine included insomnia and somnolence, although differences in side effects between groups were not significant.

Naltrexone

Naltrexone has been studied extensively in ASD, including for symptoms of hyperactivity and inattention. Some open-label studies (Campbell et al., 1988; Herman et al., 1989) suggest global benefit, but among the placebo-controlled trials, results are inconsistent. Campbell and colleagues (1993) found that hyperactivity was significantly improved according to parent and teacher ratings on the Conners Rating Scale. Willemsen-Swinkels and colleagues (1996) reported no significant improvement according to parent ratings, but teacher ratings of hyperactivity did improve. This is in contrast to Kolmen and colleagues (1995) who found significant improvement on parent ratings, but not on teacher ratings. Actometers were used to measure activity in both the Willemsen-Swinkels (1996) and the Kolmen (1995) studies, although no difference was found between the naltrexone and placebo groups. A small follow-up study by Kolmen and colleagues (1997) did not find a significant difference between naltrexone and placebo on either parent or teacher Conners ratings. Bouvard and colleagues (1995) also studied naltrexone in 10 children with ASD and found no significant improvement as compared to placebo. None of the controlled trials with naltrexone reported significant differences in side effect profiles as compared to placebo.

Summary – Attention Deficit and Hyperactivity

Methylphenidate and atomoxetine are effective in treating symptoms of ADHD in ASD. However, response rates to methylphenidate may differ in ASD compared to what is reported in typically developing children with Attention Deficit/Hyperactivity Disorder (ADHD) alone. The National Institute of Mental Health Collaborative Multisite Multimodal Treatment Study of Children with ADHD (MTA) reported response rates of 70 to 80% as compared to the 49% reported in the RUPP Autism Network trial of methylphenidate (2005). In the only controlled study of atomoxetine, results were significantly better than placebo, but the sample size was small and only 7 of 16 children (43%) were considered responders. Overall, both methylphenidate and atomoxetine appear to effectively treat ADHD-related symptoms in ASD. However, response rates may be lower in ASD than in ADHD alone, and symptoms of inattention may be less likely to respond than symptoms of hyperactivity and impulsivity. Treatment success may be limited by tolerability. A total of 18% of subjects with ASD discontinued the RUPP methylphenidate trial, while only 1.4% discontinued in the MTA study. Methylphenidate may also improve irritability in ADHD without ASD, whereas worsening irritability is a significant concern in some patients with ASD.

Many studies have demonstrated efficacy for antipsychotic medications and since the RUPP trial with risperidone (McCracken et al., 2002), this medicine in particular has consistently shown benefit for hyperactivity in ASD (Gagliano et al., 2004; Malone et al., 2002; Shea et al., 2004; Troost et al., 2005). However, significant concerns about tolerability remain and suggest that benefits of this medication must be carefully weighed against the risks. In the absence of significant aggression or behavioral problems that prevent children from being maintained in the least restrictive environment, a convincing argument could be made for reserving the use of risperidone or aripiprazole until other more benign options have failed in treating symptoms of hyperactivity and impulsivity in ASD.

Evidence from controlled studies of alpha2 receptors agonists for ADHD-related symptoms in ASD is inconsistent and response rates are relatively low. Open-label studies of guanfacine appear promising but additional controlled studies are needed. Alpha2 receptors agonists may nevertheless be a reasonable alternative or augmentation strategy and have the advantage of being relatively benign. Amantadine and other NMDA antagonists are of significant interest for the treatment of ASD symptoms, but their use has to be measured against a relative dearth of evidence and only one controlled trial to date. Trials are underway with memantine, a glutamate antagonist, but beyond promising results from open-label and retrospective reports (Chez et al., 2007; Erickson et al., 2007), results from controlled trials are still pending. Despite multiple controlled trials, results with naltrexone are inconsistent and isolated positive findings should be interpreted with caution.

Many other medications have been studied in ASD, but few specifically measured symptoms of ADHD, and no additional randomized controlled trials have found evidence to support their use for this symptom domain.

ANXIETY AND REPETITIVE BEHAVIORS

A core symptom domain of ASD is restrictive, repetitive, and stereotyped behavior. While repetitive behaviors also appear in normal development and in developmental disabilities other than ASD, several studies suggest that they occur with greater severity and frequency in ASD (Bodfish et al., 2000; Richler et al., 2007). In addition, repetitive behaviors may be among the most enduring feature of ASD in children (Lord et al., 2006). Perhaps as a result, repetitive behaviors are a frequent target for intervention, as improvement in this domain can improve overall outcomes for affected children. Although behavioral interventions are the first line treatment for repetitive behaviors in ASD, pharmacological intervention is also frequently explored. Among the various options reviewed in this section, serotonergic medications have been widely used (Fatemi et al., 1998; Hollander et al., 2000; 2005; King et al., 2009; Namerow et al., 2003), in part due to their efficacy in anxiety and obsessive-compulsive disorder, which overlap extensively with the repetitive behavior domain in ASD. Risperidone and other atypical antipsychotics with strong affinity for many serotonin receptors, particularly the 5-HT2A receptor, are also frequently used to treat this domain.

In addition, a growing body of evidence has linked ASD to abnormalities in serotonin function. Biochemical, pharmacological challenge, and genetic studies have demonstrated the importance of the serotonergic system for central nervous system function and suggest a role for serotonergic dysregulation in the etiology of autism. Schain and Freedman (1961) were the first to report elevated platelet serotonin levels in patients with ASD compared to healthy controls, and approximately one-third of patients with autism have hyperserotonemia (Anderson et al., 1987; Hranilovic et al., 2007; Ritvo et al., 1970). Further support for the role of the serotonin system in repetitive behaviors is derived from pharmacological challenge studies, in which tryptophan depletion to reduce 5-hydroxytryptamine (5HT) neurotransmission in adults with autism results in significant worsening of repetitive behaviors (McDougle et al., 1996a). Likewise, the sensitivity of the 5HT1d receptor as measured by growth hormone response during sumatriptan challenge was positively correlated with the severity of repetitive behaviors in another study (Novotny et al., 2000). Multiple genes involved in serotonin neurotransmission have also been shown to be associated with ASD, though few findings have been consistently replicated. A summary of trials of medication for repetitive behaviors is shown in Table 1.6.3.

Fluoxetine

Fluoxetine has been the most rigorously studied of the selective serotonin reuptake inhibitors (SSRIs) in autism and is frequently prescribed for the treatment of repetitive behaviors. Numerous case reports, open-label studies, and retrospective chart reviews of fluoxetine have been published, with promising results (DeLong et al., 1998; Fatemi et al., 1998; Ghaziuddin et al., 1991;

TABLE 1.6.3 Selected Controlled Trials of Serotonergic Medications for Repetitive Behaviors in Autism

Medication	Authors	Design	Sample	Measures	Results
Fluvoxamine	McDougle et al., 1996	Placebo parallel	30 adults	CGI-I	Positive
Fluvoxamine	Change to McDougle and colleagues (referenced in McDougle et al., 2000)	Placebo parallel	34 children and adolescents	CGI-I	Negative
Fluvoxamine	Fukuda et al., 2001	Placebo crossover	18 children	CGI-I	Positive
Fluoxetine	Buchsbaum et al., 2001	Placebo crossover	6 adults	CGI-I	Positive
Fluoxetine	Hollander et al., 2005	Placebo crossover	39 children and adolescents	CY-BOCS GACIM	Positive
Fluoxetine	Clinical Trials Network, unpublished	Placebo parallel	158 children and adolescents	CY-BOCS	Negative
Citalopram	King et al., 2009	Placebo parallel	149 children and adolescents	CGI-I	Negative
Clomipramine	Remington et al., 2001	Placebo crossover with haloperidol	37 children, adolescents, and adults	CARS ABC	Negative

Key: CGI-I = Clinical Global Impression – Improvement Scale; CY-BOCS = Children's Yale-Brown Obsessive Compulsive Scale; CARS = Childhood Autism Rating Scale; GACIM = Global Autism Composite Improvement Measure; ABC = Aberrant Behavior Checklist.

Koshes, 1997; Mehlinger et al., 1990; Todd, 1991). As a result of these open trials, several placebocontrolled studies were undertaken, including a crossover trial in six adults with ASD (Buchsbaum et al., 2001). Patients in the Buchsbaum trial (2001) showed significant improvement on scores of the Yale-Brown Obsessive Compulsive Scale (Y-BOCS) (Goodman et al., 1989) Obsessions subscale and the Hamilton Anxiety Scale (Hamilton, 1959). Hollander and colleagues (2005) examined the effect of fluoxetine on repetitive behaviors in 39 children with ASD, using a crossover design with 8 weeks of treatment with both placebo and fluoxetine, separated by a 4-week washout period. Fluoxetine reduced repetitive behaviors on the Children's Yale-Brown Obsessive Compulsive Scale (CY-BOCS; Scahill et al., 2006). There were no significant differences in side effects between fluoxetine and placebo. Based in part on the success of this study, Autism Speaks organized an industry-sponsored trial through its Clinical Trials Network (CTN), Study of Fluoxetine in Autism (SOFIA), for the treatment of repetitive behaviors. A total of 19 sites throughout the US enrolled 158 children and adolescents for a 14-week treatment of placebo or orally disintegrating fluoxetine. In February of 2009, Autism Speaks announced results that repetitive behaviors were reduced in both groups compared to baseline, but no significant difference existed between groups. Although possibly a function of a high placebo response rate, fluoxetine was not more efficacious than placebo for reducing repetitive behaviors.

Citalopram

Shortly before the SOFIA results were released, King and colleagues (2009) published results from a 12-week,

multi-centered, placebo-controlled trial of liquid citalopram for the treatment of repetitive behaviors in ASD sponsored by the US National Institutes of Health through the Studies to Advance Autism Research and Treatment (STAART) network. A total of 149 children and adolescents were randomized to receive citalopram or placebo; the CGI was the primary outcome measure and the CY-BOCS for Pervasive Developmental Disorders (CY-BOCS-PDD; Scahill et al., 2006) was utilized as a secondary outcome measure, although all participants had at least moderate compulsive behaviors at baseline. No significant difference in response rates on the CGI or in the CY-BOCS-PDD score were found between the citalopram and placebo group; approximately one-third of participants were rated as responders in both groups. Side effects were significantly more likely to occur among patients taking citalopram, including increased energy, impulsivity, decreased concentration, hyperactivity, stereotypy, diarrhea, insomnia, dry skin, and pruritus. These results were convincing, albeit disappointing given two previous retrospective chart reviews of citalopram (Couturier and Nicolson, 2002; Namerow et al., 2003) which suggested effectiveness for treating anxiety in ASD.

Fluvoxamine

McDougle and colleagues (1996b) published results from a 12-week placebo-controlled study of fluvoxamine which suggested efficacy for repetitive behavior, among other symptom domains, in adults with autism. Thirty adult subjects were randomized to receive either fluvoxamine or placebo and 53% of patients treated with fluvoxamine were rated as responders as compared to 0%

in the placebo group. Side effects were mild and included sedation and nausea. McDougle and colleagues (referenced in McDougle et al., 2000) did a follow-up study in 34 children and adolescents with ASD using a similar design, but in this study, only 1 of 18 fluvoxamine-treated subjects was judged a responder (compared to 0 of 16 placebo-treated subjects). There were also significantly more side effects in the children on fluvoxamine compared to the adults, including insomnia, hyperactivity, agitation, and aggression. In contrast, Fukuda et al. (2001) performed a placebo-crossover study of fluvoxamine in 19 children with ASD over four weeks, and reported improvement in 56% of subjects using the CGI among other measures. No severe side effects were observed during the Fukuda trial. Overall, results from published reports of fluvoxamine in ASD are inconsistent. From the scant data available, however, the utility of fluvoxamine is limited and it appears that this medication is more efficacious and better tolerated in adults.

There are no published placebo-controlled studies of escitalopram, sertraline, or paroxetine in ASD, but several open-label studies and case reports have been conducted which suggest improvement in a number of domains, including anxiety and repetitive behavior (Branford et al., 1998; McDougle et al., 1998; Snead et al., 1994; Steingard et al., 1997). One retrospective review documents the efficacy of venlafaxine, a serotonin-norepinephrine reuptake inhibitor, in reducing repetitive behaviors in ASD (Hollander et al., 2000). Clomipramine, a tricyclic antidepressant with serotonin reuptake inhibiting properties, has also been used with some success based on data from two small studies, one in children (McDougle et al., 1992), and one in adults (Brodkin et al., 1997). Brodkin and colleagues (1997) performed a prospective open-label study with clomipramine in 35 adults with ASD over 12 weeks, and 55% of the 33 patients who completed the trial were categorized as treatment responders on the CGI, including for repetitive behavior. A total of 13 patients had clinically significant adverse effects, such as constipation, weight gain, anorgasmia, sedation, agitation, and seizures in 3 patients (including 2 patients with seizure disorders on anticonvulsants). There were no adverse cardiovascular effects. In a double-blind placebo-controlled crossover study comparing clomipramine and haloperidol for autism-related symptoms overall and stereotypies specifically (Remington et al., 2001), only 37% of 32 subjects completed the clomipramine treatment arm, whereas 69.7% completed the haloperidol arm (65% completed the placebo arm). As such, results are difficult to interpret, but it does appear that using clomipramine in ASD is compromised by issues of tolerability. In general, results from studies with clomipramine are inconsistent and children appear more susceptible to adverse effects.

Among other serotonergic medications, mirtazapine acts as a presynaptic alpha2-adrenoreceptor antagonist and a 5-HT2 and 5-HT3 antagonist. Several investigators have published case reports documenting improvement with mirtazapine for anxiety and compulsive behaviors in ASD (Albertini et al., 2006; Coskun and Mukaddes, 2008; Coskun et al., 2009; Nguyen and Murphy, 2001), but no controlled trials have been published to date. Buspirone is a novel anxiolytic agent that acts as a 5HT-1A receptor partial agonist, dopamine-2 receptor antagonist, and is metabolized to an alpha2-adrenergic receptor antagonist. Realmuto et al. (1989) performed a small open-label trial of buspirone in 4 children with ASD and did not find any improvement on obsessive thinking. Buitelaar and colleagues (1998), on the other hand, also conducted an open-label study of buspirone in children with ASD and, after six to eight weeks of treatment, 76% of 21 children were designated responders on the CGI.

Risperidone and Aripiprazole

The efficacy of antipsychotics for treating repetitive behaviors in ASD has also been examined in secondary outcome analyses in several studies. Two of the controlled trials with risperidone reported results from the ABC Stereotypy subscale and both demonstrated significant improvement with risperidone as compared to placebo (McDougle et al., 2005; RUPP, 2002; McDougle et al., 2005; Shea et al., 2004), although one study did not correct for multiple testing (Shea et al., 2004). The RUPP study (McDougle et al., 2005) also included results from the CY-BOCS in secondary analyses and again found significant improvement with risperidone (McDougle et al., 2005). Likewise, aripiprazole has been demonstrated as efficacious in reducing repetitive behaviors in ASD according to results from secondary outcome analyses with the ABC Stereotypy subscale and CY-BOCS (Marcus et al., 2009; Owen et al., 2009). However, only the highest dose of aripiprazole, 15 mg, in the study by Marcus and colleagues (2009) showed significant improvement as compared to placebo, and not the lower doses of 5 mg or 10 mg.

Summary – Anxiety and Repetitive Behaviors

To date, there remains a paucity of controlled studies for the treatment of anxiety and repetitive behaviors in ASD and most studies focus on serotonergic medications. Fluvoxamine may be effective for repetitive and maladaptive behaviors in adults with autism (McDougle, 1996b), but not in children (Martin et al., 2003; McDougle, 2000). There is a significant amount of evidence from case studies and retrospective and prospective open-label studies to suggest that other SSRIs in general are effective for the treatment of repetitive and other maladaptive behaviors associated with ASD. Despite corroborating evidence from a few small controlled trials (Buchsbaum et al., 2001; Fukuda et al., 2001; Hollander et al., 2005; McDougle et al., 1996), results from neither of two recent, large randomized placebo-controlled trials of citalopram or fluoxetine demonstrated statistical separation from placebo (Autism Speaks, 2009; King et al., 2009).

Existing studies do seem to suggest that children with ASD may be more sensitive to SSRI-associated adverse effects than adults, and the appropriate dosing of SSRIs in children with ASD is still in question (Posey et al., 2006). In general, patients with ASD tend to respond to very low doses of SRIs and there is some evidence that the likelihood of adverse effects increases with higher doses. A mean dose of only 16.5 mg/day of liquid citalopram (King et al., 2009) caused considerable side effects including behavioral activation, increased energy level, impulsiveness, decreased concentration, hyperactivity, and stereotypies.

While atypical antipsychotics appear to be effective for reducing repetitive behaviors in ASD, their use is compromised by side effects such as sedation, weight gain, and EPS. However, in some cases, repetitive behaviors may reach levels of severity that warrant consideration of antipsychotics when safer options have been unsuccessful.

CONCLUSIONS

The field of psychopharmacological treatment in ASD has grown in recent years and significant evidence now exists to support the use of a number of different medications across many symptom domains. There has been little progress in targeting core symptoms of social and language impairment, however, and much work is still needed. Accumulating evidence suggests that delineating subpopulations of individuals with autism according to genetic etiology may be necessary in order to better understand efficacy and tolerability in ASD. Incorporating biochemical or genetic markers to further characterize ASD phenotypes will also be useful in predicting treatment response and/or side effects. Objective measurement instruments that are sensitive to change with treatment also need to be validated in order to reliably assess core symptom domains in ASD in the context of clinical trials. In addition, age, developmental status, gender, and intellectual ability may be important moderators of treatment response and tolerance, and should be examined thoroughly in future trials. In general, treatment of children and adolescents with ASD should be initiated with low starting dosages and

gradual titration schedules. These children are often exquisitely sensitive to side effects as well as paradoxical effects. Improved understanding of the nature and likelihood of medication side effects in ASD may help identify risk factors to predict in advance which individuals are most vulnerable. As with other medications, benefits (both short-term as well as long-term) must be weighed against risks, and future research with larger samples and placebo-controlled designs will aid in that calculation.

ACKNOWLEDGMENT

Dr Kolevzon would like to acknowledge Drs Mihir Parikh and Maria McCarthy for their previous contributions in researching and writing about pharmacological treatments in aggression and about serotonergic medications in ASD respectively.

References

Albertini, G., Polito, E., Sara, M., Di Gennaro, G., Onorati, P., 2006. Compulsive masturbation in infantile autism treated by mirtazapine. Pediatric Neurology 34, 417–418.

Aman, M.G., Langworthy, K.S., 2000. Pharmacotherapy for hyperactivity in children with autism and other pervasive developmental disorders. Journal of Autism and Developmental Disorders 30, 451–459.

Anderson, G.M., Freedman, D.X., Cohen, D.J., Doe, A., Doe, B., 1987. Whole blood serotonin in autistic and normal subjects. Journal of Child Psychology and Psychiatry 28, 885–900.

Anderson, G.M., Scahill, L., McCracken, J.T., McDougle, C.J., Aman, M.G., Tierney, E., et al., 2007. Effects of short- and long-term risperidone treatment on prolactin levels in children with autism. Biological Psychiatry 61, 545–550.

Anderson, L.T., Campbell, M., Adams, P., Small, A.M., Perry, R., Shell, J., 1989. The effects of haloperidol on discrimination learning and behavioral symptoms in autistic children. Journal of Autism and Developmental Disorders 19, 227–239.

Anderson, L.T., Campbell, M., Grega, D.M., Perry, R., Small, A.M., Green, W.H., 1984. Haloperidol in the treatment of infantile autism: Effects on learning and behavioral symptoms. American Journal of Psychiatry 141, 1195–1202.

Arnold, L.E., Aman, M.G., Cook, A.M., Witwer, A.N., Hall, K.L., Thompson, S., et al., 2006. Atomoxetine for hyperactivity in autism spectrum disorders: Placebo-controlled crossover pilot trial. Journal of the American Academy of Child & Adolescent Psychiatry 45, 1196–1205.

Arnold, L.E., Vitiello, B., McDougle, C.J., Scahill, L., Shah, B., Gonzalez, N.M., et al., 2003. Patient-defined target symptoms respond to risperidone in RUPP Autism Study: Customer approach to clinical trials. Journal of the American Academy of Child & Adolescent Psychiatry 42, 1443–1450.

Autism Speaks, 2009. Autism Speaks Announces Results Reported for the Study of Fluoxetine in Autism Available at. <http://www.autismspeaks.org/about-us/press-releases/autism-speaks-announces-results-reported-study-fluoxetine-autism-sofia> (accessed 08.05.12.).

Belsito, K.M., Law, P.A., Kirk, K.S., Landa, R.J., Zimmerman, A.W., 2001. Lamotrigine therapy for autistic disorder: A randomized, double-blind, placebo-controlled trial. Journal of Autism and Developmental Disorders 31, 175–181.

Berridge, C.W., Devilbiss, D.M., Andrzejewski, M.E., Arnsten, A.F., Kelley, A.E., Schmeichel, B., et al., 2006. Methylphenidate preferentially increases catecholamine neurotransmission within the prefrontal cortex at low doses that enhance cognitive function. Biological Psychiatry 60, 1111–1120.

Birmaher, B., Quintana, H., Greenhill, L., 1988. Methylphenidate treatment of hyperactive autistic children. Journal of the American Academy of Child & Adolescent Psychiatry 27, 248–251.

Bodfish, J.W., Symons, F.J., Parker, D.E., Lewis, M.H., 2000. Varieties of repetitive behavior in autism: Comparisons to mental retardation. Journal of Autism and Developmental Disorders 30, 237–243.

Bouvard, M.P., Leboyer, M., Launay, J., Recasens, C., Plumet, M., Waller-Perotte, D., et al., 1995. Low-dose naltrexone effects on plasma chemistries and clinical symptoms in autism: A double-blind, placebo-controlled study. Psychiatric Research 58, 191–201.

Branford, D., Bhaumik, S., Nalk, B., 1998. Selective serotonin re-uptake inhibitors for the treatment of perseverative and maladaptive behaviours of people with intellectual disability. Journal of Intellectual Disability Research 42, 301–306.

Brede, M., Nagy, G., Philipp, M., Sorensen, J.B., Lohse, M.J., Hein, L., 2003. Differential control of adrenal and sympathetic catecholamine release by alpha 2-adrenoceptor subtypes. Journal of Molecular Endocrinology 17, 1640–1646.

Brodkin, E.S., McDougle, C.J., Naylor, S.T., Cohen, D.J., Price, L.H., 1997. Clomipramine in adults with pervasive developmental disorders: A prospective open-label investigation. Journal of Child and Adolescent Psychopharmacology 7, 109–121.

Buchsbaum, M.S., Hollander, E., Haznedar, M.M., Tang, C., Spiegel-Cohen, J., Wei, T.C., et al., 2001. Effect of fluoxetine on regional cerebral metabolism in autistic spectrum disorders: A pilot study. International Journal of Neuropsychopharmacology 4, 119–125.

Buitelaar, J.K., Van Der Gaag, R.J., Van Der Hoeven, J., 1998. Buspirone in the management of anxiety and irritability in children with pervasive developmental disorders: Results of an open-label study. Journal of Clinical Psychiatry 59, 56–59.

Campbell, M., Adams, P., Small, A.M., Tesch, L.M., Curren, E.L., 1988. Naltrexone in infantile autism. Psychopharmacology Bulletin 24, 135–139.

Campbell, M., Anderson, L.T., Deutsch, S.I., Green, W.H., 1984. Psychopharmacological treatment of children with the syndrome of autism. Pediatric Annals 13, 309–313. 316.

Campbell, M., Anderson, L.T., Meier, M., Cohen, I.L., Small, A.M., Samit, C., et al., 1978. A comparison of haloperidol and behavior therapy and their interaction in autistic children. Journal of the American Academy of Child & Adolescent Psychiatry 17, 640–655.

Campbell, M., Anderson, L.T., Small, A.M., Adams, P., Gonzalez, N.M., Ernst, M., 1993. Naltrexone in autistic children: Behavioral symptoms and attentional learning. Journal of the American Academy of Child & Adolescent Psychiatry 32, 1283–1291.

Campbell, M., Armenteros, J.L., Malone, R.P., Adams, P.B., Eisenberg, Z.W., Overall, J.E., 1997. Neuroleptic-related dyskinesias in autistic children: A prospective, longitudinal study. Journal of the American Academy of Child & Adolescent Psychiatry 36, 835–843.

Cazzullo, A.G., Musetti, M.C., Musetti, L., Bajo, S., Sacerdote, P., Panerai, A., 1999. Beta-endorphin levels in peripheral blood mononuclear cells and long-term naltrexone treatment in autistic children. European Neuropsychopharmacology 9, 361–366.

Chen, N.C., Bedair, H.S., McKay, B., Bowers Jr., M.B., Mazure, C., 2001. Clozapine in the treatment of aggression in an adolescent with autistic disorder. Journal of Clinical Psychiatry 62, 479–480.

Chez, M.G., Burton, Q., Dowling, T., Chang, M., Khanna, P., Kramer, C., 2007 May. Memantine as adjunctive therapy in children diagnosed with autistic spectrum disorders: An observation of initial clinical response and maintenance tolerability. Journal of Child Neurology 22, 574–579.

Cohen, I.L., Campbell, M., Posner, D., Small, A.M., Triebel, D., Anderson, L.T., 1980. Behavioral effects of haloperidol in young autistic children: An objective analysis using a within-subjects reversal design. Journal of the American Academy of Child & Adolescent Psychiatry 19, 665–677.

Cohen, S.A., Fitzgerald, B.J., Khan, S.R., Khan, A., 2004. The effect of a switch to ziprasidone in an adult population with autistic disorder: Chart review of naturalistic, open-label treatment. Journal of Clinical Psychiatry 65, 110–113.

Connor, D.F., Fletcher, K.E., Swanson, J.M., 1999. A meta-analysis of clonidine for symptoms of attention-deficit hyperactivity disorder. Journal of the American Academy of Child & Adolescent Psychiatry 38, 1551–1559.

Correll, C.U., Manu, P., Olshanskiy, V., Napolitano, B., Kane, J.M., Malhotra, A.K., 2009. Cardiometabolic risk of second-generation antipsychotic medications during first-time use in children and adolescents. Journal of the American Medical Association 302, 1765–1773.

Corson, A.H., Barkenbus, J.E., Posey, D.J., Stigler, K.A., McDougle, C.J., 2004. A retrospective analysis of quetiapine in the treatment of pervasive developmental disorders. Journal of Clinical Psychiatry 65, 1531–1536.

Coskun, M., Mukaddes, N.M., 2008. Mirtazapine treatment in a subject with autistic disorder and fetishism. Journal of Child and Adolescent Psychopharmacology 18, 206–209.

Coskun, M.A., Varghese, L., Reddoch, S., Castillo, E.M., Pearson, D.A., Loveland, K.A., et al., 2009. How somatic cortical maps differ in autistic and typical brains. Neuroreport 20, 175–179.

Couturier, J.L., Nicolson, R., 2002. A retrospective assessment of citalopram in children and adolescents with pervasive developmental disorders. Journal of Child and Adolescent Psychopharmacology 12, 243–248.

Czapinski, P., Blaszczyk, B., Czuczwar, S.J., 2005. Mechanisms of action of antiepileptic drugs. Current Topics in Medicinal Chemistry 5, 3–14.

DeLong, G.R., Teague, L.A., McSwain Kamran, M., 1998. Effects of fluoxetine treatment in young children with idiopathic autism. Developmental Medicine & Child Neurology 40, 551–562.

Erickson, C.A., Posey, D.J., Stigler, K.A., Mullett, J., Katschke, A.R., McDougle, C.J., 2007. A retrospective study of memantine in children and adolescents with pervasive developmental disorders. Psychopharmacology (Berlin) 191, 141–147.

Ernst, M., Devi, L., Silva, R.R., Gonzalez, N.M., Small, A.M., Malone, R.P., et al., 1993. Plasma beta-endorphin levels, naltrexone, and haloperidol in autistic children. Psychopharmacology Bulletin 29, 221–227.

Fankhauser, M.P., Karumanchi, V.C., German, M.L., Yates, A., Karumanchi, S.D., 1992. A double-blind, placebo-controlled study of the efficacy of transdermal clonidine in autism. Journal of Clinical Psychiatry 53, 77–82.

Fatemi, S.H., Realmuto, G.M., Khan, L., Thuras, P., 1998. Fluoxetine in treatment of adolescent patients with autism: A longitudinal open trial. Journal of Autism and Developmental Disorders 28, 303–307.

FDA, 2006. FDA Approves the First Drug to Treat Irritability Associated with Autism, Risperdal. FDA News Release, October 6, 2006.

Ferrari, P.F., van Erp, A.M., Tornatzky, W., Miczek, K.A., 2003. Accumbal dopamine and serotonin in anticipation of the next aggressive episode in rats. European Journal of Neuroscience 17, 371–378.

Findling, R.L., McNamara, N.K., Gracious, B.L., O'Riordan, M.A., Reed, M.D., Demeter, C., et al., 2004. Quetiapine in nine youths with autistic disorder. Journal of Child and Adolescent Psychopharmacology 14, 287–294.

Fisman, S., Steele, M., 1996. Use of risperidone in pervasive developmental disorders: A case series. Journal of Child and Adolescent Psychopharmacology 6, 177–190.

Fukuda, T., Sugie, H., Ito, M., Sugie, Y., 2001. Clinical evaluation of treatment with fluvoxamine, a selective serotonin reuptake inhibitor in children with autistic disorder. No To Hattatsu 33, 314–318.

Gagliano, A., Germanò, E., Pustorino, G., Impallomeni, C., D'Arrigo, C., Calamoneri, F., et al., 2004. Risperidone treatment of children with autistic disorder: Effectiveness, tolerability, and pharmacokinetic implications. Journal of Child and Adolescent Psychopharmacology 14, 39–47.

Ghaziuddin, M., Tsai, L., Ghaziuddin, N., 1991. Fluoxetine in autism with depression. Journal of the American Academy of Child & Adolescent Psychiatry 30, 508–509.

Gobbi, G., Gaudreau, P.O., Leblanc, N., 2006. Efficacy of topiramate, valproate, and their combination on aggression/agitation behavior in patients with psychosis. Journal of Clinical Psychopharmacology 26, 467–473.

Gobbi, G., Pulvirenti, L., 2001. Long-term treatment with clozapine in an adult with autistic disorder accompanied by aggressive behaviour. Journal of Psychiatry & Neuroscience 26, 340–341.

Goodman, W.K., Price, L.H., Rasmussen, S.A., Mazure, C., Fleischmann, R.L., Hill, C.L., et al., 1989. The Yale-Brown obsessive compulsive scale: I. Development, use, and reliability. Archives of General Psychiatry 46, 1006–1011.

Halperin, J.M., Kalmar, J.H., Schulz, K.P., Marks, D.J., Sharma, V., Newcom, J.H., 2006. Elevated childhood serotonergic function protects against adolescent aggression in disruptive boys. Journal of the American Academy of Child & Adolescent Psychiatry 45, 833–840.

Hamilton, M., 1959. The assessment of anxiety states by rating. British Journal of Medical Psychology 32, 50–55.

Handen, B.L., Feldman, H., Gosling, A., Breaux, A.M., McAuliffe, S., 1991. Adverse side effects of Ritalin among mentally-retarded children with ADHD. Journal of the American Academy of Child & Adolescent Psychiatry 30, 241–245.

Handen, B.L., Johnson, C.R., Lubetsky, M., 2000. Efficacy of methylphenidate among children with autism and symptoms of attention-deficit hyperactivity disorder. Journal of Autism and Developmental Disorders 30, 245–255.

Hardan, A.Y., Jou, R.J., Handen, B.L., 2005. Retrospective study of quetiapine in children and adolescents with pervasive developmental disorders. Journal of Autism and Developmental Disorders 35, 387–391.

Hazell, P.L., Stuart, J.E., 2003. A randomized controlled trial of clonidine added to psychostimulant medication for hyperactive and aggressive children. Journal of the American Academy of Child & Adolescent Psychiatry 42, 886–894.

Hellings, J.A., Weckbaugh, M., Nickel, E.J., Cain, S.E., Zarcone, J.R., Reese, R.M., et al., 2005. A double-blind, placebo-controlled study of valproate for aggression in youth with pervasive developmental disorders. Journal of Child and Adolescent Psychopharmacology 15, 682–692.

Herman, B.H., Hammock, M.K., Arthur-Smith, A., Kuehl, K., Appelgate, K., 1989. Effects of acute administration of naltrexone on cardiovascular function, body temperature, body weight and serum concentrations of liver enzymes in autistic children. Development Pharmacology & Therapeutics 12, 118–127.

Hoekstra, P.J., Troost, P.W., Lahuis, B.E., Mulder, H., Mulder, E.J., Franke, B., et al., 2010. Risperidone-induced weight gain in referred children with autism spectrum disorders is associated with a common polymorphism in the 5-hydroxytryptamine 2C receptor gene. Journal of Child and Adolescent Psychopharmacology 20, 473–477.

Hoglund, E., Korzan, W.J., Watt, M.J., Forster, G.L., Summers, T.R., Johannessen, H.F., et al., 2005. Effects of L-DOPA on aggressive behavior and central monoaminergic activity in the lizard Anolis carolinensis, using a new method for drug delivery. Behavioural Brain Research 156, 53–64.

Hollander, E., Chaplin, W., Soorya, L., Wasserman, S., Novotny, S., Rusoff, J., et al., 2010. Divalproex sodium vs placebo for the treatment of irritability in children and adolescents with autism spectrum disorders. Neuropsychopharmacology 35, 990–998.

Hollander, E., Kaplan, A., Cartwright, C., Reichman, D., 2000. Venlafaxine in children, adolescents, and young adults with autism spectrum disorders: An open retrospective clinical report. Journal of Child Neurology 15, 132–135.

Hollander, E., Phillips, A., Chaplin, W., Zagursky, K., Novotny, S., Wasserman, S., et al., 2005. A placebo controlled crossover trial of liquid fluoxetine on repetitive behaviors in childhood and adolescent autism. Neuropsychopharmacology 30, 582–589.

Hollander, E., Tracy, K.A., Swann, A.C., Coccaro, E.F., McElroy, S.L., Wozniak, P., et al., 2003. Divalproex in the treatment of impulsive aggression: Efficacy in cluster B personality disorders. Neuropsychopharmacology 28, 1186–1197.

Hollander, E., Wasserman, S., Swanson, E.N., Chaplin, W., Schapiro, M.L., Zagursky, K., et al., 2006. A double-blind placebo-controlled pilot study of olanzapine in childhood/adolescent pervasive developmental disorder. Journal of Child and Adolescent Psychopharmacology 16, 541–548.

Horrigan, J.P., Barnhill, L.J., 1997. Risperidone and explosive aggressive autism. Journal of Autism and Developmental Disorders 27, 313–323.

Hoshino, Y., Kumashiro, H., Kanero, M., Takahashi, Y., 1977. The effects of methylphenidate in early infantile autism and its relation to serum serotonin levels. Folia Psyciatrica et Neurologica Japonica 31, 605–614.

Hranilovic, D., Bujas-Petkovic, Z., Vragovic, R., Vuk, T., Hock, K., Jernej, B., 2007. Hyperserotonemia in adults with autistic disorder. Journal of Autism and Developmental Disorders 37, 1934–1940.

Ihalainen, J.A., Tanila, H., 2004. In vivo regulation of dopamine and noradrenaline release by alpha2A-adrenoceptors in the mouse nucleus accumbens. Journal of Neurochemistry 91, 49–56.

Jaselskis, C.A., Cook, E.H., Fletcher, K.E., 1992. Clonidine treatment of hyperactive and impulsive children with autistic disorder. Journal of Clinical Psychopharmacology 12, 322–327.

Johansson, A.K., Bergvall, A.H., Hansen, S., 1999. Behavioral disinhibition following basal forebrain excitotoxin lesions: Alcohol consumption, defensive aggression, impulsivity, and serotonin levels. Behavioural Brain Research 102, 17–29.

Jou, R.J., Handen, B.L., Hardan, A.Y., 2005. Retrospective assessment of atomoxetine in children and adolescents with pervasive developmental disorders. Journal of Child and Adolescent Psychopharmacology 15, 325–330.

Kemner, C., Willemsen-Swinkels, S.H., de Jonge, M., Tuynman-Qua, H., van Engeland, H., 2002. Open-label study of olanzapine in children with pervasive developmental disorder. Journal of Clinical Psychopharmacology 22, 455–460.

King, B.H., 2000. Pharmacological treatment of mood disturbances, aggression, and self-injury in persons with pervasive developmental disorders. Journal of Autism and Developmental Disorders 30, 439–445.

King, B.H., Hollander, E., Sikich, L., McCracken, J.T., Scahill, L., Bregman, J.D., et al., 2009. Lack of efficacy of citalopram in children with autism spectrum disorders and high levels of repetitive behavior: Citalopram ineffective in children with autism. Archives of General Psychiatry 66, 583–590.

King, B.H., Wright, D.M., Handen, B.L., Sikich, L., Zimmerman, A.W., Mcmahon, W., et al., 2001. Double-blind, placebo-controlled study of amantadine hydrochloride in the treatment of children with autistic disorder. Journal of the American Academy of Child & Adolescent Psychiatry 40, 658–665.

Kolmen, B.K., Feldman, H.M., Handen, B.L., Janosky, J.E., 1995. Naltrexone in young autistic children: A double-blind, placebo-controlled crossover study. Journal of the American Academy of Child & Adolescent Psychiatry 34, 223–231.

Kolmen, B.K., Feldman, H.M., Handen, B.L., Janosky, J.E., 1997. Naltrexone in young autistic children: Replication study and learning measures. Journal of the American Academy of Child & Adolescent Psychiatry 36, 1570–1578.

Koshes, R.J., 1997. Use of fluoxetine for obsessive-compulsive behavior in adults with autism. American Journal of Psychiatry 154, 578.

Leboyer, M., Philippe, A., Bouvard, M., Doe, A., Doe, B., 1999. Whole blood serotonin and plasma beta-endorphin in autistic probands and their first-degree relatives. Biological Psychiatry 45, 158–163.

Lecavalier, L., 2006. Behavioral and emotional problems in young people with pervasive developmental disorders: Relative prevalence, effects of subject characteristics, and empirical classification. Journal of Autism and Developmental Disorders 36, 1101–1114.

Locascio, J.J., Malone, R.P., Small, A.M., Kafantaris, V., Ernst, M., Lynch, N.S., et al., 1991. Factors related to haloperidol response and dyskinesias in autistic children. Psychopharmacology Bulletin 27, 119–126.

Lord, C., Risi, S., DiLavore, P.S., Shulman, C., Thurm, A., Pickles, A., 2006. Autism from 2 to 9 years of age. Archives of General Psychiatry 63, 694–701.

Malone, R.P., Cater, J., Sheikh, R.M., Choudhury, M.S., Delaney, M.A., 2001. Olanzapine versus haloperidol in children with autistic disorder: An open pilot study. Journal of the American Academy of Child & Adolescent Psychiatry 40, 887–894.

Malone, R.P., Delaney, M.A., Hyman, S.B., Cater, J.R., 2007. Ziprasidone in adolescents with autism: An open-label pilot study. Journal of Child and Adolescent Psychopharmacology 17, 779–790.

Malone, R.P., Maislin, G., Choudhury, M.S., Gifford, C., Delaney, M.A., 2002. Risperidone treatment in children and adolescents with autism: Short- and long-term safety and effectiveness. Journal of the American Academy of Child & Adolescent Psychiatry 41, 140–147.

Mandell, D.S., Morales, K.H., Marcus, S.C., Stahmer, A.C., Doshi, J., Polsky, D.E., 2008. Psychotropic medication use among Medicaid-enrolled children with autism spectrum disorders. Pediatrics 121, e441–e448.

Marcus, R.N., Owen, R., Kamen, L., Manos, G., McQuade, R.D., Carson, W.H., et al., 2009. A placebo-controlled, fixed-dose study of aripiprazole in children and adolescents with irritability associated with autistic disorder. Journal of the American Academy of Child & Adolescent Psychiatry 48, 1110–1119.

Martin, A., Koenig, K., Anderson, G.M., Scahill, L., 2003. Low-dose fluvoxamine treatment of children and adolescents with pervasive developmental disorders: A prospective, open-label study. Journal of Autism and Developmental Disorders 33, 77–85.

Martin, A., Koenig, K., Scahill, L., Bregman, J., 1999. Open-label quetiapine in the treatment of children and adolescents with autistic disorder. Journal of Child and Adolescent Psychopharmacology 9, 99–107.

McCracken, J.T., McGough, J., Shah, B., Cronin, P., Hong, D., Aman, M.G., et al., 2002. For research units on pediatric psychopharmacology autism network. Risperidone in children with autism and serious behavioral problems. New England Journal of Medicine 347, 314–321.

McDougle, C.J., Brodkin, E.S., Naylor, S.T., Carlson, D.C., Cohen, D.J., Price, L.H., 1998. Sertraline in adults with pervasive developmental disorders: A prospective open-label investigation. Journal of Clinical Psychopharmacology 18, 62–66.

McDougle, C.J., Holmes, J.P., Bronson, M.R., Anderson, G.M., Volkmar, F.R., Price, L.H., et al., 1997. Risperidone treatment of children and adolescents with pervasive developmental disorders: A prospective open-label study. Journal of the American Academy of Child & Adolescent Psychiatry 36, 685–693.

McDougle, C.J., Kem, D.L., Posey, D.J., 2002. Case series: Use of ziprasidone for maladaptive symptoms in youths with autism. Journal of the American Academy of Child & Adolescent Psychiatry 41, 921–927.

McDougle, C.J., Kresch, L.E., Posey, D.J., 2000 Oct. Repetitive thoughts and behavior in pervasive developmental disorders: Treatment with serotonin reuptake inhibitors. Journal of Autism and Developmental Disorders 30, 427–435.

McDougle, C.J., Naylor, S.T., Cohen, D.J., Volkmar, F.R., Heninger, G.R., Price, L.H., 1996. A double-blind, placebo-controlled study of fluvoxamine in adults with autistic disorder. Archives of General Psychiatry 53, 1001–1008.

McDougle, C.J., Price, L.H., Volkmar, F.R., Goodman, W.K., Ward-O'Brien, D., Nielsen, J., et al., 1992. Clomipramine in autism: Preliminary evidence of efficacy. Journal of the American Academy of Child & Adolescent Psychiatry 31, 746–750.

McDougle, C.J., Scahill, L., Aman, M.G., McCracken, J.T., Tierney, E., Davies, M., et al., 2005. Risperidone for the core symptom domains of autism: Results from the study by the autism network of the research units on pediatric psychopharmacology. American Journal of Psychiatry 162, 1142–1148.

Mehlinger, R., Scheftner, W.A., Poznanski, E., 1990. Fluoxetine and Autism. Journal of the American Academy of Child & Adolescent Psychiatry 29, 985.

Miral, S., Gencer, O., Inal-Emiroglu, F.N., Baykara, B., Baykara, A., Dirik, E., 2007. Risperidone versus haloperidol in children and adolescents with AD: A randomized, controlled, double-blind trial. European Child & Adolescent Psychiatry 17, 1–8. Epub ahead of print.

Molina, V., Ciesielski, L., Gobaille, S., Mandel, P., 1986. Effects of the potentiation of the GABAergic neurotransmission in the olfactory bulbs on mouse-killing behavior. Pharmacology Biochemistry & Behavior 24, 657–664.

Nagaraj, R., Singhi, P., Malhi, P., 2006. Risperidone in children with autism: Randomized, placebo-controlled, double-blind study. Journal of Child Neurology 21, 450–455.

Namerow, L.B., Thomas, P., Bostic, J.Q., Prince, J., Monuteaux, M.C., 2003. Use of citalopram in pervasive developmental disorders. Developmental-Behavioral Pediatrics 24, 104–108.

Nguyen, M., Murphy, T., 2001. Mirtazapine for excessive masturbation in an adolescent with autism. Journal of the American Academy of Child & Adolescent 40, 868–869.

Nicolson, R., Awad, G., Sloman, L., 1998. An open trial of risperidone in young autistic children. Journal of the American Academy of Child & Adolescent Psychiatry 37, 372–376.

Niederhofer, H., Staffen, W., Mair, A., 2003. Tianeptine: A novel strategy of psychopharmacological treatment of children with autistic disorder. Human Psychopharmacology 18, 389–393.

Novotny, S., Hollander, E., Allen, A., Mosovich, S., Aronowitz, B., Cartwright, C., et al., 2000. Increased growth hormone response to sumatriptan challenge in adult autistic disorders. Psychiatric Research 94, 173–177.

Owen, R., Sikich, L., Marcus, R.N., Corey-Lisle, P., Manos, G., McQuade, R.D., et al., 2009. Aripiprazole in the treatment of irritability in children and adolescents with autistic disorder. Pediatrics 124, 1533–1540.

Pandina, G.J., Bossie, C.A., Youssef, E., Zhu, Y., Dunbar, F., 2007. Risperidone improves behavioral symptoms in children with autism in a randomized, double-blind, placebo-controlled trial. Journal of Autism and Developmental Disorders 37, 367–373.

Patel, N.C., Crismon, M.L., Hoagwood, K., Jensen, P.S., 2005. Unanswered questions regarding atypical antipsychotic use in aggressive children and adolescents. Journal of Child and Adolescent Psychopharmacology 15, 270–284.

Perry, R., Pataki, C., Munoz-Silva, D.M., Armenteros, J., Silva, R.R., 1997. Risperidone in children and adolescents with pervasive developmental disorder: Pilot trial and follow-up. Journal of Child and Adolescent Psychopharmacology 7, 167–179.

Posey, D.J., Aman, M.G., McCracken, J.T., Scahill, L., Tierney, E., Arnold, L.E., et al., 2007. Positive effects of methylphenidate on inattention and hyperactivity in pervasive developmental disorders: An analysis of secondary measures. Biological Psychiatry 61, 538–544.

Posey, D.J., Puntney, J.I., Sasher, T.M., Kem, D.L., McDougle, C.J., 2004. Guanfacine treatment of hyperactivity and inattention in pervasive developmental disorders: A retrospective analysis of 80 cases. Journal of Child and Adolescent Psychopharmacology 14, 233–241.

Posey, D.J., Wiegand, R.E., Wilkerson, J., Maynard, M., Stigler, K.A., McDougle, C.J., 2006. Open-label atomoxetine for attention-deficit/ hyperactivity disorder symptoms associated with high-functioning pervasive developmental disorders. Journal of Child and Adolescent Psychopharmacology 16, 599–610.

Potenza, M.N., Holmes, J.P., Kanes, S.J., McDougle, C.J., 1999. Olanzapine treatment of children, adolescents, and adults with pervasive developmental disorders: An open-label pilot study. Journal of Clinical Psychopharmacology 19, 37–44.

Quintana, H., Birmaher, B., Stedge, D., Lennon, S., Freed, J., Bridge, J., et al., 1995. Use of methylphenidate in the treatment of children with autistic disorder. Journal of Autism and Developmental Disorders 25, 283–294.

Realmuto, G.M., August, G.J., Garfinkel, B.D., 1989. Clinical effect of buspirone in autistic children. Journal of Clinical Psychopharmacology 9, 122–125.

Remington, G., Sloman, L., Konstantareas, M., Parker, K., Gow, R., 2001. Clomipramine versus haloperidol in the treatment of autistic disorder: A double-blind, placebo-controlled, crossover study. Journal of Clinical Psychopharmacology 21, 440–444.

Research Units on Pediatric Psychopharmacology (RUPP), 2002. Risperidone in children with autism and serious behavioral problems. New England Journal of Medicine 347, 314–321.

Research Units on Pediatric Psychopharmacology (RUPP) Autism Network, 2005. Randomized, controlled, crossover trial of methylphenidate in pervasive developmental disorders with hyperactivity. Archives of General Psychiatry 62, 1266–1274.

Retz, W., Rosler, M., Supprian, T., Retz-Junginger, P., Thome, J., 2003. Dopamine D3 receptor gene polymorphism and violent behavior: Relation to impulsiveness and ADHD-related psychopathology. Journal of Neural Transmission 110, 561–572.

Richler, J., Bishop, S.L., Kleinke, J.R., Lord, C., 2007. Restricted and repetitive behaviors in young children with autism spectrum disorders. Journal of Autism and Developmental Disorders 37, 73–85.

Ritvo, E.R., Yuwiler, A., Geller, E., Doe, A., Doe, B., 1970. Increased blood serotonin and platelets in early infantile autism. Archives of General Psychiatry 23, 566–572.

Rothenberger, A., 1993. Psychopharmacological treatment of self-injurious behavior in individuals with autism. Acta Paedopsychiatrica 56, 99–104.

Sandman, C.A., 1988. B-endorphin disregulation in autistic and self-injurious behavior: A neurodevelopmental hypothesis. Synapse 2, 193–199.

Sandman, C.A., Hetrick, W., Taylor, D., Marion, S., 2000. Uncoupling of proopiomelanocortin (POMC) fragments is related to self-injury. Peptides 21, 785–791.

Scahill, L., McDougle, C.J., Williams, S.K., Dimitropoulos, A., Aman, M.G., McCracken, J.T., et al., 2006. Research units on pediatric psychopharmacology autism network. Children's Yale-Brown obsessive compulsive scale modified for pervasive developmental disorders. Journal of the American Academy of Child & Adolescent Psychiatry 45, 1114–1123.

Schain, R.J., Freedman, D.X., 1961. Studies on 5-hydroxyindole metabolism in autistic and other mentally retarded children. Journal of Pediatric 58, 315–320.

Shea, S., Turgay, A., Carroll, A., Schulz, M., Orlik, H., Smith, I., et al., 2004. Risperidone in the treatment of disruptive behavioral symptoms in children with autistic and other pervasive developmental disorders. Pediatrics 114, e634–e641.

Sival, R.C., Duivenvoorden, H.J., Jansen, P.A., Haffmans, P.M., Duursma, S.A., Eikelenboom, P., 2004. Sodium valproate in aggressive behaviour in dementia: A twelve-week open label follow-up study. International Journal of Geriatric Psychiatry 19, 305–312.

Snead, R.W., Boon, F., Presberg, J., 1994. Paroxetine for self-injurious behavior. Journal of the American Academy of Child & Adolescent Psychiatry 33, 909–910.

Soderpalm, B., 2002. Anticonvulsants: Aspects of their mechanism of action. European Journal of Pain 6, 3–9.

Steingard, R., Biederman, J., Spencer, T., Wilens, T., Gonzalez, A., 1993. Comparison of clonidine response in the treatment of attention-deficit hyperactivity disorder with and without comorbid tic disorders. Journal of the American Academy of Child & Adolescent Psychiatry 32, 350–353.

Steingard, R.J., Zimnitzky, B., DeMaso, D.R., Bauman, M.L., Bucci, J.P., 1997. Sertraline treatment of transition-associated anxiety and agitation in children with autistic disorder. Journal of Child and Adolescent Psychopharmacology 7, 9–15.

Strayhorn, J.M., Rapp, N., Donina, W., Strain, P.S., 1988. Randomized trial of methylphenidate for an autistic child. Journal of the American Academy of Child & Adolescent Psychiatry 27, 244–247.

Sturm, H., Fernell, E., Gillberg, C., 2004. Autism spectrum disorders in children with normal intellectual levels: Associated impairments and subgroups. Developmental Medicine & Child Neurology 46, 444–447.

Sweetman, S. (Ed.), 2004. Martindale: The Complete Drug Reference. Pharmaceutical Press, London.

Todd, R.D., 1991. Fluoxetine in autism. American Journal of Psychiatry 148, 1089.

Toichi, M., Kamio, Y., 2003. Paradoxical autonomic response to mental tasks in autism. Journal of Autism and Developmental Disorders 33, 417–426.

Troost, P.W., Lahuis, B.F., Steenhuis, M., Ketelaars, C.E., Buitelaar, J.K., van Engeland, H., et al., 2005. Long-term effects of risperidone in children with autism spectrum disorders: A placebo discontinuation study. Journal of the American Academy of Child & Adolescent Psychiatry 44, 1137–1144.

Vergnes, M., Depaulis, A., Boehrer, A., Kempf, E., 1988. Selective increase of offensive behavior in the rat following intrahypothalamic 5,7-DHT-induced serotonin depletion. Behavioural Brain Research 29, 85–91.

Wasserman, S., Iyengar, R., Chaplin, W.F., Watner, D., Waldoks, S.E., Anagnostou, E., et al., 2006. Levetiracetam versus placebo in childhood and adolescent autism: A double-blind placebo-controlled study. International Clinical Psychopharmacology 21, 363–367.

Willemsen-Swinkels, S.H., Buitelaar, J.K., van Engeland, H., 1996. The effects of chronic naltrexone treatment in young autistic children: A double-blind placebo-controlled crossover study. Biological Psychiatry 39, 1023–1031.

Willemsen-Swinkels, S.H., Buitelaar, J.K., Weijnen, F.G., van Engeland, H., 1995. Placebo-controlled acute dosage naltrexone study in young autistic children. Psychiatric Research 58, 203–215.

Zuddas, A., Ledda, M.G., Fratta, A., Muglia, P., Cianchetti, C., 1996. Clinical effects of clozapine on autistic disorder. American Journal of Psychiatry 153, 738.

Novel Therapeutics in Autism Spectrum Disorders

Evdokia Anagnostou*, Caitlyn McKeever†, Azadeh Kushki*

*Bloorview Research Institute, University of Toronto, Toronto, Ontario, Canada
†Department of Psychiatry, University of Toronto, Toronto, Ontario, Canada

INTRODUCTION

There has been a surge in clinical trials in autism spectrum disorders (ASD) over the past 2 decades, in attempts to identify effective medications for children and youths with ASD. Several classes of medications have been shown to be effective for symptoms associated with autism. There is an increasing amount of data to support the use of pharmacological treatments for hyperactivity and attention deficits (both stimulants and non-stimulants) and of atypical antipsychotics for irritability and impulsive aggression (see Chapter 1.6). Although data regarding the use of SSRIs for repetitive behaviors has been disappointing, several issues related to possible subgroups may not yet have been adequately addressed. Most research done to date is based on the premise that if a symptom domain is present across neurodevelopmental disorders, these disorders must also share a common neurobiology. Based on this premise, we have essentially been borrowing medications used to treat other disorders (e.g. ADHD and OCD) and testing them in autism. Although this approach has had some successes in symptom-reduction (e.g. FDA indication for risperidone and aripiprazole for irritability), it has not yet produced successful treatments for the core symptoms of autism, nor has it furthered the goal of improving skills necessary for learning. In addition, because we have tended to use medications tested in neuropsychiatric disorders, medication trials have largely ignored symptoms associated with ASD that are not considered behavioral, such as sensory issues and motor apraxia.

Developments in the fields of the molecular genetics and neuroscience of ASD are allowing new treatments and approaches to emerge. Based on our emerging understanding of the basic science of the disorder, novel molecular targets for autism can now be identified, which have the potential, if properly manipulated, to address core ASD. This is based on the premise that processes recently identified as being involved in ASD relate to synaptic integrity and plasticity, and as such have the potential to be manipulated for symptom relief and theoretically even reversal. The ultimate goal of this process is to develop autism-tailored pharmacological treatments, which will, in combination with behavioral interventions, make it possible to modify the

The Neuroscience of Autism Spectrum Disorders.
http://dx.doi.org/10.1016/B978-0-12-391924-3.00007-7

developmental trajectories of individuals with ASD. However, this progress is not without its challenges, some of which will be outlined below.

CHALLENGES FOR NOVEL THERAPEUTICS IN ASD

Perhaps the most significant challenge to developing novel therapeutics in ASD is the heterogeneity in both the biology and the phenomenology of ASD. Large individual differences in etiology and symptom severity and expression have been repeatedly documented. As there is a relative paucity of biomarkers that identify meaningful biological subgroups, it has been particularly hard to stratify ASD participants in intervention studies. Stratification attempts have been based on symptom severity, and occasionally by the presence of intellectual disability, but have not produced exciting new insights. The identification of rare causative mutations is providing us with the exciting option of targeting known molecular targets (e.g. SHANK3, neuroligins), however, significant challenges remain related to how to design appropriate studies for disorders where the sample sizes may not allow randomized controlled trials. Single subject designs used by behavioral researchers may provide some new opportunities in this area, but ultimately we will need to identify the common metabolic pathways that are affected by such rare mutations in order to translate this knowledge into therapeutics for the majority of individuals with ASD.

From the phenomenology point of view, measurement of symptoms which vary across chronological and mental age is posing particular problems. Variation in cognitive abilities in ASD can influence measurements of symptom severity, particularly in areas such as communication. Behaviors appearing to be quite diverse, such as eye contact, peer relationships, and social approach are all grouped under a single behavioral domain and may reflect both variation in neurobiology as well as characteristics of a particular developmental stage. As such measures appropriate to capture social perception/ cognition deficits in toddlers are highly unlikely to be useful in adolescents and adults. Standardized measures may also be failing to capture the variability of performance in this area in naturalistic settings.

To further complicate an already difficult situation, the first cohorts of children who have received intensive early intervention are now becoming adults, and it is becoming apparent that we have minimal data on the efficacy of pharmacologic interventions for adults with autism, in addition to a lack of tools to measure behavioral responses relevant to autism.

The heterogeneity of ASD is further complicated by high comorbidity with other disorders. As response to treatment is likely impacted by the presence of comorbidity, measurement of comorbid symptom domains is critical. However, there is relative paucity of outcome measures validated in ASD that target comorbid psychiatric conditions (e.g. depression and anxiety), or medical comorbidities (e.g. gastrointestinal complaints, sleep disturbance). Lastly, biological heterogeneity of ASD may be impacted not only by the presence of rare but causative mutations but also the possibility that a wide range of medical conditions could be contributing to the observed phenotype. Such areas include increased oxidative stress, mitochondrial dysfunction, immune dysregulation, and metabolic disorders. At this point in time, it remains unclear whether and how, even in the absence of a diagnosable disorder, these medical issues can impact ASD symptoms, impact the risk of autism, and impact treatment response to psychopharmacologic agents (Zecavati and Spence, 2009).

TRANSLATING GENOMIC ADVANCES INTO NOVEL THERAPEUTICS

Irrespective of these challenges and gaps in research on experimental therapeutics in ASD, we are still at the threshold of exciting novel therapeutics as emerging findings from basic science are providing potential new molecular targets. The use of animal models to better understand the basic neurobiology of single gene disorders associated with human autistic behavior and cognitive impairment is proving to be fruitful. Examples include tuberous sclerosis, Fragile X syndrome, Rett syndrome and neurofibromatosis among others. Specifically, inhibitors of the protein kinase mTOR have been shown to reverse CNS changes associated with tuberous sclerosis (Ehninger et al., 2009), pharmacological or genetic reduction of mGluR5 signaling has been shown to ameliorate multiple Fragile X mutant phenotypes in both mice and fruit flies, statins may ameliorate phenotypes associated with neurofibromatosis (Acosta et al., 2006), and insulin-like growth factor 1 may reverse CNS changes associated with Rett syndrome (Tropea et al., 2009), and Phelan-McDermid Syndrome (Buxbaum J. International Congress of Human Genetics in Montreal, Canada, 2011) to name a few. Clinical trials based on findings in animal models are underway.

To further illustrate the point, we will discuss the examples of Fragile X and tuberous sclerosis (and see Chapters 4.5 and 4.8). Both disorders are single gene disorders associated with autism and intellectual disability. Both are associated with genes that regulate synaptic protein synthesis, a mechanism now suggested to be involved in both autism and intellectual disability.

Both have early data suggesting that the effect of the respective genetic changes may be reversed pharmacologically in the animal model (Auerbach et al., 2011).

Fragile X syndrome (FXS) is an X linked disorder, and the most common inherited cause of ASD and intellectual disability (Hagerman, 2006). It can manifest in humans in a variety of ways, including mental retardation, autism-like behaviors, hyperactivity, anxiety, sensory hypersensitivity, altered gastrointestinal function, and childhood epilepsy. It is caused by transcriptional silencing of a single gene, FMR1, and loss of the protein product, FMRP. The gene has been knocked out in mice and flies, to understand the functional implications of the loss of FMRP (D'Hulst and Kooy, 2009). It seems that activation of the metabotropic glutamate receptor 5 (mGluR5) has downstream consequences that relate to a variety of core deficits in these models. Of particular interest is the fact that partial inhibition of the mGluR5 has led to reversal of multiple features of Fragile X in animal models (Krueger and Bear, 2011; Dölen and Bear, 2008; Dölen et al., 2010). A series of human clinical trials are under way using compounds that either reduce glutamate release in the brain or target selectively mGluR5.

Tuberous sclerosis (TSC), like Fragile X syndrome, is a single gene disorder, caused by mutations in hamartin or tuberin (TCSC1 and TSC2 respectively) (van Slegtenhorst et al., 1998). Similarly to Fragile X, tuberous sclerosis involves genes that alter synaptic protein synthesis. ASD features are common in this disorder, although the definition of TSC is based on the presence of a combination of findings that include cortical tubers, subependymal nodules, subependymal giant cell astrocytomas, fibromas, hamartomas, hypomelanotic macules among others. It remains unclear whether the number and location of tubers correlate with cognitive deficits (Kassiri et al., 2011; Kaczorowska et al., 2011), however, disinhibition of the mTOR pathway has been shown to be related to cognitive dysfunction (Auerbach et al., 2011). This observation has raised the possibility that the mTOR inhibitors may impact on cognitive/behavioral features of the disorder. In fact, Ehninger et al., 2009 showed that rapamycin, an mTOR inhibitor, reversed spatial learning deficits and context discrimination in the animal model.

In addition, Auerbach et al., 2011 showed that although both mutations are associated with synaptic dysfunction in the hippocampus of the $Fmr1^{-/y}$ and $Tsc2^{+/-}$ mice, synaptic protein synthesis is exaggerated in the case of the Fmr1 mouse and diminished in the case of the Tsc2 mouse, suggesting that the bidirectional deviation from an optimal range of synaptic protein synthesis can lead to behavioral/cognitive impairments.

The two disorders above also illustrate a new paradigm in translational research in ASD. Unlike previous attempts to develop animal models for ASD where the behavioral deficits were replicated in the animal and validated by documenting improvements with pharmacological agents shown to be important to the human behavioral domain (e.g., depression and SSRIs), we have the ability to now engineer causative mutations of ASD in animal models and develop therapeutics based on their ability to reverse or ameliorate the biochemical, structural and/or neurological deficits. Although the disruption in brain function by a mutation may be associated with different behavioral profiles across species, understanding the physiological effects of such mutations has the potential to elucidate common pathophysiological mechanisms involved in these disorders and provide targets for therapeutics (see Chapter 4.9). In other words, although each mutation may be responsible for a small number of cases within the autism spectrum, it is possible that there are subgroups of individuals with autism that have biological deficits that are 'fragile X-like', or 'TSC-like' etc., and so treatments developed for the rare causative single mutations may be effective in the treatment of such subgroups.

OTHER POTENTIAL NOVEL PHARMACOLOGICAL TARGETS

Immune Disruption

The case of immune dysfunction in autism highlights that the fact information about biological processes involved in this disorder may not only come from genomics, and emphasizes the value of neuropathology studies. Although there are several sources of evidence that link autism to immune disruption (see Chapter 2.9), the key finding in ASD has been evidence of ongoing neuroinflammation in post-mortem brains (Vargas et al., 2005; Li et al., 2009; Morgan et al., 2010). Both micro- and astro-glial cells play critical roles in cortical organization, neuronal transmission, and synaptic plasticity, and their activation can produce significant neuronal and synaptic changes that may contribute to the CNS dysfunction observed in autism. Increased inflammatory cytokine and chemokine production in brain and CSF has been reported (Vargas et al., 2005; Li et al., 2009; Morgan et al., 2010). Immune responses in the periphery have also been reported to be dysfunctional and include increased plasma proinflammatory factors (Onore et al., 2012; Zimmerman et al., 2005; 2006; Jyonouchi et al., 2005a; 2005b; 2001; Croonenberghs et al., 2002a, b), changes that are consistent with likely a skewed T helper cell type 1 (TH1/TH2 cytokine profiles), decreased lymphocyte numbers, decreased T cell mitogen response, and the imbalance of serum immunoglobulin levels. Immunogenetic studies of the HLA genes, which are important determinants of immune function, provide further evidence of immune disruption in autism (Pardo et al., 2005). Compared to unrelated controls, individuals with autism or their mothers have been reported to have a significantly more frequent occurrence of a particular MHC haplotype (B44-Sc 30-DR4) associated with immune dysfunction. Autism has also been associated with significantly greater frequency of other immune-based genes including HLA-DRB1, complement C4 alleles (Ashwood and Wakefield, 2006), and HLA-A2 alleles (Torres et al., 2006). Finally, there is emerging evidence that that autoimmune disorders occur with significantly greater frequency in families of individuals with autism (Sweeten et al., 2003).

Although there evidence suggesting immune dysfunction in ASD, it is not clear yet whether the immune findings converge on a single immunopathology. Still, immune dysfunction is a 'drugable' target. There is preliminary evidence that some available agents may favorably modulate the immune system of children with ASD, such as omega-3s and pioglitazone. However, well-controlled studies are urgently needed to further investigate the effects of these compounds.

The Glutamate System

As previously discussed, the Fragile X model of autism illustrates that manipulation of aspects of the glutamatergic system can lead to phenotypes that may include autism-like features. As such, this system has received attention as the focus of translational work in recent years. Multiple studies have reported higher than typical levels of glutamate in plasma for individuals with autism or Asperger syndrome (Rolf et al., 1993; Moreno-Fuenmayor et al., 1996; Aldred et al., 2003; Shinohe et al., 2006), suggesting an imbalance in excitation to inhibition ratios. In addition to metabotropic receptors, there are several other possible molecular targets for pharmacological manipulation. Postmortem studies have shown reduced levels of glutamic acid decarboxylase protein (the enzyme responsible for normal conversion of glutamate to GABA in the brain) in brains of individuals with autism, suggesting increased levels of glutamate or transporter receptor density in autistic brains (Fatemi, 2002). Decreased AMPA-type glutamate receptor density in the cerebellum of autistic individuals has also been reported (Purcell et al., 2001) and related findings have been made in some mouse models of monogenic forms of ASD (for example, SHANK3-deficient mice, see Chapter 4.7). A series of genetic studies have implicated various glutamate receptor genes in ASD (Phillipe et al., 1999; Serajee et al., 2003; Barnby et al., 2005).

Studies involving compounds which affect the NMDA receptor provide preliminary evidence that encourage and support further pharmacological studies targeting the glutamate system. In particular, amantadine, shown to have NMDA non-competitive inhibitor activity, was reported to be well-tolerated, and to have modest effects on irritability and hyperactivity in a double blind placebo controlled trial in children with autism (King et al., 2001). Another non-competitive NMDA inhibitor, memantine, is reported to include improvements in irritability, lethargy, hyperactivity, inappropriate speech, stereotypy, memory, and language in four open-label studies involving a total of 186 children with autism (Owley et al., 2006; Chez et al., 2007; Niederhofer, 2007; Erickson et al., 2007). Finally, dextromethorphan, an NMDA receptor antagonist, was found to improve problem behaviors (e.g., tantrums and self-injurious behavior) as well as anxiety, motor planning, socialization, and language (Woodard et al., 2005; Welch and Sovner, 1992) in a series of case studies involving children with autism.

The aforementioned studies provide evidence which encourages pharmacological interventions targeting aspects of the glutamate system in ASD. However, the evidence remains preliminary and well-controlled studies in this area are still needed.

Oxytocin and Vasopressin

Oxytocin (OXT) and its sister peptide vasopressin (AVP) have now been shown to be important for many aspects of social cognition and affiliative behaviors, which are all important in ASD. OXT knockout mice show social recognition deficits, in the context of intact olfaction and cognitive abilities, which were reversed by intraventricular OXT – but not by AVP administration (Ferguson et al., 2000). Sala et al., (2011) reported that oxytocin receptor (OXTR) null mice demonstrated resistance to change and susceptibility to seizures in addition to the social deficits observed in OXT knockouts. Of clear interest to therapeutics, oxytocin restored social exploration and recognition deficits, and pretreatment with a selective V1a antagonist blocked the oxytocin effect, suggesting that oxytocin can exert therapeutic effects through the V1a receptor, in the case of absent or abnormal oxytocin receptors.

Whether oxytocin is involved in the pathophysiology of autism is not yet clear. A series of genetic association studies have suggested a link between the oxytocin receptor gene (Wu et al., 2005; Ylisaukko-oja et al., 2006; Jacob et al., 2007), or the V1a receptor (Kim et al., 2002; Wassink et al., 2004; Yirmiya et al., 2006) and autism. Studies of blood levels have suggested lower mean levels of oxytocin in ASD compared to typically developing, age matched controls (Modahl et al., 1998), and a failure to show to show the expected developmental decrease with age (Green et al., 2001). Intravenous administration of oxytocin has been shown to facilitate social learning during an intravenous oxytocin challenge in ASD patients (Hollander et al., 2007). Early intranasal oxytocin studies showed that this treatment promotes trust and prosocial behavior in humans (Kosfeld et al., 2005). A series of recent reviews have summarized the available data for the effects of intranasal oxytocin in typically developing young adults and ASD adults and adolescents (Green and Hollander, 2010) and suggest that there is therapeutic potential to manipulating this system. Well-controlled studies in this area are clearly needed to address issues of efficacy and safety. In the meantime, the science community needs to also provide clarification on the pharmacodynamics, mode of administration and potential outcome measures to be used in such trials.

Augmentation of Behavioral Interventions

Data reviewed above, whether it relates to synaptic protein synthesis, inhibition/excitation ratios, immune dysfunction or neuropeptides involved in social cognition, suggest that candidate brain systems have the potential to be manipulated in ways that may alter the biology of the disorder. If medications targeting these systems become available, it is likely that they will be used in combination with behavioral interventions, as the purpose of early intensive behavioral interventions is to facilitate skill acquisition important for learning and the development of social behavior and communication. If medications improve neuronal functioning, the hope is that they will help individuals with ASD become more responsive to psychoeducational interventions.

CONCLUSIONS

In summary, emerging data from genomics, animal model and neuropathology are starting to identify pathways that may be targets for pharmacological manipulation. Fragile X and tuberous sclerosis were described as two examples among many, where understanding the basic cellular processes involved in single gene disorders associated with ASD may lead to novel therapeutics for individuals with apparently idiopathic autism. Understanding the processes involved in subgroups of individuals with ASD, whether related to single gene mechanisms or representing final common pathways of a variety of biological differences, offer exciting new avenues for experimental therapeutics in developmental disorders. These studies also highlight the fact that the solutions may be more complicated that previously

suspected, as deviation in either direction from optimally regulated systems may lead to shared phenotypes, suggesting that information on phenotype alone may not be sufficient to provide safe and effective treatments.

References

Acosta, M.T., Gioia, G.A., Silva, A.J., 2006. Neurofibromatosis type 1: new insights into neurocognitive issues. Current Neurology and Neuroscience Reports 6, 136–143.

Aldred, S., Moore, K.M., Fitzgerald, M., Waring, R.H., 2003. Plasma amino acid levels in children with autism and their families. Journal of Autism and Developmental Disorders 33, 93–97.

Ashwood, P., Wakefield, A.J., 2006. Immune activation of peripheral blood and mucosal cd3+ lymphocyte cytokine profiles in children with autism and gastrointestinal symptoms. Journal of Neuroimmunology 173, 126–134.

Auerbach, B.D., Osterweil, E.K., Bear, M.F., 2011. Mutations causing syndromic autism define an axis of synaptic pathophysiology. Nature 23 , 63–68.

Barnby, G., Abbott, A., Sykes, N., Morris, A., Weeks, D.E., Mott, R., et al., 2005. Candidate-gene screening and association analysis at the autism-susceptibility locus on chromosome16p: evidence of association at GRIN2A and ABAT. American Journal of Human Genetics 76, 950–966.

Chez, M., Burton, Q., Dowling, T., Chang, M., Khanna, P., Kramer, C., 2007. Memantine as adjunctive therapy in children diagnosed with ASD. Journal of Child Neurology 22, 574–579.

Croonenberghs, J., Bosmans, E., Deboutte, D., Kenis, G., Maes, M., 2002. Activation of the inflammatory response system in autism. Neuropsychobiology 45, 1–6.

Croonenberghs, J., Wauters, A., Devreese, K., Verkerk, R., Scharpe, S., Bosmans, E., et al., 2002. Increased serum albumin, gamma globulin, immunoglobulin IgG, and IgG2 and IgG4 in autism. Psychological Medicine 32 , 1457–1463.

D'Hulst, C., Kooy, R.F., 2009. Fragile X syndrome: from molecular genetics to therapy. Journal of Medical Genetics 46, 577–584.

Dölen, G., Bear, M.F., 2008. Role for metabotropic glutamate receptor 5 (mGluR5) in the pathogenesis of fragile X syndrome. Journal of Physiology 586, 1503–1508.

Dölen, G., Carpenter, R.L., Ocain, T.D., Bear, M.F., 2010. Mechanism-based approaches to treating fragile X. Pharmacology & Therapeutics 127 , 78–93.

Ehninger, D., de Vries, P.J., Silva, A.J., 2009. From mTOR to cognition: molecular and cellular mechanisms of cognitive impairments in tuberous sclerosis. Journal of Intellectual Disability Research 53, 838–851.

Erickson, C.A., Posey, D.J., Stigler, K.A., Mullett, J., Katschke, A.R., McDougle, C.J., 2007. A retrospective study of memantine in children and adolescents with PDD. Psychopharmacology191, 141–147.

Fatemi, S.H., 2002. The role of Reelin in pathology of autism. Molecular Psychiatry 7, 919–920.

Ferguson, J.N., Young, L.J., Hearn, E.F., Matzuk, M.M., Insel, T.R., Winslow, J.T., 2000. Social amnesia in mice lacking the oxytocin gene. Nature Genetics 25, 284–288.

Green, J.J., Hollander, E., 2010. Autism and oxytocin: new developments in translational approaches to therapeutics. Neurotherapeutics 7 , 250–257.

Green, L., Fein, D., Modahl, C., Feinstein, C., Waterhouse, L., Morris, M., 2001. Oxytocin and autistic disorder: alterations in peptide forms. Biological Psychiatry 50, 609–613.

Hagerman, R.J., 2006. Lessons from fragile X regarding neurobiology, autism, and neurodegeneration. Journal of Developmental & Behavioral Pediatrics 27 , 63–74.

Hollander, E., Bartz, J., Chaplin, W., Phillips, A., Sumner, J., Soorya, L., et al., 2007. Oxytocin increases retention of social cognition in autism. *Biological Psychiatry.* Biological Psychiatry 61 , 498–503.

Jacob, S., Brunea, C.W., Carter, C.S., Leventhal, B.L., Lord, C., Cook, E.H., 2007. Association of the Oxytocin Receptor Gene (OXTR) in Caucasian Children and Adolescents with Autism. Neuroscience Letters.

Jyonouchi, H., Geng, L., Ruby, A., Reddy, C., Zimmerman-Bier, B., 2005. Evaluation of an association between gastrointestinal symptoms and cytokine production against common dietary proteins in children with autism spectrum disorders. Journal of Pediatrics 146, 605–610.

Jyonouchi, H., Geng, L., Ruby, A., Zimmerman-Bier, B., 2005. Dysregulated innate immune responses in young children with autism spectrum disorders: Their relationship to gastrointestinal symptoms and dietary intervention. Neuropsychobiology 51, 77–85.

Jyonouchi, H., Sun, S., Le, H., 2001. Proinflammatory and regulatory cytokine production associated with innate and adaptive immune responses in children with autism spectrum disorders and developmental regression. Journal of Neuroimmunology 120, 170–179.

Kaczorowska, M., Jurkiewicz, E., Domańska-Pakieła, D., Syczewska, M., Lojszczyk, B., Chmielewski, D., et al., 2011. Cerebral tuber count and its impact on mental outcome of patients with tuberous sclerosis complex. Epilepsia 52 , 22–27.

Kassiri, J., Snyder, T.J., Bhargava, R., Wheatley, B.M., Sinclair, D.B., 2011. Cortical tubers, cognition, and epilepsy in tuberous sclerosis. Pediatric Neurology 44 , 328–332.

Kim, S.J., Young, L.J., Gonen, D., Veenstra-VanderWeele, J., Courchesne, R., Courchesne, E., et al., 2001. Double-blind, placebo-controlled study of amantadine hydrochloride in the treatment of children with autistic disorder. Journal of the American Academy of Child & Adolescent Psychiatry 6, 658–665. 40.

Kosfeld, M., Heinrichs, M., Zak, P.J., Fischbacher, U., Fehr, E., 2005. Oxytocin increases trust in humans. Nature 435 , 673–676.

Krueger, D.D., Bear, M.F., 2011. Toward fulfilling the promise of molecular medicine in fragile X syndrome. Annual Review of Medicine 62, 411–429.

Li, X., Chauhan, A., Sheikh, A.M., Patil, S., Chauhan, V., Li, X.M., et al., 2009. Elevated immune response in the brain of autistic patients. Journal of Neuroimmunology 207, 111–116.

Lord, C., Leventhal, B.L., Cook, E.H., Insel, T.R., 2002. Transmission disequilibrium testing of arginine vasopressin receptor 1A (AVPR1A) polymorphisms in autism. Molecular Psychiatry 7 , 503–507.

Modahl, C., Green, L., Fein, D., Morris, M., Waterhouse, L., Feinstein, C., et al., 1998. Plasma oxytocin levels in autistic children. Biological Psychiatry 43, 270–277.

Moreno-Fuenmayor, H., Borjas, L., Arrieta, A., Valera, V., Socorro-Candanoza, L., 1996. Plasma excitatory amino acids in autism. Investigación. clínica. 37, 113–128.

Morgan, J.T., Chana, G., Pardo, C.A., Achim, C., Semendeferi, K., Buckwalter, J., et al., 2010. Microglial activation and increased microglial density observed in the dorsolateral prefrontal cortex in autism. Biological Psychiatry 15, 368–376.

Niederhofer, H., 2007. Glutamate antagonists seem to be slightly effective in osychopharmacologic treatment of autism. Journal of Clinical Psychopharmacology 27, 317.

Onore, C., Careaga, M., Ashwood, P., 2012. The role of immune dysfunction in the pathophysiology of autism. Brain, Behavior, and Immunity 26 , 383–392.

Owley, T., Salt, J., Guter, S., Grieve, A., Walton, L., Ayuyao, N., et al., 2006. A prospective, open label trial of memantine in the treatment of cognitive, behavioral and memory dysfunction in pervasive developmental disorders. Journal of Child and Adolescent Psychopharmacology 16, 517–524.

Pardo, C.A., Vargas, D.L., Zimmerman, A.W., 2005. Immunity, neuroglia and neuroinflammation in autism. International Review of Psychiatry 17, 485–495.

Phillipe, A., Martinez, M., Guilloud-Bataille, M., Gillberg, C., Rastam, M., Sponheim, E., et al., 1999. Genome-wide scan for autism susceptibility genes. Paris Autism Research International Sibpair Study. Human Molecular Genetics 8, 805–812.

Purcell, A.E., Jeon, O.H., Zimmerman, A.W., Blue, M.E., Pevsner, J., 2001. Postmortem brain abnormalities of the glutamate neurotransmitter system in autism. Neurology 57, 1618–1628.

Rolf, L.H., Haarmann, F.Y., Grotemeyer, K.H., Kehrer, H., 1993. Serotonin and amino acid content in platelets of autistic children. Acta Psychiatrica Scandinavica 87, 312–316.

Sala, M., Braida, D., Lentini, D., Busnelli, M., Bulgheroni, E., Capurro, V., et al., 2011. Pharmacologic Rescue of Impaired Cognitive Flexibility, Social Deficits, Increased Aggression, and Seizure Susceptibility in Oxytocin Receptor Null Mice: A Neurobehavioral Model of Autism. Biological Psychiatry Feb 17.

Serajee, F.J., Zhong, H., Nabi, R., Huq, A.H., 2003. The metabotropic glutamate receptor 8 gene at 7q31: partial duplication and possible association with autism. Journal of Medical Genetics 40, 42.

Shinohe, A., Hashimoto, K., Nakamura, K., Tsujii, M., Iwata, Y., Tsuchiya, K.J., et al., 2006. Increased serum levels of glutamate in adult patients with autism. Progress in Neuro-Psychopharmacology and Biological Psychiatry 30 , 1472–1477.

Sweeten, T.L., Bowyer, S.L., Posey, D.J., Halberstadt, G.M., McDougle, C.J., 2003. Increased prevalence of familial autoimmunity in probands with pervasive developmental disorders. Pediatrics 112 e420.

Torres, A.R., Sweeten, T.L., Cutler, A., Bedke, B.J., Fillmore, M., Stubbs, E.G., et al., 2006. The association and linkage of the hla-a2 class i allele with autism. Human Immunology 67, 346–351.

Tropea, D., Giacometti, E., Wilson, N.R., Beard, C., McCurry, C., Fu, D.D., et al., 2009. Partial reversal of Rett Syndrome-like symptoms in MeCP2 mutant mice. Proceedings of the National Academy of Sciences USA 106, 2029–2034.

Van Slegtenhorst, M., Nellist, M., Nagelkerken, B., Cheadle, J., Snell, R., van den Ouweland, A., et al., 1998. Interaction between hamartin and tuberin, the TSC1 and TSC2 gene products. Human Molecular Genetics 7 , 1053–1057.

Vargas, D.L., Nascimbene, C., Krishnan, C., Zimmerman, A.W., Pardo, C.A., 2005. Neuroglial activation and neuroinflammation in the brain of patients with autism. Annals of Neurology 57, 67–81.

Wassink, T.H., Piven, J., Vieland, V.J., Pietila, J., Goedken, R.J., Folstein, S.E., et al., 2004. Examination of AVPR1a as an autism susceptibility gene. Molecular Psychiatry 9 , 968–972.

Welch, L., Sovner, R., 1992. The treatment of a chronic organic mental disorder with dextromethorphan in a man with severe mental retardation. British Journal of Psychiatry 161, 118–120.

Woodard, C., Groden, J., Goodwin, M., Shanower, C., Bianco, J., 2005. The treatment of the behavioral sequelae of autism with dextromethorphan: a case report. Journal of Autism and Developmental Disorders 35, 515–518.

Wu, S., Jia, M., Ruan, Y., Liu, J., Guo, Y., Shuang, M., et al., 2005. Positive association of the oxytocin receptor gene (OXTR) with autism in the Chinese Han population. Biological Psychiatry 58 , 74–77.

Yirmiya, N., Rosenberg, C., Levi, S., Salomon, S., Shulman, C., Nemanov, L., et al., 2006. Association between the arginine vasopressin 1a receptor (AVPR1a) gene and autism in a family-based study: mediation by socialization skills. Molecular Psychiatry 11 , 488–494.

Ylisaukko-oja, T., Alarcón, M., Cantor, R.M., Auranen, M., Vanhala, R., Kempas, E., et al., 2006. Search for autism loci by combined analysis of autism genetic resource exchange and finnish families. Annals of Neurology 59, 145–155.

Zecavati, N., Spence, S.J., 2009. Neurometabolic disorders and dysfunction in autism psectrum disorders. Current Neurology and Neuroscience Reports 9 , 129–136.

Zimmerman, A., Connors, S.L., Pardo-Villamizar, C.A., 2006. Neuroimmunology and neurotransmitters in autism. Autism: A Neurological Disorder of Early Brain Development, 141–159.

Zimmerman, A.W., Jyonouchi, H., Comi, A.M., Connors, S.L., Milstien, S., Varsou, A., et al., 2005. Cerebrospinal fluid and serum markers of inflammation in autism. Pediatric Neurology 33, 195–201.

ETIOLOGY OF AUTISM SPECTRUM DISORDERS

Joseph D. Buxbaum

There have been eight twin studies in autism spectrum disorders (ASD) and all show increased concordance between monozygotic twins, compared to dizygotic twins. These findings are strong evidence for an important role for genetics in ASD 'ACE' modeling, which derives its name from an attempt to divide risk into three components, termed **A** (additive genetics), **C** (common twin environment), and **E** (unique twin environment), gives estimates of heritability amongst the highest in psychiatry when applied to these twin studies. Additional family studies also provide strong support for a genetic risk for ASD. Genes and their gene products provide a molecular window into disease pathogenesis, are readily translated into model systems, and are ideal targets for drug development.

There is also evidence from the twin studies for what has been called 'environmental' risk for ASD. ACE modeling was established years ago, before other mechanisms were considered in detail, and it is important to understand that the historical titles associated with each category (broadly 'genetic' and 'environmental') are imprecise, with 'genetic' including things in addition to germline genetic changes, and 'environment' covering things including genetic and non-genetic factors. For example, in modern epidemiology one can consider *de novo* germline mutation, epigenetics, somatic mutation, epistatic interactions between loci, stochastic phenomena – including random X chromosome inactivation, monoallelic expression of some genes, mitochondrial effects, parent-of-origin effects, gene–environment interaction and gene–environment correlation, maternal/fetal effects, and likely additional mechanisms. Where each of these mechanisms fall in ACE modeling is not always well studied, but suffice to say that many of these mechanisms will fall into 'genetic' or 'environmental' categories. In short, what proportion of positive values for A, C or E reflect some of these other mechanisms cannot be determined from ACE modelling, and the field is only now beginning to grapple with some of these mechanisms, as represented in several of the chapters in this section.

In spite of the etiological complexity of ASD, there have been enormous efforts in genetic and environmental risk factor discovery with significant successes in identifying high-risk ASD genes and loci (Betancur and Coleman) and high-risk ASD copy number variants (Marshall, Lionel, and Scherer).

There has been considerably less success in identifying common single nucleotide polymorphisms (SNPs) in ASD (Anney), although sample sizes are very small compared to other complex disorders such as schizophrenia, and the ASD studies are underpowered for realistic effect sizes. Given the estimates of the large number of ASD genes and loci (many hundreds), methods of massively parallel (next-generation) sequencing will likely be an important means for gene discovery in ASD, with some important results already emerging (Cai and Buxbaum).

Some of the additional risk for ASD can be encompassed by mitochondrial effects (Naviaux), prenatal and perinatal risk factors (Sandin, Kolevzon, Levine, Hultman, and Reichenberg), and other environmental influences (Lyall, Schmidt, and Hertz-Picciotto). In addition, some of the genetic and non-genetic risk can be mediated by hormonal influences (Auyeung and Baron-Cohen) and immune abnormalities (Eloi, Heuer, and Van de Water).

While not exhaustive as to potential processes that can contribute to ASD risk, this section provides an up-to-date survey of recent findings in ASD risk and mediators of ASD risk. The role of the nuclear genome in ASD has been validated through ongoing gene discovery. In addition, the contributions of other risk factors and mediators of risk are supported by a growing body of evidence. The next few years promises to bring an explosion of discovery in the etiology of ASD.

Etiological Heterogeneity in Autism Spectrum Disorders: Role of Rare Variants

Catalina Betancur*, Mary Coleman[†]

*INSERM U952, CNRS UMR 7224 and Pierre and Marie Curie University, Paris, France
[†]Foundation for Autism Research, Sarasota, FL, USA

INTRODUCTION

Autism spectrum disorders (ASD) encompass a group of behaviorally defined developmental disabilities characterized by marked clinical and etiological heterogeneity. ASD can be associated with intellectual disability (ID) of varying degrees ($\sim$70%), epilepsy ($\sim$30%), and dysmorphic features and congenital malformations ($\sim$20%) (Coleman and Gillberg, 2012). ASD can thus be considered syndromic (i.e., associated with dysmorphic, neuromuscular, metabolic or other distinctive clinical features, including structural brain abnormalities) or nonsyndromic, similar to the division of ID into syndromic and nonsyndromic forms (Gecz et al., 2009).[1]

The genetic architecture of ASD is highly heterogeneous (Abrahams and Geschwind, 2008; Betancur, 2011; State, 2010). About 20% of individuals have an identified genetic etiology. Cytogenetically visible chromosomal aberrations have been reported in $\sim$5% of cases, involving many different loci on all chromosomes. The most frequent abnormalities are maternally derived 15q11–q13 duplications, involving the imprinted Prader–Willi/Angelman region and detected in $\sim$1%. ASD, can also be due to mutations of numerous single-genes involved in autosomal dominant, autosomal recessive and X-linked disorders. The most common single gene defect identified in ASD is fragile X syndrome (*FMR1*), present in $\sim$2% of cases (Kielinen

[1]Note that the term 'syndromic' autism refers to the clinical presentation of the patient and not to the fact that a genetic disorder or syndrome has been identified in the patient. Genetic defects can be associated with syndromic or nonsyndromic clinical presentations. Furthermore, note that the term 'idiopathic' autism means that a specific etiology has not been identified in that patient (i.e., unexplained autism); the term 'idiopathic' should not be used in lieu of nonsyndromic or isolated autism. Finally, the use of the terms 'primary' and 'secondary' autism to refer to nonsyndromic and syndromic forms, respectively, is inappropriate, since all cases of autism, regardless of the associated phenotype, are secondary to disruption of normal brain development.

The Neuroscience of Autism Spectrum Disorders.
http://dx.doi.org/10.1016/B978-0-12-391924-3.00008-9

et al., 2004) (Chapter 4.5). Other monogenic disorders described in ASD include tuberous sclerosis (*TSC1*, *TSC2*) (Chapter 4.8), Angelman syndrome (*UBE3A*), Rett syndrome (*MECP2*) (Chapter 4.6), and *PTEN* mutations in patients with macrocephaly and autism (Chapter 4.8). Rare mutations have been identified in multiple synaptic genes, including *NLGN3*, *NLGN4X* (Jamain et al., 2003), *SHANK3* (Durand et al., 2007), and *SHANK2* (Berkel et al., 2010; Pinto et al., 2010) (Chapter 4.7). Recent genome-wide microarray studies in large ASD samples have highlighted the important contribution of rare submicroscopic deletions and duplications, called copy number variation (CNV), to the etiology of ASD, including *de novo* events in 5–10% of cases (Marshall et al., 2008; Pinto et al., 2010; Sanders et al., 2011; Sebat et al., 2007) (Chapter 2.2). Most recently, the first whole-exome sequencing studies in ASD have shown an increased rate of rare *de novo* point mutations and confirmed a high degree of locus heterogeneity (Neale et al., 2012; O'Roak et al., 2011; 2012; Sanders et al., 2012) (Chapter 2.4).

The constantly increasing number of distinct, individually rare genetic causes of ASD and the substantial contribution of *de novo* events indicates that the genetic architecture of ASD resembles that of ID, with hundreds of genetic and genomic disorders involved, each accounting for a very small fraction of cases. In fact, all the known genetic causes of ASD are also causes of ID, indicating that these two neurodevelopmental disorders share common genetic bases.

We recently performed an exhaustive review of all the genetic and genomic disorders reported in subjects with ASD or autistic behavior, and identified 103 disease genes and 44 recurrent genomic imbalances (Betancur, 2011), and the numbers have continued to grow. These findings are in stark contrast to a persisting claim among the autism research community that we know very little about the etiology of autism, and that there are only a modest number of autism loci known. Here, rather than listing all the genetic and genomic disorders involved in ASD, we review what we can learn about the profound etiological heterogeneity underlying ASD.

The most obvious conclusion we can draw is that, when examined from an etiological perspective, ASD is not a single disease entity but a behavioral manifestation of many hundreds of single-gene and genomic disorders. In addition, it is emerging that *de novo* variants are an important part of the architecture of ASD, consistent with purifying selection against deleterious genetic variants of major effect. One of the most important observations is that there is considerable overlap in high-risk genes and loci for ASD, ID, and epilepsy. Similarly, many of the rare recurrent CNVs identified recently have been found to confer risk for a broad range of neurological and psychiatric phenotypes, including

not only ID, ASD, and epilepsy, but also schizophrenia and attention deficit/hyperactivity disorder (ADHD). This highlights how disruption of core neurodevelopmental processes can give rise to a wide range of clinical manifestations, and that greater attention should be placed on the neurobiological processes of brain development and function rather than on the precise behavioral manifestation. Finally, we show how some of the genes implicate specific pathways, subcellular organelles, or systems in the pathophysiology of ASD, which can lead to biological and neurobiological insights into disease mechanisms.

GENETIC DISORDERS STRONGLY ASSOCIATED WITH ASD

Table 2.1.1 shows genetic and genomic disorders in which ASD is a common manifestation. For some of these disorders, ASD is among the clinical hallmarks, including Phelan-McDermid syndrome (22q13 deletion syndrome/*SHANK3* mutations), maternal 15q11–q13 duplications, Rett syndrome (*MECP2*) and *MECP2* duplication syndrome, fragile X syndrome (*FMR1*), tuberous sclerosis (*TSC1*, *TSC2*), adenylosuccinate lyase deficiency (*ADSL*), Timothy syndrome (*CACNA1C*), cortical dysplasia-focal epilepsy syndrome (*CNTNAP2*), Smith–Lemli–Opitz syndrome (*DHCR7*), Smith–Magenis syndrome (17p11.2 deletion, *RAI1* mutations), and Potocki–Lupski syndrome (17p11.2 duplication) (see Table 2.1.1 for references). Another disorder strongly associated with ASD is the recently described 2q23.1 microdeletion syndrome, caused by haploinsufficiency of the methyl-CpG-binding domain 5 (*MBD5*) gene. An analysis of 65 individuals with deletions or translocations involving *MBD5* reported that all had 'autistic-like' behaviors (Talkowski et al., 2011). If these findings were confirmed using standardized diagnostic assessments, this would constitute the first genetic disorder exhibiting fully penetrant ASD. However, this appears unlikely, given that none of the disorders implicated in ASD to date are associated with ASD in 100% of cases, reflecting the variable expressivity of many genetic conditions.

Other disorders with common ASD manifestations are brain creatine deficiency (*SLC6A8*, *GAMT*, *GATM*), Cornelia de Lange syndrome (*NIPBL*, *SMC1A*), CHARGE syndrome (*CHD7*), Cohen syndrome (*VPS13B*), Joubert syndrome and related syndromes (*AHI1*, *NPHP1*, *CEP290*, *RPGRIP1L*), myotonic dystrophy type 1 (*DMPK*), X-linked female-limited epilepsy and ID (*PCDH19*), 2q37 deletion syndrome, Cri du Chat syndrome (5p deletion), Williams syndrome (7q11.23 deletion), 7q11.23 duplication syndrome, 8p23.1 deletion syndrome, WAGR syndrome (11p13 deletion),

TABLE 2.1.1 Genetic Disorders Strongly Associated with ASD

Disorder (prevalence)[a]	Gene (locus); inheritance	Mutations	Prevalence in ASD	Proportion with ASD	Clinical features	Selected references[b]
Fragile X syndrome (1:4,000 males, 1:6,000 females)	FMR1 (Xq27.3); X-linked	Trinucleotide repeat expansion	~2%	~60% males and ~20% females with the full mutation have ASD. Among premutation carriers, 15% males and 5% females have ASD	ID, ASD, ADHD, characteristic facial appearance, macroorchidism. Females are generally less affected than males.	Clifford et al., 2007; Hagerman et al., 2010; Kielinen et al., 2004
22q13 deletion syndrome/Phelan-McDermid syndrome (>800 cases diagnosed)	SHANK3 (22q13.33); dominant	22q13 deletion, mutation	~0.5%	55% (6/11) individuals with 22q13 deletions had autistic behavior; among subjects with ring chromosome 22 including a 22q13 deletion, 44% (12/27) had a clinical diagnosis of ASD and 85% (23/27) had autistic traits	ID, absent or severely delayed speech, autistic behavior, seizures, hypotonia, decreased sensitivity to pain, mouthing/chewing, dysplastic toenails	Durand et al., 2007; Jeffries et al., 2005; Manning et al., 2004
Rett syndrome (1:8,500 females); MECP2 duplication syndrome (~1% in males with ID)	MECP2 (Xq28); X-linked	Mutation, deletion, duplication	~1% in females, rare in males	ASD/autistic features are frequent in girls with Rett syndrome; 76% (13/17) males with MECP2 duplication have autism/autistic features	MECP2 mutations or deletions cause Rett syndrome in females (severe ID and speech impairment, loss of purposeful hand use, ataxia, hyperventilation), and are often fatal in males; MECP2 duplication syndrome occurs mostly in males	Carney et al., 2003; Ramocki et al., 2010
15q11–q13 duplication syndrome (1:20,000–30,000)	UBE3A (15q11.2); dominant; imprinted	Interstitial duplication or isodicentric chromosome 15, usually of maternal origin	~1%	81% (44/54) with isodicentric chromosome 15 met criteria for autism and 92% (50/54) for ASD	ID, language impairment, seizures, mild dysmorphism, infantile hypotonia. Maternally derived duplications confer a high risk of ASD, whereas duplications of paternal origin usually remain phenotypically silent but can lead to ASD/ID	Depienne et al., 2009; Hogart et al., 2010

(Continued)

TABLE 2.1.1   Genetic Disorders Strongly Associated with ASD – cont'd

Disorder (prevalence)[a]	Gene (locus); inheritance	Mutations	Prevalence in ASD	Proportion with ASD	Clinical features	Selected references[b]
Angelman syndrome (1:12,000–20,000)	UBE3A (15q11.2); dominant; imprinted	Maternal 15q11–q13 deletion, paternal uniparental disomy, mutation, imprinting defect	Rare	63% (38/60) ASD (range 50–81%)	ID, lack of speech, inappropriate laughter, seizures, microcephaly, ataxia	Sahoo et al., 2006; Trillingsgaard and Østergaard, 2004
Prader–Willi syndrome (1:10,000–25,000)	HBII-85 snoRNA cluster (15q11.2); dominant; imprinted	Paternal 15q11–q13 deletion, maternal uniparental disomy, imprinting defect	Rare	23% (49/209) ASD (range 19–25%)	ID, obsessive-compulsive behavior, skin picking, psychosis, hypotonia, obesity, hypogonadism, short stature	Descheemaeker et al., 2006; Veltman et al., 2005
Smith–Magenis syndrome (1:15,000)	RAI1 (17p11.2); dominant	17p11.2 deletion, mutation	Rare	90% (18/20) ASD	ID, hyperactivity, sleep disorder, seizures, self-mutilation, hoarse voice, brachydactyly, hypotonia	Laje et al., 2010
Potocki–Lupski syndrome (1:20,000)	RAI1 (17p11.2); dominant	17p11.2 duplication	Rare	Autistic features are present in the majority; 67% (10/15) meet criteria for ASD	ID, ASD, ADHD, infantile hypotonia, failure to thrive, sleep apnea, cardiovascular abnormalities	Treadwell-Deering et al., 2010
Tuberous sclerosis (1:5,800)	TSC1 (9q34.13), TSC2 (16p13.3); dominant	Mutation, deletion	~1%	40% ASD (20–60%)	ID, non-malignant tumors in the brain, kidneys, heart, eyes, lungs, and skin, seizures	Numis et al., 2011
Adenylosuccinate lyase deficiency (<100 cases reported)	ADSL (22q13.1); recessive	Mutation	Extremely rare	~50% autism/autistic features	Disorder of purine metabolism characterized by ID, epilepsy, and autistic features	Spiegel et al., 2006
Smith–Lemli–Opitz syndrome (1:20,000–40,000)	DHCR7 (11q13.4); recessive	Mutation	Rare	53% (9/17) autism, 71% (10/14) ASD	Inborn error of metabolism affecting cholesterol biosynthesis characterized by growth retardation, microcephaly, ID, and multiple malformations of variable severity	Sikora et al., 2006; Tierney et al., 2006
CHARGE syndrome (1:10,000)	CHD7 (8q12.2); dominant	Mutation, deletion (rare)	Rare	68% (17/25) ASD/autistic traits (including 48% with ASD)	ID, coloboma, heart anomaly, choanal atresia, genital and ear anomalies	Johansson et al., 2006

Syndrome	Gene/locus; inheritance	Type of mutation	Prevalence	% ASD	Clinical features	Reference
Timothy syndrome (<20 individuals reported)	*CACNA1C* (12p13.33); dominant	Mutation	Extremely rare	80% (4/5) ASD	ID, ASD, cardiac abnormalities (long QT syndrome, malformations), hand/foot syndactyly, facial dysmorphism, seizures	Splawski et al., 2004
Cortical dysplasia-focal epilepsy syndrome (10 individuals reported)	*CNTNAP2* (7q35); recessive	Mutation	Extremely rare	67% (6/9) autism or ASD	Severe intractable seizures, ID, ASD, and focal brain malformations in Amish children	Strauss et al., 2006
Brain creatine transporter deficiency syndrome (>150 individuals diagnosed; 45 families reported)	*SLC6A8* (Xq28); X-linked	Mutation	Very rare	Frequent ASD/autistic features	Inborn error of creatine metabolism characterized by ID, speech delay, autistic behavior and seizures	Longo et al., 2011
2q23.1 microdeletion syndrome (65 individuals reported)	*MBD5* (2q23.1); dominant	2q23.1 deletion	0.17% (7/4061)	100% (65/65) subjects with deletions or translocations involving *MBD5* had autistic features	Angelman-like phenotype including ID, severe speech impairment, seizures, behavioral problems, microcephaly, mild dysmorphism, short stature, ataxic gait	Talkowski et al., 2011
8p23.1 deletion syndrome (1:10,000–30,000)	? (8p23.1); dominant	8p23.1 deletion	Rare	57% (4/7) autism	Congenital heart defects, congenital diaphragmatic hernia, mild facial dysmorphism, ID, hyperactivity	Fisch et al., 2010
Cohen syndrome (500–1000 individuals diagnosed)	*VPS13B* (8q22.2); recessive	Mutation, deletion	Very rare	49% (22/45) autism	ID, typical facial dysmorphism, retinal dystrophy, neutropenia, obesity, microcephaly	Howlin et al., 2005
Cornelia de Lange syndrome (1:50,000)	*NIPBL* (5p13.2); dominant *SMC1A* (Xp11.22); X-linked	Mutation, deletion (rare)	Very rare	47–67% autism	ID, facial dysmorphism, upper limb malformations, growth retardation	Bhuiyan et al., 2006; Moss et al., 2008; Oliver et al., 2008
Myotonic dystrophy 1/Steinert disease (1:20,000)	*DMPK* (19q13.32); dominant	Trinucleotide repeat expansion	Unknown	49% (28/57) ASD (including 35% with autism)	Muscle weakness, myotonia (sustained muscle contraction), cataract, cardiac arrhythmia, variable degrees of ID	Ekstrom et al., 2008

(Continued)

TABLE 2.1.1   Genetic Disorders Strongly Associated with ASD — cont'd

Disorder (prevalence)[a]	Gene (locus); inheritance	Mutations	Prevalence in ASD	Proportion with ASD	Clinical features	Selected references[b]
Williams–Beuren syndrome (1:7,500–20,000)	Contiguous gene syndrome (7q11.23); dominant	7q11.23 deletion	Rare	50% (15/30) ASD	ID, ADHD, characteristic neurobehavioral profile (poor visuospatial skills and strengths in selected language skills), aortic stenosis, distinctive facial features, connective tissue abnormalities, endocrine abnormalities	Klein-Tasman et al., 2009; Tordjman et al., 2012
7q11.23 duplication (unknown)	Contiguous gene syndrome (7q11.23); dominant	7q11.23 duplication	Rare	40% (11/27) autism	ID, speech delay, expressive language impairment, ASD, ADHD, seizures, mild dysmorphic features, congenital heart defects, brain MRI abnormalities	Depienne et al., 2007; Van der Aa et al., 2009
WAGR syndrome (1:100,000)	Contiguous gene syndrome (11p13); dominant	11p13 deletion	Very rare	52% (16/31) ASD (including 14 with autism)	ID, Wilms tumor, aniridia, genitourinary anomalies	Xu et al., 2008
16p11.2 microdeletion (1:3,500–5,000)	Contiguous gene syndrome (16p11.2); dominant	16p11.2 deletion	~0.5%	33% (7/21) ASD; 19% (3/16) autism	ID, ASD, language impairment, behavioral problems, epilepsy, dysmorphism, macrocephaly, congenital abnormalities, obesity	Hanson et al., 2010; Shinawi et al., 2010; Weiss et al., 2008
16p11.2 microduplication (1:3,500–5,000)	Contiguous gene syndrome (16p11.2); dominant	16p11.2 duplication	~0.5%	20% (2/10) autistic features; several cases reported with autism/ASD	ID, ASD, SCZ, ADHD, speech delay, epilepsy, dysmorphism, microcephaly, congenital abnormalities, underweight	Shinawi et al., 2010; Weiss et al., 2008
22q11 deletion syndrome/DiGeorge syndrome/ velocardiofacial syndrome (1:4,000–6,000)	TBX1 + others (22q11.21); dominant	22q11.2 deletion, mutation	Rare	28% (84/299) ASD (range 14–50%)	ID, ASD, OCD, ADHD, SCZ, speech delay, epilepsy, facial abnormalities, velopharyngeal insufficiency, cleft palate, heart defects, renal anomalies, immune deficiency, hypocalcemia	Antshel et al., 2007; Fine et al., 2005; Niklasson et al., 2009; Vorstman et al., 2006

Syndrome	Gene(s)/inheritance	Mutation type	Frequency	ASD	Features	References
Joubert syndrome (1:100,000)	AHI1 (6q23.3), NPHP1 (2q13), CEP290 (12q21.32), RPGRIP1L (16q12.2): recessive	Mutation, deletion	Very rare	13–36% ASD	ID, distinctive cerebellar and brainstem malformation (molar tooth sign on MRI), ataxia, breathing abnormalities, some times retinal dystrophy and renal disease. Only 4 of 16 genes implicated in Joubert syndrome so far have been reported to be mutated in subjects with ASD	Ozonoff et al., 1999; Takahashi et al., 2005
Female-limited epilepsy and ID (unknown)	PCDH19 (Xq22.1); X-linked	Mutation, deletion	Rare	30% (12/40) autistic features/ASD	Unique pattern of X-linked inheritance with male sparing; early infantile epileptic encephalopathy, variable ID	Dibbens et al., 2008; Marini et al., 2010; Scheffer et al., 2008
2q37 deletion syndrome (estimated at 1:12,000)	HDAC4 + other(s) (2q37); dominant	2q37 deletion	Rare	24% (16/66) autistic behavior; in a smaller study, 63% (5/8) had autism	Mild-moderate ID, brachydactyly, characteristic facial appearance, short stature, obesity, hypotonia, ASD, and seizures. Haploinsufficiency of HDAC4 causes the core manifestations, including brachydactyly and ID, but other genes yet to be identified contribute to the phenotype in individuals with terminal deletions distal to HDAC4	Devillard et al., 2010; Falk and Casas, 2007; Fisch et al., 2010
Cri du Chat syndrome/5p deletion syndrome (1:15,000–50,000)	? (candidates SEMAF, CTNND2) (5p15.2-p15.33); dominant	5p deletion	Rare	39% (9/23) ASD	ID, high-pitched cat-like cry, microcephaly, dysmorphic facial features	Moss et al., 2008
9q subtelomeric deletion syndrome/Kleefstra syndrome (unknown)	EHMT1 (9q34.3); dominant	9q deletion, mutation	Rare	23% (5/22) ASD/autistic features	ID, childhood hypotonia, distinctive facial features, severe speech impairment, seizures, congenital defects	Kleefstra et al., 2009

(Continued)

TABLE 2.1.1 Genetic Disorders Strongly Associated with ASD – cont'd

Disorder (prevalence)[a]	Gene (locus); inheritance	Mutations	Prevalence in ASD	Proportion with ASD	Clinical features	Selected references[b]
PTEN-related syndromes (unknown, likely underdiagnosed)	*PTEN* (10q23.31); dominant	Mutation, deletion	7% among 99 individuals with ASD and macrocephaly tested clinically for *PTEN* mutations	15% (4/26) ASD	Marked macrocephaly, ASD, ID. The penetrance of other manifestations of *PTEN* hamartoma–tumor syndrome (Bannayan–Riley–Ruvalcaba syndrome and Cowden syndrome) increases with age and includes benign and malignant tumors and mucocutaneous lesions	McBride et al., 2010; Tan et al., 2007
Klinefelter syndrome (XXY) (1:500–1,000 males)	Many	Extra X chromosome	~0.5%	48% (15/31) had significant autism traits; in 2 studies, 11% (2/19) and 27% (14/51) met criteria for ASD	Tall stature, hypogonadism, infertility, ID, speech impairments	Bishop et al., 2011; Bruining et al., 2009; Kielinen et al., 2004; van Rijn et al., 2008
XYY syndrome (1:1,000 males)	Many	Extra Y chromosome	~0.5%	19% (11/58) ASD	Tall stature, hypogonadism, infertility, language impairment	Bishop et al., 2011; Kielinen et al., 2004
XXYY syndrome (1:18,000–40,000 males)	Many	Extra X and Y chromosomes	Rare	28% (26/92) ASD (6 autism, 20 PDD-NOS)	Tall stature, hypogonadism, infertility, learning disabilities, ID, ADHD	Tartaglia et al., 2008
Down syndrome (1:800)	Many	Trisomy 21	3% (1.7–3.7%) in epidemiological studies; considerably less (<0.5%) in clinical or research samples	15% ASD (5% autism and 10% PDD-NOS)	ID, facial dysmorphism, hypotonia, joint laxity, short stature, heart defects	Fombonne et al., 1997; Kielinen et al., 2004; Lowenthal et al., 2007; Oliveira et al., 2007

[a]The prevalence of many of these disorders is likely underestimated, due to lack of systematic surveillance and because individuals with atypical, milder features are not diagnosed.

[b]Additional references implicating these disorders in ASD can be found in Betancur (2011).

ADHD = attention deficit/hyperactivity disorder; ASD = autism spectrum disorder; ID = intellectual disability; MRI = magnetic resonance imaging; OCD = obsessive-compulsive disorder; PDD-NOS = pervasive developmental disorder not otherwise specified; SCZ = schizophrenia.

Angelman syndrome (maternal 15q11–q13 deletion), 16p11.2 microdeletion, and 22q11 deletion syndrome (velocardiofacial/DiGeorge syndrome).

In other disorders, ASD appear to be somewhat less frequent but still at much higher rates than in the general population, such as in *PTEN*-related syndromes, Kleefstra syndrome (9q subtelomeric deletion syndrome/*EHMT1* mutations), Prader–Willi syndrome (paternal 15q11–q13 deletion), 15q24 microdeletion syndrome, and 16p11.2 microduplication. Finally, certain chromosomal aneuploidies are associated with an increased risk for ASD, including Down syndrome, Klinefelter syndrome (XXY), XYY syndrome, and XXYY syndrome.

Note that for most genetic disorders, no reliable estimates of the frequency of ASD among affected individuals or the frequency of the disorder among patients with ASD are available. Even in disorders for which such studies have been conducted, the samples are usually quite small and few are population-based. While it is assumed that these genetic syndromes are rare, some could be underdiagnosed, since only a minority of patients with ASD has been screened for most of these conditions. Several genetic disorders have been described only recently and their prevalence is unknown. Furthermore, the methods employed to diagnose ASD in these studies are very variable, and in some instances no standardized diagnostic assessments were used. Clearly, more data are needed on the prevalence of specific genetic disorders in ASD, and of ASD in genetic disorders, using reliable diagnostic assessment tools in large samples. The frequencies cited in Table 2.1.1 should serve to give an idea of the association between ASD and certain genetic disorders but should not be considered precise. Most of the disorders associated with a high risk for ASD are rare or very rare; apart from fragile X syndrome (~2%), only a few account for at most ~0.5–1% of ASD cases (Table 2.1.1).

GENETIC OVERLAP BETWEEN ASD AND INTELLECTUAL DISABILITY

Like ASD, ID is a common and highly heterogeneous neurodevelopmental disorder, affecting 2–3% of the population. Like in ASD, chromosomal abnormalities detected with conventional karyotyping account for about 5% of cases of ID, while novel microarray-based methods have a diagnostic yield of 10–15%, underscoring the major role of submicroscopic CNVs as causes of ID. Down syndrome (trisomy 21) is the most frequent chromosomal cause of ID, and has also been identified as a relatively frequent cause of autism in several epidemiological studies (Table 2.1.1). The most common single-gene defect in male patients with ID is fragile X syndrome, with full mutations identified in 2.6% of

patients; the combined frequency in males and females with ID is 2% (Michelson et al., 2011), like in ASD. In females with moderate to severe ID, *MECP2* testing is diagnostic in 1.5% (Michelson et al., 2011). At least 93 genes have been identified that are implicated in X-linked ID; 52 are associated with syndromic ID, while 41 genes have been found to be associated with nonsyndromic ID (Figure 2.1.1) (Gecz et al., 2009; Ropers, 2010). The distinction between syndromic and nonsyndromic ID is not precise, and many genes initially identified in syndromic conditions were later reported in subjects with nonsyndromic forms. Among the 93 genes involved in X-linked ID, 45 have also been implicated in ASD (Figure 2.1.1), demonstrating the profound etiological overlap between these phenotypes. In addition, numerous autosomal genes, either due to dominant, usually *de novo* mutations or to recessive gene defects, have been implicated in ID (and ASD), but many more remain unidentified.

Table 2.1.2 shows several recently identified recurrent microdeletions and microduplications reported in individuals with ID, ASD, and other neurodevelopmental or neuropsychiatric disorders. Some of these novel recurrent CNVs have a recognizable phenotype, such as the 17q21.31 microdeletion syndrome, with a distinctive facial dysmorphism. Others, such as CNVs at 1q21.1, 15q13.3, 16p13.11, and 16p11.2, give rise to less consistent phenotypes (variable expressivity) and have been identified in cohorts of patients ascertained for ID, epilepsy, ASD, or schizophrenia, blurring the current nosological boundaries of these disorders. Several of these aberrations show incomplete penetrance, as demonstrated by their presence in clinically unaffected relatives and in controls. These CNVs have been studied in very large samples of subjects with various neurocognitive and neuropsychiatric conditions, and there appears to be a clear increased frequency in affected subjects versus controls for some of them, suggesting that they act as risk factors; for other CNVs, particularly those that appear to be relatively more frequent in controls, the clinical significance is still uncertain (e.g., 15q13.3 and 16p13.11 duplications).

When reviewing these studies, it is clear that not all 'intellectual disability genes and loci' are necessarily associated with ID. As shown in Box 2.1.1, several genetic and genomic disorders have been reported in individuals with higher function ASD (Asperger syndrome). Similarly, not all genetic defects involved in the etiology of ID and ASD are identified in individuals presenting with marked dysmorphic features or other congenital malformations. In fact, many disease genes implicated in ASD can be associated with nonsyndromic presentations (Box 2.1.2).

It should be clear when looking at the genetic and genomic disorders for which ASD is a manifestation

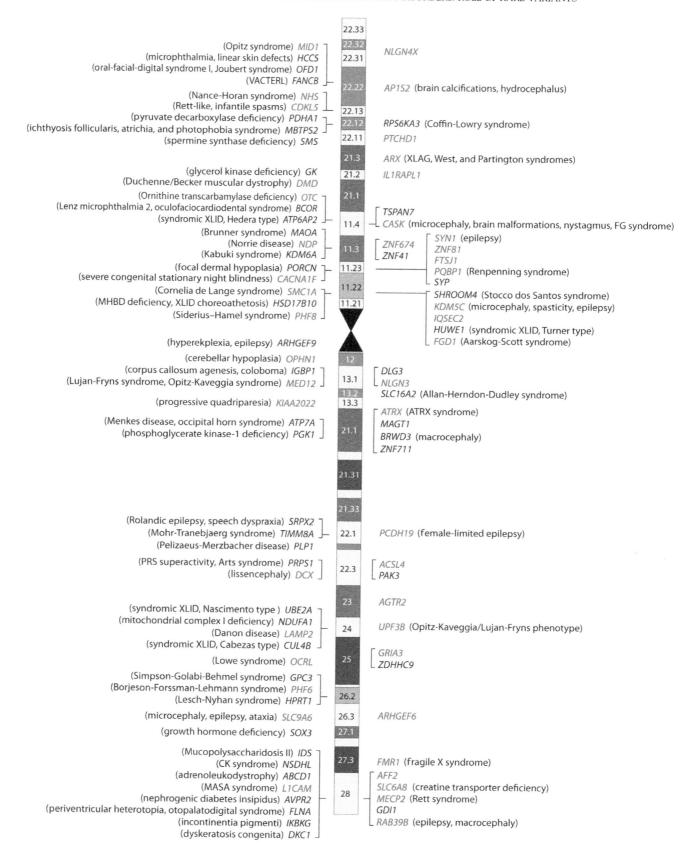

that variable expressivity is the rule rather than the exception, and none will invariably present with ASD. This point is important to consider from a neurobiological perspective. There is, for example, an emphasis on studying ASD-like behaviors in rodent and primate models of ASD; if mutations in the underlying genes do not reliably lead to ASD in humans, other intermediate neurobiological phenotypes are perhaps equally or even more relevant to understanding disease pathogenesis (Section 4).

GENETIC OVERLAP BETWEEN ASD AND EPILEPSY

Epilepsies are common and etiologically heterogeneous disorders, affecting up to 3% of the population. About 30% of children with epilepsy have ASD, and conversely, epilepsy is observed in about a third of ASD individuals. Many well-known genetic disorders share ID, ASD, and epilepsy as prominent phenotypic features, including fragile X syndrome, tuberous sclerosis, Rett syndrome, and Angelman syndrome. In addition, monogenic forms involving mutations in genes encoding voltage-gated or ligand-gated ion channels, referred to as 'channelopathies' have been identified in epilepsy, and increasingly in ASD, such as the neuronal voltage-gated sodium channel genes *SCN1A* and *SCN2A* (Table 2.1.3). Both genes have been implicated in various forms of epilepsy, including early-onset epileptic encephalopathies. This group of severe epilepsies is characterized by progressive intellectual deficits or regression, and includes West syndrome (infantile spasms), Dravet syndrome (severe myoclonic epilepsy of infancy), and Ohtahara syndrome (early infantile epileptic encephalopathy with burst-suppression) (Mastrangelo and Leuzzi, 2012; Paciorkowski et al., 2011). Table 2.1.3 shows several genes involved in early infantile epileptic encephalopathies that can also manifest with ASD (e.g., *ARX*, *CDKL5*, *MECP2*, *MEF2C*, *FOXG1*, *STXBP1*, and *PCDH19*).

Like *MECP2*, mutations in the X-linked cyclin-dependent kinase-like 5 (*CDKL5*) gene are more common in girls and are associated with a Rett-like phenotype with infantile spasms and ID; several cases have been described with autism (Table 2.1.3). Another X-linked gene, protocadherin 19 (*PCDH19*), was recently implicated in 'epilepsy and mental retardation limited to females,' a familial disorder with an unusual mode of inheritance, since only heterozygous females are affected and transmitting males are asymptomatic. *PCDH19* mutations, mostly occurring *de novo*, have also been shown to be a frequent cause of sporadic infantile-onset epileptic encephalopathy in females, and have been reported in females with epilepsy without cognitive impairment (Depienne and Leguern, 2012). ASD or autistic features appear to be frequent among patients with *PCDH19* mutations, with rates of 22–38% (Table 2.1.1). Interestingly, a *PCDH19* mutation was reported in a female with Asperger syndrome and normal IQ, with a history of infantile-onset seizures (Hynes et al., 2010). The female-limited expression is explained by a phenomenon called cellular interference; random X inactivation in mutated females leads to tissue mosaicism, with PCDH19-positive and PCDH19-negative cells, with altered interactions between the two populations (Depienne and Leguern, 2012). In contrast, complete absence of the protein, as seen in mutated males, is not deleterious. The only affected male reported to date was shown to be mosaic for the *PCDH19* deletion in skin fibroblasts (Depienne and Leguern, 2012).

In addition to the genes involved in early-onset epilepsy and ASD listed in Table 2.1.3, many other genes implicated in ASD and ID are associated with epilepsy, including those involved in metabolic disorders (Table 2.1.3), Joubert syndrome and related disorders (Table 2.1.3), and disorders of the RAS/mitogen-activated protein kinase (MAPK) pathway (Table 2.1.4). Moreover, several recently discovered recurrent CNVs associated with ID and ASD, such as 15q13.3 and 16p13.11 deletions, increase risk for various forms of epilepsy (Table 2.1.2). Large, rare non-recurrent CNVs also play a role in the genetic etiology of epilepsy (Mulley and Mefford, 2011), similarly to what has been observed in ID, ASD, and other neuropsychiatric disorders.

The strong association between ASD and epilepsy suggests that they share common mechanisms of synaptic dysfunction. From the neurobiological perspective, understanding this shared vulnerability is an important direction and the model of excitatory/inhibitory imbalance, first developed in epilepsy, is now being considered in forms of ASD (Chapter 3.9).

FIGURE 2.1.1   Genes implicated in syndromic and/or nonsyndromic forms of X-linked intellectual disability (XLID) and their localization on the X chromosome. Genes reported to be mutated in ASD are highlighted in red. Genes that cause syndromic forms of XLID are shown on the left; those that can cause nonsyndromic forms are on the right. The distinction between syndromic and nonsyndromic genes is not always clear-cut, and several genes on the right have been involved in syndromic as well as nonsyndromic XLID; the syndromic presentation is indicated in parentheses. Abbreviations: ATRX (alpha thalassemia, mental retardation syndrome, X-linked) syndrome; MASA (mental retardation, aphasia, shuffling gait, and adducted thumbs) syndrome; MHBD (2-methyl-3-hydroxybutyryl-CoA dehydrogenase) deficiency; PRS (phosphoribosylpyrophosphate synthetase) superactivity; VACTERL (vertebral anomalies, anal atresia, cardiac malformations, tracheoesophageal fistula, renal anomalies, and limb anomalies); XLAG (X-linked lissencephaly and abnormal genitalia) syndrome. *This figure is an updated version of the one originally published in Betancur (2011), copyright 2011, with permission from Elsevier.*

TABLE 2.1.2 Novel Microdeletion and Microduplication Syndromes Reported in Individuals with ASD and Other Neurodevelopmental Disorders

Disorder	Cytoband	Position (Mb)[a]	Comment	References reporting ASD
1q21.1 microdeletion/ microduplication syndrome	1q21.1	146.5–147.7	Neurodevelopmental disorders (ID, learning disability, ASD, schizophrenia, ADHD, epilepsy), dysmorphic features, congenital abnormalities, microcephaly (deletions) or macrocephaly (duplications). Both deletions and duplications exhibit incomplete penetrance (reported in unaffected parents and controls)	Brunetti-Pierri et al., 2008; Mefford et al., 2008; Pinto et al., 2010; Szatmari et al., 2007
2p15–p16.1 microdeletion syndrome	2p15–p16.1	57.7–61.7	ID, growth retardation, microcephaly, dysmorphic features, congenital abnormalities; 4 of 6 subjects reported with the microdeletion have ASD/autistic behavior	Liang et al., 2009; Rajcan-Separovic et al., 2007
3q29 microdeletion/ microduplication syndrome	3q29	195.7–197.5	3q29 deletions are associated with reduced head size, mild dysmorphic features, and multiple congenital anomalies and have been reported in patients with ID, ASD (including one with Asperger syndrome and another one with autism and normal IQ), and schizophrenia. No microduplications have been described thus far in ASD	Ballif et al., 2008; Quintero-Rivera et al., 2010; Willatt et al., 2005
10q22–q23 deletion	10q22.3–q23.2	81.7–88.9	Recurrent 10q22–q23 deletions of varying sizes have been associated with cognitive and behavioral abnormalities including ASD and hyperactivity	Alliman et al., 2010; Balciuniene et al., 2007
15q13.3 microdeletion syndrome/15q13.3 microduplication	15q13.2–q13.3	30.8–32.7	Microdeletion syndrome associated with highly variable phenotype and incomplete penetrance, including ID, seizures, subtle facial dysmorphism, and neuropsychiatric disorders; 44% (15/34) have ASD. Males are more likely to be symptomatic. Reciprocal duplications have been reported in association with ID, ASD, and ADHD, as well as in controls and unaffected parents, and their clinical significance is uncertain at present. The CNVs span CHRNA7, a candidate gene for epilepsy	Ben-Shachar et al., 2009; Miller et al., 2009; Pinto et al., 2010; Sharp et al., 2008; van Bon et al., 2009
15q24 microdeletion syndrome	15q24.1–q24.2	74.4–76.2	Microdeletion syndrome characterized by ID, typical facial characteristics, and mild hand and genital anomalies. 23% (8/35) of reported cases have ASD	Marshall et al., 2008; McInnes et al., 2010; Mefford et al., 2012
16p13.11 microdeletion/ microduplication	16p13.11	15.5–16.3	Recurrent 16p13.11 microdeletions are associated with a variable phenotype and incomplete penetrance, and have been reported in subjects with ID, ASD, congenital anomalies, epilepsy, and schizophrenia, sometimes inherited from unaffected parents. Duplications have been reported in ID, autism, schizophrenia, and in controls, and their clinical significance is unclear at present	Pinto et al., 2010; Ullmann et al., 2007

16p11.2–p12.2 microdeletion/ microduplication syndrome	16p11.2–p12.2	21.6–29.0	Newly recognized microdeletion syndrome; 6 deletions reported in subjects with ID, severe language impairment, and distinct dysmorphic features (without ASD); 5 reciprocal duplications described, the only feature shared by all patients is ASD	Tabet et al., 2012
16p11.2 microdeletion/ microduplication syndrome	16p11.2	29.5–30.2	16p11.2 microdeletions/microduplications have been reported in ASD, ID, schizophrenia, epilepsy, ADHD, and in healthy subjects; both types are associated with incomplete penetrance and variable expressivity, particularly in the case of duplications. Deletions are associated with obesity and duplications with being underweight	Hanson et al., 2010; Rosenfeld et al., 2010; Shinawi et al., 2010; Weiss et al., 2008
17p13.3 microdeletion (Miller–Dieker syndrome, isolated lissencephaly), 17p13.3 microduplication	17p13.3	1–2.5	17p13.3 deletions encompassing PAFAH1B1 cause isolated lissencephaly; larger deletions including YWHAE cause Miller–Dieker syndrome, characterized by severe lissencephaly and additional dysmorphic features and malformations. Microduplications of the Miller–Dieker region as well as smaller duplications affecting PAFAH1B1 or YWHAE have been described recently, including in ASD	Bi et al., 2009; Bruno et al., 2010
17q12 deletion/ duplication syndrome	17q12	34.8–36.2	17q12 deletions encompassing the HNF1B gene cause renal cysts and diabetes syndrome, with ID, ASD, schizophrenia, seizures, and brain abnormalities; the reciprocal duplications are associated with ID and epilepsy, and are less penetrant than deletions. The gene responsible for the neuropsychiatric phenotypes is unknown	Moreno-De-Luca et al., 2010
17q21.31 microdeletion/ microduplication syndrome	17q21.31	43.6–44.2	The 17q21.3 microdeletion syndrome is characterized by ID, hypotonia, and facial dysmorphism; only 2 cases with ASD have been identified. 17q21.31 microduplications have been reported in several ASD cases. KANSL1 was recently identified as the causative gene	Cooper et al., 2011; Grisart et al., 2009
Xq28 duplication syndrome (MECP2 duplication syndrome)	Xq28	152.7–153.4	The Xq28 duplication syndrome is caused by the duplication of MECP2; it is mostly reported in males (females are protected by X inactivation) and is often associated with ASD or autistic features	Ramocki et al., 2010

[a]Human reference genome hg19, NCBI 37 (February 2009).
ADHD = attention deficit/hyperactivity disorder; ASD = autism spectrum disorder; ID = intellectual disability.

BOX 2.1.1

GENETIC DISORDERS REPORTED IN ASPERGER SYNDROME

Although all the genetic disorders identified thus far in subjects with ASD are also established causes of intellectual disability (ID), this does not mean that they are invariably associated with ID. For instance, tuberous sclerosis is associated with ID in only 30% of patients, and Williams syndrome (7q11.23 deletion) in 75%, although almost all affected subjects have neuropsychiatric problems. Thus, it is not surprising that genetic and genomic mutations are found in higher functioning patients, and not exclusively in patients with autism and ID. Several disorders have been identified in individuals without ID, including subjects with Asperger syndrome (see table below).

Genetic disorder	References
NRXN1 deletion (2p16.3)	Wisniowiecka-Kowalnik et al., 2010
3q29 microdeletion	Baynam et al., 2006
Williams syndrome (7q11.23 deletion)	Kilincaslan et al., 2011
Bannayan–Riley–Ruvalcaba syndrome (PTEN mutation, 10q23.31)	Lynch et al., 2009
LEOPARD syndrome (PTPN11 mutation, 12q24.13)	Watanabe et al., 2011
15q13.3 microdeletion	Ben-Shachar et al., 2009
16p11.2 microdeletion	Rosenfeld et al., 2010; Sebat et al., 2007
Myotonic dystrophy 1 (DMPK mutation, 19q13.32)	Blondis et al., 1996; Paul and Allington-Smith, 1997
22q11.2 deletion syndrome (DiGeorge/velocardiofacial syndrome)	Gothelf et al., 2004; Pinto et al., 2010
Velocardiofacial syndrome (TBX1 mutation, 22q11.21)	Paylor et al., 2006
22q13.33 duplication including SHANK3	Durand et al., 2007
NLGN4X mutation (Xp22.31-p22.32)	Jamain et al., 2003
Nance–Horan syndrome (NHS deletion, Xp22.13)	PARIS study, unpublished
IL1RAPL1 mutation (Xp21.2-p21.3)	Piton et al., 2008
Lujan–Fryns syndrome (MED12 mutation, Xq13.1)	Schwartz et al., 2007
NLGN3 mutation (Xq13.1)	Jamain et al., 2003
Female-limited epilepsy and ID (PCDH19 mutation, Xq22.1)	Hynes et al., 2010
Fragile X syndrome (FMR1 mutation, Xq27.3)	Hagerman et al., 1994
Fragile X premutation (FMR1 premutation, Xq27.3)	Aziz et al., 2003
Klinefelter syndrome (XXY)	van Rijn et al., 2008
XYY syndrome	Gillberg, 1989
45,X/46,XY mosaicism	Fontenelle et al., 2004
Mitochondrial disorder (A3243G mutation)	Pons et al., 2004

METABOLIC DISORDERS ASSOCIATED WITH ASD

Several metabolic disorders have been associated with an autistic phenotype (Table 2.1.3). Although inborn errors of metabolism are rare and probably account for a small proportion of individuals with ASD, their diagnosis is important because some are potentially treatable. Metabolic disorders may be suspected on the basis of parental consanguinity, affected family members, early seizures, episodic decompensation, developmental regression, and coarse facial features. However, many recently described disorders can present as nonsyndromic ID and/or ASD and should therefore be considered in the etiological diagnosis of ASD (Kayser, 2008).

Phenylketonuria was identified as a relatively common cause of ASD in older studies, but since the

BOX 2.1.2

GENES INVOLVED IN NONSYNDROMIC ASD

There is a widely spread misconception that genetic disorders are only identified in individuals with ASD that have a syndromic presentation, i.e., that exhibit facial dysmorphism, congenital malformations, and/or neurologic abnormalities such as microcephaly or structural brain malformations. However, the evidence is clear that many genetic defects can be observed in children that present only with ASD, with no apparent physical abnormalities. For example, many genes involved in X-linked or autosomal nonsyndromic ID have also been implicated in nonsyndromic ASD (see table below and Figure 2.1.1). In addition, many other genes have been implicated in both syndromic as well as nonsyndromic forms of ASD/ID. The table below summarizes examples of genes for which nonsyndromic cases have been reported. For genes for which both nonsyndromic and syndromic cases have been reported, this is noted.

Gene	Gene name	Cytoband	Presentation	References
AUTOSOMAL DOMINANT				
FOXP1	forkhead box P1	3p14.1	Nonsyndromic	Hamdan et al., 2010; O'Roak et al., 2011
SYNGAP1	synaptic Ras GTPase-activating protein 1	6p21.32	Nonsyndromic	Hamdan et al., 2011; Pinto et al., 2010
SHANK2	SH3 and multiple ankyrin repeat domains 2	11q13.3	Nonsyndromic	Berkel et al., 2010; Pinto et al., 2010
GRIN2B	glutamate receptor, ionotropic, N-methyl D-aspartate 2B	12p13.1	Nonsyndromic/syndromic	Endele et al., 2010; O'Roak et al., 2011
SHANK3	SH3 and multiple ankyrin repeat domains 3	22q13.33	Nonsyndromic/syndromic	Durand et al., 2007; Moessner et al., 2007
AUTOSOMAL RECESSIVE				
PRSS12	protease, serine, 12 (neurotrypsin)	4q26	Nonsyndromic	(PARIS study, unpublished)
X-LINKED				
NLGN4X	neuroligin 4, X-linked	Xp22.31−p22.32	Nonsyndromic	Jamain et al., 2003; Laumonnier et al., 2004
AP1S2	adaptor-related protein complex 1, sigma 2 subunit	Xp22.2	Nonsyndromic/syndromic	Borck et al., 2008
PTCHD1	patched domain containing 1	Xp22.11	Nonsyndromic	Noor et al., 2010; Pinto et al., 2010
ARX	aristaless-related homeobox	Xp21.3	Nonsyndromic/syndromic	Partington et al., 2004; Turner et al., 2002
IL1RAPL1	interleukin 1 receptor accessory protein-like 1	Xp21.2−p21.3	Nonsyndromic	Pinto et al., 2010; Piton et al., 2008
CASK	calcium/calmodulin-dependent serine protein kinase	Xp11.4	Nonsyndromic/syndromic	Hackett et al., 2010
ZNF674	zinc finger protein 674	Xp11.3	Nonsyndromic	Lugtenberg et al., 2006
SYN1	synapsin I	Xp11.23	Nonsyndromic/syndromic	Fassio et al., 2011
ZNF81	zinc finger protein 81	Xp11.23	Nonsyndromic	Kleefstra et al., 2004
FTSJ1	FtsJ homolog 1	Xp11.23	Nonsyndromic	Froyen et al., 2007

<u>BOX 2.1.2— (cont'd)</u>

Gene	Gene name	Cytoband	Presentation	References
PQBP1	polyglutamine binding protein 1	Xq11.23	Nonsyndromic/syndromic	Cossee et al., 2006; Stevenson et al., 2005
KDM5C	lysine (K)-specific demethylase 5C	Xp11.22	Nonsyndromic/syndromic	Adegbola et al., 2008
IQSEC2	IQ motif and Sec7 domain 2	Xp11.22	Nonsyndromic	Shoubridge et al., 2010
FGD1	FYVE, RhoGEF and PH domain-containing 1	Xp11.22	Nonsyndromic/syndromic	Assumpcao et al., 1999
NLGN3	neuroligin 3	Xq13.1	Nonsyndromic	Jamain et al., 2003
ATRX	alpha thalassemia/mental retardation syndrome X-linked	Xq21.1	Nonsyndromic/syndromic	Wada and Gibbons, 2003
PCDH19	protocadherin 19	Xq22.1	Nonsyndromic/syndromic	Hynes et al., 2010; Marini et al., 2010
ACSL4	acyl-CoA synthetase long-chain family member 4	Xq22.3	Nonsyndromic	Longo et al., 2003; Meloni et al., 2002
AGTR2	angiotensin II receptor, type 2	Xq23	Nonsyndromic	Vervoort et al., 2002
UPF3B	UPF3 regulator of nonsense transcripts homolog B	Xq24	Nonsyndromic	Addington et al., 2011; Laumonnier et al., 2010
GRIA3	glutamate receptor, ionotrophic, AMPA 3	Xq25	Nonsyndromic	Chiyonobu et al., 2007; Wu et al., 2007
ARHGEF6	Rac/Cdc42 guanine nucleotide exchange factor 6	Xq26.3	Nonsyndromic	Kutsche et al., 2000
FMR1	fragile X mental retardation 1	Xq27.3	Nonsyndromic/syndromic	Hagerman et al., 2010
AFF2	AF4/FMR2 family, member 2	Xq28	Nonsyndromic	Stettner et al., 2011
SLC6A8	solute carrier family 6 (neurotransmitter transporter, creatine), member 8	Xq28	Nonsyndromic/syndromic	Poo-Arguelles et al., 2006; Sempere et al., 2009a
MECP2	methyl CpG binding protein 2	Xq28	Nonsyndromic/syndromic	Carney et al., 2003
RAB39B	RAB39B, member RAS oncogene family	Xq28	Nonsyndromic/syndromic	Giannandrea et al., 2010

introduction of newborn screening programs and with early dietary intervention, affected children can now expect to lead relatively normal lives (Baieli et al., 2003). Unfortunately, phenylketonuria is still identified among patients with ASD in emerging countries without neonatal testing or among subjects born before these screening programs were started (Steiner et al., 2007).

Cerebral creatine deficiency syndromes may be due to two disorders of creatine synthesis, arginine:glycine amidinotransferase deficiency (GATM) and guanidinoacetate methyltransferase deficiency (GAMT), inherited as autosomal recessive traits, or to creatine transporter deficiency (SLC6A8), an X-linked disorder (Longo et al., 2011). All three deficiencies are characterized by ID, severe speech impairment, epilepsy and autistic behavior (Table 2.1.3). Although GATM and GAMT mutations are very rare, creatine transporter deficiency could account for up to 1% of unexplained

TABLE 2.1.3 Disease Genes and Genetic Disorders Reported in Individuals with ASD: Examples of Clinical and Etiological Subgroups

Gene	Gene name	Cytoband	Disorder	Inheritance pattern	References reporting ASD
EARLY-ONSET EPILEPSY					
SCN1A	sodium channel, voltage-gated, type I, alpha subunit	2q24.3	Severe myoclonic epilepsy of infancy (Dravet syndrome)	Dominant	Marini et al., 2009; O'Roak et al., 2011
SCN2A	sodium channel, voltage-gated, type II, alpha subunit	2q24.3	Early infantile epileptic encephalopathy; benign familial infantile seizures	Dominant	Neale et al., 2012; Sanders et al., 2012
MEF2C	myocyte enhancer factor 2C	5q14.3	5q14.3 microdeletion syndrome	Dominant	Novara et al., 2010
ALDH7A1	aldehyde dehydrogenase 7 family, member A1	5q23.2	Pyridoxine-dependent epilepsy	Recessive	Burd et al., 2000; Mills et al., 2010
CNTNAP2	contactin associated protein-like 2	7q35–q36.1	Cortical dysplasia-focal epilepsy syndrome; Pitt–Hopkins-like syndrome-1	Recessive	Strauss et al., 2006; Zweier et al., 2009
STXBP1	syntaxin binding protein 1	9q34.11	Early infantile epileptic encephalopathy	Dominant	Milh et al., 2011; Neale et al., 2012
FOXG1	forkhead box G1	14q12	Congenital variant of Rett syndrome	Dominant	Brunetti-Pierri et al., 2011; Philippe et al., 2010
PAFAH1B1	platelet-activating factor acetylhydrolase 1b, regulatory subunit 1	17p13.3	Isolated lissencephaly	Dominant	Saillour et al., 2009
CDKL5	cyclin-dependent kinase-like 5	Xp22.13	Early infantile epileptic encephalopathy	X-linked	Archer et al., 2006; Russo et al., 2009
ARX	aristaless-related homeobox	Xp21.3	Early infantile epileptic encephalopathy; brain malformations with abnormal genitalia; nonsyndromic ID	X-linked	Partington et al., 2004; Turner et al., 2002
SYN1	synapsin I	Xp11.23	X-linked epilepsy with variable learning disabilities and behavior disorders	X-linked	Fassio et al., 2011; Garcia et al., 2004
PCDH19	protocadherin 19	Xq22.1	X-linked female-limited epilepsy and cognitive impairment; early infantile epileptic encephalopathy	X-linked	Hynes et al., 2010; Marini et al., 2010
DCX	doublecortin	Xq22.3	X-linked lissencephaly	X-linked	Leger et al., 2008
SLC9A6	solute carrier family 9 (sodium/hydrogen exchanger), member 6	Xq26.3	Syndromic X-linked ID, Christianson type (ID, microcephaly, epilepsy, and ataxia)	X-linked	Garbern et al., 2010
RAB39B	RAB39B, member RAS oncogene family	Xq28	X-linked ID associated with autism, epilepsy, and macrocephaly	X-linked	Giannandrea et al., 2010
METABOLIC DISORDERS					
Disorders of purine and pyrimidine metabolism					
ADSL	adenylosuccinate lyase	22q13.1	Adenylosuccinate lyase deficiency (purine synthesis disorder)	Recessive	Spiegel et al., 2006

(Continued)

TABLE 2.1.3 Disease Genes and Genetic Disorders Reported in Individuals with ASD: Examples of Clinical and Etiological Subgroups — cont'd

Gene	Gene name	Cytoband	Disorder	Inheritance pattern	References reporting ASD
DPYD	dihydropyrimidine dehydrogenase	1p21.3	Dihydropyrimidine dehydrogenase deficiency (disorder of the pyrimidine degradation pathway)	Recessive	van Kuilenburg et al., 2009; Van Kuilenburg et al., 1999)
Creatine deficiency syndromes					
SLC6A8	solute carrier family 6 (neurotransmitter transporter, creatine), member 8	Xq28	Brain creatine deficiency can be caused by mutation in the creatine transporter gene *SLC6A8*, or by defects in the biosynthesis of creatine (*GAMT* and *GATM* genes)	X-linked	Poo-Arguelles et al., 2006; Sempere et al., 2009a
GATM	glycine amidinotransferase	15q21.1	Arginine:glycine amidinotransferase (AGAT) deficiency	Recessive	Battini et al., 2002
GAMT	guanidinoacetate N-methyltransferase	19p13.3	Guanidinoacetate methyltransferase (GAMT) deficiency	Recessive	Sempere et al., 2009b
Disorder of cholesterol synthesis					
DHCR7	7-dehydrocholesterol reductase	11q13.4	Smith–Lemli–Opitz syndrome	Recessive	Sikora et al., 2006; Tierney et al., 2006
Defect of phenylalanine metabolism					
PAH	phenylalanine hydroxylase	12q23.2	Phenylketonuria	Recessive	Baieli et al., 2003; Steiner et al., 2007
Disorders of vitamin metabolism					
BTD	biotinidase	3p24.3	Biotinidase deficiency (defect in the recycling of the vitamin biotin)	Recessive	Zaffanello et al., 2003
ALDH7A1	aldehyde dehydrogenase 7 family, member A1	5q23.2	Pyridoxine-dependent epilepsy (vitamin B6)	Recessive	Burd et al., 2000; Mills et al., 2010
Defect of GABA catabolism					
ALDH5A1	aldehyde dehydrogenase 5 family, member A1	6p22.2	Succinic semialdehyde dehydrogenase deficiency (gamma-hydroxybutyric aciduria)	Recessive	Knerr et al., 2008; Pearl et al., 2003
Lysosomal storage disorders					
SGSH	N-sulfoglucosamine sulfohydrolase	17q25.3	Mucopolysaccharidosis IIIA (Sanfilippo syndrome A)	Recessive	Petit et al., 1996; Wolanczyk et al., 2000
NAGLU	N-acetylglucosaminidase, alpha	17q21.31	Mucopolysaccharidosis IIIB (Sanfilippo syndrome B)	Recessive	Heron et al., 2011
HGSNAT	heparan-alpha-glucosaminide N-acetyltransferase	8p11.21	Mucopolysaccharidosis IIIC (Sanfilippo syndrome C)	Recessive	Heron et al., 2011
GNS	glucosamine (N-acetyl)-6-sulfatase	12q14.3	Mucopolysaccharidosis IIID (Sanfilippo syndrome D)	Recessive	Heron et al., 2011

Folate deficiency syndrome

Gene	Full name	Location	Disorder	Inheritance	Reference
FOLR1	folate receptor 1	11q13.4	Cerebral folate transport deficiency	Recessive	Cario et al., 2009
Urea cycle disorder					
OTC	ornithine carbamoyltransferase	Xp11.4	Ornithine transcarbamylase deficiency	X-linked	Gorker and Tuzun, 2005
Defect of amino acid metabolism					
MUT	methylmalonyl CoA mutase	6p12.3	Methylmalonic aciduria	Recessive	de Baulny et al., 2005
JOUBERT SYNDROME AND RELATED CILIOPATHIES					
AHI1	Abelson helper integration site 1	6q23.3	Joubert syndrome 3	Recessive	Ozonoff et al., 1999; Takahashi et al., 2005
NPHP1	nephronophthisis 1	2q13	Joubert syndrome 4; nephronophthisis 1, juvenile	Recessive	Tory et al., 2007
CEP290	centrosomal protein 290kDa	12q21.32	Joubert syndrome 5; Leber congenital amaurosis 10; Bardet–Biedl syndrome 14	Recessive	Coppieters et al., 2010; Perrault et al., 2007; Tory et al., 2007
RPGRIP1L	RPGRIP1-like (retinitis pigmentosa GTPase regulator-like)	16q12.2	Joubert syndrome 7	Recessive	Doherty et al., 2010
GUCY2D	guanylate cyclase 2D, membrane	17p13.1	Leber congenital amaurosis 1	Recessive	Coppieters et al., 2010
RPE65	retinal pigment epithelium-specific protein 65kDa	1p31.3	Leber congenital amaurosis 2	Recessive	Coppieters et al., 2010; Yzer et al., 2003
MKKS	McKusick–Kaufman syndrome	20p12.2	Bardet–Biedl syndrome 6; McKusick–Kaufman syndrome	Recessive	Barnett et al., 2002; Moore et al., 2005
BBS10	Bardet–Biedl syndrome 10	12q21.2	Bardet–Biedl syndrome 10	Recessive	Deveault et al., 2011
MUSCULAR DYSTROPHIES					
DMD	dystrophin	Xp21.2–p21.1	Muscular dystrophy, Duchenne and Becker types	X-linked	Hinton et al., 2009; Young et al., 2008
DMPK	dystrophia myotonica-protein kinase	19q13.32	Myotonic dystrophy 1 (Steinert disease)	Dominant	Ekstrom et al., 2008
POMGNT1	protein-O-linked mannose beta1,2-N-acetylglucosaminyltransferase	1p34.1	Muscle-eye-brain disease (congenital muscular dystrophy, structural eye abnormalities and lissencephaly)	Recessive	Haliloglu et al., 2004; Hehr et al., 2007
POMT1	protein-O-mannosyltransferase 1	9q34.13	Limb-girdle muscular dystrophy with ID; Walker–Warburg syndrome	Recessive	D'Amico et al., 2006

ID = intellectual disability.

TABLE 2.1.4 Disease Genes and Genetic Disorders Reported in Individuals with ASD: Examples of Functional Pathways

Gene	Gene name	Cytoband	Disorder	Inheritance pattern	References reporting ASD
RAS/MAPK SIGNALING PATHWAY[a]					
BRAF	v-raf murine sarcoma viral oncogene homolog B1 (BRAF, serine/threonine kinase)	7q34	Cardio-facio-cutaneous syndrome, Noonan syndrome, LEOPARD syndrome	Dominant	Nava et al., 2007; Nystrom et al., 2008
KRAS	v-Ki-ras2 Kirsten rat sarcoma viral oncogene homolog (KRAS, small G-protein)	12p12.1	Cardio-facio-cutaneous syndrome, Noonan syndrome	Dominant	Nava et al., 2007; Nystrom et al., 2008
MAP2K1	mitogen-activated protein kinase kinase 1 (MEK1, tyrosine/serine/threonine kinase)	15q22.31	Cardio-facio-cutaneous syndrome	Dominant	Nava et al., 2007
PTPN11	protein tyrosine phosphatase, non-receptor type 11 (SHP2, tyrosine phosphatase)	12q24.13	Noonan syndrome, LEOPARD syndrome	Dominant	Pierpont et al., 2009; Watanabe et al., 2011
HRAS	v-Ha-ras Harvey rat sarcoma viral oncogene homolog (HRAS, small G-protein)	11p15.5	Costello syndrome	Dominant	Kerr et al., 2006
NF1	neurofibromin 1 (neurofibromin, RAS-GTPase activator protein)	17q11.2	Neurofibromatosis type 1	Dominant	Williams and Hersh, 1998
SPRED1	sprouty-related, EVH1 domain-containing 1 (SPRED1, inhibitor of Raf activation by Ras)	15q14	Neurofibromatosis type 1-like syndrome (Legius syndrome)	Dominant	Laycock-van Spyk et al., 2011
SYNGAP1	synaptic Ras GTPase-activating protein 1 (SYNGAP1, RAS-GTPase activator protein)	6p21.32	Nonsyndromic ID	Dominant	Hamdan et al., 2011; Pinto et al., 2010
CHANNELOPATHIES					
SCN1A	sodium channel, voltage-gated, type I, alpha	2q24.3	Severe myoclonic epilepsy of infancy (Dravet syndrome)	Dominant	Marini et al., 2009; O'Roak et al., 2011
SCN2A	sodium channel, voltage-gated, type II, alpha	2q24.3	Early infantile epileptic encephalopathy; benign familial infantile seizures	Dominant	Neale et al., 2012; Sanders et al., 2012
CACNA1C	calcium channel, voltage-dependent, L type, alpha 1C subunit	12p13.33	Timothy syndrome (long QT syndrome with syndactyly)	Dominant	Splawski et al., 2004
CACNA1F	calcium channel, voltage-dependent, L type, alpha 1F subunit	Xp11.23	X-linked incomplete congenital stationary night blindness, severe form	X-linked	Hemara-Wahanui et al., 2005
KCNJ11	potassium inwardly-rectifying channel, subfamily J, member 11	11p15.1	DEND syndrome (developmental delay, epilepsy, and neonatal diabetes)	Dominant	Flanagan et al., 2007; Tonini et al., 2006
CELL-ADHESION MOLECULES					
NRXN1	neurexin 1	2p16.3	Disrupted in ASD, ID, and other neurodevelopmental and psychiatric disorders (dominant?); Pitt–Hopkins-like syndrome-2 (recessive)	Dominant?/ recessive	Ching et al., 2010; Pinto et al., 2010; Szatmari et al., 2007; Zweier et al., 2009

Gene	Protein	Locus	Phenotype	Inheritance	References
CNTNAP2	contactin-associated protein-like 2	7q35–q36.1	Cortical dysplasia-focal epilepsy syndrome and Pitt–Hopkins-like syndrome-1 (recessive). Deletions or chromosomal rearrangements disrupting a *single* copy of CNTNAP2 have been reported in patients with ASD, ID, epilepsy, schizophrenia, and bipolar disorder as well as in healthy subjects; their clinical significance is unknown	Recessive	Strauss et al., 2006; Zweier et al., 2009
HEPACAM	hepatic and glial cell adhesion molecule	11q24.2	Megalencephalic leukoencephalopathy with subcortical cysts	Recessive	Lopez-Hernandez et al., 2011
NLGN4X	neuroligin 4, X-linked	Xp22.31–p22.32	Nonsyndromic X-linked ASD and/or ID	X-linked	Jamain et al., 2003; Laumonnier et al., 2004
NLGN3	neuroligin 3	Xq13.1	Nonsyndromic X-linked ASD and/or ID	X-linked	Jamain et al., 2003
PCDH19	protocadherin 19	Xq22.1	X-linked female-limited epilepsy and cognitive impairment	X-linked	Hynes et al., 2010; Marini et al., 2010
L1CAM	L1 cell adhesion molecule	Xq28	Syndromic X-linked ID with hydrocephalus, MASA (mental retardation, aphasia, shuffling gait, and adducted thumbs) syndrome	X-linked	Simonati et al., 2006
mTOR SIGNALING PATHWAY[b]					
PTEN	phosphatase and tensin homolog (tyrosine phosphatase)	10q23.31	PTEN hamartoma-tumor syndrome (including Bannayan–Riley–Ruvalcaba syndrome and Cowden syndrome); macrocephaly/autism syndrome	Dominant	Butler et al., 2005; Buxbaum et al., 2007; McBride et al., 2010
TSC1	tuberous sclerosis 1 (tumor suppressor protein)	9q34.13	Tuberous sclerosis complex	Dominant	Numis et al., 2011
TSC2	tuberous sclerosis 2 (tumor suppressor protein)	16p13.3	Tuberous sclerosis complex	Dominant	Numis et al., 2011
EPIGENETIC REGULATION[c]					
MBD5	methyl-CpG-binding domain protein 5 (methyl DNA binding)	2q23.1	2q23.1 microdeletion syndrome (ID, severe speech impairment, seizures, short stature, microcephaly, and mild dysmorphic features)	Dominant	Talkowski et al., 2011
NSD1	nuclear receptor-binding SET domain protein 1 (histone methyltransferase)	5q35.2–q35.3	Sotos syndrome (overgrowth syndrome characterized by macrocephaly, advanced bone age, characteristic facial features and learning disabilities)	Dominant	Schaefer and Lutz, 2006; Ververi et al., 2012
ARID1B	AT-rich interactive domain 1B, SWI1-like (chromatin remodeling)	6q25.3	ID, speech impairment, autism, corpus callosum abnormalities, Coffin–Siris syndrome	Dominant	Halgren et al., 2011; Santen et al., 2012

(Continued)

TABLE 2.1.4 Disease Genes and Genetic Disorders Reported in Individuals with ASD: Examples of Functional Pathways – cont'd

Gene	Gene name	Cytoband	Disorder	Inheritance pattern	References reporting ASD
CHD7	chromodomain helicase DNA-binding protein 7 (ATPase/helicase)	8q12.2	CHARGE syndrome (coloboma, heart anomaly, choanal atresia, retardation, genital and ear anomalies)	Dominant	Johansson et al., 2006
SMARCA2	SWI/SNF-related matrix-associated (ATPase/helicase)	9p24.3	Nicolaides–Baraitser syndrome, Coffin–Siris syndrome	Dominant	Sousa et al., 2009; Van Houdt et al., 2012
EHMT1	euchromatic histone-lysine N-methyltransferase 1 (histone methyltransferase)	9q34.3	Kleefstra syndrome/9q subtelomeric deletion syndrome (ID, distinctive facial features, microcephaly, and hypotonia)	Dominant	Kleefstra et al., 2009
FOXG1	forkhead box G1 (transcription regulation)	14q12	Congenital variant of Rett syndrome	Dominant	Brunetti-Pierri et al., 2011; Philippe et al., 2010
CREBBP	CREB-binding protein (histone acetyltransferase)	16p13.3	Rubinstein–Taybi syndrome (ID, characteristic facial features, broad thumbs and big toes)	Dominant	Schorry et al., 2008
SRCAP	Snf2-related CREBBP activator protein (chromatin remodeling)	16p11.2	Floating–Harbor syndrome	Dominant	Hood et al., 2012; White et al., 2010
CDKL5	cyclin-dependent kinase-like 5 (kinase)	Xp22.13	Early infantile epileptic encephalopathy	X-linked	Archer et al., 2006; Russo et al., 2009
ZNF674	zinc finger family member 674 (DNA binding)	Xp11.3	Nonsyndromic X-linked ID	X-linked	Lugtenberg et al., 2006
KDM5C JARID1C	lysine (K)-specific demethylase 5C (histone demethylase)	Xp11.22	Large spectrum of phenotypes including ID with microcephaly, spasticity, short stature, epilepsy, and facial anomalies, as well as nonsyndromic ID	X-linked	Adegbola et al., 2008
PHF8	PHD finger protein 8 (histone demethylase)	Xp11.22	Siderius–Hamel syndrome (ID with cleft lip or cleft palate)	X-linked	Qiao et al., 2008
MED12	mediator complex subunit 12 (transcription regulation)	Xq13.1	Lujan–Fryns syndrome (X-linked ID with marfanoid habitus)	X-linked	Lerma-Carrillo et al., 2006; Schwartz et al., 2007
ATRX	transcriptional regulator ATRX (ATPase/ helicase)	Xq21.1	Large spectrum of phenotypes including ATRX syndrome (alpha thalassemia/ mental retardation syndrome X-linked) and nonsyndromic ID	X-linked	Wada and Gibbons, 2003
PHF6	PHD finger protein 6 (histone binding)	Xq26.2	Borjeson–Forssman–Lehmann syndrome (ID, epilepsy, and hypogonadism)	X-linked	de Winter et al., 2009
MECP2	methyl-CpG-binding protein 2 (methyl DNA binding)	Xq28	Rett syndrome in females; congenital encephalopathy or nonsyndromic ID in males; MECP2 duplication syndrome, mostly in males	X-linked	Carney et al., 2003; Ramocki et al., 2010

[a]The protein name and its function are indicated in parentheses after the gene name.
[b]The protein function is indicated in parentheses after the gene name.
[c]The epigenetic function is indicated in parentheses after the gene name.
ASD = autism spectrum disorder; ID = intellectual disability.

ID in males (Clark et al., 2006). Because the presentation is nonsyndromic and autistic behavior is common, this condition could be underdiagnosed in populations of lower functioning males with ASD.

Autism may also occur in the context of mitochondrial disorders, resulting either from mutations in mitochondrial DNA or, more commonly, in nuclear DNA genes encoding mitochondrial-targeted proteins (see Chapter 2.5). Mitochondrial disorders can present with a vast range of symptoms, severity, age of onset, and outcome, with a minimum prevalence estimated at 1:5,000.

Understanding how metabolic disorders affect brain development and function can lead to a better understanding of the pathophysiology of ASD. At the same time, the frequently indirect nature of this relationship may make such studies more challenging than, for example, studying how synaptic genes alter brain functioning. However, because many metabolic disorders are treatable, understanding the range of metabolic disorders associated with ASD and testing for them can provide immediate clinical benefits, and allow for genetic counseling.

OTHER EXAMPLES OF ETIOLOGICAL SUBGROUPS ASSOCIATED WITH ASD

Joubert syndrome is a clinically and genetically heterogeneous group of disorders characterized by a distinctive cerebellar and brainstem malformation, cerebellar ataxia, ID, and breathing abnormalities, sometimes including retinal dystrophy and renal disease. ASD is a relatively frequent finding in individuals with Joubert syndrome, present in 13–36% of patients (Table 2.1.1). Sixteen genes have been implicated in Joubert syndrome, the majority very recently; thus, it is not surprising that so far only four of these genes have been reported to be mutated in subjects with ASD/autistic traits (Table 2.1.3). Joubert syndrome and related disorders arise from ciliary dysfunction and are collectively termed ciliopathies. Other ciliopathies reported in subjects with ASD include Leber congenital amaurosis and Bardet–Biedl syndrome, both of which exhibit phenotypic overlap with Joubert syndrome (Table 2.1.3). The means by which cilia are involved in neurodevelopmental processes, and by which ciliopathies lead to neurodevelopmental disorders, are areas of active research. One exciting emerging finding is that primary (or nonmotile) cilia, found on most neurons and astrocytes, play roles as modulators of signal transduction during both brain development and homeostasis (Lee and Gleeson, 2011). The primary cilia can mediate signaling through sonic hedgehog, wingless, planar cell polarity, and fibroblast growth factor pathways.

Another group of disorders that can be associated with ASD is muscular dystrophies (Table 2.1.3). Duchenne and Becker muscular dystrophies are caused by deficient expression of the cytoskeletal protein dystrophin, coded by the *DMD* gene on chromosome Xp21.2–p21.1. One-third of the children with Duchenne muscular dystrophy and about 12% of those with the Becker type also have ID. A small subgroup of these boys with both of these disorders also have ASD, with frequencies varying between 3% and 19% (Hinton et al., 2009; Kumagai et al., 2001; Wu et al., 2005). Several maternally inherited exonic duplications of *DMD* have been identified in males ascertained for ASD, with no documented muscle disease (Pagnamenta et al., 2011; Pinto et al., 2010), suggestive of the mild end of the spectrum of dystrophinopathies seen in Becker muscular dystrophy, with later onset or subclinical muscle involvement. Another form of muscular dystrophy that includes cases with autistic features is myotonic dystrophy type 1, also known as Steinert disease, caused by expansion of a CTG trinucleotide repeat in the 3'-untranslated region in the *DMPK* gene (Table 2.1.3). The clinical findings span a continuum from mild to severe. In a study of 57 children with myotonic dystrophy type 1, 49% were found to have ASD; the more clinically severe the myotonic dystrophy, the higher the frequency of children with autistic features (Ekstrom et al., 2008). This may be an underdiagnosed disease entity in autistic populations (Coleman and Gillberg, 2012).

Dysregulation of the RAS/MAPK cascade is the common molecular basis for multiple congenital anomaly syndromes known as neuro-cardio-facio-cutaneous syndromes, characterized by a distinctive facial appearance, heart defects, musculocutaneous abnormalities, and ID, including Noonan syndrome, LEOPARD syndrome (lentigines, electrocardiogram abnormalities, ocular hypertelorism, pulmonic valvular stenosis, abnormalities of genitalia, retardation of growth, and deafness), cardio-facio-cutaneous syndrome, and Costello syndrome (Table 2.1.4) (Samuels et al., 2009). These overlapping phenotypes can arise from heterozygous mutations in many genes, including *PTPN11*, *BRAF*, *RAF1*, *KRAS*, *HRAS*, *MAP2K1*, *MAP2K2*, *SOS1*, and *SHOC2*. Neurofibromatosis type I and neurofibromatosis type I-like syndrome, which are caused by loss-of-function mutations of *NF1* and *SPRED1*, respectively, can also be included in the same disease entity (Aoki et al., 2008). As shown in Table 2.1.3, all these disorders have been reported in subjects with ASD. In particular, ASD was observed in 8% of 65 children with Noonan syndrome (Pierpont et al., 2009), as well as in several patients with cardio-facio-cutaneous syndrome or

Noonan syndrome with *BRAF*, *KRAS* or *MAP2K1* mutations (Nava et al., 2007; Nystrom et al., 2008).

MYRIAD BIOLOGICAL PATHWAYS

When considering genes involved in autism, neurobiologists usually think about synaptic genes such as those coding for the postsynaptic cell adhesion molecules neuroligins 3 and 4 (*NLGN3*, *NLGN4X*), their presynaptic partner neurexin 1 (*NRXN1*), and the postsynaptic scaffolding proteins *SHANK2* and *SHANK3* (Betancur et al., 2009). In addition to this pathway (described in Chapter 4.7), further evidence implicating synaptic dysfunction in the pathogenesis of ASD has come from the study of genetic disorders with increased rates of ASD, such as fragile X syndrome (*FRM1*), Rett syndrome (*MECP2*), tuberous sclerosis (*TSC1* and *TSC2*) and Angelman syndrome (*UBE3A*). Rare mutations in numerous other genes encoding pre- and postsynaptic proteins have also been reported in ID and ASD, including *STXBP1* and *SYNGAP*, as well as the X-linked genes *AP1S2*, *ARHGEF6*, *CASK*, *GRIA3*, *FGD1*, *IQSEC2*, *IL1RAPL1*, *OPHN1*, *RAB39B*, and *SYN1* (Figure 2.1.1) (for references implicating these genes in ASD, see Betancur, 2011; for a general review, see van Bokhoven, 2011).

Although the focus on the synaptic pathway in recent years has contributed to our understanding of the patho-physiology of autism, there are dozens of other non-synaptic genes that have been implicated in ASD and which encompass a wide range of biological functions and cellular processes. Mechanisms by which such genes disrupt brain and neuronal development and function will provide a deeper understanding of ASD pathogenesis. Some examples of biological pathways and organelles recurrently implicated in ASD are highlighted in Tables 2.1.3 and 2.1.4. In addition to the genes involved in ciliopathies (Table 2.1.3) and the RAS/MAPK signaling pathway (Table 2.1.4) mentioned above, Table 2.1.4 shows genes involved in channelopathies, genes coding for cell-adhesion molecules and genes implicated in the protein kinase mammalian target of rapamycin (mTOR) signaling pathway. Hyperactivation of mTOR as a consequence of loss-of-function mutations in the genes *TSC1*, *TSC2*, and *PTEN* is responsible for the development of tuberous sclerosis, *PTEN* hamartoma-tumor syndrome (including Cowden syndrome, Bannayan–Riley–Ruvalcaba syndrome, and Proteus syndrome), and macrocephaly/autism syndrome (for review, see de Vries, 2010). Molecularly targeted treatments using mTOR inhibitors (such as rapamycin) are currently in clinical trials, providing great promise and hope.

Another emerging pathway involves ASD/ID genes that encode regulators of chromatin structure and of chromatin-mediated transcription (for review, see van Bokhoven and Kramer, 2010). Table 2.1.4 shows the genes mutated in ASD involved in epigenetic regulation of neuronal gene expression. Prominent examples of epigenetic ASD/ID genes include *MECP2*, *CHD7* (CHARGE sydrome), *EHMT1* (Kleefstra syndrome), and the recently implicated gene *MBD5* (2q23.1 microdeletion syndrome), all listed in Table 2.1.1 as being frequently associated with ASD.

CONCLUSION

The findings discussed in this review clearly indicate that autism represents the final common pathway for hundreds of genetic and genomic disorders. Despite the abundant evidence, this etiological heterogeneity is still not widely recognized by autism researchers, and most studies fail to take it into account. The genetic overlap and the frequent comorbidity of ASD, ID, and epilepsy indicate that the disruption of essential neurodevelopmental processes can give rise to a wide range of manifestations, where the final outcome is likely modulated by the genetic background of each individual as well as other factors including possibly environmental and stochastic factors. Increased understanding of the common genetic, molecular, and cellular mechanisms underlying these neurodevelopmental disorders may provide a framework for novel therapeutic interventions.

Chromosome microarray analysis has revolutionized the molecular diagnostic process in ASD and other neuro-developmental conditions and is now recommended as a first-line test in the genetic workup of these children, providing an etiological diagnosis in 10 to 15% of cases. Novel high-throughput whole-exome and whole-genome sequencing technologies have hugely accelerated the mutation finding process for Mendelian disorders in the past two years, and hopefully will soon become a first-line approach in the etiological exploration of patients with ASD, replacing targeted sequencing of candidate disease genes (Chapter 2.4).

Currently the most applicable benefit of genetic testing is family planning. A prospective longitudinal study of 664 infants with an older biological sibling with ASD found that 18.7% developed ASD (Ozonoff et al., 2011). Although many of the mutations associated with autism so far identified are *de novo*, future siblings are at risk in the cases where the variant is inherited from a parent, such as in autosomal dominant disorders with variable expressivity inherited from mildly affected parents (e.g., tuberous sclerosis, *PTEN* related syndromes, 22q11 deletion syndrome), autosomal recessive disorders or maternally transmitted X-linked disorders (or even a paternally transmitted X-linked disorder, as for *PCDH19*). Germinal mosaicism in one of the parents can also explain rare instances of familial recurrence. This mechanism has been implicated in a surprising number of cases of siblings with ASD carrying apparently *de novo* mutations, not found in the parents' DNA (e.g., *SHANK3* mutations, and deletions, *NRXN1* deletions, *NLGN4X* mutation, 16p11.2 deletion, 2q23.1 deletion, Rett syndrome and tuberous sclerosis) and may remain unrecognized in sporadic cases in small families.

An etiological diagnosis has important benefits for the patients with ASD and their families. For the patients, it can help anticipate and manage associated medical and behavioral comorbidities. For the parents, the benefits include relieving anxiety and uncertainty, limiting further costly or invasive diagnostic testing, improving understanding of treatment and prognosis, genetic counseling regarding recurrence risk as well as preventing recurrence through screening for carriers and prenatal testing. A specific disease diagnosis can be empowering to parents who wish to become involved in more targeted support and research groups. For the medical and research community, each child who is accurately diagnosed adds to our presently limited understanding of the pathological cascades which result in autistic features; undoubtedly new findings will include previously unrecognized disease mechanisms. For the neurobiologist especially, the myriad genetic findings in ASD offer a rich source of targets for further study, providing a window into brain and neuronal development and function. The deeper understanding of these brain and neuronal processes will ultimately lead to better outcomes in ASD and other neurodevelopmental disorders.

References

Abrahams, B.S., Geschwind, D.H., 2008. Advances in autism genetics: On the threshold of a new neurobiology. Nature Reviews Genetics 9, 341–355.

Addington, A.M., Gauthier, J., Piton, A., Hamdan, F.F., Raymond, A., Gogtay, N., et al., 2011. A novel frameshift mutation in UPF3B identified in brothers affected with childhood onset schizophrenia and autism spectrum disorders. Molecular Psychiatry 16, 238–239.

Adegbola, A., Gao, H., Sommer, S., Browning, M., 2008. A novel mutation in JARID1C/SMCX in a patient with autism spectrum disorder (ASD). American Journal of Medical Genetics Part A 146A, 505–511.

Alliman, S., Coppinger, J., Marcadier, J., Thiese, H., Brock, P., Shafer, S., et al., 2010. Clinical and molecular characterization of individuals with recurrent genomic disorder at 10q22.3q23.2. Clinical Genetics 78, 162–168.

Antshel, K.M., Aneja, A., Strunge, L., Peebles, J., Fremont, W.P., Stallone, K., et al., 2007. Autistic spectrum disorders in velo-cardio facial syndrome (22q11.2 deletion). Journal of Autism and Developmental Disorders 37, 1776–1786.

Aoki, Y., Niihori, T., Narumi, Y., Kure, S., Matsubara, Y., 2008. The RAS/MAPK syndromes: Novel roles of the RAS pathway in human genetic disorders. Human Mutation 29, 992–1006.

Archer, H.L., Evans, J., Edwards, S., Colley, J., Newbury-Ecob, R., O'Callaghan, F., et al., 2006. CDKL5 mutations cause infantile spasms, early onset seizures, and severe mental retardation in female patients. Journal of Medical Genetics 43, 729–734.

Assumpcao, F., Santos, R.C., Rosario, M., Mercadante, M., 1999. Brief report: Autism and Aarskog syndrome. Journal of Autism and Developmental Disorders 29, 179–181.

Aziz, M., Stathopulu, E., Callias, M., Taylor, C., Turk, J., Oostra, B., et al., 2003. Clinical features of boys with fragile X premutations and intermediate alleles. American Journal of Medical Genetics Part B: Neuropsychiatric Genetics 121B, 119–127.

Baieli, S., Pavone, L., Meli, C., Fiumara, A., Coleman, M., 2003. Autism and phenylketonuria. Journal of Autism and Developmental Disorders 33, 201–204.

Balciuniene, J., Feng, N., Iyadurai, K., Hirsch, B., Charnas, L., Bill, B.R., et al., 2007. Recurrent 10q22-q23 deletions: A genomic disorder on 10q associated with cognitive and behavioral abnormalities. American Journal of Human Genetics 80, 938–947.

Ballif, B.C., Theisen, A., Coppinger, J., Gowans, G.C., Hersh, J.H., Madan-Khetarpal, S., et al., 2008. Expanding the clinical phenotype of the 3q29 microdeletion syndrome and characterization of the reciprocal microduplication. Molecular Cytogenetics 1, 8.

Barnett, S., Reilly, S., Carr, L., Ojo, I., Beales, P.L., Charman, T., 2002. Behavioural phenotype of Bardet-Biedl syndrome. Journal of Medical Genetics 39, e76.

Battini, R., Leuzzi, V., Carducci, C., Tosetti, M., Bianchi, M.C., Item, C.B., et al., 2002. Creatine depletion in a new case with AGAT deficiency: Clinical and genetic study in a large pedigree. Molecular Genetics and Metabolism 77, 326–331.

Baynam, G., Goldblatt, J., Townshend, S., 2006. A case of 3q29 microdeletion with novel features and a review of cytogenetically visible terminal 3q deletions. Clinical Dysmorphology 15, 145–148.

Ben-Shachar, S., Lanpher, B., German, J.R., Qasaymeh, M., Potocki, L., Nagamani, S.C., et al., 2009. Microdeletion 15q13.3: A locus with incomplete penetrance for autism, mental retardation, and psychiatric disorders. Journal of Medical Genetics 46, 382–388.

Berkel, S., Marshall, C.R., Weiss, B., Howe, J., Roeth, R., Moog, U., et al., 2010. Mutations in the SHANK2 synaptic scaffolding gene in autism spectrum disorder and mental retardation. Nature Genetics 42, 489–491.

Betancur, C., 2011. Etiological heterogeneity in autism spectrum disorders: More than 100 genetic and genomic disorders and still counting. Brain Research 1380, 42–77.

Betancur, C., Sakurai, T., Buxbaum, J.D., 2009. The emerging role of synaptic cell-adhesion pathways in the pathogenesis of autism spectrum disorders. Trends Neuroscience 32, 402–412.

Bhuiyan, Z.A., Klein, M., Hammond, P., van Haeringen, A., Mannens, M.M., Van Berckelaer-Onnes, I., et al., 2006. Genotype-phenotype correlations of 39 patients with Cornelia De Lange syndrome: The Dutch experience. Journal of Medical Genetics 43, 568–575.

Bi, W., Sapir, T., Shchelochkov, O.A., Zhang, F., Withers, M.A., Hunter, J.V., et al., 2009. Increased LIS1 expression affects human and mouse brain development. Nature Genetics 41, 168–177.

Bishop, D.V., Jacobs, P.A., Lachlan, K., Wellesley, D., Barnicoat, A., Boyd, P.A., et al., 2011. Autism, language and communication in children with sex chromosome trisomies. Archives of Disease in Childhood 96, 954–959.

Blondis, T.A., Cook Jr., E., Koza-Taylor, P., Finn, T., 1996. Asperger syndrome associated with Steinert's myotonic dystrophy. Developmental Medicine & Child Neurology 38, 840–847.

Borck, G., Molla-Herman, A., Boddaert, N., Encha-Razavi, F., Philippe, A., Robel, L., et al., 2008. Clinical, cellular, and neuropathological consequences of AP1S2 mutations: Further delineation of a recognizable X-linked mental retardation syndrome. Human Mutation 29, 966–974.

Bruining, H., Swaab, H., Kas, M., van Engeland, H., 2009. Psychiatric characteristics in a self-selected sample of boys with Klinefelter syndrome. Pediatrics 123, e865–e870.

Brunetti-Pierri, N., Berg, J.S., Scaglia, F., Belmont, J., Bacino, C.A., Sahoo, T., et al., 2008. Recurrent reciprocal 1q21.1 deletions and duplications associated with microcephaly or macrocephaly and developmental and behavioral abnormalities. Nature Genetics 40, 1466–1471.

Brunetti-Pierri, N., Paciorkowski, A.R., Ciccone, R., Mina, E.D., Bonaglia, M.C., Borgatti, R., et al., 2011. Duplications of FOXG1 in 14q12 are associated with developmental epilepsy, mental retardation, and severe speech impairment. European Journal of Human Genetics 19, 102–107.

Bruno, D.L., Anderlid, B.M., Lindstrand, A., van Ravenswaaij-Arts, C., Ganesamoorthy, D., Lundin, J., et al., 2010. Further molecular and clinical delineation of co-locating 17p13.3 microdeletions and microduplications that show distinctive phenotypes. Journal of Medical Genetics 47, 299–311.

Burd, L., Stenehjem, A., Franceschini, L.A., Kerbeshian, J., 2000. A 15-year follow-up of a boy with pyridoxine (vitamin B6)-dependent seizures with autism, breath holding, and severe mental retardation. Journal of Child Neurology 15, 763–765.

Butler, M.G., Dasouki, M.J., Zhou, X.P., Talebizadeh, Z., Brown, M., Takahashi, T.N., et al., 2005. Subset of individuals with autism spectrum disorders and extreme macrocephaly associated with germline PTEN tumour suppressor gene mutations. Journal of Medical Genetics 42, 318–321.

Buxbaum, J.D., Cai, G., Chaste, P., Nygren, G., Goldsmith, J., Reichert, J., et al., 2007. Mutation screening of the PTEN gene in patients with autism spectrum disorders and macrocephaly. American Journal of Medical Genetics Part B: Neuropsychiatric Genetics 144B, 484–491.

Cario, H., Bode, H., Debatin, K.M., Opladen, T., Schwarz, K., 2009. Congenital null mutations of the FOLR1 gene: A progressive neurologic disease and its treatment. Neurology 73, 2127–2129.

Carney, R.M., Wolpert, C.M., Ravan, S.A., Shahbazian, M., Ashley-Koch, A., Cuccaro, M.L., et al., 2003. Identification of MeCP2 mutations in a series of females with autistic disorder. Pediatric Neurology 28, 205–211.

Ching, M.S., Shen, Y., Tan, W.H., Jeste, S.S., Morrow, E.M., Chen, X., et al., 2010. Deletions of NRXN1 (neurexin-1) predispose to a wide spectrum of developmental disorders. American Journal of Medical Genetics Part B: Neuropsychiatric Genetics 153B, 937–947.

Chiyonobu, T., Hayashi, S., Kobayashi, K., Morimoto, M., Miyanomae, Y., Nishimura, A., et al., 2007. Partial tandem duplication of GRIA3 in a male with mental retardation. American Journal of Medical Genetics Part A 143A, 1448–1455.

Clark, A.J., Rosenberg, E.H., Almeida, L.S., Wood, T.C., Jakobs, C., Stevenson, R.E., et al., 2006. X-linked creatine transporter (SLC6A8) mutations in about 1% of males with mental retardation of unknown etiology. Human Genetics 119, 604–610.

Clifford, S., Dissanayake, C., Bui, Q.M., Huggins, R., Taylor, A.K., Loesch, D.Z., 2007. Autism spectrum phenotype in males and females with fragile X full mutation and premutation. Journal of Autism and Developmental Disorders 37, 738–747.

Coleman, M., Gillberg, C., 2012. The Autisms. Oxford University Press, New York.

Cooper, G.M., Coe, B.P., Girirajan, S., Rosenfeld, J.A., Vu, T.H., Baker, C., et al., 2011. A copy number variation morbidity map of developmental delay. Nature Genetics 43, 838–846.

Coppieters, F., Casteels, I., Meire, F., De Jaegere, S., Hooghe, S., van Regemorter, N., et al., 2010. Genetic screening of LCA in Belgium: Predominance of CEP290 and identification of potential modifier alleles in AHI1 of CEP290-related phenotypes. Human Mutation 31, E1709–E1766.

Cossee, M., Demeer, B., Blanchet, P., Echenne, B., Singh, D., Hagens, O., et al., 2006. Exonic microdeletions in the X-linked PQBP1 gene in mentally retarded patients: A pathogenic mutation and in-frame deletions of uncertain effect. European Journal of Human Genetics 14, 418–425.

D'Amico, A., Tessa, A., Bruno, C., Petrini, S., Biancheri, R., Pane, M., et al., 2006. Expanding the clinical spectrum of POMT1 phenotype. Neurology 66, 1564–1567.

de Baulny, H.O., Benoist, J.F., Rigal, O., Touati, G., Rabier, D., Saudubray, J.M., 2005. Methylmalonic and propionic acidaemias: Management and outcome. Journal of Inherited Metabolic Disease 28, 415–423.

Depienne, C., Heron, D., Betancur, C., Benyahia, B., Trouillard, O., Bouteiller, D., et al., 2007. Autism, language delay and mental retardation in a patient with 7q11 duplication. Journal of Medical Genetics 44, 452–458.

Depienne, C., Leguern, E., 2012. PCDH19-related infantile epileptic encephalopathy: An unusual X-linked inheritance disorder. Human Mutation 33, 627–634.

Depienne, C., Moreno-De-Luca, D., Heron, D., Bouteiller, D., Gennetier, A., Delorme, R., et al., 2009. Screening for genomic rearrangements and methylation abnormalities of the 15q11-q13 region in autism spectrum disorders. Biological Psychiatry 66, 349–359.

Descheemaeker, M.J., Govers, V., Vermeulen, P., Fryns, J.P., 2006. Pervasive developmental disorders in Prader-Willi syndrome: The Leuven experience in 59 subjects and controls. American Journal of Medical Genetics Part A 140, 1136–1142.

Deveault, C., Billingsley, G., Duncan, J.L., Bin, J., Theal, R., Vincent, A., et al., 2011. BBS genotype-phenotype assessment of a multiethnic patient cohort calls for a revision of the disease definition. Human Mutation 32, 610–619.

Devillard, F., Guinchat, V., Moreno-De-Luca, D., Tabet, A.C., Gruchy, N., Guillem, P., et al., 2010. Paracentric inversion of chromosome 2 associated with cryptic duplication of 2q14 and deletion of 2q37 in a patient with autism. American Journal of Medical Genetics Part A 152A, 2346–2354.

de Vries, P.J., 2010. Targeted treatments for cognitive and neurodevelopmental disorders in tuberous sclerosis complex. Neurotherapeutics 7, 275–282.

de Winter, C.F., van Dijk, F., Stolker, J.J., Hennekam, R.C., 2009. Behavioural phenotype in Borjeson-Forssman-Lehmann syndrome. Journal of Intellectual Disability Research 53, 319–328.

Dibbens, L.M., Tarpey, P.S., Hynes, K., Bayly, M.A., Scheffer, I.E., Smith, R., et al., 2008. X-linked protocadherin 19 mutations cause female-limited epilepsy and cognitive impairment. Nature Genetics 40, 776–781.

Doherty, D., Parisi, M.A., Finn, L.S., Gunay-Aygun, M., Al-Mateen, M., Bates, D., et al., 2010. Mutations in 3 genes (MKS3, CC2D2A and RPGRIP1L) cause COACH syndrome (Joubert syndrome with congenital hepatic fibrosis). Journal of Medical Genetics 47, 8–21.

Durand, C.M., Betancur, C., Boeckers, T.M., Bockmann, J., Chaste, P., Fauchereau, F., et al., 2007. Mutations in the gene encoding the synaptic scaffolding protein SHANK3 are associated with autism spectrum disorders. Nature Genetics 39, 25–27.

Ekstrom, A.B., Hakenas-Plate, L., Samuelsson, L., Tulinius, M., Wentz, E., 2008. Autism spectrum conditions in myotonic dystrophy type 1: A study on 57 individuals with congenital and childhood forms. American Journal of Medical Genetics Part B: Neuropsychiatric Genetics 147B, 918–926.

Endele, S., Rosenberger, G., Geider, K., Popp, B., Tamer, C., Stefanova, I., et al., 2010. Mutations in GRIN2A and GRIN2B encoding regulatory subunits of NMDA receptors cause variable neurodevelopmental phenotypes. Nature Genetics 42, 1021–1026.

Falk, R.E., Casas, K.A., 2007. Chromosome 2q37 deletion: Clinical and molecular aspects. American Journal of Medical Genetics. Part C, Seminars in Medical Genetics 145C, 357–371.

Fassio, A., Patry, L., Congia, S., Onofri, F., Piton, A., Gauthier, J., et al., 2011. SYN1 loss-of-function mutations in autism and partial epilepsy cause impaired synaptic function. Human Molecular Genetics 20, 2297–2307.

Fine, S.E., Weissman, A., Gerdes, M., Pinto-Martin, J., Zackai, E.H., McDonald-McGinn, D.M., et al., 2005. Autism spectrum disorders and symptoms in children with molecularly confirmed 22q11.2 deletion syndrome. Journal of Autism and Developmental Disorders 35, 461–470.

Fisch, G.S., Grossfeld, P., Falk, R., Battaglia, A., Youngblom, J., Simensen, R., 2010. Cognitive-behavioral features of Wolf-Hirschhorn syndrome and other subtelomeric microdeletions. American Journal of Medical Genetics. Part C, Seminars in Medical Genetics 154C, 417–426.

Flanagan, S.E., Patch, A.M., Mackay, D.J., Edghill, E.L., Gloyn, A.L., Robinson, D., et al., 2007. Mutations in ATP-sensitive K$^+$ channel genes cause transient neonatal diabetes and permanent diabetes in childhood or adulthood. Diabetes 56, 1930–1937.

Fombonne, E., Du Mazaubrun, C., Cans, C., Grandjean, H., 1997. Autism and associated medical disorders in a French epidemiological survey. Journal of the American Academy of Child and Adolescent Psychiatry 36, 1561–1569.

Fontenelle, L.F., Mendlowicz, M.V., Bezerra de Menezes, G., dos Santos Martins, R.R., Versiani, M., 2004. Asperger Syndrome, obsessive-compulsive disorder, and major depression in a patient with 45, X/46, XY mosaicism. Psychopathology 37, 105–109.

Froyen, G., Bauters, M., Boyle, J., Van Esch, H., Govaerts, K., van Bokhoven, H., et al., 2007. Loss of SLC38A5 and FTSJ1 at Xp11.23 in three brothers with non-syndromic mental retardation due to a microdeletion in an unstable genomic region. Human Genetics 121, 539–547.

Garbern, J.Y., Neumann, M., Trojanowski, J.Q., Lee, V.M., Feldman, G., Norris, J.W., et al., 2010. A mutation affecting the sodium/proton exchanger, SLC9A6, causes mental retardation with tau deposition. Brain 133, 1391–1402.

Garcia, C.C., Blair, H.J., Seager, M., Coulthard, A., Tennant, S., Buddles, M., et al., 2004. Identification of a mutation in synapsin I, a synaptic vesicle protein, in a family with epilepsy. Journal of Medical Genetics 41, 183–186.

Gecz, J., Shoubridge, C., Corbett, M., 2009. The genetic landscape of intellectual disability arising from chromosome X. Trends in Genetics 25, 308–316.

Giannandrea, M., Bianchi, V., Mignogna, M.L., Sirri, A., Carrabino, S., D'Elia, E., et al., 2010. Mutations in the small GTPase gene RAB39B are responsible for X-linked mental retardation associated with autism, epilepsy, and macrocephaly. American Journal of Human Genetics 86, 185–195.

Gillberg, C., 1989. Asperger syndrome in 23 Swedish children. Developmental Medicine & Child Neurology 31, 520–531.

Gorker, I., Tuzun, U., 2005. Autistic-like findings associated with a urea cycle disorder in a 4-year-old girl. Journal of Psychiatry & Neuroscience 30, 133–135.

Gothelf, D., Presburger, G., Zohar, A.H., Burg, M., Nahmani, A., Frydman, M., et al., 2004. Obsessive-compulsive disorder in patients with velocardiofacial (22q11 deletion) syndrome.

American Journal of Medical Genetics Part B: Neuropsychiatric Genetics 126B, 99–105.

Grisart, B., Willatt, L., Destree, A., Fryns, J.P., Rack, K., de Ravel, T., et al., 2009. 17q21.31 microduplication patients are characterised by behavioural problems and poor social interaction. Journal of Medical Genetics 46, 524–530.

Hackett, A., Tarpey, P.S., Licata, A., Cox, J., Whibley, A., Boyle, J., et al., 2010. CASK mutations are frequent in males and cause X-linked nystagmus and variable XLMR phenotypes. European Journal of Human Genetics 18, 544–552.

Hagerman, R., Hoem, G., Hagerman, P., 2010. Fragile X and autism: Intertwined at the molecular level leading to targeted treatments. Molecular Autism 1, 12.

Hagerman, R.J., Hull, C.E., Safanda, J.F., Carpenter, I., Staley, L.W., O'Connor, R.A., et al., 1994. High functioning fragile X males: Demonstration of an unmethylated fully expanded FMR-1 mutation associated with protein expression. American Journal of Medical Genetics 51, 298–308.

Halgren, C., Kjaergaard, S., Bak, M., Hansen, C., El-Schich, Z., Anderson, C., et al., 2011. Corpus callosum abnormalities, intellectual disability, speech impairment, and autism in patients with haploinsufficiency of ARID1B. Clinical Genetics.

Haliloglu, G., Gross, C., Senbil, N., Talim, B., Hehr, U., Uyanik, G., et al., 2004. Clinical spectrum of muscle-eye-brain disease: From the typical presentation to severe autistic features. Acta Myol 23, 137–139.

Hamdan, F.F., Daoud, H., Piton, A., Gauthier, J., Dobrzeniecka, S., Krebs, M.O., et al., 2011. De novo SYNGAP1 mutations in non-syndromic intellectual disability and autism. Biological Psychiatry 69, 898–901.

Hamdan, F.F., Daoud, H., Rochefort, D., Piton, A., Gauthier, J., Langlois, M., et al., 2010. De novo mutations in FOXP1 in cases with intellectual disability, autism, and language impairment. American Journal of Human Genetics 87, 671–678.

Hanson, E., Nasir, R.H., Fong, A., Lian, A., Hundley, R., Shen, Y., et al., 2010. Cognitive and behavioral characterization of 16p11.2 deletion syndrome. Journal of Developmental & Behavioral Pediatrics 31, 649–657.

Hehr, U., Uyanik, G., Gross, C., Walter, M.C., Bohring, A., Cohen, M., et al., 2007. Novel POMGnT1 mutations define broader phenotypic spectrum of muscle-eye-brain disease. Neurogenetics 8, 279–288.

Hemara-Wahanui, A., Berjukow, S., Hope, C.I., Dearden, P.K., Wu, S.B., Wilson-Wheeler, J., et al., 2005. A CACNA1F mutation identified in an X-linked retinal disorder shifts the voltage dependence of Cav1.4 channel activation. Proceedings of the National Academy of Sciences USA 102, 7553–7558.

Heron, B., Mikaeloff, Y., Froissart, R., Caridade, G., Maire, I., Caillaud, C., et al., 2011. Incidence and natural history of mucopolysaccharidosis type III in France and comparison with United Kingdom and Greece. American Journal of Medical Genetics Part A 155A, 58–68.

Hinton, V.J., Cyrulnik, S.E., Fee, R.J., Batchelder, A., Kiefel, J.M., Goldstein, E.M., et al., 2009. Association of autistic spectrum disorders with dystrophinopathies. Pediatric Neurology 41, 339–346.

Hogart, A., Wu, D., LaSalle, J.M., Schanen, N.C., 2010. The comorbidity of autism with the genomic disorders of chromosome 15q11.2-q13. Neurobiology of Disease 38, 181–191.

Hood, R.L., Lines, M.A., Nikkel, S.M., Schwartzentruber, J., Beaulieu, C., Nowaczyk, M.J., et al., 2012. Mutations in SRCAP, encoding SNF2-related CREBBP activator protein, cause Floating-Harbor syndrome. American Journal of Human Genetics 90, 308–313.

Howlin, P., Karpf, J., Turk, J., 2005. Behavioural characteristics and autistic features in individuals with Cohen Syndrome. European Child & Adolescent Psychiatry 14, 57–64.

Hynes, K., Tarpey, P., Dibbens, L.M., Bayly, M.A., Berkovic, S.F., Smith, R., et al., 2010. Epilepsy and mental retardation limited to females with PCDH19 mutations can present de novo or in single generation families. Journal of Medical Genetics 47, 211–216.

Jamain, S., Quach, H., Betancur, C., Rastam, M., Colineaux, C., Gillberg, I.C., et al., 2003. Mutations of the X-linked genes encoding neuroligins NLGN3 and NLGN4 are associated with autism. Nature Genetics 34, 27–29.

Jeffries, A.R., Curran, S., Elmslie, F., Sharma, A., Wenger, S., Hummel, M., et al., 2005. Molecular and phenotypic characterization of ring chromosome 22. American Journal of Medical Genetics Part A 137, 139–147.

Johansson, M., Rastam, M., Billstedt, E., Danielsson, S., Stromland, K., Miller, M., et al., 2006. Autism spectrum disorders and underlying brain pathology in CHARGE association. Developmental Medicine & Child Neurology 48, 40–50.

Kayser, M.A., 2008. Inherited metabolic diseases in neurodevelopmental and neurobehavioral disorders. Semin Pediatric Neurology 15, 127–131.

Kerr, B., Delrue, M.A., Sigaudy, S., Perveen, R., Marche, M., Burgelin, I., et al., 2006. Genotype-phenotype correlation in Costello syndrome: HRAS mutation analysis in 43 cases. Journal of Medical Genetics 43, 401–405.

Kielinen, M., Rantala, H., Timonen, E., Linna, S.L., Moilanen, I., 2004. Associated medical disorders and disabilities in children with autistic disorder: A population-based study. Autism 8, 49–60.

Kilincaslan, A., Tanidir, C., Tutkunkardas, M.D., Mukaddes, N.M., 2011. Asperger's disorder and Williams syndrome: A case report. Turkish Journal of Pediatrics 53, 352–355.

Kleefstra, T., van Zelst-Stams, W.A., Nillesen, W.M., Cormier-Daire, V., Houge, G., Foulds, N., et al., 2009. Further clinical and molecular delineation of the 9q subtelomeric deletion syndrome supports a major contribution of EHMT1 haploinsufficiency to the core phenotype. Journal of Medical Genetics 46, 598–606.

Kleefstra, T., Yntema, H.G., Oudakker, A.R., Banning, M.J., Kalscheuer, V.M., Chelly, J., et al., 2004. Zinc finger 81 (ZNF81) mutations associated with X-linked mental retardation. Journal of Medical Genetics 41, 394–399.

Klein-Tasman, B.P., Phillips, K.D., Lord, C., Mervis, C.B., Gallo, F.J., 2009. Overlap with the autism spectrum in young children with Williams syndrome. Journal of Developmental & Behavioral Pediatrics 30, 289–299.

Knerr, I., Gibson, K.M., Jakobs, C., Pearl, P.L., 2008. Neuropsychiatric morbidity in adolescent and adult succinic semialdehyde dehydrogenase deficiency patients. CNS Spectrums 13, 598–605.

Kumagai, T., Miura, K., Ohki, T., Matsumoto, A., Miyazaki, S., Nakamura, M., et al., 2001. [Central nervous system involvements in Duchenne/Becker muscular dystrophy]. No To Hattatsu 33, 480–486.

Kutsche, K., Yntema, H., Brandt, A., Jantke, I., Nothwang, H.G., Orth, U., et al., 2000. Mutations in ARHGEF6, encoding a guanine nucleotide exchange factor for Rho GTPases, in patients with X-linked mental retardation. Nature Genetics 26, 247–250.

Laje, G., Morse, R., Richter, W., Ball, J., Pao, M., Smith, A.C., 2010. Autism spectrum features in Smith-Magenis syndrome. American Journal of Medical Genetics. Part C, Seminars in Medical Genetics 154C, 456–462.

Laumonnier, F., Bonnet-Brilhault, F., Gomot, M., Blanc, R., David, A., Moizard, M.P., et al., 2004. X-linked mental retardation and autism are associated with a mutation in the NLGN4 gene, a member of the neuroligin family. American Journal of Human Genetics 74, 552–557.

Laumonnier, F., Shoubridge, C., Antar, C., Nguyen, L.S., Van Esch, H., Kleefstra, T., et al., 2010. Mutations of the UPF3B gene, which encodes a protein widely expressed in neurons, are associated with nonspecific mental retardation with or without autism. Molecular Psychiatry 15, 767–776.

Laycock-van Spyk, S., Jim, H.P., Thomas, L., Spurlock, G., Fares, L., Palmer-Smith, S., et al., 2011. Identification of five novel SPRED1 germline mutations in Legius syndrome. Clinical Genetics 80, 93–96.

Lee, J.E., Gleeson, J.G., 2011. Cilia in the nervous system: Linking cilia function and neurodevelopmental disorders. Current Opinion in Neurology 24, 98–105.

Leger, P.L., Souville, I., Boddaert, N., Elie, C., Pinard, J.M., Plouin, P., et al., 2008. The location of DCX mutations predicts malformation severity in X-linked lissencephaly. Neurogenetics 9, 277–285.

Lerma-Carrillo, I., Molina, J.D., Cuevas-Duran, T., Julve-Correcher, C., Espejo-Saavedra, J.M., Andrade-Rosa, C., et al., 2006. Psychopathology in the Lujan-Fryns syndrome: Report of two patients and review. American Journal of Medical Genetics Part A 140, 2807–2811.

Liang, J.S., Shimojima, K., Ohno, K., Sugiura, C., Une, Y., Ohno, K., et al., 2009. A newly recognised microdeletion syndrome of 2p15-16.1 manifesting moderate developmental delay, autistic behaviour, short stature, microcephaly, and dysmorphic features: A new patient with 3.2 Mb deletion. Journal of Medical Genetics 46, 645–647.

Longo, N., Ardon, O., Vanzo, R., Schwartz, E., Pasquali, M., 2011. Disorders of creatine transport and metabolism. American Journal of Medical Genetics. Part C, Seminars in Medical Genetics 157, 72–78.

Longo, I., Frints, S.G., Fryns, J.P., Meloni, I., Pescucci, C., Ariani, F., et al., 2003. A third MRX family (MRX68) is the result of mutation in the long chain fatty acid-CoA ligase 4 (FACL4) gene: Proposal of a rapid enzymatic assay for screening mentally retarded patients. Journal of Medical Genetics 40, 11–17.

Lopez-Hernandez, T., Ridder, M.C., Montolio, M., Capdevila-Nortes, X., Polder, E., Sirisi, S., et al., 2011. Mutant GlialCAM causes megalencephalic leukoencephalopathy with subcortical cysts, benign familial macrocephaly, and macrocephaly with retardation and autism. American Journal of Human Genetics 88, 422–432.

Lowenthal, R., Paula, C.S., Schwartzman, J.S., Brunoni, D., Mercadante, M.T., 2007. Prevalence of pervasive developmental disorder in Down's syndrome. Journal of Autism and Developmental Disorders 37, 1394–1395.

Lugtenberg, D., Yntema, H.G., Banning, M.J., Oudakker, A.R., Firth, H.V., Willatt, L., et al., 2006. ZNF674: A new kruppel-associated box-containing zinc-finger gene involved in nonsyndromic X-linked mental retardation. American Journal of Human Genetics 78, 265–278.

Lynch, N.E., Lynch, S.A., McMenamin, J., Webb, D., 2009. Bannayan-Riley-Ruvalcaba syndrome: A cause of extreme macrocephaly and neurodevelopmental delay. Archives of Disease in Childhood 94, 553–554.

Manning, M.A., Cassidy, S.B., Clericuzio, C., Cherry, A.M., Schwartz, S., Hudgins, L., et al., 2004. Terminal 22q deletion syndrome: A newly recognized cause of speech and language disability in the autism spectrum. Pediatrics 114, 451–457.

Marini, C., Mei, D., Parmeggiani, L., Norci, V., Calado, E., Ferrari, A., et al., 2010. Protocadherin 19 mutations in girls with infantile-onset epilepsy. Neurology 75, 646–653.

Marini, C., Scheffer, I.E., Nabbout, R., Mei, D., Cox, K., Dibbens, L.M., et al., 2009. SCN1A duplications and deletions detected in Dravet syndrome: Implications for molecular diagnosis. Epilepsia 50, 1670–1678.

Marshall, C.R., Noor, A., Vincent, J.B., Lionel, A.C., Feuk, L., Skaug, J., et al., 2008. Structural variation of chromosomes in autism spectrum disorder. American Journal of Human Genetics 82, 477–488.

Mastrangelo, M., Leuzzi, V., 2012. Genes of early-onset epileptic encephalopathies: From genotype to phenotype. Pediatr Neurol 46, 24–31.

McBride, K.L., Varga, E.A., Pastore, M.T., Prior, T.W., Manickam, K., Atkin, J.F., et al., 2010. Confirmation study of PTEN mutations among individuals with autism or developmental delays/mental retardation and macrocephaly. Autism Research 3, 137–141.

McInnes, L.A., Nakamine, A., Pilorge, M., Brandt, T., Jimenez Gonzalez, P., Fallas, M., et al., 2010. A large-scale survey of the novel 15q24 microdeletion syndrome in autism spectrum disorders identifies an atypical deletion that narrows the critical region. Molecular Autism 1, 5.

Mefford, H.C., Rosenfeld, J.A., Shur, N., Slavotinek, A.M., Cox, V.A., Hennekam, R.C., et al., 2012. Further clinical and molecular delineation of the 15q24 microdeletion syndrome. Journal of Medical Genetics 49, 110–118.

Mefford, H.C., Sharp, A.J., Baker, C., Itsara, A., Jiang, Z., Buysse, K., et al., 2008. Recurrent rearrangements of chromosome 1q21.1 and variable pediatric phenotypes. New England Journal of Medicine 359, 1685–1699.

Meloni, I., Muscettola, M., Raynaud, M., Longo, I., Bruttini, M., Moizard, M.P., et al., 2002. FACL4, encoding fatty acid-CoA ligase 4, is mutated in nonspecific X-linked mental retardation. Nature Genetics 30, 436–440.

Michelson, D.J., Shevell, M.I., Sherr, E.H., Moeschler, J.B., Gropman, A.L., Ashwal, S., 2011. Evidence report: Genetic and metabolic testing on children with global developmental delay: Report of the Quality Standards Subcommittee of the American Academy of Neurology and the Practice Committee of the Child Neurology Society. Neurology 77, 1629–1635.

Milh, M., Villeneuve, N., Chouchane, M., Kaminska, A., Laroche, C., Barthez, M.A., et al., 2011. Epileptic and nonepileptic features in patients with early onset epileptic encephalopathy and STXBP1 mutations. Epilepsia 52, 1828–1834.

Miller, D.T., Shen, Y., Weiss, L.A., Korn, J., Anselm, I., Bridgemohan, C., et al., 2009. Microdeletion/duplication at 15q13.2q13.3 among individuals with features of autism and other neuropsychiatric disorders. Journal of Medical Genetics 46, 242–248.

Mills, P.B., Footitt, E.J., Mills, K.A., Tuschl, K., Aylett, S., Varadkar, S., et al., 2010. Genotypic and phenotypic spectrum of pyridoxine-dependent epilepsy (ALDH7A1 deficiency). Brain 133, 2148–2159.

Moessner, R., Marshall, C.R., Sutcliffe, J.S., Skaug, J., Pinto, D., Vincent, J., et al., 2007. Contribution of SHANK3 mutations to autism spectrum disorder. American Journal of Human Genetics 81, 1289–1297.

Moore, S.J., Green, J.S., Fan, Y., Bhogal, A.K., Dicks, E., Fernandez, B.A., et al., 2005. Clinical and genetic epidemiology of Bardet-Biedl syndrome in Newfoundland: A 22-year prospective, population-based, cohort study. American Journal of Medical Genetics Part A 132, 352–360.

Moreno-De-Luca, D., Mulle, J.G., Kaminsky, E.B., Sanders, S.J., Myers, S.M., Adam, M.P., et al., 2010. Deletion 17q12 is a recurrent copy number variant that confers high risk of autism and schizophrenia. American Journal of Human Genetics 87, 618–630.

Moss, J.F., Oliver, C., Berg, K., Kaur, G., Jephcott, L., Cornish, K., 2008. Prevalence of autism spectrum phenomenology in Cornelia de Lange and Cri du Chat syndromes. American Journal Of Mental Retardation 113, 278–291.

Mulley, J.C., Mefford, H.C., 2011. Epilepsy and the new cytogenetics. Epilepsia 52, 423–432.

Nava, C., Hanna, N., Michot, C., Pereira, S., Pouvreau, N., Niihori, T., et al., 2007. Cardio-facio-cutaneous and Noonan syndromes due to mutations in the RAS/MAPK signalling pathway: Genotype-phenotype relationships and overlap with Costello syndrome. Journal of Medical Genetics 44, 763–771.

Neale, B.M., Kou, Y., Liu, L., Ma'ayan, A., Samocha, K.E., Sabo, A., et al., 2012. Patterns and rates of exonic de novo mutations in autism spectrum disorders. Nature 485, 242–245.

Niklasson, L., Rasmussen, P., Oskarsdottir, S., Gillberg, C., 2009. Autism, ADHD, mental retardation and behavior problems in 100 individuals with 22q11 deletion syndrome. Research in Developmental Disabilities 30, 763–773.

Noor, A., Whibley, A., Marshall, C.R., Gianakopoulos, P.J., Piton, A., Carson, A.R., et al., 2010. Disruption at the PTCHD1 locus on Xp22.11 in autism spectrum disorder and intellectual disability. Science Translational Medicine 2, 49ra68.

Novara, F., Beri, S., Giorda, R., Ortibus, E., Nageshappa, S., Darra, F., et al., 2010. Refining the phenotype associated with MEF2C haploinsufficiency. Clinical Genetics 78, 471–477.

Numis, A.L., Major, P., Montenegro, M.A., Muzykewicz, D.A., Pulsifer, M.B., Thiele, E.A., 2011. Identification of risk factors for autism spectrum disorders in tuberous sclerosis complex. Neurology 76, 981–987.

Nystrom, A.M., Ekvall, S., Berglund, E., Bjorkqvist, M., Braathen, G., Duchen, K., et al., 2008. Noonan and cardio-facio-cutaneous syndromes: Two clinically and genetically overlapping disorders. Journal of Medical Genetics 45, 500–506.

Oliveira, G., Ataide, A., Marques, C., Miguel, T.S., Coutinho, A.M., Mota-Vieira, L., et al., 2007. Epidemiology of autism spectrum disorder in Portugal: Prevalence, clinical characterization, and medical conditions. Developmental Medicine & Child Neurology 49, 726–733.

Oliver, C., Arron, K., Sloneem, J., Hall, S., 2008. Behavioural phenotype of Cornelia de Lange syndrome: Case-control study. British Journal of Psychiatry 193, 466–470.

O'Roak, B.J., Deriziotis, P., Lee, C., Vives, L., Schwartz, J.J., Girirajan, S., et al., 2011. Exome sequencing in sporadic autism spectrum disorders identifies severe de novo mutations. Nature Genetics 43, 585–589.

O'Roak, B.J., Vives, L., Girirajan, S., Karakoc, E., Krumm, N., Coe, B.P., et al., 2012. Sporadic autism exomes reveal a highly interconnected protein network of de novo mutations. Nature 485, 246–250.

Ozonoff, S., Williams, B.J., Gale, S., Miller, J.N., 1999. Autism and autistic behavior in Joubert syndrome. Journal of Child Neurology 14, 636–641.

Ozonoff, S., Young, G.S., Carter, A., Messinger, D., Yirmiya, N., Zwaigenbaum, L., et al., 2011. Recurrence risk for autism spectrum disorders: A baby siblings research consortium study. Pediatrics 128, e488–e495.

Paciorkowski, A.R., Thio, L.L., Dobyns, W.B., 2011. Genetic and biologic classification of infantile spasms. Pediatric Neurology 45, 355–367.

Pagnamenta, A.T., Holt, R., Yusuf, M., Pinto, D., Wing, K., Betancur, C., et al., 2011. A family with autism and rare copy number variants disrupting the Duchenne/Becker muscular dystrophy gene DMD and TRPM3. Journal of Neurodevelopmental Disorders 3, 124–131.

Partington, M.W., Turner, G., Boyle, J., Gecz, J., 2004. Three new families with X-linked mental retardation caused by the 428-451dup(24bp) mutation in ARX. Clinical Genetics 66, 39–45.

Paul, M., Allington-Smith, P., 1997. Asperger syndrome associated with Steinert's myotonic dystrophy. Developmental Medicine & Child Neurology 39, 280–281.

Paylor, R., Glaser, B., Mupo, A., Ataliotis, P., Spencer, C., Sobotka, A., et al., 2006. Tbx1 haploinsufficiency is linked to behavioral disorders in mice and humans: Implications for 22q11 deletion syndrome. Proceedings of the National Academy of Sciences USA 103, 7729–7734.

Pearl, P.L., Gibson, K.M., Acosta, M.T., Vezina, L.G., Theodore, W.H., Rogawski, M.A., et al., 2003. Clinical spectrum of succinic semialdehyde dehydrogenase deficiency. Neurology 60, 1413–1417.

Perrault, I., Delphin, N., Hanein, S., Gerber, S., Dufier, J.L., Roche, O., et al., 2007. Spectrum of NPHP6/CEP290 mutations in Leber congenital amaurosis and delineation of the associated phenotype. Human Mutation 28, 416.

Petit, E., Herault, J., Raynaud, M., Cherpi, C., Perrot, A., Barthelemy, C., et al., 1996. X chromosome and infantile autism. Biological Psychiatry 40, 457–464.

Philippe, C., Amsallem, D., Francannet, C., Lambert, L., Saunier, A., Verneau, F., et al., 2010. Phenotypic variability in Rett syndrome associated with FOXG1 mutations in females. Journal of Medical Genetics 47, 59–65.

Pierpont, E.I., Pierpont, M.E., Mendelsohn, N.J., Roberts, A.E., Tworog-Dube, E., Seidenberg, M.S., 2009. Genotype differences in cognitive functioning in Noonan syndrome. Genes, Brain and Behavior 8, 275–282.

Pinto, D., Pagnamenta, A.T., Klei, L., Anney, R., Merico, D., Regan, R., et al., 2010. Functional impact of global rare copy number variation in autism spectrum disorders. Nature 466, 368–372.

Piton, A., Michaud, J.L., Peng, H., Aradhya, S., Gauthier, J., Mottron, L., et al., 2008. Mutations in the calcium-related gene IL1RAPL1 are associated with autism. Human Molecular Genetics 17, 3965–3974.

Pons, R., Andreu, A.L., Checcarelli, N., Vila, M.R., Engelstad, K., Sue, C.M., et al., 2004. Mitochondrial DNA abnormalities and autistic spectrum disorders. Journal of Pediatrics 144, 81–85.

Poo-Arguelles, P., Arias, A., Vilaseca, M.A., Ribes, A., Artuch, R., Sans-Fito, A., et al., 2006. X-linked creatine transporter deficiency in two patients with severe mental retardation and autism. Journal of Inherited Metabolic Disease 29, 220–223.

Qiao, Y., Liu, X., Harvard, C., Hildebrand, M.J., Rajcan-Separovic, E., Holden, J.J., et al., 2008. Autism-associated familial microdeletion of Xp11.22. Clinical Genetics 74, 134–144.

Quintero-Rivera, F., Sharifi-Hannauer, P., Martinez-Agosto, J.A., 2010. Autistic and psychiatric findings associated with the 3q29 microdeletion syndrome: Case report and review. American Journal of Medical Genetics Part A 152A, 2459–2467.

Rajcan-Separovic, E., Harvard, C., Liu, X., McGillivray, B., Hall, J.G., Qiao, Y., et al., 2007. Clinical and molecular cytogenetic characterisation of a newly recognised microdeletion syndrome involving 2p15-16.1. Journal of Medical Genetics 44, 269–276.

Ramocki, M.B., Tavyev, Y.J., Peters, S.U., 2010. The MECP2 duplication syndrome. American Journal of Medical Genetics Part A 152A, 1079–1088.

Ropers, H.H., 2010. Genetics of early onset cognitive impairment. Annual Review of Genomics and Human Genetics 11, 161–187.

Rosenfeld, J.A., Coppinger, J., Bejjani, B.A., Girirajan, S., Eichler, E.E., Shaffer, L.G., et al., 2010. Speech delays and behavioral problems are the predominant features in individuals with developmental delays and 16p11.2 microdeletions and microduplications. Journal of Neurodevelopmental Disorders 2, 26–38.

Russo, S., Marchi, M., Cogliati, F., Bonati, M.T., Pintaudi, M., Veneselli, E., et al., 2009. Novel mutations in the CDKL5 gene, predicted effects and associated phenotypes. Neurogenetics 10, 241–250.

Sahoo, T., Peters, S.U., Madduri, N.S., Glaze, D.G., German, J.R., Bird, L.M., et al., 2006. Microarray based comparative genomic hybridization testing in deletion bearing patients with Angelman syndrome: Genotype-phenotype correlations. Journal of Medical Genetics 43, 512–516.

Saillour, Y., Carion, N., Quelin, C., Leger, P.L., Boddaert, N., Elie, C., et al., 2009. LIS1-related isolated lissencephaly: Spectrum of mutations and relationships with malformation severity. Archives of Neurology 66, 1007–1015.

Samuels, I.S., Saitta, S.C., Landreth, G.E., 2009. MAP'ing CNS development and cognition: An ERKsome process. Neuron 61, 160–167.

Sanders, S.J., Ercan-Sencicek, A.G., Hus, V., Luo, R., Murtha, M.T., Moreno-De-Luca, D., et al., 2011. Multiple recurrent de novo CNVs, including duplications of the 7q11.23 Williams syndrome region, are strongly associated with autism. Neuron 70, 863–885.

Sanders, S.J., Murtha, M.T., Gupta, A.R., Murdoch, J.D., Raubeson, M.J., Willsey, A.J., et al., 2012. De novo mutations revealed by whole-exome sequencing are strongly associated with autism. Nature 485, 237–241.

Santen, G.W., Aten, E., Sun, Y., Almomani, R., Gilissen, C., Nielsen, M., et al., 2012. Mutations in SWI/SNF chromatin remodeling complex gene ARID1B cause Coffin-Siris syndrome. Nature Genetics 44, 379–380.

Schaefer, G.B., Lutz, R.E., 2006. Diagnostic yield in the clinical genetic evaluation of autism spectrum disorders. Genetics in Medicine 8, 549–556.

Scheffer, I.E., Turner, S.J., Dibbens, L.M., Bayly, M.A., Friend, K., Hodgson, B., et al., 2008. Epilepsy and mental retardation limited to females: An under-recognized disorder. Brain 131, 918–927.

Schorry, E.K., Keddache, M., Lanphear, N., Rubinstein, J.H., Srodulski, S., Fletcher, D., et al., 2008. Genotype-phenotype correlations in Rubinstein-Taybi syndrome. American Journal of Medical Genetics Part A 146A, 2512–2519.

Schwartz, C.E., Tarpey, P.S., Lubs, H.A., Verloes, A., May, M.M., Risheg, H., et al., 2007. The original Lujan syndrome family has a novel missense mutation (p.N1007S) in the MED12 gene. Journal of Medical Genetics 44, 472–477.

Sebat, J., Lakshmi, B., Malhotra, D., Troge, J., Lese-Martin, C., Walsh, T., et al., 2007. Strong association of de novo copy number mutations with autism. Science 316, 445–449.

Sempere, A., Fons, C., Arias, A., Rodriguez-Pombo, P., Colomer, R., Merinero, B., et al., 2009. Creatine transporter deficiency in two adult patients with static encephalopathy. Journal of Inherited Metabolic Disease Short report #158. [Online].

Sempere, A., Fons, C., Arias, A., Rodriguez-Pombo, P., Merinero, B., Alcaide, P., et al., 2009. [Cerebral creatine deficiency: First Spanish patients harbouring mutations in GAMT gene]. Medicina Clìnica (Barc) 133, 745–749.

Sharp, A.J., Mefford, H.C., Li, K., Baker, C., Skinner, C., Stevenson, R.E., et al., 2008. A recurrent 15q13.3 microdeletion syndrome associated with mental retardation and seizures. Nature Genetics 40, 322–328.

Shinawi, M., Liu, P., Kang, S.H., Shen, J., Belmont, J.W., Scott, D.A., et al., 2010. Recurrent reciprocal 16p11.2 rearrangements associated with global developmental delay, behavioural problems, dysmorphism, epilepsy, and abnormal head size. Journal of Medical Genetics 47, 332–341.

Shoubridge, C., Tarpey, P.S., Abidi, F., Ramsden, S.L., Rujirabanjerd, S., Murphy, J.A., et al., 2010. Mutations in the guanine nucleotide exchange factor gene IQSEC2 cause nonsyndromic intellectual disability. Nature Genetics 42, 486–488.

Sikora, D.M., Pettit-Kekel, K., Penfield, J., Merkens, L.S., Steiner, R.D., 2006. The near universal presence of autism spectrum disorders in children with Smith-Lemli-Opitz syndrome. American Journal of Medical Genetics Part A 140, 1511–1518.

Simonati, A., Boaretto, F., Vettori, A., Dabrilli, P., Criscuolo, L., Rizzuto, N., et al., 2006. A novel missense mutation in the L1CAM gene in a boy with L1 disease. Neurological Sciences 27, 114–117.

Sousa, S.B., Abdul-Rahman, O.A., Bottani, A., Cormier-Daire, V., Fryer, A., Gillessen-Kaesbach, G., et al., 2009. Nicolaides-Baraitser syndrome: Delineation of the phenotype. American Journal of Medical Genetics Part A 149A, 1628–1640.

Spiegel, E.K., Colman, R.F., Patterson, D., 2006. Adenylosuccinate lyase deficiency. Molecular Genetics and Metabolism 89, 19–31.

Splawski, I., Timothy, K.W., Sharpe, L.M., Decher, N., Kumar, P., Bloise, R., et al., 2004. Ca(V)1.2 calcium channel dysfunction causes a multisystem disorder including arrhythmia and autism. Cell 119, 19–31.

State, M.W., 2010. The genetics of child psychiatric disorders: Focus on autism and Tourette syndrome. Neuron 68, 254–269.

Steiner, C.E., Acosta, A.X., Guerreiro, M.M., Marques-de-Faria, A.P., 2007. Genotype and natural history in unrelated individuals with phenylketonuria and autistic behavior. Arq Neuropsiquiatr 65, 202–205.

Stettner, G.M., Shoukier, M., Hoger, C., Brockmann, K., Auber, B., 2011. Familial intellectual disability and autistic behavior caused by a small FMR2 gene deletion. American Journal of Medical Genetics Part A 155A, 2003–2007.

Stevenson, R.E., Bennett, C.W., Abidi, F., Kleefstra, T., Porteous, M., Simensen, R.J., et al., 2005. Renpenning syndrome comes into focus. American Journal of Medical Genetics Part A 134, 415–421.

Strauss, K.A., Puffenberger, E.G., Huentelman, M.J., Gottlieb, S., Dobrin, S.E., Parod, J.M., et al., 2006. Recessive symptomatic focal epilepsy and mutant contactin-associated protein-like 2. New England Journal of Medicine 354, 1370–1377.

Szatmari, P., Paterson, A.D., Zwaigenbaum, L., Roberts, W., Brian, J., Liu, X.Q., et al., 2007. Mapping autism risk loci using genetic linkage and chromosomal rearrangements. Nature Genetics 39, 319–328.

Tabet, A.C., Pilorge, M., Delorme, R., Amsellem, F., Pinard, J.M., Leboyer, M., et al., 2012. Autism multiplex family with 16p11.2p12.2 microduplication syndrome in monozygotic twins and distal 16p11.2 deletion in their brother. European Journal of Human Genetics 20, 540–546.

Takahashi, T.N., Farmer, J.E., Deidrick, K.K., Hsu, B.S., Miles, J.H., Maria, B.L., 2005. Joubert syndrome is not a cause of classical autism. American Journal of Medical Genetics Part A 132, 347–351.

Talkowski, M.E., Mullegama, S.V., Rosenfeld, J.A., van Bon, B.W., Shen, Y., Repnikova, E.A., et al., 2011. Assessment of 2q23.1 microdeletion syndrome implicates MBD5 as a single causal locus of intellectual disability, epilepsy, and autism spectrum disorder. American Journal of Human Genetics 89, 551–563.

Tan, W.H., Baris, H.N., Burrows, P.E., Robson, C.D., Alomari, A.I., Mulliken, J.B., et al., 2007. The spectrum of vascular anomalies in patients with PTEN mutations: Implications for diagnosis and management. Journal of Medical Genetics 44, 594–602.

Tartaglia, N., Davis, S., Hench, A., Nimishakavi, S., Beauregard, R., Reynolds, A., et al., 2008. A new look at XXYY syndrome: Medical and psychological features. American Journal of Medical Genetics Part A 146A, 1509–1522.

Tierney, E., Bukelis, I., Thompson, R.E., Ahmed, K., Aneja, A., Kratz, L., et al., 2006. Abnormalities of cholesterol metabolism in autism spectrum disorders. American Journal of Medical Genetics Part B: Neuropsychiatric Genetics 141B, 666–668.

Tonini, G., Bizzarri, C., Bonfanti, R., Vanelli, M., Cerutti, F., Faleschini, E., et al., 2006. Sulfonylurea treatment outweighs insulin therapy in short-term metabolic control of patients with permanent neonatal diabetes mellitus due to activating mutations of the KCNJ11 (KIR6.2) gene. Diabetologia 49, 2210–2213.

Tordjman, S., Anderson, G.M., Botbol, M., Toutain, A., Sarda, P., Carlier, M., et al., 2012. Autistic disorder in patients with Williams-Beuren syndrome: A reconsideration of the Williams-Beuren syndrome phenotype. PLoS One 7, e30778.

Tory, K., Lacoste, T., Burglen, L., Moriniere, V., Boddaert, N., Macher, M.A., et al., 2007. High NPHP1 and NPHP6 mutation rate in patients with Joubert syndrome and nephronophthisis: Potential epistatic effect of NPHP6 and AHI1 mutations in patients with NPHP1 mutations. Journal of the American Society of Nephrology 18, 1566–1575.

Treadwell-Deering, D.E., Powell, M.P., Potocki, L., 2010. Cognitive and behavioral characterization of the Potocki-Lupski syndrome (duplication 17p11.2). Journal of Developmental & Behavioral Pediatrics 31, 137–143.

Trillingsgaard, A., Østergaard, J., 2004. Autism in Angelman syndrome: An exploration of comorbidity. Autism 8, 163–174.

Turner, G., Partington, M., Kerr, B., Mangelsdorf, M., Gecz, J., 2002. Variable expression of mental retardation, autism, seizures, and dystonic hand movements in two families with an identical ARX gene mutation. American Journal of Medical Genetics 112, 405–411.

Ullmann, R., Turner, G., Kirchhoff, M., Chen, W., Tonge, B., Rosenberg, C., et al., 2007. Array CGH identifies reciprocal 16p13.1 duplications and deletions that predispose to autism and/or mental retardation. Human Mutation 28, 674–682.

van Bokhoven, H., 2011. Genetic and epigenetic networks in intellectual disabilities. Annual Review of Genetics 45, 81–104.

van Bokhoven, H., Kramer, J.M., 2010. Disruption of the epigenetic code: An emerging mechanism in mental retardation. Neurobiology of Disease 39, 3–12.

van Bon, B.W., Mefford, H.C., Menten, B., Koolen, D.A., Sharp, A.J., Nillesen, W.M., et al., 2009. Further delineation of the 15q13 microdeletion and duplication syndromes: A clinical spectrum varying from non-pathogenic to a severe outcome. Journal of Medical Genetics 46, 511–523.

Van der Aa, N., Rooms, L., Vandeweyer, G., van den Ende, J., Reyniers, E., Fichera, M., et al., 2009. Fourteen new cases contribute to the characterization of the 7q11.23 microduplication syndrome. European Journal of Medical Genetics 52, 94–100.

Van Houdt, J.K., Nowakowska, B.A., Sousa, S.B., van Schaik, B.D., Seuntjens, E., Avonce, N., et al., 2012. Heterozygous missense mutations in SMARCA2 cause Nicolaides-Baraitser syndrome. Nature Genetics 44, 445–449.

Van Kuilenburg, A.B., Meijer, J., Mul, A.N., Hennekam, R.C., Hoovers, J.M., de Die-Smulders, C.E., et al., 2009. Analysis of severely affected patients with dihydropyrimidine dehydrogenase deficiency reveals large intragenic rearrangements of DPYD and a de novo interstitial deletion del(1)(p13.3p21.3). Human Genetics 125, 581–590.

Van Kuilenburg, A.B., Vreken, P., Abeling, N.G., Bakker, H.D., Meinsma, R., Van Lenthe, H., et al., 1999. Genotype and phenotype in patients with dihydropyrimidine dehydrogenase deficiency. Human Genetics 104, 1–9.

van Rijn, S., Swaab, H., Aleman, A., Kahn, R.S., 2008. Social behavior and autism traits in a sex chromosomal disorder: Klinefelter (47XXY) syndrome. Journal of Autism and Developmental Disorders 38, 1634–1641.

Veltman, M.W., Craig, E.E., Bolton, P.F., 2005. Autism spectrum disorders in Prader-Willi and Angelman syndromes: A systematic review. Psychiatric Genetics 15, 243–254.

Ververi, A., Vargiami, E., Papadopoulou, V., Tryfonas, D., Zafeiriou, D.I., 2012. Clinical and laboratory data in a sample of Greek children with autism spectrum disorders. Journal of Autism and Developmental Disorders 42, 1470–1476.

Vervoort, V.S., Beachem, M.A., Edwards, P.S., Ladd, S., Miller, K.E., de Mollerat, X., et al., 2002. AGTR2 mutations in X-linked mental retardation. Science 296, 2401–2403.

Vorstman, J.A., Morcus, M.E., Duijff, S.N., Klaassen, P.W., Heineman-de Boer, J.A., Beemer, F.A., et al., 2006. The 22q11.2 deletion in children: High rate of autistic disorders and early onset of psychotic symptoms. Journal of the American Academy of Child and Adolescent Psychiatry 45, 1104–1113.

Wada, T., Gibbons, R.J., 2003. ATR-X syndrome. In: Fisch, G.S. (Ed.), Genetics and Genomics of Neurobehavioral Disorders. Humana Press, Totowa, NJ, pp. 309–334.

Watanabe, Y., Yano, S., Niihori, T., Aoki, Y., Matsubara, Y., Yoshino, M., et al., 2011. A familial case of LEOPARD syndrome associated with a high-functioning autism spectrum disorder. Brain & Development 33, 576–579.

Weiss, L.A., Shen, Y., Korn, J.M., Arking, D.E., Miller, D.T., Fossdal, R., et al., 2008. Association between microdeletion and microduplication at 16p11.2 and autism. New England Journal of Medicine 358, 667–675.

White, S.M., Morgan, A., Da Costa, A., Lacombe, D., Knight, S.J., Houlston, R., et al., 2010. The phenotype of Floating-Harbor syndrome in 10 patients. American Journal of Medical Genetics Part A 152A, 821–829.

Willatt, L., Cox, J., Barber, J., Cabanas, E.D., Collins, A., Donnai, D., et al., 2005. 3q29 microdeletion syndrome: Clinical and molecular characterization of a new syndrome. American Journal of Human Genetics 77, 154–160.

Williams, P.G., Hersh, J.H., 1998. Brief report: The association of neurofibromatosis type 1 and autism. Journal of Autism and Developmental Disorders 28, 567–571.

Wisniowiecka-Kowalnik, B., Nesteruk, M., Peters, S.U., Xia, Z., Cooper, M.L., Savage, S., et al., 2010. Intragenic rearrangements in NRXN1 in three families with autism spectrum disorder, developmental delay, and speech delay. American Journal of Medical Genetics Part B: Neuropsychiatric Genetics 153B, 983–993.

Wolanczyk, T., Banaszkiewicz, A., Mierzewska, H., Czartoryska, B., Zdziennicka, E., 2000. [Hyperactivity and behavioral disorders in Sanfilippo A (mucopolysaccharidosis type IIIA) – case report and review of the literature]. Psychiatr Pol 34, 831–837.

Wu, J.Y., Kuban, K.C., Allred, E., Shapiro, F., Darras, B.T., 2005. Association of Duchenne muscular dystrophy with autism spectrum disorder. Journal of Child Neurology 20, 790–795.

Wu, Y., Arai, A.C., Rumbaugh, G., Srivastava, A.K., Turner, G., Hayashi, T., et al., 2007. Mutations in ionotropic AMPA receptor 3 alter channel properties and are associated with moderate cognitive impairment in humans. Proceedings of the National Academy of Sciences USA 104, 18,163–18,168.

Xu, S., Han, J.C., Morales, A., Menzie, C.M., Williams, K., Fan, Y.S., 2008. Characterization of 11p14-p12 deletion in WAGR syndrome by array CGH for identifying genes contributing to mental retardation and autism. Cytogenetic and Genome Research 122, 181–187.

Young, H.K., Barton, B.A., Waisbren, S., Portales Dale, L., Ryan, M.M., Webster, R.I., et al., 2008. Cognitive and psychological profile of males with Becker muscular dystrophy. Journal of Child Neurology 23, 155–162.

Yzer, S., van den Born, L.I., Schuil, J., Kroes, H.Y., van Genderen, M.M., Boonstra, F.N., et al., 2003. A Tyr368His RPE65 founder mutation is associated with variable expression and progression of early onset retinal dystrophy in 10 families of a genetically isolated population. Journal of Medical Genetics 40, 709–713.

Zaffanello, M., Zamboni, G., Fontana, E., Zoccante, L., Tato, L., 2003. A case of partial biotinidase deficiency associated with autism. Child Neuropsychol 9, 184–188.

Zweier, C., de Jong, E.K., Zweier, M., Orrico, A., Ousager, L.B., Collins, A.L., et al., 2009. CNTNAP2 and NRXN1 are mutated in autosomal-recessive Pitt-Hopkins-like mental retardation and determine the level of a common synaptic protein in Drosophila. American Journal of Human Genetics 85, 655–666.

Copy Number Variation in Autism Spectrum Disorders

Christian R. Marshall*, Anath C. Lionel*,†, Stephen W. Scherer*

*The Center for Applied Genomics, The Hospital for Sick Children, and McLaughlin Center and Department of Molecular Genetics, University of Toronto, Ontario, Canada †Program in Genetics and Genome Biology, The Hospital for Sick Children, Ontario, Canada

INTRODUCTION AND BACKGROUND

Autism is the prototypic form of a spectrum of conditions officially known as pervasive developmental disorders (PDD), but more widely referred to as autism spectrum disorders (ASD). Other subtypes within ASD include Asperger syndrome and pervasive developmental disorder not otherwise specified (PDD-NOS). ASD are characterized by challenges in communication, impaired social function, repetitive behaviors, and restricted interests with onset before the age of three (American Psychiatric Association, 2000). Signs and symptoms can present with a range of severity and in a variety of combinations often along with developmental disability/intellectual disability (DD/ID), sleep difficulties, seizure, and other neurological and behavioral issues. Upwards of 40% of ASD cases have DD/ID (O'Brien and Pearson, 2004) while other common neurodevelopment comorbidities include atypical schizophrenia (SZ) (0.5–5%) (Hofvander et al., 2009; Sporn et al., 2004), attention deficit/hyperactivity disorder (ADHD) (59–75%) (Goldstein and Schwebach, 2004; Rommelse et al., 2010) and obsessive-compulsive disorder (OCD) (60%) (Leyfer et al., 2006; Ruta et al., 2010; see also Section 1).

The latest estimates put the population prevalence of ASD at approximately 1 in 110 (Autism and Developmental Disabilities Monitoring Network, 2009; see also Chapter 1.1), likely 10 times that of classically defined autism. Incidence appears to be independent of ancestry and demographics, with similar rates being found on a global scale when the same diagnostic tools are used (Fombonne, 2009). A feature of ASD is a gender bias, with males four times more likely than females to receive a diagnosis. However there is variability as it may rise to 11:1 when considering Asperger disorder and fall to 1:1 when considering severe syndromic cases arising from *de novo* mutations (Gillberg et al., 2006).

The genetic factors involved in ASD are beginning to be illuminated, although it took decades after the disorder was first described (Kanner, 1946) to recognize the importance of heritability in ASD (Folstein and

The Neuroscience of Autism Spectrum Disorders.
http://dx.doi.org/10.1016/B978-0-12-391924-3.00009-0

Rosen-Sheidley, 2001). With heritability estimates from family studies as high as 90%, ASD is one of the neurodevelopmental disorders most influenced by genetics. The development of high-throughput, high-resolution, genome-wide scanning technologies coupled with the availability of large case cohorts has led to significant progress in delineating the genomic architecture underlying the ASD phenotype. One area that has benefitted greatly from the evolving technology is the study of copy number variation (CNV) through microarray analysis. CNV, defined as segments of DNA duplicated or deleted when comparing individuals, is now established as a prevalent source of genomic variation (Iafrate et al., 2004; Redon et al., 2006; Sebat et al., 2004).

CNV may be benign and part of normal genetic variation or may be associated with risk of a disease (Lee and Scherer, 2010). Screening for copy number variants (CNVs), has proven to be one of the more successful strategies for the discovery of ASD candidate loci over the last five years (Cook and Scherer, 2008; State, 2010b). The identification of very rare *de novo* or inherited CNVs of high penetrance in ASD has in part given rise to a paradigm shift away from common variant models of ASD genetic architecture to one suggesting a role for multiple rare and distinct genetic risk factors (see also Chapter 2.1). With a lack of consensus in results from recent genome-wide association (GWA) studies in ASD, it is reasonable to conclude few common polymorphisms are likely to contribute a high relative risk in ASD (Devlin et al., 2011; see also Chapter 2.3). The other central observation is that the same or overlapping CNVs are being identified as risk factors across different neurodevelopmental disorders (Carroll and Owen, 2009; Guilmatre et al., 2009; Pinto et al., 2010) – perhaps not surprisingly given the overlap in phenotype across conditions. In this chapter we provide an overview of the latest in CNV analysis techniques and discuss the latest CNVs associated with ASD, discoveries that have impacted diagnostic tools and clinical definitions.

GENETICS OF ASD

Family studies have provided strong evidence for the contribution of complex genetic factors in ASD etiology. Early studies showed a recurrence risk in siblings of ASD probands of 8–10% (Szatmari et al., 1998; Zwaigenbaum et al., 2005) with more recent studies observing as many as 25% of siblings affected (Constantino et al., 2010; Ozonoff et al., 2011). The latter observation puts risk in siblings of an ASD child at roughly 20 times higher than the general population risk. A recent study looking at the differential in ASD diagnosis in siblings found the recurrence rate was approximately twice in full siblings compared to that among half siblings (Constantino et al., 2012) further demonstrating the large genetic component to ASD etiology. Although familial clustering may point to environmental factors, twin studies point to a substantial genetic contribution that cannot be explained solely by the environment. Estimates of heritability from twin studies range from 37 to 90% (Bailey et al., 1995; Hallmayer et al., 2011; Le Couteur et al., 1996; Rosenberg et al., 2009; Steffenburg et al., 1989). The most recent twin study showed much lower heritability (37%) compared to earlier studies when using a strict autism cutoff, although the confidence interval was wide (8–84%) (Hallmayer et al., 2011). When considering a broader spectrum of related cognitive or social abnormalities, upwards of 92% of monozygotic (MZ) twins were concordant for phenotype in contrast with ~ 10% in dizygotic (DZ) twins (Bailey et al., 1995; Constantino et al., 2010). This difference in concordance between MZ and DZ twins suggests ASD is a multi-locus disorder (Risch et al., 1999) and that the phenotype likely extends to a subclinical, broader autism phenotype (BAP) (Losh et al., 2008).

ASD-RELATED SYNDROMES AND CHROMOSOMAL ABNORMALITIES

Current estimates suggest that approximately 15% of ASD cases are associated with known Mendelian or genetic syndromes. These include microscopically visible chromosomal abnormalities, in some instances large, cytogenetically visible CNV (Abrahams and Geschwind, 2008; Veenstra-Vanderweele et al., 2004; Chapter 2.1). Mutations causing fragile X (~ 1–2%), tuberous sclerosis (~ 1%), Rett syndrome (~ 0.5%) and neurofibromatosis (< 1%) are the Mendelian conditions most frequently cited. ASD has been associated with other rare disorders including Sotos, Cowden, Moebius, Smith–Lemli–Opitz, and Timothy syndromes. More broadly, a recent review showed that over 103 genes implicated in ID/DD have been associated with ASD, strengthening the observed genetic overlap among neurodevelopmental disorders (Betancur, 2011). Microscopically visible abnormalities detected by high-resolution karyotyping are observed in close to 5% of ASD cases. A early survey of 15 studies found the mean rate of karyotypically visible anomalies to be 7.4% (129/1749) with a range of 0–54% (Xu et al., 2004). A more recent clinical survey of idiopathic ASD found a considerably lower rate of karyotypic changes, with positive results in 2.2% (19/852) cases (Shen et al., 2010). The differences in these rates is likely due to ascertainment, as those ASD cases with accompanying dysmorphology and/or severe ID are more likely to harbor a large unbalanced change detectable by karyotyping. Although large structural changes have been found on all chromosomes, most are so rare that association with ASD is difficult to prove. One of the few exceptions, and the most common karyotypic change found in individuals with ASD (at a frequency of ~ 1%), is a 15q11–13 duplication (of the maternal allele) of the Prader–Willi/Angelman syndrome region (Baker et al., 1994).

COPY NUMBER VARIATION: TECHNOLOGICAL METHODS AND INTERPRETATION

CNV analysis is inherently challenging, and before examining CNV in ASD, a discussion of CNV detection methods and interpretation is warranted. The most common method for high-throughput genome-wide detection of CNVs is microarray analysis, which is capable of genotyping millions of genomic loci simultaneously. Commercially available microarray platforms generally fall into two categories. The first is comparative genomic hybridization (CGH) arrays, which uses competitive hybridization of differentially labeled reference and test DNA to an array of oligonucleotide probes. Copy number is measured as the relative difference in fluorescence after scanning, allowing for a direct comparison of copy number. Commercial suppliers of CGH arrays include Roche NimbleGen and Agilent Technologies. The second category of platforms comprises single nucleotide polymorphism (SNP)-genotyping microarrays, which are primarily designed to interrogate millions of SNP genotypes from a single individual for GWA studies. In these experiments, the reference must be built from other experiments in order to analyze for copy number, since only a single DNA sample is hybridized to the array. The main commercial suppliers of SNP-genotyping arrays include companies such as Affymetrix and Illumina.

Most ASD CNV studies have used SNP-genotyping arrays mainly because the primary study design was GWA. The advantage of a SNP-based platform is that the SNP genotype information can be used for population structure analysis, quality control checks, determination of allele-specific copy number changes, and confirmation of deletions (i.e., through genotype homozygosity or loss of heterozygosity (LOH)). For both microarray techniques there are a host of algorithms available for CNV analysis, either developed commercially or independently, some of which can be used across platforms. A non-exhaustive list of the more common analysis programs we use includes PennCNV (Wang et al., 2007), QuantiSNP (Colella et al., 2007), iPattern (Pinto et al., 2011), Birdsuite (Korn et al., 2008) for SNP arrays and DNA analytics (Agilent), and DNA copy (Venkatraman and Olshen, 2007) for CGH arrays.

Although both CGH and SNP microarrays are capable of providing excellent CNV data, there is no one combination of platform and algorithm that is best, and use of several strategies can be complementary, with the caveat that algorithms developed specifically for a certain data type (e.g., Birdsuite for Affymetrix 6.0 and DNA Analytics for Agilent data) generally perform better (Pinto et al., 2011). To maximize CNV discovery while allowing for a simple prioritization using a combination of calling algorithms is the best strategy in our experience (Pinto et al., 2011). We have observed that using multiple algorithms typically yields > 50 high-confidence CNV calls using a million plus feature array and, further, that calls made by more than one algorithm validate at a rate of > 90% using an independent laboratory technique like quantitative polymerase chain reaction (PCR) (Lionel et al., 2011; Marshall et al., 2008; Pinto et al., 2010).

Equally important in an effective strategy for CNV calling is a way to prioritize biologically relevant variants for follow-up, as depicted in Figure 2.2.1. There are several different schemes, but comparison with CNV data from large control cohorts is essential for pinpointing rare CNVs in ASD cases. Ideally, the CNVs from controls would be analyzed in the same manner as the cases, due to the challenges in CNV calling described above. We tend to prioritize CNVs for follow-up based on:

1. CNVs known to be associated with a neurodevelopmental disorder (e.g., 1q21.1, 16p11.2);
2. Parental transmission, with priority given to those rare CNVs overlapping genes that are *de novo* in origin;
3. Rare overlapping or recurrent CNVs that affect genes and are present at a low (< 0.1%) frequency in control cohorts.

Other factors such as prioritization based on genomic size and position, deletion versus duplication, and overlap with known candidate genes are applicable across the broader categories above.

COPY NUMBER VARIATION IN ASD

The combined observations of evidence for a strong genetic contribution to ASD from family studies, an increase in cytogenetically visible abnormalities in ASD cases compared to controls, and a lack of reproducible common variants associated with ASD led to the hypothesis that rare submicroscopic variants in the form of CNVs contribute to the genetic architecture of ASD. As discussed in the section below, CNV

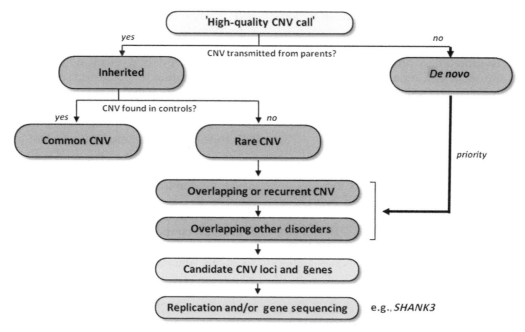

FIGURE 2.2.1   General analyses and prioritization workflow for discovery of rare CNVs associated with ASD. Microarray data is analyzed for CNV using multiple algorithms to maximize CNV discovery and create a high-quality CNV dataset. CNV prioritization (red boxes) is based on several criteria with *de novo* CNVs typically given highest priority for follow-up. For rare inherited CNVs not found in controls, parameters such as recurrence in cases and overlap with other neurodevelopmental disorders help define candidate CNVs and genes for follow-up (orange box). These can be replicated in other cohorts or, if a single gene is implicated, can be sequenced to find other mutations (blue box).

detection has proven an effective strategy for identifying ASD candidate genes. However, although not the focus of this chapter, it should be noted that the most powerful strategy for discovery of ASD candidate genes involves CNV analysis coupled with follow-up exon resequencing for identification of potentially damaging sequence-level mutations (see Chapter 2.4). Combinations of strategies have led to the discovery of both CNVs and nonsense mutations resulting in haploinsufficiency of genes such as *SHANK3* (Durand et al., 2007; Gauthier et al., 2009; Moessner et al., 2007) and *SHANK2* (Berkel et al., 2010; Leblond et al., 2012) in ASD cases (described in further detail in Chapter 4.7).

The analysis of a small cohort of syndromic ASD cases using a bacterial artificial chromosome (BAC)-CGH array (Jacquemont et al., 2006) and low-resolution 10K SNP data from a linkage study (Szatmari et al., 2007) provided some of the first evidence that CNVs contribute to ASD risk. In the five years since this discovery, a series of large studies using a mixture of high-resolution microarrays has further examined the role of CNVs in ASD (Bucan et al., 2009; Christian et al., 2008; Gai et al., 2011; Glessner et al., 2009; Levy et al., 2011; Marshall et al., 2008; Morrow et al., 2008; Pinto et al., 2010; Rosenfeld et al., 2010a; Sanders et al., 2011; Sebat et al., 2007; Weiss et al., 2008). The design of these studies varies but typically involves CNV

analysis of probands and in many cases parents for examination of *de novo* rate. Adjudication of ASD risk CNVs generally involved a similar strategy to that outlined in the previous section, with particular emphasis on *de novo* variants, which have been repeatedly highlighted in the ASD literature for defining CNVs of high risk.

The most relevant findings from the collection of CNV screens in ASD include:

1. Upwards of 10% of ASD cases harbor a rare CNV that may confer risk for ASD.
2. The CNV *de novo* rate in ASD is roughly three to seven times that in controls (Levy et al., 2011; Marshall et al., 2008; Pinto et al., 2010; Sanders et al., 2011; Sebat et al., 2007) and has been reported to be higher in simplex compared to multiplex families (Marshall et al., 2008; Sebat et al., 2007) although this is not always the case (Pinto et al., 2010).
3. Some cases have multiple *de novo* variants presenting with a more complex and syndromic form of ASD.
4. Rare *de novo* and inherited variants implicate the same genes, indicating that transmitted variants are clearly risk factors in some families and may display incomplete penetrance (Fernandez et al., 2010; Vaags et al., 2012).
5. Although many CNVs act in an apparently dominant manner, some transmission is clearly recessive in

consanguineous ASD families with rare homozygous deletions (Morrow et al., 2008).

6. Many rare overlapping CNVs involve genes implicated in other neurodevelopmental disorders and ID/DD, indicating some ASD loci are likely pleiotropic with variable expressivity (Cook and Scherer, 2008; Guilmatre et al., 2009; Lionel et al., 2011).

7. Pathway analysis shows enrichment of particular gene sets including GTPase/Ras (Pinto et al., 2010); ubiquitin degradation genes (Glessner et al., 2009); genes involved in synapse development, axon targeting, and neuron motility (Gilman et al., 2011); and genes in the TSC/SHANK network (Sakai et al., 2011).

It is clear that CNV analysis focused on rare variants in general, both *de novo* and inherited, has led to discovery of dozens of ASD susceptibility loci, where the CNV defines a locus with several genes or points to involvement of a single gene. Table 2.2.1 summarizes some of the most interesting ASD CNVs from two of the more comprehensive studies conducted to date (Pinto et al. 2010; Sanders et al., 2011). One of the most common recurrent CNVs in studies of idiopathic ASD is the ~ 550 kb microdeletion/duplication at 16p11.2 observed in ~ 0.8% of cases (Kumar et al., 2008; Marshall et al., 2008; Weiss et al., 2008). With screening of additional patient populations, since its discovery the phenotype associated with this CNV has expanded to include ASD cases with dysmorphology (Fernandez et al., 2010), as well as cases with general developmental delay (Rosenfeld et al., 2010b; Shinawi et al., 2010), obesity (Bochukova et al., 2010; Jacquemont et al., 2011; Walters et al., 2010), other neurodevelopmental disorders (Lionel et al., 2011; McCarthy et al., 2009), and some unaffected individuals (Bijlsma et al., 2009). We and others have observed that 16p11.2 deletions appear nearly 100% penetrant for a phenotype whereas duplications display reduced penetrance and are more likely to be inherited (Fernandez et al., 2010).

One intriguing locus that may be a model for beginning to explain the skewed male ASD diagnosis is the discovery of CNVs associated with ASD at the *PTCHD1/PTCHD1AS2* locus at Xp22.11 (Marshall et al., 2008; Noor et al., 2010; Pinto et al., 2010). The initial discovery included maternally inherited exonic deletions in ASD that segregated in two affected brothers (Marshall et al., 2008). Later, deletions in ASD males disrupting a non-coding RNA gene (*PTCHD1AS2*) in the 5' region upstream from *PTCHD1* (Noor et al., 2010) were observed. Other studies (Filges et al., 2011; Sanders et al., 2011) have found equivalent deletions, and combined data suggests ~ 0.5% of males with ASD have a deletion at this locus.

Another consistent observation across multiple CNV screening studies is the involvement of individually rare variants overlapping genes important for development and function of neuronal circuits (Bourgeron, 2009; Ramocki and Zoghbi, 2008), especially those located at the synaptic complex (State, 2010a; Toro et al., 2010). Before CNV analysis was widely used, candidate gene sequencing approaches pointed to the involvement of single synaptic complex genes in ASD risk, with rare functional mutations detected in other X-linked genes such as *NLGN4X* and *NLGN3* (Jamain et al., 2003; Laumonnier et al., 2004). At the synaptic membranes, neuroligins (NLGNs) bind with neurexins (NRXNs) and together function as major organizers of excitatory glutamatergic synapses (Sudhof, 2008). While CNVs

TABLE 2.2.1 Autism Spectrum Disorder Risk Loci from CNV Studies

Cytoband	CNV locus and genes	Combined number of events in cases/controls[1]		P-value (cases vs. controls)[2]	Frequency in ASD (males)
		Case (n = 2120)	Control (n = 2159)		
2p16.3	*NRXN1*	9	1	0.011	0.4%
11q13.3	*SHANK2*	2	0	0.245	0.1%
15q11−q13	5 Mb and 12 genes	2	0	0.245	0.1%
15q13.3	1.5 Mb and 6 genes	5	0	0.030	0.2%
16p11.2	550 kb and 30 genes	18	3	0.001	0.8%
22q13.33	*SHANK3*	1	0	0.495	0.05%
Xp22.11	*PTCHD1/PTCHD1AS2*	10/1807 males	0/786 males	0.038	0.5% (0.6%)
Xp22.3	*NLGN4X*	1/1807 males	0/786 males	1	0.05% (0.06%)
Xq13.1	*NLGN3*	1/1807 males	0/786 males	1	0.05% (0.06%)

[1] *From Pinto et al. (2010) and Sanders et al. (2011).*
[2] *Fisher's exact 2-sided p-value.*

TABLE 2.2.2   Summary of Exonic *NRXN1* Deletions in Autism Spectrum Disorder

	Case*		Control	
	n	Exonic deletion	n	Exonic deletion
Szatmari et al., 2007	196	1	–	–
Glessner et al., 2009	2,195	6	2,519	0
Pinto et al., 2010	996	3	4,964	0
Shen et al., 2010	848	1	–	–
Guilmatre et al., 2009	260	2	236	0
Sanders et al., 2011	1,124	3	–	–
Bremer et al., 2011	223	1	–	–
Total	**5,842**	**17**	**7,719**	**0**

* Deletions are significantly associated with ASD: Fischer's exact test $P < 6 \times 10^{-6}$.

overlapping NLGNs appear to be very uncommon in any disorder, rare exonic *NXRN1* deletions have been consistently found in ASD CNV screens (Reichelt et al., 2011).

The first observation of an *NXRN1* deletion in ASD was found in a low-resolution Affymetrix 10K genome-wide linkage scan (Szatmari et al., 2007). Higher-resolution scans have found exonic deletions in ASD cases and not controls (Ching et al., 2010; Glessner et al., 2009; Kim et al., 2008; Pinto et al., 2010; Sanders et al., 2011; Shen et al., 2010), but often the association does not reach statistical significance due to small sample numbers and the fact that these deletions are individually very rare. It is only by performing a meta-analysis across several studies that we observe a highly significant ($P < 6 \times 10^{-6}$) association of *NRXN1* deletions in ASD compared to controls, as shown in Table 2.2.2 and

Figure 2.2.2. It is now apparent that all three members of the NRXN family may be implicated in ASD, as recent CNV (Vaags et al., 2012) and candidate gene sequencing (Gauthier et al., 2011) studies have found rare mutations in *NRXN3* and *NRXN2*, respectively, in ASD cases. CNVs have also implicated genes expressed at the postsynaptic density (PSD) in ASD etiology, most notably genes for scaffolding proteins such as *SHANK2* (Berkel et al., 2010; 2012; Leblond et al., 2012), *SHANK3* (Durand et al., 2007; Moessner et al., 2007), and *DLGAP2* (Pinto et al., 2010). The SHANK proteins are crucial components of the PSD and complex with the NLGNs which, in turn, bind with the trans-synaptic NRXNs (State, 2010a; Chapter 4.7). Although the association of larger 22q13.3 terminal deletions have been associated with an ASD phenotype for some time (Goizet et al., 2000; Manning et al., 2004), it was not until more recently that CNVs and mutations specific to *SHANK3* were shown to be associated with ASD (Durand et al., 2007; Gauthier et al., 2009; Moessner et al., 2007). More recent studies have identified multiple *de novo* CNVs in unrelated ASD cases overlapping the paralogue *SHANK2* (Berkel et al., 2010), a finding that has recently been replicated (Leblond et al., 2012).

Finally, CNVs in several genes important for axonal growth have been linked to ASD. Contactin proteins form connections between axons and glial cells and are also important for axonal guidance. CNVs in ASD cases have been found at *CNTN4* (Cottrell et al., 2011; Roohi et al., 2009) and the contactin-associated protein gene *CNTNAP2* (Nord et al., 2011). Other cell adhesion proteins have also been implicated in ASD by CNV analysis, including the cadherins *CDH8* (Pagnamenta et al., 2011b) and CDH13 (Sanders et al., 2011), and protocadherins PCDH9 (Marshall et al., 2008) and PCDH10 (Morrow et al., 2008).

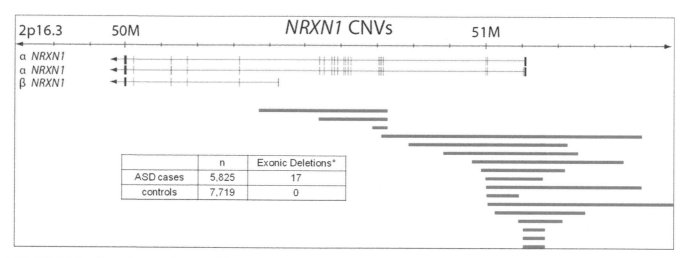

FIGURE 2.2.2   Genomic map of exonic deletions (red bars) in seven CNV studies outlined in Table 2.2.2. Exonic deletions of *NRXN1* are significantly associated with ASD (Fischer's exact test $P < 6 \times 10^{-6}$).

The penetrance of a CNV for ASD will depend on the dosage sensitivity and function of the gene(s) affected (Cook and Scherer, 2008). Some CNVs affecting single (e.g., *SHANK* deletions) or multiple (e.g., 16p11.2 deletions) genes will likely be sufficient to cause ASD on their own and represent highly penetrant forms of the disorder. These CNVs will typically be *de novo* in origin, cause a more severe clinical presentation, and be more prevalent in sporadic forms of ASD. Other CNVs may contribute to the phenotype but in most cases would require other genetic or non-genetic factors in order to reach the threshold of an ASD diagnosis (Cook and Scherer, 2008). These CNVs of reduced penetrance are often inherited and may be observed in non-ASD family members (parents or siblings) and in population controls, or display pleiotropy in contributing to other neurodevelopmental disorders. It is clear in the present field that there is a general lack of data allowing a more cohesive understanding of the genotype and phenotype relationship in ASD for most of the candidate CNVs, particularly the ones that are inherited with variable penetrance. Part of the challenge is that most of these CNVs are inherently rare, an issue that will be partially solved through CNV analysis of more cases. The other key is the ability to go back to the family to collect more detailed clinical information. A comparison of detailed phenotype measures across individuals (ASD and non-ASD) harboring a specific candidate CNV will be crucial for determining association with ASD.

CONCLUSIONS AND FUTURE STUDIES

Arguably, the emergence of CNV analysis as an unbiased genome-wide strategy for discovery of candidate genes represents an important advance in the study of rare variation underlying ASD etiology. This strategy has benefitted greatly from the rapid development of microarray technology, particularly with increased genomic resolution (i.e., now up to 5 million probes in a single experiment) allowing reliable detection of unbalanced changes larger than 1 kb in size. CNVs have proven useful in pinpointing single genes (e.g. those from SHANK and NRXN families) and multigenic loci (e.g., 16p11.2 and 1q21.1). Although these loci are individually rare in a cohort, one may now expect to find a putative pathogenic CNV in upwards of ~ 10% of ASD cases using the latest high-resolution platforms. Many of these will be *de novo* in origin as the literature has consistently shown an important role for *de novo* CNVs in ASD (Levy et al., 2011; Marshall et al., 2008; Pinto et al., 2010; Sanders et al., 2011; Sebat et al., 2007). For these new mutations to persist in the population

and contribute to inherited forms of ASD, they would need to be shielded from negative selection (Zhao et al., 2007). As genome scanning resolution increases, one may also expect the rate of *de novo* events found to be associated with ASD to increase. Indeed, recent CNV studies examining the frequencies and distribution of *de novo* events estimate that there are as many as 300 *de novo* risk loci related to ASD across the genome (Levy et al., 2011; Pinto et al., 2010; Sanders et al., 2011).

Although *de novo* CNVs can explain some of the genetic architecture underlying ASD risk, the mechanism is inconsistent with the high estimates of ASD heritability from family and twin studies. Some of the more highly penetrant ASD CNVs that are transmitted from unaffected parents may be explained by a difference in gender expression through parent-of-origin effects (e.g., 15q11–13 duplications of the maternal allele), or recessive (Morrow et al., 2008) or X-linked transmission in males (Jamain et al., 2003; Noor et al., 2010). It has been suggested that gene–gene or gene–environment interactions may explain the inheritance patterns of ASD (Risch et al., 1999). More recent research has pointed to the possible involvement of multiple CNVs conferring ASD risk in single individuals (Pagnamenta et al., 2011a; Vorstman et al., 2011) suggesting a multigenic threshold model for ASD. It is clear that there is considerable work to be done in defining the risk associated with rare inherited CNVs in ASD, for which a detailed clinical phenotype will be essential. This information will also be important to tease out subtle phenotypes that are similar across disorders.

One emerging trend in the field that was not discussed in detail here is the finding of the same CNV as a risk factor in multiple neuropsychiatric disorders (Carroll and Owen, 2009; Guilmatre et al., 2009; Saus et al., 2010; Sebat et al., 2009). For example, a recent study of ours found rare CNVs at *ASTN2* associated with both ASD and ADHD patients (Lionel et al., 2011). Moreover, other genes such as *NRXN1* and *CNTNAP2* have been observed to be affected by rare CNVs in patients with a diverse spectrum of neurocognitive phenotypes (Gregor et al., 2011).

The success of CNV analysis in uncovering many of the variants associated with ASD has raised expectations in the clinical community and in the public (Scherer and Dawson, 2011). Although microarray technology is still the primary technique for CNV detection, the rapid decrease in next-generation sequencing costs will soon make CNV detection through whole-genome sequencing feasible, presenting further challenges for data interpretation. As a larger catalogue of ASD risk CNVs is generated, the translation of research findings into clinical practice will aid early detection and treatment of ASD.

ACKNOWLEDGMENTS

The authors wish to thank Dr Daisuke Sato for assistance. SWS holds the GlaxoSmithKline Canadian Institutes of Health Research (CIHR) Endowed Chair in Genome Sciences.

References

Abrahams, B.S., Geschwind, D.H., 2008. Advances in Autism genetics: On the threshold of a new neurobiology. Nature Reviews Genetics 9, 341–355.

American Psychiatric Association, 2000. Diagnostic and Statistical Manual of Mental Disorders, Fourth Edition - Text Revision (DSMIV-TR). Washington DC, American Psychiatric Association.

Autism and Developmental Disabilities Monitoring Network, 2009. Prevalence of Autism spectrum disorders - Autism and Developmental Disabilities Monitoring Network, United States, 2006. Morbidity and Mortality Weekly Report. Surveillance Summaries 58, 1–20.

Bailey, A., Le Couteur, A., Gottesman, I., Bolton, P., Simonoff, E., Yuzda, E., et al., 1995. Autism as a strongly genetic disorder: Evidence from a British twin study. Psychological Medicine 25, 63–77.

Baker, P., Piven, J., Schwartz, S., Patil, S., 1994. Brief report: Duplication of chromosome 15q11-13 in two individuals with autistic disorder. Journal of Autism & Developmental Disorders 24, 529–535.

Berkel, S., Marshall, C.R., Weiss, B., Howe, J., Roeth, R., Moog, U., et al., 2010. Mutations in the SHANK2 synaptic scaffolding gene in Autism spectrum disorder and mental retardation. Nature Genetics 42, 489–491.

Berkel, S., Tang, W., Trevino, M., Vogt, M., Obenhaus, H.A., Gass, P., et al., 2012. Inherited and de novo SHANK2 variants associated with Autism spectrum disorder impair neuronal morphogenesis and physiology. Human Molecular Genetics 21, 344–357.

Betancur, C., 2011. Etiological heterogeneity in Autism spectrum disorders: More than 100 genetic and genomic disorders and still counting. Brain Research 1380, 42–77.

Bijlsma, E.K., Gijsbers, A.C., Schuurs-Hoeijmakers, J.H., van Haeringen, A., Fransen van de Putte, D.E., Anderlid, B.M., et al., 2009. Extending the phenotype of recurrent rearrangements of 16p11.2: Deletions in mentally retarded patients without Autism and in normal individuals. European Journal of Medical Genetics 52, 77–87.

Bochukova, E.G., Huang, N., Keogh, J., Henning, E., Purmann, C., Blaszczyk, K., et al., 2010. Large, rare chromosomal deletions associated with severe early-onset obesity. Nature 463, 666–670.

Bourgeron, T., 2009. A synaptic trek to Autism. Current Opinion in Neurobiology 19, 231–234.

Bremer, A., Giacobini, M., Eriksson, M., Gustavsson, P., Nordin, V., Fernell, E., et al., 2011. Copy number variation characteristics in subpopulations of patients with Autism spectrum disorders. American Journal of Medical Genetics Part B: Neuropsychiatric 156, 115–124.

Bucan, M., Abrahams, B.S., Wang, K., Glessner, J.T., Herman, E.I., Sonnenblick, L.I., et al., 2009. Genome-wide analyses of exonic copy number variants in a family-based study point to novel Autism susceptibility genes. PLoS Genetics 5, e1000536.

Carroll, L.S., Owen, M.J., 2009. Genetic overlap between Autism schizophrenia and bipolar disorder. Genome Medicine 1, 102.

Ching, M.S., Shen, Y., Tan, W.H., Jeste, S.S., Morrow, E.M., Chen, X., et al., 2010. Deletions of NRXN1 (neurexin-1) predispose to a wide spectrum of developmental disorders. American Journal of Medical Genetics Part B: Neuropsychiatric 153B, 937–947.

Christian, S.L., Brune, C.W., Sudi, J., Kumar, R.A., Liu, S., Karamohamed, S., et al., 2008. Novel submicroscopic chromosomal abnormalities detected in Autism spectrum disorder. Biological Psychiatry 63, 1111–1117.

Colella, S., Yau, C., Taylor, J.M., Mirza, G., Butler, H., Clouston, P., et al., 2007. QuantiSNP: An Objective Bayes Hidden-Markov Model to detect and accurately map copy number variation using SNP genotyping data. Nucleic Acids Research 35, 2013–2025.

Constantino, J.N., Todorov, A., Hilton, C., Law, P., Zhang, Y., Molloy, E., et al., 2012. Autism recurrence in half siblings: Strong support for genetic mechanisms of transmission in ASD. Molecular Psychiatry.

Constantino, J.N., Zhang, Y., Frazier, T., Abbacchi, A.M., Law, P., 2010. Sibling recurrence and the genetic epidemiology of Autism. American Journal of Psychiatry 167, 1349–1356.

Cook Jr., E.H., Scherer, S.W., 2008. Copy-number variations associated with neuropsychiatric conditions. Nature 455, 919–923.

Cottrell, C.E., Bir, N., Varga, E., Alvarez, C.E., Bouyain, S., Zernzach, R., et al., 2011. Contactin 4 as an Autism susceptibility locus. Autism Research 4, 189–199.

Devlin, B., Melhem, N., Roeder, K., 2011. Do common variants play a role in risk for Autism Evidence and theoretical musings. Brain Research 1380, 78–84.

Durand, C.M., Betancur, C., Boeckers, T.M., Bockmann, J., Chaste, P., Fauchereau, F., et al., 2007. Mutations in the gene encoding the synaptic scaffolding protein SHANK3 are associated with Autism spectrum disorders. Nature Genetics 39, 25–27.

Fernandez, B.A., Roberts, W., Chung, B., Weksberg, R., Meyn, S., Szatmari, P., et al., 2010. Phenotypic spectrum associated with de novo and inherited deletions and duplications at 16p11.2 in individuals ascertained for diagnosis of Autism spectrum disorder. Journal of Medical Genetics 47, 195–203.

Filges, I., Rothlisberger, B., Blattner, A., Boesch, N., Demougin, P., Wenzel, F., et al., 2011. Deletion in Xp22.11: PTCHD1 is a candidate gene for X-linked intellectual disability with or without Autism. Clinical Genetics 79, 79–85.

Folstein, S.E., Rosen-Sheidley, B., 2001. Genetics of Autism: Complex aetiology for a heterogeneous disorder. Nature Reviews Genetics 2, 943–955.

Fombonne, E., 2009. Epidemiology of pervasive developmental disorders. Pediatric Research 65, 591–598.

Gai, X., Xie, H.M., Perin, J.C., Takahashi, N., Murphy, K., Wenocur, A.S., et al., 2011. Rare structural variation of synapse and neurotransmission genes in Autism. Molecular Psychiatry.

Gauthier, J., Siddiqui, T., Huashan, P., Yokomaku, D., Hamdan, F., Champagne, N., et al., 2011. Truncating mutations in NRXN2 and NRXN1 in Autism spectrum disorders and schizophrenia. Human Genetics 130, 563–573.

Gauthier, J., Spiegelman, D., Piton, A., Lafreniere, R.G., Laurent, S., St-Onge, J., et al., 2009. Novel de novo SHANK3 mutation in autistic patients. American Journal of Medical Genetics Part B: Neuropsychiatric 150B, 421–424.

Gillberg, C., Cederlund, M., Lamberg, K., Zeijlon, L., 2006. Brief report: "The Autism epidemic". The registered prevalence of Autism in a Swedish urban area. Journal of Autism & Developmental Disorders 36, 429–435.

Gilman, S.R., Iossifov, I., Levy, D., Ronemus, M., Wigler, M., Vitkup, D., 2011. Rare de novo variants associated with Autism implicate a large functional network of genes involved in formation and function of synapses. Neuron 70, 898–907.

Glessner, J.T., Wang, K., Cai, G., Korvatska, O., Kim, C.E., Wood, S., et al., 2009. Autism genome-wide copy number variation reveals ubiquitin and neuronal genes. Nature 459, 569–573.

Goizet, C., Excoffier, E., Taine, L., Taupiac, E., El Moneim, A.A., Arveiler, B., et al., 2000. Case with autistic syndrome and chromosome 22q13.3 deletion detected by FISH. American Journal of Medical Genetics 96, 839–844.

Goldstein, S., Schwebach, A.J., 2004. The comorbidity of pervasive developmental disorder and attention deficit hyperactivity disorder: Results of a retrospective chart review. Journal of Autism & Developmental Disorders 34, 329–339.

Gregor, A., Albrecht, B., Bader, I., Bijlsma, E.K., Ekici, A.B., Engels, H., et al., 2011. Expanding the clinical spectrum associated with defects in CNTNAP2 and NRXN1. BMC Medical Genetics 12, 106.

Guilmatre, A., Dubourg, C., Mosca, A.L., Legallic, S., Goldenberg, A., Drouin-Garraud, V., et al., 2009. Recurrent rearrangements in synaptic and neurodevelopmental genes and shared biologic pathways in schizophrenia, Autism and mental retardation. Archives of General Psychiatry 66, 947–956.

Hallmayer, J., Cleveland, S., Torres, A., Phillips, J., Cohen, B., Torigoe, T., et al., 2011. Genetic heritability and shared environmental factors among twin pairs with Autism. Archives of General Psychiatry 68, 1095–1102.

Hofvander, B., Delorme, R., Chaste, P., Nyden, A., Wentz, E., Stahlberg, O., et al., 2009. Psychiatric and psychosocial problems in adults with normal-intelligence Autism spectrum disorders. BMC Psychiatry 9, 35.

Iafrate, A.J., Feuk, L., Rivera, M.N., Listewnik, M.L., Donahoe, P.K., Qi, Y., et al., 2004. Detection of large-scale variation in the human genome. Nature Genetics 36, 949–951.

Jacquemont, M.L., Sanlaville, D., Redon, R., Raoul, O., Cormier-Daire, V., Lyonnet, S., et al., 2006. Array-based comparative genomic hybridisation identifies high frequency of cryptic chromosomal rearrangements in patients with syndromic Autism spectrum disorders. Journal of Medical Genetics 43, 843–849.

Jacquemont, S., Reymond, A., Zufferey, F., Harewood, L., Walters, R.G., Kutalik, Z., et al., 2011. Mirror extreme BMI phenotypes associated with gene dosage at the chromosome 16p11.2 locus. Nature 478, 97–102.

Jamain, S., Quach, H., Betancur, C., Rastam, M., Colineaux, C., Gillberg, I.C., et al., 2003. Mutations of the X-linked genes encoding neuroligins NLGN3 and NLGN4 are associated with Autism. Nature Genetics 34, 27–29.

Kanner, L., 1946. Child psychiatry; mental deficiency. American Journal of Psychiatry 102, 520–522.

Kim, H.G., Kishikawa, S., Higgins, A.W., Seong, I.S., Donovan, D.J., Shen, Y., et al., 2008. Disruption of neurexin 1 associated with Autism spectrum disorder. American Journal of Human Genetics 82, 199–207.

Korn, J.M., Kuruvilla, F.G., McCarroll, S.A., Wysoker, A., Nemesh, J., Cawley, S., et al., 2008. Integrated genotype calling and association analysis of SNPs, common copy number polymorphisms and rare CNVs. Nature Genetics 40, 1253–1260.

Kumar, R.A., KaraMohamed, S., Sudi, J., Conrad, D.F., Brune, C., Badner, J.A., et al., 2008. Recurrent 16p11.2 microdeletions in Autism. Human Molecular Genetics 17, 628–638.

Laumonnier, F., Bonnet-Brilhault, F., Gomot, M., Blanc, R., David, A., Moizard, M.P., et al., 2004. X-linked mental retardation and Autism are associated with a mutation in the NLGN4 gene, a member of the neuroligin family. American Journal of Human Genetics 74, 552–557.

Leblond, C.S., Heinrich, J., Delorme, R., Proepper, C., Betancur, C., Huguet, G., et al., 2012. Genetic and functional analyses of *SHANK2* mutations suggest a multiple hit model of autism spectrum disorders. PLoS Genetics 8, e1002521.

Le Couteur, A., Bailey, A., Goode, S., Pickles, A., Robertson, S., Gottesman, I., et al., 1996. A broader phenotype of Autism: The clinical spectrum in twins. Journal of Child Psychology and Psychiatry 37, 785–801.

Lee, C., Scherer, S.W., 2010. The clinical context of copy number variation in the human genome. Expert Reviews in Molecular Medicine 12, e8.

Levy, D., Ronemus, M., Yamrom, B., Lee, Y.H., Leotta, A., Kendall, J., et al., 2011. Rare de novo and transmitted copy-number variation in autistic spectrum disorders. Neuron 70, 886–897.

Leyfer, O.T., Folstein, S.E., Bacalman, S., Davis, N.O., Dinh, E., Morgan, J., et al., 2006. Comorbid psychiatric disorders in children with Autism: Interview development and rates of disorders. Journal of Autism & Developmental Disorders 36, 849–861.

Lionel, A.C., Crosbie, J., Barbosa, N., Goodale, T., Thiruvahindrapuram, B., Rickaby, J., et al., 2011. Rare copy number variation discovery and cross-disorder comparisons identify risk genes for ADHD. Science Translational Medicine 3, 95ra75.

Losh, M., Childress, D., Lam, K., Piven, J., 2008. Defining key features of the broad Autism phenotype: A comparison across parents of multiple- and single-incidence Autism families. American Journal of Medical Genetics B. Neuropsychiatr. Genet. 147B, 424–433.

Manning, M.A., Cassidy, S.B., Clericuzio, C., Cherry, A.M., Schwartz, S., Hudgins, L., et al., 2004. Terminal 22q deletion syndrome: A newly recognized cause of speech and language disability in the Autism spectrum. Pediatrics 114, 451–457.

Marshall, C.R., Noor, A., Vincent, J.B., Lionel, A.C., Feuk, L., Skaug, J., et al., 2008. Structural variation of chromosomes in Autism spectrum disorder. American Journal of Human Genetics 82, 477–488.

McCarthy, S.E., Makarov, V., Kirov, G., Addington, A.M., McClellan, J., Yoon, S., et al., 2009. Microduplications of 16p11.2 are associated with schizophrenia. Nature Genetics 41, 1223–1227.

Moessner, R., Marshall, C.R., Sutcliffe, J.S., Skaug, J., Pinto, D., Vincent, J., et al., 2007. Contribution of SHANK3 mutations to Autism spectrum disorder. American Journal of Human Genetics 81, 1289–1297.

Morrow, E.M., Yoo, S.Y., Flavell, S.W., Kim, T.K., Lin, Y., Hill, R.S., et al., 2008. Identifying Autism loci and genes by tracing recent shared ancestry. Science 321, 218–223.

Noor, A., Whibley, A., Marshall, C.R., Gianakopoulos, P.J., Piton, A., Carson, A.R., et al., 2010. Disruption at the PTCHD1 Locus on Xp22.11 in Autism spectrum disorder and intellectual disability. Science Translational Medicine 2, 49ra68.

Nord, A.S., Roeb, W., Dickel, D.E., Walsh, T., Kusenda, M., O'Connor, K.L., et al., 2011. Reduced transcript expression of genes affected by inherited and de novo CNVs in Autism. European Journal of Human Genetics 19, 727–731.

O'Brien, G., Pearson, J., 2004. Autism and learning disability. Autism 8, 125–140.

Ozonoff, S., Young, G.S., Carter, A., Messinger, D., Yirmiya, N., Zwaigenbaum, L., et al., 2011. Recurrence risk for autism spectrum disorders: A Baby Siblings Research Consortium study. Pediatrics.

Pagnamenta, A.T., Holt, R., Yusuf, M., Pinto, D., Wing, K., Betancur, C., et al., 2011. A family with Autism and rare copy number variants disrupting the Duchenne/Becker muscular dystrophy gene DMD and TRPM3. Journal of Neurodevelopmental Disorders 3, 124–131.

Pagnamenta, A.T., Khan, H., Walker, S., Gerrelli, D., Wing, K., Bonaglia, M.C., et al., 2011. Rare familial 16q21 microdeletions under a linkage peak implicate cadherin 8 (CDH8) in susceptibility to Autism and learning disability. Journal of Medical Genetics 48, 48–54.

Pinto, D., Darvishi, K., Shi, X., Rajan, D., Rigler, D., Fitzgerald, T., et al., 2011. Comprehensive assessment of array-based platforms and calling algorithms for detection of copy number variants. Nature Biotechnology 29, 512–520.

Pinto, D., Pagnamenta, A.T., Klei, L., Anney, R., Merico, D., Regan, R., et al., 2010. Functional impact of global rare copy number variation in Autism spectrum disorders. Nature 466, 368–372.

Ramocki, M.B., Zoghbi, H.Y., 2008. Failure of neuronal homeostasis results in common neuropsychiatric phenotypes. Nature 455, 912–918.

Redon, R., Ishikawa, S., Fitch, K.R., Feuk, L., Perry, G.H., Andrews, T.D., et al., 2006. Global variation in copy number in the human genome. Nature 444, 444–454.

Reichelt, A.C., Rodgers, R.J., Clapcote, S.J., 2011. The role of neurexins in schizophrenia and autistic spectrum disorder. Neuropharmacology.

Risch, N., Spiker, D., Lotspeich, L., Nouri, N., Hinds, D., Hallmayer, J., et al., 1999. A genomic screen of Autism: Evidence for a multilocus etiology. American Journal of Human Genetics 65, 493–507.

Rommelse, N.N., Franke, B., Geurts, H.M., Hartman, C.A., Buitelaar, J.K., 2010. Shared heritability of attention-deficit/hyperactivity disorder and Autism spectrum disorder. European Child & Adolescent Psychiatry 19, 281–295.

Roohi, J., Montagna, C., Tegay, D.H., Palmer, L.E., DeVincent, C., Pomeroy, J.C., et al., 2009. Disruption of contactin 4 in three subjects with Autism spectrum disorder. Journal of Medical Genetics 46, 176–182.

Rosenberg, R.E., Law, J.K., Yenokyan, G., McGready, J., Kaufmann, W.E., Law, P.A., 2009. Characteristics and concordance of Autism spectrum disorders among 277 twin pairs. Archives of Pediatrics & Adolescent Medicine 163, 907–914.

Rosenfeld, J.A., Ballif, B.C., Torchia, B.S., Sahoo, T., Ravnan, J.B., Schultz, R., et al., 2010. Copy number variations associated with Autism spectrum disorders contribute to a spectrum of neurodevelopmental disorders. Genetics in Medicine 12, 694–702.

Rosenfeld, J.A., Coppinger, J., Bejjani, B.A., Girirajan, S., Eichler, E.E., Shaffer, L.G., et al., 2010. Speech delays and behavioral problems are the predominant features in individuals with developmental delays and 16p11.2 microdeletions and microduplications. Journal of Neurodevelopmental Disorders 2, 26–38.

Ruta, L., Mugno, D., D'Arrigo, V.G., Vitiello, B., Mazzone, L., 2010. Obsessive-compulsive traits in children and adolescents with Asperger syndrome. European Child & Adolescent Psychiatry 19, 17–24.

Sakai, Y., Shaw, C.A., Dawson, B.C., Dugas, D.V., Al-Mohtaseb, Z., Hill, D.E., et al., 2011. Protein interactome reveals converging molecular pathways among Autism disorders. Science Translational Medicine 3, 86ra49.

Sanders, S.J., Ercan-Sencicek, A.G., Hus, V., Luo, R., Murtha, M.T., Moreno-De-Luca, D., et al., 2011. Multiple recurrent de novo CNVs, including duplications of the 7q11.23 Williams syndrome region, are strongly associated with Autism. Neuron 70, 863–885.

Saus, E., Brunet, A., Armengol, L., Alonso, P., Crespo, J.M., Fernandez-Aranda, F., et al., 2010. Comprehensive copy number variant (CNV) analysis of neuronal pathways genes in psychiatric disorders identifies rare variants within patients. Journal of Psychiatric Research 44, 971–978.

Scherer, S.W., Dawson, G., 2011. Risk factors for Autism: Translating genomic discoveries into diagnostics. Human Genetics 130, 123–148.

Sebat, J., Lakshmi, B., Malhotra, D., Troge, J., Lese-Martin, C., Walsh, T., et al., 2007. Strong association of de novo copy number mutations with Autism. Science 316, 445–449.

Sebat, J., Lakshmi, B., Troge, J., Alexander, J., Young, J., Lundin, P., et al., 2004. Large-scale copy number polymorphism in the human genome. Science 305, 525–528.

Sebat, J., Levy, D.L., McCarthy, S.E., 2009. Rare structural variants in schizophrenia: One disorder, multiple mutations; one mutation, multiple disorders. Trends in Genetics 25, 528–535.

Shen, Y., Dies, K.A., Holm, I.A., Bridgemohan, C., Sobeih, M.M., Caronna, E.B., et al., 2010. Clinical genetic testing for patients with Autism spectrum disorders. Pediatrics 125, e727–e735.

Shinawi, M., Liu, P., Kang, S.H., Shen, J., Belmont, J.W., Scott, D.A., et al., 2010. Recurrent reciprocal 16p11.2 rearrangements associated with global developmental delay, behavioural problems, dysmorphism, epilepsy, and abnormal head size. Journal of Medical Genetics 47, 332–341.

Sporn, A.L., Addington, A.M., Gogtay, N., Ordonez, A.E., Gornick, M., Clasen, L., et al., 2004. Pervasive developmental disorder and childhood-onset schizophrenia: Comorbid disorder or a phenotypic variant of a very early onset illness? Biological Psychiatry 55, 989–994.

State, M.W., 2010. Another piece of the Autism puzzle. Nature Genetics 42, 478–479.

State, M.W., 2010. The genetics of child psychiatric disorders: Focus on Autism and Tourette syndrome. Neuron 68, 254–269.

Steffenburg, S., Gillberg, C., Hellgren, L., Andersson, L., Gillberg, I.C., Jakobsson, G., et al., 1989. A twin study of Autism in Denmark, Finland, Iceland, Norway and Sweden. Journal of Child Psychology and Psychiatry 30, 405–416.

Sudhof, T.C., 2008. Neuroligins and neurexins link synaptic function to cognitive disease. Nature 455, 903–911.

Szatmari, P., Jones, M.B., Zwaigenbaum, L., MacLean, J.E., 1998. Genetics of Autism: Overview and new directions. Journal of Autism & Developmental Disorders 28, 351–368.

Szatmari, P., Paterson, A.D., Zwaigenbaum, L., Roberts, W., Brian, J., Liu, X.Q., et al., 2007. Mapping Autism risk loci using genetic linkage and chromosomal rearrangements. Nature Genetics 39, 319–328.

Toro, R., Konyukh, M., Delorme, R., Leblond, C., Chaste, P., Fauchereau, F., et al., 2010. Key role for gene dosage and synaptic homeostasis in Autism spectrum disorders. Trends in Genetics 26, 363–372.

Vaags, A.K., Lionel, A.C., Sato, D., Goodenberger, M., Stein, Q.P., Curran, S., et al., 2012. Rare deletions at the neurexin 3 locus in Autism spectrum disorder. American Journal of Human Genetics 90, 133–141.

Veenstra-Vanderweele, J., Christian, S.L., Cook Jr., E.H., 2004. Autism as a paradigmatic complex genetic disorder. Annual Review of Genomics and Human Genetics 5, 379–405.

Venkatraman, E.S., Olshen, A.B., 2007. A faster circular binary segmentation algorithm for the analysis of array CGH data. Bioinformatics 23, 657–663.

Vorstman, J.A., van Daalen, E., Jalali, G.R., Schmidt, E.R., Pasterkamp, R.J., de Jonge, M., et al., 2011. A double hit implicates DIAPH3 as an Autism risk gene. Molecular Psychiatry 16, 442–451.

Walters, R.G., Jacquemont, S., Valsesia, A., de Smith, A.J., Martinet, D., Andersson, J., et al., 2010. A new highly penetrant form of obesity due to deletions on chromosome 16p11.2. Nature 463, 671–675.

Wang, K., Li, M., Hadley, D., Liu, R., Glessner, J., Grant, S.F., et al., 2007. PennCNV: An integrated hidden Markov model designed for high-resolution copy number variation detection in whole-genome SNP genotyping data. Genome Research 17, 1665–1674.

Weiss, L.A., Shen, Y., Korn, J.M., Arking, D.E., Miller, D.T., Fossdal, R., et al., 2008. Association between microdeletion and microduplication at 16p11.2 and Autism. New England Journal of Medicine 358, 667–675.

Xu, J., Zwaigenbaum, L., Szatmari, P., Scherer, S.W., 2004. Molecular cytogenetics of autism. Current Genomics. 5, 347–364.

Zhao, X., Leotta, A., Kustanovich, V., Lajonchere, C., Geschwind, D.H., Law, K., et al., 2007. A unified genetic theory for sporadic and inherited Autism. Proceedings of the National Academy of Sciences USA 104, 12,831–12,836.

Zwaigenbaum, L., Bryson, S., Rogers, T., Roberts, W., Brian, J., Szatmari, P., 2005. Behavioral manifestations of Autism in the first year of life. International Journal of Developmental Neuroscience 23, 143–152.

Common Genetic Variants in Autism Spectrum Disorders

Richard J.L. Anney

Department of Psychiatry and Neuropsychiatric Genetics Research Group, Trinity College Dublin, Dublin, Ireland

INTRODUCTION

The prevalence of autism has been estimated at approximately 15–20 per 10,000 people (Fombonne, 2009), with the more inclusive diagnosis of autism spectrum disorders (ASD) estimated at 60 in 10,000 children (Fernell and Gillberg, 2010; Fombonne, 2009). ASD have been established as highly familial disorders with siblings of a proband showing at least 25-fold higher prevalence than that of the general population (Bailey et al., 1995). Additional evidence from twin studies indicates that the etiology of ASD includes a strongly heritable component (Abrahams and Geschwind, 2008). Historically, ASD have been highlighted as the most heritable of the neurodevelopmental disorders, supported by the oft-cited estimate of 0.9 presented by the British Twin Study (Bailey et al., 1995). Two recent reports of ASD and ASD symptoms suggest a smaller genetic component. Examining 202 twin pairs from the California Twin Registry, Hallmayer and colleagues estimated that the variance explained by the additive genetic risk was a more modest 0.4, with the majority of the variance explained by the shared environment (Hallmayer et al., 2011). Closely following this report, Robinson and colleagues from Twins Early Development Study (TEDS) reported their examination of ASD traits in a 12-year-old twin population. Using an extreme trait design from a population of 5,944 twin-pairs, a group of 192 twin-pairs with at least one ASD-affected twin was selected. A strong additive genetic component was observed for each of the three core autism domains: social interaction (0.72), communication impairment (0.76), and restrictive-repetitive behaviors (0.76) (Robinson et al., 2011). Interestingly, the authors highlight that there is a considerable, greater than 50%, unique genetic component within each domain.

Given the evidence supporting a genetic component, researchers have employed a variety of approaches ranging from family-based linkage, candidate gene, and genome-wide array, to, more recently, high-throughput sequencing studies to gain a better understanding of the specific genetic risk underpinning the heritability of ASD.

The Neuroscience of Autism Spectrum Disorders.
http://dx.doi.org/10.1016/B978-0-12-391924-3.00010-7

LINKAGE STUDIES IN AUTISM

The success of positional cloning in identifying genes responsible for Mendelian disorders has encouraged the application of linkage approaches to more complex traits, such as ASD. Based on the criteria of Lander and Kruglyak (1995) many regions of the genome have been highlighted as being *suggestive*, namely providing:

statistical evidence that would be expected to occur one time at random in a genome scan.

Only a few scans have highlighted loci with *significant* linkage; that is:

statistical evidence expected to occur only 0.05 times in a genome scan (that is with a probability of 5%).

To date, none of the significant linkage peaks have been established as *confirmed*, namely:

significant linkage from one or a combination of initial studies that has subsequently been confirmed in a further sample, preferably by an independent group of investigators. For confirmation, a nominal P value of 0.01 should be required.

The first genome-wide linkage study of autism by the International Molecular Genetic Study of Autism Consortium (IMGSAC) (IMGSAC, 1998) was performed using a two-stage genome search in 87 affected sib-pairs plus 12 non-sib affected relative-pairs. A total of six regions were highlighted as showing linkage at multi-point maximum logarithmic odds (LOD) score > 1, including *significant* linkage arising on chromosome 7q32–q34. A subsequent analysis of 170 multiplex IMGSAC families provided additional support for a 7q locus at 7q22 in UK and non-UK families (IMGSAC and Bailey, 2001). A further IMGSAC analysis including 83 sib-pairs with autism provided additional *suggestive* support for linkages on chromosomes 7q22 and 16p13, alongside novel *significant* linkage to chromosome 2q31 (IMGSAC and Monaco, 2001). A subsequent linkage study of 95 families, collected by the Autism Genome Research Exchange (AGRE) consortium and the Seaver Autism Center, with two or more individuals with autism or related disorders, provided supporting evidence of linkage to 2q31–q32, which is enriched when the analyses are restricted to individuals with speech-language delay (Buxbaum et al., 2001).

A number of linkage studies quickly followed that of the IMGSAC consortium. The Paris Autism Research International Sibpair (PARIS) study (Philippe et al., 1999) reported a linkage study in 51 multiplex families recruited from Sweden, France, Norway, the USA, Italy, Austria, and Belgium. The PARIS study highlighted 11 regions that gave nominal linkage of $P < 0.05$ or lower, 4 of which overlap to some extent with regions

on chromosomes 2q31–q32, 7q31, 16p13, and 19p13 identified by IMGSAC. The strongest finding from this report was a *suggestive* linkage on chromosome 6q16. Secondly, Risch and colleagues (1999) performed a two-stage genome-wide scan including 139 multiplex sibships, with parents, containing 147 independent affected sib-pairs. The largest LOD score highlighted a *suggestive* linkage to a novel locus on chromosome 1p21. The Collaborative Linkage Study of Autism (CLSA) (Barrett et al., 1999) reported on 75 families ascertained through an affected sib-pair. *Suggestive* linkage was identified for two regions on chromosome 13q22 and 13q12 in addition to supporting data for linkage on 7q at 7q21 – building on the evidence surrounding the long arm of chromosome 7. Additional support for these loci was provided by a genome-wide linkage scan using affected sib-pairs from the Collaborative Program for Excellence in Autism (CPEA) collection, which highlighted their strongest linkage to a marker on 7q32 (Schellenberg et al., 2006).

Liu and colleagues (2001) examined 335 microsatellite markers in 110 multiplex families with autism from the AGRE. *Suggestive* linkage was observed on chromosomes 5p13, Xq26–qtel, and 19q12 alongside modest support for the previously reported linkage on 7q (7q31 and 7q36) and 16p13. A follow-up analysis increasing the microsatellite density and sample size to 345 multiplex families (Yonan et al., 2003), including 235 new multiplex families, resulted in *suggestive* evidence for linkage at chromosomes 17q11, 5p13, 11p11–p13, 4q21–q22, and 8q24.

Auranen and colleagues (2002) performed a two-stage genome-wide scan approach in 38 Finnish families with case diagnoses including autism, infantile autism, Asperger syndrome (AS), and developmental dysphasia. *Significant* linkage was found on chromosome 3q25–q27 using infantile autism and AS as an affection status. Ylisaukko-oja and colleagues (2004) performed a two-stage genome-wide scan in Finnish families ascertained for AS with a strictly defined phenotype. Fine mapping highlighted *significant* linkage on chromosome 1q21–q22, with suggestive evidence at 3q25–q27 and 3p14–p24, both of which had previously been highlighted as autism loci in the Finnish population (Auranen et al., 2002; 2003). Additional confirmation of the 3q25–q27 peak was observed in a single large extended Utah pedigree of northern European ancestry (Coon et al., 2005).

Using the Affymetrix 10K single nucleotide polymorphism (SNP) array, the Autism Genome Project (AGP) examined linkage in a much larger collection of 1,168 multiply affected families. The AGP collection examined in this linkage analysis represented a combination of four existing ASD research collections: IMGSAC, AGRE, the Autism Genetics Cooperative (AGC – incorporating families from the CLSA, Seaver Autism Center, CANA-GEN and PARIS collections), and the CPEA collection (Szatmari et al., 2007). This study yielded *suggestive* linkage to chromosome 11p12–p13 and a large region on chromosome 15q23–q25. Of the regions that featured prominently in previous linkage analyses, there was also modest support for previously highlighted linkage regions on chromosomes 2q31 (female autism probands) and 7q22 (male ASD probands) from families of European ancestry.

The advancement to SNP-based linkage designs continued with a linkage study by Weiss and colleagues (2009) using 16,581 independent markers from the Affymetrix 500K/5.0 array in a sample derived from the AGRE and NIMH (National Institute of Mental Health) collections. A total of 1,031 families including 1,553 affected offspring were used in analyses. Two novel loci were highlighted as showing *suggestive* and *significant* linkage, on chromosomes 6p27 and 20p13, respectively.

ASSOCIATION STUDIES IN AUTISM

In the mid-1990s Risch and Merikangas demonstrated that where genetic variants have only small effect on risk, the association study is a more powerful approach than linkage to identify genetic risk (Risch and Merikangas, 1996). In essence, an association study calculates the significance of the relationship between variation at a genetic marker and a trait. There are two classical designs used to determine the statistical association with the candidate variation, namely the case-control design and the family-based association test. In the case-control design, the researcher examines the statistical association of a variant within a gene of interest, to test whether specified alleles are observed more often than by chance alone in individuals with a disease compared to those without. For neurodevelopmental disorders, family-based association tests such as the transmission-disequilibrium test (TDT) have been widely used. The basic principle of the TDT design is to determine whether there is non-random transmission of alleles from the parents to the child (Spielman et al., 1993). Under the null hypothesis of no association, variants which are heterozygous at a particular allele in the parent will have equal likelihood to be transmitted to the child. In the event that there is a deviation from the null for a given allele, there is said to be transmission-disequilibrium.

The application of the association study design in ASD, like many other complex traits, has been governed by fiscal and technological limitations. Ideally, one would examine all points of common variation within the genome for association with ASD. Despite the

application of this approach looking more feasible in the coming years given the rapid advances being made in genomic technologies, studies initiated little over a decade ago were restricted by our limited knowledge of variation across the genome and by the low to modest throughput of the available genotyping methods used to examine variation. Early association studies focused on candidate loci inspired by evidence regarding the putative location of risk variation from linkage and cytogenetic studies (positional candidate genes). Additional candidate loci were explored based on our hypotheses of the biological processes underpinning ASD. The combination of positional and biological candidate genes enabled researchers to restrict and focus resources to fewer, more plausible, regions of the genome to search for association with ASD. More recently, technologies have been developed that enable higher-throughput genotyping, which have given rise to studies that explore variation across the whole genome without the requirement for any *a priori* knowledge of genes or loci.

Positional Candidate Gene Studies

The identification of many *significant* and *suggestive* loci from linkage studies encouraged fine mapping and candidate gene association studies to determine the genes underpinning these linkage signals. These linkage findings highlighted autism susceptibility loci across many chromosomes, including *significant* linkage to loci at 2q, 3q, 7q, and 20p. From the perspective of regional follow-up for positional candidate genes, the linkage regions on chromosomes 2q and 7q have received the greatest interest.

2q31–q32

The identification of *significant* linkage to 2q31–q32 (Buxbaum et al., 2001; IMGSAC and Monaco, 2001) led to a number of candidate-gene-based investigations. Subsequent fine mapping of the region underlined genes *SLC25A12*, *STK39*, and *ITGA4* as putative risk genes in the region.

SLC25A12 (mitochondrial aspartate/glutamate carrier) was highlighted in an extensive mutation screen of 82 known exons in nine genes (*GAD1*, *FLJ13096*, *FLJ13984*, PRO2037, *FLJ23462*, *HAT-1*, *DNC12*, *DLX2*, and *SLC25A12*) spanning the 2q32 region (Ramoz et al., 2004). Using both single-stranded conformational polymorphism (SSCP) and denaturing high-performance liquid chromatography (dHPLC) on 35–47 individuals from families showing linkage to the 2q region, the authors identified 29 SNPs, including 2 SNPs in *SLC25A12* that showed significant transmission disequilibrium in an extended cohort of 197 autism families from the Seaver Autism Center/AGRE collections (rs2056202, P = 0.001; rs2292813, P = 0.01). A subsequent study by this group in 334 families extended the fine mapping of the 2q31 region to include 2q24–q33, identifying significant associations for SNPs in *SLC25A12* (rs2056202; P = 0.006), *STK39* (rs1807984; P = 0.007), and *ITGA4* (rs2305586; P = 0.009) (Ramoz et al., 2008). Subsequent validation studies for variants in *SLC25A12* both support (Kim et al., 2011; Segurado et al., 2005; Turunen et al., 2008) and refute (Blasi et al., 2006; Chien et al., 2010; Correia et al., 2006; Rabionet et al., 2006) the role of *SLC25A12* as a risk factor in ASD and ASD traits.

The positional candidature of 2q31–q32 was further supported by a case study of a young Irish male with high-functioning autism with a complex translocation traversing chromosome 2q32 (46,XY,t(9;2)(q31.1; q32.2q31.3)) (Gallagher et al., 2003). Subsequent association mapping with microsatellite and SNP markers identified association at SNPs within the *ITGA4* gene (Conroy et al., 2009). Mutation screening revealed a synonymous variation within the splice donor sequence of exon 16 that which showed modest association with autism in a sample of 548 trios from the Irish Autism Collection, the Vanderbilt University Autism Collection, and the AGRE collection (rs12690517; odds ratio (OR) = 1.3; P = 0.008). Additional association studies of *ITGA4* and autism have also been reported for haplotypes (0.00053 < P < 0.022) in a study of 164 parents-proband Portuguese trios (Correia et al., 2009).

7q

The many linkage signals along the long arm of chromosome 7 has led to study of candidate genes at three loci: q21, q31–q32, and q35–q36. Positive associations with genes within these regions have led to further investigations in an attempt to confirm risk genes and variants for autism.

7q21

RELN (7q22) encodes the extracellular matrix protein reelin. Reelin plays a pivotal role in the development of laminar structures including the cerebral cortex, cerebellum, and hippocampus. Persico and colleagues (2001) identified five polymorphisms across the *RELN* gene locus, including a GGC repeat located immediately 5' of the *RELN* ATG translation initiator codon. Using both case-control and family-based designs, the authors identified a nominal association with this repeat polymorphism. The association with the 5' untranslated region (UTR) triplet-repeat polymorphism was replicated in a combined collection of families from Duke, Vanderbilt, and AGRE (Skaar et al., 2005). Subsequent studies provided only weak support (Ashley-Koch et al., 2007; Holt et al., 2010; Kelemenova et al., 2010; Li et al., 2008; Serajee et al., 2006; Zhang et al, 2002) or refutation (Bonora et al., 2003; Devlin et al., 2004; Dutta et al.,

2008; He et al., 2011; Krebs et al., 2002; Li et al., 2004) of the role of *RELN* as a risk factor in ASD.

7q31–q32

Like *RELN*, *MET* (7q31) is also a strong biological candidate gene for autism. MET receptor tyrosine kinase signaling is involved in brain growth and maturation, immune function, and gastrointestinal repair. In a family-based study of autism including 1,231 cases, Campbell and colleagues observed a strong association between rs1858830 and autism (P < 0.00005) (Campbell et al., 2006). The rs1858830 association was subsequently replicated, albeit not to a similar strength, in an independent collection of 101 families from the same group (P = 0.033) (Campbell et al., 2008) and 174 patients from the South Carolina Autism Project (P < 0.05) (Jackson et al., 2009). Two additional studies failed to garner additional support for association at the rs1858830 variant, but did find support for other *MET* SNPs, namely rs38845; P < 0.004; Sousa et al., 2009 and rs38841 (P < 0.044; replication P < 0.0006; Thanseem et al., 2010). Despite the lack of replication, it is of interest that all three SNPs, rs1858830, rs38845, and rs38841, span a 9.4 kb region in the 5' region of the gene.

7q35–q36

The *CNTNAP2* (7q35) gene encodes the contactin-associated protein-like 2 protein, which is a member of the neurexin family and thought to play a role in axonal differentiation and guidance. *CNTNAP2* is one of the largest genes in the human genome, encompassing approximately 1.5% of chromosome 7. The position and biological candidature of this gene has led to three fine-mapping and association studies of the *CNTNAP2* region. Arking and colleagues observed an association at *CNTNAP2* using a two-stage design including 137 affected probands in the stage-1 analyses and 1,219 stage-2 analyses of families from the NIMH/AGRE collection. The main association observed was for rs7794745, located in intron 2 of the gene (P1 = 0.00002, P2 = 0.005) (Arking et al., 2008). A subsequent study of 185 Han Chinese families reported weak supporting evidence for a haplotype containing the rs7794745 SNP (Li et al., 2010).

Another extensively studied positional candidate gene on 7q is the homeobox gene *EN2* (7q36). In a study that predates the linkage findings, Petit and colleagues reported on a case-control study of 100 patients with autism and 100 controls, which indicated an association with a GC/−− insert deletion restriction fragment length polymorphism (rs34808376; *PvuII*) in the 5'-flanking region of the *EN2* gene (Petit et al., 1995). Following on from the linkage findings, Zhong and colleagues (2003) explored the rs34808376 association in addition to an extra coding variant (rs3735653), but failed to find association in 204 families from the AGRE collection. Gharani and colleagues (2004) followed this to report an association with two intronic SNPs (rs1861972, P = 0.0018; rs1861973, P = 0.0003) in a collection of 167 ASD families. In a study containing an additional 351 AGRE/NIMH families, a strong association was observed for the rs1861972–rs1861973 haplotype in the combined 518 families (P = 0.00000035) (Benayed et al., 2005). A recent report by Sen and colleagues (2010) confirmed the rs1861973 association in 48 narrowly defined ASD families from Guwhati, India (P = 0.006). Although a number of other studies have reported positive associations with variants at the EN2 locus (Benayed et al., 2005; Brune et al., 2008; Gharani et al., 2004; Wang et al., 2008; Yang et al., 2008), the reported associations should be considered with caution, as the strengths of the associations are weak, the number of markers and haplotype comparisons can be extensive, and therefore the associations do not withstand correction for multiple comparisons.

Biological Candidate Genes

In addition to positional candidature, candidate gene studies are motivated by biological evidence which supports the putative roles of the gene in the etiology of the disease. These hypotheses may include the correlation of components of metabolic pathways with the disorder, known drug targets, animal models, of disease traits (e.g., AVPR1A) and related single-gene disorders which share traits and outcomes (e.g., ASD-enriched disorders such as fragile X mental retardation (FMR1), Rett's syndrome (MECP2), and tuberous sclerosis complex (TSC1, TSC2)). Positional and biological candidature is not mutually exclusive, in reality it is quite the opposite, whereby biological candidates are prioritized within positional data.

Social Cognition Candidate Genes

Alongside communication and repetitive behaviors, social interaction is a core area of deficit in ASD. The biological processes underpinning social interaction and social cognition have become an increasing focus of ASD research. Individuals with ASD often show deficits of social cognition encompassing personality; trust; altruism; social bonding; cooperation; and the ability to recognize, interpret, and respond appropriately to other people's social cues. Evidence from animal models has highlighted the neuropeptides oxytocin (OT) and vasopressin (AVP) as being important in social cognition; affecting individual differences in parenting behavior, social recognition, and affiliate behaviors (reviewed by Skuse and Gallagher, 2011).

The genes that encode the oxytocin and arginine-vasopressin neuropeptides, OXT and AVP, reside in a 15 kb window on the short arm of chromosome 20 (20p13). Despite evidence of linkage to 20p13 (Weiss et al., 2009), to date, candidate gene studies do not support a strong role for genetic variation at the OXT-AVP gene region in autism (Kelemenova et al., 2010; Tansey et al., unpublished data; Yrigollen et al., 2008). The focus of association studies for these social cognition genes has been on the neuropeptide receptors for OT and AVP. The OT receptor gene (OXTR) is localized to chromosome 3p25 and encodes a G-protein coupled receptor. Seven reports have been published that examine association in the OXTR gene (Jacob et al., 2007; Lerer et al., 2008; Liu et al., 2010; Tansey et al., 2010; Wermter et al., 2010; Wu et al., 2005; Yrigollen et al., 2008). Most of the reported associations are weak (0.01 < P < 0.05) and uncorrected for multiple testing. Of the six studies that tested the marker rs2254298, three report nominal association with autism (P = 0.03: Jacob et al., 2007; P = 0.001: Liu et al., 2010; P = 0.02: Wu et al., 2005). However, the weak association strength, inconsistency in the risk allele, and lack of validation in three other studies (Lerer et al., 2008; Tansey et al., 2010; Wermter et al., 2010) indicate that these observations should be interpreted with caution. The AVP receptor (AVPR1A) offers a similar story of weak and inconsistent association within a cluster of functional variation in the 5′ region of the gene. A number of studies have described association for the RS1 and RS3 elements of the AVPR1A gene in autism. However, these multi-allelic markers do not show consistency in the risk allele (Kim et al., 2002; Tansey et al., 2011; Wassink et al., 2004; Yang et al., 2010a,b). Additional associations have been observed at other 5′ variants such as the AVR (Yirmiya et al., 2006) and rs11174815 SNP (Tansey et al., 2011). Therefore, despite the strong biological plausibility of the OXT-AVP system being important in social cognition, the evidence from association analyses in autism per se is weak. This does not preclude a role for these genes within specific biological processes involved in social cognition.

Neurotransmitter-Related Candidate Genes

In recent years, advances in molecular techniques have led to the highlighting of the role of structural variation in individuals with ASD. Multiple rare chromosomal rearrangements (each individually < 1% frequency), also known as copy number variation (CNV), are thought to cause at least 20% of cases of ASD. The identification of CNV in individuals with autism has helped to focus positional and biological candidate gene analyses. Following the observation that individuals with duplications of the Prader–Willi/Angelman syndrome critical region (15q11–13) presented with ASD symptoms, Cook and colleagues fine-mapped the region to identify genes that may be associated with autism (Cook et al., 1998). Association was observed between the *GABRB3* microsatellite marker GABRB3 155CA-2 (P = 0.0014), and replicated, although for a different allele, by Buxbaum and colleagues (P = 0.0039: Buxbaum et al., 2002). Additional nominal associations were reported for SNP markers in the DUKE and AGRE families (P < 0.02: Menold et al., 2001), the TUFTS/AGRE collection (P < 0.02: McCauley et al., 2004a), but not in additional collections from IMGSAC (Maestrini et al., 1999), Stanford (Salmon et al., 1999), DUKE/AGRE (Ashley-Koch et al., 2006), or the United Kingdom (Curran et al., 2005). More recently, Delahanty and colleagues have shown that maternal origin of the associated allele may also of importance (Delahanty et al., 2011).

The glutamate receptor, ionotropic kainate 2 receptor gene, *GRIK2* (GluR6), was also initially identified through positional data. *GRIK2* is localized under 6q16.3–q21, one of the 11 highlighted linkage regions identified by the PARIS study (Philippe et al., 1999). Subsequent fine mapping of the region highlighted an association with maternally transmitted alleles between intron 14 and exon 16 of the *GRIK2* gene (0.007 < P < 0.02): Jamain et al., 2002). Nominal associations were reported for the exon 15 SNP rs2227283 in Han Chinese (P = 0.032: Shuang et al., 2004), but not replicated in families from India (Dutta et al., 2007). A second association signal has since been highlighted by Holt and colleagues (2010), as part of the EU Autism MOLGEN Consortium, who observed an association in exon 1 of *GRIK2* (rs2518261; P = 0.008) but not at the intron 14 to exon 16 region of the gene.

Considerable attention has been focused on the serotonergic system, supported by the observation that up to one-third of individuals with ASD show hyperserotonemia. A number of studies have reported an increase in platelet serotonin in individuals with autism (Campbell et al., 1974; Hoshino et al., 1984; Minderaa et al., 1989; Ritvo et al., 1970; Schain and Freedman, 1961), with variation in serotonin levels observed in younger age groups with ASD (McBride et al., 1998). Serotonin levels peak at 200% of adult levels at age 5, then decrease over time for typically developing children (Chugani, 2002). For individuals with autism, serotonin levels gradually increase to 150% adult levels between the ages of 2 to 11, suggesting that humans undergo a period of high brain serotonin synthesis during childhood, and this developmental process is disrupted in ASD children (Chugani, 2002). In addition, pharmacological interventions using selective serotonergic reuptake inhibitors (SSRIs) have been used to reduce restricted repetitive behaviors and stereotypical/compulsive behaviors associated with autism (McCracken et al., 2002;

McDougle et al., 1996). SSRIs target the serotonin transporter protein encoded by the gene *SLC6A4* (solute carrier family 6 (neurotransmitter transporter, serotonin), member 4). A number of studies have examined genetic variation in the *SLC6A4* gene and autism. Cook and colleagues (1997) reported a weak association with the short allele of the HTTLPR promoter polymorphism (P = 0.03). This initial association was confirmed at the allele-level by others (Conroy et al., 2004; Devlin et al., 2005; Kim et al., 2002; McCauley et al., 2004b; Sutcliffe et al., 2005). However, a meta-analysis of independent published studies failed to support a role for the *SLC6A4* HTTLPR variant in autism (Huang and Santangelo, 2008).

Genome-Wide Association Studies in Autism

Although not obsolete, the candidate gene approach was superseded in prominence by the genome-wide association study (GWAS), in the late 2000s. Advances in our understanding of common SNP variation across the human genome, combined with the development of high-throughput array-based genotyping platforms, enabled hypothesis-free GWAS to be performed. These approaches allow the interrogation of many hundreds of thousands of SNP markers across the genome in many thousands of individuals. Many GWAS have been performed that examine genetic risk of psychiatric disorders, including four examining autism spectrum disorders.

The interpretation of an association signal in GWAS generally uses frequentist approaches, based on the arbitrary 1 in 20, or P < 0.05, threshold. Due to the large number of SNPs tested simultaneously in GWAS, a conventional statistical significance threshold of P = 0.05, would be far too lenient, and result in many thousands of false positive findings. A traditional Bonferroni correction, whereby the significance threshold is adjusted according to the number of independent tests, suggests a single GWAS threshold of $\sim 1 \times 10^{-8}$ to 5×10^{-8} for studies using markers with a minor allele frequency greater than 5% (Hoggart et al., 2008). If a lower minor allele frequency threshold is used then the number of independent tests will increase and a more stringent correction should be applied.

Wang and colleagues (2009) performed a family-based GWAS on 780 AGRE families, a case-control-based GWAS on 1,204 cases from the ACC (Autism Case-Control) collection, and an additional 6,491 CHOP (Children's Hospital of Philadelphia) controls genotyped on the Illumina HumanHap550 BeadChip. All individuals were defined as having European ancestry. Neither family-based nor case-control analysis yielded GW-significant findings. A combined analysis yielded one GW-significant finding on chromosome 5p14.1 (rs4307059; $P = 3.4 \times 10^{-8}$) and a number of suggestive signals on chromosomes 13q33.3, 14q21.1, and Xp22.32. A round of validation of the chromosome 5p14.1 region was performed using a 477 families of European ancestry from the family-based CAP (Collaborative Autism Project) and 108 cases from the CART (Center for Autism Research and Treatment) study, together with 540 non-disease controls from the Illumina iControlDB. The authors highlight modest to strong replication of the association signal on chromosome 5p14.1 with a maximum combined association signal across all four studies of 2.1×10^{-8} (rs4307059). The 5p14.1 region highlighted by Wang and colleagues is a gene desert. The index association signal (rs4307059) is approximately 1 Mb from the closest genes, where it is approximately equidistant from the centomeric *CDH9* and telomeric *CDH10* genes.

Ma and colleagues (Ma et al., 2009) performed a family-based GWAS on 438 ASD families from the CAP project with a validation set of 457 families from the AGRE collection. All samples were genotyped on the Illumina 1M Beadchip. None of the markers investigated were shown to be GW-significant in the discovery, validation, or combined analyses. This report was a parallel and reciprocal collaboration with the work published by Wang and colleagues (described above) albeit using a higher-density genotyping array. Despite subtle differences in sample composition across the reports, the authors retain a strong association signal on chromosome 5p14.1. The index associations of Ma and colleagues in the 5p14.1 are not identical to those of Wang and colleagues; however they do occur within markers showing strong LD with those markers highlighted by Wang and colleagues. Although these two reports highlight the 5p14.1 region, their non-independence does not proffer additional support for this region.

Weiss and colleagues (2009) performed a family-based GWAS in a combination of AGRE and NIMH families genotyped on the Affymetrix 500K/5.0 array. A total of 1,031 families and 1,553 affected offspring were used for association studies. In the initial scan the authors did not find any GW-significant associations. Additional supplementation of the family-based studies was made with a case-control set derived from 90 probands without parental data, that were subsequently matched to controls from the NIMH collection. This garnered some additional signal for the top hits. A replication consortium of more than 2,000 trios was genotyped for 45 SNPs across all of the top associated regions. The replication consortium included families enrolled in the Autism Genome Project Consortium, the Homozygosity Mapping Collaborative for Autism, the Massachusetts General Hospital, the Children's

Hospital of Boston Autism Collection, the Montreal Autism Collection, the Finnish Autism Collection, and others. The only marker that showed evidence of replication resides on the short arm of chromosome 5 at 5p15. Although, like that of Ma and colleagues (2009), this report has considerable overlap with the AGRE families reported by Wang and colleagues (2009), Weiss and colleagues did not see association at 5p14.1. The chromosome 5p association lies in close proximity to *TAS2R1*. The *TAS2R1* gene encodes a G-protein coupled receptor that is involved in bitter taste recognition. The authors highlight a more biologically plausible ASD candidate gene approximately 80 kb telomeric, *SEMA5A*. *SEMA5A* encodes a gene important in axonal guidance that is shown to be down-regulated in the occipital lobe cortex, lymphoblast cell lines, and lymphocytes of individuals with autism.

Finally, a GWAS from the AGP (Anney et al., 2010) was performed using a family-based design and genotyped on the Illumina 1M Beadchip. A total of 1,369 families, containing 1,385 affected offspring, passed quality control and were used in the association analysis. From the primary analyses, a single GW-significant finding was observed on chromosome 20 at position 20p12 within the *MACROD2* gene locus (rs4141463; $P = 2.1 \times 10^{-8}$). A validation dataset was drawn from 595 AGRE families (1,086 probands) not already present in the AGP primary analyses. To enhance the power of the study, a supplementary control sample collected from the Study of Addiction Genetics (SAGE), was also genotyped using the Illumina 1M Beadchip and was incorporated into a case-control design with the AGP probands. Weak statistical support was observed for *MACROD2* in the AGRE validation sample, albeit showing the same direction of effect for the risk allele. Combined analysis of the AGP, AGRE, and SAGE datasets all show a GW-significant effect. The role of *MACROD2* is largely unknown. Previously named *C20orf133*, *MACROD2* is one of the largest genes in the genome, spanning over 2 Mb. *MACROD2* (MACRO-domain containing 2) is so named because of the MACRO-domain in the protein. This domain is an ADP-ribose-binding module (Karras et al., 2005) that has been implicated in the ADP-ribosylation of proteins, an important post-translational modification that occurs in a variety of biological processes such as DNA repair, transcription, chromatin biology, and long-term memory formation (Cohen-Armon et al., 2004). Direct evidence has shown that the MACROD2 protein has a role in DNA repair (Timinszky et al., 2009) and possible roles in heterochromatin formation, histone modification, and sirtuin biology (Chen et al., 2011; Hoff and Wolberger, 2005; Liou et al., 2005). Of note, the association signal observed in the AGP, albeit tagged to the *MACROD2* gene, resides in an intronic region near an intragenic non-protein-coding RNA *NCRNA00186*.

When examining the three largest GWAS studies to date – those of Wang and colleagues (2009), Weiss and colleagues (2009), and Anney and colleagues (2010) – there is no support for the highlighted loci of each manuscript in the subsequent investigations. Evaluations of these studies suggest that a combination of these data would result in the diminishment of the association signals and a loss of evidence, making them non-significant (Devlin et al., 2011). Therefore, the conclusion of these early studies is that common variation examined on the respective arrays does not impart modest effect on the risk of developing ASD.

One of the phrases that has become commonly applied to loci where there is a failure to replicate a given finding is *'the winner's curse.'* This is a scenario where the *'winners,'* or top results from a study, achieved their position at the top of the pile through somewhat favorable events in the sampling and experimental procedures (e.g., favorable genotyping errors). It is assumed that in reality the true effect size in the population is towards the more conservative boundaries of the confidence intervals for these markers. In order to better identify those markers influenced by the *winner's* and, presumably, the *loser's* curses, it is important to reduce the impact of these biases by improving our estimates of the true effect sizes. Although sample size will improve the power of a study to observe an effect, it is not the only factor that can do this. Other influences on the power of a genetic association study are the significance threshold, the linkage disequilibrium between the test and causative marker, the allele frequency of the test marker, and the magnitude of the effect.

In practice, one may be able to reduce the threshold required to meet significance by reducing the burden of multiple testing. This approach moves the study design away from the hypothesis-free GWAS approach and towards hypothesis-testing designs based on specific genes and groups of genes. For example, one might predict that genes involved in axon guidance and synapse are important in the etiology of ASD. Examining only the genes involved in these processes or expressed in these structures would in effect reduce the number of tests and subsequent multiple testing burden.

Linkage disequilibrium, the phenomenon whereby one marker is co-inherited with another marker, has been used to identify risk variants in disease without having to directly test the true causative marker. Instead, a marker that is highly correlated to the risk variant can be examined as a proxy for the risk variant. Microarrays for use in GWAS are designed to cover the entire genome, by taking advantage of linkage disequilibrium to reduce marker redundancy and maximizing correlation with un-typed markers. However, this does not result in perfect coverage of the genome and may limit discovery or the strength of the association signal for the true risk variant. To reduce the influence of linkage disequilibrium researchers can:

1. Directly examine more markers through more densely populated microarrays (e.g., the Illumina HumanOmni5-Quad which contains ~ 4.3M markers);
2. Directly examine more markers through sequencing approaches which are not limited to predefined marker lists;
3. Indirectly examine more markers through imputation of missing data (Marchini and Howie, 2010).

The genotype imputation approaches are considerably more attractive to researchers examining pre-genotyped data as they do not require the considerable costs of re-genotyping. Genotype imputation routines take information on the haplotype structure of a reference panel of individuals genotyped on a large set of markers to infer missing genotypes in the test dataset. In addition to imputing part missing data, these methods can impute missing markers in studies that utilize data from different genotyping platforms, and in family-based designs can be extended to the imputation of missing individuals (Li et al., 2009). Reference haplotype panels derived from the HapMap project (http://www.hapmap.org) and the 1,000 genomes project (http://www.1000genomes.org) are currently available to increase the coverage of common variation in GWAS. These reference panels can in principle increase marker coverage to greater than 20 million SNPs, albeit with the requirements of non-trivial computational time.

Theoretically, one can attempt to influence the allele frequency in the test population under investigation and in turn increase the effect size by examining more homogenous clinical populations. The heterogeneous presentation of the ASD population highlights the possibility that there may be some merit in identifying individuals with similar clinical presentations to putatively enrich the study for genetic identity. One might predict that in clinically similar individuals the genetic underpinnings are more likely to be analogous, therefore putatively enriching the allele frequency and effect size in the test population. In this *enriched* population, there is a requirement for fewer individuals to observe an effect than in an admixed population. Across the linkage, candidate gene, and GWAS literature, researchers have explored this approach in groups of ASD individuals with a range of hypothesis-driven constraints, including gender, ancestry, and diagnostic classifiers such as level of language, cognitive function, and clinical and statistical clustering of trait data (e.g., Anney et al., 2010; Liu et al., 2011; Salyakina et al., 2010) albeit without the desired improvement in association signal above what might be expected given the increased multiple testing burden.

Finally, as noted above, one can improve the power of a study by increasing the number of individuals examined in the study. A mega- and meta-analysis of available ASD GWAS data is currently underway as part of the Psychiatric GWAS Consortium ASD Working Group. This study includes data from families reported in the published GWAS alongside additional families and patients from the Autism Genome Project, Simons Simplex Collection, and the Finnish Autism Collection. The combined analyses will include data from approximately 5,600 individuals with ASD. These combined collections will provide the most robust examination of candidate genes to date. Moreover, they will do so without ambiguity to the non-independence of studies. The collaborative nature of the ASD genetics field has often led to the sharing of resources between studies. This is highlighted by the inclusion, to a varying degree, of individuals from the AGRE (http://www.agre.org) collection in either the discovery phase or replication phase of many genetics studies. Mega-analyses using raw genotype data have enabled the identification of these individuals and also those who have enrolled in research programs at more than one site. Sources of cryptic overlap in sampling have the potential to lead to misinterpretation of findings, such as inflated association and false-replication. The combining of datasets can therefore provide a clearer picture to the involvement of candidate genes without the confounding of non-independence.

CONCLUSIONS

In parallel to the examination of common variation in autism, there has been considerable effort to identify rare and private risk variation. Rare and private structural and sequence variations are being identified that may explain the origins of ASD within some families. This conglomeration of rare variant data offers insight into biological pathways that may underpin autism. Moreover, recurrent different rare mutations within genes and loci may identify a group of individuals with specific 'autisms' defined through their genetic architecture. Further studies of the clinical characteristics of these families may enable opportunities for better diagnosis and treatment of individuals presenting with these mutations.

The identification of rare variants that are likely to be causative in ASD may also help identify novel candidate genes and pathways. Early GWAS studies in ASD have realistically been powered only to identify 'low hanging fruit' using single-marker designs, in clinically and sometimes ethnically heterogeneous samples. The

return to hypothesis-driven biological candidate gene approaches within these higher-resolution datasets, where the examination of genes is informed by evidence from rare-variant studies, may be better powered than genome-wide studies to identify association in more discrete clinical groups. Moreover, without considerable increases in study sizes, hypothesis-driven designs are the only feasible avenue at present to robustly examine more complex genetic models, such as haplotype, gene–gene and gene–environment interactions in ASD.

The identification of rare structural and sequence variations in ASD, combined with the lack of unambiguous risk or protective loci from association studies, has led researchers to question whether there is a role for common variation in autism. Devlin and colleagues (2011) explored this using published GWAS data, to examine whether there was statistical evidence to support a role for common variants in ASD. The authors conclude that the data collected thus far would suggest that common variation is 'unlikely' but not 'implausible.' Moreover, a pragmatic interpretation of the GWAS data is that there are no common variations of modest effect implicated in ASD. That is not to say that common variations of small effect are unlikely to influence development of ASD. A recent analysis of approximately 3,000 families from the GWAS from the Autism Genome Project reveals a modest polygenic association signal from many thousands of associated loci, indicating that common variation *en masse* cannot be excluded from the disease model and does account, in part, for the variance in ASD (Anney, Autism Genome Project, personal communication).

Nevertheless, the overall disappointing pattern of GWAS and candidate gene association results, not unique to ASD research, has exposed a number of the challenges facing the ASD research community in its endeavor to identify common variation that contributes to ASD. Most notable is the low statistical power of current studies to observe association with variants of small effect. Noting that if the early 'failures' in psychiatric genetics are merely due to low power, Sullivan and colleagues (2011) argue that:

> if samples are sufficient, GWAS can deliver fundamental knowledge about genetic architecture, identify specific loci for biological follow-up and localize pathways altered in disease.

Subsequently, this was borne out in recent successes in mega-analyses of GWAS-level data in studies of schizophrenia (Ripke et al., 2011) and bipolar disorder (Sklar et al., 2011). These studies from the Psychiatric GWAS Consortium address the sample size directly, identifying ~ 15 loci meeting GW-significant association through two-stage meta-analyses of approximately 18,000 individuals with schizophrenia and 12,000 individuals with bipolar disorder, respectively. Sullivan (2011) calculates that further increasing these samples three- to four-fold could lead to unambiguous identification of at least 60 loci implicated in these disorders. The sample size in the upcoming Psychiatric GWAS Consortium ASD study is still less than those used to identify risk variants in schizophrenia and bipolar disorder, and therefore it is anticipated that there will be a need to continue to invest in larger, well-phenotyped ASD collections for genetics research. However, the encouraging data regarding the polygenic signature in ASD alongside data from other mega-analyses give optimism that there is merit to the ongoing endeavors of the ASD research community in searching for common risk variation of small effect.

References

Abrahams, B.S., Geschwind, D.H., et al., 2008. Advances in Autism-genetics: On the threshold of a new neurobiology. Nature Reviews Genetics 9, 341–355.

Anney, R., Klei, L., Pinto, D., et al., 2010. A genome-wide scan for common alleles affecting risk for Autism. Human Molecular Genetics 19, 4072–4082.

Arking, D.E., Cutler, D.J., Brune, C.W., et al., 2008. A common genetic variant in the neurexin superfamily member CNTNAP2 increases familial risk of Autism. American Journal of Human Genetics 82, 160–164.

Ashley-Koch, A.E., Jaworski, J., Ma de, Q., et al., 2007. Investigation of potential gene-gene interactions between APOE and RELN contributing to Autism risk. Psychiatric Genetics 17, 221–226.

Ashley-Koch, A.E., Mei, H., Jaworski, J., et al., 2006. An analysis paradigm for investigating multi-locus effects in complex disease: Examination of three GABA receptor subunit genes on 15q11-q13 as risk factors for autistic disorder. Annals of Human Genetics 70, 281–292.

Auranen, M., Vanhala, R., Varilo, T., et al., 2002. A genomewide screen for Autism-spectrum disorders: Evidence for a major susceptibility locus on chromosome 3q25-27. American Journal of Human Genetics 71, 777–790.

Auranen, M., Varilo, T., Alen, R., et al., 2003. Evidence for allelic association on chromosome 3q25-27 in families with Autism spectrum disorders originating from a subisolate of Finland. Archives of General Psychiatry 8, 879–884.

Bailey, A., Le Couteur, A., Gottesman, I., et al., 1995. Autism as a strongly genetic disorder: Evidence from a British twin study. Psychological Medicine 25, 63–77.

Barrett, S., Beck, J.C., Bernier, R., et al., 1999. An autosomal genomic screen for Autism Collaborative linkage study of Autism. American Journal of Medical Genetics 88, 609–615.

Benayed, R., Gharani, N., Rossman, I., et al., 2005. Support for the homeobox transcription factor gene ENGRAILED 2 as an Autism spectrum disorder susceptibility locus. American Journal of Human Genetics 77, 851–868.

Blasi, F., Bacchelli, E., Carone, S., et al., 2006. SLC25A12 and CMYA3 gene variants are not associated with Autism in the IMGSAC multiplex family sample. European Journal of Human Genetics 14, 123–126.

Bonora, E., Beyer, K.S., Lamb, J.A., et al., 2003. Analysis of reelin as a candidate gene for Autism. Archives of General Psychiatry 8, 885–892.

Brune, C.W., Korvatska, E., Allen-Brady, K., et al., 2008. Heterogeneous association between engrailed-2 and Autism in the CPEA network. American Journal of Medical Genetics B. NeuroPsychiatric Genetics 147B, 187–193.

Buxbaum, J.D., Silverman, J.M., Smith, C.J., et al., 2001. Evidence for a susceptibility gene for Autism on chromosome 2 and for genetic heterogeneity. American Journal of Human Genetics 68, 1514–1520.

Buxbaum, J.D., Silverman, J.M., Smith, C.J., et al., 2002. Association between a GABRB3 polymorphism and Autism. Archives of General Psychiatry 7, 311–316.

Campbell, D.B., Li, C., Sutcliffe, J.S., et al., 2008. Genetic evidence implicating multiple genes in the MET receptor tyrosine kinase pathway in Autism spectrum disorder. Autism Research 1, 159–168.

Campbell, D.B., Sutcliffe, J.S., Ebert, P.J., 2006. A genetic variant that disrupts MET transcription is associated with Autism. Proceedings of the National Academy of Sciences USA 103, 16,834–16,839.

Campbell, M., Friedman, E., DeVito, E., et al., 1974. Blood serotonin in psychotic and brain damaged children. Journal Autism Children Schizophr 4, 33–41.

Chen, D., Vollmar, M., Rossi, M.N., et al., 2011. Identification of macrodomain proteins as novel O-acetyl-ADP-ribose deacetylases. Journal of Biological Chemistry 286, 13,261–13,271.

Chien, W.H., Wu, Y.Y., Gau, S.S., et al., 2010. Association study of the SLC25A12 gene and Autism in Han Chinese in Taiwan. Prog. Neuropsychopharmacol Biological Archives of General 34, 189–192.

Chugani, D.C., 2002. Role of altered brain serotonin mechanisms in Autism. Archives of General Psychiatry 7, S16–S17.

Cohen-Armon, M., Visochek, L., Katzoff, A., et al., 2004. Long-term memory requires polyADP-ribosylation. Science 304, 1820–1822.

Conroy, J., Cochrane, L., Anney, R.J., 2009. Fine mapping and association studies in a candidate region for Autism on chromosome 2q31-q32. American Journal of Medical Genetics B. NeuroPsychiatric Genetics 150B, 535–544.

Conroy, J., Meally, E., Kearney, G., et al., 2004. Serotonin transporter gene and Autism: A haplotype analysis in an Irish autistic population. Archives of General Psychiatry 9, 587–593.

Cook Jr., E.H., Courchesne, R., Lord, C., et al., 1997. Evidence of linkage between the serotonin transporter and autistic disorder. Archives of General Psychiatry 2, 247–250.

Cook Jr., E.H., Courchesne, R.Y., Cox, N.J., et al., 1998. Linkage-disequilibrium mapping of autistic disorder, with 15q11-13 markers. American Journal of Human Genetics 62, 1077–1083.

Coon, H., Matsunami, N., Stevens, J., et al., 2005. Evidence for linkage on chromosome 3q25-27 in a large Autism extended pedigree. Human Heredity 60, 220–226.

Correia, C., Coutinho, A.M., Almeida, J., et al., 2009. Association of the alpha4 integrin subunit gene (ITGA4) with Autism. American Journal of Medical Genetics B. Neuropsychiatric. Genetics.

Correia, C., Coutinho, A.M., Diogo, L., 2006. Brief report: High frequency of biochemical markers for mitochondrial dysfunction in Autism – no association with the mitochondrial aspartate/glutamate carrier SLC25A12 gene. Journal of Autism and Developmental Disorders 36, 1137–1140.

Curran, S., Roberts, S., Thomas, S., 2005. An association analysis of microsatellite markers across the Prader-Willi/Angelman critical region on chromosome 15 (q11-13) and Autism spectrum disorder. American Journal of Medical Genetics B. NeuroPsychiatric Genetics 137B, 25–28.

Delahanty, R.J., Kang, J.Q., Brune, C.W., 2011. Maternal transmission of a rare GABRB3 signal peptide variant is associated with Autism. Archives of General Psychiatry 16, 86–96.

Devlin, B., Bennett, P., Dawson, G., 2004. Alleles of a reelin CGG repeat do not convey liability to Autism in a sample from the

CPEA network. American Journal of Medical Genetics B. Neuro-Psychiatric Genetics 126B, 46–50.

Devlin, B., Cook Jr., E.H., Coon, H., et al., 2005. Autism and the serotonin transporter: The long and short of it. Archives of General Psychiatry 10, 1110–1116.

Devlin, B., Melhem, N., Roeder, K., et al., 2011. Do common variants play a role in risk for Autism Evidence and theoretical musings. Brain Research 1380, 78–84.

Dutta, S., Das, S., Guhathakurta, S., et al., 2007. Glutamate receptor 6 gene (GluR6 or GRIK2) polymorphisms in the Indian population: A genetic association study on Autism spectrum disorder. Cellular and Molecular Neurobiology 27, 1035–1047.

Dutta, S., Sinha, S., Ghosh, S., 2008. Genetic analysis of reelin gene (RELN) SNPs: No association with Autism spectrum disorder in the Indian population. Neuroscience Letters 441, 56–60.

Fernell, E., Gillberg, C., 2010. Autism spectrum disorder diagnoses in Stockholm preschoolers. Research In Developmental Disabilities 31, 680–685.

Fombonne, E., 2009. Epidemiology of pervasive developmental disorders. Pediatric Research 65, 591–598.

Gallagher, L., Becker, K., Kearney, G., et al., 2003. Brief report: A case of Autism associated with del(2)(q32.1q32.2) or (q32.2q32.3). Journal of Autism and Developmental Disorders 33, 105–108.

Gharani, N., Benayed, R., Mancuso, V., et al., 2004. Association of the homeobox transcription factor, ENGRAILED 2, 3, with Autism spectrum disorder. Archives of General Psychiatry 9, 474–484.

Hallmayer, J., Cleveland, S., Torres, A., et al., 2011. Genetic heritability and shared environmental factors among twin pairs with autism. Archives of General Psychiatry.

He, Y., Xun, G., Xia, K., et al., 2011. No significant association between RELN polymorphism and Autism in case-control and family-based association study in Chinese Han population. Archives of General Research 187, 462–464.

Hoff, K.G., Wolberger, C., 2005. Getting a grip on O-acetyl-ADP-ribose. Nature Structural & Molecular Biology 12, 560–561.

Hoggart, C.J., Clark, T.G., De Lorio, M., 2008. Genome-wide significance for dense SNP and resequencing data. Genetic Epidemiology 32, 179–185.

Holt, R., Barnby, G., Maestrini, E., et al., 2010. Linkage and candidate gene studies of Autism spectrum disorders in European populations. European Journal of Human Genetics 18, 1013–1019.

Hoshino, Y., Yamamoto, T., Kaneko, M., 1984. Blood serotonin and free tryptophan concentration in autistic children. Neuropsychobiology 11, 22–27.

Huang, C.H., Santangelo, S.L., 2008. Autism and serotonin transporter gene polymorphisms: A systematic review and meta-analysis. American Journal of Medical Genetics B. NeuroPsychiatric Genetics 147B, 903–913.

International Molecular Genetic Study of Autism Consortium (IMGSAC), 1998. A full genome screen for Autism with evidence for linkage to a region on chromosome 7q. Human Molecular Genetics 7, 571–578.

International Molecular Genetic Study of Autism Consortium (IMGSAC), Bailey, A., et al., 2001. Further characterization of the Autism susceptibility locus AUTS1 on chromosome 7q. Human Molecular Genetics 10, 973–982.

International Molecular Genetic Study of Autism Consortium (IMGSAC), Monaco, A.P., 2001. A genomewide screen for Autism: strong evidence for linkage to chromosomes 2q, 7q, and 16p. American Journal of Human Genetics 69, 570–581.

Jackson, P.B., Boccuto, L., Skinner, C., et al., 2009. Further evidence that the rs1858830 C variant in the promoter region of the MET gene is associated with autistic disorder. Autism Research 2, 232–236.

Jacob, S., Brune, C.W., Carter, C.S., et al., 2007. Association of the oxytocin receptor gene (OXTR) in Caucasian children and adolescents with Autism. Neuroscience Letters 417, 6–9.

Jamain, S., Betancur, C., Quach, H., et al., 2002. Linkage and association of the glutamate receptor 6 gene with Autism. Archives of General Psychiatry 7, 302–310.

Karras, G.I., Kustatscher, G., Buhecha, H.R., et al., 2005. The macro domain is an ADP-ribose binding module. EMBO JOURNAL 24, 1911–1920.

Kelemenova, S., Schmidtova, E., Ficek, A., 2010. Polymorphisms of candidate genes in Slovak autistic patients. Psychiatric Genetics 20, 137–139.

Kim, S.J., Cox, N., Courchesne, R., et al., 2002. Transmission disequilibrium mapping at the serotonin transporter gene (SLC6A4) region in autistic disorder. Archives of General Psychiatry 7, 278–288.

Kim, S.J., Silva, R.M., Flores, C.G., 2011. A quantitative association study of SLC25A12 and restricted repetitive behavior traits in Autism spectrum disorders. Molecular Autism 2, 8.

Kim, S.J., Young, L.J., Gonen, D., et al., 2002. Transmission disequilibrium testing of arginine vasopressin receptor 1A (AVPR1A) polymorphisms in Autism. Archives of General Psychiatry 7, 503–507.

Krebs, M.O., Betancur, C., Leroy, S., et al., 2002. Absence of association between a polymorphic GGC repeat in the 5′ untranslated region of the reelin gene and Autism. Archives of General Psychiatry 7, 801–804.

Lander, E., Kruglyak, L., 1995. Genetic dissection of complex traits: Guidelines for interpreting and reporting linkage results. Nature Genetics 11, 241–247.

Lerer, E., Levi, S., Salomon, S., et al., 2008. Association between the oxytocin receptor (OXTR) gene and Autism relationship to Vineland Adaptive Behavior Scales and cognition. Archives of General Psychiatry 13, 980–988.

Li, H., Li, Y., Shao, J., et al., 2008. The association analysis of RELN and GRM8 genes with autistic spectrum disorder in Chinese Han population. American Journal of Medical Genetics B. NeuroPsychiatric Genetics 147B, 194–200.

Li, J., Nguyen, L., Gleason, C., et al., 2004. Lack of evidence for an association between WNT2 and RELN polymorphisms and Autism. American Journal of Medical Genetics B. NeuroPsychiatric Genetics 126B, 51–57.

Li, X., Hu, Z., He, Y., et al., 2010. Association analysis of CNTNAP2 polymorphisms with Autism in the Chinese Han population. Psychiatric Genetics 20, 113–117.

Li, Y., Willer, C., Sanna, S., et al., 2009. Genotype imputation. Annual Review of Genomics Human Genetics 10, 387–406.

Liou, G.G., Tanny, J.C., Kruger, R.G., et al., 2005. Assembly of the SIR complex and its regulation by O-acetyl-ADP-ribose, a product of NAD-dependent histone deacetylation. Cell 121, 515–527.

Liu, J., Nyholt, D.R., Magnussen, P., et al., 2001. A genomewide screen for Autism susceptibility loci. American Journal of Human Genetics 69, 327–340.

Liu, X., Kawamura, Y., Shimada, T., 2010. Association of the oxytocin receptor (OXTR) gene polymorphisms with Autism spectrum disorder (ASD) in the Japanese population. Journal of Human Genetics 55, 137–141.

Liu, X.Q., Georgiades, S., Duku, E., et al., 2011. Identification of genetic loci underlying the phenotypic constructs of Autism spectrum disorders. Journal of the American Academy of Child and Adolescent Archives of General 50, 687–696. e613.

Ma, D., Salyakina, D., Jaworski, J.M., et al., 2009. A genome-wide association study of Autism reveals a common novel risk locus at 5p14.1. Annals of Human Genetics 73, 263–273.

Maestrini, E., Lai, C., Marlow, A., et al., 1999. Serotonin transporter (5-HTT) and gamma-aminobutyric acid receptor subunit beta3

(GABRB3) gene polymorphisms are not associated with Autism in the IMGSA families. The International Molecular Genetic Study of Autism Consortium. American Journal of Medical Genetics 88, 492–496.

Marchini, J., Howie, B., 2010. Genotype imputation for genome-wide association studies. Nature Reviews Genetics 11, 499–511.

McBride, P.A., Anderson, G.M., Hertzig, M.E., et al., 1998. Effects of diagnosis, race, and puberty on platelet serotonin levels in Autism and mental retardation. Journal of the American Academy of Child and Adolescent Archives of General 37, 767–776.

McCauley, J.L., Olson, L.M., Delahanty, R., et al., 2004. A linkage disequilibrium map of the 1-Mb 15q12 GABA(A) receptor subunit cluster and association to Autism. American Journal of Medical Genetics B. NeuroPsychiatric Genetics 131B, 51–59.

McCauley, J.L., Olson, L.M., Dowd, M., et al., 2004. Linkage and association analysis at the serotonin transporter (SLC6A4) locus in a rigid-compulsive subset of Autism. American Journal of Medical Genetics B. NeuroPsychiatric Genetics 127B, 104–112.

McCracken, J.T., McGough, J., Shah, B., et al., 2002. Risperidone in children with Autism and serious behavioral problems. New England Journal of Medicine 347, 314–321.

McDougle, C.J., Naylor, S.T., Cohen, D.J., et al., 1996. A double-blind, placebo-controlled study of fluvoxamine in adults with autistic disorder. Archives of General Psychiatry 53, 1001–1008.

Menold, M.M., Shao, Y., Wolpert, C.M., et al., 2001. Association analysis of chromosome 15 gabaa receptor subunit genes in autistic disorder. Journal of Neurogenetics 15, 245–259.

Minderaa, R.B., Anderson, G.M., Volkmar, F.R., et al., 1989. Whole blood serotonin and tryptophan in Autism: Temporal stability and the effects of medication. Journal of Autism and Developmental Disorders 19, 129–136.

Persico, A.M., D'Agruma, L., Maiorano, N., et al., 2001. Reelin gene alleles and haplotypes as a factor predisposing to autistic disorder. Archives of General Psychiatry 6, 150–159.

Petit, E., Herault, J., Martineau, J., et al., 1995. Association study with two markers of a human homeogene in infantile Autism. Journal of Medical Genetics 32, 269–274.

Philippe, A., Martinez, M., Guilloud-Bataille, M., et al., 1999. Genome-wide scan for Autism susceptibility genes. Paris Autism Research International Sibpair Study. Human Molecular Genetics 8, 805–812.

Rabionet, R., McCauley, J.L., Jaworski, J.M., et al., 2006. Lack of association between Autism and SLC25A12. American Journal Archives of General 163, 929–931.

Ramoz, N., Cai, G., Reichert, J.G., et al., 2008. An analysis of candidate Autism loci on chromosome 2q24-q33: Evidence for association to the STK39 gene. American Journal of Medical Genetics B. NeuroPsychiatric Genetics 147B, 1152–1158.

Ramoz, N., Reichert, J.G., Smith, C.J., et al., 2004. Linkage and association of the mitochondrial aspartate/glutamate carrier SLC25A12 gene with Autism. American Journal Archives of General 161, 662–669.

Ripke, S., Sanders, A.R., Kendler, K.S., et al., 2011. Genome-wide association study identifies five new schizophrenia loci. Nature Genetics 43, 969–976.

Risch, N., Merikangas, K., 1996. The future of genetic studies of complex human diseases. Science 273, 1516–1517.

Risch, N., Spiker, D., Lotspeich, L., et al., 1999. A genomic screen of Autism: Evidence for a multilocus etiology. American Journal of Human Genetics 65, 493–507.

Ritvo, E.R., Yuwiler, A., Geller, E., et al., 1970. Increased blood serotonin and platelets in early infantile Autism. Archives of General 23, 566–572.

Robinson, E.B., Koenen, K.C., McCormick, M.C., 2011. A multivariate twin study of autistic traits in 12-year-olds: Testing the fractionable autism triad hypothesis. Behavior Genetics.

Salmon, B., Hallmayer, J., Rogers, T., et al., 1999. Absence of linkage and linkage disequilibrium to chromosome 15q11-q13 markers in 139 multiplex families with Autism. American Journal of Medical Genetics 88, 551–556.

Salyakina, D., Ma, D.Q., Jaworski, J.M., et al., 2010. Variants in several genomic regions associated with Asperger disorder. Autism Research 3, 303–310.

Schain, R.J., Freedman, D.X., 1961. Studies on 5-hydroxyindole metabolism in autistic and other mentally retarded children. Journal of Pediatrics 58, 315–320.

Schellenberg, G.D., Dawson, G., Sung, Y.J., et al., 2006. Evidence for multiple loci from a genome scan of Autism kindreds. Archives of General Psychiatry 11, 1049–1060. 1979.

Segurado, R., Conroy, J., Meally, E., et al., 2005. Confirmation of association between Autism and the mitochondrial aspartate/glutamate carrier SLC25A12 gene on chromosome 2q31. American Journal Archives of General 162, 2182–2184.

Sen, B., Singh, A.S., Sinha, S., et al., 2010. Family-based studies indicate association of Engrailed 2 gene with Autism in an Indian population. Genes, Brain and Behavior 9, 248–255.

Serajee, F.J., Zhong, H., Mahbubul Huq, A.H., et al., 2006. Association of Reelin gene polymorphisms with Autism. Genomics 87, 75–83.

Shuang, M., Liu, J., Jia, M.X., et al., 2004. Family-based association study between Autism and glutamate receptor 6 gene in Chinese Han trios. American Journal of Medical Genetics B. NeuroPsychiatric Genetics 131B, 48–50.

Skaar, D.A., Shao, Y., Haines, J.L., et al., 2005. Analysis of the RELN gene as a genetic risk factor for Autism. Archives of General Psychiatry 10, 563–571.

Sklar, P., Ripke, S., Scott, L.J., et al., 2011. Large-scale genome-wide association analysis of bipolar disorder identifies a new susceptibility locus near ODZ4. Nature Genetics 43, 977–983.

Skuse, D.H., Gallagher, L., 2011. Genetic influences on social cognition. Pediatric Research 69, 85R–91R.

Sousa, I., Clark, T.G., Toma, C., et al., 2009. MET and Autism susceptibility: Family and case-control studies. European Journal of Human Genetics 17, 749–758.

Spielman, R.S., McGinnis, R.E., Ewens, W.J., et al., 1993. Transmission test for linkage disequilibrium: The insulin gene region and insulin-dependent diabetes mellitus (IDDM). American Journal of Human Genetics 52, 506–516.

Sullivan, P., 2011. Don't give up on GWAS. Molecular Psychiatry.

Sutcliffe, J.S., Delahanty, R.J., Prasad, H.C., et al., 2005. Allelic heterogeneity at the serotonin transporter locus (SLC6A4) confers susceptibility to Autism and rigid-compulsive behaviors. American Journal of Human Genetics 77, 265–279.

Szatmari, P., Paterson, A.D., Zwaigenbaum, L., et al., 2007. Mapping Autism risk loci using genetic linkage and chromosomal rearrangements. Nature Genetics 39, 319–328.

Tansey, K.E., Brookes, K.J., Hill, M.J., et al., 2010. Oxytocin receptor (OXTR) does not play a major role in the aetiology of Autism: Genetic and molecular studies. Neuroscience Letters 474, 163–167.

Tansey, K.E., Hill, M.J., Cochrane, L.E., et al., 2011. Functionality of promoter microsatellites of arginine vasopressin receptor 1A (AVPR1A): Implications for Autism. Molecular Autism 2, 3.

Thanseem, I., Nakamura, K., Miyachi, T., et al., 2010. Further evidence for the role of MET in Autism susceptibility. Neuroscience Research 68, 137–141.

Timinszky, G., Till, S., Hassa, P.O., et al., 2009. A macrodomain-containing histone rearranges chromatin upon sensing PARP1 activation. Nature Structural & Molecular Biology 16, 923–929.

Turunen, J.A., Rehnstrom, K., Kilpinen, H., et al., 2008. Mitochondrial aspartate/glutamate carrier SLC25A12 gene is associated with Autism. Autism Research 1, 189–192.

Wang, K., Zhang, H., Ma, D., et al., 2009. Common genetic variants on 5p14.1 associate with Autism spectrum disorders. Nature 459, 528–533.

Wang, L., Jia, M., Yue, W., 2008. Association of the ENGRAILED 2 (EN2) gene with Autism in Chinese Han population. American Journal of Medical Genetics B. NeuroPsychiatric Genetics 147B, 434–438.

Wassink, T.H., Piven, J., Vieland, V.J., et al., 2004. Examination of AVPR1a as an Autism susceptibility gene. Molecular Psychiatry 9, 968–972.

Weiss, L.A., Arking, D.E., Daly, M.J., et al., 2009. A genome-wide linkage and association scan reveals novel loci for Autism. Nature 461, 802–808.

Wermter, A.K., Kamp-Becker, I., Hesse, P., et al., 2010. Evidence for the involvement of genetic variation in the oxytocin receptor gene (OXTR) in the etiology of autistic disorders on high-functioning level. American Journal of Medical Genetics B. NeuroPsychiatric Genetics 153B, 629–639.

Wu, S., Jia, M., Ruan, Y., et al., 2005. Positive association of the oxytocin receptor gene (OXTR) with Autism in the Chinese Han population. Biological Psychiatry 58, 74–77.

Yang, P., Lung, F.W., Jong, Y.J., et al., 2008. Association of the homeobox transcription factor gene ENGRAILED 2 with autistic disorder in Chinese children. Neuropsychobiology 57, 3–8.

Yang, S.Y., Cho, S.C., Yoo, H.J., et al., 2010. Association study between single nucleotide polymorphisms in promoter region of AVPR1A and Korean Autism spectrum disorders. Neuroscience Letters 479, 197–200.

Yang, S.Y., Cho, S.C., Yoo, H.J., et al., 2010. Family-based association study of microsatellites in the 5′ flanking region of AVPR1A with Autism spectrum disorder in the Korean population. Psychiatry Research 178, 199–201.

Yirmiya, N., Rosenberg, C., Levi, S., et al., 2006. Association between the arginine vasopressin 1a receptor (AVPR1a) gene and Autism in a family-based study: Mediation by socialization skills. Molecular Psychiatry 11, 488–494.

Ylisaukko-oja, T., Nieminen-von Wendt, T., Kempas, E., et al., 2004. Genome-wide scan for loci of Asperger syndrome. Molecular Psychiatry 9, 161–168.

Yonan, A.L., Alarcon, M., Cheng, R., et al., 2003. A genomewide screen of 345 families for Autism susceptibility loci. American Journal of Human Genetics 73, 886–897.

Yrigollen, C.M., Han, S.S., Kochetkova, A., et al., 2008. Genes controlling affiliative behavior as candidate genes for Autism. Biological Psychiatry 63, 911–916.

Zhang, H., Liu, X., Zhang, C., et al., 2002. Reelin gene alleles and susceptibility to Autism spectrum disorders. Molecular Psychiatry 7, 1012–1017.

Zhong, H., Serajee, F.J., Nabi, R., et al., 2003. No association between the EN2 gene and autistic disorder. Journal of Medical Genetics 40, e4.

2.4

Next-Generation Sequencing For Gene and Pathway Discovery and Analysis in Autism Spectrum Disorders

Guiqing Cai*, Joseph D. Buxbaum†

*Seaver Autism Center for Research and Treatment, Laboratory of Molecular Neuropsychiatry, Department of Psychiatry, Friedman Brain Institute, Mount Sinai School of Medicine, New York, NY, USA †as above, and Departments of Psychiatry, Neuroscience, and Genetics and Genomic Sciences, Friedman Brain Institute, Mount Sinai School of Medicine, New York, NY, USA

INTRODUCTION

Multiple twin and family studies have shown that there is a very strong genetic basis to autism spectrum disorders (ASD) (Bailey et al., 1995; Jorde et al., 1991), and many genetic and genomic disorders caused by rare mutations are associated with ASD (Betancur, 2011). Fragile X syndrome is thought to be one of the most common monogenic forms of ASD, with estimates of 1–2% of subjects with ASD having an *FMR1* mutation (Abrahams and Geschwind, 2008). Other more common monogenic forms of ASD include mutations in *SHANK3* (Phelan–McDermid syndrome), *TSC1* and

TSC2 (tuberous sclerosis), *NF1* (neurofibromatosis), *UBE3A* (Angelman syndrome), and *MECP2* (Rett syndrome).

Although they are individually rare, identifying such mutations identifies novel therapeutic targets and points to biological pathways involved in ASD. For example, SHANK3 is located in the postsynaptic density, and mutation of this gene indicates a role for glutamate synaptic function in the etiology of ASD (Durand et al., 2007; Gauthier et al., 2010; Moessner et al., 2007; for more details see Chapter 5.6). Similarly, the X-linked genes neuroligin 4 and 3 (*NLGN4* and *NLGN3*) point to disruption of excitatory transmission in ASD. Mutations of these genes were identified in patients with autism, Asperger syndrome, and/or intellectual disability in several families (Jamain et al., 2003; Laumonnier et al., 2004). Other examples of disrupted pathways and subcellular compartments in ASD can be found in Chapter 2.1.

Current estimates indicate that there are many hundreds of loci as yet undiscovered in ASD (see below) and each represents an opportunity for clinical dissection, pathway analysis, and even experimental therapeutics (Wink et al., 2010). However, traditional sequencing had been a bottleneck for finding mutations on a genomic scale. New sequencing technologies developed in recent years will bring an explosion of genetic findings to ASD and will dramatically advance our understanding of ASD pathogenesis, and expand treatment options.

NEXT-GENERATION SEQUENCING TECHNOLOGIES

Traditional ('first-generation') sequencing came into very widespread use following the methods developed in parallel by Sanger and by Maxam and Gilbert (Maxam and Gilbert, 1977; Sanger et al., 1977;). Sanger sequencing uses chain-termination methods where, during the sequencing by synthesis, a proportion of each sequencing reaction is terminated by adding one of four dideoxynucleotides (ddATP, ddGTP, ddCTP, or ddTTP) generating a ladder of products differing from the next by a single base. These fragments can be separated by electrophoresis with the sequence of template DNA decoded. This chain-termination approach, when combined with automated capillary electrophoresis, yielded vastly improved speed and accuracy. Technical simplicity, high accuracy of raw reads, and read length of about 800–1000 bp, made this the dominant technology for DNA sequencing for over two decades, and the successful completion of the human genome sequencing project was a tour de force which relied on this technology. However, the international 10-year effort and high cost for sequencing the first human genome reflected its major limitations.

Next-generation sequencing (NGS) emerged early in 2000, when Lynx Therapeutics published a massively parallel signature sequencing (MPSS) method in *Nature Biotechnology* (Brenner et al., 2000). In 2005, NGS approaches became more available with the publication of the sequence-by-synthesis technology developed by 454 Life Sciences (Margulies et al., 2005) and of the multiplex polony sequencing protocol of George Church's lab (Shendure et al., 2005). Additional NGS sequencing technologies have been developed and many are commercially available. These methods differ in template preparation, sequencing chemistry, sequencing platform, imaging, and data analysis. Four NGS technologies will be briefly described in the following sections to highlight their relevant advantages.

PYROSEQUENCING

Pyrosequencing was originally developed on the basis of the sequencing-by-synthesis principle, but it relies on the detection of pyrophosphate release on nucleotide incorporation, rather than chain termination with dideoxynucleotides (Ronaghi et al., 1996; 1998). One example of pyrosequencing is in use on the Roche/454 NGS platform. The DNA library is first generated through random fragmentation of genomic DNA and an emulsion polymerase chain reaction (PCR) is used to prepare the template library by clonal amplification of template DNA in single aqueous droplet-encapsulated reaction beads and DNA complexes. The surface of the beads contains oligonucleotide probes with sequences that are complementary to the adaptors binding the DNA fragments. Thousands of copies of the same template sequence are clonally amplified. Emulsion PCR beads can be chemically attached to a glass slide or deposited into PicoTiterPlate wells (Margulies et al., 2005). Addition of nucleotides complementary to the template strand, in enzymatic reactions including DNA polymerase and luciferase, results in a chemiluminescent signal recorded by a CCD camera within the instrument. Software then identifies the location of the beads and correlates the light flashes with each type of nucleotide that was incorporated into the synthesized DNA. About 1 million reads at lengths of average 400 bases can be generated per run at this time.

Cyclic Reversible Termination

Cyclic reversible termination was developed as the basis of a new non-Sanger DNA sequencing method. An important feature of this method is the termination of DNA synthesis after the addition of a single nucleotide. The Illumina/Solexa system uses this method combined with a process called 'bridge PCR' amplification, which is used to yield thousands of copies of each fragment in a cluster on the surface of a flow cell. Template DNA is fragmented and captured by adaptor ligation to corresponding primers, which are covalently attached to a solid phase on flow cells. By adding unlabeled nucleotides and enzymes, amplification proceeds in cycles. The enzyme incorporates nucleotides to build double-stranded bridges on the solid-phase substrate. Denaturation leaves single-stranded template with one end of each bridge tethered to the surface. Several million dense clusters of double-stranded DNA are generated in each channel of the flow cell. During sequencing, each of the four deoxynucleotides is labeled with a different fluorescent dye and one fluorescently-labeled nucleotide is added to the 3′ end of each growing strand. Fluorescence from each cluster on the flow cell is captured upon laser excitation. The dye and terminating group are chemically cleaved and a new cycle of nucleotide incorporation and fluorescent imaging is carried out (Metzker, 2010; Shendure et al., 2011). One limitation of this system is the length of fragment sequenced: The initial sequence length per read was 36 nt but now 100 nt is achieved on Illumina's HiSeq2000. This platform is widely used for re-sequencing projects and whole-genome or whole-exome re-sequencing, as well as other applications such as RNA-seq, ChIP-seq and Methyl-seq (discussed later in this chapter).

Sequencing by Ligation

Sequencing by ligation followed by emulsion PCR template preparation is used on the Applied Biosystems (now Life Technologies) SOLiD platform. Like the 454 technology, the DNA template fragments are clonally amplified on beads, however the beads are placed on the solid-phase of a flow cell so greater density is achieved than in other approaches. In sequencing by ligation, a mixture of different fluorescently labeled dinucleotide probes is pumped into the flow cell. As the correct dinucleotide probe incorporates the template DNA, it is ligated onto the pre-built primer on the solid-phase. After wash-out of the unincorporated probes, fluorescence is captured and recorded. Each fluorescence wavelength corresponds to a particular dinucleotide combination. Then the fluorescent dye is removed and washed and the next sequencing cycle starts. Although 1 billion reads from a single run can be achieved, the limitation of this system is the short sequence read length (50 nt), however accuracy is very high.

Single-Molecule Sequencing

The recent emergence of single-molecule sequencing technologies in the NGS field expands sequencing capabilities enormously. As it represents a qualitative improvement from the technologies noted above, some have taken to calling it third-generation sequencing. Unlike the second-generation sequencing technologies discussed above, single-molecule sequencing interrogates a single molecule of DNA or RNA template in real time. No clonal amplification of DNA or RNA template is required, which overcomes biases introduced by PCR amplification. Single-molecule sequencing can also radically reduce sequencing costs and provide much increased read lengths, however, the most important advantages of this technology are the capacity for real-time measurements of DNA or RNA composition and detection of base modifications such as DNA methylation (Schadt et al., 2010).

The first commercially available single-molecule sequencer was from Helicos Biosciences using a proprietary technology (Bowers et al., 2009). Sample preparation started with fragmentation of genomic DNA, adding a 3′ poly(A) tail, and capturing these single-stranded templates on a flow cell surface with covalently bound 5′ dT oligonucleotides. The flow cell with these single-stranded molecules was assembled into the HeliScope sequencer, where specially designed fluorescently labeled nucleotide analogues were pumped in one at a time. Through sequencing by synthesis in the presence of polymerase, templates with corresponding nucleotides were identified and the surface was scanned for the fluorescence label. The incorporated fluorescent moiety was then removed, the next fluorescent nucleotide pumped in and the process was repeated (Ozsolak et al., 2009; Shendure et al., 2011). Since this method uses a wash-and-scan process, the total sequencing time can be as long as that of other second-generation sequencing technologies (Schadt et al., 2010).

A more widely deployed single-molecule technology is that of Pacific Biosciences, known as single-molecule real-time sequencing (SMRT). A critical part of this system is called zero-mode waveguide (ZMW), where a single DNA polymerase enzyme with a single molecule of a DNA template is immobilized at the bottom of a ZMW detector. Each of the four DNA bases, attached to one of four different fluorescent dyes, is flooded above an array of ZMWs. When the correct nucleotide is detected by the polymerase, it is incorporated into the growing DNA strand and the phospho-linked fluorescent tag is cleaved off and diffuses out of the observation area of the ZMW. A detector registers the fluorescent signal of nucleotide incorporation, and the base call is made according to the corresponding fluorescence of the dye (Schadt et al., 2010). Very importantly, the kinetics of nucleotide incorporation can provide information on chemical modification of the template, providing epigenetic information (Song et al., 2011). The SMRT system shows many desirable features of single-molecule sequencing: much faster sequencing times, long reads, small amounts of starting material, low sequencing costs, and the ability to detect epigenetic modifications directly.

Other technologies for single-molecule sequencing are emerging. Oxford Nanopore technology uses a nanopore through which single-stranded DNA molecules are electrophoretically driven. When each nucleotide on the DNA molecule partially obstructs the nanopore, it alters the pore's electrical properties to a different degree and the change is then recorded as corresponding to that particular nucleotide (Branton et al., 2008; Kasianowicz et al., 1996). Halcyon Molecular uses transmission electron microscopy to directly image and chemically detect atoms of unique nucleotides. They developed annular dark-field imaging in an aberration-corrected scanning which can identify the chemical type of every atom in a monolayer of hexagonal boron nitride containing substitutional defects (Krivanek et al., 2010). Ion Torrent by Life Technologies uses a semiconductor circuit to perform non-optical DNA sequencing of genomes directly. Sequence data are obtained by directly sensing the ions produced by template-directed DNA polymerase synthesis using all-natural nucleotides on a massively parallel semiconductor-sensing device or ion chip (Rothberg et al., 2011). VisiGen Biotechnologies uses an engineered DNA polymerase tagged with a fluorophore. When it binds to a donor nucleotide with the fluorophore label, a fluorescence resonant energy transfer occurs and this signal is detected in real time. All of these technologies show promise and further enhancements will soon lead to profound changes in NGS, providing a further revolution in gene and pathway discovery and analysis.

APPLICATION OF NEXT-GENERATION SEQUENCING TECHNOLOGIES IN HUMAN DISEASE

The rapid development of the next-generation sequencing technologies has given unprecedented power to solve problems in multiple fields of molecular biology, resulting in many discoveries and new insights. With the emergence of new library preparation methods, computing pipelines for processing the huge volumes of sequencing data, and enhanced analysis strategies, NGS is being applied in many areas. In this section, some of the major applications of NGS will be discussed in the context of human health.

Whole-Genome Sequencing

NGS demonstrated its profound power with the sequencing of James D. Watson's genome using the Roche/454 NGS platform (Wheeler et al., 2008). The sequence was completed in two months, at approximately one-hundredth the cost of traditional Sanger automated sequencing methods. This work was quickly followed by five additional genomes sequenced using different NGS platforms: a Yoruban individual (NA18507) was sequenced on the Illumina/Solexa platform (Bentley et al., 2008) and on the Applied Biosystems SOLiD platform (McKernan et al., 2009), a Chinese genome (YH) and two Korean genomes (AK1 and SJK) were sequenced on the Illumina/Solexa platform (Ahn et al., 2009; Kim et al., 2009; Wang et al.,

2008), and one genome (Stephen R. Quake) was sequenced using the single-molecule method by Helicos Biosciences (Pushkarev et al., 2009).

One objective of genomic sequencing is to relate single nucleotide variants (SNVs), indels, and structural variations (SVs) to relevant phenotypes. When compared with the reference human genome, about 3–3.5 million SNVs were identified in each individual genome mentioned above. In 2010, the 1,000 Genomes Project was initiated with the aim of providing a deep characterization of human genome sequence variation as a foundation for investigating genotype and phenotype relationships (1,000 Genomes Project Consortium, 2010). This project is now moving quickly to complete its current goal of sequencing and analyzing the genomes of 2,500 individuals from seven populations worldwide. Recently, the UK10K was announced, funded by the Wellcome Trust, which aims to sequence the whole genomes of 4,000 people in the general population, as well as whole exomes of 6,000 individuals with extreme phenotypes or rare disease, including autism (http://www.uk10k.org/goals.html).

The first disease mutation identified by whole-genome sequencing was reported in a family with a recessive form of Charcot–Marie–Tooth disease (Lupski et al., 2010). Patient DNA was first sequenced by ligation on an Applied Biosystems SOLiD NGS platform and about 3.4 million SNVs were identified. Filtering against single nucleotide polymorphisms or SNVs in public databases was carried out to identify the particular mutation responsible for the observed phenotypes in this family. By further examining segregation of remaining functional variants in all family members, two mutations in *SH3TC2* (SH3 domain and tetratricopeptide repeats 2) were identified as being responsible for the separate subclinical phenotypes in this family. A similar strategy has been used in another family with two children affected with Miller syndrome. Mutation in the *DHODH* gene was identified as the primary cause of Miller syndrome, while mutation in *DNAH5* was identified as a cause of primary ciliary dyskinesia in the patients (Roach et al., 2010). A third report concerned the identification of mutations in *SPR*, which encodes sepiapterin reductase, in a 14-year-old fraternal twin-pair diagnosed with DOPA-responsive dystonia (DRD). The discovery led to clinical interventions targeting both dopamine (with L-DOPA) and serotonin (with 5-hydroxytryptophan supplementation), which led to clinical improvements (Bainbridge et al., 2011). This list is growing rapidly and will continue to provide both etiological diagnosis and new therapeutic strategies in the care of patients.

Whole-genome sequencing has special importance for sequencing the cancer genome. By comparing the genome in cancer biopsies with that of healthy cells from the same patient, genes critical in the development of the cancer can be identified. For example, Mardis and colleagues sequenced an acute myeloid leukemia genome and a matched normal skin genome from the same patient using the Illumina/Solexa platform, and identified recurring mutations which were relevant to cancer pathogenesis (Mardis et al., 2009). Welch and colleagues used whole-genome sequencing to aid in the diagnosis of a specific leukemia subtype leading to treatment modifications in a patient (Welch et al., 2011). With the ultimate goal of developing much-improved strategies to better diagnose and treat various cancers, the US National Institutes of Health (NIH) Cancer Genome Atlas project (http:// cancergenome.nih.gov/) is characterizing more than 20 tumor types at genomic and other levels using NGS technology.

NGS-based whole-genome sequencing is revolutionizing our ability to rapidly characterize microbial strains related to life-threatening infectious disease. In 2011, origins of the strain causing a cholera outbreak in Haiti and the *E. coli* strain causing an outbreak of hemolytic-uremic syndrome in Germany were quickly identified using NGS technology, including single-molecule sequencing (Chin et al., 2011; Mellmann et al., 2011; Rasko et al., 2011).

Whole-Exome Sequencing

Whole-exome sequencing was developed as an efficient and inexpensive means of capturing the subgenome that is directly related to coding regions of the genome. By using target selection and enrichment approaches, only the protein-coding regions of the genome are sequenced on the NGS platform. As protein-coding regions constitute only ~ 1.5% of the human genome and cover only ~ 30–40 megabases (Mb) of sequence, this allows for many more samples to be probed in a given NGS experiment. As a proof-of-concept, Ng and colleagues did whole-exome sequencing in four unrelated individuals with a rare autosome dominant inherited disorder (Miller syndrome) and showed that this approach was very cost-efficient as a means of identifying causal variants of rare disorders (Ng et al., 2009).

Though a variety of methods for whole-exome library preparation have been developed, solution-based target enrichment is becoming the most prevalent, because of its simplicity and ease of automation. Briefly, a pool of oligonucleotides probes (DNA or RNA) is synthesized to selectively hybridize to the targeted exonic regions of genomic DNA. The probes include tags for pull-down with beads, such that the hybridized probe-target fragments can be isolated and the unbound regions of genomic DNA washed away. The targeted genomic fragments are then sequenced on an NGS platform (Kahvejian et al., 2008).

Whole-exome sequencing focuses on what is thought to be the most medically relevant part of the human genome, as this reduces the overhead of both the molecular and analytical aspects. This approach has been broadly applied to identifying the genes that underlie rare disorders. In only the past two years, causal genes or alleles have been identified for more than two dozen Mendelian disorders, and the approach is now being used to identify rare etiologically relevant variants underlying complex traits, such as schizophrenia and autism (Bamshad et al., 2011). An example of early success is the whole-exome sequencing of 10 individuals with unexplained mental retardation in whom pathogenic *de novo* mutations were identified (Vissers et al., 2010).

Transcriptome Sequencing (RNA-seq)

Understanding the transcriptome is an essential step in interpreting functional elements of the genome, revealing the molecular constituents of cells and tissues, and understanding changes associated with development and disease. Using NGS technology for transcriptome sequencing (RNA-seq) allows RNA to be directly sequenced in a high-throughput and quantitative manner (Wang et al., 2009). For most current RNA-seq applications, a population of RNA (e.g., mRNA) is converted to complementary DNA (cDNA) and then double-stranded cDNA is synthesized for library preparation for NGS. However, reverse transcription and library amplification steps introduce biases and artifacts (and increase costs). For this reason there is great interest in using single-molecule sequencing technology, where RNA can be directly sequenced with reverse transcriptase (Schadt et al., 2010).

Epigenome Sequencing

The epigenome is the overall epigenetic state of a given genomic sample, and for a given individual genome there may be many hundreds of stable epigenomes, depending on the stability of the chromatin states (Park, 2009). DNA methylation and histone modification are epigenetic modifications that can be mapped genome-wide with NGS technologies at single-nucleotide resolution (Hawkins et al., 2010). Methods developed for genome-wide DNA methylation analysis include bisulfite conversion followed by capture and sequencing (BC-seq), methylated DNA immunoprecipitation-based sequencing (MeDIP), and methylation-sensitive-restriction-enzyme-dependent library preparation and sequencing (Methyl-seq, HELP-seq) (Laird, 2010). As noted above, single-molecule RNA sequencing can also detect methylated DNA, as well as additional modification of DNA (Ozsolak and Milos, 2011; Song et al., 2011).

Methods for histone modification analysis include chromatin immunoprecipitation followed by sequencing (ChIP-seq), and DNase I hypersensitivity site footprinting coupled with NGS (DNase-seq). Specific DNA sites in direct physical interaction with transcription factors and other proteins can be isolated by immunoprecipitation and then subjected to NGS sequencing (Laird, 2010). NGS-based ChIP-seq is able to analyze the interaction pattern of any protein that binds DNA, thus allowing us to study these interactions on a genomic scale (Johnson et al., 2007).

NEXT-GENERATION SEQUENCING IN AUTISM SPECTRUM DISORDERS

Whole-Exome Sequencing In ASD

ASD are common neurodevelopmental disorders often associated with a large burden on the affected individual, the family, and on society. Rare genetic or genomic mutations are clearly implicated in ASD (the rare nature of such variation is due to purifying selection acting on deleterious variation), and there is also likely an as-yet-undefined role for common genetic variation in ASD (O'Roak and State, 2008). ASD are highly heterogeneous from the perspective of genetic etiology, and only about 10–20% of individuals currently have an identified genetic cause. At the same time, more than 100 genetic and genomic loci have been reported in subjects with ASD, showing the success of ongoing efforts but also underscoring the fact that whole-exome and whole-genome sequencing will be critical approaches for identifying ASD genes and loci (Betancur, 2011).

The first whole-exome study of ASD was published in 2011. In this study, 20 individuals with sporadic ASD and their parents were sequenced for *de novo* mutations of major effect (O'Roak et al., 2011). Four potentially causative *de novo* events were identified, in *FOXP1*, *GRIN2B*, *SCN1A*, and *LAMC3*. The study showed that family-based exome sequencing was a powerful approach for identifying new candidate genes for ASD, especially if there was a focus on *de novo* variation.

Several large-scale whole-exome sequencing projects have been initiated in the past two years. One collaborative project received support from the NIMH to sequence several hundred trios, as well as 1,000 cases and carefully matched controls. In the first stage of this project, whole-exome sequencing was performed in a total of 175 ASD trios (Neale et al., 2012). The overall rate of *de novo* mutation was only slightly higher than the expected rate, however, there was significantly

enriched connectivity among the proteins encoded by genes harboring *de novo* missense or nonsense mutations, as well as excess connectivity to prior ASD genes of major effect, indicating that a subset of observed events were relevant to ASD risk. Moreover, analysis of *de novo* variation in this and parallel studies (described below) and the case-control data provided evidence in favor of *CHD8* and *KATNAL2* as genuine autism risk genes.

A second ongoing large exome-sequencing project, supported by the Simons Foundation, is focused on the Simons Simplex Collection (SSC). A unique feature of the SSC is that each family is comprised of a proband, unaffected parents, and, in most kindreds, an unaffected sibling, which allows researchers to use these unaffected siblings as an important control group (Fischbach and Lord, 2010; Sanders et al., 2011). Three studies totalling ca 750 SSC trios have been completed (Iossifov et al., 2012; O'Roak et al., 2012 Sanders et al., 2012). In one study (Sanders et al., 2012), where the unaffected sibling was also sequenced, it was clear that deleterious *de novo* mutations were significantly elevated in affected as compared to unaffected siblings, and this was more pronounced when the authors considered *de novo* mutations present in brain-expressed genes. The authors conclude that ca 45% of *de novo* deleterious variants in brain-expressed genes carry risk of ASD in these families. Moreover, based on two independent nonsense substitutions disrupting the same gene, this study identifies *SCN2A* (sodium channel, voltage-gated, type II, alpha subunit), as a bona fide ASD gene.

A second completed SSC study identified *CHD8* and *NTNG1* as ASD genes (O'Roak et al., 2012). This study (as well as the other studies noted above) shows very clearly that *de novo* point mutations are positively correlated with paternal age, consistent with an increased risk of developing ASD for children of older fathers. O'Roak and colleagues also show that *de novo* point mutations are overwhelmingly paternal in origin (5:1 bias) consistent with this hypothesis. Finally, Iossifov et al. show that there is an enrichment of likely ASD genes amongst genes regulated by the Fragile-X-syndrome associated FMR1 protein.

Importantly, examining all four studies together, one can estimate both the numbers of ASD genes that can be identified by these approaches (ca 500), as well as the rate of gene discovery as a function of trios sequenced (see Sanders et al., 2012). For example, using as criteria recurrent *de novo* loss-of-function variants, analyses showed that for 6,000 families (approximately what is available now in US repositories) a threshold of three or more such variants is sufficient to declare genome-wide significance and 20–50 ASD genes would be identified by this criterion alone. Using two or more *de novo* loss-of-function variants as the criterion would identify 60–120 likely ASD genes with an FDR of 0.1. In addition, other forms of discovery, such as recessive loci, would lead to additional gene discovery.

Additional whole-exome projects include those led by researchers at the Hospital for Sick Children at Toronto, which aims to create whole-exome sequences for a cohort of 1,000 Canadian patients (Walker et al., 2011). Meanwhile, the UK10K project is currently performing whole-exome sequencing of about 600 ASD subjects (http://www.uk10k.org/goals.html). Supported by a NIMH Grand Opportunity grant, the Broad Institute and Harvard Medical School are also conducting a study of whole-exome and eventually whole-genome sequencing of Middle Eastern patients with a recessive form of autism whose parents share a common ancestry.

An analysis of the 1,000 cases and matched controls from the NIMH-funded initiative show clearly that there is a roughly two-fold elevation in individuals with homozygous loss-of-function variation in ASD (Lim et al., submitted), and examination of recessive forms of ASD with NGS will likely identify many additional ASD loci.

Whole-Genome Sequencing in ASD

There are several whole-genome projects ongoing at pilot scale. Moreover, in October 2011, Autism Speaks and Beijing Genome Institute (BGI) in China jointly announced a commitment to a collaborative project to perform whole-genome sequencing over a two-year period on more than 2,000 participating families who have two or more children on the autism spectrum. This project would create the world's largest library of sequenced genomes of individuals with ASD and will add substantially to ongoing efforts in gene discovery in ASD.

Transcriptome and Epigenome Sequencing in ASD

Transcriptome sequencing represents an invaluable means of exploring the biology of ASD, but there are current limitations due to the availability of sufficient numbers of high-quality postmortem brain samples. In one study in postmortem ASD brains, researchers made use of RNA-seq as validation data for gene expression arrays. RNA-seq validated changes in groups of genes identified by co-expression analysis, and provided further evidence for a convergence of transcriptional and alternative-splicing abnormalities in the synaptic and signaling pathogenesis of ASD (Voineagu et al., 2011). RNA-seq in postmortem brain samples, peripheral samples, and inducible pluripotent stem cells differentiated into neural cells will be an important avenue in ASD research.

To characterize epigenetic signatures of ASD in prefrontal cortex neurons, Shulha and colleagues performed genome-wide mapping of the histone marker H3K4me3 in neuronal and non-neuronal nuclei from postmortem ASD brain samples. ASD cases showed altered H3K4me3 peaks for numerous genes regulating neuronal connectivity, social behaviors, and cognition, often in conjunction with altered expression of the corresponding transcripts (Shulha et al., 2011). Although a small number of samples were used in these studies, the findings show the power of NGS for ASD research. Again, this approach, when applied to additional postmortem brain samples, peripheral samples, and inducible pluripotent stem cells differentiated into neural cells, will provide insights into the pathways which are disrupted in ASD.

CONCLUSION

Next-generation sequencing technologies allow us to interrogate the human genome base by base physically and functionally in an efficient and affordable way. It is likely that whole-exome and whole-genome sequencing will be widely applied in the clinical setting to facilitate genetic diagnosis and inform therapy (Bamshad et al., 2011). However, there are many challenges in identifying disease variants or genes responsible for clinical phenotypes. Characterizing the human genome at the individual and population levels is a fundamental requirement for clarifying the contribution of genetic variation to human phenotypic traits, including those that are disease-related. For example, it was recently estimated that an individual human genome typically contains about 100 loss-of-function variants with about 20 genes completely inactivated, based on systematic investigation of whole-genome sequencing data from 180 subjects in four different populations (MacArthur et al., 2012). Careful application of NGS techniques will help us to identify rare genetic variants in ASD, assess their relative contribution, and ultimately lead to improved diagnosis and treatment. As ASD involves core abnormalities in social cognition and language, both of which are central to what makes us human, these findings will have broad ramifications in the neurosciences (Geschwind, 2011).

References

1000 Genomes Project Consortium, 2010. A map of human genome variation from population-scale sequencing. Nature 467, 1061–1073.

Abrahams, B.S., Geschwind, D.H., 2008. Advances in Autism genetics: On the threshold of a new neurobiology. Nature Reviews Genetics 9, 341–355.

Ahn, S.M., Kim, T.H., Lee, S., Kim, D., Ghang, H., Kim, D.S., et al., 2009. The first Korean genome sequence and analysis: Full genome sequencing for a socio-ethnic group. Genome Research 19, 1622–1629.

Bailey, A., Le Couteur, A., Gottesman, I., Bolton, P., Simonoff, E., Yuzda, E., et al., 1995. Autism as a strongly genetic disorder: Evidence from a British twin study. Psychological Medicine 25, 63–77.

Bainbridge, M.N., Wiszniewski, W., Murdock, D.R., Friedman, J., Gonzaga-Jauregui, C., Newsham, I., et al., 2011. Whole-genome sequencing for optimized patient management. Science Translational Medicine 3, 87re3.

Bamshad, M.J., Ng, S.B., Bigham, A.W., Tabor, H.K., Emond, M.J., Nickerson, D.A., et al., 2011. Exome sequencing as a tool for Mendelian disease gene discovery. Nature Reviews Genetics 12, 745–755.

Bentley, D.R., Balasubramanian, S., Swerdlow, H.P., Smith, G.P., Milton, J., Brown, C.G., et al., 2008. Accurate whole human genome sequencing using reversible terminator chemistry. Nature 456, 53–59.

Betancur, C., 2011. Etiological heterogeneity in Autism spectrum disorders: More than 100 genetic and genomic disorders and still counting. Brain Research 1380, 42–77.

Bowers, J., Mitchell, J., Beer, E., Buzby, P.R., Causey, M., Efcavitch, J.W., et al., 2009. Virtual terminator nucleotides for next-generation DNA sequencing. Nature Methods 6, 593–595.

Branton, D., Deamer, D.W., Marziali, A., Bayley, H., Benner, S.A., Butler, T., et al., 2008. The potential and challenges of nanopore sequencing. Nature Biotechnology 26, 1146–1153.

Brenner, S., Johnson, M., Bridgham, J., Golda, G., Lloyd, D.H., Johnson, D., et al., 2000. Gene expression analysis by massively parallel signature sequencing (MPSS) on microbead arrays. Nature Biotechnology 18, 630–634.

Chin, C.S., Sorenson, J., Harris, J.B., Robins, W.P., Charles, R.C., Jean-Charles, R.R., et al., 2011. The origin of the Haitian cholera outbreak strain. New England Journal of Medicine 364, 33–42.

Durand, C.M., Betancur, C., Boeckers, T.M., Bockmann, J., Chaste, P., Fauchereau, F., et al., 2007. Mutations in the gene encoding the synaptic scaffolding protein SHANK3 are associated with Autism spectrum disorders. Nature Genetics 39, 25–27.

Fischbach, G.D., Lord, C., 2010. The Simons Simplex Collection: A resource for identification of Autism genetic risk factors. Neuron 68, 192–195.

Gauthier, J., Champagne, N., Lafreniere, R.G., Xiong, L., Spiegelman, D., Brustein, E., et al., 2010. De novo mutations in the gene encoding the synaptic scaffolding protein SHANK3 in patients ascertained for schizophrenia. Proceedings of the National Academy of Sciences USA 107, 7863–7868.

Geschwind, D.H., 2011. Genetics of Autism spectrum disorders. Trends in Cognitive Sciences 15, 409–416.

Hawkins, R.D., Hon, G.C., Ren, B., 2010. Next-generation genomics: An integrative approach. Nature Reviews Genetics 11, 476–486.

Iossifov, I., Ronemus, M., Levy, D., Wang, Z., Hakker, I., Rosenbaum, J., et al., 2012. De novo gene disruptions in children on the autistic spectrum. Neuron 74, 285–299.

Jamain, S., Quach, H., Betancur, C., Rastam, M., Colineaux, C., Gillberg, I.C., et al., 2003. Mutations of the X-linked genes encoding neuroligins NLGN3 and NLGN4 are associated with Autism. Nature Genetics 34, 27–29.

Johnson, D.S., Mortazavi, A., Myers, R.M., Wold, B., 2007. Genome-wide mapping of in vivo protein-DNA interactions. Science 316, 1497–1502.

Jorde, L.B., Hasstedt, S.J., Ritvo, E.R., Mason-Brothers, A., Freeman, B.J., Pingree, C., et al., 1991. Complex segregation analysis of Autism. American Journal of Human Genetics 49, 932–938.

Kahvejian, A., Quackenbush, J., Thompson, J.F., 2008. What would you do if you could sequence everything? Nature Biotechnology 26, 1125–1133.

Kasianowicz, J.J., Brandin, E., Branton, D., Deamer, D.W., 1996. Characterization of individual polynucleotide molecules using a membrane channel. Proceedings of the National Academy of Sciences USA 93, 13,770–13,773.

Kim, J.I., Ju, Y.S., Park, H., Kim, S., Lee, S., Yi, J.H., et al., 2009. A highly annotated whole-genome sequence of a Korean individual. Nature 460, 1011–1015.

Krivanek, O.L., Chisholm, M.F., Nicolosi, V., Pennycook, T.J., Corbin, G.J., Dellby, N., et al., 2010. Atom-by-atom structural and chemical analysis by annular dark-field electron microscopy. Nature 464, 571–574.

Laird, P.W., 2010. Principles and challenges of genomewide DNA methylation analysis. Nature Reviews Genetics 11, 191–203.

Laumonnier, F., Bonnet-Brilhault, F., Gomot, M., Blanc, R., David, A., Moizard, M.P., et al., 2004. X-linked mental retardation and Autism are associated with a mutation in the NLGN4 gene, a member of the neuroligin family. American Journal of Human Genetics 74, 552–557.

Lim, E.T., Raychaudhuri, S., Stevens, C., Sabo, A., Neale, B.M., Sanders, S.J., et al., 2012. Enrichment of low-frequency two-hit loss-of-function events in cases suggests recessive component in Autism.

Lupski, J.R., Reid, J.G., Gonzaga-Jauregui, C., Rio Deiros, D., Chen, D.C., Nazareth, L., et al., 2010. Whole-genome sequencing in a patient with Charcot-Marie-Tooth neuropathy. New England Journal of Medicine 362, 1181–1191.

MacArthur, D.G., Balasubramanian, S., Frankish, A., Huang, N., Morris, J., Walter, K., et al., 2012. A systematic survey of loss-of-function variants in human protein-coding genes. Science 335, 823–828.

Mardis, E.R., Ding, L., Dooling, D.J., Larson, D.E., McLellan, M.D., Chen, K., et al., 2009. Recurring mutations found by sequencing an acute myeloid leukemia genome. New England Journal of Medicine 361, 1058–1066.

Margulies, M., Egholm, M., Altman, W.E., Attiya, S., Bader, J.S., Bemben, L.A., et al., 2005. Genome sequencing in microfabricated high-density picolitre reactors. Nature 437, 376–380.

Maxam, A.M., Gilbert, W., 1977. A new method for sequencing DNA. Proceedings of the National Academy of Sciences USA 74, 560–564.

McKernan, K.J., Peckham, H.E., Costa, G.L., McLaughlin, S.F., Fu, Y., Tsung, E.F., et al., 2009. Sequence and structural variation in a human genome uncovered by short-read, massively parallel ligation sequencing using two-base encoding. Genome Research 19, 1527–1541.

Mellmann, A., Harmsen, D., Cummings, C.A., Zentz, E.B., Leopold, S.R., Rico, A., et al., 2011. Prospective genomic characterization of the German enterohemorrhagic Escherichia coli O104:H4 outbreak by rapid next generation sequencing technology. PLoS One 6, e22751.

Metzker, M.L., 2010. Sequencing technologies - the next generation. Nature Reviews Genetics 11, 31–46.

Moessner, R., Marshall, C.R., Sutcliffe, J.S., Skaug, J., Pinto, D., Vincent, J., et al., 2007. Contribution of SHANK3 mutations to Autism spectrum disorder. American Journal of Human Genetics 81, 1289–1297.

Neale, B.M., Kou, Y., Liu, L., Ma'ayan, A., Samocha, K.E., Sabo, A., et al., 2012. Patterns and rates of exonic de novo mutations in Autism spectrum disorders. Nature 485, 242–245.

Ng, S.B., Turner, E.H., Robertson, P.D., Flygare, S.D., Bigham, A.W., Lee, C., et al., 2009. Targeted capture and massively parallel sequencing of 12 human exomes. Nature 461, 272–276.

O'Roak, B.J., Deriziotis, P., Lee, C., Vives, L., Schwartz, J.J., Girirajan, S., et al., 2011. Exome sequencing in sporadic Autism spectrum disorders identifies severe de novo mutations. Nature Genetics 43, 585–589.

O'Roak, B.J., State, M.W., 2008. Autism genetics: Strategies, challenges, and opportunities. Autism Research 1, 4–17.

O'Roak, B.J., Vives, L., Girirajan, S., Karakoc, E., Krumm, N., Coe, B.P., et al., 2012. Sporadic Autism exomes reveal a highly interconnected protein network of de novo mutations. Nature 485, 246–250.

Ozsolak, F., Milos, P.M., 2011. Transcriptome profiling using single-molecule direct RNA sequencing. Methods in Molecular Biology 733, 51–61.

Ozsolak, F., Platt, A.R., Jones, D.R., Reifenberger, J.G., Sass, L.E., McInerney, P., et al., 2009. Direct RNA sequencing. Nature 461, 814–818.

Park, P.J., 2009. ChIP-seq: Advantages and challenges of a maturing technology. Nature Reviews Genetics 10, 669–680.

Pushkarev, D., Neff, N.F., Quake, S.R., 2009. Single-molecule sequencing of an individual human genome. Nature Biotechnology 27, 847–850.

Rasko, D.A., Webster, D.R., Sahl, J.W., Bashir, A., Boisen, N., Scheutz, F., et al., 2011. Origins of the E. coli strain causing an outbreak of hemolytic-uremic syndrome in Germany. New England Journal of Medicine 365, 709–717.

Roach, J.C., Glusman, G., Smit, A.F., Huff, C.D., Hubley, R., Shannon, P.T., et al., 2010. Analysis of genetic inheritance in a family quartet by whole-genome sequencing. Science 328, 636–639.

Ronaghi, M., Karamohamed, S., Pettersson, B., Uhlen, M., Nyren, P., 1996. Real-time DNA sequencing using detection of pyrophosphate release. Analytical Biochemistry 242, 84–89.

Ronaghi, M., Uhlen, M., Nyren, P., 1998. A sequencing method based on real-time pyrophosphate. Science 281, 363–365.

Rothberg, J.M., Hinz, W., Rearick, T.M., Schultz, J., Mileski, W., Davey, M., et al., 2011. An integrated semiconductor device enabling non-optical genome sequencing. Nature 475, 348–352.

Sanders, S.J., Ercan-Sencicek, A.G., Hus, V., Luo, R., Murtha, M.T., Moreno-De-Luca, D., et al., 2011. Multiple recurrent de novo CNVs, including duplications of the 7q11.23 Williams syndrome region, are strongly associated with Autism. Neuron 70, 863–885.

Sanders, S.J., Murtha, M.T., Gupta, A.R., Murdoch, J.D., Raubeson, M.J., Willsey, A.J., et al., 2012. De novo mutations revealed by whole-exome sequencing are strongly associated with Autism. Nature 485, 237–241.

Sanger, F., Nicklen, S., Coulson, A.R., 1977. DNA sequencing with chain-terminating inhibitors. Proceedings of the National Academy of Sciences USA 74, 5463–5467.

Schadt, E.E., Turner, S., Kasarskis, A., 2010. A window into third-generation sequencing. Human Molecular Genetics 19, R227–R240.

Shendure, J.A., Porreca, G.J., Church, G.M., Gardner, A.F., Hendrickson, C.L., Kieleczawa, J., et al., 2011. Overview of DNA sequencing strategies. Current Protocols in Molecular Biology.

Shendure, J., Porreca, G.J., Reppas, N.B., Lin, X., McCutcheon, J.P., Rosenbaum, A.M., et al., 2005. Accurate multiplex polony sequencing of an evolved bacterial genome. Science 309, 1728–1732.

Shulha, H.P., Cheung, I., Whittle, C., Wang, J., Virgil, D., Lin, C.L., et al., 2011. Epigenetic signatures of autism Trimethylated H3K4 landscapes in prefrontal neurons. Archives of GeneralArchives of General .

Song, C.X., Clark, T.A., Lu, X.Y., Kislyuk, A., Dai, Q., Turner, S.W., et al., 2011. Sensitive and specific single-molecule sequencing of 5-hydroxymethylcytosine. Nature Methods 9, 75–77.

Vissers, L.E., de Ligt, J., Gilissen, C., Janssen, I., Steehouwer, M., de Vries, P., et al., 2010. A de novo paradigm for mental retardation. Nature Genetics 42, 1109–1112.

Voineagu, I., Wang, X., Johnston, P., Lowe, J.K., Tian, Y., Horvath, S., et al., 2011. Transcriptomic analysis of autistic brain reveals convergent molecular pathology. Nature 474, 380–384.

Walker, S., Prasad, A., Marshall, C.R., Pereira, S.L., Lau, L., Foong, J., et al., 2011. Exome Sequencing in Autism Spectrum Disorder ASHG annual meeting, poster# 875T.

Wang, J., Wang, W., Li, R., Li, Y., Tian, G., Goodman, L., et al., 2008. The diploid genome sequence of an Asian individual. Nature 456, 60–65.

Wang, Z., Gerstein, M., Snyder, M., 2009. RNA-Seq: A revolutionary tool for transcriptomics. Nature Reviews Genetics 10, 57–63.

Welch, J.S., Westervelt, P., Ding, L., Larson, D.E., Klco, J.M., Kulkarni, S., et al., 2011. Use of whole-genome sequencing to diagnose a cryptic fusion oncogene. Journal of the American Medical Association 305, 1577–1584.

Wheeler, D.A., Srinivasan, M., Egholm, M., Shen, Y., Chen, L., McGuire, A., et al., 2008. The complete genome of an individual by massively parallel DNA sequencing. Nature 452, 872–876.

Wink, L.K., Plawecki, M.H., Erickson, C.A., Stigler, K.A., McDougle, C.J., 2010. Emerging drugs for the treatment of symptoms associated with Autism spectrum disorders. Expert Opinion on Emerging Drugs 15, 481–494.

Mitochondria and Autism Spectrum Disorders

Robert K. Naviaux

The Mitochondrial and Metabolic Disease Center, Departments of Medicine, Pediatrics, Pathology,
University of California, San Diego School of Medicine, San Diego, CA, USA

THE BIRTH OF MITOCHONDRIAL MEDICINE

The first clinical and biochemical description of mitochondrial disease was reported by Rolf Luft in 1962 (Luft et al., 1962). Only two patients with Luft disease have been described to date (DiMauro et al., 1976). Both were interesting examples of intellectually normal adults (both women) with a rare form of mitochondrial over-function associated with high oxygen consumption rates, hypermetabolism, heat intolerance, resting tachycardia, hyperhidrosis, and death in middle age from respiratory muscle failure. Although mitochondria were first reported to contain their own DNA in 1963 by Margit and Sylvan Nass (Nass and Nass, 1963), it was another 25 years before the first DNA mutations were found that caused mitochondrial disease. We date the dawn of the molecular age of mitochondrial medicine to 1988, when Doug Wallace and colleagues reported the first mitochondrial DNA (mtDNA) mutations that cause disease (Wallace et al., 1988a, b). In the same year, Holt (1988) and Zeviani (1988) and their colleagues reported the first disease-associated deletions in mtDNA. Today, we know of more than 300 clinically, biochemically, or molecularly distinct forms of mitochondrial disease (Naviaux, 2004).

WHAT IS DEFINITE MITOCHONDRIAL DISEASE?

Mitochondrial disorders are among the most difficult diseases to diagnose in all of medicine. They constitute a large group of clinically heterogeneous disorders that have defied all efforts to find a universal biomarker or universal symptom. In most cases, a child with mitochondrial disease is completely healthy at birth, but develops symptoms in a step-wise fashion, weeks to years later. In rare cases, symptoms may not appear until 70 years of age (Weiss and Saneto, 2010). New symptoms typically appear over time, so that at any one time early in the disease, not all symptoms are present. This makes early diagnosis challenging or impossible. Mitochondrial diseases share the one fact that they are fundamentally bioenergetic and metabolic disorders that result from defects (under-function) in oxidative phosphorylation – the ability to make ATP in mitochondria from electrons, hydrogen, and oxygen. This clinical heterogeneity has led to the widely quoted axiom that mitochondrial disease can produce any symptom, in any organ, at any age (Munnich et al., 1996).

Mitochondrial under-function and over-function disorders are clinically distinct. Historically, the field of mitochondrial medicine has focused on the disorders of under-function. The disorders of over-function will be addressed later in this chapter. Mitochondrial under-function diseases can be divided into primary and secondary forms. Primary mitochondrial diseases are genetic disorders caused by mutations in either nuclear or mitochondrial DNA that affect the proteins of the mitochondrial respiratory chain. For this reason, they are sometimes call respiratory chain (RC) disorders. Secondary mitochondrial diseases are ecogenetic disorders that result from a combination of environmental and genetic factors. The distinction between primary and secondary mitochondrial disorders is clinically important because it carries implications for genetic counseling. Primary disorders are monogenic and carry recurrence risks associated with known Mendelian and maternal patterns of genetic transmission. Secondary disorders are rarely monogenic and require exposure to one or more environmental factors such as a drug, toxicant, or viral infection. Counseling for recurrence risks of secondary mitochondrial and other ecogenetic disorders is empiric.

When a single biomarker, sign, or symptom is unable to establish a disease diagnosis in a deterministic manner, medicine has historically developed probabilistic methods for diagnosis. The modified Walker criteria (Bernier et al., 2002) have been widely adopted to group or stratify patients according to the likelihood of genetic forms of mitochondrial disease. Using these criteria, patients are given a diagnosis of definite, probable, or possible mitochondrial disease (Table 2.5.1). If a causal DNA mutation is not found, a muscle biopsy is typically required to confirm a definite diagnosis of mitochondrial disease. The criteria for 'definite' mitochondrial disease have been used

TABLE 2.5.1   Modified Walker Criteria for the Diagnosis of Mitochondrial Disease*

Mitochondrial disease diagnosis	Diagnostic requirements
Definite	$\geq$ 2 major, or 1 major + 2 minor criteria
Probable	1 major + 1 minor, or $\geq$ 3 minor criteria
Possible	1 major, or 1 minor clinical + 1 other minor criterion
Major criteria	**Minor criteria**
Clinical: Classic multisystem mitochondrial phenotype with progressive clinical course, or positive family history	Clinical: Incomplete mitochondrial phenotype
Histology: $\geq$ 2% Ragged-red fibers (RRF)	Histology: 1—2% RRF if 30—50 years old, or any RRF if < 30 years, or widespread ultrastructural abnormalities
Enzymology: $\geq$ 2% COX-negative fibers if < 50 yrs old; or $\geq$ 5% COX-negative fibers if $\geq$ 50 yrs old; or < 20% any respiratory chain (RC) enzyme or polarographic activity; or < 30% in cell culture, or 20—30% in $\geq$ 2 different tissues	Enzymology: Antibody-based demonstration of defective RC subunit expression, or 20—30% RC activity in a tissue, or 30—40% RC activity in a cell line, or 30—40% RC activity in $\geq$ 2 tissues
Functional: Fibroblast ATP synthesis $\geq$ 3 SD below the mean	Functional: Fibroblast ATP synthesis 2—3 SD below the mean, or unable to grow in galactose
Molecular: Pathogenic mtDNA or nuclear DNA abnormality	Molecular: mtDNA or nuclear DNA abnormality of probable pathogenicity
	Metabolic: $\geq$ 1 Abnormal metabolic indicator of RC function (eg., lactate, 31P-MRS)

* *Tables summarized from Bernier et al., 2002.*

to determine the epidemiology of mitochondrial disease.

EPIDEMIOLOGY OF MITOCHONDRIAL DISEASE

The epidemiology of mitochondrial disease has evolved rapidly over the past 15 years. The first estimates of its prevalence were as low as 1:33,000 (Applegarth et al., 2000). These lower estimates were hampered by the absence of consistent standards for diagnosis and early stages of the rapidly growing awareness of the clinical heterogeneity of mitochondrial diseases. Most children with mitochondrial disease before the year 2000 died without a proper diagnosis. The best figures now available are that 1 in 2,000 children born each year in the US will develop definite mitochondrial disease in their lifetimes. About half of these children (1:4,000) will develop symptoms in the first 10 years of life (Naviaux, 2004). The other half (1:4,000) will remain healthy, without any symptoms until after age 10. Many adult mitochondrial disorders do not manifest until 20–50 years of age, and in rare cases not until the 70s (Weiss and Saneto, 2010). About half of adult mitochondrial disease is caused by mtDNA mutations and half by nuclear DNA mutations. A recent study of mitochondrial disease among adults in the UK found about 1 in 4,000 adults (25.7 per 100,000) had or were at risk for mtDNA-based disease (Schaefer et al., 2008). The growing awareness that mutations in nuclear DNA can lead to many different adult mitochondrial disorders with many different symptoms (Cohen and Naviaux, 2010; Saneto and Naviaux, 2010) means that the prevalence figures for adult mitochondrial disorders may continue to rise over the next few years.

About 15% of pediatric mitochondrial disease is caused by mtDNA mutations (Rotig et al., 2004) and 85% is caused by nuclear DNA mutations that are inherited in a Mendelian fashion. Most of these are inherited as autosomal recessive disorders, but X-linked and dominant forms are also well known. Over 200 point mutations and 400 deletion break points have been described in mitochondrial DNA that lead to disease (DiMauro et al., 2006) and over 60 nuclear genes have been identified with well over 500 disease-causing mutations (Falk, 2010; Haas et al., 2008; Wong, 2010). Excellent diagnostic algorithms have recently been published to assist physicians in choosing which genes to select for DNA testing to best explain a particular clinical presentation (Wong, 2010; Wong et al., 2010). When an mtDNA mutation is suspected, full mitochondrial DNA sequencing by NextGen methods is now available and recommended (Kauffman et al., 2012). When a Mendelian pattern of transmission is identified in a pedigree and the probability of finding one of the more common nuclear gene causes is low, exome capture and NextGen sequencing of 362 to 524 nuclear mitochondrial genes is available (Shen et al., 2011; Vasta et al., 2009).

DEFINITE MITOCHONDRIAL DISEASE IS A RARE CAUSE OF AUTISM SPECTRUM DISORDERS

The first evidence of a mitochondrial DNA mutation that could cause autism spectrum disorders (ASD) was published in 2000 (Graf et al., 2000). In this report, the authors found a heteroplasmic point mutation in the mitochondrial tRNA for lysine (G8362A) that was the cause of Leigh syndrome in a 6-year-old girl with a history of normal development in the first year of life, with the onset of ataxia and myoclonus at 15 months of age. She had classic, symmetric T2 signal abnormalities in the basal ganglia and brain stem, characteristic of Leigh syndrome. Her speech and language were normal except for dysarthria and moderate intellectual impairment. The mtDNA mutation was associated with a respiratory chain defect in muscle complex IV. Her younger brother was diagnosed with ASD after developmental regression at 1.5–2 years of age. By 3.5 years of age, he had no functional speech or language, was hyperactive, and displayed bouts of self-injurious behavior. He carried the same tRNA lysine mutation as his older sister, but at lower level of heteroplasmy (61% vs. 86%). In sharp contrast to his older sister with Leigh syndrome, the muscle biopsy of the brother with autism showed a paradoxical hyperactivity in complex I that was 250% of normal (200.6 vs. 81; SD of 29.4; normalized for citrate synthase activity) (Graf et al., 2000). Recently, a group of children with hyperactivity of complex IV and autism has been described (Frye and Naviaux, 2011). Some patients with complex IV hyperactivity and autism have been found to have a mutation in the mitochondrial calcium-regulated aspartate-glutamate carrier (AGC1) (Palmieri et al., 2010).

In March 2008, the connection between mitochondria and autism was catapulted into the national spotlight when news media picked up the story of Hannah Poling (Stobbe, 2008; Wallis, 2008), a little girl who had mitochondrial disease and developed an ASD within weeks of receiving several immunizations at 1.5 years of age in 2000 (Poling et al., 2006). In June 2008, the US National Institute of Mental Health (NIMH), National Institute of Child Health and Human Development (NICHD), Centers for Disease Control and Prevention (CDC), and Food and Drug Administration (FDA) rapidly organized a public, special topic symposium on Mitochondrial Disease and Autism in Indianapolis, IN, in conjunction with the annual meeting of the United Mitochondrial Disease Foundation (UMDF) (Gorski, 2008). This case is unusual for definite forms of mitochondrial diseases, which typically do not show regression after routine immunizations (Verity et al., 2010; 2011).

Now, in 2012, the connection between mitochondrial dysfunction and ASD (Haas, 2010; Rossignol and Frye, 2011) remains one of the freshest new leads in nearly 70 years of autism research since autism was first identified as a childhood disease by Leo Kanner in 1943 (Kanner, 1943). However, as evidenced in an epidemiological study in mainland Portugal and the Azores, only 5% of children with ASD have definite forms of mitochondrial disease (Oliveira et al., 2007), and this estimate would benefit from replication in independent epidemiological cohorts. The classic forms of primary mitochondrial disease have a very different clinical character to that found in children with ASD. Mitochondrial disease patients often have devastating, multi-organ system disorders with mortalities as high as 10–50% per year after the onset of the first symptoms (Cohen and Naviaux, 2010; Naviaux, 1997; Rahman et al., 1996). This mortality far exceeds the rate of 0.2% deaths per year (26 of 342 ASD patients studied over 36 years) observed in ASD (Mouridsen et al., 2008). In addition, children with mitochondrial disease are often found to have decreased sensitivity to sound, touch, and light, decreased muscle strength, decreased activity, with normal social engagement. Hyperactivity and repetitive movements are rare in definite mitochondrial disease. These symptoms are in sharp contrast to those found in children with ASD.

The weight of the evidence collected since 2000 now points to a more subtle connection between mitochondrial function and ASD. Simple mitochondrial under-function does not cause either narrowly defined autism or ASD, with rare exceptions (Shoffner et al., 2010; Weissman et al., 2008). Several cases of mitochondrial respiratory chain over-function and ASD have now been described (Frye and Naviaux, 2011; Graf et al., 2000). This is likely to be an under-reported phenomenon, since most specialists in mitochondrial medicine dismiss respiratory chain enzyme hyperactivity ($\geq$ 165% of controls) as incidental, or as compensation for another, often unmeasured, defect. In either case, respiratory chain over-function is not a cause of primary mitochondrial disease. The relative proportions and overlaps between children with autism and mitochondrial disease are summarized in Figure 2.5.1.

MITOCHONDRIAL DISEASE AND AUTISM RESPOND DIFFERENTLY TO THE SAME TREATMENTS

If two diseases have the same cause, they should respond similarly to the same treatments. The fact that this is not the case with definite mitochondrial disease and ASD is further evidence that these disorders should not be lumped together. Table 2.5.2 lists four cases that distinguish mitochondrial disease on the one hand and ASD on the other. Valproic acid (depakote, divalproex) is an 8-carbon branched-chain fatty acid that is widely used to treat seizures and other disorders in ASD (Hollander et al., 2010), but is known to produce mitochondrial toxicity in the large majority of patients with mitochondrial disease (Saneto et al., 2010). The only case of mitochondrial disease in which valproic acid therapy is usually well tolerated and effective is in MERRF (myoclonus, epilepsy, with

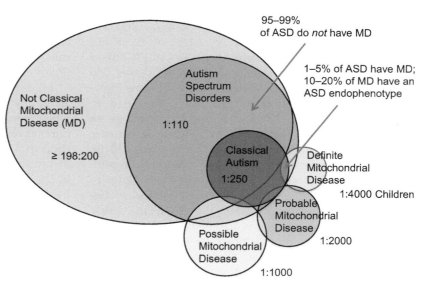

FIGURE 2.5.1   The majority of children with autism do not have classic forms of mitochondrial disease (MD). Epidemiologic studies show that fewer than 5% of children with autism spectrum disorders have classical mitochondrial disease. Other forms of mitochondrial dysfunction, such as a persistent danger response, or segmental over-function of certain mitochondrial functions in innate immunity, may be more common and impair cellular communication by effects on metabolism. These non-oxidative-phosphorylation functions of mitochondria are not routinely measured in the evaluation of children for classic forms of mitochondrial disease.

TABLE 2.5.2 Definite Mitochondrial Disease and Autism Respond Differently to the Same Treatments

Treatment or feature	Definite mitochondrial disease	Autism spectrum disorders	Reference
Valproate	Deterioration (except MERRF)	71% improved	Hollander et al., 2010
Fever	Deterioration (fade response)	83% improved	Curran et al., 2007
Hyperbaric O_2	Deterioration	30–80% improved, or no net benefit	Jepson et al., 2011; Rossignol et al., 2009
Recovery (spontaneous or therapy-associated)	Very rare (LHON, reversible COX tRNA-Glu)	3–25%	Helt et al., 2008

LHON = Leber's hereditary optic neuropathy.

ragged-red fibers) when given with L-carnitine supplementation. This is a form of mitochondrial disease that is characterized by massive mitochondrial proliferation and may have some symptoms that result from an element of metabolic hyperfunction, in addition to the known oxidative phosphorylation deficiency.

The response to fever is also different in mitochondrial disease patients and most patients with ASD. Infections and fever caused over 70% of the neurodegenerative events observed in children with mitochondrial disease (Edmonds et al., 2002). However, in a prospective study of 30 children with autism and 30 controls, Andy Zimmerman and his colleagues at the Kennedy Krieger Institute found that 83% (25 of 30) of the children with ASD improved in at least one area related to hyperactivity, stereotypy, or speech, although lethargy scores were worse (Curran et al., 2007) (Table 2.5.2). The curious 'awakening' of ASD during fever is short-lived, as the children returned to their previous state with the resolution of the infection and fever. Infection and fever are also known to produce transient improvements in some patients with schizophrenia. The history of the role of fever, cytokines, and innate immunity in the pathogenesis of disease has been reviewed (Patterson, 2009). How can fever be involved both in the cause of autism and in its transient improvement? We will return to this question later in this chapter in the sections on innate immunity and mitochondrial hormesis.

Hyperbaric oxygen treatment was shown to have neutral (Jepson et al., 2011) or beneficial (Rossignol et al., 2009) effects on children with ASD. This would be in sharp contrast to the experience of definite mitochondrial disease patients who can suffer catastrophic neurodegeneration and sometimes death associated with hyperbaric oxygen therapy (Table 2.5.2). The question of hyperbaric oxygen therapy for mitochondrial disease was addressed by the scientific advisory board of the United Mitochondrial Disease Foundation in 2007 (UMDF, 2007). Classic mitochondrial disease is caused

by an inherited inability of the cell to use oxygen. The forcible delivery of increased levels of oxygen in classic forms of mitochondrial disease does not improve mitochondrial function. Instead, it results in a deleterious increase in damaging reactive oxygen species (ROS), which can further damage mitochondrial membranes, enzymes, and DNA and lead to neurodegeneration. This difference in the clinical response to hyperbaric oxygen further differentiates the major mechanisms of pathogenesis that underlie ASD and mitochondrial disease and underscores the risk of hyperbaric oxygen in ASD unless mitochondrial disease is ruled out.

Recovery or partial recovery has been reported in 3–25% of children with ASD (Helt et al., 2008) (Table 2.5.2). In most cases this has occurred in association with intensive behavioral and/or biomedical therapy. Recoveries in mitochondrial disease are virtually unheard of. There are two rare exceptions that in total constitute less than 1% of all mitochondrial disease. These are spontaneous or treatment-associated recovery of vision in certain forms of Leber's hereditary optic neuropathy (LHON) (Sadun et al., 2011) and spontaneous recovery in a rare form of cytochrome oxidase deficiency (Mimaki et al., 2010). In all other cases of mitochondrial disease, the natural history typically involves step-wise or gradual deterioration over months to years after the onset of symptoms. In many cases, this leads to early death. Multiple organ systems eventually become involved.

Single-gene defects cause the classic forms of mitochondrial disease. In contrast, most ASD is thought to be multifactorial, with genes of major and minor effect interacting with environmental and additional factors (see other chapters in this section). Where genes meet the environment is metabolism, and mitochondria are the hub of the wheel of metabolism. The remainder of this chapter focuses on the metabolic functions of mitochondria that are involved in innate immunity. Cellular defense is one of the most ancient functions of mitochondria. By considering the responses of genes and metabolic processes to danger signals in the environment, we can get a little closer to understanding the complex link between mitochondria and ASD.

NUCLEAR MITOCHONDRIAL GENOCARTOGRAPHY AND CNVS

The mitochondrial proteome consists of about 1,500 proteins (Pagliarini et al., 2008) encoded by over 1,000 nuclear genes (Figure 2.5.2) and 13 proteins made by mtDNA. Every one of the 10^{14} cells of the body contains different mitochondria, that are specialized to meet the metabolic demands of that cell. Therefore, there is a different mitochondrial network, with a different proteome, with different post-translational modifications for every different cell in the body. This remarkable feat is accomplished by regulating both nuclear and mitochondrial gene expression in tissue-specific ways (Johnson et al., 2007), and by making dozens of post-translational modifications in proteins that fine-tune metabolism according to the time of day, availability of nutrients, toxin exposure, microbial infection, and even the season of the year (Staples and Brown, 2008; Zhao et al., 2011). The chromosomal location of each of these 1,500 proteins can be mapped. On average, each of our 23 chromosomes contains about 20–70 mitochondrial genes (Figure 2.5.2).

Recent studies have shown that about 4% of children with autism have rare DNA copy number variations (CNVs) that might contribute to disease, compared to just 2% of typically developing, age-matched controls (e.g., Pinto et al., 2010; see also Chapters 2.1 and 2.2). Most of these CNVs were duplications, not deletions, although there is good evidence that deletions are more likely associated with ASD and other neurodevelopmental disorders. Interestingly, the same CNVs found to be associated with ASD have also been found to be enriched in patients with schizophrenia (e.g., Guilmatre et al., 2009; see also Chapters 2.1 and 2.2), suggesting that disruption of brain development by CNV can contribute to a myriad of neurodevelopmental disorders, likely in concert with other genetic or environmental factors (see Chapter 2.1). Analysis of the genes affected by recurrent CNVs and single-gene defects in ASD highlights the complex etiology of ASD with

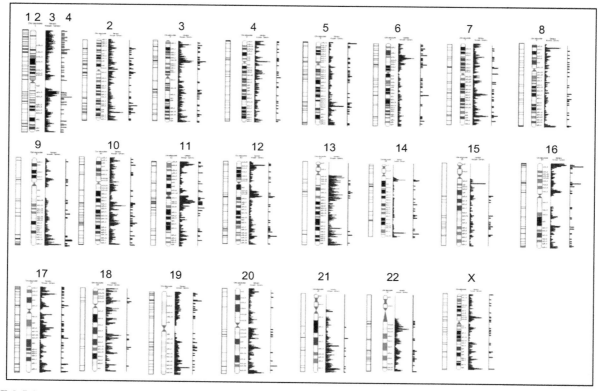

FIGURE 2.5.2   Mitochondrial genocartography. Each of the 23 human chromosomes illustrated is associated with four vertical bars (labeled 1–4 over chromosome 1). Bar #1 in blue illustrates the number and position of nuclear mitochondrial genes. Over 1,000 of these are known. Bar #2 illustrates the conventional G-banding pattern of each chromosome. Bar #3 illustrates the density of non-mitochondrial genes on the chromosome. Bar #4 illustrates the density of mitochondrial genes on the chromosome. Each chromosome contains 20–70 mitochondrial genes. When copy number variations (CNVs) occur, the mitochondrial genes in the affected areas are also varied, leading to gene dose effects that can alter any of over 500 bioenergetic and metabolic functions of mitochondria in the cell.

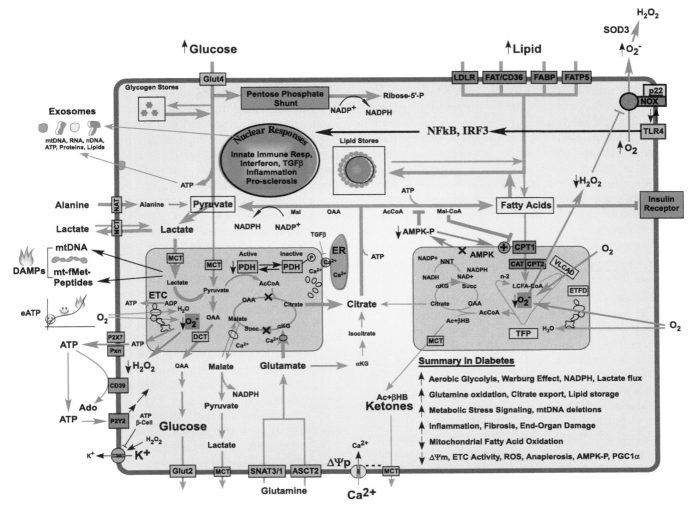

FIGURE 2.5.3 The language of the cell is metabolism. Cells communicate with neighboring and distant cells in the body by exchanging small molecule metabolites like nucleotides, organic acids, amino acids, and lipids. This ancient language of the cell is still largely untranslated. New methods in mass spectrometry are revealing how cells communicate messages about stress, danger, health, and disease. The cell above is a liver cell adapting to nutrient excess in diabetes. Mitochondria are illustrated as the two blue boxes in the center, receiving pyruvate on the left and fatty acids on the right. Cells in affected tissues of patients with autism speak a different message but use the same vocabulary of chemical words. The most common developmental and chronic diseases in medicine can be understood as disorders of cellular communication.

multiple organelles and systems implicated (Chapter 2.1). The interpretation of duplication CNVs is complicated, because typically developing children can have the same CNVs, consistent with reduced impact and/or penetrance of duplications (Pinto et al., 2010).

MITOCHONDRIA AND THE CONTROL OF CNVs, DNA INSTABILITY, AND REPAIR

Gene duplication and deletion events are regulated by cross-over events that lead to mitotic recombination (Matos et al., 2011). It is known that changes in mitochondrial DNA copy number have dramatic effects on nuclear DNA repair and genomic instability (Singh et al., 2005). What are some of the factors that control mtDNA copy number in cells? TLR4 signaling after LPS signaling associated with bacterial infection leads to mtDNA damage and depletion (Suliman et al., 2005). Significant amounts of free fatty acids can also act as endogenous ligands of the TLR4 receptor during periods of metabolic mismatch associated with disorders like diabetes (Schaeffler et al., 2009). Interferon released during infections activates the cellular RNAse L that can traffic to mitochondria and destroy mitochondrial RNA (Chandrasekaran et al., 2004). Even certain viruses, like herpes simplex virus, encode a special DNAse (UL12.5) that travels to mitochondria and produces mitochondrial DNA damage and depletion (Corcoran et al., 2009). It turns out that many infectious agents target mitochondria in an effort to downregulate oxygen consumption, which inhibits DNA synthesis and replication.

A spectrum of environmental neurotoxicants such as bisphenol A (BPA), polychlorinated biphenyls (PCBs) (Jolous-Jamshidi et al., 2010), and certain polybrominated diphenyl ethers (PBDEs) (Ashwood et al., 2009), known to cause autism-like behaviors in mouse and rat models, also can regulate mitochondrial function either directly or indirectly via alterations in cellular calcium handling (Coburn et al., 2008). Although it has not yet been experimentally verified, it seems plausible that infection, environmental neurotoxicants, and/or metabolic stress can each produce changes in mitochondrial function that might alter the somatic control of mitotic recombination and CNV formation rates during embryogenesis and early childhood development. Acutely this can produce a transient increase in somatic CNV formation.

MITOCELLULAR HORMESIS

Chronically, mitochondria are known to help the cell adapt to past metabolic stresses by producing long-term changes in cellular reactivity in a process called mitochondrial hormesis (Ristow and Zarse, 2010). When both mitochondrial and cellular mechanisms adapt, the result is mitocellular hormesis. Mitocellular hormesis in response to xenobiotics produces long-term up-regulation of cellular oxidation, inactivation, and excretion pathways like cytochrome P450, sulfation, and glucuronidation (Xu et al., 2005). Mitocellular hormesis in response to infectious or inflammatory agents activates innate immune pathways that increase reactive oxygen species (ROS) production, activate cell signaling and cytokine responses, alter folate, B12, and other vitamin metabolism, and change the gene expression and epigenetic programs of the cell. The response to cellular stress is invariably biphasic. First there is an acute inhibition, followed by long-term adaptation, much like the metabolic memory response associated with exercise (Ji et al., 2006). When the triggering stimulus is inhibitory, or surpasses the mitochondrial capacity to process the resulting metabolites, then mitochondrial proliferation and hyperfunction results (Sano and Fukuda, 2008). If proliferation and mitochondrial hyperfunction occur in neurons or microglia in the brain, then persistent low-level excitotoxicity and neuroinflammation can result. What is the final common denominator that maintains this cycle of metabolic innate immune activation, excitotoxicity, and inflammation?

MITOCHONDRIAL FUNCTIONS IN METABOLISM

Mitochondria are located at the hub of the wheel of metabolism. They perform over 500 different functions in the cell. Respiratory chain proteins constitute about 10–20% of the mitochondrial proteome (Pagliarini et al., 2008). The other 80–90% of mitochondrial proteins play roles in hundreds of other pathways, including in innate immunity, cellular defense, amino acid transport, calcium metabolism, iron metabolism, copper metabolism, reductive and oxidative stress metabolism, hydrogen sulfide and nitric oxide metabolism, fuel sensing, translation, protein folding and assembly, autophagy, microtubule association, folate metabolism, porphyrin metabolism, steroid metabolism, glycolate metabolism, and DNA repair. None of these non-oxidative phosphorylation functions is routinely measured when a child is evaluated for mitochondrial disease. Therefore, a large part of mitochondrial function has never been systematically measured in children with ASD because it relates to functions outside the respiratory chain, and produces symptoms that are not characteristic of definite mitochondrial disease.

It can be stated simply that metabolism is the language of the cell. Figure 2.5.2 illustrates some of the metabolic pathways that characterize a liver cell. The methods of mass spectrometry and metabolomics have allowed investigators to 'eavesdrop' on the collective conversation of cells in ASD. These early studies have identified abnormalities in glutathione (James et al., 2004), taurine, glutamate, hippurate (Yap et al., 2010), and polyunsaturated phospholipid metabolism (Pastural et al., 2009). The language of metabolism is spoken using small molecule metabolites as the words. This is a universal language of life on Earth, with many dialects that reflect the specialization of organisms adapting to their environment. Despite its universal usage, this language of metabolism is still largely untranslated. Future studies using the tools of mass spectrometry will help expand our lexicon of metabolites and their meanings, and help us to interpret the conversation of metabolism in children with ASD.

MITOCHONDRIAL FUNCTIONS IN INNATE IMMUNITY

One of the most ancient functions of mitochondria is in cell defense. I have called this the 'secret life of mitochondria' because it is largely separate from oxidative phosphorylation. When a cell is attacked by a virus, a cascade of events is initiated that is designed to protect the cell from injury, limit viral replication, and warn neighboring cells of the intrusion. Healthy cells can increase or decrease their response to a given infection or inflammatory stimulus by a process of priming. Primed cells have adopted a more defensive set-point, sacrificing certain differentiated cell functions for the ability to respond rapidly to an attack. When this happens in the brain, excitotoxicity and inflammation can result. When it happens in gut-associated lymphoid tissue (GALT), then abnormally aggressive responses to the normal gut microbiome can result. If a cell is injured or broken in the attack, then a large number of molecules are released into the extracellular space as 'danger' signals. Many of these are present in high concentrations within mitochondria. These danger signals are collectively called damage-associated molecular patterns (DAMPS). ATP is a DAMP (Zhang et al., 2010). Inside the cell, ATP concentrations range from 1–5 mM depending on the cell type. Each cell maintains a pericellular halo of ATP in the 1–5 µM range that interacts with a family of ancient cell-surface proteins called purinergic receptors. The possible role of purinergic signaling in ASD will be discussed in a later section.

Another reason that a number of mitochondrial molecules act as DAMPs is the evolutionary origin of mitochondria as the ancestors of ancient, free-living gram-negative bacteria (Cavalier-Smith, 2006). Mitochondrial DNA itself contains unmethylated CpG dinucleotides that resemble bacterial DNA and activate TLR9. Proteins synthesized in mitochondria start with a bacteria-like formyl-methionine. N-formyl-methionine-containing peptides from mitochondria bind the formyl peptide receptor (FPR1, and FPRL1) and activate innate immunity (West et al., 2011). The regulation of intracellular calcium release from the endoplasmic reticulum to mitochondria through the IP3 receptor and ryanodine receptor channel is a crucial point of regulation of the metabolic response to infection and stress (Zecchini et al., 2007). Recent studies have suggested that abnormalities in mitochondrial calcium handling (Gellerich et al., 2010) may be a common denominator in ASD (Napolioni et al., 2011).

REGRESSION

Regression is common in mitochondrial disease in response to infection. The first report to quantify the risk of neurodegeneration with infection in definite mitochondrial disease was published in 2002 (Edmonds et al., 2002). The authors of this paper found that 60% of children with mitochondrial disease suffered neurodegenerative events (regressions). A total of 72% of the regression events were associated with infections that occurred within two weeks before the onset of regression. None of the regression events in children with mitochondrial disease were associated with childhood immunizations. A total of 28% of the regressions

occurred spontaneously, with no identifiable trigger. Regressions occurred at any age, and were not confined to the first two to three years of life. The form of regression was one of a 'fade' response that occurred 2–10 days after the peak fever associated with the illness. Most often the neurodegeneration occurred during an otherwise normal recovery period after a common childhood infectious illness. Over a period of a few days, the child became obtunded or encephalopathic, or experienced a stroke-like episode, new-onset seizures, or lost the ability to walk or talk, lost vision, developed swallowing problems or gastrointestinal dysmotility, or lost other developmental milestones. In most cases, the child was able to make a slow and sometimes complete recovery over several months, but often there were residual deficits. In less common cases, there was a slow progression to encephalopathy, coma, and death over two to three months.

Regression is less common in ASD and more subject to large differences in estimates of its prevalence based on small differences in the definition of regression. Regression occurred in 15% of 333 children 2–5 years of age with ASD reported by Hansen et al. (2008). The criteria for regression were loss of both language and social skills. The loss of social skills was found to be a more sensitive indicator for regression and 26% of children had either language loss or loss of social skills. 59% percent of the 333 children in this CHARGE study had no history of regression. The severity of the neurological regressions in ASD was much less, and their character was different to those in mitochondrial disease. Strokes and permanent weakness are rare in ASD, and no deaths were reported.

The role of mitochondrial dysfunction as a risk factor for regression in a subgroup of children with ASD was recently highlighted in a paper by Shoffner et al. (2010). A group of 28 children with both mitochondrial respiratory chain disease and ASD were selected for retrospective analysis. The authors found that 61% had a history of a neurodegenerative episode that eventually grew into the features of ASD. 39% of children developed ASD gradually, without a history of regression. When regression occurred, 71% happened within two weeks of a fever of over 101°F. These proportions were similar to those originally reported by Edmonds et al. in children without autism (Edmonds et al., 2002). In four children (14% of the 28), the fever occurred after routine vaccination. In the remaining eight children, fever came with a routine infection or was a fever of unknown origin. This study emphasizes the fragile nature of children with mitochondrial disease. The observation that four children regressed after immunization is rare in mitochondrial disease in general. Most children with classic forms of mitochondrial disease tolerate immunization well.

TABLE 2.5.3   Careful Attention to the Timing and Symptoms of an Adverse Reaction After Infection or Immunization Provides Insights into the Underlying Cause

| | Character of the adverse reaction | | |
	STORM	FLARE	FADE
Timing	2–12 hrs, or 2–6 days after exposure	Peaks at 48–72 hrs – coincides with peak symptoms of infection	Peaks at 2–10 days after peak symptoms of infection
Symptoms	Fever, HA, abd/low back pain, T-cell activation, widespread apoptosis, TNFα/IFNγ synergy, +/− ADCC, complement C5a, shock, histamine, DIC, hemorrhage	Stereotyped 'sickness behavior'; or high fever ≥ 10°2F, hyper-irritability, inconsolability, intermittent high-pitched screaming, delirium, opisthotonous, GI hypermotility with diarrhea	No fever or low-grade fever, ataxia, gastroparesis, aphasia or hypophasia, stroke-like episodes, change in muscle tone (hypo- or transient hypertonia 2' to CNS hypofunction)
Sequelae	Death in 4–14 days; or slow recovery over 2–6 months, sometimes with permanent disability	Self-limited course, normal vaccination conversion rate; or loss of milestones, with appearance of autism spectrum behaviors over 3–6 months. May improve transiently with fever later.	Self-limited neurodegeneration, poor vaccination conversion rate, slow recovery; or progressive complications and multi-organ system dysfunction, leading to death in 1–4 months
Mechanism	Anamnestic response	Exaggerated innate immune response, possible mitochondrial hyperfunction	Mitochondrial failure
Examples	Jesse Gelsinger (Wilson, 2009); Dengue shock (Pang et al., 2007)	Hannah Poling (Poling et al., 2006)	Reye syndrome (Partin, 1994) Definite mitochondrial disease after infection (Edmonds et al., 2002)

Abd = abdominal; CNS = central nervous system; GI = gastrointestinal; IFN = interferon; TNF = tumor necrosis factor.

STORM, FLARE, AND FADE RESPONSES

Careful attention to the timing and character of an adverse reaction to infection or immunization can provide crucial insight into the cellular mechanisms involved. Table 2.5.3 illustrates the three classes of adverse response. The cytokine 'storm' response requires prior immunization with the triggering antigen. Perhaps the most famous example is the tragic case of Jesse Gelsinger who developed a cytokine storm within hours of receiving gene therapy with an adenovirus vector and died two days later (Wilson, 2009). Another widely recognized example of a perfect storm of cytokines occurs with Dengue shock syndrome (Pang et al., 2007), in which a second exposure to Dengue virus produces a severe memory, or anamnestic, response that can lead to shock and death.

When children with the common forms of mitochondrial disease suffer a regression, it is most often a 'fade' response (Table 2.5.3). The fade response is typically delayed for 2–10 days *after* a fever resolves (Edmonds et al., 2002), similar to the time course found in Reye syndrome in the 1980s (Partin, 1994). In the case of Reye syndrome, the early metabolic profile of highly elevated short chain fatty acids that are normally fully metabolized in mitochondria is evidence that mitochondria are catastrophically downregulated early in the disease process. Recovery from Reye syndrome was associated with the removal of short chain fatty acids like propionate, isobutyrate, and isovalerate (Trauner et al., 1977) indicating that mitochondrial function was restored. Parents of children with mitochondrial disease will typically report that their child was getting better from their cold or flu, when, suddenly, their consciousness fades. The child can become difficult to fully awaken, or will stop walking, stop talking, stiffen or lose muscle tone, or have a seizure, or a stroke-like episode. The fade response involves an energy failure, and can lead to a series of neurodegenerative events and even death over the next two to three months, or to a self-limited event like a stroke-like episode that gradually gets better.

In contrast, autistic regression that is associated with unrecognized mitochondrial dysfunction appears to be more of a 'flare' response, similar to that suffered by Hannah Poling and described in the scientific literature (Poling et al., 2006). A flare response typically occurs early, at the peak of the fever and inflammatory response, within two to three days of infection (Table 2.5.3). During a flare response, there is a high fever, often over 102°F, with hyper-irritablilty, crying, inconsolability, a disrupted sleep-wake cycle, and a refusal to walk in children who might otherwise appear to be physically able to walk, choosing rather to crawl (Poling et al.,

2006). Following a flare response, there can be a gradual evolution of other problems from persistent gastrointestinal problems and diarrhea, a gradual loss of language over two to three months, with the onset of repetitive movements, to gaze and social avoidance (Poling et al., 2006). It must be emphasized that a flare response is not simply a high fever, or even a dramatic reaction to a high fever, like a febrile seizure. It is a multisystem inflammatory response that carries a risk of autistic regression in genetically susceptible children. Is it possible that an unusually high fever is because of a primed state of innate immunity associated with an element of mitochondrial hyperfunction? Mutations in the ryanodine receptor known to cause calcium release and mitochondrial heat production by uncoupling in malignant hyperthermia result from induction of primed mitochondria (Yuen et al., 2012). Systemic inflammation not only triggers calcium release, but is a known trigger of excitotoxic amounts of ATP in the brain (Gourine et al., 2007).

THE POSSIBLE ROLE OF PURINERGIC SIGNALING IN AUTISM SPECTRUM DISORDERS

How might all of the facts about the complex connection between mitochondria and ASD be integrated into a unified theory of pathogenesis? One possibility might be called a purinergic theory of autism. The metabolism of a child adjusts dynamically during development to match the changing environment by the process of metabolic matching. Changes in nutrition, infectious agents, environmental toxicants, and activity each cause metabolic mismatch that permits the cells and tissues to adapt to the current environment, and to strengthen the response to future encounters. Rebound growth after transient metabolic inhibition can result in changes in the time-dependent choreography of brain development. Mitocellular hormesis to severe stress can produce a chronic and pathological increase in many components of mitochondrial metabolism, and to an increase in extracellular ATP (eATP). eATP is a damage-associated molecular pattern (DAMP) that binds to purinergic receptors (P2X and P2Y) on all cells, triggering innate immunity and inflammation, alters brain synapse formation, and contributes to neurochemically mediated excitotoxicity. When this happens during vulnerable periods of brain development, between the late first trimester and the first two years of life, the risk of ASD might be increased.

Several excellent reviews on extracellular nucleotide signaling via purinergic receptors have recently appeared (Abbracchio et al., 2009; Burnstock and Verkhratsky, 2009; Surprenant and North, 2009). P2X receptors are ATP-gated cation channels that regulate calcium conductance. These are known as the ionotropic purinergic receptors. P2Y receptors are G-protein coupled receptors (GPCRs), collectively called the metabotropic purinergic receptors. In humans, there are seven subclasses of P2X receptor, designated P2X1–7. There are eight subclasses of P2Y receptor,

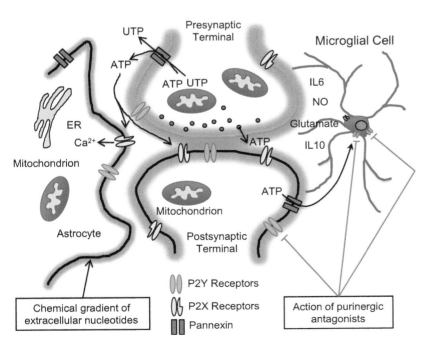

FIGURE 2.5.4 Purinergic regulation of synaptogenesis. ATP is a co-neurotransmitter at every synapse studied to date. Mitochondria are the ultimate source of extracellular ATP (eATP). The activity and usage of each synapse regulates that concentration of eATP surrounding the synaptic junction. Microglial cells monitor synaptic activity and respond to eATP to either stabilize or inhibit synapse formation. Excitotoxicity results in excessive eATP that binds to microglial purinergic receptors and stimulates neuroinflammation. ER = endoplasmic reticulum; IL = interleukin; NO = nitric oxide.

designated P2Y1, 2, 4, 6, 11, 12, 13, and 14 (P2Y 3, 5, 7, 8, 9, and 10 were subsequently removed from the list) (Jacobson and Boeynaems, 2010). P2X receptors are all ATP-gated. P2Y agonists differ according to subtype. ATP, UTP, ADP, UDP, and UDP-glucose are used selectively by different subtypes. $EC_{50}s$ are typically in the micromolar range. Nucleotide signaling via P2X and P2Y receptors mediates a large number of biological phenomena of relevance to autism. These include normal synaptogenesis and brain development (Abbracchio et al., 2009), regulation of the PI3K/AKT pathway (Franke et al., 2009), control of immune responses and chronic inflammation (Pelegrin, 2008), gut motility (Gallego et al., 2008), gut permeability (Matos et al., 2007), taste chemosensory transduction (Surprenant and North, 2009), sensitivity to food allergies (Leng et al., 2008), hearing (Housley et al., 2002), innate immune signaling, neuroinflammation, antiviral signaling, microglial activation, neutrophil chemotaxis, autophagy, and chronic pain syndromes (Abbracchio et al., 2009). Figure 2.5.4 illustrates the role of purinergic receptors in the types of cell which play a role in normal synapse formation. The role of purinergic signaling in ASD has not yet been reported but is under active investigation in the author's laboratory. From the perspective of brain development and function, purinergic signaling represents an important new area for study in ASD as it has direct effects on pathways implicated in ASD (see Section 4).

SUMMARY

Recently, the connections between mitochondria and ASD have become increasingly clear. The nature of this connection is more complex than previously thought. Simple reduction in mitochondrial function does not cause ASD. A small, but informative, fraction of autism is caused by single-gene defects or DNA copy number variations. The large majority of ASD is the result of variation in hundreds of genes and loci interacting with environmental and other factors. The crossroads of genes and environment is metabolism. Mitocellular hormesis is the adaptation of cellular and mitochondrial metabolism to environmental change. Changes in nutrition, infectious agents, environmental toxicants, intellectual attention, and physical activity each play a role in mitocellular hormesis during children's development. Definite mitochondrial disease is responsible for as much as 5% of ASD. However, pathological disturbances in mitochondrial metabolism leading to excitotoxicity may lie at the heart of a larger proportion of ASD and this is an important area for future studies.

ACKNOWLEDGMENTS

RKN thanks the UCSD Christini Fund, the Wright Foundation, the Lennox Foundation, the Jane Botsford Johnson Foundation, and the Hailey's Wish Foundation for their support. RKN thanks Roman Sasik, Gary Hardiman, and Narimene Lakmine for assistance in creating the chromosomal map of mitochondrial proteins.

References

Abbracchio, M.P., Burnstock, G., Verkhratsky, A., Zimmermann, H., 2009. Purinergic signalling in the nervous system: An overview. Trends In Neurosciences 32, 19–29.

Applegarth, D.A., Toone, J.R., Lowry, R.B., 2000. Incidence of inborn errors of metabolism in British Columbia, 1969-1996. Pediatrics 105, e10.

Ashwood, P., Schauer, J., Pessah IN, Van de Water, J., 2009. Preliminary evidence of the in vitro effects of BDE-47 on innate immune responses in children with Autism spectrum disorders. Journal of Neuroimmunology 208, 130–135.

Bernier, F.P., Boneh, A., Dennett, X., Chow, C.W., Cleary, M.A., Thorburn, D.R., 2002. Diagnostic criteria for respiratory chain disorders in adults and children. Neurology 59, 1406–1411.

Burnstock, G., Verkhratsky, A., 2009. Evolutionary origins of the purinergic signalling system. Acta Physiologica (Oxford) 195, 415–447.

Cavalier-Smith, T., 2006. Origin of mitochondria by intracellular enslavement of a photosynthetic purple bacterium. Proceedings Biological Sciences 273, 1943–1952.

Chandrasekaran, K., Mehrabian, Z., Li, X.L., Hassel, B., 2004. RNase-L regulates the stability of mitochondrial DNA-encoded mRNAs in mouse embryo fibroblasts. Biochemical and Biophysical Research Communications 325, 18–23.

Coburn, C.G., Curras-Collazo, M.C., Kodavanti, P.R., 2008. In vitro effects of environmentally relevant polybrominated diphenyl ether (PBDE) congeners on calcium buffering mechanisms in rat brain. Neurochemical Research 33, 355–364.

Cohen, B.H., Naviaux, R.K., 2010. The clinical diagnosis of POLG disease and other mitochondrial DNA depletion disorders. Methods 51, 364–373.

Corcoran, J.A., Saffran, H.A., Duguay, B.A., Smiley, J.R., 2009. Herpes simplex virus UL12.5 targets mitochondria through a mitochondrial localization sequence proximal to the N terminus. Journal of Virology 83, 2601–2610.

Curran, L.K., Newschaffer, C.J., Lee, L.C., Crawford, S.O., Johnston, M.V., Zimmerman, A.W., 2007. Behaviors associated with fever in children with Autism spectrum disorders. Pediatrics 120, e1386–1392.

DiMauro, S., Bonilla, E., Lee, C.P., Schotland, D.L., Scarpa, A., Conn H., Jr., et al., 1976. Luft's disease: Further biochemical and ultrastructural studies of skeletal muscle in the second case. Journal of the Neurological Sciences 27, 217–232.

DiMauro, S., Hirano, M., Schon, E.A., 2006. Mitochondrial Medicine. Informa Healthcare.

Edmonds, J.L., Kirse, D.J., Kearns, D., Deutsch, R., Spruijt, L., Naviaux, R.K., 2002. The otolaryngological manifestations of mitochondrial disease and the risk of neurodegeneration with infection. Archives of Otolaryngology 128, 355–362.

Falk, M.J., 2010. Neurodevelopmental manifestations of mitochondrial disease. Journal of Developmental and Behavioral Pediatrics 31, 610–621.

Franke, H., Sauer, C., Rudolph, C., Krugel, U., Hengstler, J.G., Illes, P., 2009. P2 receptor-mediated stimulation of the PI3-K/Akt-pathway in vivo. Glia 57, 1031–1045.

Frye, R.E., Naviaux, R.K., 2011. Autistic disorder with complex IV overactivity: A new mitochondrial syndrome. Journal of Pediatric Neurology 9, 427–434.

Gallego, D., Vanden Berghe, P., Farre, R., Tack, J., Jimenez, M., 2008. P2Y1 receptors mediate inhibitory neuromuscular transmission and enteric neuronal activation in small intestine. Neurogastroenterology and Motility 20, 159–168.

Gellerich, F.N., Gizatullina, Z., Trumbeckaite, S., Nguyen, H.P., Pallas, T., Arandarcikaite, O., et al., 2010. The regulation of OXPHOS by extramitochondrial calcium. Biochimica et Biophysica Acta 1797, 1018–1027.

Gorski, C., 2008. Dialogue about the potential links between mitochondrial disease and Autism spectrum disorders begins at Indy. UMDF News Release, June 17.

Gourine, A.V., Dale, N., Llaudet, E., Poputnikov, D.M., Spyer, K.M., Gourine, V.N., 2007. Release of ATP in the central nervous system during systemic inflammation: Real-time measurement in the hypothalamus of conscious rabbits. Journal of Physiology 585, 305–316.

Graf, W.D., Marin-Garcia, J., Gao, H.G., Pizzo, S., Naviaux, R.K., Markusic, D., et al., 2000. Autism associated with the mitochondrial DNA G8363A transfer RNA(Lys) mutation. Journal of Child Neurology 15, 357–361.

Guilmatre, A., Dubourg, C., Mosca, A.L., Legallic, S., Goldenberg, A., Drouin-Garraud, V., et al., 2009. Recurrent rearrangements in synaptic and neurodevelopmental genes and shared biologic pathways in schizophrenia, Autism and mental retardation. Archives of General Psychiatry 66, 947–956.

Haas, R.H., 2010. Autism and mitochondrial disease. Developmental Disabilities Research Reviews 16, 144–153.

Haas, R.H., Parikh, S., Falk, M.J., Saneto, R.P., Wolf, N.I., Darin, N., et al., 2008. The in-depth evaluation of suspected mitochondrial disease. Molecular Genetics and Metabolism.

Hansen, R.L., Ozonoff, S., Krakowiak, P., Angkustsiri, K., Jones, C., Deprey, L.J., et al., 2008. Regression in Autism Prevalence and associated factors in the CHARGE Study. Ambulatory Pediatrics 8, 25–31.

Helt, M., Kelley, E., Kinsbourne, M., Pandey, J., Boorstein, H., Herbert, M., et al., 2008. Can children with Autism recover? If so, how? Neuropsychology Review 18, 339–366.

Hollander, E., Chaplin, W., Soorya, L., Wasserman, S., Novotny, S., Rusoff, J., et al., 2010. Divalproex sodium vs placebo for the treatment of irritability in children and adolescents with Autismspectrum disorders. Neuropsychopharmacology 35, 990–998.

Holt, I.J., Harding, A.E., Morgan-Hughes, J.A., 1988. Deletions of muscle mitochondrial DNA in patients with mitochondrial myopathies. Nature 331, 717–719.

Housley, G.D., Jagger, D.J., Greenwood, D., Raybould, N.P., Salih, S.G., Jarlebark, L.E., et al., 2002. Purinergic regulation of sound transduction and auditory neurotransmission. Audiology and Neurotology 7, 55–61.

Jacobson, K.A., Boeynaems, J.M., 2010. P2Y nucleotide receptors: Promise of therapeutic applications. Drug Discovery Today 15, 570–578.

James, S.J., Cutler, P., Melnyk, S., Jernigan, S., Janak, L., Gaylor, D.W., et al., 2004. Metabolic biomarkers of increased oxidative stress and impaired methylation capacity in children with Autism. The American Journal of Clinical Nutrition 80, 1611–1617.

Jepson, B., Granpeesheh, D., Tarbox, J., Olive, M.L., Stott, C., Braud, S., et al., 2011. Controlled evaluation of the effects of hyperbaric oxygen therapy on the behavior of 16 children with Autism

spectrum disorders. Journal of Autism and Developmental Disorders 41, 575–588.

Ji, L.L., Gomez-Cabrera, M.C., Vina, J., 2006. Exercise and hormesis: Activation of cellular antioxidant signaling pathway. Annals of the New York Academy of Sciences 1067, 425–435.

Johnson, D.T., Harris, R.A., Blair, P.V., Balaban, R.S., 2007. Functional consequences of mitochondrial proteome heterogeneity. American Journal of Physiology - Cell Physiology 292, C698–C707.

Jolous-Jamshidi, B., Cromwell, H.C., McFarland, A.M., Meserve, L.A., 2010. Perinatal exposure to polychlorinated biphenyls alters social behaviors in rats. Toxicology Letters 199, 136–143.

Kanner, L., 1943. Autistic distubances of affective contact. The Nervous Child 2, 217–250.

Kauffman, M.A., Gonzalez-Moron, D., Consalvo, D., Westergaard, G., Vazquez, M., Mancini, E., et al., 2012. Diagnosis of mitochondrial disorders applying massive pyrosequencing. Molecular Biology Reports.

Leng, Y., Yamamoto, T., Kadowaki, M., 2008. Alteration of cholinergic, purinergic and sensory neurotransmission in the mouse colon of food allergy model. Neuroscience Letters 445, 195–198.

Luft, R., Ikkos, D., Palmieri, G., Ernster, L., Afzelius, B., 1962. A case of severe hypermetabolism of nonthyroid origin with a defect in the maintenance of mitochondrial respiratory control: A correlated clinical, biochemical, and morphological study. Journal of Clinical Investigation 41, 1776–1804.

Matos, J., Blanco, M.G., Maslen, S., Skehel, J.M., West, S.C., 2011. Regulatory control of the resolution of DNA recombination intermediates during meiosis and mitosis. Cell 147, 158–172.

Matos, J.E., Sorensen, M.V., Geyti, C.S., Robaye, B., Boeynaems, J.M., Leipziger, J., 2007. Distal colonic Na(+) absorption inhibited by luminal P2Y(2) receptors. Pflügers Arch 454, 977–987.

Mimaki, M., Hatakeyama, H., Komaki, H., Yokoyama, M., Arai, H., Kirino, Y., et al., 2010. Reversible infantile respiratory chain deficiency: A clinical and molecular study. Annals of Neurology 68, 845–854.

Mouridsen, S.E., Bronnum-Hansen, H., Rich, B., Isager, T., 2008. Mortality and causes of death in Autism spectrum disorders: An update. Autism 12, 403–414.

Munnich, A., Rotig, A., Chretien, D., Cormier, V., Bourgeron, T., Bonnefont, J.P., et al., 1996. Clinical presentation of mitochondrial disorders in childhood. Journal of Inherited Metabolic Disease 19, 521–527.

Napolioni, V., Persico, A.M., Porcelli, V., Palmieri, L., 2011. The mitochondrial aspartate/glutamate carrier AGC1 and calcium homeostasis: Physiological links and abnormalities in Autism. Molecular Neurobiology 44, 83–92.

Nass, M.M., Nass, S., 1963. Intramitochondrial fibers with DNA characteristics. I. Fixation and electron staining reactions. The Journal of Cell Biology 19, 593–611.

Naviaux, R.K., 1997. The spectrum of mitochondrial disease. In: Mitochondrial and metabolic disorders: a primary care phsycian's guide. Psy-Ed Corporation, Oradell, NJ, pp. 3–10.

Naviaux, R.K., 2004. Developing a systematic approach to the diagnosis and classification of mitochondrial disease. Mitochondrion 4, 351–361.

Oliveira, G., Ataide, A., Marques, C., Miguel, T.S., Coutinho, A.M., Mota-Vieira, L., et al., 2007. Epidemiology of Autismspectrum disorder in Portugal: Prevalence, clinical characterization, and medical conditions. Developmental Medicine & Child Neurology 49, 726–733.

Pagliarini, D.J., Calvo, S.E., Chang, B., Sheth, S.A., Vafai, S.B., Ong, S.E., et al., 2008. A mitochondrial protein compendium elucidates complex I disease biology. Cell 134, 112–123.

Palmieri, L., Papaleo, V., Porcelli, V., Scarcia, P., Gaita, L., Sacco, R., et al., 2010. Altered calcium homeostasis in Autismspectrum disorders: Evidence from biochemical and genetic studies of the mitochondrial aspartate/glutamate carrier AGC1. Molecular Archives of General 15, 38–52.

Pang, T., Cardosa, M.J., Guzman, M.G., 2007. Of cascades and perfect storms: The immunopathogenesis of Dengue haemorrhagic fever-Dengue shock syndrome (DHF/DSS). Immunology & Cell Biology 85, 43–45.

Partin, J.C., 1994. Reye's Syndrome. In: Suchy, F. (Ed.), Liver Disease in Children. Mosby, St. Louis, MO, pp. 653–671.

Pastural, E., Ritchie, S., Lu, Y., Jin, W., Kavianpour, A., Khine Su-Myat, K., et al., 2009. Novel plasma phospholipid biomarkers of Autism: Mitochondrial dysfunction as a putative causative mechanism. Prostaglandins Leukot Essent Fatty Acids 81, 253–264.

Patterson, P.H., 2009. Immune involvement in schizophrenia and Autism: Etiology, pathology and animal models. Behavioural Brain Research 204, 313–321.

Pelegrin, P., 2008. Targeting interleukin-1 signaling in chronic inflammation: Focus on P2X(7) receptor and Pannexin-1. Drug News Perspect 21, 424–433.

Pinto, D., Pagnamenta, A.T., Klei, L., Anney, R., Merico, D., Regan, R., et al., 2010. Functional impact of global rare copy number variation in Autism spectrum disorders. Nature 466, 368–372.

Poling, J.S., Frye, R.E., Shoffner, J., Zimmerman, A.W., 2006. Developmental regression and mitochondrial dysfunction in a child with Autism. Journal of Child Neurology 21, 170–172.

Rahman, S., Blok, R.B., Dahl, H.H., Danks, D.M., Kirby, D.M., Chow, C.W., et al., 1996. Leigh syndrome: Clinical features and biochemical and DNA abnormalities. Annals of Neurology 39, 343–351.

Ristow, M., Zarse, K., 2010. How increased oxidative stress promotes longevity and metabolic health: The concept of mitochondrial hormesis (mitohormesis). Experimental Gerontology 45, 410–418.

Rossignol, D.A., Frye, R.E., 2011. Mitochondrial dysfunction in Autism spectrum disorders: A systematic review and meta-analysis. Molecular Psychiatry.

Rossignol, D.A., Rossignol, L.W., Smith, S., Schneider, C., Logerquist, S., Usman, A., et al., 2009. Hyperbaric treatment for children with Autism A multicenter, randomized, double-blind, controlled trial. BMC Pediatrics 9, 21.

Rotig, A., Lebon, S., Zinovieva, E., Mollet, J., Sarzi, E., Bonnefont, J.P., et al., 2004. Molecular diagnostics of mitochondrial disorders. Biochimica et Biophysica Acta 1659, 129–135.

Sadun, A.A., La Morgia, C., Carelli, V., 2011. Leber's Hereditary Optic Neuropathy. Current Treatment Options in Neurology 13, 109–117.

Saneto, R.P., Naviaux, R.K., 2010. Polymerase gamma disease through the ages. Developmental Disabilities Research Reviews 16, 163–174.

Saneto, R.P., Lee, I.C., Koenig, M.K., Bao, X., Weng, S.W., Naviaux, R.K., et al., 2010. POLG DNA testing as an emerging standard of care before instituting valproic acid therapy for pediatric seizure disorders. Seizure 19, 140–146.

Sano, M., Fukuda, K., 2008. Activation of mitochondrial biogenesis by hormesis. Circulation Research 103, 1191–1193.

Schaefer, A.M., McFarland, R., Blakely, E.L., He, L., Whittaker, R.G., Taylor, R.W., et al., 2008. Prevalence of mitochondrial DNA disease in adults. Annals of Neurology 63, 35–39.

Schaeffler, A., Gross, P., Buettner, R., Bollheimer, C., Buechler, C., Neumeier, M., et al., 2009. Fatty acid-induced induction of Toll-like receptor-4/nuclear factor-kappaB pathway in adipocytes links nutritional signalling with innate immunity. Immunology 126, 233–245.

Shen, P., Wang, W., Krishnakumar, S., Palm, C., Chi, A.K., Enns, G.M., et al., 2011. High-quality DNA sequence capture of 524 disease candidate genes. Proceedings of the National Academy of Sciences USA 108, 6549–6554.

Shoffner, J., Hyams, L., Langley, G.N., Cossette, S., Mylacraine, L., Dale, J., et al., 2010. Fever plus mitochondrial disease could be risk factors for autistic regression. Journal of Child Neurology 25, 429–434.

Singh, K.K., Kulawiec, M., Still, I., Desouki, M.M., Geradts, J., Matsui, S., 2005. Inter-genomic cross talk between mitochondria and the nucleus plays an important role in tumorigenesis. Gene 354, 140–146.

Staples, J.F., Brown, J.C., 2008. Mitochondrial metabolism in hibernation and daily torpor: A review. Journal of Comparative Physiology B. Biochemical, Systemic, and Environmental Physiology 178, 811–827.

Stobbe, M., 2008. Parents Speak Out on Vaccine Settlement. In: Washington Post, March 6. Associated Press, Washington, DC.

Suliman, H.B., Welty-Wolf, K.E., Carraway, M.S., Schwartz, D.A., Hollingsworth, J.W., Piantadosi, C.A., 2005. Toll-like receptor 4 mediates mitochondrial DNA damage and biogenic responses after heat-inactivated E. coli. FASEB Journal 19, 1531–1533.

Surprenant, A., North, R.A., 2009. Signaling at purinergic P2X receptors. Annual Review of Physiology 71, 333–359.

Trauner, D., Sweetman, L., Holm, J., Kulovich, S., Nyhan, W.L., 1977. Biochemical correlates of illness and recovery in Reye's syndrome. Annals of Neurology 2, 238–241.

UMDF, 2007. United Mitochondrial Disease Foundation (UMDF) Scientific & Medical Advisory Board statement on hyperbaric oxygen Therapy. Mitochondrial News 12, 1–20.

Vasta, V., Ng, S.B., Turner, E.H., Shendure, J., Hahn, S.H., 2009. Next generation sequence analysis for mitochondrial disorders. Genome Medicine 1, 100.

Verity, C.M., Stellitano, L.S., Winstone, A.M., 2011. The PIND study found no association between vaccination and Autism in mitochondrial disease – correction. Developmental Medicine & Child Neurology 53, 477.

Verity, C.M., Winstone, A.M., Stellitano, L., Krishnakumar, D., Will, R., McFarland, R., 2010. The clinical presentation of mitochondrial diseases in children with progressive intellectual and neurological deterioration: A national, prospective, population-based study. Developmental Medicine & Child Neurology 52, 434–440.

Wallace, D.C., Singh, G., Lott, M.T., Hodge, J.A., Schurr, T.G., Lezza, A.M., et al., 1988. Mitochondrial DNA mutation associated with Leber's hereditary optic neuropathy. Science 242, 1427–1430.

Wallace, D.C., Zheng, X.X., Lott, M.T., Shoffner, J.M., Hodge, J.A., Kelley, R.I., et al., 1988. Familial mitochondrial encephalomyopathy (MERRF): Genetic, pathophysiological, and biochemical characterization of a mitochondrial DNA disease. Cell 55, 601–610.

Wallis C (2008) Case Study: Autism and Vaccines Time Magazine, March 10. Available at: <http://www.time.com/time/health/article/0, 8599, 1721109,00.html> (accessed 24.05.12).

Weiss, M.D., Saneto, R.P., 2010. Sensory ataxic neuropathy with dysarthria and ophthalmoparesis (SANDO) in late life due to compound heterozygous POLG mutations. Muscle and Nerve 41, 882–885.

Weissman, J.R., Kelley, R.I., Bauman, M.L., Cohen, B.H., Murray, K.F., Mitchell, R.L., et al., 2008. Mitochondrial disease in Autism spectrum disorder patients: A cohort analysis. PLoS ONE 3, e3815.

West, A.P., Shadel, G.S., Ghosh, S., 2011. Mitochondria in innate immune responses. Nature Reviews Immunology 11, 389–402.

Wilson, J.M., 2009. Lessons learned from the gene therapy trial for ornithine transcarbamylase deficiency. Molecular Genetics and Metabolism 96, 151–157.

Wong, L.J., 2010. Molecular genetics of mitochondrial disorders. Developmental Disabilities Research Reviews 16, 154–162.

Wong, L.J., Scaglia, F., Graham, B.H., Craigen, W.J., 2010. Current molecular diagnostic algorithm for mitochondrial disorders. Molecular Genetics and Metabolism 100, 111–117.

Xu, C., Li, C.Y., Kong, A.N., 2005. Induction of phase I, II and III drug metabolism/transport by xenobiotics. Archives of Pharmacal Research 28, 249–268.

Yap, I.K., Angley, M., Veselkov, K.A., Holmes, E., Lindon, J.C., Nicholson, J.K., 2010. Urinary metabolic phenotyping differentiates children with Autismfrom their unaffected siblings and age-matched controls. Journal of Proteomic Research 9, 2996–3004.

Yuen, B., Boncompagni, S., Feng, W., Yang, T., Lopez, J.R., Matthaei, K.I., et al., 2012. Mice expressing T4826I-RYR1 are viable but exhibit sex- and genotype-dependent susceptibility to malignant hyperthermia and muscle damage. FASEB Journal 26, 1311–1322.

Zecchini, E., Siviero, R., Giorgi, C., Rizzuto, R., Pinton, P., 2007. Mitochondrial calcium signalling: Message of life and death. The Italian Journal of Biochemistry 56, 235–242.

Zeviani, M., Moraes, C.T., DiMauro, S., Nakase, H., Bonilla, E., Schon, E.A., et al., 1988. Deletions of mitochondrial DNA in Kearns-Sayre syndrome. Neurology 38, 1339–1346.

Zhang, Q., Raoof, M., Chen, Y., Sumi, Y., Sursal, T., Junger, W., et al., 2010. Circulating mitochondrial DAMPs cause inflammatory responses to injury. Nature 464, 104–107.

Zhao, X., Leon, I.R., Bak, S., Mogensen, M., Wrzesinski, K., Hojlund, K., et al., 2011. Phosphoproteome analysis of functional mitochondria isolated from resting human muscle reveals extensive phosphorylation of inner membrane protein complexes and enzymes. Molecular & Cellular Proteomics 10, M110.000299.

Parental and Perinatal Risk Factors for Autism: Epidemiological Findings and Potential Mechanisms

Sven Sandin*,†, Alexander Kolevzon**, Stephen Z. Levine‡, Christina M. Hultman†, Abraham Reichenberg*,**

*Department of Psychosis Studies, Institute of Psychiatry, King's College London, London, UK
†Department of Medical Epidemiology and Biostatistics, Karolinska Institutet, Stockholm, Sweden
**Department of Psychiatry, Mount Sinai School of Medicine, New York, NY, USA
‡Department of Community Mental Health, Faculty of Social Welfare and Health Sciences, University of Haifa, Israel

INTRODUCTION

Etiological models and research in autism and autism spectrum disorders (ASD) focus predominantly on the substantial role of genetic factors (Bailey et al., 1995). Yet, there is evidence that non-heritable pre- or perinatal events, and/or environmental exposures, are likely to also have a significant etiological role (Bristol et al., 1996). For example, studies of twins (Bailey et al., 1995; Smalley et al., 1988) indicate that

no more than 70% of monozygotic twin-pairs are fully concordant for autism, however, approximately 90% are concordant for a broader spectrum of related cognitive or social abnormalities. A recent twin study from California reported that shared environmental factors are a major component of ASD risk (Hallmayer et al., 2011). Moreover, recent estimates of the rates of ASD in relatives of autistic individuals are higher than previously reported (Constantino et al., 2010; Ozonoff et al., 2011).

The Neuroscience of Autism Spectrum Disorders.
http://dx.doi.org/10.1016/B978-0-12-391924-3.00013-2

Parental, perinatal, and obstetric conditions have been associated with several neurological and psychiatric disorders with established genetic etiologies, including Down's syndrome, dyslexia, intellectual disability, and schizophrenia (Cannon et al., 2002; Croen et al., 2001; Durkin et al., 1976; Malaspina et al., 2001; Moster et al., 2008; Penrose, 1967), as well as with developmental difficulties, such as speech and language problems, internalizing problems, attention problems, social problems, and hyperactivity (Aram et al., 1991; Hack et al., 1994; Moster et al., 2008; Pharoah et al., 1994; Schothorst and van Engeland, 1996; Veen et al., 1991). A large number of potential non-heritable factors have thus also been examined in relation to ASD, including parental and familial demographic characteristics, various obstetric complications, prenatal or intrapartum use of medications, and parental preconception chemical exposures (see Chapters 2.7–2.9 as well as Kolevzon et al., 2007).

Despite the significant research into the association between pregnancy and birth conditions and complications and ASD, the causal nature of these associations is still disputed. This may be due to several methodological limitations in the studies to date that have examined associations between parental characteristics, obstetric conditions, and risk of autism. First, many earlier studies of perinatal risk factors for ASD had small sample sizes (Lord et al., 1991; Piven et al., 1993) and therefore lacked statistical power to detect meaningful differences. Acknowledging this limitation, studies often used aggregated scores of perinatal and obstetric conditions, such as 'obstetric suboptimality.' However, different perinatal conditions may have different roles in the etiology of autism. Furthermore, such aggregation of conditions might increase the likelihood of non-differential misclassfication of exposure, and possibly attenuate the estimate of true associations. Second, most studies used clinical rather than epidemiological samples. Study designs that rely on clinical samples are especially prone to selection and ascertainment bias. Finally, some investigators relied on crude prenatal exposure data, such as maternal retrospective reporting of events that occurred during pregnancy. Maternal recall is prone to bias, because mothers of cases are more likely to recall pre- and perinatal events than mothers of controls. This differential recall is likely to bias the true measure of association away from the null hypothesis and lead to spurious positive results. Even when misclassification of exposure by the parent is not conditioned on whether or not the child has autism, it may still bias the results and attenuate a true association.

We chose to focus this chapter on two groups of risk factors: advancing parental age and indicators of intra-uterine growth. We chose those factors for several reasons. First, parental age and indicators of intrauterine growth (e.g., birth weight) are particularly attractive markers for investigation in relation to developmental outcomes because they can be measured accurately and are routinely recorded across years and cultures. Hence results are less prone to selection bias or misclassification of exposure. Second, there are plausible biological mechanisms that could underlie an association with ASD, and help elucidate possible etiologies. Third, animal models of such 'exposure' can be developed, allowing for direct back-translation to animal models. Finally, prevalence estimates of autism have increased dramatically during the past two decades. The increase is in part due to changes in diagnostic criteria and improved diagnostic accuracy and awareness (see Chapter 1.1). Yet it may also reflect a true increase in the incidence of ASD. If there is indeed a true increase in its incidence, then factors which affect risk of autism should also show an increase in incidence. The factors we discuss in this chapter show such an increase: age of parenting has been increasing in the United States and Europe in recent decades (Bray et al., 2006; Martin et al., 2005). Advances in perinatal care have dramatically increased the number of low-birth babies and babies born prematurely who survive (Wood et al., 2000).

ADVANCING PARENTAL AGE AND RISK OF ASD

Advanced maternal age was found to be associated with several developmental disorders, including Down's syndrome (Penrose, 1967), and mental retardation of unknown cause (Croen et al., 2001). Brain damage during pregnancy may also be more likely to occur in offspring of older mothers (Durkin et al., 1976). Advanced paternal age has been associated with adult-onset non-familial schizophrenia (Brown et al., 2002; El-Saadi et al., 2004; Malaspina et al., 2001; Torrey et al., 2009), bipolar disorder (Frans et al., 2008), and with decreased intellectual capacities in the offspring (Malaspina et al., 2005; Saha et al., 2009). Advanced paternal age has also been associated with several congenital disorders including Apert's syndrome, cleft lip and/or palate, hydrocephalus, neural tube defects, and Down's syndrome (Kolevzon et al., 2007; Reichenberg et al., 2006). Advanced maternal age and advanced paternal age are two of the most frequently studied risk factors for ASD (Hultman et al., 2011; Kolevzon et al., 2007; Sandin et al., 2012). However, despite extensive research, the results from the individual studies are mixed and the presence of associations is still disputed (Reichenberg et al., 2010).

GROWTH RESTRICTION AND PRETERM BIRTH

Low birth weight, defined as birth weight less than 2,500 grams, is considered a marker for newborns at high risk for later neurological, psychiatric, and neuropsychological problems (Hack et al., 2005). It has been associated with a variety of cognitive difficulties and psychiatric outcomes in children, including speech and language, internalizing, attention and social problems, hyperactivity, and learning disabilities (Kolevzon et al., 2007). However, low-birth-weight newborns represent a heterogeneous group in term of etiology, and low birth weight is often an indicator of earlier, intrauterine factors. The birth weight of premature babies is usually low. Thus, it may be particularly informative to consider gestational age. Similar to low birth weight, gestational age, and particularly short gestation (birth before 37 weeks), has also been associated with adverse health outcomes, including developmental delays and later intellectual impairments in childhood and adolescence (Moster et al., 2008; Schothorst and van Engeland, 1996; Wood et al., 2000). Compared to birth weight, gestational age is less accurately measured and more often unrecorded, thereby necessitating more careful data checking and cleaning. Despite being studied frequently (Kolevzon et al., 2007), research results that relate birth weight and gestational age and risk of ASD from individual studies are mixed, and the strength of the associations is still disputed (Buchmayer et al., 2009).

INTEGRATION OF STUDY RESULTS: A META-ANALYSIS OF EPIDEMIOLOGICAL STUDIES OF PARENTAL AGE, PRETERM BIRTH AND GROWTH RESTRICTION, AND RISK OF ASD

One way of resolving study discrepancies and obtaining a more reliable estimate of the true association between an exposure and an outcome is by integrating study results and applying meta-analytical methods.

In this chapter we describe a systematic review and meta-analysis of population-based epidemiological studies published up to January 2012, which was conducted in order to elucidate the association between advancing maternal age, advancing paternal age, preterm birth, intrauterine growth, and risk of ASD. We identified published peer-reviewed studies through a search of PUBMED, using the keywords 'autism' together with 'maternal,' 'paternal,' 'parental,' 'obstetric' or 'perinatal' together with the words 'risk' or 'association' or 'associated'. We included papers published in English from 1 January 1990 to 31 December 2011. We screened the resulting abstracts and obtained full text versions of potentially relevant studies. We used the following inclusion criteria:

1. A well-defined sample of cases drawn from population-based registry or cohort;
2. Comparison subjects drawn from the general population with information on parental age obtained from the same source;
3. Use of a standardized format for presentation of data, allowing for comparisons between studies and calculation of relative risk measures;
4. Presentation of results for maternal age *and* paternal age, *and* indicators of growth restriction and preterm birth (i.e., birth weight and/or gestational age and/or being small for gestational age).

Table 2.6.1 presents the characteristics of five studies from the US (Durkin et al., 2008; Grether et al., 2009), Denmark (Larsson et al., 2005; Maimburg and Vaeth, 2006), and Sweden (Hultman et al., 2011) which fulfilled **all** inclusion criteria and were included in the meta-analysis. The five studies included in the analysis had a total of 23,983 ASD cases and 7,816,709 subjects without an ASD diagnosis.

ADVANCING MATERNAL AGE

Table 2.6.2 presents the results of the meta-analysis examining the association between advancing maternal

TABLE 2.6.1 List of Studies and Study Characteristics Identified for Meta-Analysis of Maternal and Paternal Age at the Time of Birth of the Offspring and Intrauterine Growth and Risk of ASD in the Offspring

Study	Diagnostic method	Birth year/s	Sex ratio (M/F)	Design	Cases	Non-cases
Grether et al., 2009; US (California)	DSM III/IV	1989–2002	4.9	Cohort	20,701	6,506,555
Durkin et al., 2008; US (10 states)	DSM-IV	1994	4.5	Case-cohort	1,251	253,347
Larsson et al., 2005; Denmark	ICD 8/10	1973–1999	3.2	Case-control (nested)	698	17,450
Hultman et al., 2011; Sweden	ICD 9/10	1983–1992	3.2	Cohort	860	1,034,627
Maimburg and Vaeth, 2006; Denmark	ICD 8/10	1990–1999	4.1	Case-control (nested)	473	4,730

TABLE 2.6.2   Association Between Advancing Maternal and Paternal Age at the Time of Birth of the Offspring and Risk of ASD in the Offspring. Presented are the Adjusted Risk Ratios and Accompanying 95% Confidence Intervals

Study	Maternal age (35 or 40 and older)	Paternal age (40 or older)	Paternal age (50 or older)
Grether et al., 2009; US (California)	1.4 (1.3−1.6)	1.4 (1.3−1.5)	1.5 (1.3−1.8)
Durkin et al., 2008; US (10 states)	1.3 (1.1−1.6)	1.4 (1.1−1.8)	NA
Larsson et al., 2005; Denmark	1.6 (0.9−2.7)	1.4 (0.9−1.9)	NA
Hultman et al., 2011; Sweden	1.2 (0.9−1.5)	1.4 (1.1−1.9)	2.2 (1.3−3.9)
Maimburg and Vaeth, 2006; Denmark	1.3 (1.2−1.7)	1.2 (0.9−1.7)	NA
Pooled meta-analysis estimate	1.3 (1.2−1.4)	1.4 (1.3−1.5)	1.7 (1.2−2.3)

NA: not available.
Note: All studies adjusted for other parent's age, intrauterine growth (gestational age, weight for gestational age, or birth weight), and sex. Additional adjustment varied between studies and covariates included birth order, socioeconomic status (paternal and/or maternal education, source of payment of delivery), perinatal conditions (prenatal fetal distress, Apgar score, congenital malformations, fetal position), family psychiatric history (maternal and/or paternal psychiatric history), and ethnicity (maternal/paternal race or country of origin).

age and risk of ASD. The results support an increased risk of ASD in the offspring of older mothers. After adjustment for potential confounding covariates including paternal age, indicators of intrauterine growth, sex, and parental socio-demographic characteristics, the random-effect pooled estimate of the risk of ASD in the offspring of mothers aged 35 or older compared with mothers aged 25–29 years was 1.3 (95% confidence intervals: 1.2–1.4).

ADVANCING PATERNAL AGE

Table 2.6.2 also presents the results of the meta-analysis examining the association between advancing paternal age and risk for ASD. The results showed support for an increased risk of ASD in the offspring of older fathers. After adjustment for potential

confounding covariates including maternal age, indicators of intrauterine growth, sex, and parental socio-demographic characteristics, the random-effect pooled estimate of the risk of ASD in the offspring of fathers aged 40 or older compared with fathers aged 20–29 years was 1.4 (95% confidence intervals: 1.3–1.5). There was also evidence for a monotonic increase in risk of ASD with increasing paternal age categories. The random-effect pooled estimate of the risk of ASD in the offspring of fathers aged 50 or older compared with fathers aged 20–29 years was 1.7 (95% confidence intervals: 1.2–2.3).

GROWTH RESTRICTION AND PRETERM BIRTH

Table 2.6.3 presents the results of the meta-analysis examining the association between indicators of growth

TABLE 2.6.3   Association Between Indicators of Intrauterine Growth and Risk of ASD in the Offspring. Presented are the Adjusted Risk Ratios and Accompanying 95% Confidence Intervals

Study	Low birth weight (< 2,500 grams)	Preterm birth (< 37 weeks)	Growth restriction (small for gestational age)
Grether et al., 2009; US (California)	1.4 (1.1−1.7)	1.4 (1.2−1.6)	NA
Durkin et al., 2008; US (10 states)	NA	1.4 (1.2−1.7)	1.1 (0.7−1.6)
Larsson et al., 2005; Denmark	NA	2.5 (1.6−3.9)	1.3 (1.0−1.7)
Hultman et al., 2011; Sweden	1.0 (0.7−1.5)	NA	2.1 (1.5−3.0)
Maimburg and Vaeth, 2006; Denmark	3.0 (1.7−5.1)	1.7 (0.6−4.4)	1.4 (1.1−1.9)
Pooled meta-analysis estimate	1.5 (1.0−2.5)	1.5 (1.3−1.9)	1.4 (1.1−1.8)

NA: not available.
Note: All studies adjusted for parents, age and sex. Additional adjustment varied between studies and covariates included birth order, socioeconomic status (paternal and/or maternal education, source of payment of delivery), perinatal conditions (prenatal fetal distress, Apgar score, Aongenital malformations, fetal position), family psychiatric history (maternal and/or paternal psychiatric history), and ethnicity (maternal/paternal race or country of origin). Criteria for being born small for gestational age varied between studies. In studies from Sweden and the US two standard deviations below the mean birth weight for a given week of gestation was used. In Denmark, <10th decile of birth weight for a given week of gestational was used.

restriction and preterm birth and risk of ASD. The results showed support for an association between growth restriction and risk of ASD. After adjustment for potential confounding covariates including paternal age, maternal age, sex, and parental socio-demographic characteristics, the random-effect pooled estimate of the risk of ASD in low- (< 2,500 grams) birth-weight individuals compared with individuals born at normal birth weight ($\geq$ 2,500 grams) was 1.5 (95% confidence intervals: 1.0–2.5). For individuals born preterm (before week 37) the random-effect pooled estimate of the risk of ASD was 1.5 (95% confidence intervals: 1.3–1.9). Fetal growth restriction (being born small for gestational age) was also associated with increased risk of ASD. The random-effect pooled estimate of the risk of ASD in individuals born small for gestational age was 1.4 (95% confidence intervals: 1.1–1.8).

SUMMARY OF META-ANALYSIS

This meta-analysis supports the assertion that advancing maternal age and advancing paternal age at the time of birth are associated with an increasing risk of ASD in the offspring. It also supports an association between intrauterine growth restriction and preterm birth and an increased risk of ASD. The associations between advancing maternal age, advancing paternal age, and abnormal intrauterine growth and preterm birth, and risk of ASD were robust to adjustment for confounding covariates including, obstetric complications, birth year, birth order, parental psychiatric history, and markers of socioeconomic status. Importantly, the association between each of the variables examined and risk of ASD persisted after the effects of all other variables had been considered, supporting an independent relation between maternal age, paternal age, intrauterine growth restriction, preterm birth, and autism. The meta-analysis suggests that offspring of mothers older than 35 have 30% increased risk of developing ASD. Offspring of fathers older than 40 have 40% increased risk of developing ASD. Being born less than 2,500 grams, before week 37, or being born small for gestational age were associated with a 50%, 50%, and 40% increased risk of developing ASD, respectively.

POTENTIAL ETIOLOGICAL MECHANISMS

Etiological Mechanisms of Advancing Paternal and Maternal Age

One possible explanation for the paternal age and maternal age effects is an increased occurrence of spontaneous genomic alterations. It is thought that the spermatogonial stem cell divisions occurring over the life-course result in higher mutational rates and cytogenetic abnormalities (Buwe et al., 2005; Crow, 2000) in the sperm of older men. Maternal age is also an important factor in the etiology of chromosome anomalies (Ginsburg et al., 2000; Martin, 2008), and genomic modifications et al., 1997; Orr and Zoghbi, 2007).

Numerous neurological and psychiatric disorders have been related to genomic alterations (Reichenberg et al., 2009). Interestingly, a number of studies have uncovered an increased prevalence of *de novo* copy number variants (CNVs), and other forms of genomic alterations, in children with ASD (see Chapters 2.1 and 2.2 as well as Christian et al., 2008; Marshall et al., 2008; Sebat et al., 2007), supporting the notion that novel mutational events may be important in the pathogenesis of autism. Whether these events are also related to advancing paternal or maternal age requires further examination, however, recent studies provide very clear evidence for increased rate of *de novo* single nucleotide variation in children of older parents (Neale et al., 2012), providing a clear mechanism by which advanced parental age can influence ASD risk.

An additional mechanism is that epigenetic dysfunction underlies some parental age effects. 'Epigenetics' refers to the heritable, but reversible, regulation of gene expression (Henikoff and Matzke, 1997). Epigenetic dysfunction has been associated with several neuropsychiatric disorders (Mill et al., 2008), and is also implicated in single-gene disorders, including Rett and fragile X syndromes, characterized by ASD-like features in some patients (Reichenberg et al., 2009). A study by Flanagan and colleagues (2006) reported intra- and inter-individual epigenetic variability in the male germline, and found a number of genes that demonstrated age-related DNA-methylation changes. In addition, it is possible that the accumulated exposure to various environmental toxins over the life-course could result in genomic and/or epigenetic alterations in the germ cells of older parents. Toxins have been shown to induce DNA damage, germline mutations, and global hypermethylation (Yauk et al., 2008) in germ cells, and have long-term developmental consequences in offspring (Williams and Ross, 2007).

Etiological Mechanisms of Growth Restriction and Preterm Birth

Birth weight is affected by multiple genetic and environmental factors, as well as duration of the pregnancy and rate of fetal growth. Maternal and prenatal conditions associated with low birth weight and preterm birth are likely to be heterogeneous in etiology. Thus, it is unknown whether the intrauterine disturbances may directly compromise the fetus and result in ASD, or whether they reflect the effects of a fetus compromised by other factors. One study that examined the relationship between perinatal complications and ASD showed increased perinatal complications in siblings of individuals with ASD, and concluded that perinatal complications in ASD reflect the effects of a fetus compromised by other factors, most likely underlying genetic factors or their interaction with the environment (Glasson et al., 2004).

Preterm birth has been associated with maternal infections, high blood pressure, maternal diabetes, and preeclampsia (March-of-Dimes Foundation). However, in about half of all cases of preterm birth, the causes cannot be determined (March-of-Dimes Foundation). A number of prenatal conditions are known to be associated with growth restriction. Placental problems can reduce blood flow and nutrients to the fetus, limiting growth. Maternal nutritional problems during pregnancy may also effect *in utero* growth (Feigin et al., 2003). Finally, infections in the fetus have also been associated with abnormal growth (Feigin et al., 2003). Maternal infections (Maimburg and Vaeth, 2006), maternal diabetes, hypertension (Hultman et al., 2002), and placental abnormalities (Eaton et al., 2001; Glasson et al., 2004) have been only sporadically examined in relation to ASD, and it is therefore unclear whether they could explain the association between growth restriction and ASD.

CONCLUSIONS AND FUTURE DIRECTIONS

According to current evidence from epidemiological studies, two parental characteristics and two obstetric conditions consistently emerge as potential risk factors for autism, namely, advancing paternal age (age at birth of offspring $\geq$ 40), advancing maternal age (age at birth of offspring $\geq$ 35), and preterm birth and intrauterine growth restriction. In a meta-analysis that adjusted for confounding variables, these factors remained statistically significant. Future studies should continue to explore whether parental characteristics and obstetric conditions are associated with an increased risk of ASD. Given the inconsistency present in some results, large multisite and/or multi-registry epidemiological studies are likely to be particularly important. This is firstly because some of the risk factors are extremely rare (e.g., very low birth weights of < 1,000 grams) and only very large studies will allow a reliable examination of risk association. Secondly, potential effect modifiers or confounders such as gender, birth order, and cohort effects can only be reliably examined in such large-scale designs. Finally, large epidemiological studies will allow determination of whether different risk factors act independently, additively, or multiplicatively.

There was insufficient information in already published studies to reliably distinguish between autistic disorder and autism spectrum disorders. Distinguishing between common and unique risk factors for autistic disorder and spectrum disorders may be important for identifying shared and non-shared etiologies. A broader autism phenotype, with characteristic social, language, and behavioral impairments has been described. Future studies may also seek to assess the impact of parental characteristics and obstetric conditions identified through this review on dimensional outcomes related to the broader phenotype in the general population.

Perhaps the most important potential confounder to consider is genetic susceptibility to ASD. Genetic susceptibility may be associated with obstetric suboptimality, e.g., older parental age, maternal stress, or poor fetal growth. To determine whether parental or perinatal exposures are independent risk factors for ASD, a measure of genetic susceptibility should be included in future studies. This would allow for the assessment of genetic susceptibility as a confounder, and could also help examine the interaction of ASD genetic susceptibility (more broadly defined) with non-heritable, potentially preventable pre- and perinatal risk factors for ASD. To this goal, registry-based epidemiological studies could be particularly useful, as has been recently demonstrated (Daniels et al., 2008; Lauritsen et al., 2005). Registry-based epidemiological studies could also be utilized to distinguish familial from environmental effects on pre- and perinatal risk factors for ASD (Svensson et al., 2009). If biological samples are available, specific gene(s) by environment interactions could be reliably examined.

ACKNOWLEDGMENTS

This work was supported by grants from Autism Speaks, by a Margaret Temple award from the British Medical Association, and by the Beatrice and Samuel A. Seaver Foundation.

References

Aram, D.M., Hack, M., Hawkins, S., Weissman, B.M., Borawski-Clark, E., 1991. Very-low-birthweight children and speech and language development. Journal of Speech, Language, and Hearing Research 34, 1169–1179.

Bailey, A., Le Couteur, A., Gottesman, I., Bolton, P., Simonoff, E., Yuzda, E., et al., 1995. Autism as a strongly genetic disorder: Evidence from a British twin study. Psychological Medicine 25, 63–77.

Bray, I., Gunnell, D., Davey Smith, G., 2006. Advanced paternal age: How old is too old? Journal of Epidemiology & Community Health 60, 851–853.

Bristol, M.M., Cohen, D.J., Costello, E.J., Denckla, M., Eckberg, T.J., Kallen, R., et al., 1996. State of the science in autism: Report to the

National Institutes Health. Journal of Autism and Developmental Disorders 26, 121–154.

Brown, A.S., Schaefer, C.A., Wyatt, R.J., Begg, M.D., Goetz, R., Bresnahan, M.A., et al., 2002. Paternal age and risk of schizophrenia in adult offspring. American Journal of Psychiatry 159, 1528–1533.

Buchmayer, S., Johansson, S., Johansson, A., Hultman, C.M., Sparen, P., Cnattingius, S., 2009. Can association between preterm birth and autism be explained by maternal or neonatal morbidity? Pediatrics.

Buwe, A., Guttenbach, M., Schmid, M., 2005. Effect of paternal age on the frequency of cytogenetic abnormalities in human spermatozoa. Cytogenetic and Genome Research 111, 213–228.

Cannon, M., Jones, P.B., Murray, R.M., 2002. Obstetric complications and schizophrenia: Historical and meta-analytic review. American Journal of Psychiatry 159, 1080–1092.

Christian, S.L., Brune, C.W., Sudi, J., Kumar, R.A., Liu, S., Karamohamed, S., et al., 2008. Novel submicroscopic chromosomal abnormalities detected in autism spectrum disorder. Biological Psychiatry 63, 1111–1117.

Constantino, J.N., Zhang, Y., Frazier, T., Abbacchi, A.M., Law, P., 2010. Sibling recurrence and the genetic epidemiology of autism. American Journal of Psychiatry 167, 1349–1356.

Croen, L.A., Grether, J.K., Selvin, S., 2001. The epidemiology of mental retardation of unknown cause. Pediatrics 107, E86.

Crow, J.F., 2000. The origins, patterns and implications of human spontaneous mutation. Nature Reviews Genetics 1, 40–47.

Daniels, J.L., Forssen, U., Hultman, C.M., Cnattingius, S., Savitz, D.A., Feychting, M., et al., 2008. Parental psychiatric disorders associated with autism spectrum disorders in the offspring. Pediatrics 121, e1357–e1362.

Durkin, M.S., Maenner, M.J., Newschaffer, C.J., Lee, L.C., Cunniff, C.M., Daniels, J.L., et al., 2008. Advanced parental age and the risk of autism spectrum disorder. American Journal of Epidemiology 168, 1268–1276.

Durkin, M.V., Kaveggia, E.G., Pendleton, E., Neuhauser, G., Opitz, J.M., 1976. Analysis of etiologic factors in cerebral palsy with severe mental retardation. I. Analysis of gestational, parturitional and neonatal data. European Journal of Pediatrics 123, 67–81.

Eaton, W.W., Mortensen, P.B., Thomsen, P.H., Frydenberg, M., 2001. Obstetric complications and risk for severe psychopathology in childhood. Journal of Autism & Developmental Disorders 31, 279–285.

El-Saadi, O., Pedersen, C.B., McNeil, T.F., Saha, S., Welham, J., O'Callaghan, E., et al., 2004. Paternal and maternal age as risk factors for psychosis: Findings from Denmark, Sweden and Australia. Schizophrenia Research 67, 227–236.

Feigin, R.D., Cherry, J., Demmler, G., Kaplan, S., 2003. In: Textbook of Pediatric Infectious Diseases. Saunders.

Flanagan, J.M., Popendikyte, V., Pozdniakovaite, N., Sobolev, M., Assadzadeh, A., Schumacher, A., et al., 2006. Intra- and interindividual epigenetic variation in human germ cells. American Journal of Human Genetics 79, 67–84.

Frans, E.M., Sandin, S., Reichenberg, A., Lichtenstein, P., Langstrom, N., Hultman, C.M., 2008. Advancing paternal age and bipolar disorder. Archives of General Psychiatry 65, 1034–1040.

Ginsburg, C., Fokstuen, S., Schinzel, A., 2000. The contribution of uniparental disomy to congenital development defects in children born to mothers at advanced childbearing age. American Journal of Medical Genetics 95, 454–460.

Glasson, E.J., Bower, C., Petterson, B., de Klerk, N., Chaney, G., Hallmayer, J.F., 2004. Perinatal factors and the development of autism: A population study. Archives of General Psychiatry 61, 618–627.

Grether, J.K., Anderson, M.C., Croen, L.A., Smith, D., Windham, G.C., 2009. Risk of autism and increasing maternal and paternal age in a large North American population. American Journal of Epidemiology 170, 1118–1126.

Hack, M., Taylor, H.G., Drotar, D., Schluchter, M., Cartar, L., Andreias, L., et al., 2005. Chronic conditions, functional limitations, and special health care needs of school-aged children born with extremely low-birth-weight in the 1990s. Journal of the American Medical Association 294, 318–325.

Hack, M., Taylor, H.G., Klein, N., Eiben, R., Schatschneider, C., Mercuri-Minich, N., 1994. School-age outcomes in children with birth weights under 750 g. New England Journal of Medicine 331, 753–759.

Hallmayer, J., Cleveland, S., Torres, A., Phillips, J., Cohen, B., Torigoe, T., et al., 2011. Genetic heritability and shared environmental factors among twin pairs with autism. Archives of General Psychiatry 68, 1095–1102.

Henikoff, S., Matzke, M.A., 1997. Exploring and explaining epigenetic effects. Trends in Genetics 13, 293–295.

Hultman, C.M., Sandin, S., Levine, S.Z., Lichtenstein, P., Reichenberg, A., 2011. Advancing paternal age and risk of autism: New evidence from a population-based study and a meta-analysis of epidemiological studies. Molecular Psychiatry 16, 1203–1212.

Hultman, C.M., Sparen, P., Cnattingius, S., 2002. Perinatal risk factors for infantile autism. Epidemiology 13, 417–423.

Kaytor, M.D., Burright, E.N., Duvick, L.A., Zoghbi, H.Y., Orr, H.T., 1997. Increased trinucleotide repeat instability with advanced maternal age. Human Molecular Genetics 6, 2135–2139.

Kolevzon, A., Gross, R., Reichenberg, A., 2007. Prenatal and perinatal risk factors for autism: A review and integration of findings. Archives of Pediatrics & Adolescent Medicine 161, 326–333.

Larsson, H.J., Eaton, W.W., Madsen, K.M., Vestergaard, M., Olesen, A.V., Agerbo, E., et al., 2005. Risk factors for autism: Perinatal factors, parental psychiatric history, and socioeconomic status. American Journal of Epidemiology 161, 916–925.

Lauritsen, M.B., Pedersen, C.B., Mortensen, P.B., 2005. Effects of familial risk factors and place of birth on the risk of autism: A nationwide register-based study. Journal of Child Psychology & Psychiatry 46, 963–971.

Lord, C., Mulloy, C., Wendelboe, M., Schopler, E., 1991. Pre- and perinatal factors in high-functioning females and males with autism. Journal of Autism & Developmental Disorders 21, 197–209.

Maimburg, R.D., Vaeth, M., 2006. Perinatal risk factors and infantile autism. Acta Psychiatrica Scandinavica 114, 257–264.

Malaspina, D., Harlap, S., Fennig, S., Heiman, D., Nahon, D., Feldman, D., et al., 2001. Advancing paternal age and the risk of schizophrenia. Archives of General Psychiatry 58, 361–367.

Malaspina, D., Reichenberg, A., Weiser, M., Fennig, S., Davidson, M., Harlap, S., et al., 2005. Paternal age and intelligence: Implications for age-related genomic changes in male germ cells. Psychiatric Genetics 15, 117–125.

March-of-Dimes. March of Dimes Foundation: Medical References. Retrieved Nov 26, 2009, from: <http:\\www.marchofdimes.com/professionals/14332_1157.asp>

Marshall, C.R., Noor, A., Vincent, J.B., Lionel, A.C., Feuk, L., Skaug, J., et al., 2008. Structural variation of chromosomes in autism spectrum disorder. American Journal of Human Genetics 82, 477–488.

Martin, J.A., Hamilton, B.E., Sutton, P.D., Ventura, S.J., Menacker, F., Munson, M.L., 2005. Births: Final data for 2003. National Vital Statistics Reports 54, 1–116.

Martin, R.H., 2008. Meiotic errors in human oogenesis and spermatogenesis. Reproductive BioMedicine. Online 16, 523–531.

Mill, J., Tang, T., Kaminsky, Z., Khare, T., Yazdanpanah, S., Bouchard, L., et al., 2008. Epigenomic profiling reveals DNA-methylation changes associated with major psychosis. American Journal of Human Genetics 82, 696–711.

Moster, D., Lie, R.T., Markestad, T., 2008. Long-term medical and social consequences of preterm birth. New England Journal of Medicine 359, 262–273.

Neale, B.M., Kou, Y., Liu, L., Ma'ayan, A., Samocha, K.E., Sabo, A., et al., 2012. Patterns and rates of exonic de novo mutations in autism spectrum disorders. Nature 485, 242–245.

Orr, H.T., Zoghbi, H.Y., 2007. Trinucleotide repeat disorders. Annual Review of Neuroscience 30, 575–621.

Ozonoff, S., Young, G.S., Carter, A., Messinger, D., Yirmiya, N., Zwaigenbaum, L., et al., 2011. Recurrence risk for autism spectrum disorders: A baby siblings research consortium study. Pediatrics 128, e488–e495.

Penrose, L.S., 1967. The effects of change in maternal age distribution upon the incidence of mongolism. Journal of Mental Deficiency Research 11, 54–57.

Pharoah, P.O., Stevenson, C.J., Cooke, R.W., Stevenson, R.C., 1994. Prevalence of behaviour disorders in low birthweight infants. Archives of Disease in Childhood 70, 271–274.

Piven, J., Simon, J., Chase, G.A., Wzorek, M., Landa, R., Gayle, J., et al., 1993. The etiology of autism: Pre-, peri- and neonatal factors. Journal of the American Academy of Child & Adolescent Psychiatry 32, 1256–1263.

Reichenberg, A., Gross, R., Sandin, S., Susser, E.S., 2010. Advancing paternal and maternal age are both important for autism risk. American Journal of Public Health 100, 772–773.

Reichenberg, A., Gross, R., Weiser, M., Bresnahan, M., Silverman, J., Harlap, S., et al., 2006. Advancing paternal age and autism. Archives of General Psychiatry 63, 1026–1032.

Reichenberg, A., Mill, J., MacCabe, J.H., 2009. Epigenetics, genomic mutations and cognitive function. Cognitive Neuropsychiatry 14, 377–390.

Saha, S., Barnett, A.G., Foldi, C., Burne, T.H., Eyles, D.W., Buka, S.L., et al., 2009. Advanced paternal age is associated with impaired neurocognitive outcomes during infancy and childhood. PLoS Medicine 6, e40.

Sandin, S., Hultman, C.M., Kolevzon, A., Gross, R., MacCabe, J.H., Reichenberg, A. Advancing maternal age is associated with increasing risk for autism - a review and meta analysis. Journal of the American Academy of Child and Adolescent Psychiatry 51, 477–486.

Schothorst, P.F., van Engeland, H., 1996. Long-term behavioral sequelae of prematurity. Journal of the American Academy of Child & Adolescent Psychiatry 35, 175–183.

Sebat, J., Lakshmi, B., Malhotra, D., Troge, J., Lese-Martin, C., Walsh, T., et al., 2007. Strong association of de novo copy number mutations with autism. Science 316, 445–449.

Smalley, S.L., Asarnow, R.F., Spence, M.A., 1988. Autism and genetics. A decade of research. Archives of General Psychiatry 45, 953–961.

Svensson, A.C., Sandin, S., Cnattingius, S., Reilly, M., Pawitan, Y., Hultman, C.M., et al., 2009. Maternal effects for preterm birth: A genetic epidemiologic study of 630,000 families. American Journal of Epidemiology 170, 1365–1372.

Torrey, E.F., Buka, S., Cannon, T.D., Goldstein, J.M., Seidman, L.J., Liu, T., et al., 2009. Paternal age as a risk factor for schizophrenia: How important is it? Schizophrenia Research 114, 1–5.

Veen, S., Ens-Dokkum, M.H., Schreuder, A.M., Verloove-Vanhorick, S.P., Brand, R., Ruys, J.H., 1991. Impairments, disabilities, and handicaps of very preterm and very-low-birthweight infants at five years of age. The collaborative project on preterm and small for gestational age infants (POPS) in the Netherlands. Lancet 338, 33–36.

Williams, J.H., Ross, L., 2007. Consequences of prenatal toxin exposure for mental health in children and adolescents: A systematic review. European Child & Adolescent Psychiatry 16, 243–253.

Wood, N.S., Marlow, N., Costeloe, K., Gibson, A.T., Wilkinson, A.R., 2000. Neurologic and developmental disability after extremely preterm birth. EPICure Study Group. New England Journal of Medicine 343, 378–384.

Yauk, C., Polyzos, A., Rowan-Carroll, A., Somers, C.M., Godschalk, R.W., Van Schooten, F.J., et al., 2008. Germ-line mutations, DNA damage, and global hypermethylation in mice exposed to particulate air pollution in an urban/industrial location. Proceedings of the National Academy of Sciences of the USA 105, 605–610.

The Environment in Autism Spectrum Disorders

Kristen Lyall*, Rebecca J. Schmidt[†], Irva Hertz-Picciotto[†]

*MIND Institute, University of California, Davis, Sacramento, CA, USA [†]Department of Public Health Sciences, The MIND Institute, University of California, Davis, CA, USA

BACKGROUND

Autism spectrum disorders (ASD) are complex, etiologically heterogeneous conditions. Early on, the finding that monozygotic twin concordance was less than 100% (Folstein and Rutter, 1977; Steffenburg et al., 1989) demonstrated that non-genetic factors, i.e., the environment, can influence the risk of having these behavioral disorders. Estimates of the relative contribution from such factors is under active study, with a recent large twin study finding that non-genetic factors accounted for 55% of the variance in autism risk (Hallmayer et al., 2011; see also Chapter 2.3).

The sharp rise in prevalence of autism over a few decades is partially attributable to changes in diagnostic criteria, awareness, and attitudes, but several analyses indicate that these artifacts may not explain all of the increase in incidence/prevalence observed (Hertz-Picciotto and Delwiche, 2009; King and Bearman 2009; see also Chapter 1.1). For this reason, environmental contributions to the rise in autism should be considered. Not only environmental factors that have increased over time may play a role; since many cases of autism were likely missed in the past, exposures that have been stable over time may also be involved. Additionally, because our environment is constantly changing, with some neurodevelopmental toxins decreasing and others increasing, a wide range of temporal patterns for a given exposure could be consistent with the trends in autism incidence, and even exposures that have been declining cannot be precluded as risk factors. Finally, interactions among various environmental factors can result in altered patterns over time that will not be explained by the calendar-time trend of any one contributor.

Environmental contributors to autism are defined broadly as all non-genetic factors, from viruses, to medications, to chemicals, to social influences. These likely interact with genetic factors through epigenetic, metabolic, and other mechanisms. This chapter discusses known and suspected environmental exposures that

The Neuroscience of Autism Spectrum Disorders.
http://dx.doi.org/10.1016/B978-0-12-391924-3.00014-4

alter risk of autism, with a focus on exogenous agents that act during the preconception and prenatal periods. Endogenous perinatal factors such as pregnancy complications are not covered here, but are covered in Chapter 2.6. Exposures are grouped into medically related factors, maternal lifestyle, and environmental chemicals. We conclude with future research directions for identifying environmental contributions to autism.

EXOGENOUS MEDICALLY RELATED FACTORS

Infections

Some of the earliest clues regarding non-genetic etiological factors in autism concern infectious agents. An epidemic of rubella in the 1960s revealed that children whose mothers were infected during pregnancy had a remarkably high autism prevalence of 4–7% (Chess 1971; 1978). Congenital cytomegalovirus exposure has also been associated with autism (Sweeten et al., 2004; Yamashita et al., 2003). These and other investigations of prenatal exposures highlight gestation as a critical period in aberrant brain development in autism. Though these viruses are unlikely to account for current cases of autism, maternal infections of relevance to today's children have also been linked to increased risk. Maternal fever and influenza have been associated with autism in some, but not all, studies (Gardener et al., 2009). Maternally reported fever during pregnancy was associated with increased odds of autism in a case-control study (Zerbo et al., 2012). Despite limitations in many earlier studies (including lack of control for potential confounders), a meta-analysis of prenatal factors calculated the summary estimate for the association between maternal infection and autism in the four studies that did adjust for confounders to be odds ratio (OR) = 1.82, (95% confidence interval (CI) 1.01, 3.30). Significant heterogeneity, however, was observed across studies (Gardener et al., 2009). Variations in definition, timing, and method of assessment of exposure may have contributed to discrepant results.

A role of maternal infection or maternal immune response during pregnancy is supported by animal models of autistic behaviors that rely on poly I:C (viral) injections during pregnancy (Boksa, 2010; Smith et al., 2007), and by evidence of maternal autoantibodies to fetal brain proteins in a subset of mothers of children with autism (Braunschweig et al., 2008). These topics are further discussed in Chapter 2.9 (Immune Abnormalities and Autism Spectrum Disorders).

Other evidence bearing on the infection/immune hypothesis comes from the literature on seasonality. Season of both birth and conception have been examined. The largest and most methodologically rigorous such study to date, including nearly 20,000 autism cases and over 6 million births in California, found a modest but statistically significant increase in risk of autism (adjusted OR = 1.06, 95% CI 1.02–1.10) for children conceived in the winter months (December, January, February, March) compared to the summer; when alternatively analyzed by month of birth, August–December deliveries were associated with an increased risk of autism, but only November births remained significant after adjustment for year of birth, maternal education, and child ethnicity (Zerbo et al., 2011). Although previous results are somewhat inconsistent, and some showed no seasonality (Hultman et al., 2002; Kolevzon et al., 2006; Landau et al., 1999), many prior studies suggested higher autism risk with birth in March (Barak et al., 1995; Mouridsen et al., 1994). Differences in results may be due to small sample sizes, different time periods and regions studied, inappropriate comparison group, or inadequate control of confounding variables, particularly calendar time.

While season could represent a surrogate for influenza epidemic or other infectious agents, it also could be a proxy for other environmental agents such as nutritional factors and use of pesticides. Because pesticide use (discussed below), maternal infections, and even nutritional factors may also vary by location, discrepancies in seasonality studies may stem from spatial variability, or contributions from several of these factors. Further, each seasonal risk factor may affect autism risk by acting at a different critical period in early development. Additional research on the effects of timing of these and other environmental exposures is needed.

Maternal Medications

Thalidomide, a medication used primarily for morning sickness during the 1950s and 60s, was found to increase the risk of having a child with autism in mothers using the drug at days 20–24 post-conception (Stromland et al.,1994). Among 100 mothers using thalidomide, 4 of their children had autism (Lotter, 1966), an occurrence 100 times higher than the estimate of 4 in 10,000 from that era (Fombonne, 2009). Valproic acid has also been associated with a substantial increase in autism risk. In mothers using this anti-epileptic drug during pregnancy, prevalence of autism increased to ~ 5–8% in two separate clinical investigations (Moore et al., 2000; Rasalam et al., 2005). These studies also suggested a high prevalence of developmental delays or broadly defined autistic behaviors (60–77%) in children whose mothers used this and other anti-epileptic drugs. Though maternal use of valproic acid and thalidomide cannot account for a large proportion of autism cases, these associations demonstrate that pharmacological

child (Steegers-Theunissen et al., 2009), which alters epigenetic regulation of gene expression. As an exposure with established gene–environment interactions, epigenetic effects, and neurodevelopmental consequences, prenatal nutritional status should be explored further in relation to ASD etiology.

Alcohol

Few rigorous studies of alcohol and autism have been conducted. A pedigree analysis found a higher prevalence of reported alcoholism among first- and second-degree female relatives of children with autism, which the authors concluded suggested a shared genetic influence for psychiatric comorbidity (Miles et al., 2003). A nested case-control study in Sweden of autism in relation to inpatient hospital diagnoses of psychiatric disorders among parents, including alcohol and drug addiction/abuse, found no association (Daniels et al., 2008). However, these studies did not address maternal alcohol intake during pregnancy.

More recently, Eliasen et al. (2010) studied the association between prenatal alcohol exposure and the risk of ASD in a population-based prospective study of 80,552 children and their mothers. Participants were enrolled in the Danish National Birth Cohort study from 1996 to 2002, and alcohol consumption was obtained by self-report during pregnancy. From the Danish Central Psychiatry Register, 401 children had an ASD diagnosis, of which 157 had infantile autism. No association was found between average alcohol consumption and either ASD or infantile autism. No trend was observed with increasing number (0, 1, 2, 3, or 4+) of binge (5 or more drinks on one occasion) episodes during pregnancy. Selection bias (participation rate was ~30%) and reporting bias may explain both this anomalous finding and the lack of association with heavy alcohol drinking. Because of its size and prospective design, this study provides the best research to date on maternal alcohol intake and ASD, and suggests no increased risk from light to moderate maternal alcohol use. Nevertheless, given that high prenatal alcohol exposure impairs neurodevelopment in humans (Eliasen et al., 2010; Jacobson and Jacobson, 2002) and produces structural brain anomalies in animal studies congruent with those observed in children with ASD (Casanova, 2007), further research is warranted, although obtaining accurate information on alcohol consumption is challenging in any epidemiological study.

Cigarette Smoking

As reviewed by Button et al. (2007), several longitudinal studies have linked maternal cigarette smoking and risk for psychiatric sequelae and behavioral disorders, including social problems, in the child. The first study to report an association between maternal daily smoking during early pregnancy and autism was a population-based case-control study of perinatal risk factors for autism in Sweden (Hultman et al., 2002). Though the study suggested an association between maternal smoking and ICD-9 diagnosis of autism, inappropriate adjustment for mediators, lack of adjustment for socioeconomic status, and possible selection bias call into question the validity of these findings.

A number of other studies have assessed maternal smoking in association with autism, each with limitations. In a small population-based prospective study (Indredavik et al., 2007) of 84 adolescents at 14 years, maternally reported smoking during pregnancy was strongly associated with social problems as measured by the Autism Spectrum Screening Questionnaire (ASSQ) (Ehlers et al., 1999). Another study, including 72 children with ASD among 4,779 children aged 6–8 years, examined indoor environmental contributions to autism and found a significant association between maternal smoking and parentally reported ASD in the child (Larsson et al., 2009). Self-reported smoking exposure was prospectively collected, thereby eliminating recall bias, and several socio-demographic factors were considered as potential confounders of the association; however, the number of cases exposed to environmental tobacco smoke was relatively small (n = 21).

In a cohort study that included maternal smoking as a potential confounder, a higher percentage of mothers who smoked during pregnancy had children with ASD (Hvidtjorn et al., 2011), although the difference could have been be confounded by socioeconomic status. In children with attention-deficit/hyperactivity disorder (ADHD), researchers reported an interaction of maternal smoking with both catechol O-methyltransferase and serotonin transporter genes in relation to ASD symptoms (Nijmeijer et al., 2010). A recent retrospective study also identified maternal smoking as a shared predictor of ASD and ADHD in children who also experienced fetal hypokinesia in early pregnancy (Habek and Kovacevic, 2011).

Mechanisms underlying an association between maternal smoking and ASD and other neurobehavioral outcomes have been hypothesized based on limited human research and animal studies, and include reduced blood flow to the brain due to placental insufficiency and oxygen deprivation (Albuquerque et al., 2004), alteration of gene expression in the fetal brain, (Luck et al., 1985), and alteration of nicotinic receptors that develop in the first trimester of pregnancy and influence brain development (Williams et al., 1998). Further, prenatal nicotine exposure has been shown to lead to changes in neurotransmitter activity and turnover that can persist into adulthood (Muneoka et al.,

2001; Roy and Sabherwal, 1998). In addition, prenatal smoking may indicate underlying psychological conditions in the mother that are inherited by the offspring (Fergusson et al., 1998).

Given conflicting results for an association between maternal smoking and autism, and the biological plausibility for an effect of nicotine on the developing fetal brain, there is a need for more rigorously designed studies of maternal smoking in relation to ASD.

ENVIRONMENTAL CHEMICALS

Background

Environmental chemicals in air, food, water, and personal care or household products represent a potential hazard for the developing organism. This is in part because regulations for testing adverse health effects are weak with regard to neurodevelopment. After thalidomide was shown to cause phocomelia (absent or severely stunted limbs) in humans, regulations began to address teratogenicity, which includes gross physical malformations during organogenesis, but most testing requirements do not cover long-term behavioral aberrations or cognitive deficits from prenatal exposures. Thus, it took decades after the problem of low-level lead effects on child brain development was demonstrated (Needleman and Leviton, 1979) for action to be taken on lead exposure, and it is not uncommon for lead-containing products that pose a hazard to children to enter the market (Norman et al., 1997). Other recognized neurodevelopmental toxins include mercury and organophosphates, and a growing literature suggests neurobehavioral effects from polychlorinated biphenyls and other endocrine-disrupting compounds.

Endocrine-Disrupting Chemicals (EDCs)

Polychlorinated biphenyls (PCBs) are a class of persistent halogenated compound used in coolant fluids, plasticizers, and adhesives. Because of their persistence in the environment, they are included as POPs (Persistent Organic Pollutants) under the Stockholm Convention (Secretariat of the Stockholm Convention). Two accidents in which PCBs were introduced into rice oil resulted in poisoned populations with serious health effects in Japan in 1968, and Taiwan in 1979 (Masuda, 1985). Children born years after their mothers had been poisoned showed serious developmental problems. Some PCBs share structural similarity to dioxin, a highly toxic substance, while various other PCBs exhibit estrogenic, anti-estrogenic, androgenic, or anti-androgenic properties, suggesting that different forms, defined according to their chemical structure

and activity, may have differing health risks (Park et al., 2010). Industrial use of PCBs was banned in 1976. Food and breast milk continue to be sources of exposure due to bioaccumulation of PCBs through the food chain (Hertz-Picciotto et al., 2008), but body burdens in the general population have declined steadily and markedly over the last few decades..

To date, no study has specifically examined PCB exposure in association with autism. However, cognitive deficits have been observed in numerous human studies (Korrick and Sagiv, 2008), as have attention problems and ADHD-like behaviors (Sagiv et al., 2010; Verner et al., 2010), particularly in boys (Sagiv et al., 2012). In addition, one study suggested timing-specific effects for different outcomes, with attention problems associated with prenatal PCB exposure, and child activity level associated with postnatal (lactational) exposure (Sagiv et al., 2010). In a community with chronic exposures from a chemical manufacturing plant, decades after production ceased, Bayley scores were significantly lower in children whose mothers had higher levels of mono-ortho-substituted (dioxin-like) PCBs (Park et al., 2010), or their hydroxylated metabolites (Park et al., 2009), suggesting that prenatal dioxin-like PCB exposure in particular may influence *in utero* brain development (Wilhelm et al., 2008). Thyroid disruption has been suggested to contribute to the prenatal effects on brain development (Parent et al., 2011).

Whereas PCB levels have been declining, human exposures to polybrominated diphenyl ethers (PBDEs), another class of endocrine-disrupting chemicals, began to increase dramatically in the 1990s through the early 2000s. These compounds are added as flame retardants to foam in furniture, children's clothing, and other household materials. While penta- and octa- forms of PBDEs are no longer produced in the United States, deca- formulations continue to be manufactured. PBDEs exhibit similar toxicities to PCBs, including findings of thyroid dysregulation and neurocognitive deficits (Herbstman et al., 2010; Rose et al., 2010; Viberg et al., 2008). Despite banned production, levels of PBDEs in humans are high (Frederiksen et al., 2009), as these chemicals bioaccumulate; furthermore, unlike PCBs, the highest levels of PBDEs are found in the youngest individuals (Rose et al., 2010).

The only investigation of PBDEs in relation to autism was a pilot study within the CHARGE case-control population. This study did not show any differences in PBDE levels between 51 cases and 49 controls (Hertz-Picciotto et al., 2011), though diet did influence PBDE levels. Given that PBDE measurements were conducted on samples taken from the child at age 3–5 (as a surrogate for prenatal exposure), this work does not preclude an impact of PBDEs on autism from a more relevant time frame, namely, during gestation and early stages of brain development. A birth cohort study conducted in Menorca, Spain, found that measures of poor social competence, measured on the California Preschool Social Competence Scale, were associated with greater serum PBDE-47 concentrations at 4 years of age (Gascon et al., 2010). In comparison, a study that examined cord blood concentrations of congeners of PBDEs in association with child cognitive and behavioral scores at 12–48 and 72 months found that those children with higher PBDE levels had lower scores on mental and psychomotor development tests (including the Mental Development Index and Wechsler IQ test) in adjusted analyses (Herbstman et al., 2010). In addition, another study found that maternal PBDE levels measured late in pregnancy were associated with decreased fine motor skill and increased attention problems in offspring (Roze et al., 2009). Investigation of PBDEs during critical time periods of development and subsequent risk of ASD is warranted. Animal studies show that PBDEs produce hyperactivity and altered motor behavior and development in rodents (Gee and Moser, 2008; Suvorov et al., 2009).

Both bisphenol A (BPA) and phthalates have been shown to be endocrine disruptors. BPA is a plasticizer found in plastic drink containers, the lining of food cans and plastic food wrappings, dental appliances and resins, and baby bottles, among other things. It has estrogenic properties. BPA and other endocrine disruptors have been associated with attention problems in children, and have also been associated with schizophrenia (Brown, 2009; Masuo et al., 2004). Phthalates are used in cosmetics, lotions, fragrances, vinyl flooring, and a variety of plastics, and have anti-androgenic properties. A recent study investigating indoor environmental factors found an unexpected doubling of risk of autism in children whose homes had vinyl (PVC) flooring in the child and parent bedrooms (Larsson et al., 2009). PVC flooring is a significant source of airborne phthalates. Replication and continued investigation of these short-lived endocrine-disrupting chemicals in association with neurodevelopment and autism in particular are needed.

One plausible mechanism by which EDCs may alter brain development and increase risk of autism is through disruption of thyroid homeostasis during pregnancy. The fetus depends on maternal thyroid hormones (T3 and T4) during the first part of pregnancy. Adequate levels are required for fetal neurodevelopment, including neuronal growth, cell migration, and differentiation in the hippocampus, cerebral cortex, and cerebellum (Boas et al., 2011). Dioxins, PCBs, PBDEs, BPA, and phthalates have all been shown to disrupt thyroid function in some manner (Hertz-Picciotto et al., 2008; Hougaard et al., 2008; Pocar et al., 2011; Windham et al., 2006; Zhou et al., 2002). Changes in thyroid hormone levels affect dendritic development of Purkinje cells (Kimura-Kuroda et al., 2007), which is of note given that Purkinje cell loss is a highly replicated finding in children with autism (Amaral, 2008). In rodents, thyroid disruption has been shown to be a major pathway for neurodevelopmental toxicity (Goldey and Crofton, 1998). There is also evidence that EDCs alter molecular signaling, including calcium (Shafer et al., 2005; Wong et al., 1997). These chemicals may also have direct effects on neural development or the placental or blood–brain barriers. Additionally, the strong male:female ratio in autism of about four could be a clue that effects of EDCs on steroid hormones might play a role in autism etiology, as testosterone and estradiol influence fetal brain development.

As with the nutritional factors, these EDCs may interact with genes to influence autism risk. Animal studies of PBDE exposure demonstrate disruption of levels of brain-derived neurotrophic factor (BDNF) (Viberg et al., 2008), and polymorphisms in the BDNF gene have been linked with autism. PCBs appear to influence expression of a wide range of genes (Mitra et al., 2012). To date, very little research has addressed either the influence of environment on gene expression relevant to neurodevelopment or the modification of environmental effects on neurodevelopment by genotype.

Pesticides

By design, pesticides are neurotoxic, usually acting on neurotransmission. Further, some pesticides have been shown to be EDCs or POPs (Korrick and Sagiv, 2008), suggesting similar mechanisms to those discussed above. In the 1950s, organochlorine pesticides (DDT, heptachlor) came into widespread use, in, for instance, major efforts to eradicate malaria through mosquito control. After discoveries of persistence and adverse effects on wildlife, less persistent compounds, such as the organophosphates, were developed. Nevertheless, some organochlorines continue to be used, and one of the first reports on pesticides and autism found a strong association with residential proximity to agricultural applications of endosulfan and dicofol during the first trimester (Roberts et al., 2007). Another study found higher metabolites of organophosphate pesticides to be associated with poorer scores on a subscale of the Child Behavior Checklist representing symptoms of pervasive developmental disorder (Eskenazi et al., 2007). Other epidemiological investigations have found deficits in motor coordination, visuospatial performance, and memory (Harari et al., 2010), and higher risk of ADHD (Engel et al., 2011). In addition, a gene involved in metabolizing these chemicals, Paraoxonase 1 (PON1), may be a susceptibility factor for the association (Engel et al., 2011).

The organophosphates were banned from use in household products by the US Environmental

Protection Agency (EPA) in the late 1990s, but continue to be used in commercial applications. Since then, use of pyrethroid pesticides in the home has increased. As of 2009, over 3,500 registered products contain synthetic pyrethroids or their naturally derived counterparts, pyrethrins. Despite relatively short half-lives, pyrethroid metabolites have been found in over 70% of adults in the United States (Barr et al., 2010), likely due to their common usage and ubiquitous presence in household products. Preliminary work from the CHARGE case-control study suggested increased risk of autism with increasing reported use of products containing pyrethroids (Hertz-Picciotto et al., in review); however, as this is the only study currently available that assessed the association, further studies are needed to determine whether pyrethroid exposure influences risk of autism.

Depending on the type of compound, pesticides could influence neurodevelopment through a variety of mechanisms, including interference with establishment of serotonergic systems, changes in activity of monoamine oxidase or acetylcholinesterase, altered GABA function, endocrine disruption, immune dysregulation, and altered lipid metabolism; and, like PBDEs, pesticides have also been associated with calcium signaling (Lawrence and Casida, 1983; Malaviya et al., 1993).

Air Pollution and Proximity to Freeways

Several investigators report links between air pollution and risk of autism, using a variety of methods for estimating exposure (Kalkbrenner et al., 2010; Palmer et al., 2009; Volk et al., 2011; Windham et al., 2006). The first investigation, conducted in California by Windham and colleagues, included 284 children with autism and 657 controls, and used census tract-based estimates derived by the US Environmental Protection Agency (EPA) for 19 hazardous air pollutant (HAP) chemicals (Windham et al., 2006). In adjusted analyses, individuals in the top quartile of exposure to chlorinated solvents and heavy metals were 50% more likely to have autism compared to those in the lowest two quartiles (combined for the reference group). Specific compounds significantly associated with autism were trichloroethylene and vinyl chloride, and the metals cadmium, mercury, and nickel. Diesel particulate matter was also significantly associated with autism (OR for top quartile = 1.44, 95% CI 1.03–2.02). However, exposures in this study were based on modeled estimates of HAPs in census tracts of birth residence that pertained to those locations two years after the birth, and thus did not capture prenatal exposure.

A study of children in North Carolina and West Virginia also found significantly elevated risk of autism for a number of air pollutants, including diesel, mercury, nickel, styrene, and beryllium in unadjusted analyses (Kalkbrenner et al., 2010), though no statistically significant associations were found when adjusting for demographic factors. However, the range of concentrations for certain pollutants was small, and the exposure assessment corresponded to the year of birth for only a fraction of the children.

Proximity to a major freeway during gestation has also been associated with increased risk for autism in analyses of 304 autism cases and 259 controls from the CHARGE study (Volk et al., 2011). In contrast to studies described above, Volk and colleagues used geocoded residences for each mother at time of delivery and calculated distance to freeways as a surrogate for air pollution. Exposure groups were defined as living within the closest 10%, the next 15% and the next 25%, of the distribution of distance from freeway, with those in the farthest 50% (corresponding to 0.9 miles or more) serving as the referent group. The association was also examined according to trimester of pregnancy, though there was a high correlation across time points. In analyses adjusted for socio-demographic factors and maternal smoking, significant associations were found for maternal residence at time of delivery and for residence during the third trimester. Residence within 309 meters of a freeway at time of delivery compared to greater than 1,419 meters was associated with nearly a doubling in odds of having a child with autism (OR = 1.86, 95% CI 1.04–3.45), while residence in third trimester for the same contrast in distance categories was associated with over twice the odds of having a child with autism (95% CI 1.16–4.42). Intermediate distances did not show associations with autism, nor did proximity to smaller roadways, which is consistent with high concentration of pollutants near major freeways and decline in particulate matter to background levels beyond 300 meters from a major freeway. Given that socio-demographic factors were adjusted for, these results suggest that chemicals in air pollution may account for the observed association. Further analyses utilizing estimates of traffic-related pollution using the CALINE4 line-source air-quality dispersion model, and regional air pollutant measures based on EPA's Air Quality System data, also demonstrated significant associations with autism (Volk et al., in press).

Thus, a growing body of work suggests potential associations between air pollutants and autism risk. Air pollution is a highly complex and variable mixture of particles of different sizes, metals, and volatile organic compounds. Identifying the specific constituents responsible for the association is a challenge due to the high correlation among the HAPs.

The associations seen between chemicals in air pollution and autism may act through a number of potential biological pathways. Studies have shown alterations in blood–brain barrier signaling through oxidative stress and inflammation in mice exposed to diesel particulates (Hartz et al., 2008), suggesting the potential for an immune-mediated pathway or for more direct effects on neural development. Rats exposed prenatally to ozone, benzo[a]pyrene, and other HAPs have been found to have a range of neurological aberrations with relevance to autism, including alterations in neural circuitry, decreased neuronal plasticity, reduced glutamate receptor development, reduced expression of serotonin receptors, and behavioral deficits (Bouayed et al., 2009; Brown et al. 2007).

Endocrine disruption may also be a pathway for a HAP–autism association, as many of the chemicals identified in air pollution, including diesel particulates, mercury, and other metals, have been shown to influence levels of thyroid hormone (Tasker et al., 2005). Continued research investigating specific air contaminants and air pollution generally is needed to confirm the relationship with autism and to elucidate potential etiological pathways of these associations.

SUMMARY AND FUTURE DIRECTIONS

The etiology of autism remains elusive, but growing evidence supports a role, in at least some cases, for maternal lifestyle factors, preconception or prenatal maternal nutrition, maternal infections and medications, and exposure to environmental chemicals such as constituents of ambient air pollution. It is evident that large gene–environment studies will be required to capture the complexity of this disorder, and that increased focus on identifying specific environmental factors and time periods is needed. It is also clear that there is no one cause of autism; rather, many environmental and genetic factors are likely involved, and the specific subsets of factors may be different for different individuals. Promising directions for future research include determination of critical etiological windows for environmental exposures (which likely vary by type of exposure), and continued investigation into maternal factors during the preconception, prenatal, and perinatal periods. Further, parallel mechanistic investigations are needed to unravel the pathways by which exogenous factors might alter the course of brain development and contribute to autism.

ACKNOWLEDGMENTS

This work was supported in part by NIH grants R01-ES015359, R01-ES020392, P01-ES011269, U.S. EPA grant #R833292. The Whiteley Center is gratefully acknowledged as the locus of a scholarly retreat where the review of literature that formed the basis for this chapter was initiated.

References

Albuquerque, C.A., Smith, K.R., Johnson, C., et al., 2004. Influence of maternal tobacco smoking during pregnancy on uterine, umbilical and fetal cerebral artery blood flows. Early Human Development 80, 31–42.

Amaral, D.G., Schumann, C.M., Nordahl, C.W., 2008. Neuroanatomy of autism. Trends in Neurosciences 31, 137–145.

Barak, Y., Ring, A., Sulkes, J., et al., 1995. Season of birth and autistic disorder in Israel. American Journal of Psychiatry 152, 798–800.

Barr, D.B., Olsson, A.O., Wong, L.Y., et al., 2010. Urinary concentrations of metabolites of pyrethroid insecticides in the general U.S. population: National Health and Nutrition Examination Survey 1999-2002. Environmental Health Perspectives 118, 742–748.

Boas, M., Feldt-Rasmussen, U., Main, K.M., 2011. Thyroid effects of endocrine disrupting chemicals. Molecular and Cellular Endocrinology.

Boksa, P., 2010. Effects of prenatal infection on brain development and behavior: A review of findings from animal models. Brain, Behavior, and Immunity 24, 881–897.

Bouayed, J., Desor, F., Rammal, H., et al., 2009. Effects of lactational exposure to benzo[alpha]pyrene (B[alpha]P) on postnatal neurodevelopment, neuronal receptor gene expression and behaviour in mice. Toxicology 259, 97–106.

Braunschweig, D., Ashwood, P., Krakowiak, P., Hertz-Picciotto, I., Hansen, R., Croen, L.A., et al., 2008. Autism: Maternally derived antibodies specific for fetal brain proteins. Neurotoxicology 29, 226–231.

Brown Jr., J.S., 2009. Effects of bisphenol-A and other endocrine disruptors compared with abnormalities of schizophrenia: An endocrine-disruption theory of schizophrenia. Schizophr Bull 35, 256–278.

Brown, L.A., Khousbouei, H., Goodwin, J.S., et al., 2007. Down-regulation of early ionotrophic glutamate receptor subunit developmental expression as a mechanism for observed plasticity deficits following gestational exposure to benzo(a)pyrene. Neurotoxicology 28, 965–978.

Button, T.M., Maughan, B., McGuffin, P., 2007. The relationship of maternal smoking to psychological problems in the offspring. Early Human Development 83, 727–732.

Casanova, M.F., 2007. The neuropathology of autism. Brain Pathology 17, 422–433.

Cheslack-Postava, K., Liu, K., Bearman, P.S., 2011. Closely spaced pregnancies are associated with increased odds of autism in California sibling births. Pediatrics 127, 246–253.

Chess, S., 1971. Autism in children with congenital rubella. Journal of Autism Child Schizophrenin 1, 33–47.

Chess, S., Fernandez, P., Korn, S., 1978. Behavioral consequences of congenital rubella. Journal of Pediatrics 93, 699–703.

Conde-Agudelo, A., Rosas-Bermúdez, A., Kafury-Goeta, A.C., 2006. Birth spacing and risk of adverse perinatal outcomes: A meta-analysis. Journal of the American Medical Association 295, 1809–1823.

Croen, L.A., Grether, J.K., Yoshida, C.K., et al., 2011. Antidepressant use during pregnancy and childhood autism spectrum disorders. Archives of General Psychiatry 68, 1104–1112.

Czeizel, A.E., 2000. Primary prevention of neural-tube defects and some other major congenital abnormalities: Recommendations for the appropriate use of folic acid during pregnancy. Paediatric Drugs 2, 437–449.

Daniels, J.L., Forssen, U., Hultman, C.M., et al., 2008. Parental psychiatric disorders associated with autism spectrum disorders in the offspring. Pediatrics 121, e1357–e1362.

Deykin, E.Y., MacMahon, B., 1980. Pregnancy, delivery, and neonatal complications among autistic children. American Journal of Diseases of Children 134, 860–864.

Ehlers, S., Gillberg, C., Wing, L., 1999. A screening questionnaire for Asperger syndrome and other high-functioning autism spectrum disorders in school age children. Journal of Autism and Developmental Disorders 29, 129–141.

Eliasen, M., Tolstrup, J.S., Nybo Andersen, A.M., et al., 2010. Prenatal alcohol exposure and autistic spectrum disorders – a population-based prospective study of 80,552 children and their mothers. International Journal of Epidemiology 39, 1074–1081.

Engel, S.M., Wetmur, J., Chen, J., et al., 2011. Prenatal exposure to organophosphates, paraoxonase 1, and cognitive development in childhood. Environmental Health Perspectives 119, 1182–1188.

Eskenazi, B., Marks, A.R., Bradman, A., et al., 2007. Organophosphate pesticide exposure and neurodevelopment in young Mexican-American children. Environmental Health Perspectives 115, 792–798.

Fergusson, D.M., Woodward, L.J., Horwood, L.J., 1998. Maternal smoking during pregnancy and psychiatric adjustment in late adolescence. Archives of General Psychiatry 55, 721–727.

Fernández-Gonzalez, R., Moreira, P., Bilbao, A., et al., 2004. Long-term effect of *in vitro* culture of mouse embryos with serum on mRNA expression of imprinting genes, development, and behavior. Proceedings of the National Academy of Sciences of the USA 101, 5880–5885.

Folstein, S., Rutter, M., 1977. Infantile autism: A genetic study of 21 twin pairs. Journal of Child Psychology and Psychiatry 18, 297–321.

Fombonne, E., 2009. Epidemiology of pervasive developmental disorders. Pediatric Research 65, 591–598.

Frederiksen, M., Vorkamp, K., Thomsen, M., et al., 2009. Human internal and external exposure to PBDEs – a review of levels and sources. International Journal of Hygiene and Environmental Health 212, 109–134.

Gardener, H., Spiegelman, D., Buka, S., 2009. Prenatal risk factors for autism: Comprehensive meta-analysis. British Journal of Psychiatry 195, 7–14.

Gascon, M., Vrijheid, M., Martínez, D., et al., 2011. Effects of pre- and postnatal exposure to low levels of polybromodiphenyl ethers on neurodevelopment and thyroid hormone levels at 4 years of age. Environment International 37, 605–611, doi: 10.1016/j.envint.2010.12.005.

Gee, J.R., Moser, V.C., 2008. Acute postnatal exposure to brominated diphenylether 47 delays neuromotor ontogeny and alters motor activity in mice. Neurotoxicology and Teratology 30, 79–87.

Gillberg, C., Gillberg, C., 1983. Infantile autism: A total population study of reduced optimality in the pre-, peri-, and neonatal period. Journal of Autism and Developmental Disorders 13, 153–166.

Goldey, E.S., Crofton, K.M., 1998. Thyroxine replacement attenuates hypothyroxinemia, hearing loss, and motor deficits following developmental exposure to Aroclor 1254 in rats. Toxicology Science 45, 94–105.

Habek, D., Kovacevic, M., 2011. Adverse pregnancy outcomes and long-term morbidity after early fetal hypokinesia in maternal smoking pregnancies. Archives of Gynecology and Obstetrics 283, 491–495.

Hallmayer, J., Cleveland, S., Torres, A., Phillips, J., Cohen, B., Torigoe, T., et al., 2011. Genetic heritability and shared environmental factors among twin pairs with autism. Archives of General Psychiatry.

Harari, R., Julvez, J., Murata, K., et al., 2010. Neurobehavioral deficits and increased blood pressure in school-age children prenatally exposed to pesticides. Environmental Health Perspectives 118, 890–896.

Hartz, A.M., Bauer, B., Block, M.L., et al., 2008. Diesel exhaust particles induce oxidative stress, proinflammatory signaling, and P-glyco-protein up-regulation at the blood-brain barrier. FASEB Journal 22, 2723–2733.

Herbstman, J.B., Sjödin, A., Kurzon, M., et al., 2010. Prenatal exposure to PBDEs and neurodevelopment. Environmental Health Perspectives 118, 712–719.

Hertz-Picciotto, I., Bergman, A., Fängström, B., et al., 2011. Polybrominated diphenyl ethers in relation to autism and developmental delay: A case-control study. Environmental Health 10, 1.

Hertz-Picciotto, I., Croen, L.A., Hansen, R., Jones, C.R., van de Water, J., Pessah, I.N., 2006. The CHARGE study: An epidemiologic investigation of genetic and environmental factors contributing to autism. Environmental Health Perspectives 114, 1119–1125.

Hertz-Picciotto, I., Delwiche, L., 2009. The rise in autism and the role of age at diagnosis. Epidemiology 20, 84–90.

Hertz-Picciotto, I., Park, H.Y., Dostal, M., et al., 2008. Prenatal exposures to persistent and non-persistent organic compounds and effects on immune system development. Basic & Clinical Pharmacology & Toxicology 102, 146–154.

Hertz-Picciotto, I, Tassone, F, Delwiche, L, Hansen, R, Pessah, I. Autism in relation to early life pyrethrin or pyrethroid exposures, and interaction with MAOA genotype. In review.

Hougaard, K.S., Jensen, K.A., Nordly, P., et al., 2008. Effects of prenatal exposure to diesel exhaust particles on postnatal development, behavior, genotoxicity and inflammation in mice. Particle and Fibre Toxicology 5, 3.

Hultman, C.M., Sparén, P., Cnattingius, S., et al., 2002. Perinatal risk factors for infantile autism. Epidemiology 13, 417–423.

Hvidtjørn, D., Grove, J., Schendel, D., Schieve, L.A., Sværke, C., Ernst, E., et al., 2011. Risk of autism spectrum disorders in children born after assisted conception: A population-based follow-up study. Journal of Epidemiology & Community Health 65, 497–502.

Hvidtjørn, D., Schieve, L., Schendel, D., Jacobsson, B., Sværke, C., Thorsen, P., 2009. Cerebral palsy, autism spectrum disorders, and developmental delay in children born after assisted conception: A systematic review and meta-analysis. Archives of Pediatrics & Adolescent Medicine 163, 72–83.

Indredavik, M.S., Brubakk, A.-M., Romundstad, P., et al., 2007. Prenatal smoking exposure and psychiatric symptoms in adolescence. Acta Paediatrica 96, 377–382.

Institute of Medicine, 1990. Nutrition during Pregnancy 1990. National Academy Press, Washington, DC.

Jacobson, J.L., Jacobson, S.W., 2002. Effects of prenatal alcohol exposure on child development. Alcohol Research and Health 26, 282–286.

James, S.J., Melnyk, S., Jernigan, S., et al., 2010. A functional polymorphism in the reduced folate carrier gene and DNA hypomethylation in mothers of children with autism. American Journal of Medical Genetics Part B: Neuropsychiatric Genetics 153B, 1209–1220.

Julvez, J., Fortuny, J., Mendez, M., 2009. Maternal use of folic acid supplements during pregnancy and four-year-old neurodevelopment in a population-based birth cohort. Paediatric and Perinatal Epidemiology 23, 199–206.

Kalkbrenner, A.E., Daniels, J.L., Chen, J.C., et al., 2010. Perinatal exposure to hazardous air pollutants and autism spectrum disorders at age 8. Epidemiology 21, 631–641.

Kimura-Kuroda, J., Nagata, I., Kuroda, Y., 2007. Disrupting effects of hydroxy-polychlorinated biphenyl (PCB) congeners on neuronal development of cerebellar Purkinje cells: A possible causal factor for developmental brain disorders? Chemosphere 67, S412–S420.

King, M., Bearman, P., 2009. Diagnostic change and the increased prevalence of autism. International Journal of Epidemiology 38, 1224–1234.

Kolevzon, A., Weiser, M., Gross, R., et al., 2006. Effects of season of birth on autism spectrum disorders: Fact or fiction? American Journal of Psychiatry 163, 1288–1290.

Korrick, S.A., Sagiv, S.K., 2008. Polychlorinated biphenyls, organochlorine pesticides and neurodevelopment. Current Opinion in Pediatrics 20, 198–204.

Landau, E.C., Cicchetti, D.V., Klin, A., et al., 1999. Season of birth in autism: A fiction revisited. Journal of Autism and Developmental Disorders 29, 385–393.

Larsson, H.J., Eaton, W.W., Madsen, K.M., Vestergaard, M., Olesen, A.V., Agerbo, E., et al., 2005. Risk factors for autism: Perinatal factors, parental psychiatric history, and socioeconomic status. American Journal of Epidemiology 161, 916–925. discussion 926–918.

Larsson, M., Weiss, B., Janson, S., et al., 2009. Associations between indoor environmental factors and parental-reported autistic spectrum disorders in children 6-8 years of age. Neurotoxicology 30, 822–831.

Lawrence, L.J., Casida, J.E., 1983. Stereospecific action of pyrethroid insecticides on the gamma-aminobutyric acid receptor-ionophore complex. Science 221, 1399–1401.

Lotter, V., 1966. Epidemiology of autistic conditions in young children: Some characteristics of the parents and children. Social Psychiatry 1, 124–137.

Luck, W., Nau, H., Hansen, R., et al., 1985. Extent of nicotine and cotinine transfer to the human fetus, placenta and amniotic fluid of smoking mothers. Dev Pharmacol Therapy 8, 384–395.

Lyall, K., Pauls, D.L., Santangelo, S.L., et al., 2012. (Manuscript accepted for publication) Infertility and fertility therapies in association with autism spectrum disorders in children of the Nurses' Health Study II. Paediatric and Perinatal Epidemiology.

Maimburg, R.D., Vaeth, M., 2006. Perinatal risk factors and infantile autism. Acta Psychiatrica Scandinavica 114, 257–264.

Malaviya, M., Husain, R., Seth, P.K., et al., 1993. Perinatal effects of two pyrethroid insecticides on brain neurotransmitter function in the neonatal rat. Veterinary & Human Toxicology 35, 119–122.

Masuda, Y., 1985. Health status of Japanese and Taiwanese after exposure to contaminated rice oil. Environmental Health Perspectives 60, 321–325.

Masuo, Y., Morita, M., Oka, S., et al., 2004. Motor hyperactivity caused by a deficit in dopaminergic neurons and the effects of endocrine disruptors: A study inspired by the physiological roles of PACAP in the brain. Regulatory Peptides 123, 225–234.

Matsuishi, T., Yamashita, Y., Ohtani, Y., et al., 1999. Brief report: Incidence of and risk factors for autistic disorder in neonatal intensive care unit survivors. Journal of Autism and Developmental Disorders 29, 161–166.

Miles, J.H., Takahashi, T.N., Haber, A., Hadden, L., 2003. Autism families with a high incidence of alcoholism. Journal of Autism and Developmental Disorders 33, 403–415.

Milman, N., Byg, K.E., Hvas, A.M., et al., 2006. Erythrocyte folate, plasma folate and plasma homocysteine during normal pregnancy and postpartum: A longitudinal study comprising 404 Danish women. European Journal of Haematology 76, 200–205.

Mitra, P.S., Ghosh, S., Zang, S., et al., 2012. Analysis of the toxicogenomic effects of exposure to persistent organic pollutants (POPs) in Slovakian girls: Correlations between gene expression and disease risk. Environment International 39, 188–199.

Moore, S.J., Turnpenny, P., Quinn, A., et al., 2000. A clinical study of 57 children with fetal anticonvulsant syndromes. Journal of Medical Genetics 37, 489–497.

Mouridsen, S.E., Nielsen, S., Rich, B., et al., 1994. Season of birth in infantile autism and other types of childhood psychoses. Child Psychiatry & Human Development 25, 31–43.

MRC Vitamin Study Research Group, 1991. Prevention of neural tube defects: Results of the Medical Research Council Vitamin Study. Lancet 338, 131–137.

Muneoka, K., Ogawa, T., Kamei, K., et al., 2001. Nicotine exposure during pregnancy is a factor which influences serotonin transporter density in the rat brain. European Journal of Pharmacology 411, 279–282.

Needleman, H.L., Leviton, A., 1979. Neurologic effects of exposure to lead. Journal of Pediatrics 94, 505–506.

Nijmeijer, J.S., Hartman, C.A., Rommelse, N.N., et al., 2010. Perinatal risk factors interacting with catechol O-methyltransferase and the serotonin transporter gene predict ASD symptoms in children with ADHD. Journal of Child Psychology and Psychiatry 51, 1242–1250.

Norman, E.H., Hertz-Picciotto, I., Salmen, D.A., et al., 1997. Childhood lead poisoning and vinyl miniblind exposure. Archives of Pediatrics & Adolescent Medicine 151, 1033–1037.

O'Rourke, K.M., Redlinger, T.E., Waller, D.K., 2000. Declining levels of erythrocyte folate during the postpartum period among Hispanic women living on the Texas-Mexico border. Journal of Women's Health and Gender-Based Medicine 9, 397–403.

Palmer, R.F., Blanchard, S., Wood, R., 2009. Proximity to point sources of environmental mercury release as a predictor of autism prevalence. Health Place 15, 18–24.

Parent, A.S., Naveau, E., Gerard, A., et al., 2011. Early developmental actions of endocrine disruptors on the hypothalamus, hippocampus, and cerebral cortex. Journal of Toxicology and Environmental Health Part B: Critical Reviews 14, 328–345.

Park, H.Y., Hertz-Picciotto, I., Sovcikova, E., et al., 2010. Neurodevelopmental toxicity of prenatal polychlorinated biphenyls (PCBs) by chemical structure and activity: A birth cohort study. Environmental Health 9, 51.

Park, H.Y., Park, J.S., Sovcikova, E., et al., 2009. Exposure to hydroxylated polychlorinated biphenyls (OH-PCBs) in the prenatal period and subsequent neurodevelopment in eastern Slovakia. Environmental Health Perspectives 117, 1600–1606.

Picciano, M.F., 2003. Pregnancy and lactation: Physiological adjustments, nutritional requirements and the role of dietary supplements. Journal of Nutrition 133, 1997S–2002S.

Piven, J., Simon, J., Chase, G.A., Wzorek, M., Landa, R., Gayle, J., et al., 1993. The etiology of autism: Pre-, peri-, and neonatal factors. Journal of the American Academy of Child and Adolescent Psychiatry 32, 1256–1263.

Pocar, P., Fiandanese, N., Secchi, C., et al., 2011. Exposure to di(2-ethyl-hexyl) phthalate (DEHP) *in utero* and during lactation causes long-term pituitary-gonadal axis disruption in male and female mouse offspring. Endocrinology. 153 [E pub a head of print].

Rasalam, A.D., Hailey, H., Williams, J.H., et al., 2005. Characteristics of fetal anticonvulsant syndrome associated autistic disorder. Developmental Medicine & Child Neurology 47, 551–555.

Roberts, E.M., English, P.B., Grether, J.K., et al., 2007. Maternal residence near agricultural pesticide applications and autism spectrum disorders among children in the California Central Valley. Environmental Health Perspectives 115, 1482–1489.

Rose, M., Bennett, D.H., Bergman, A., et al., 2010. PBDEs in 2-5 year-old children from California and associations with diet and indoor environment. Environmental Science & Technology 44, 2648–2653.

Roy, T.S., Sabherwal, U., 1998. Effects of gestational nicotine exposure on hippocampal morphology. Neurotoxicology and Teratology 20, 465–473.

Roza, S.J., van Batenburg-Eddes, T., Steegers, E.A., Jaddoe, V.W., Mackenbach, J.P., Hofman, A., et al., 2010. Maternal folic acid supplement use in early pregnancy and child behavioural problems: The Generation R Study. British Journal of Nutrition 103, 445–452.

Roze, E., Meijer, L., Bakker, A., et al., 2009. Prenatal exposure to organohalogens, including brominated flame retardants, influences motor, cognitive, and behavioral performance at school age. Environmental Health Perspectives 117, 1953–1958.

Sagiv, S.K., Thurston, S.W., Bellinger, D.C., et al., 2010. Prenatal organochlorine exposure and behaviors associated with attention deficit hyperactivity disorder in school-aged children. American Journal of Epidemiology 171, 593–601.

Sagiv, S.K., Thurston, S.W., Bellinger, D.C., et al., 2012. Neuropsychological measures of attention and impulse control among 8-year-old children exposed prenatally to organochlorines. Environmental Health Perspectives [E pub a head of print].

Sato, A., Otsu, E., Negishi, H., et al., 2007. Aberrant DNA methylation of imprinted loci in superovulated oocytes. Human Reproduction 22, 26–35.

Schanen, N.C., 2006. Epigenetics of autism spectrum disorders. Human Molecular Genetics (15 Spec. No 2), R138–R150.

Schlotz, W., Jones, A., Phillips, D.I., et al., 2010. Lower maternal folate status in early pregnancy is associated with childhood hyperactivity and peer problems in offspring. Journal of Child Psychology and Psychiatry 51, 594–602.

Schmidt, R.J., Hansen, R.L., Hartiala, J., et al., 2011. Prenatal vitamins, one-carbon metabolism gene variants, and risk for autism. Epidemiology 22, 476–485.

Schmidt, R.J., Tancredi, D.J., Ozonoff, S., et al., 2012. Maternal periconceptional folic acid intake and risk of autism spectrum disorders and developmental delay in the CHARGE (CHildhood Autism Risks from Genetics and Environment) case-control study. American Journal of Clinical Nutrition 96, 80–89.

Secretariat of the Stockholm Convention, 2009. Measures to reduce or eliminate POPs. Available at: http://www.pops.int Retrieved June 12, 2009. Geneva.

Shafer, T.J., Meyer, D.A., Crofton, K.M., 2005. Developmental neurotoxicity of pyrethroid insecticides: Critical review and future research needs. Environmental Health Perspectives 113, 123–136.

Smith, S.E., Li, J., Garbett, K., et al., 2007. Maternal immune activation alters fetal brain development through interleukin-6. Journal of Neuroscience 27, 10,695–10,702.

Smits, L.J., Essed, G.G., 2001. Short interpregnancy intervals and unfavourable pregnancy outcome: Role of folate depletion. Lancet 358, 2074–2077.

Steegers-Theunissen, R.P., Obermann-Borst, S.A., Kremer, D., et al., 2009. Periconceptional maternal folic acid use of 400 microg per day is related to increased methylation of the IGF2 gene in the very young child. PLoS ONE 4, e7845.

Steffenburg, S., Gillberg, C., Hellgren, L., et al., 1989. A twin study of autism in Denmark, Finland, Iceland, Norway and Sweden. Journal of Child Psychology and Psychiatry 30, 405–416.

Stromland, K., Nordin, V., Miller, M., Akerstrom, B., Gillberg, C., 1994. Autism in thalidomide embryopathy: A population study. Developmental Medicine & Child Neurology 36, 351–356.

Suvorov, A., Girard, S., Lachapelle, S., Abdelouahab, N., Sebire, G., Takser, L., 2009. Perinatal exposure to low-dose BDE-47, an emergent environmental contaminant, causes hyperactivity in rat offspring. Neonatology 95, 203–209.

Sweeten, T.L., Posey, D.J., McDougle, C.J., 2004. Brief report: Autistic disorder in three children with cytomegalovirus infection. Journal of Autism and Developmental Disorders 34, 583–586.

Tasker, L., Mergler, D., Baldwin, M., et al., 2005. Thyroid hormones in pregnancy in relation to environmental exposure to organochlorine compounds and mercury. Environmental Health Perspectives 113, 1039–1045.

Thomas, P., Zahorodny, W., Peng, B., et al., 2011. The association of autism diagnosis with socioeconomic status. Autism 16, 201–213.

United States Environmental Protection Agency, 2012. Pyrethroids and Pyrethrins. Available at:http://www.epa.gov/oppsrrd1/reevaluation/pyrethroids-pyrethrins.html Retrieved January 2012.

van Eijsden, M., Smits, L.J., van der Wal, M.F., et al., 2008. Association between short interpregnancy intervals and term birth weight: The role of folate depletion. American Journal of Clinical Nutrition 88, 147–153.

Verner, M.A., Plusquellec, P., Muckle, G., et al., 2010. Alteration of infant attention and activity by polychlorinated biphenyls: Unravelling critical windows of susceptibility using physiologically based pharmacokinetic modeling. Neurotoxicology 31, 424–431.

Viberg, H., Mundy, W., Eriksson, P., 2008. Neonatal exposure to decabrominated diphenyl ether (PBDE 209) results in changes in BDNF, CaMKII and GAP-43, biochemical substrates of neuronal survival, growth, and synaptogenesis. Neurotoxicology 29, 152–159.

Volk, H.E., Hertz-Picciotto, I., Delwiche, L., et al., 2011. Residential proximity to freeways and autism in the CHARGE study. Environmental Health Perspectives 119, 873–877.

Volk, H.E; Lurmann, F; Penfold, B; Hertz-Picciotto, I; McConnell, R; Traffic related air pollution, particulate matter, and autism. Archives of General Psychiatry. In press.

Wallace, A., Anderson, G., Dubrow, R., 2008. Obstetric and parental psychiatric variables as potential predictors of autism severity. Journal of Autism and Developmental Disorders 38, 1542–1554.

Wilhelm, M., Wittsiepe, J., Lemm, F., et al., 2008. The Duisburg birth cohort study: Influence of the prenatal exposure to PCDD/Fs and dioxin-like PCBs on thyroid hormone status in newborns and neurodevelopment of infants until the age of 24 months. Mutation Research 659, 83–92.

Williams, G.M., O'Callaghan, M., Najman, J.M., et al., 1998. Maternal cigarette smoking and child psychiatric morbidity: A longitudinal study. Pediatrics 102, e11.

Windham, G.C., Zhang, L., Gunier, R., et al., 2006. Autism spectrum disorders in relation to distribution of hazardous air pollutants in the San Francisco Bay area. Environmental Health Perspectives 114, 1438–1444.

Wong, P.W., Joy, R.M., Albertson, T.E., et al., 1997. Ortho-substituted 2,2′,3,5′,6-pentachlorobiphenyl (PCB 95) alters rat hippocampal ryanodine receptors and neuroplasticity in vitro: Evidence for altered hippocampal function. Neurotoxicology 18, 443–456.

Yamashita, Y., Fujimoto, C., Nakajima, E., et al., 2003. Possible association between congenital cytomegalovirus infection and autistic disorder. Journal of Autism and Developmental Disorders 33, 455–459.

Zerbo, O., Iosif, A.M., Delwiche, L., et al., 2011. Month of conception and risk of autism. Epidemiology 22, 469–475.

Zerbo, O., Iosif, A.M., Walker, C., Ozonoff, S., Hansen, R.L., Hertz-Picciotto, I., 2012. Is maternal influenza or fever during pregnancy associated with autism or developmental delays? Results from the CHARGE Study. Journal of Autism and Developmental Disorders [E pub ahead of print].

Zhou, T., Taylor, M.M., DeVito, M.J., et al., 2002. Developmental exposure to brominated diphenyl ethers results in thyroid hormone disruption. Toxicology Science 66, 105–116.

Zhu, B.P., 2005. Effect of interpregnancy interval on birth outcomes: Findings from three recent US studies. International Journal of Gynecology & Obstetrics 89, S25–S33.

Hormonal Influences in Typical Development: Implications for Autism

Bonnie Auyeung, Simon Baron-Cohen

Autism Research Centre, Department of Psychiatry, University of Cambridge, Cambridge, UK

OUTLINE

SEX BIASES IN CLINICAL CONDITIONS

Many clinical conditions occur in males more often than females, including autism, dyslexia, specific language impairment, attention-deficit hyperactivity disorder (ADHD), and early-onset persistent antisocial behavior (Rutter et al., 2003). Depression, anorexia, and anxiety disorders tend to show a female bias in sex ratio, raising the question of whether there are sex-linked or sex-limiting factors involved in the etiology of conditions that do exhibit a sex bias.

Autism, high-functioning autism, Asperger syndrome, and Pervasive Developmental Disorder (not otherwise specified; PDD-NOS) are here referred to as Autism

The Neuroscience of Autism Spectrum Disorders.
http://dx.doi.org/10.1016/B978-0-12-391924-3.00015-6

Spectrum Conditions (ASC)[1], and are considered to lie on the same continuum. Individuals with an ASC diagnosis are impaired in reciprocal social interaction and communication, and show strongly repetitive behaviors and unusually narrow interests (APA, 1994). The prevalence of ASC in children is estimated to be 116.1 per 10,000 (Baird et al., 2006) and 94 per 10,000 (Baird et al., 2006; Baron-Cohen et al., 2009) in two British populations. A large multi-center regional study in North America has estimated the prevalence of ASC to be approximately 91 per 10,000 (Autism and Developmental Disabilities Monitoring Network Surveillance Year 2006 Principal Investigators, Centers for Disease Control and Prevention, 2009). There is also a clear male to female ratio in ASC, estimated at 4:1 for classic autism (Chakrabarti and Fombonne, 2005) and as high as 10.8:1 in individuals with Asperger Syndrome (Gillberg et al., 2006).

The striking sex ratio in ASC might reflect difficulties in the diagnosis of ASC in females (Ernsperger et al., 2007; Lai et al., 2011), however, this is unlikely to account for the male sex bias entirely and instead it may provide important clues to the etiology of the condition (Baron-Cohen et al., 2005; Baron-Cohen, 2002). ASC have strong neurobiological and genetic components (Geschwind, 2009; Stodgell et al., 2001), however the specific factors (hormonal, genetic, or environmental) that are responsible for the higher male prevalence in the conditions remain unclear. Recent evidence is consistent with the idea that sex steroid hormones, and in particular, prenatal exposure to testosterone, is related to the development of autistic traits (Baron-Cohen et al., 2004).

ASC in particular has been described as an extreme manifestation of certain sexually dimorphic traits or a consequence of an 'extreme male brain' (EMB) (Baron-Cohen et al., 2005; Baron-Cohen, 2002). Hormones have been shown to have a clear role in physical and behavioral sexual differentiation (Hines, 2004). In this chapter, we review evidence suggesting a role for prenatal exposure to hormones in the development of cognitive sex differences and traits associated with ASC, and we consider future directions.

TYPICAL SEX DIFFERENCES AND ASC

It is widely accepted that males and females show significant differences in their neuroanatomy, cognition and behavior from an early age. In early development, female infants show a stronger preference for looking at social stimuli (faces) from 24 hours after birth (Connellan et al., 2000). Girls also make more eye contact immediately after birth (Hittelman and Dickes, 1979), at 12 months of age (Lutchmaya et al., 2002a) and at 2 and 4 years of age (Podrouzek and Furrow, 1988). Studies examining play preferences point towards more interest in mechanical and constructional play in boys, demonstrated by a preference for playing with toy vehicles or construction sets, while girls are more likely to choose to play with dolls or toy animals (Berenbaum and Hines, 1992; Liss, 1979; Servin et al., 1999; Smith and Daglish, 1977). In addition, sex differences in spatial ability favoring males have been found in infants as young as 3–4 months of age (Quinn and Liben, 2008) and 5 months of age (Moore and Johnson, 2008) and remain consistent throughout development (Voyer et al., 1995).

The EMB theory of ASC was first defined using evidence from psychological measures, and proposes that individuals with ASC are impaired in empathy (the drive to identify another person's emotions and thoughts, and to respond to these with an appropriate emotion), while being average or even superior in systemizing (the drive to analyze, explore and construct a system). The Empathy Quotient (EQ) and Systemizing Quotient (SQ) were developed in order to examine trends in gender-typical behavior (Baron-Cohen et al., 2003; Baron-Cohen and Wheelwright, 2004). Findings from the EQ in children and adults have shown that on average females score significantly higher than males (Auyeung et al., 2009; Baron-Cohen and Wheelwright, 2004; Carroll and Chiew, 2006; Wheelwright et al., 2006). SQ results indicate that on average males score significantly higher than females (Auyeung et al., 2009; Baron-Cohen et al., 2003; Carroll and Chiew, 2006; Wheelwright et al., 2006). Performance in individuals with ASC have shown an extreme of the typical male performance, with adults and children scoring lower than typical males on the EQ and higher than typical males on the SQ (Auyeung et al., 2009; Baron-Cohen et al., 2003; Baron-Cohen and Wheelwright, 2004; Wheelwright et al., 2006).

Using standardized scores on the EQ and SQ, a series of cognitive 'brain types' can be calculated, where individuals are described as being 'balanced' (Type B), better at empathy (Type E) or better at systemizing (Type S). 'Extreme' Type E (Extreme E) or Type S (Extreme S)

---

[1]The American Psychiatric Association uses the term ASD for Autism Spectrum Disorders. We prefer the use of the term ASC as those at the higher-functioning end of the autistic spectrum do not necessarily see themselves as having a 'disorder', and the profile of strengths and difficulties in ASC can be conceptualized as atypical but not necessarily disordered. ASC remains a medical diagnosis, hence the use of the term 'condition', which signals that such individuals need support. Use of the term ASC is we feel both more respectful to differences; recognizes that the profile in question does not fit a simple 'disease' model but includes areas of strength (e.g., in attention to detail) as well as areas of disability; and does not identify the individual purely in terms of the latter.

are also assigned, in which an individual shows a significantly larger discrepancy in a given direction (Goldenfeld et al., 2005; Wheelwright et al., 2006). Type S (S > E) is more common in males, while Type E (E > S) is more common in females. Extreme types are also found, and a large proportion of children (47.2%) and adults (61.6%) with ASC fall in the Extreme S (S >> E), compared to approximately 5% of typical males and 1% of typical females (Auyeung et al., 2009; Wheelwright et al., 2006).

Since specific normative sex differences appear exaggerated in autism, this suggests that mechanisms related to sexual differentiation may overlap with the mechanisms involved in autism. For example, in addition to findings using the EQ, individuals with ASC tend to show impairment in empathy-related tasks in which females score more highly, such as the 'Social Stories Questionnaire' (Lawson et al., 2004), the 'Reading the Mind in the Eyes' task (Baron-Cohen et al., 1997) and the recognition of 'faux pas' in short stories (Baron-Cohen et al., 1999). Adults with ASC score lower on the Friendship and Relationship Questionnaire, which assesses empathic styles of relationships (Baron-Cohen and Wheelwright, 2003). Children with autism perform less well than controls on the 'Feshbach and Powell Audiovisual Test for Empathy', a measure of empathy and emotional responsiveness (Yirmiya et al., 1992). Children with ASC also have more difficulties passing 'theory of mind' tests compared to typically developing children (Baron-Cohen, 1995; Baron-Cohen et al., 1985; Happé, 1995). Cognitive empathy (synonymous with 'mentalizing' or 'theory of mind') appears to be more universally impaired in ASC, whilst affective empathy may be intact (Dziobek et al., 2008), or may define a subgroup.

In non-social tasks, individuals with ASC are superior to typical controls on tasks that involve systemizing (Lawson et al., 2004) and on certain visuo-spatial tasks that normally give rise to male superiority, such as figure disembedding (Falter et al., 2008; Jolliffe and Baron-Cohen, 1997; Ropar and Mitchell, 2001; Shah and Frith, 1983), block design (Ropar and Mitchell, 2001; Shah and Frith, 1993) and mental rotation (Brosnan et al., 2009; Falter et al., 2008).

A study of toddlers as young as 14 months with an ASC spent significantly more time fixating on dynamic geometric images, whereas typically developing toddlers showed longer looking times at social stimuli. Further, if a toddler spent more than 69% of his or her time fixating on geometric patterns, then the positive predictive value for accurately classifying that toddler as having an ASD was 100% (Pierce et al., 2010). These findings suggest that these looking preferences can be found very early in life and used to differentiate toddlers with ASC from typically developing toddlers,

and again this data suggests an EMB profile in autism, since looking preferences show significant sex differences at birth (Connellan et al., 2000) and in the first year of life (Lutchmaya and Baron-Cohen, 2002).

However, the EMB theory does not apply to all measures showing a male advantage. For example, Falter et al., (2008) found that children with autism do not show superior performance on a measure of targeting ability compared to typically developing boys. It is possible that problems with motor coordination (dyspraxia) in the ASC group may have affected performance on this task (Knickmeyer et al., 2008). It is worth emphasizing that the EMB theory predicts intact or superior performance on measures of systemizing in ASC, and a discrepancy between an individual's empathy and systemizing abilities.

In addition to the evidence at the behavioral level, it has been suggested that characteristics of neurodevelopment in autism, such as larger overall brain volumes and greater growth of the amygdala during childhood may also represent an exaggeration of typical sex differences in brain development (Baron-Cohen et al., 2005). Studies using fMRI indicate that typical females show increased activity in the extrastriate cortex during the Embedded Figures Test and increased activity bilaterally in the inferior frontal cortex during the 'Reading the Mind in the Eyes' task. Parents of children with ASC also tend to show hyper-masculinization of brain activity, suggesting that hyper-masculinization may be part of the broader autism phenotype (Baron-Cohen et al., 2006). An extensive review of the EMB theory at both the behavioral and neural level can be found elsewhere (Baron-Cohen et al., 2005; 2011).

HUMAN BEHAVIORAL SEX DIFFERENCES AND EXPOSURE TO HORMONES

With regard to the effect of sex hormones, there is now considerable evidence from human and non-human studies that prenatal exposure to hormones can have lasting effects on later behavior and development. Hormones are essential for reproduction, growth and development, maintenance of the internal environment and the production, use and storage of energy (Knickmeyer and Baron-Cohen, 2006a). There are marked physical and behavioral consequences of exposure to hormones throughout life. Prenatally, the presence or absence of specific hormones (or their receptors) is essential for the sexual differentiation of the fetus (De Vries and Simerly, 2002; Ehrhardt and Meyer-Bahlburg, 1981; Goy and McEwen, 1980). In addition to stimulating the development of physical characteristics such as genitalia (Fuchs and Klopper,

1983; Hines, 2004; Kimura, 1999; Novy and Resko, 1981; Tulchinsky and Little, 1994), there is increasing evidence that prenatal hormones have a substantial effect on gender-typical aspects of behavior (Cohen-Bendahan et al., 2005; Hines, 2004). Sex hormones also have an epigenetic role in changing gene expression throughout development and likely interact with sex chromosome effects on sexual differentiation (McCarthy and Arnold, 2011; McCarthy et al., 2009).

Timing

The timing of hormonal effects is crucial when studying lasting effects on development. There are thought to be two general types of hormonal effect: organizational and activational (Phoenix et al., 1959). Organizational effects are most likely to occur during early development when most neural structures are being established, producing permanent changes in the brain (Phoenix et al., 1959), whereas activational effects are short term and are dependent on current hormone levels. Since many neurodevelopmental conditions are typically persistent with an early onset, any hormonal influence on the development of neurodevelopmental conditions such as ASC is likely to be organizational in nature.

It is widely thought that organizational effects are maximal during sensitive/critical periods of development. These are hypothetical windows of time in which a tissue can be formed (Hines, 2004). Outside the sensitive period, the effect of the hormone will be limited, protecting the animal from disruptive influences. This means, for example, that the circulating sex hormones necessary for adult sexual functioning do not cause unwanted alterations to tissues, even though the same hormones might have been essential in laying down cellular organization during the initial development of those tissues.

In animal models, the critical period for sexual differentiation of the brain occurs when differences between the sexes in serum testosterone are highest (Smith and Hines, 2000). Therefore it is likely that this is an important period for sexual differentiation of the human brain as well. For typical human males, there is believed to be a surge in fetal testosterone (fT) levels at around weeks 8–24 of gestation (Baron-Cohen et al., 2004; Collaer and Hines, 1995; Hines, 2004; Smail et al., 1981). During this period, male fetuses produce more than 2.5 times the levels observed in females (Beck-Peccoz et al., 1991). There is then a decline to barely detectable levels from the end of this period until birth. As a result, any effects of fT on development are most likely to take place during this period. For typical human females, levels are generally very low throughout pregnancy and childhood (Hines, 2004).

In addition to the fetal surge, two other periods of elevated testosterone have been observed in typical males. The first takes place shortly after birth and reaches a peak at approximately 3–4 months of age (Smail et al., 1981), after which measurements return to very low levels until puberty. Figure 2.8.1 shows the circulating levels of testosterone during the prenatal and neonatal period.

The role of prenatal hormone levels in the development of later behavior in non-human mammals has been explored in experiments comparing castrated males, normal males, normal females, and females treated with androgens. Castrated males usually show feminized neural development, cognition and behavior, while females treated with androgen show masculinized neural development, cognition and behavior in a number of species (Arnold and Gorski, 1984; Clark et al., 1996; Williams and Meck, 1991).

The direct manipulation of fT levels is not possible in humans for ethical reasons. The investigation of prenatal hormone exposure and its relation to development in humans has therefore been investigated in naturally occurring abnormal environments, such as in individuals with Congenital Adrenal Hyperplasia (CAH) – a genetic disorder that causes excess adrenal androgen production, beginning prenatally, in both males and females (New, 1998). Studies of individuals with CAH have generally found that girls with CAH show masculinization of performance in activities such as spatial orientation, visualization, targeting, personality, cognitive abilities and sexuality (Hampson et al., 1998; Hines et al., 2003; Resnick et al., 1986). Girls with CAH exhibit more autistic traits, measured using the Autism Spectrum Quotient (AQ), than their unaffected sisters (Knickmeyer et al., 2006). While CAH provides an interesting opportunity to investigate the effects of additional androgen exposure, the relatively rare occurrence of CAH in conjunction with ASC makes it difficult to obtain large enough sample sizes for generalization of research findings to the wider population. Researchers have also suggested that CAH-related disease characteristics, rather than prenatal androgen exposure, could be responsible for the atypical cognitive profiles observed in this population (Fausto-Sterling, 1992; Quadagno et al., 1977).

The ratio between the length of the 2nd and 4th digit (2D:4D) is sexually dimorphic, being lower in males than in females, and may be a useful proxy measure for fT production in humans during the first trimester of gestation (Manning et al., 1998). However, the use of this physical measurement has shown inconsistent results (Valla and Ceci, 2011).

Studies researching fetal hand development have observed the sex difference in 2D:4D ratio in fetuses between 9–40 weeks of gestation (Malas et al., 2006).

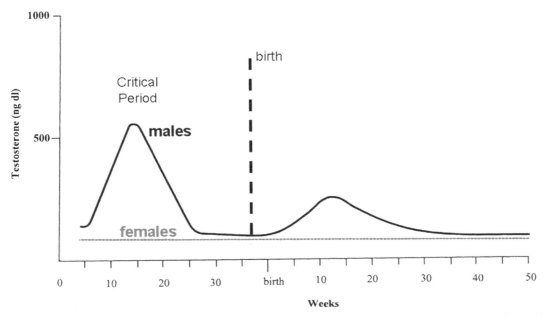

FIGURE 2.8.1 **Circulating levels of testosterone in the human fetus and neonate.** Note: Males (blue line) have higher levels of testosterone than females (red dashed line), particularly from about weeks 8–24 of gestation and weeks 2–26 of postnatal life. *Figure adapted from: Hines, (2004).*

2D:4D ratio has been found to be negatively associated with the ratio of fT to fetal estrogen (Lutchmaya et al., 2004). Lower (i.e., hyper-masculinized) digit ratios have been found in children with autism compared to typically developing children. This pattern was also found in the siblings and parents of children with autism, suggesting a genetic basis for the elevated fT levels in autism (Manning et al., 2001; Milne et al., 2006). If 2D:4D ratio does reflect prenatal exposure to testosterone, this evidence suggests children with ASC may have been exposed to higher than average levels of fT.

There is now substantial literature on the effect of prenatal (fetal) testosterone on postnatal development. Due to the dangers of directly sampling fetal hormone levels, these studies generally measure fT levels through amniocentesis samples, obtained for clinical purposes (e.g. in order to detect genetic abnormalities in the fetus). Amniocentesis is typically performed during a relatively narrow time window which is thought to coincide with the hypothesized critical period for human sexual differentiation (between approximately weeks 8 and 24 of gestation) (Hines, 2004). Human male and female fetuses produce testosterone, with male fetuses producing more than 2.5 times the levels observed in females (Beck-Peccoz et al., 1991). In early prenatal life, testosterone enters the amniotic fluid via diffusion through the fetal skin, and later enters the fluid via fetal urination (Robinson et al., 1977). Males are exposed to testosterone from the fetal adrenals and testes. The female fetus is also exposed

to androgens, but at lower levels. A small proportion may come from the fetal adrenals (a by-product of the production of corticosteroids) and some comes from the maternal adrenals, ovaries and fat (Martin, 1985). The underproduction of aromatase could also result in higher fT levels by impairing conversion of testosterone to estrogen (Abramovich, 1974). Dihydrotestosterone (DHT) is produced from testosterone and may be a stronger activator of the androgen receptor than testosterone itself. Therefore overproduction of 5α-reductase could also produce masculinization of certain characteristics (Larsen et al., 2002).

A number of studies have linked elevated levels of fT in the amniotic fluid with the masculinization of certain behaviors, beginning shortly after birth. fT levels in amniotic fluid are measured by radioimmunoassay. Amniotic fluid is extracted with diethylether.

THE ROLE OF FETAL TESTOSTERONE IN COGNITIVE SEX DIFFERENCES AND AUTISTIC TRAITS

The Cambridge Child Development Project is an ongoing longitudinal study investigating the relationship between prenatal hormone levels and the development of behaviors relating to ASC (Baron-Cohen et al., 2004; Knickmeyer and Baron-Cohen, 2006b). Mothers of participating children had all undergone amniocentesis for clinical reasons between 1996 and 2005 and gave birth to healthy singleton infants. To date, these children have been tested postnatally at several time points and the findings of these studies will now be discussed.

Eye Contact at 12 Months

Reduced eye contact is a characteristic common in children with autism (Lutchmaya et al., 2002a; Swettenham et al., 1998). The first study aimed to measure fT and estradiol levels in relation to eye contact in a sample of 70 typically developing, 12-month old children (Lutchmaya et al., 2002a). Frequency and duration of eye contact were measured using videotaped sessions. Sex differences were found, with girls making significantly more eye contact than boys. The amount of eye contact varied with fT levels when the sexes were combined. Within the sexes, a relationship was only found for boys (Lutchmaya et al., 2002a). No relationships were observed between the outcome and estradiol levels. Results were taken to indicate that fT may play a role in shaping the neural mechanisms underlying social development (Lutchmaya et al., 2002a).

Vocabulary Size at 18–24 Months

In some subgroups within ASC, such as classic autism, vocabulary development is also delayed (Rutter, 1978). Another study (of 87 children) focused on the relationship between vocabulary size in relation to fT and estradiol levels from amniocentesis. Vocabulary size was measured using the Communicative Development Inventory, which is a self-administered checklist of words for parents to complete (Hamilton et al., 2000). Girls were found to have significantly larger vocabularies than boys at both time points (Lutchmaya et al., 2002b). Results showed that levels of fT inversely predicted the rate of vocabulary development in typically developing children between the ages of 18 and 24 months (Lutchmaya et al., 2002b). Within sex analyses showed no significant relationships in boys or girls, which the authors believe may have been due to the relatively small sample sizes. No relationships between estradiol and vocabulary size were found. Despite the lack of significant results within sex, the significant findings in the combined sample suggest that fT may be involved in communicative development (Lutchmaya et al., 2002b).

Intentional Language at 4 Years

Thirty-eight children completed a 'moving geometric shapes' task at age 4 where they were asked to describe cartoons with two moving triangles whose interaction with each other suggested social relationships and psychological motivations (Knickmeyer et al., 2006).

Sex differences were observed with girls using more mental and affective state terms to describe the cartoons compared to boys, however no relationships between fT levels and mental or affective state terms were observed. Girls were found to use more intentional propositions than males, and a negative relationship between fT levels and frequency of intentional propositions was observed when the sexes were combined and in boys. Boys used more neutral propositions than females, and fT was related to the frequency of neutral propositions when the sexes were combined. However, no significant relationships were observed when boys and girls were examined separately. No relationships with estradiol were observed. These results are consistent with the EMB theory, since other studies have found that individuals with ASC show worse performance than typical males on a similar moving geometric shapes task (Klin, 2000).

Restricted Interests and Social Relationships at Age 4 Years

Individuals with ASC demonstrate more restricted interests as well as difficulties with social relationships (APA, 1994). A follow-up at 4 years of age in this cohort of children utilized the Children's Communication Checklist (Bishop, 1998). The quality of social relationships subscale demonstrated an association between higher fT levels and poorer quality of social relationships for both sexes combined but not individually. A lack of significant correlations within each sex was thought to be a result of the small sample size (n = 58).

Levels of fT were also associated with more narrow interests when the sexes were combined and in boys only (Knickmeyer et al., 2005). Sex differences were reported, with males scoring higher (i.e. having more narrow interests) than females (Knickmeyer et al., 2005).

Gender-Typical Play at 5–9 Years

Girls with ASC have been shown to exhibit a more masculinized play style, and that boys with ASC also show a play preference consistent with their sex (Knickmeyer et al., 2007). At 5 years of age, the mothers of the children were asked to complete a modified version of the Child Game Participation Questionnaire (Bates and Bentler, 1973). No significant relationship between levels of fT and game participation were observed when the entire group was included in the analysis, or when boys and girls were examined separately. These findings may reflect a relatively small sample size (n = 53) or perhaps an insufficiently sensitive behavioral measure. However, at 6–9 years of age, higher fT levels predicted more male-typical scores on the Pre-School Activities Inventory, which is a standardized questionnaire measure of gender-typical play in both boys and girls. This relationship was significant in both boys and girls (Auyeung et al., 2009).

Gender-Role Behavior at 6–9 Years

The Bem Sex Role Inventory is a questionnaire developed to measure feminine and masculine personality traits. The dimensions of Masculinity and Femininity are considered to be independent of each other (Bem, 1974). Items were selected as masculine or feminine on the basis of cultural definitions of sex-typed social desirability (Bem, 1974). Examination of scores on this measured showed that higher fT levels were associated with higher masculinity scores on the BSRI when boys and girls were examined together, and when girls were examined alone. No relationships were found between fT levels and scores on the femininity scale. Within sex results suggest that girls exposed to higher testosterone levels *in utero* are perceived as exhibiting more masculinized behavior (Auyeung, 2008). Therefore, these studies relating amniotic fluid testosterone to subsequent behavior may be useful for elucidating the role of prenatal hormonal exposure in gender-typical behavioral development.

Intelligence Quotient (IQ) and Block Design at 6–10 Years

The Wechsler Abbreviated Scale of Intelligence (WASI) was used to measure IQ (Wechsler, 1999). The WASI provides scores for Verbal IQ, Performance IQ and Full Scale IQ. The relationship between fT and the Block Design component of the WASI was investigated. Block Design performance shows sexual dimorphism in adulthood (male advantage) (Lynn, 1998; Lynn et al., 2005; Rönnlund and Nilsson, 2006). Individuals with ASC have also shown superior performance on this subscale (Happé, 1994; Shah and Frith, 1993). No significant sex-differences were found between boys and girls for Full Scale IQ, Performance IQ, Verbal IQ or Block Design scores. In addition, no significant correlations were found between fT levels and Full Scale IQ, Performance IQ, Verbal IQ and Block Design scores (Auyeung et al., 2009). These findings suggest that fT levels are not related to IQ and it would be beneficial for other studies to examine whether these results are replicated in larger samples and in different age groups.

Visuospatial Ability at 7–10 Years

The relationship between prenatal hormone levels measured from amniotic fluid (collected during the second trimester of pregnancy) and performance in three areas of visuospatial ability that have previously shown significant sex differences has been examined. EFT scores showed a clear advantage for boys, consistent with previous research showing superior male performance on this task (Nebot, 1988), although not all studies of this age group have found this sex difference (Bigelow, 1971). As previously mentioned, individuals with ASC perform better on this task compared to controls (Falter et al., 2008; Jolliffe and Baron-Cohen, 1997; Ropar and Mitchell, 2001; Shah and Frith, 1983). fT levels were found to be a significant predictor of EFT scores for all participants together and also when boys and girls were examined separately (Auyeung et al., 2012).

For the mental rotation test, a significant sex difference favoring males was found in the number of correct items the child attained. However, no significant relationship was observed between mental rotation ability and fT levels when all participants were examined together or when examined separately by sex or rotation strategy. In targeting ability no significant sex differences or associations with fT were found.

At first glance, all three of these tasks examine areas of visuospatial ability that have previously shown sex differences. However, the design of tasks for children is often very difficult. In the case of the EFT, the specific task used in this study has been widely employed and is non-computerized. The other tasks, however, were adapted versions of measures used by other researchers. The finding that amniotic fluid fT level was significantly related to EFT score but not the other tasks examined in this study also requires further investigation. These findings underline the importance of task method and participant selection, including factors such as control group used, age at testing, and sample sizes (for detailed reviews, see Hines, 2004; Puts et al., 2008).

Mind Reading at 6–9 Years

Mind reading is the ability to put oneself into the mind of another person and infer what the person is thinking or feeling. It is also referred to as theory of mind (Leslie, 1987) or mentalizing (Frith et al., 1991). The child version of the 'Reading the Mind in the Eyes' Test consists of 28 pictures of the eye region of the face, each depicting a mental state, including subtle emotions (Baron-Cohen et al., 2001). Results revealed a significant negative correlation with fT suggesting that higher levels predicted worse mind reading ability. Within sex analyses revealed there was also a significant negative correlation between fT and the eyes test for both boys and the girls (Chapman et al., 2006).

Empathy and Systemizing at 6–8 Years

Below average empathy, alongside an intact or strong drive to systemize appears to be characteristic of ASC (Baron-Cohen, 2002). Using the children's versions of the Systemizing Quotient (SQ-C) and Empathizing Quotient (EQ-C), boys scored higher than girls on the SQ-C, and levels of fT positively predicted SQ-C scores in boys and girls individually (Auyeung et al., 2006). Sex differences were observed in EQ-C scores, with girls scoring higher than boys. A significant negative correlation between fT levels and EQ-C was observed when the sexes were combined and within boys. For the EQ-C a main effect of sex was found, but no main effect of fT. However, the effect of fT cannot be disregarded, since sex and fT are strongly correlated (Chapman et al., 2006).

Autistic Traits in Toddlers at 18–24 Months

In light of the above results, a more direct approach to evaluating the links between autistic traits and fT was implemented. The relationships between fT levels, fetal estradiol (FE) levels and neonatal testosterone (NT) levels measured from saliva at 3–4 months of age, and their relationship to the development of autistic traits, measured using the Quantitative Checklist for Autism in Toddlers (Q-CHAT), were examined. The Q-CHAT revealed a significant sex difference in autistic traits, with boys scoring higher (indicating more autistic traits) than girls. Q-CHAT scores were predicted by fT levels only, with both Sex and the FT/Sex interaction excluded from the model (Auyeung et al., 2010).

The relationships between fT levels, FE levels, NT levels and autistic traits were investigated in a subset of children (n = 35). No relationships between FE, NT levels and Q-CHAT scores were observed. However, sample size for this study was small and it would be interesting to see if similar results were reported for larger sample sizes. In addition, FE and NT levels showed no sex differences or relationships with fT levels. A relationship between fT and Q-CHAT was also observed in this subset of children whose mothers agreed to bring their child in for salivary sample collection (Auyeung, 2008).

Autistic Traits at 6–9 Years of Age

In this study, effects of fT were directly evaluated against autistic traits as measured by the Childhood Autism Spectrum Test (CAST) (Scott et al., 2002; Williams et al., 2005) and the Child Autism Spectrum Quotient (AQ-Child) (Auyeung et al., 2008).

fT levels were positively associated with higher scores (indicating greater number of autistic traits) on the CAST as well as on the AQ-Child. For the AQ-Child, this relationship was seen within sex as well as when the sexes were combined, suggesting this is an effect of fT rather than an effect of sex. The relationship between CAST scores and fT was also seen within males, but not within females (Auyeung et al., 2009). These findings are consistent with the notion that higher levels of fT may be associated with the development of autistic traits.

SUMMARY OF THE CAMBRIDGE CHILD DEVELOPMENT PROJECT

Table 2.8.1 describes the measures used in the Cambridge Child Development Project to identify sex differences in behavior and the links with fT for boys and girls together. For each measure, Table 2.8.1 shows the direction of the sex differences (if present) and the effect size obtained in this sample, calculated using Cohen's d. The final columns indicate the correlation obtained with fT and whether fT levels (independent of sex) was a significant predictor in the regression analyses.

Within Sex Relationships

Levels of fT are typically much higher in boys than girls. If increased exposure to fT is sufficiently responsible for changes in sex-typical behavior, it may be possible to observe a link between behavior and fT level using within-sex analyses. Table 2.8.2 shows a summary of results within each sex for variables that demonstrated a significant correlation with fT in Table 2.8.1.

Table 2.8.2 shows that within sex correlations with fT levels were seen for most of the variables that show a sex difference. The table also shows that for the variables with larger sample sizes, within sex effects of fT were observed more often in girls than boys. Other studies have also reported relationships between fT and behavior in girls and not boys. The current findings are consistent with previous studies in samples such as CAH, which have generally found stronger correlations between hormone levels and male-typical behavior in girls rather than boys (Berenbaum and Hines, 1992; Berenbaum and Snyder, 1995; Berenbaum, 1999; Ehrhardt and Baker, 1974; Hines et al., 2004). An exception to this was found in earlier studies where the samples sizes were smaller as well as with the CAST scores that demonstrated a correlation in boys only.

Several reasons might account for the bias of within sex correlations towards girls. Females might be particularly sensitive to changes in fT level or androgen levels may need to be very high before sex-typed activity preference is masculinized in boys. It has also been proposed that elevated fT exposure may produce increased

TABLE 2.8.1 Cambridge Child Development Project Results

Characteristic	Measure	Child age	Sex diff.	Cohen's d	Correlation with FT	FT sig, predictor
Eye Contact	Frequency	12 months	Yes (F>M)	0.53	−0.30*	Yes
Vocabulary Size	Communicative Development Inventory	18–24 months	Yes (F>M)	0.66	−0.20	Yes
Intentional Language	Intentional Propositions	4 years	Yes (F>M)	0.62	—	Yes
Restricted Interests	Children's Communication Checklist	4 years	Yes (F<M)	0.64	—	Yes
Social Relationships	Children's Communication Checklist	4 years	Yes (F>M)	0.47	−0.30*	Yes
Gender-typical Play	Pre-School Activities Inventory	6–9 years	Yes (F<M)	2.79	0.63**	Yes
Gender-role Behavior	Bem Sex Role Inventory Femininity Total	6–9 years	Yes (F>M)	0.54	−0.05	—
	Bem Sex Role Inventory Masculinity Total		Yes (F<M)	0.35	0.27**	Yes
Full Scale IQ	WASI – Total	6–10 years	No	0.48	0.10	—
Block Design	WASI – Block Design Subscale	6–10 years	No	0.27	0.19	—
Visuospatial Ability	Embedded Figures Test	7–10 years	Yes (F<M)	1.15	0.54**	Yes
	Ball-Throwing Task	7–10 years	No	0.34	0.10	—
	Correct items	7–10 years	Yes (F<M)	0.60	0.10	—
Mind Reading	Reading the Mind in the Eyes	6–9 years	No	0.31	−0.43**	Yes
Empathy	Empathy Quotient	6–9 years	Yes (F>M)	0.76	−0.28**	No
Systemising	Systemizing Quotient	6–9 years	Yes (F<M)	0.49	0.31**	Yes
Autistic traits	Q-CHAT	18–24 months	Yes (F<M)	0.46	0.40**	Yes
Autistic traits	AQ-Child	6–10 years	Yes (F<M)	0.87	0.41**	Yes
Autistic traits	CAST	6–10 years	Yes (F<M)	0.30	0.25**	Yes

Note: Effect sizes for sex differences were computed using Cohen's d where a d value of 0.2 is considered a small effect size, a d of 0.5 is considered a medium effect size, and a d greater than 0.8 is considered a large effect size (Cohen, 1988).
Correlations are reported for both sexes combined.
– denotes that a regression analysis was not conducted.

masculinization up to a certain dose, but additional exposure may cause demasculinization (Knickmeyer et al., 2007).

A common feature of all the studies presented in Table 2.8.2 is that they focus on typically developing children. Children with ASC have not been included in the analyses, since a much larger sample in which to measure fetal hormone levels would be needed. A further possible explanation for the lack of correlation between behaviors and fT levels in boys is that 'male extreme' hormone levels may result in ASC and are excluded by default, since only typically developing children were included in these studies (see Figure 2.8.2). In contrast, 'female extremes' of fT level simply result in 'masculinized' female behavior and are included in the samples. Exclusion of boys with very high fT levels might be expected to reduce within sex differences in boys.

fT and the Brain

Results from the current studies suggest that higher prenatal hormone levels could be responsible for greater

TABLE 2.8.2   Within Sex Results, Outcome Variables and Sample Sizes

Measure	Child age	FT sig. predictor for all cases	FT sig. predictor for boys	FT sig. predictor for girls	Study n (n boys, n girls)
Eye Contact	12 months	Yes	Yes	No	71 (41 boys, 29 girls)
Vocabulary Size	18–24 months	Yes	No	No	87 (47 boys, 40 girls)
Intentional Language	4 years	Yes	No	No	38 (24 boys, 14 girls)
Restricted Interests	4 years	Yes	No	No	58 (35 boys, 24 girls)
Social Relationships	4 years	Yes	No	No	58 (35 boys, 24 girls)
PSAI Total	6–9 years	Yes	No	Yes	212 (112 boys, 100 girls)
BSRI Masculinity		Yes	No	Yes	207 (107 boys, 100 girls)
Embedded Figures	7–10 years	Yes	Yes	Yes	64 (35 boys, 29 girls)
Mind Reading	6–9 years	Yes	Yes	Yes	78 (40 boys, 38 girls)
Systemising	6–9 years	Yes	No	Yes	204 (111 boys, 93 girls)
Q-CHAT	18–24 months	Yes	Yes	Yes	129 (66 boys, 63 girls)
AQ-Child	6–10 years	Yes	Yes	Yes	235 (118 boys, 117 girls)
CAST	6–10 years	Yes	Yes	No	235 (118 boys, 117 girls)

Note: Only outcome variables with significant FT correlations are shown.
Variables included in regression analysis are reported for both sexes combined.
n indicates sample sizes.

masculinization of behavior. However, it is clear that fT, measured during the second trimester of pregnancy is not the only factor contributing to the behaviors examined. We know this because it only accounts for a proportion of the variance (summarized in Table 2.8.2 between 0–67%, depending on the behavior and on sex).

Other evidence supporting the role for fT in human development comes from physical studies of brain structure. If hormones are a risk factor for ASC, then one could hypothesize that there may be an overlap between areas of the human brain that show sexual dimorphism because of their density of androgen receptors, and those that are atypical in individuals with ASC. Table 2.8.3 shows Knickmeyer and Baron-Cohen's (2006) comparison of brain regions that are sexually dimorphic, those that are atypical in autism and those that contain the most androgen receptors. While this points to

some overlap (especially in the amygdala, corpus callosum, temporal and frontal cortex), it is important to recognize that this approach does not prove that sexual dimorphism is due to the density of androgen receptors, or that the abnormalities in ASC are necessarily associated with androgen receptors. Such overlap could be purely coincidental and will require direct testing of any causal factors.

Recently, we have extended investigation into how fT may affect brain development. Increased fT levels have also been shown to affect brain morphology, showing a significant relationship with increased rightward asymmetry (e.g., Right > Left) of a posterior subsection of the callosum (Chura et al., 2010). We have also found that fT influences later cortical gray matter volume, which is observed to be sexually dimorphic (Lombardo et al., in press). Increases in fT predicted increased gray matter

FIGURE 2.8.2   Hypothetical fetal testosterone levels in typical and ASC populations.

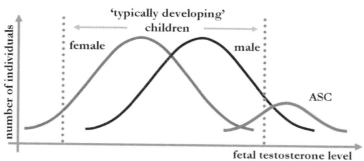

TABLE 2.8.3 Comparison of Brain Regions Implicated in Autism with those Showing Gross Anatomical Sex Differences and those Expressing Androgen Receptors

Autism	Androgen receptors	Sexually dimorphic (gross anatomical level)
Parietal-temporal lobe	Temporal lobe	Parietal and Temporal lobe
Cerebellum	Cerebellum	
Amygdala	Amygdala	Amygdala
Hippocampus		
Corpus callosum	Corpus callosum	Corpus callosum
Frontal cortex	Frontal cortex	Frontal cortex
	Hypothalamus	Hypothalamus
	Cingulate Cortex	

Table from: Knickmeyer and Baron-Cohen (2006a).

in the right temporo-parietal junction, and this brain region shows a Male > Female pattern of sexual dimorphism. Similarly, gray matter in the planum temporale and posterior lateral orbitofrontal cortex are inversely related to fT levels, and show a Female > Male pattern of sexual dimorphism. Thus, fT predicts development of gray matter in directions that are congruent with observed sexual dimorphism and is indicative of the organizational nature of its influence on sexually dimorphic brain development.

ADDITIONAL CONSIDERATIONS

The relationships between prenatal hormones and behaviors that show sex differences in humans are likely to be dependent on many factors and these studies only report correlations with hormone levels measured at a single time point. Research in animals has generally shown that hormonal effects on sexually dimorphic behavior may be dose and time-dependent, with increased masculinization occurring for higher levels of androgen exposure (Cohen-Bendahan et al., 2005; Hines, 2004). The present results in humans are generally in line with findings in individuals with CAH showing that fT masculinizes behavior in domains that show sex differences in girls. The current results also tend to suggest that using measures sensitive to 'extreme' forms of male behavior, elevated fT exposure may also be related to masculinization in girls and perhaps 'hyper-masculinization' in boys.

The effects of fT may also be non-linear. Previous studies have shown non-linear relationships with prenatal hormones and behavior in humans (Lutchmaya et al., 2002a). Research in nonhumans also suggests that

the hormone levels required to affect development also differ across behaviors (Goy and McEwen, 1980). Moreover, the presence of one hormone may also promote or prevent the effects of another (Cohen-Bendahan et al., 2005; Goy and McEwen, 1980). Finally, the effect of hormones is also dependent on the availability of receptors, as seen when examining individuals with Complete or Partial Androgen Insensitivity Syndrome.

The influence of all these hormonal factors on later behavioral development is outside the scope of these studies. These differing relationships in boys versus girls as well as the differing amounts of variability that fT accounts for (as shown in Tables 2.8.1 and 2.8.2), bring attention to the many factors that must be considered when exploring hormone-behavior relations in humans.

The Role of Social Factors in the Development of Sex Differences

Social interactions undoubtedly play an important role in the development of gender-typical play and toy choices. Gender-based expectations may cause parents, teachers or caregivers to elicit and reinforce expected behavior from children (Stern and Karraker, 1989), thus shaping the child's behavior. It has been shown that infant gender labeling as male or female often elicits sex-stereotypic responses from adults and children (Stern and Karraker, 1989). It has also been suggested that girls are encouraged to be more sensitive and caring towards others than boys (Gilligan, 1982). Findings from studies examining play preferences have indicated that boys are encouraged by parents to play with masculine-typical toys and discouraged from playing with feminine-typical toys (Fagot, 1978; Fagot and Hagan, 1991). Girls, on the other hand, are also encouraged to play with feminine-typical toys but not necessarily discouraged from playing with masculine-typical toys (Fagot, 1978; Fagot and Hagan, 1991). While these factors might influence the behavior exhibited by typically developing children, studies examining eye contact (Hittelman and Dickes, 1979) and preference for social stimuli in newborn children (Connellan et al., 2000) provide convincing evidence for a biological basis for some sex differences. It is not clear how such social factors might apply to the ASC group.

Factors That Influence fT Levels

A number of studies have examined factors such as stress, which influence testosterone levels both pre- and post-natally. Prenatal stress in male rats has been found to demasculinize and feminize adult sexual behavior (Ward, 1977). Testosterone levels in newborn male rats are also observed to be reduced in stressed compared to non-stressed controls. There are also potentially consistent findings in humans, such as homosexual men reporting more maternal stressors (such as bereavement) during pregnancy, relative to controls (Dorner et al., 1983). In females, there is some evidence that prenatal stress is associated with masculinized gender role and sexual behavior (Hines et al., 2002).

Gitau et al. (2005) found that fT levels measured from fetal plasma samples correlated positively with both fetal cortisol (assumed to be a reflection of stress levels) and maternal testosterone concentrations in 44 human fetuses. Maternal plasma testosterone and fetal plasma cortisol were independently correlated with fetal plasma testosterone in both sexes. Unlike the norm in the adult, where testosterone production is often inhibited by cortisol, in the fetus a positive association has been observed (Gitau et al., 2005). One small scale study (n = 12) showed that children with autism showed a more variable circadian rhythm as well as significant elevations in cortisol (indicating increased stress) following exposure to a novel, non-social stimulus compared to typical children (Corbett et al., 2006).

It is difficult to control for emotional stress, and further studies could also control for cortisol levels when examining the effects of hormones such as testosterone on later behavior. Additionally, future research examining whether relationships exist between serum fT and cortisol levels or amniotic fT and cortisol levels would be useful. It would also be interesting to investigate the effects of prenatal levels of cortisol on later behavior and in children with ASC. However, this would require a longitudinal strategy in large samples.

Hormone levels during pregnancy may also be influenced by the timing of previous maternal birth history. A study of umbilical cord blood has shown that first-born children of both sexes have higher levels of estrogen, progesterone and testosterone (Maccoby et al., 1979). This finding was independent of maternal age, length of labor or birth weight. When childbirths are spaced closely together (within 4 years), results show that hormone levels are lower than normal. After 4 years, levels return to first-born levels or above. The effects of sibling spacing has also been observed to be greater on boys than girls (Maccoby et al., 1979). It is unclear how such factors might affect the results in this study, or whether these differences are replicated in fetal testosterone levels.

Genetic sex is determined at conception. However, it is accepted that genetic variation has an important role in the development of ASC (Folstein and Rosen-Sheidley, 2001; Gupta and State, 2007; Lauritsen and Ewald, 2001). This is clear from the high degree of heritability observed in autism (Bailey et al., 1995; Ritvo et al., 1985). The degree to which genetic variation is coupled with changes in hormone exposure is also unknown,

and it may be that changes in hormone levels are simply a manifestation of a genetic influence. This would be an interesting area for future research, since investigations of current testosterone levels have shown rates of heritability between 50% and 66% (Harris et al., 1998; Hoekstra et al., 2006).

LIMITATIONS OF MEASURING PRENATAL EXPOSURE TO HORMONES IN AMNIOTIC FLUID

The use of amniotic fluid to measure prenatal hormonal exposure has several limitations. Ideally, it would be best to make direct measurements of testosterone at regular intervals throughout gestation and into postnatal life. However, it would be extremely hazardous to attempt direct measurements from the fetus itself for purely research purposes. It is not possible to obtain repeated samples of fT because amniocentesis itself carries a risk of causing miscarriage (of about 1%) (d'Ercole et al., 2003; Sangalli et al., 2004). As a result, obtaining amniotic fT measures are opportunistic, when the procedure is being carried out for clinical reasons, with never more than a single measurement of fT at one time-point although it is known that hormones fluctuate during the day and between days, even in fetuses (Seron-Ferre et al., 1993; Walsh et al., 1984). The representativeness of a single sample of fT thus remains unclear, but would be difficult to explore in an ethical manner.

In addition, given the reported time course of testosterone secretion, the most promising time to measure fT is probably at prenatal weeks 8 to 24 (Smail et al., 1981), but this is still a relatively wide range. In addition, research in non-human primates has shown that androgens masculinize different behaviors at different times during gestation, suggesting different behaviors may also have different sensitive periods for development (Goy et al., 1988). For all these reasons, the inferences we can therefore draw about the single measurement of fT are necessarily limited. However, where a significant correlation between amniotic fT and a behavior is observed this should represent a very conservative estimate of the correlation between overall fT levels and that behavior.

Human behavior is complex, and biological, social or cultural factors are continuously interacting, making it challenging to investigate the causes of behavior. To the extent that social factors have been considered within the experiments presented in this chapter, these have been restricted to certain demographic variables (such as maternal age, parental education, and number of siblings), and it is acknowledged that behaviors and traits are likely to be influenced by a range of social factors that have not been measured in these studies.

Results from these studies suggest that variations in fT levels are related to aspects of sexually dimorphic behavior and cognition in typically developing children. However, extrapolating these results to individuals with a formal diagnosis of ASC needs to be done with caution. The sample sizes of the current studies are too small to be able to test whether fT levels are elevated in formally diagnosed cases of ASC. Since these have a prevalence rate of about 1% (Baird et al., 2006), a sample size of thousands would be required. A large-scale UK-Danish collaboration is currently under way to increase sample sizes sufficiently to compare fT levels in cases of ASC versus controls.

Against these limitations, the strength of the amniocentesis design is that it provides a quantifiable measure of fetal exposure to testosterone from the prenatal environment, while avoiding unnecessary additional risk associated with serum sample collection during a period in which it is hypothesized that masculinization of the brain occurs. Some previous studies investigating the relationship between fT and cognitive development in humans have relied on individuals with abnormal hormonal environments during pregnancy, such as those with CAH, or those exposed to drugs that mimic or block natural hormones (Hines et al., 2003; Knickmeyer et al., 2006; Pasterski et al., 2005; Servin et al., 2003). In these cases it is difficult to differentiate between the effects of the hormonal environment, a genetic abnormality associated with the disorder, or any additional effects that drugs may produce. It is probable that the current sample is more representative of the general population than studies based on abnormal environments.

FURTHER EVIDENCE IMPLICATING TESTOSTERONE IN AUTISM

Genetic influences may interact with prenatal hormone levels in the development of ASC. Evidence of a genetic link to sex steroid hormones and ASC comes from a study which shows that genes regulating sex steroids are associated with autistic traits, as measured by scores on the Autism Spectrum Quotient (AQ), in a typical adult sample (Chakrabarti et al., 2009). A parallel study also showed that genes regulating sex steroids are associated with a diagnosis of Asperger Syndrome in a case-control sample (Chakrabarti et al., 2009). Other genes such as the SRD5A1 and Androgen Receptor (AR) genes have been associated with ASC (Henningsson et al., 2009; Hu et al., 2009).

Using a different line of evidence, a number of studies have also found *current* androgen dysregulation in those with ASC or in their relatives, or an association between androgen-related genes and ASC. Androgen-related medical conditions such as polycystic ovary syndrome (PCOS), ovarian growths, and hirsutism occur at elevated rates in women with Asperger Syndrome, and in mothers of children with autism (Ingudomnukul et al., 2007). A subset of male adolescents with autism show hyper-androgeny, or elevated levels of androgens, and precocious puberty (Tordjman et al., 1997). Delayed menarche has also been found in females with ASC (Ingudomnukul et al., 2007; Knickmeyer et al., 2006). Puberty timing reflects hormonal programming of the hypothalamic-pituitary-gonadal axis during gestation (Grumbach and Styne, 1998).

In addition, left-handedness and ambidexterity are more common in typical males (Peters, 1991) and individuals with autism (Gillberg, 1983). Increased fT is implicated in left-handedness and asymmetric lateralization (Fein et al., 1985; McManus et al., 1992; Satz et al., 1985; Soper et al., 1986). The typical male brain is also heavier than the female brain, a difference that in animals is partly due to fT. Individuals with autism have even heavier brains than typical males (Hardan et al., 2001).

FUTURE DIRECTIONS

There is converging evidence supporting a role for prenatal hormones in the development of sexually dimorphic behavior. It is possible that genetic influences are responsible for or interact with the prenatal hormone levels that lead to the development of ASC. Considering the current support for a role for fT in the development of autistic traits, it would be beneficial for future studies to examine the relationships between fT levels, genetic variation and the development of autistic traits.

The replication of the current results in larger sample sizes would also help to increase the range of fT levels observed in these studies and assist in identifying any factors that are linked with levels in the extreme ranges. Future studies could assess whether relationships between fT levels and the development of autistic traits are consistent for individuals with a clinical diagnosis of ASC, since the current samples only included typically developing children.

It would also be valuable to further establish the relationships between direct measures of hormones (e.g. amniotic fluid or serum measures) and physical characteristics (e.g. 2D:4D ratio or dermatoglyphics) which have been used as proxy measures of hormone exposure. The benefit of using these types of measurements is that they are easy to obtain and have also been linked to multiple areas of human development. However, limited evidence exists for a relationship between these proxy measures and exposure to prenatal hormones. If such a link was confirmed using direct measures of hormones, it could simplify future investigations of hormone effects.

The EMB theory of autism has been developed from studies in typically developing and high-functioning individuals. It would be interesting to extend the scope of this theory by an examination of individuals with more severe forms of ASC.

CONCLUSIONS

Autism Spectrum Conditions (ASC) are characterized by social impairments, restricted and repetitive interests accompanied by language delay. ASC are believed to lie on a spectrum, reflecting the range of individual ability in each of these areas. Some of the behaviors that are characteristic of ASC have been linked to extremes of certain male-typical behaviors. Evidence includes superior performance on a range of tasks where male individuals typically outperform females and impairment on tasks which show female superiority.

Research suggests that gender-typical behaviors may be affected by gonadal hormones, in particular fetal exposure to testosterone. The objective of the current studies was to examine the link between fT levels (measured in amniotic fluid) and a series of sexually dimorphic behaviors. Results suggest that prenatal exposure to elevated fT levels enhances masculinization of certain behaviors. In addition, direct measurement of autistic traits was used to examine whether these measures of behavior are consistent with the EMB theory of autism. It was striking that on all three measures (CAST, AQ-Child, and Q-CHAT), fT positively predicted number of autistic traits.

In summary, fT levels have been found to be significantly related to some, but not all, male-typical traits, and lend further support for a role of fT levels in the development of behaviors related to sex differences. The findings presented also lend support to the EMB theory of ASC and to a further relationship with fetal testosterone levels. Although higher levels of fT are unlikely to be the sole the cause of autism, the studies reported here provide evidence for a role of fT in the development of autistic traits in typically developing children. This remains to be tested in clinical samples. It is hoped that results from this series of studies may enable further understanding of the etiology of ASC and of typical variation in sexually dimorphic behavior.

References

Abramovich, D.R., 1974. Human sexual differentiation - *in utero* influences. Journal of Obstetrics and Gynecology 81, 448–453.

American Psychiatric Association (APA), 1994. DSM-IV Diagnostic and Statistical Manual of Mental Disorders, fourth ed. American Psychiatric Association, Washington DC.

Arnold, A.P., Gorski, R.A., 1984. Gonadal steroid induction of structural sex differences in the central nervous system. Annual Review of Neuroscience 7, 413–442.

Autism and Developmental Disabilities Monitoring Network Surveillance Year 2006 Principal Investigators, Centers for Disease Control and Prevention, 2009. Prevalence of autism spectrum disorders - Autism and Developmental Disabilities Monitoring Network, United States, 2006. Morbidity and Mortality Weekly Report Surveillance Summary 58, 1–20.

Auyeung, B., 2008. Foetal testosterone, cognitive sex differences and autistic traits. University of Cambridge, Cambridge, United Kingdom.

Auyeung, B., Baron-Cohen, S., Ashwin, E., Knickmeyer, R., Taylor, K., Hackett, G., et al., 2009. Fetal testosterone predicts sexually differentiated childhood behavior in girls and in boys. Psychological Science 20, 144–148.

Auyeung, B., Baron-Cohen, S., Chapman, E., Knickmeyer, R., Taylor, K., Hackett, G., 2006. Foetal testosterone and the child systemizing quotient. European Journal of Endocrinology 155, S123–S130.

Auyeung, B., Baron-Cohen, S., Chapman, E., Knickmeyer, R., Taylor, K., Hackett, G., 2009. Fetal testosterone and autistic traits. British Journal of Psychiatry 100, 1–22.

Auyeung, B., Baron-Cohen, S., Wheelwright, S., Allison, C., 2008. The autism spectrum quotient: Children's version (AQ-Child). Journal of Autism and Developmental Disorders 38, 1230–1240.

Auyeung, B., Baron-Cohen, S., Wheelwright, S., Samarawickrema, N., Atkinson, M., 2009. The children's empathy quotient (EQ-C) and systemizing quotient (SQ-C): Sex differences in typical development and of autism spectrum conditions. Journal of Autism and Developmental Disorders 39, 1509–1521.

Auyeung, B., Knickmeyer, R., Ashwin, E., Taylor, K., Hackett, G., Baron-Cohen, S., 2012. Effects of fetal testosterone on visuospatial ability. Archives of Sexual Behavior 41, 571–581.

Auyeung, B., Taylor, K., Hackett, G., Baron-Cohen, S., 2010. Foetal testosterone and autistic traits in 18 to 24-month-old children. Molecular Autism 1.

Bailey, A., Le Couteur, A., Gottesman, I., Bolton, P., Simonoff, E., Yuzda, E., et al., 1995. Autism as a strongly genetic disorder: Evidence from a British twin study. Psychological Medicine 25, 63–77.

Baird, G., Simonoff, E., Pickles, A., Chandler, S., Loucas, T., Meldrum, D., et al., 2006. Prevalence of disorders of the autism spectrum in a population cohort of children in South Thames: The Special Needs and Autism Project (SNAP). Lancet 368, 210–215.

Baron-Cohen, S., 1995. Mindblindness: An essay on autism and theory of mind. Learning, development, and conceptual change. The MIT Press, Cambridge, MA, US. 171.

Baron-Cohen, S., 2002. The extreme male brain theory of autism. Trends in Cognitive Sciences 6, 248–254.

Baron-Cohen, S., Wheelwright, S., 2003. The Friendship Questionnaire: An investigation of adults with Asperger syndrome or high-functioning autism, and normal sex differences. Journal of Autism and Developmental Disorders 33, 509–517.

Baron-Cohen, S., Wheelwright, S., 2004. The Empathy Quotient: An investigation of adults with Asperger syndrome or high functioning autism, and normal sex differences. Journal of Autism and Developmental Disorders 34, 163–175.

Baron-Cohen, S., Jolliffe, T., Mortimore, C., Robertson, M., 1997. Another advanced test of theory of mind: Evidence from very high functioning adults with autism or Asperger Syndrome. Journal of Child Psychology and Psychiatry 38, 813–822.

Baron-Cohen, S., Knickmeyer, R., Belmonte, M.K., 2005. Sex differences in the brain: Implications for explaining autism. Science 310, 819–823.

Baron-Cohen, S., Leslie, A.M., Frith, U., 1985. Does the autistic child have a theory of mind? Cognition 21, 37–46.

Baron-Cohen, S., Lombardo, M.V., Auyeung, B., Ashwin, E., Chakrabarti, B., Knickmeyer, R., 2011. Why are autism spectrum conditions more prevalent in males? PLoS Biology 9.

Baron-Cohen, S., Lutchmaya, S., Knickmeyer, R., 2004. Prenatal testosterone in mind. The MIT Press, Cambridge, Massachusetts.

Baron-Cohen, S., O'Riordan, M., Stone, V., Jones, R., Plaisted, K., 1999. Recognition of faux pas by normally developing children and children with Asperger syndrome or high-functioning autism. Journal of Autism and Developmental Disorders 29, 407–418.

Baron-Cohen, S., Richler, J., Bisarya, D., Gurunathan, N., Wheelwright, S., 2003. The Systemizing Quotient: An investigation of adults with Asperger syndrome or high functioning autism, and normal sex differences. Philosophical Transactions of the Royal Society London 358, 361–374.

Baron-Cohen, S., Ring, H., Chitnis, X., Wheelwright, S., Gregory, L., Williams, S., et al., 2006. fMRI of parents of children with Asperger Syndrome: A pilot study. Brain Cognition 61, 122–130.

Baron-Cohen, S., Scott, F.J., Allison, C., Williams, J., Bolton, P., Matthews, F.E., et al., 2009. Prevalence of autism-spectrum conditions: UK school-based population study. British Journal of Psychiatry 194, 500–509.

Baron-Cohen, S., Wheelwright, S., Spong, A., Scahill, L., Lawson, J., 2001. Are intuitive physics and intuitive psychology independent? A test with children with Asperger syndrome. Journal of Developmental and Learning Disorders 5, 47–78.

Bates, J.E., Bentler, P.M., 1973. Play activities of normal and effeminate boys. Developmental Psychology 9, 20–27.

Beck-Peccoz, P., Padmanabhan, V., Baggiani, A.M., Cortelazzi, D., Buscaglia, M., Medri, G., et al., 1991. Maturation of hypothalamic-pituitary-gonadal function in normal human fetuses: Circulating levels of gonadotropins, their common alpha-subunit and free testosterone, and discrepancy between immunological and biological activities of circulating follicle-stimulating hormone. Journal of Clinical Endocrinology and Metabolism 73, 525–532.

Bem, S.L., 1974. The measurement of psychological androgyny. Journal of Consulting and Clinical Psychology 42, 155–162.

Berenbaum, S.A., 1999. Effects of early androgens on sex-typed activities and interests in adolescents with congenital adrenal hyperplasia. Hormones and Behavior 35, 102–110.

Berenbaum, S.A., Hines, M., 1992. Early androgens are related to childhood sex-typed toy preferences. Psychological Science 3, 203–206.

Berenbaum, S.A., Snyder, E., 1995. Early hormonal influences on childhood sex-typed activity and playmate preferences: Implications for the development of sexual orientation. Developmental Psychology 31, 31–42.

Bigelow, G., 1971. Field dependence-field independence. Journal of Educational Research 64, 397–400.

Bishop, D.V.M., 1998. Development of the children's communication checklist (CCC): A method for assessing qualitative aspects of communicative impairment in children. Journal of Child Psychology and Psychiatry 6, 879–891.

Brosnan, M., Daggar, R., Collomosse, J., 2009. The relationship between systemising and mental rotation and the implications for the extreme male brain theory of autism. Journal of Autism and Developmental Disorders.

Carroll, J.M., Chiew, K.Y., 2006. Sex and discipline differences in empathising, systemising and autistic symptomatology: Evidence from a student population. Journal of Autism and Developmental Disorders 36, 949–957.

Chakrabarti, B., Dudbridge, F., Kent, L., Wheelwright, S., Hill-Cawthorne, G., Allison, C., et al., 2009. Genes related to sex steroids, neural growth, and social-emotional behavior are associated with autistic traits, empathy, and Asperger syndrome. Autism Resource 2, 157–177.

Chakrabarti, S., Fombonne, E., 2005. Pervasive developmental disorders in preschool children: Confirmation of high prevalence. American Journal of Psychiatry 162, 1133–1141.

Chapman, E., Baron-Cohen, S., Auyeung, B., Knickmeyer, R., Taylor, K., Hackett, G., 2006. Fetal testosterone and empathy: Evidence from the Empathy Quotient (EQ) and the 'Reading the Mind in the Eyes' test. Society for Neuroscience 1, 135–148.

Chura, L.R., Lombardo, M.V., Ashwin, E., Auyeung, B., Chakrabarti, B., Bullmore, E.T., et al., 2010. Organizational effects of fetal testosterone on human corpus callosum size and asymmetry. Psychoneuroendocrinology 35, 122–132.

Clark, M.M., Robertson, R.K., Galef, B.G., 1996. Effects of perinatal testosterone on handedness of gerbils: Support for part of the Geschwind-Galaburda hypothesis. Behavioural Neuroscience 110, 413–417.

Cohen, J., 1988. Statistical power analysis for the behavioral sciences, Second ed. Lawrence Erlbaum Associates, Hillsdale, NJ.

Cohen-Bendahan, C.C., van de Beek, C., Berenbaum, S.A., 2005. Prenatal sex hormone effects on child and adult sex-typed behavior: Methods and findings. Neuroscience and Biobehavioral Reviews 29, 353–384.

Collaer, M.L., Hines, M., 1995. Human behavioural sex differences: A role for gonadal hormones during early development? Psychological Bulletin 118, 55–107.

Connellan, J., Baron-Cohen, S., Wheelwright, S., Batki, A., Ahluwalia, J., 2000. Sex differences in human neonatal social perception. Infant Behavior and Development 23, 113–118.

Corbett, B.A., Mendoza, S., Abdullah, M., Wegelin, J.A., Levine, S., 2006. Cortisol circadian rhythms and response to stress in children with autism. Psychoneuroendocrinology 31, 59–68.

d'Ercole, C., Shojai, R., Desbriere, R., Chau, C., Bretelle, F., Piechon, L., et al., 2003. Prenatal screening: Invasive diagnostic approaches. Child's Nervous System 19, 444–447.

De Vries, G.J., Simerly, R.B., 2002. Anatomy, development, and function of sexually dimorphic neural circuits in the mammalian brain. In: Pfaff, D.W., Arnold, A.E., Etgen, A.M., Fahrbach, S.E., Rubin, R.T. (Eds.), Hormone Brain Behavior, vol. 4. Academic Press, San Diego, CA, pp. 137–191.

Dorner, G., Schenk, B., Schmiedel, B., Ahrens, L., 1983. Stressful events in prenatal life of bi- and homosexual men. Experimental Clinical Endocrinology 81, 83–87.

Dziobek, I., Rogers, K., Fleck, S., Bahnemann, M., Heekeren, H.R., Wolf, O.T., et al., 2008. Dissociation of cognitive and emotional empathy in adults with Asperger syndrome using the Multifaceted Empathy Test (MET). Journal of Autism and Developmental Disorders 38, 464–473.

Ehrhardt, A.A., Baker, S.W., 1974. Fetal androgens, human central nervous system differentiation, and behavior sex differences. In: Friedman, R.C., Richart, R.R., Vande Wiele, R.L. (Eds.), Sex Differences in Behavior. Wiley, New York, pp. 33–51.

Ehrhardt, A.A., Meyer-Bahlburg, H.F., 1981. Effects of prenatal sex hormones on gender-related behavior. Science 211, 1312–1318.

Ernsperger, L., Wendel, D., Willey, L.H., 2007. Girls under the umbrella of autism spectrum disorders. Autism Asperger Publishing Company, Shawnee Mission, Kansas.

Fagot, B.I., 1978. The influence of sex of child on parental reactions to toddler children. Child Development 49, 459–465.

Fagot, B.I., Hagan, R., 1991. Observations of parent reactions to sex-stereotyped behaviors: Age and sex effects. Child Development 62, 617–628.

Falter, C.M., Plaisted, K.C., Davis, G., 2008. Visuo-spatial processing in autism-Testing the predictions of extreme male brain theory. Journal of Autism and Developmental Disorders 38, 507–515.

Fausto-Sterling, A., 1992. Myths of gender. Basic Books, New York.

Fein, D., Waterhouse, L., Lucci, D., Pennington, B., Humes, M., 1985. Handedness and cognitve functions in pervasive developmental disorders. Journal of Autism and Developmental Disorders 15, 323–333.

Folstein, S.E., Rosen-Sheidley, B., 2001. Genetics of autism: Complex aetiology for a heterogeneous disorder. Nature Reviews Genetics 2, 943–955.

Frith, U., Morton, J., Leslie, A.M., 1991. The cognitive basis of a biological disorder: Autism. Trends in Neurosciences 14, 433–438.

Fuchs, F., Klopper, A., 1983. Endocrinology of Pregnancy. Harper & Row, Philadelphia.

Geschwind, D.H., 2009. Advances in autism. Annual Review of Medicine 60, 367–380.

Gillberg, C., 1983. Autistic children's hand preferences: Results from an epidemiological study of infantile autism. Psychiatry Research 10, 21–30.

Gillberg, C., Cederlund, M., Lamberg, K., Zeijlon, L., 2006. Brief report: The autism epidemic. The registered prevalence of autism in a Swedish urban area. Journal of Autism and Developmental Disorders 36, 429–435.

Gilligan, C., 1982. In a different voice: Psychological theory and women's development. Harvard University Press, Cambridge, Massachusetts.

Gitau, R., Adams, D., Fisk, N.M., Glover, V., 2005. Fetal plasma testosterone correlates positively with cortisol. archives of disease in childhood. Fetal and Neonatal Edition 90, F166–169.

Goldenfeld, N., Baron-Cohen, S., Wheelwright, S., 2005. Empathizing and systemizing in males, females and autism. International Journal of Clinical Neuropsychology 2, 338–345.

Goy, R.W., McEwen, B.S., 1980. Sexual Differentiation of the Brain. The MIT Press, Cambridge, MA.

Goy, R.W., Bercovitch, F.B., McBrair, M.C., 1988. Behavioral masculinization is independent of genital masculinization in prenatally androgenized female rhesus macaques. Hormones and Behavior 22, 552–571.

Grumbach, M.M., Styne, D.M., 1998. Puberty: Ontogeny, neuroendocrinology, physiology and disorders. In: Foster, W. (Ed.), Williams Textbook of Endocrinology. W.B. Saunders, Philadelphia.

Gupta, A.R., State, M.W., 2007. Recent advances in the genetics of autism. Biological Psychiatry 61, 429–437.

Hamilton, A., Plunkett, K., Shafer, G., 2000. Infant vocabulary development assessed with a british communicative inventory: Lower scores in the UK than the USA. Journal of Child Language 27, 689–705.

Hampson, E., Rovet, J.F., Altmann, D., 1998. Spatial reasoning in children with congenital adrenal hyperplasia due to 21-hydroxylase deficiency. Developmental Neuropsychology 14, 299–320.

Happé, F.G., 1994. Wechsler IQ profile and theory of mind in autism: A research note. Journal of Child Psychology and Psychiatry 35, 1461–1471.

Happé, F.G., 1995. The role of age and verbal ability in the theory of mind task performance of subjects with autism. Child Development 66, 843–855.

Hardan, A.Y., Minshew, N.J., Mallikarjuhn, M., Keshavan, M.S., 2001. Brain volume in autism. Journal of Child Neurology 16, 421–424.

Harris, J.A., Vernon, P.A., Boomsma, D.I., 1998. The heritability of testosterone: A study of Dutch adolescent twins and their parents. Behavior Genetics 28, 165–171.

Henningsson, S., Jonsson, L., Ljunggren, E., Westberg, L., Gillberg, C., Rastam, M., et al., 2009. Possible association between the androgen receptor gene and autism spectrum disorder. Psychoneuroendocrinology 34, 752–761.

Hines, M., 2004. Brain gender. Oxford University Press, Inc, New York.

Hines, M., Brook, C., Conway, G.S., 2004. Androgen and psychosexual development: Core gender identity, sexual orientation and recalled childhood gender role behavior in women and men with congenital adrenal hyperplasia (CAH). Journal of Sex Research 41, 75–81.

Hines, M., Fane, B.A., Pasterski, V.L., Matthews, G.A., Conway, G.S., Brook, C., 2003. Spatial abilities following prenatal androgen abnormality: Targeting and mental rotations performance in individuals with congenital adrenal hyperplasia. Psychoneuroendocrinology 28, 1010–1026.

Hines, M., Johnston, K.J., Golombok, S., Rust, J., Stevens, M., Golding, J., 2002. Prenatal stress and gender role behavior in girls and boys: A longitudinal, population study. Hormones and Behavior 42, 126–134.

Hittelman, J.H., Dickes, R., 1979. Sex differences in neonatal eye contact time. Merrill-Palmer Quarterly 25, 171–184.

Hoekstra, R., Bartels, M., Boomsma, D.I., 2006. Heritability of testosterone levels in 12-year-old twins and its relation to pubertal development. Twin Research and Human Genetics 9, 558–565.

Hu, V.W., Sarachana, T., Kim, K.S., Nguyen, A., Kulkarni, S., Steinberg, M.E., et al., 2009. Gene expression profiling differentiates autism case-controls and phenotypic variants of autism spectrum disorders: Evidence for circadian rhythm dysfunction in severe autism. Autism Resource 2, 78–97.

Ingudomnukul, E., Baron-Cohen, S., Knickmeyer, R., Wheelwright, S., 2007. Elevated rates of testosterone-related disorders in a sample of women with autism spectrum conditions. Hormones and Behavior 51, 597–604.

Jolliffe, T., Baron-Cohen, S., 1997. Are people with autism and asperger syndrome faster than normal on the Embedded figures test? Journal of Child Psychology and Psychiatry 38, 527–534.

Kimura, D., 1999. Sex and Cognition. The MIT Press, Cambridge, MA.

Klin, Ami, 2000. Attributing social meaning to ambiguous visual stimuli in higher-functioning autism and Asperger syndrome: The Social Attribution Task. Journal of Child Psychology and Psychiatry 7, 831–846.

Knickmeyer, R.C., Baron-Cohen, S., 2006. Fetal testosterone and sex differences in typical social development and in autism. Journal of Child Neurology 21, 825–845.

Knickmeyer, R.C., Baron-Cohen, S., 2006. Fetal testosterone and sex differences. Early Human Development 82, 755–760.

Knickmeyer, R.C., Baron-Cohen, S., Auyeung, B., Ashwin, E., 2008. How to test the extreme male brain theory of autism in terms of foetal androgens? Journal of Autism and Developmental Disorders 38, 995–996.

Knickmeyer, R., Baron-Cohen, S., Fane, B.A., Wheelwright, S., Mathews, G.A., Conway, G.S., et al., 2006. Androgens and autistic traits: A study of individuals with congenital adrenal hyperplasia. Hormones and Behavior 50, 148–153.

Knickmeyer, R., Baron-Cohen, S., Hoekstra, R., Wheelwright, S., 2006. Age of menarche in females with autism spectrum conditions. Developmental Medicine and Child Neurology 48, 1007–1008.

Knickmeyer, R., Baron-Cohen, S., Raggatt, P., Taylor, K., Hackett, G., 2006. Fetal testosterone and empathy. Hormones and Behavior 49, 282–292.

Knickmeyer, R., Baron-Cohen, S., Raggatt, P., Taylor, K., 2005. Foetal testosterone, social relationships, and restricted interests in children. Journal of Child Psychology and Psychiatry 46, 198–210.

Knickmeyer, R.C., Wheelwright, S., Baron-Cohen, S.B., 2007. Sextypical play: Masculinization/defeminization in girls with an autism spectrum condition. Journal of Autism and Developmental Disorders.

Lai, M.C., Lombardo, M.V., Pasco, G., Ruigrok, A.N., Wheelwright, S.J., Sadek, S.A., et al., 2011. A behavioral comparison of male and female adults with high functioning autism spectrum conditions. PLoS ONE 6 e20835.

Larsen, P.R., Kronenberg, H.M., Melmed, S., Polonsky, K.S., 2002. Williams Textbook of Endocrinology, tenth ed. Saunders, Philadelphia.

Lauritsen, M., Ewald, H., 2001. The genetics of autism. Acta Psychiatrica Scandinavica 103, 411–427.

Lawson, J., Baron-Cohen, S., Wheelwright, S., 2004. Empathising and systemising in adults with and without Asperger syndrome. Journal of Autism and Developmental Disorders 34, 301–310.

Leslie, A.M., 1987. Pretence and representation: The origins of "theory of mind". Psychological Review 94, 412–426.

Liss, M.B., 1979. Variables influencing modeling and sex-typed play. Psychological Reports 44, 1107–1115.

Lombardo, M.V., Ashwin, E., Auyeung, B., Chakrabarti, B., Taylor, K., Hackett, G., et al., 2012. Fetal testosterone influences sexually dimorphic gray matter in the human brain. Journal of Neuroscience 32, 674–680.

Lutchmaya, S., Baron-Cohen, S., 2002. Human sex differences in social and non-social looking preferences, at 12 months of age. Infant Behavior & Development 25, 319–325.

Lutchmaya, S., Baron-Cohen, S., Raggatt, P., 2002. Foetal testosterone and eye contact in 12 month old infants. Infant Behavior & Development 25, 327–335.

Lutchmaya, S., Baron-Cohen, S., Raggatt, P., 2002. Foetal testosterone and vocabulary size in 18- and 24-month-old infants. Infant Behavior & Development 24, 418–424.

Lutchmaya, S., Baron-Cohen, S., Raggatt, P., Knickmeyer, R., Manning, J.T., 2004. 2nd to 4th digit ratios, fetal testosterone and estradiol. Early Human Development 77, 23–28.

Lynn, R., 1998. Sex differences in intelligence: Data from a Scottish standardisation of the WAIS-R. Personality and Individual Differences 24, 289–290.

Lynn, R., Raine, A., Venables, P.H., Mednick, S.A., Irwing, P., 2005. Sex differences on the WISC-R in Mauritius. Intelligence 33, 527–533.

Maccoby, E.E., Doering, C.H., Jacklin, C.N., Kraemer, H., 1979. Concentrations of sex hormones in umbilical cord blood: Their relation to sex and birth order of infants. Child Development 50, 632–642.

Malas, M.A., Dogan, S., Evcil, E.H., Desdicioglu, K., 2006. Fetal development of the hand, digits and digit ratio (2D:4D). Early Human Development 82, 469–475.

Manning, J.T., Baron-Cohen, S., Wheelwright, S., Sanders, G., 2001. The 2nd to 4th digit ratio and autism. Developmental Medicine & Child Neurology 43, 160–164.

Manning, J.T., Scutt, D., Wilson, J., Lewis-Jones, D.I., 1998. The ratio of 2nd to 4th digit length: A predictor of sperm numbers and concentrations of testosterone, luteinizing hormone and oestrogen. Human Reproduction 13, 3000–3004.

Martin, C.R., 1985. Endocrine Physiology. Oxford University Press, New York.

McCarthy, M.M., Arnold, A.P., 2011. Reframing sexual differentiation of the brain. Nature Neuroscience 14, 677–683.

McCarthy, M.M., Auger, A.P., Bale, T.L., De Vries, G.J., Dunn, G.A., Forger, N.G., et al., 2009. The epigenetics of sex differences in the brain. Journal of Neuroscience 29, 12815–12823.

McManus, I.C., Murray, B., Doyle, K., Baron-Cohen, S., 1992. Handedness in childhood autism shows a dissociation of skill and preference. Cortex 28, 373–381.

Milne, E., White, S., Campbell, R., Swettenham, J., Hansen, P., Ramus, F., 2006. Motion and form coherence detection in autistic spectrum disorder: Relationship to motor control and 2:4 digit ratio. Journal of Autism and Developmental Disorders 36, 225–237.

Moore, D.S., Johnson, S.P., 2008. Mental rotation in human infants: A sex difference. Psychological Science 19, 1063–1066.

Nebot, T.K., 1988. Sex differences among children on embedded tasks. Perceptual and Motor Skills 67, 972–974.

New, M.I., 1998. Diagnosis and management of congenital adrenal hyperplasia. Annual Review of Medicine 49, 311–328.

Novy, M.J., Resko, J.A. (Eds.), 1981. Fetal Endocrinology. Academic Press, New York.

Pasterski, V.L., Geffner, M.E., Brain, C., Hindmarsh, P., Brook, C., Hines, M., 2005. Prenatal hormones and postnatal socialization by parents as determinants of male-typical toy play in girls with congenital adrenal hyperplasia. Child Development 76, 264–278.

Peters, M., 1991. Sex differences in human brain size and the general meaning of differences in brain size. Canadian Journal of Psychology 45, 507–522.

Phoenix, C.H., Goy, R.W., Gerall, A.A., Young, W.C., 1959. Organizing action of prenatally administered testosterone propionate on the tissues mediating mating behavior in the female guinea pig. Endocrinology 65, 369–382.

Pierce, K., Conant, D., Hazin, R., Stoner, R., Desmond, J., 2010. Preference for geometric patterns early in life as a risk factor for autism. Archives of General Psychiatry 68, 101–109.

Podrouzek, W., Furrow, D., 1988. Preschoolers' use of eye contact while speaking: The influence of sex, age, and conversational partner. Journal of Psycholinguistic Research 17, 89–98.

Puts, D.A., McDaniel, M.A., Jordan, C.L., Breedlove, S.M., 2008. Spatial ability and prenatal androgens: Meta-analyses of congenital adrenal hyperplasia and digit ratio (2D:4D) studies. Archives of Sexual Behavior 37, 100–111.

Quadagno, D.M., Briscoe, R., Quadagno, J.S., 1977. Effects of perinatal gonadal hormones on selected nonsexual behavior patterns: A critical assessment of the nonhuman and human literature. Psychological Bulletin 84, 62–80.

Quinn, P.C., Liben, L.S., 2008. A sex difference in mental rotation in young infants. Psychological Science 19, 1067–1070.

Resnick, S.M., Berenbaum, S.A., Gottesman, I.I., Bouchard, T.J., 1986. Early hormonal influences on cognitive functioning in congenital adrenal hyperplasia. Developmental Psychology 22, 191–198.

Ritvo, E.R., Freeman, B.J., Mason-Brothers, A., Mo, A., Ritvo, A.M., 1985. Concordance for the syndrome of autism in 40 pairs of afflicted twins. American Journal of Psychiatry 142, 74–77.

Robinson, J., Judd, H., Young, P., Jones, D., Yen, S., 1977. Amniotic fluid androgens and estrogens in midgestation. Journal of Clinical Endocrinology 45, 755–761.

Rönnlund, M., Nilsson, L., 2006. Adult life-span patterns in WAIS-R Block Design performance: Cross-sectional versus longitudinal age gradients and relations to demographic factors. Intelligence 34, 63–78.

Ropar, D., Mitchell, P., 2001. Susceptibility to illusions and performance on visuospatial tasks in individuals with autism. Journal of Child Psychology and Psychiatry 42, 539–549.

Rutter, M., 1978. Diagnosis and definition. In: Rutter, M., Schopler, E. (Eds.), Autism: A Reappraisal of Concepts and Treatment. Plenum Press, New York, pp. 1–26.

Rutter, M., Caspi, A., Moffitt, T.E., 2003. Using sex differences in psychopathology to study causal mechanisms: Unifying issues and research strategies. Journal of Child Psychology and Psychiatry 44, 1092–1115.

Sangalli, M., Langdana, F., Thurlow, C., 2004. Pregnancy loss rate following routine genetic amniocentesis at Wellington Hospital. New Zealand Medical Journal 117, U818.

Satz, P., Soper, H., Orsini, D., Henry, R., Zvi, J., 1985. Handedness subtypes in autism. Psychiatric Annals 15, 447–451.

Scott, F.J., Baron-Cohen, S., Bolton, P., Brayne, C., 2002. The CAST (Childhood Asperger Syndrome Test): Preliminary development of a UK screen for mainstream primary-school-age children. Autism 6, 9–13.

Seron-Ferre, M., Ducsay, C.A., Valenzuela, G.J., 1993. Circadian rhythms during pregnancy. Endocrine Reviews 14, 594–609.

Servin, A., Bohlin, G., Berlin, D., 1999. Sex differences in 1-, 3-, and 5-year-olds' toy-choice in a structured play session. Scandinavian Journal of Psychology 40, 43–48.

Servin, A., Nordenström, A., Larsson, A., Bohlin, G., 2003. Prenatal androgens and gender-typed behavior: A study of girls with mild and severe forms of congenital adrenal hyperplasia. Developmental Psychology 39, 440–450.

Shah, A., Frith, U., 1983. An islet of ability in autistic children: A research note. Journal of Child Psychology and Psychiatry 24, 613–620.

Shah, A., Frith, C., 1993. Why do autistic individuals show superior performance on the block design task? Journal of Child Psychology and Psychiatry 34, 1351–1364.

Smail, P.J., Reyes, F.I., Winter, J.S.D., Faiman, C., 1981. The fetal hormonal environment and its effect on the morphogenesis of the genital system. In: Kogan, S.J., Hafez, E.S.E. (Eds.), Pediatric Andrology. Martinus Nijhoff, Boston, pp. 9–19.

Smith, L.L., Hines, M., 2000. Language lateralization and handedness in women prenatally exposed to diethylstilbestrol (DES). Psychoneuroendocrinology 25, 497–512.

Smith, P.K., Daglish, L., 1977. Sex differences in parent and infant behavior in the home. Child Development 48, 1250–1254.

Soper, H., Satz, P., Orsini, D., Henry, R., Zvi, J., Schulman, M., 1986. Handedness patterns in autism suggest subtypes. Journal of Autism and Developmental Disorders 16, 155–167.

Stern, M., Karraker, K.H., 1989. Sex stereotyping of infants: A review of gender labeling studies. Sex Roles 20, 501–522.

Stodgell, C.J., Ingram, J.I., Hyman, S.L., 2001. The role of candidate genes in unraveling the genetics of autism. Int. Rev. Res. Ment. Ret. 23, 57–81.

Swettenham, J., Baron-Cohen, S., Charman, T., Cox, A., Baird, G., Drew, A., et al., 1998. The frequency and distribution of spontaneous attention shifts between social and non-social stimuli in autistic, typically developing, and non-autistic developmentally delayed infants. Journal of Child Psychology and Psychiatry 9, 747–753.

Tordjman, A., Ferrari, P., Sulmont, V., Duyme, M., Roubertoux, P., 1997. Androgenic activity in autism. American Journal of Psychiatry 154, 11.

Tulchinsky, D., Little, A.B., 1994. Maternal-fetal endocrinology, Second ed. W.B. Saunders, Philadelphia; London.

Valla, J., Ceci, S.J., 2011. Can sex differences in science be tied to the long reach of prenatal hormones? Brain organization theory, digit ratio (2D/4D), and sex differences in preferences and cognition. Perspectives on Psychological Science 6, 134–136.

Voyer, D., Voyer, S., Bryden, M.P., 1995. Magnitude of sex differences in spatial abilities: A meta-analysis and consideration of critical variables. Psychological Bulletin 117, 250–270.

Walsh, S.W., Ducsay, C.A., Novy, M.J., 1984. Circadian hormonal interactions among the mother, fetus, and amniotic fluid. Journal of Obstetrics and Gynecology 150, 745–753.

Ward, I.L., 1977. Exogenous androgen activates female behavior in noncopulating, prenatally stressed male rats. Journal of Comparative Physiology and Psychology 91, 465–471.

Wechsler, D., 1999. Wechsler Abbreviated Scale of Intelligence. The Psychological Corporation & Harcourt Brace, San Antonio, TX.

Wheelwright, S., Baron-Cohen, S., Goldenfeld, N., Delaney, J., Fine, D., Smith, R., et al., 2006. Predicting Autism Spectrum Quotient (AQ) from the Systemizing Quotient-Revised (SQ-R) and Empathy Quotient (EQ). Brain Research 1079, 47–56.

Williams, C.L., Meck, W.H., 1991. The organizational effects of gonadal steroids on sexually dimorphic spatial ability. Psychoneuroendocrinology 16, 155–176.

Williams, J., Scott, F., Stott, C., Allison, C., Bolton, P., Baron-Cohen, S., et al., 2005. The CAST (Childhood Asperger Syndrome Test): Test accuracy. Autism 9, 45–68.

Yirmiya, N., Sigman, M.D., Kasari, C., Mundy, P., 1992. Empathy and cognition in high-functioning children with autism. Child Development 63, 150–160.

2.9

Immune Abnormalities and Autism Spectrum Disorders

Majannie Eloi Akintude*, Luke Heuer*, Judy Van de Water†

*University of California, Davis, CA, USA †Department of Internationl Medicine and the UC Davis MIND Institute, Davis, CA, USA

O U T L I N E

HISTORICAL RELATIONSHIP OF IMMUNE ABNORMALITIES WITH ASD

Autism spectrum disorders (ASD) are characterized by difficulties in social interactions, impairment in verbal and/or nonverbal communication, and in the development of stereotyped behaviors and restricted interest (Lord et al., 2000; APA, 2000). Over the past twenty-five years the prevalence of ASD has increased rapidly for a variety of reasons (see Chapter 1.1). The Center for Disease and Control (CDC) estimates that 1 to 110 live births in the United States is diagnosed with ASD ((CDC), 2006; Boyle et al., 2011; Investigators and (CDC), 2009). The increased prevalence of ASD is suggested to be the result of increased awareness, more effective diagnosis and classification approaches, as well as due to truly higher incidence rates (Hertz-Picciotto and Delwiche, 2009). Autism is typically diagnosed between the ages of 2–3 years, and has a male to female ratio of 4:1. Currently, the factors leading to autism are not completely known and there is no biological marker common to all forms of the syndrome. Because of the diversity in phenotypes and the differences in the severity of the symptoms among individuals with ASD, it is a referred to as a spectrum disorder which is presumably caused by different etiologies (Altevogt et al., 2008). Genetic and environmental factors are both suggested as having a role in the etiology of ASD. Genetic studies on individuals diagnosed with ASD have demonstrated that while many different genes are implicated in ASD, there is extreme genetic and genomic heterogeneity [see Chapters 2.1–2.4, also (Zhao et al., 2007)]. In addition, there is now a growing body of research suggesting that abnormalities in the immune system may also be a contributing factor in the etiology of ASD (Ashwood et al., 2006).

The Neuroscience of Autism Spectrum Disorders.
http://dx.doi.org/10.1016/B978-0-12-391924-3.00016-8

As autism is a spectrum disorder, a better understanding of the immune abnormalities noted in these individuals is critical, since immune profiling could be used in the future to identify subpopulations of ASD patients. Investigation of the immune response in children with autism is a new and growing research field that has developed tremendously over the past 30 years. Despite a somewhat rocky start, numerous recent studies now provide us with strong evidence indicating immune abnormalities in children with autism, and understanding these abnormalities might make available new tools for enhanced diagnosis and treatment of ASD.

First described in 1977, investigators demonstrated that children with autism had a decrease in their immune response after immune challenge (Stubbs and Crawford, 1977). Over the next 30 years, multiple studies continued to describe immune anomalies in individuals with ASD. There were early issues with poorly controlled studies, but as the field has matured, investigators have consistently demonstrated immune abnormalities in children with ASD, as well as in immediate family members. Some of the most compelling recent research is the presence of neuroinflammation, skewed cytokine profiles, altered lymphocyte activation, elevated circulating monocytes and autoimmune phenomena in children with autism and their mothers (Ashwood et al., 2006; Braunschweig et al., 2008; Enstrom et al., 2009b; Heuer et al., 2008; Vargas et al., 2005). Research to understand the direct relationship between immune dysfunction and autism continues, and such investigations could lead to a better understanding of the interplay between the immune and nervous systems. The following chapter will attempt to describe the current state of immune-related research in autism, and to explain how, through this research, there is the potential for a better understanding of this enigmatic disorder.

INTRODUCTION TO THE IMMUNE SYSTEM

To understand the potential role of the immune system relative to ASD, one must first be introduced to the major players involved in the immune system. The immune system as the body's defense mechanism against invaders is a very complex structure known to interact with many other systems in the body, including the endocrine and nervous systems (Carpentier and Palmer, 2009; Deverman and Patterson, 2009; McAllister and Van de Water, 2009). Upon invasion or infection with a pathogen, the immune system reacts by removal of the agent and develops immunological memory to prevent reoccurrence of infection, which is a major

strength of the immune response. The development of immunological memory helps the host by establishing a mechanism to quickly remove invaders in subsequent infections. Immune cell memory relies upon an intricate web of interaction between multiple immune factors and cell subtypes. A proper immunological response may only be achieved when all the immunological factors are well balanced, and thus in a homeostatic state. However, in disease states such as autoimmunity, the immune system may respond to 'self-protein', seeing it as the foreign antigen, thus creating a chronic activation or inflammatory atmosphere (Murphy, 2011). In other cases, the immune system may be unable to mount a proper immune response due to the depletion or dysfunction of the immune cells, such as in the case of HIV/AIDS. Overall, the immune system is solely responsible for the host's defense and is controlled and maintained by the delicate interplay between several immunological factors that can be simply divided into two arms; the innate immune and the adaptive immune response.

The innate immune response is a first-line defense system and is non-specific in its response to pathogens. These cells recognize non-specific pathogens by generic receptors on innate immune cells. This mechanism provides the host with a generic way to quickly identify certain component patterns derived from bacterial and viral particles that activate particular receptors when mounting an immune response (Murphy, 2011). These responses subsequently lead to the activation of the more specific adaptive immune response that requires presentation of processed antigens to other immune cells. Major players in the innate immune response include the monocyte/macrophage lineage, which plays a significant role in phagocytosis, the NK cells which are important in viral infections and tumor destruction, immunoglobins and the complement molecules, which both play a role in the clearance of pathogens.

The adaptive immune system is a highly specialized group of cells that respond specifically to eliminate or prevent reoccurrence of pathogens by immunological memory. Its strength arises from its ability to recognize and remember specific pathogens (Murphy, 2011). The major cell types of the adaptive immune system include the B and T lymphocytes. B-lymphocytes, or B cells, differentiate into plasma cells to secrete antibodies upon stimulation and activation, an extremely important component of the humoral immune response. T lymphocytes, or T cells, are the major effector cells of the adaptive immune system and are responsible for the elimination of infectious agents (Murphy, 2011). Mediators of both the innate and adaptive arms of the immune system exist in the form of cytokines and chemokines. Cytokines are released from immune cells and signal to other cells for activation, replication, and

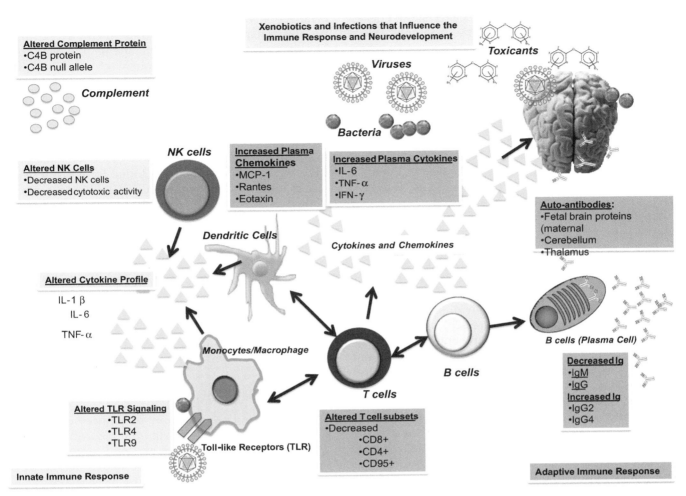

FIGURE 2.9.1 **Overview of immune abnormalities in children with autism.** Research has shown children with autism have various impairments in both the innate and adaptive immune response. In the innate immune response, research has shown the presence of altered complement protein levels, reduced NK cell activity, and changes in both the Toll-like Receptor (TLR) signaling pathways in monocytes, as well as cytokine and chemokine dysreguation. For the adaptive immune response, effector cells such as T cells have also been shown to have cytokine and chemokine dysregulation. Decreased IgG and IgM, as well as auto-antibodies brain proteins have been described in children with autism, and maternal auto-antibodies to fetal brain proteins are highly specific for ASD. Xenobiotic exposure and/or infections are also suggested to influence the immune response in children with autism. Taken together, alterations in the immune response are strongly indicated in children with autism.

killing. Chemokines are involved in directing the immune cells to migrate to sites of infection (Murphy, 2011). Each of the above-described systems has been implicated to play a role in the pathogenesis of autism. They are discussed in further detail in the following sections, and summarized in Figure 2.9.1.

ABNORMALITIES IN INNATE IMMUNITY IN ASD

Various studies have indicated differences in the innate immune response between children with ASD and unaffected individuals. As mentioned earlier, the innate immune system is the host's first line of defense.

The differences described in innate immunity in children with ASD compared to unaffected individuals include changes in monocytes/macrophages and natural killer (NK) cell activation and cell numbers (Enstrom et al., 2009b; 2010; Onore et al., 2011). Complement levels have also been reported to be altered in ASD (Mostafa and Shehab, 2010; Warren et al., 1991). An overview of the innate immune abnormalities found in children with ASD is given in the next section.

Monocytes/Macrophages

Monocytes are major players in the innate immune response. Upon infection, peripheral blood monocytes differentiate into macrophages in the tissue and travel to the site of infection. As the most prominent effector cells in the innate immune response, macrophages are involved in identifying pathogens, phagocytosing them, and activating the adaptive immune response through antigen presentation via the MHC (major histocompatibility complex) (Murphy, 2011). Macrophages express TLRs, which broadly recognize common PAMPS on viruses and bacteria. Altered monocyte/macropaghe numbers and activation levels have been indicated in children with autism. A study that examined the absolute leukocyte counts in age- and gender-matched healthy children compared to those with ASD showed a significantly higher monocyte count in the latter group, with no difference in the absolute leukocyte counts (Sweeten et al., 2003b). This is an interesting finding since high blood monocyte counts are often associated with autoimmune disorders and some infectious diseases (Sweeten et al., 2003b). This study indicated that the immune system of children with autism might operate at a higher level of activation compared to healthy children. Thus, this increased activation may lead to alterations in neurodevelopment.

In an attempt to examine the function and activation of monocytes in a well-characterized group of children with autism, Enstrom et al. examined monocyte signaling via TLR-2, TLR-4, and TLR-9. Monocytes were cultured and activated with mitogens specific for each signaling pathway and resulted in altered TLR signaling in ASD compared to controls. TLR-2 activated monocytes demonstrated an increase in pro-inflammatory cytokines, IL-1b, IL-6 and TNF-α, while TLR-4 activation also showed an increase in IL-1 β (Enstrom et al., 2010). TLR-9 activation resulted in a decrease in IL-1b, IL-6, GMCSF and TNF-α. These findings are intriguing as pro-inflammatory cytokines are thought to affect neurodevelopment (Aly et al., 2006; Doherty, 2007). Therefore, the innate immune system might have an impact on the function and development of the nervous system, which may lead to changes in behavioral outcomes. These results also indicated that children with autism have a dysfunction in monocyte signaling that may lead to long-term problems in their response to infection. Therefore, it is important to continue the investigations of monocyte function and cytokine expression in children with ASD.

Several reports demonstrate disturbances in gastrointestinal activity in children with autism (Ashwood and Wakefield, 2006; Maenner et al. 2011; Wasilewska et al., 2009). One study examining monocyte activation levels in the blood of children with autism with persistent gastrointestinal abnormalities indicated that these children had innate immune abnormalities (Ashwood et al., 2003). Monocytes were isolated from the children and activated via mitogen stimulation. The results suggested that children with gastrointestinal problems in conjunction with ASD produced lower amounts of the pro-inflammatory cytokines IL-6, IL-1β, IL-12, IL-23 and the counter-regulatory cytokine IL-10 when monocytes were stimulated (Jyonouchi et al., 2011). This impaired signaling was in response to Toll-like receptor agonists for TLR2/6 and TLR 7/8, which are intracellular receptors for ssRNA. The authors suggested that impaired innate signaling might be an indication of an increased vulnerability to common microbial infections in children with autism who have gastrointestinal problems. Overall, the authors concluded from this research that this sub-group of children with ASD and gastrointestinal problems may be more vulnerable to common microbial infections and that classical monocytes may play a role in disease pathogenesis in children with ASD and gastrointestinal co-morbidities (Jyonouchi et al., 2011).

As much research is still needed in the area of monoctye activity in children with ASD, it would be intriguing to consider abnormalities in monocyte signaling and activation as a potential biomarker for altered immune function in a sub-group of children with autism.

Natural Killer Cells (NK)

NK cells are a unique subset of lympocytes that walk a fine line between the innate immune system and the adaptive immune system. NK cells only represent a small number of total lymphocytes in peripheral blood and do not express the traditional specific receptors as their T and B lymphocyte counterparts (Schleinitz et al., 2010). NK cells have been shown to play a role in immunity against parasitic and viral infections, cancer, and have a suggested role in autoimmunity. These cells are found in abundance in both the human liver and uterus (Schleinitz et al., 2010), and are the most prominent lymphocyte subset found in the uterus during pregnancy. Further, research has shown a link between low numbers of NK cells and miscarriage recurrence (Tang et al., 2011). Therefore researchers have explored the link between pregnancy, autoimmunity, and NK cell function as a possible mechanism for tolerance induction. An imbalance between inhibitory and activating NK cells has been implicated in several autoimmune disorders, such as systemic lupus erythematosus (SLE), multiple sclerosis, diabetes, rheumatoid arthritis (RA), and the neurodevelopmental disorder, autism (Enstrom et al., 2009b; Schleinitz et al., 2010).

Over two decades ago Warren et al., (1987) described a decrease in NK cell function in children with autism. A more recent study examined mRNA expression in peripheral blood of children with ASD and found an increase in expression of NK cell associated genes (Gregg et al., 2008). In another study, which examined a large population of autism subjects, lower NK cell activity was found in about 45% of a subset of children with ASD (Vojdani et al., 2008). In an expansion of the study by Gregg et al. (2008), Enstrom et al. (2009b), examined NK cell activity in children with ASD together with age-matched typically developing controls, and looked for changes in activation and killing. Using microarray analysis, the researchers profiled NK gene expression and a performed functional analysis on NK cells isolated from peripheral blood. Results showed that after stimulation, there was a decrease in NK cell cytotoxic activity compared to age-matched controls. In addition, there was an up-regulation in RNA expression of NK cell receptors and effector molecules (Enstrom et al., 2009b).

There has been one report of an infection model for autism using mice that implicates an alteration in NK cell numbers (Hsiao and Patterson, 2011). In a rodent model of maternal immune activation (MIA), which mimics viral infection using a synthetic double-stranded RNA (poly(I:C)) and leads to autism-related behaviors in offspring, examination of the placentas following infection revealed an increase in uterine NK cells (Hsiao and Patterson, 2011). This is an important finding, as an alteration in the NK cells located in the placenta during fetal development might have a negative impact on neurodevelopment. Thus, it will be interesting to further investigate NK cell activity in the placenta and uterus during pregnancy. Abnormalities in NK cells, such as described above, may represent a susceptibility factor in ASD, and may predispose to the development of autoimmunity and/or adverse neuroimmune interactions during critical periods of development.

Research findings highlighted in this section suggest that abnormalities in the innate immune response are prevalent in children with ASD. As the innate immune system is the body's first line of defense, it is critical to fully understand why children with ASD have such abnormalities. As a fully functional innate immune response is necessary for the adaptive immune response to occur, abnormalities in the innate response will affect the subsequent adaptive immune response, which may result in children with ASD having increased adaptive immune abnormalities – as described in the next section.

Humoral Immunity

Immunoglobins

In addition to cell-mediated immunity, the humoral immune response makes up the other functional arm of the immune system. Humoral immunity involves the substances found in the humors or body fluid, and is primary comprised of antibodies and components of the complement system. Antibodies are secreted by B cells, which receive co-stimulation from CD4+ helper T cells as well as antigen presenting cells, such as the dendritic cells. Antibodies or immunoglobulins (Ig) are 'Y'-shaped glycoproteins that are found in the blood and tissue. In humans, there are four major types of antibodies; IgM which is produced first, IgA, which is found in mucosal tissue, IgE, which plays a role in the allergy response, and IgG which makes up the bulk of immunoglobulin in the circulation and is also known to cross the placenta during gestation. Each Ig has a different biological function and property for a specific immune defense. Ig acts by priming macrophages for phagocytosis and neutralization of foreign objects such as bacteria and viruses (Murphy, 2011). It may also cause agglutination and precipitation of antigen-antibody complexes and stimulation of the complement pathway.

Several studies have examined circulating immunoglobulin levels in autism. One such study showed decreased levels of IgM and IgG in plasma from children with autism, which correlated with more aberrant behaviors (Heuer et al., 2008). In another study, increased levels of the atypical isotypes, IgG2 and IgG4 were reported in the plasma of children with autism (Croonenberghs et al., 2002b; Enstrom et al., 2009a). Immunoglobulin levels are the result of the complex interaction between antigen presenting cells, T cells and B cells. In addition, Ig levels are extremely low at birth and take up to 10 years to reach adult levels. As such, these levels may be a useful measure of normal development of the humoral immune system.

The finding that children with ASD have lower overall levels that correlate with behavioral symptoms might indicate a common factor that affects the development of both the immune and nervous systems. Identification of this common defect would be instrumental in defining at least one pathological pathway in ASD.

Complement

The complement pathway plays a critical role in both the innate and adaptive immune response. Composed of three different distinct pathways including classical, mannose binding lectin (MBL), and alternative (Murphy, 2011), complement is involved in the lysis and removal of infectious organisms from the blood, and is suggested to be involved in cellular apoptosis in the brain (Corbett et al., 2007). The complement pathway activates over 25 proteins and protein fragments that can opsonize pathogens, induce inflammation, and form antibody-antigen complexes.

Research has proved that an association exists between complement levels and some autoimmune disorders (Mostafa and Shehab, 2010; Samano et al., 2004). Since recent studies have indicated an autoimmune phenomenon in autism, investigators have sought to identify a potential role for the complement system in autism; the complement component C4 has been studied most extensively. Complement component C4 commences the initial step of activation in the classical pathway of complement activation and humoral defense and is determined by two pairs of allotypes, C4A and C4B (Samano et al., 2004; Warren et al., 1994). The plasma C4 protein is composed of the protein products of the C4A and C4B genes, which are localized in the middle of the class III region of the MHC molecule (Martinez et al., 2001). Deficiency in the C4 allotype has been associated with several autoimmune-associated diseases such as SLE, and has also been linked with autism (Onore et al., 2011; Samano et al., 2004). Research has shown that individuals with autism had a significant increase in the frequency of the null allele at the C4B locus compared to controls (Warren et al., 1991). A more recent study also linked the C4B null allele to autism and a family history of autoimmunity (Mostafa and Shehab, 2010). Results indicated that the presence of the C4B null allele was significantly higher in children with autism (37%) compared to controls (8%) (Mostafa and Shehab, 2010). In addition, the increased presence of the C4B null allele had a significantly higher association with autism, and a family history of autoimmunity (Mostafa and Shehab, 2010; Sweeten et al., 2008; Warren et al., 1995). Taken together, these studies indicate a possible link between the C4B null allele and autoimmunity in association with autism.

Research findings have also indicated that C4B null alleles have an increased frequency in children with autism independent of autoimmunity (Odell et al., 2005; Sweeten et al., 2003a). Investigators discovered that an increased frequency of the C4B null allele in subjects with the human leukocyte antigen class III C4BQ0 had an increased risk of developing autism (Odell et al., 2005). In this study, the researchers examined families with and without ASD. An estimated 42.4% of subjects with autism were carriers compared to only 14.5% of controls. The investigators concluded that this genetic trait leads to a relative risk of 4.33 of developing autism (Odell et al., 2005). In another study, researchers examined the association of the C4B null allele with a common mutation in CYP21A2, a gene located 3Kb downstream of C4 that encodes for an enzyme important in the synthesis of cortisol and the maintenance of proper androgen levels (Sweeten et al., 2003a). This association was investigated due to concurrent deletions of the C4B null allele and the CYP21A2 gene (Carroll et al., 1985). However, no association between the C4B null allele and CYP21A2 genetic mutation was noted for autism (Sweeten et al., 2008).

Other, early, studies describing the levels of the C4B protein in serum from children with autism compared to control subjects indicated that activated T lymphocytes were inversely correlated with decreased plasma levels of C4B protein (Warren et al., 1995).

Another study by the same group indicated a decrease in C4B protein concentration in the plasma of autistic patients compared to that of normal subjects (Warren et al., 1994). A more recent case-control proteomic study, which examined serum from children with autism compared to typical control subjects, found a differential expression of proteins in apolipoprotein, complement factor H related protein (FHRI), complement C1q, and fibronectin 1 (FN1). In addition, complement deposition has been indicated in both brain and gastrointestinal tissue from children with autism (Torrente et al., 2002; Vargas et al., 2005).

Studies using brain tissue taken from individuals with ASD are limited, due to the rare availability of these tissue samples from young children. However, in one seminal study, Vargas and colleagues examined post-mortem brain tissue samples from children with autism. Using immunocytochemistry, the investigators found deposition of complement proteins in the cerebellum that was absent in control brains (Vargas et al., 2005). The complement complexes were located in the Purkinje cells as well as the microglia, which are the macrophage-like cells of the nervous system. The presence of complement protein in these tissue sections suggests that complement activation might play a role in tissue destruction in the brains of these individuals. Of great interest, the complement deposits were not found to be co-localized with immunoglobulin in the brain. Thus, there may be an alternative role for complement in the brain, especially when found near microglia. A role for C1q in axonal pruning has been described in the developing brain, and perhaps the increased C1q levels in the autistic brain represent an attempt at repair or remodeling (Amler et al., 2006).

In addition to looking for complement components in the brain, researchers have also examined duodenal biopsies from children with regressive autism and compared them to children with various autoimmune disorders such as celiac disease, cerebral palsy, mental retardation, as well as to normal controls. Using immunohistochemistry, an increase in the deposition of the complement protein C1q was found on the epithelial surface, co-localized with IgG in biopsy samples from children with regressive autism (Torrente et al., 2002). The presence of C1q deposits co-localized with IgG suggests immune activation in gut lesions in children with regressive autism. This provides further evidence of possible immune-mediated pathology in autism.

Evidence of changes in blood complement component levels, now noted by several groups, as well as tissue deposition of C1q, strengthens the notion that complement may in some way be associated with pathological changes in a subgroup of individuals with autism. However, additional studies are needed to determine the exact mechanism, if any, of the relationship between components of the complement system and the development of autism.

ABNORMALITIES IN THE ADAPTIVE IMMUNE RESPONSE IN ASD

In addition to abnormalities in the innate arm of the immune system, abnormalities in the cells and components that comprise the adaptive immune system have been noted in some individuals with autism. We will highlight the major findings in this section.

Cellular Immunity

T Lymphocytes (T cells)

T lymphocytes, or T cells, play a major role in cell-mediated immunity as effector cells of the adaptive immune response. They are distinguished from other lymphocytes, such as B cells, by the T cell receptor (TCR) on the cell surface. T cells can further be divided by the expression of TCR accessory proteins such as CD4 and CD8 on the cell surface. CD4 positive cells are helper T cells (Th) that become activated upon recognition of a specific peptide in conjunction with MHC class II molecules located on antigen-presenting cells. Once activated, the cells differentiate into specific Th subtypes depending on what cytokines are secreted by the antigen presenting cell. Each subtype has a specific role in directing the immune system according to the type of pathogen encountered. T helper-1 cells protect against intracellular pathogens, T helper-2 cells protect against multi-cellular parasitic pathogens, and T helper-17 cells protect against extra-cellular bacteria at mucosal surfaces. In addition, there are CD4+ subsets like Th0, Th3, and Tregs that protect against excessive inflammation during infection, or the perpetuation of autoimmunity. These different subsets of the T helper lineage secrete different cytokines to facilitate different actions within the immune response, and are usually defined by both their cell surface molecule expression and the cytokines they secrete. The CD8-positive T cells, or cytotoxic T cells (CTL), play an important role in viral immunity and cancer defense. These cells are presented with antigen via MHC class I molecules, which are present on almost every cell type within the body, including the neurons of the brain (Murphy, 2011; Needleman et al., 2010).

Over the course of autism research, several studies have indicated abnormalities in T cell immunity in children with autism compared to healthy controls. In addition to the original Stubbs and Crawford study in 1977 that examined decreased lymphocytes counts in children with ASD, a subsequent study, which examined a group of children aged 7–15 with autism, cultured lymphocytes challenged with PHA displayed a decrease in the percentages of T helper cells following stimulation, and a lower suppressor cell ratio as determined by flow cytometry (Denney et al., 1996). In a more recent paper, utilizing a well-characterized population of children with autism compared to age-matched controls, peripheral blood mononuclear cells (PBMCs) were isolated and challenged with PHA or tetanus, and cytokine profiles from the cellular response were determined. Children with autism exhibited an increase in GM-CSF, TNF-α and IL-13 expression and a decrease in IL-12p40 expression. Of great interest, cytokine expression was associated with altered behaviors in children with autism. For example, an increase in T helper-1 cytokines was associated with greater impairments in core features of autism and aberrant behaviors (Ashwood et al., 2011b). As for cellular markers on T cells, there was a significant decrease in the expression of CD3, CD4, and CD8 T cells, which may partially explain the altered cytokine profiles in children with autism (Ashwood et al., 2011b).

The Fas receptor (FasR), also referred to as the cell surface marker CD95, has also been associated with ASD. The Fas receptor serves as a death receptor, which upon ligation with Fas ligand, initiates programmed cells death or apoptosis. Within the immune system, the Fas receptor is involved with maintaining immunological tolerance (Stranges et al., 2007). This is likely achieved by limiting lymphocyte proliferation and attenuation of CD95 signaling may play a role in autoimmunity (Stranges et al., 2007). CD4+ T lymphocytes from children with autism showed a decreased expression of CD95. This suggests that children with autism might have difficulty in regulating the cellular immune response (Stranges et al., 2007).

Regulatory T cells play an important role in immunological self-tolerance and the prevention of autoimmunity. T regulatory cells are identified by expression of CD4 and CD25 on their cell surface, as wells as the intracellular expression of the transcription factor FOXP3. A study examining regulatory cells indicated that children with autism had a significantly lower frequency of CD4+ CD25+ T regulatory cells compared to controls (Mostafa et al., 2010). Results also indicated lower T regulatory cell frequencies in children with autism that had allergic manifestations and a family history of autoimmunity. Thus, the decreased frequency of T regulatory cells in children with autism may be a contributing factor to autoimmunity in a subgroup of autistic subjects (Mostafa et al., 2010).

T cells are critical components of the adaptive immune response. Thus, abnormalities in this cell type may lead to disruption in other aspects of the adaptive immune response. It is therefore important to fully comprehend the abnormalities found in both T cell numbers and function, in order to better understand the mechanisms of immune dysfunction in ASD.

B Lymphocytes (B cells)

B cells also serve an important role in the adaptive immune response, specifically the humoral immune response. B cells recognize invading pathogens through the B cell receptor, a membrane bound version of immunoglobulin. This recognition triggers phagocytosis, degradation of the pathogen, and presentation of peptide fragments through MHC II molecule to helper T cells. Depending on the type of T cell help provided, B cells can proliferate and class switch to the appropriate immunoglobulin for fighting the particular pathogen encountered (IgG, IgA, IgE, or remain IgM). Of this population of activated B cells, some will differentiate into plasma cells that migrate to the bone marrow and secrete large quantities of antigen-specific immunoglobulin, or they will become long-lived memory B cells that serve as a primer for a secondary response if the same pathogen is encountered a second time.

Despite the preponderance of studies examining immunoglobulin levels in children with autism, very few studies have investigated either B cell function or peripheral prevalence. One study examined the total lymphocyte counts using flow cytometry. Results indicated a decrease in circulating CD20+ B cells in children with autism compared to healthy controls and siblings (Yonk et al., 1990). A more recent study has demonstrated a 20% increase in the number of B cells per volume of blood in children with autism (Ashwood et al., 2011a). In addition, of the cellular activation markers measured, CD38 was significantly higher in children with autism compared to controls.

While these studies indicate a possible change in the B cell population of the immune system, further studies are needed to address the relationship between these findings and the etiology of autism. Later in this chapter we will describe the autoimmune phenomena of auto-antibodies directed against brain proteins in children with ASD, as well as antibodies to fetal brain proteins in the blood of their mothers. It will be important to fully understand the role of the humoral and innate immune systems in the production of these auto-antibodies.

Cytokines and Chemokines

Cytokines and chemokines play a very important role in intercellular communication through autocrine, paracrine, and/or endocrine action. While the term cytokine/chemokine has come to describe most small extracellular signaling molecules, which are used in nearly every tissue including the nervous system, the term has its origins in the immune system. Historically, as well as in modern immune nomenclature, the cytokines expressed by cells of the immune system are used not only to distinguish the cells phenotypically, but to describe their function as well. For example, T helper-1 cells are promoted by the presence of IL-12 and IFN-γ, and in turn secrete IFN-γ, a major player in the inflammatory response and critical for defense against intracellular bacteria. T helper-2 cells are promoted by IL-4 and secrete IL-5, IL4, and IL-13, major players in defense against multi-cellular parasites and the development of allergies. T helper-17 cells secrete IL-17 and IL-23, and regulate bacterial invasion at mucosal surfaces, while regulatory T cells secrete IL-10 and TGF-β to promote tolerance to self-proteins, as well as regulate the inflammatory response. Elevated cytokines in plasma or following cellular activation may be indicative of a disease state or the presence of an inflammatory process. Therefore, measuring cytokines as well as chemokine levels is an excellent indicator of immune status. As such, they may serve in the future as potential biomarkers to identify immune dysfunction in children with autism.

There are a plethora of studies examining the levels of cytokines and chemokines in the plasma of individuals with autism (Table 2.9.1). Subjects with autism have been reported to have a significant increase in IFN-γ and IL-1RA with a trend towards increased IL-6 and TNF-α (Croonenberghs et al., 2002a). More recently, one study indicated an increase in IL-1RA as well as IL-1β, IL-5, IL-8, IL-12(p70), IL-13, IL-17 and Gro-alpha in the plasma of ASD subjects compared to age-matched controls (Suzuki et al., 2011). Another study demonstrated an increase in IL-1β, IL-6, IL-8 and IL-12(p40) in subjects with autism, which was associated with children that had a regressive form of ASD and impaired communication and aberrant behaviors (Ashwood et al., 2011b). Elevated chemokine levels have also been indicated in children with autism. A recent study described an increase in plasma levels of MCP-1, Rantes, and eotaxin, which were all associated with higher aberrant behavioral scores and more impaired development and adaptive function (Ashwood et al., 2011c). While most of the cytokines reported to be increased in ASD are of a pro-inflammatory nature, the levels of regulatory cytokines have also been investigated. Results indicated that children with autism have decreased plasma levels of TGF-β compared to age-matched, typically developing controls and demonstrate a correlation between lower TGF-β cytokine levels and adaptive behavioral symptoms (Ashwood et al., 2008a; Okada et al., 2007).

Plasma cytokine levels provide information regarding the current immune status of the individual. By understanding which cytokine is elevated provides information about what cell type or cellular process might be abnormal. An over-activated immune system,

TABLE 2.9.1 Comprehensive Studies of Cytokine and Chemokine Profiles in Autism

Source	Study description	Reference
Plasma	Elevated levels of IL-1, IL-6, IL-8 and IL-12p40. Associated with regression	(Ashwood et al., 2011b)
	Increase in chemokine MCP-1, Rantes and Eotaxin levels in ASD subjects compared to age-matched typically developing controls. An association between increased chemokines levels with aberrant behaviors.	(Ashwood et al., 2011c)
	In male ASD subjects, an increase in cytokines IL-1β, IL-1RA, IL-5, IL-8, IL-12(p70), IL-13, IL-17 and GRO-α.	(Suzuki et al., 2011)
	Increase in leptin levels in ASD subjects compared to age-matched controls.	(Ashwood et al., 2008b)
	Increase in macrophage migration inhibitory factor (MIF) in ASD subjects compared to age-matched controls.	(Grigorenko et al., 2008)
	Decrease in TGF-β in subjects with ASD compared to controls.	(Ashwood et al., 2008a; Okada et al., 2007)
	Increase in IL-12 and IFN-γ in ASD subjects compared to age-matched controls.	(Singh, 1996)
Cytokine and chemokine expression in cell cultures	In isolated PBMCs stimulated with PHA, increase in GM-CSF, TNF-α and IL-13. A decrease in IL-12(p40) in ASD subjects compared to age-matched controls.	(Ashwood et al., 2011d)
	Stimulation of various TLR with ligands on monocytes isolated from subjects with ASD compared to age-matched controls. Increase in IL-1β, IL-6, TNF-α, with stimulation of TLR2. Increase in IL-1β, with stimulation of TLR4. Decrease in IL-1β, IL-6, GMCSF, TNF-α with TLR9.	(Enstrom et al., 2010)
	Increase in IFN-γ in NK cells from subjects with ASD.	(Enstrom et al., 2009b)
	Increased production of cytokines from Th1 and Th2 cytokines in ASD subjects compared to age-matched controls.	(Molloy et al., 2006)
	Increase in IL-12 and TNF-α in ASD subject with GI symptoms.	(Jyonouchi et al., 2005)
	Increase in IFN-γ and TNF-α in isolated PBMCs from ASD subjects compared to age-matched controls stimulated with LPS.	(Jyonouchi et al., 2002)
	Unstimulated whole blood cultures from subjects with ASD compared to age-matched controls had increased production of IFN-γ and IL-1RA with a trend towards higher IL-6 and TNF-α.	(Croonenberghs et al., 2002a)
	PBMCs isolated from ASD subjects unstimulated produced higher levels of TNF-α, IL-1β, and IL-6 compared to controls. PBMCs stimulated with LPS, PHA and tetanus produced increase levels of IL-12 and IL-1β.	(Jyonouchi et al., 2002)

resulting in elevated cytokine and chemokine levels, may promote cellular processes to occur that are dysregulated, and may go on unchecked. In other words, elevated cytokine and chemokine levels might have a negative effect on other biological processes in the developing body, such as the nervous system (McAllister and Van de Water, 2009). Understanding which cytokines and chemokines are elevated in plasma could provide clues that aid in the understanding of immune dysfunction in children with autism and how these might relate to changes in neurodevelopment.

As mentioned above, plasma cytokine levels provide information on the subjects' current immune status at the time of blood draw. However, in a human population, it is difficult to measure the response to immune challenge following infection. Through the use of cell culture systems, peripheral immune cells may be isolated from subjects to measure the *in vitro* immune response to global cell stimulation molecules (mitogens) as well as recall antigens such as vaccine proteins. By exposing immune cells to mitogenic challenge, investigators have shown that subjects with autism exhibit an increase in IL-13/IL-10 and IFN-γ/IL-10 ratios compared to control subjects (Molloy et al., 2006). The authors concluded that autism subjects have increased activation of both Th1 and Th2 cytokines with a predominance of Th2 (Molloy et al., 2006).

In a more recent study, *in vitro* stimulation of PBMCs with PHA (a T mitogen) and tetanus toxoid produced an increase in GM-CSF, TNF-α, and IL-13, and a decrease in IL-12(p40). The investigators interpreted this as a possible skewing toward a T helper-2 cytokine profile in children with ASD and away from a T helper-1 cytokine profile. A major strength of this research study was that the investigators coupled behavioral analysis with cytokine profiles. An association was found between the proinflammatory cytokines, TNF-α and IL-8, the T helper-1 cytokine, IFN-γ, and the severity of certain core behavior measurements (Ashwood et al., 2011b). From these results, the authors suggest that T helper-1 skewing was associated with a more impaired behavior, and the T helper-2 cytokine response was associated with improved levels of adaptive function in children with autism.

Although the above-described results indicate changes in the immune response in individuals with autism, these studies provide only a snapshot of the immune system at a particular time point. To fully evaluate the immune response in children with ASD, a longitudinal study using repeated cytokine measurements would be necessary. Finally, while it is not entirely clear exactly how cytokine levels might influence behavior, a better understanding of the mechanisms leading to immune dysfunction would provide information that could result in potential therapeutic intervention. Thus, it remains important to grasp the full extent of the relationship between cytokine markers of immune dysfunction and behavior in children with autism.

AUTOIMMUNITY

Auto-Antibodies – Children

Several investigators have proposed an autoimmune-based etiology for a subset of children with autism. The principal evidence in support of this hypothesis has been the discovery of auto-antibodies directed against various brain components (Connolly et al., 2006; Connolly et al., 1999; Goines et al., 2011; Wills et al., 2007; 2009; 2011). While still poorly understood, these auto-antibodies have the potential to be pathologically significant. Auto-antibodies may interfere with neuro-development by acting as a ligand for a target such as a receptor, by blocking receptor function, or by inducing cellular damage and/or activation of neuronal cells (Diamond et al., 2009). While it has been proposed that these auto-antibodies may have pathological consequences, they could simply be an epiphenomenon resulting from tissue destruction. Numerous studies have indicated that children with autism have antibodies against serotonin receptors, heat shock proteins, glial filament proteins and myelin basic protein, and other proteins with significant neurological relevance (Evers et al., 2002; Mostafa and AL-ayadhi, 2011a; Singh et al., 1997a, b; 1993; Vojdani et al., 2002). Although the findings in these studies are interesting, many lacked

proper controls and have some shortcomings. For example, the Singh et al. study involved subjects having large age (Singh et al., 1997b), from 4 to 30 years in those with autism, and from 5 to 48 years in healthy controls. Such studies should be viewed with caution, as the immune system of a child differs vastly from that of an adult. In addition, some of these studies did not have a verified diagnosis for the children with autism. Despite these possible issues, several recent reports, with proper control groups and diagnostic methods, continue to report the presence of auto-antibodies in plasma of children with autism.

It has been suggested that the presence of auto-antibodies in children with autism might be a phenotype of a subgroup of ASD (Careaga et al., 2010). Perhaps these auto-antibodies are a consequence of a previous damaging events, which may have occurred during brain development (Careaga et al., 2010). Some of the most compelling work to date has been the characterization of auto-antibodies directed against adult brain proteins using western blot analysis and immunohistochemistry in brain tissue sections (Cabanlit et al., 2007; Goines et al., 2011; Rossi et al., 2011; Wills et al., 2011). For example, a large well-characterized study using western blot analysis found that the blood of a subset of children with autism contains antibodies directed against human hypothalamus and thalamus (Cabanlit et al., 2007). This study revealed that 13/63 (21%) of subjects with ASD possessed antibodies that demonstrated specific reactivity to a cerebellar protein with an apparent molecular weight of approximately 45 kDa compared with only 1/63 (2%) of the typically developing controls. In a follow-up study, cerebellum-specific antibodies were also assessed by immunohistochemical (IHC) staining of sections from macue monkey cerebellum. Intense immunoreactivity to what was determined morphologically to be Golgi cells of the cerebellum was noted for 7/34 (21%) of subjects with ASD, compared with 0/23 of the typically-developing controls. Furthermore, there was a strong association between the presence of antibodies reactive to the 45kDa protein by western blot with positive immunohistochemical staining of cerebellar Golgi cells in the ASD group, but not controls. More recently, a study by Wills et al. established that the auto-antibodies are immunoreactive with GABAergic neurons, which are distributed throughout a number of brain regions (Wills et al., 2011).

In a subsequent study, further characterization of the behavioral phenotypes associated with these auto-antibodies showed that auto-antibodies specific for a 45kDa cerebellar protein in children were associated with a diagnosis of autism, while auto-antibodies directed towards a 62kDa protein were associated with the broader diagnosis of ASD (Goines et al., 2011). Of great interest, children with auto-antibodies directed against the 45kDa protein demonstrated more severe scores on the ABC (Aberrant Behaviors Checklist) Lethargy subscale, the ABC Stereotypy subscale, MSEL (Mullen Scales of Early Learning) test, as well as the VABS (Vineland Adaptive Behavioral Scale), in comparison to children without auto-antibody reactivity (Goines et al., 2011). Children with reactivity to the 62kDa protein demonstrated impaired scores on the ABC Inappropriate Speech subscale. Therefore, children with reactivity to proteins at 62kDa and 45kDa had lower adaptive and cognitive function, as well as increased aberrant behaviors when compared to children without these antibodies (Goines et al., 2011).

Collectively, this research indicates that auto-antibodies specific to brain proteins in children are associated with lower adaptive and cognitive function as well as core behavioral deficits associated with autism. The exact mechanism of these auto-antibodies has not been determined. The authors suggest that the difference in these reactivity patterns could result from the target proteins being involved in alternate pathways, each having a different biological outcome with respect to behavior. Currently, studies to determine the identity of these antigens are underway. Their identification will provide clues to which specific brain pathways are targeted, and how these pathways relate to the behavioral changes noted in children with autism.

The question remains regarding the pathological significance of these auto-antibodies. Under normal healthy conditions, antibodies are too large to cross the blood-brain barrier (BBB) and enter the brain. However, in various disease states and with certain infections, the BBB may become permeable and large molecules such as antibodies may cross this barrier (Diamond et al., 2009). Such states include hypertension, infections, toxin stress, and the presence of bacterial toxins such as pertussin toxin (Kuang et al., 2004; Kugler et al., 2007). Once the antibody enters the brain, it may act as a ligand for a receptor, or block receptor function. In addition, they may be able to fix complement, which can later lead to immune activation and tissue destruction (Diamond et al., 2009). One example of an autoimmune disorder in which auto-antibodies are able to cross the BBB barrier and lead to tissue destruction is the case of systemic lupus erythematosis (SLE) with associated cognitive and neuropsychiatric symptoms. Research has demonstrated that auto-antibodies cross the BBB and act as the NMDA receptor for glutamate through molecular mimicry (Kowal et al., 2004). This phenomenon was also proven in an animal model in which the auto-antibodies were administered to mice, leading cognitive impairment and neuronal cell death (Huerta et al., 2006). This is an excellent example of a neurodevelopmental disorder in which auto-antibodies are known to lead to brain destruction.

Studies have also indicated that children with autism have antibodies directed against transglutaminase. Rosenspire et al. have recently reported that:

1) A sub-population of ASD children (~25–30%) express a significantly higher than expected autoimmune response directed to transglutaminase II (anti-TG2), and

2) That expression of high levels of anti-TG2 are significantly linked in to the (HLA)-DR3, Q2 and DR7, DQ2 haplotypes (Rosenspire et al., 2011).

TG2 is a multifunctional enzyme of about 80 kDa perhaps best known for its ability to catalyze the covalent cross linking of a γ-glutaminyl residue of a protein/peptide substrate to an ε-lysl residue of a protein/peptide co-substrate (De Vivo et al., 2009). TG2 is important for normal neural development, as transglutaminase activity typically increases during early development, especially in the cerebellar cortex (Ruan and Johnson, 2007). During development, TG activity is associated with enhanced neurite outgrowth (Maccioni and Seeds, 1986; Mahoney et al., 1996), and the stabilization of CNS synapses through TG2 mediated formation of protease resistance cross-linking between synaptic proteins (Festoff et al., 2001). Due to the critical role of TG in neurodevelopment, it will be important to determine the pathological significance of these auto-antibodies in the etiology of autism.

Gangliosides have recently become another protein of interest in autism. These are sialylated glycosphingolipids located on the outer leaflets of the plasma membrane found in all vertebrates. Ganglioside proteins are abundant in the nervous system and are involved in neurotransmission, and as such play an important role in neural function (Ariga et al., 2008; Zitman et al., 2010). Ganglioside MI is the most abundant ganglioside in the neural membrane. In a recent study, children with autism had a significantly higher frequency of serum anti-ganglioside MI antibodies as measured by ELISA (Mostafa and AL-ayadhi, 2011b).

While there are several intriguing clues regarding auto-antibodies and their potential role in autism, we still have a long way to go with respect to proving their pathological significance, and in some cases, identifying the target antigens. However, there may come a time when, at least for a sub-group of individuals, we may have strong biomarkers of autism risk, and the potential for future therapeutic intervention.

Auto-Antibodies – Maternal

In addition to the presence of auto-antibodies in children with autism, the presence of auto-antibodies has also been indicated in some mothers of children with autism. The presence of maternal antibodies in autism were first described by Dalton et al., and were thought to affect behavior in a rodent model (Dalton et al., 2003). Since then, several studies have expanded upon this earlier work to more fully characterize these antibodies. For example, in one large well-characterized population study, plasma from a subset of mothers of children with autism demonstrated antibody reactivity against fetal and adult brain proteins for two bands at 37 and 73 kDa in about 12% of mothers (Braunschweig et al., 2008). This reactivity was not found in plasma from mothers of typically-developing children. In an expanded study of the same population, Braunschweig, et al. profiled fetal-brain reactive auto-antibodies for an additional 338 mothers, including 215 mothers of children diagnosed with an ASD, and 123 mothers of typically developing children (Braunschweig et al., 2011). Highly significant associations between the presence of IgG reactivity to fetal brain proteins at 37 kDa and 73kDa and a childhood diagnosis of full autism (AU) ($p = 0.0005$) was maintained in this follow up study. Interestingly, the 37/73 kDa band pattern was associated with lower scores on measures of expressive language ($p = 0.005$). Additionally, the authors reported paired reactivity to proteins at 39 kDa and 73 kDa, which correlated strongly with a broader diagnosis of ASD ($p = 0.0007$); this pattern was significantly associated with increased irritability on the Aberrant Behavioral Checklist ($p = 0.05$). Further characterization of the maternal antibody targets revealed conserved expression of both antigen pairs in late-gestation Rhesus brain as well as variable presence in human fetal CNS and non-CNS tissues. This study provides strong evidence for more than one pattern of reactivity to fetal brain proteins by maternal antibodies associated with ASDs, and such reactivity appears to have a relationship with certain behaviors characteristic of ASD.

Other research groups have also demonstrated serum auto-antibody reactivity to brain proteins. In a smaller study using only 11 mothers, Zimmerman and colleagues tested serum reactivity to prenatal, postnatal and adult rat brain using western blot analysis from mothers of children with autism (Zimmerman et al., 2007). Auto-antibody reactivity to fetal brain protein from mothers of children with autism was present for 2 to 18 years after birth. In another slightly larger study, using 100 mothers of children with autism and 100 mothers of typically developing controls, serum auto-antibody reactivity was tested via western blot analysis against rodent embryonic brain tissue and human fetal brain tissue (Singer et al., 2008). A predominant banding pattern was observed in samples from mothers of children with autism at 36kDa and 39kDa. Although the identity of the target antigens remains under investigation in the above studies, the researchers suggest that the presence of such IgG antibodies in the blood during gestation might cross the BBB potentially leading to alterations in fetal brain development.

In order to determine whether these auto-antibodies do indeed have pathological significance, various animal model studies have been conducted. A pilot non-human primate study was conducted, wherein Rhesus monkey dams were exposed during pregnancy to IgG from mothers with fetal brain-specific antibodies, or to IgG from control mothers with no reactivity. The offspring of these monkeys were evaluated for specific social, communication, and stereotypic behaviors that are characteristic of autism. The results indicated that the monkeys exposed to IgG from the mothers of children with autism showed increases in stereotypical and hyperactive behaviors (Martin et al., 2008). Another study used a mouse model to determine the possible mechanism of the auto-antibodies from mothers of children with autism. In this model, pregnant mice were administered with IgG from mothers of children with autism, and from typical controls, at embryonic days 13 through 18. Behavioral testing demonstrated that mice exposed to IgG from mothers of children with autism displayed anxiety-like behaviors and alterations in sociability (Singer et al., 2009) providing an additional example of behavioral consequences in offspring exposed to these antibodies. This is an extremely intriguing finding, as the presence of these auto-antibodies in the serum of mothers might be used as a biomarker to determine susceptibility to having a child with autism. In addition, once the target antigens are fully characterized, therapeutic interventions could be developed to prevent a subset of autism.

One must also consider the risk factors that lead to the presence of maternal antibodies to fetal brain proteins. One such risk factor is the genetic susceptibility to the production of auto-antibodies through a polymorphism in the tyrosine kinase MET receptor (Campbell et al., 2006; 2007; 2008; Eagleson et al., 2011). In an initial population case-controlled study of over 500 autism families, researchers found a genetic association between the MET 'C' allele in the promoter region of the MET gene. A relative risk of 2.27 was from autism diagnosis associated with a CC genotype and a risk of only 1.67 associated for the CG genotype compared to the GG genotype (Campbell et al., 2006). MET signaling is involved in neurodevelopment and gastrointestinal repair (Campbell et al., 2006) and a polymorphism affecting cell surface expression of this receptor could have long-lasting effects on neurodevelopment. MET also plays an important role in the immune system as a negative regulator, through control of the level of activation of antigen-presenting cells such as dendritic cells, macrophages, and B cells (Beilmann et al., 1997; 2000; Okunishi et al., 2005). Thus, alteration in this receptor may lead to immune abnormalities, such as a lack of immune regulation, thereby setting the stage for auto-antibody production. A very strong association between the presence of the MET 'C' allele and maternal auto-antibodies to fetal brain proteins was in fact noted in a recent study by Heuer et al. (2011). In a sample of 365 mothers, including 202 mothers of children with ASD, the functional *MET* promoter variant rs1858830 C allele was strongly associated with presence of an ASD-specific 37 kD + 73 kD band pattern of maternal auto-antibodies to fetal brain proteins (P = 0.003). To determine the mechanism of this genetic association, MET protein and cytokine production were measured in freshly prepared peripheral blood mononuclear cells from 76 mothers of ASD and TD children. The *MET* rs1858830 C allele was significantly associated with MET protein expression (P = 0.025). Moreover, decreased expression of the regulatory cytokine IL-10 was associated with both the *MET* gene C allele (P = 0.001) and reduced MET protein levels (P = 0.002) (Heuer et al., 2011). These results indicate genetic distinction among mothers who produce ASD-associated antibodies to fetal brain proteins, and suggest a potential mechanism for how a genetically determined decrease in MET protein production may lead to a reduction in immune regulation. Thus, this study was the first to describe a genetic susceptibility factor associated with autism, and a functional outcome of that factor. Identification of a pre-disposing genetic factor such as MET should contribute greatly towards the understanding of the mechanisms involved in a subset of ASD cases.

CONCLUSIONS

In conclusion, there is a great deal of convincing evidence suggesting that abnormalities of the immune system are frequently found in children with autism. We have described herein several studies supporting the concept that children with autism have dysfunction in both the innate and adaptive immune systems. These abnormalities include alterations in monocyte activity, complement levels, NK cell number and function, immune cellular signaling patterns, and auto-antibodies found in both the children as well as their mothers. Much progress has been made in the field of immunity and autism since the first paper describing immune abnormalities in autism was published in 1977 (Stubbs and Crawford, 1977). ASD is still a serious health concern, and the numbers of affected children have expanded dramatically in recent years. Therefore, it is essential to understand the exact mechanisms behind these various immune abnormalities and how they might serve as a biological marker of neuroimmune anomalies. It is also critical to determine how the various

immune biomarkers associate with behavioral outcome. It is through this research that we might finally elucidate delete some of the etiological mechanisms that lead to this enigmatic disorder.

References

Altevogt, B.M., Hanson, S.L., Leshner, A.I., 2008. Autism and the environment: challenges and opportunities for research. Pediatrics 121, 1225–1229.

Aly, H., Khashaba, M.T., El-Ayouty, M., El-Sayed, O., Hasanein, B.M., 2006. IL-1β, IL-6 and TNF-α and outcomes of neonatal hypoxic ischemic encephalopathy. Brain Development 28, 178–182.

American Psychiatric Association (APA), 2000. Diagnostic and statistical manual of mental disorders: DSM-IV text revision. American Psychiatric Association, Washington, DC.

Amler, R.W., Barone Jr., S., Belger, A., Berlin Jr., C.M., Cox, C., Frank, H., et al., 2006. Hershey Medical Center Technical Workshop Report: Optimizing the design and interpretation of epidemiologic studies for assessing neurodevelopmental effects from in utero chemical exposure. Neurotoxicology 27, 861–874.

Ariga, T., McDonald, M.P., Yu, R.K., 2008. Role of ganglioside metabolism in the pathogenesis of Alzheimer's disease—a review. Journal of Lipid Research 49, 1157–1175.

Ashwood, P., Wakefield, A.J., 2006. Immune activation of peripheral blood and mucosal CD3+ lymphocyte cytokine profiles in children with autism and gastrointestinal symptoms. Journal of Neuroimmunology 173, 126–134.

Ashwood, P., Anthony, A., Pellicer, A.A., Torrente, F., Walker-Smith, J.A., Wakefield, A.J., 2003. Intestinal lymphocyte populations in children with regressive autism: Evidence for extensive mucosal immunopathology. Journal of Clinical Immunology 23, 504–517.

Ashwood, P., Corbett, B.A., Kantor, A., Schulman, H., Van de Water, J., Amaral, D.G., 2011. In search of cellular immunophenotypes in the blood of children with autism. PLoS ONE 6, e19299.

Ashwood, P., Enstrom, A., Krakowiak, P., Hertz-Picciotto, I., Hansen, R.L., Croen, L.A., et al., 2008. Decreased transforming growth factor β1 in autism: A potential link between immune dysregulation and impairment in clinical behavioral outcomes. Journal of Neuroimmunology 204, 149–153.

Ashwood, P., Krakowiak, P., Hertz-Picciotto, I., Hansen, R., Pessah, I., Van de Water, J., 2011. Elevated plasma cytokines in autism spectrum disorders provide evidence of immune dysfunction and are associated with impaired behavioral outcome. Brain, Behavior and Immunity 25, 40–45.

Ashwood, P., Krakowiak, P., Hertz-Picciotto, I., Hansen, R., Pessah, I.N., Van de Water, J., 2011. Associations of impaired behaviors with elevated plasma chemokines in autism spectrum disorders. Journal of Neuroimmunology 232, 196–199.

Ashwood, P., Krakowiak, P., Hertz-Picciotto, I., Hansen, R., Pessah, I.N., Van de Water, J., 2011. Altered T cell responses in children with autism. Brain, Behavior and Immunity 25, 840–849.

Ashwood, P., Kwong, C., Hansen, R., Hertz-Picciotto, I., Croen, L., Krakowiak, P., et al., 2008. Brief report: Plasma leptin levels are elevated in autism: Association with early onset phenotype? Journal of Autism and Developmental Disorders 38, 169–175.

Ashwood, P., Wills, S., Van de Water, J., 2006. The immune response in autism: A new frontier for autism research. Journal of Leukocyte Biology 80, 1–15.

Beilmann, M., Odenthal, M., Jung, W., Vande Woude, G.F., Dienes, H.P., Schirmacher, P., 1997. Neoexpression of the c-met/hepatocyte growth factor-scatter factor receptor gene in activated monocytes. Blood 90, 4450–4458.

Beilmann, M., Vande Woude, G.F., Dienes, H.P., Schirmacher, P., 2000. Hepatocyte growth factor-stimulated invasiveness of monocytes. Blood 95, 3964–3969.

Boyle, C.A., Boulet, S., Schieve, L.A., Cohen, R.A., Blumberg, S.J., Yeargin-Allsopp, M., et al., 2011. Trends in the prevalence of developmental disabilities in US children, 1997-2008. Pediatrics 127, 1034–1042.

Braunschweig, D., Ashwood, P., Krakowiak, P., Hertz-Picciotto, I., Hansen, R., Croen, L.A., et al., 2008. Autism: Maternally derived antibodies specific for fetal brain proteins. Neurotoxicology 29, 226–231.

Braunschweig, D., Duncanson, P., Boyce, R., Hansen, R., Ashwood, P., Pessah, I.N., et al., 2011. Behavioral correlates of maternal antibody status among children with autism. Journal of Autism and Developmental Disorders [E-Pub. ahead of print].

Cabanlit, M., Wills, S., Goines, P., Ashwood, P., Van de Water, J., 2007. Brain-specific autoantibodies in the plasma of subjects with autistic spectrum disorder. Annals of the New York Academy of Sciences 1107, 92–103.

Campbell, D.B., D'Oronzio, R., Garbett, K., Ebert, P.J., Mirnics, K., Levitt, P., et al., 2007. Disruption of cerebral cortex MET signaling in autism spectrum disorder. Annals of Neurology 62, 243–250.

Campbell, D.B., Li, C., Sutcliffe, J.S., Persico, A.M., Levitt, P., 2008. Genetic evidence implicating multiple genes in the MET receptor tyrosine kinase pathway in autism spectrum disorder. Autism Research 1, 159–168.

Campbell, D.B., Sutcliffe, J.S., Ebert, P.J., Militerni, R., Bravaccio, C., Trillo, S., et al., 2006. A genetic variant that disrupts MET transcription is associated with autism. Proceedings of the National Academy of Sciences of the United States of America 103, 16834–16839.

Careaga, M., Van de Water, J., Ashwood, P., 2010. Immune dysfunction in autism: A pathway to treatment. Neurotherapeutics 7, 283–292.

Carpentier, P.A., Palmer, T.D., 2009. Immune influence on adult neural stem cell regulation and function. Neuron 64, 79–92.

Carroll, M.C., Palsdottir, A., Belt, K.T., Porter, R.R., 1985. Deletion of complement C4 and steroid 21-hydroxylase genes in the HLA class III region. EMBO Journal 4, 2547–2552.

Center for Disease and Control (CDC), C.f.D.C.a.P., 2006. Mental health in the United States: Parental report of diagnosed autism in children aged 4-17 years—United States, 2003-2004. Morbidity and Mortal Weekly Report 55, 481–486.

Investigators, A.a.D.D.M.N.S.Y.P., Center for Disease and Control (CDC), C.f.D.C.a.P., 2009. Prevalence of autism spectrum disorders - Autism and Developmental Disabilities Monitoring Network, United States, 2006. Morbidity & Mortal Weekly Report, Surveillance Summaries 58, 1–20.

Connolly, A.M., Chez, M.G., Pestronk, A., Arnold, S.T., Mehta, S., Deuel, R.K., 1999. Serum autoantibodies to brain in Landau-Kleffner variant, autism, and other neurologic disorders. Journal of Pediatrics 134, 607–613.

Connolly, A.M., Chez, M., Streif, E.M., Keeling, R.M., Golumbek, P.T., Kwon, J.M., et al., 2006. Brain-derived neurotrophic factor and autoantibodies to neural antigens in sera of children with autistic spectrum disorders, Landau-Kleffner syndrome, and epilepsy. Biological Psychiatry 59, 354–363.

Corbett, B.A., Kantor, A.B., Schulman, H., Walker, W.L., Lit, L., Ashwood, P., et al., 2007. A proteomic study of serum from children with autism showing differential expression of apolipoproteins and complement proteins. Molecular Psychiatry 12, 292–306.

Croonenberghs, J., Bosmans, E., Deboutte, D., Kenis, G., Maes, M., 2002. Activation of the inflammatory response system in autism. Neuropsychobiology 45, 1–6.

Croonenberghs, J., Wauters, A., Devreese, K., Verkerk, R., Scharpe, S., Bosmans, E., et al., 2002. Increased serum albumin, gamma globulin, immunoglobulin IgG, and IgG2 and IgG4 in autism. Psychological Medicine 32, 1457–1463.

Dalton, P., Deacon, R., Blamire, A., Pike, M., McKinlay, I., Stein, J., et al., 2003. Maternal neuronal antibodies associated with autism and a language disorder. Annals of Neurology 53, 533–537.

Denney, D.R., Frei, B.W., Gaffney, G.R., 1996. Lymphocyte subsets and interleukin-2 receptors in autistic children. Journal of Autism and Developmental Disorders 26, 87–97.

Deverman, B.E., Patterson, P.H., 2009. Cytokines and CNS development. Neuron 64, 61–78.

De Vivo, G., Di Lorenzo, R., Ricotta, M., Gentile, V., 2009. Role of the transglutaminase enzymes in the nervous system and their possible involvement in neurodegenerative diseases. Current Medicinal Chemistry 16, 4767–4773.

Diamond, B., Huerta, P.T., Mina-Osorio, P., Kowal, C., Volpe, B.T., 2009. Losing your nerves? Maybe it's the antibodies. Nature Reviews Immunology 9, 449–456.

Doherty, G.H., 2007. Developmental switch in the effects of TNFα on ventral midbrain dopaminergic neurons. Neuroscience Research 57, 296–305.

Eagleson, K.L., Campbell, D.B., Thompson, B.L., Bergman, M.Y., Levitt, P., 2011. The autism risk genes MET and PLAUR differentially impact cortical development. Autism Research 4, 68–83.

Enstrom, A., Krakowiak, P., Onore, C., Pessah, I.N., Hertz-Picciotto, I., Hansen, R.L., et al., 2009. Increased IgG4 levels in children with autism disorder. Brain, Behavior and Immunity 23, 389–395.

Enstrom, A.M., Lit, L., Onore, C.E., Gregg, J.P., Hansen, R.L., Pessah, I.N., et al., 2009. Altered gene expression and function of peripheral blood natural killer cells in children with autism. Brain, Behavior and Immunity 23, 124–133.

Enstrom, A.M., Onore, C.E., Van de Water, J.A., Ashwood, P., 2010. Differential monocyte responses to TLR ligands in children with autism spectrum disorders. Brain, Behavior and Immunity 24, 64–71.

Evers, M., Cunningham-Rundles, C., Hollander, E., 2002. Heat shock protein 90 antibodies in autism. Molecular Psychiatry 2, S26–S28.

Festoff, B.W., Suo, Z., Citron, B.A., 2001. Plasticity and stabilization of neuromuscular and CNS synapses: Interactions between thrombin protease signaling pathways and tissue transglutaminase. International Review of Cytology 211, 153–177.

Goines, P., Haapanen, L., Boyce, R., Duncanson, P., Braunschweig, D., Delwiche, L., et al., 2011. Autoantibodies to cerebellum in children with autism associate with behavior. Brain, Behavior and Immunity 25, 514–523.

Gregg, J.P., Lit, L., Baron, C.A., Hertz-Picciotto, I., Walker, W., Davis, R.A., et al., 2008. Gene expression changes in children with autism. Genomics 91, 22–29.

Grigorenko, E.L., Han, S.S., Yrigollen, C.M., Leng, L., Mizue, Y., Anderson, G.M., et al., 2008. Macrophage migration inhibitory factor and autism spectrum disorders. Pediatrics 122, e438–e445.

Hertz-Picciotto, I., Delwiche, L., 2009. The rise in autism and the role of age at diagnosis. Epidemiology 20, 84–90.

Heuer, L., Schauer, J., Goines, P., Ashwood, P., Hertz-Picciotto, I., Hansen, R., et al., 2008. Reduced levels of immunoglobulin in children with autism correlates with behavioral symptoms. Autism Research 1, 275–283.

Heuer, L., Braunschweig, D., Ashwood, P., Van de Water, J., Campbell, D.B., 2011. Association of a MET genetic variant with autism-associated maternal autoantibodies to fetal brain proteins and cytokine expression. Translational Psychiatry E-Pub. e48.

Hsiao, E.Y., Patterson, P.H., 2011. Activation of the maternal immune system induces endocrine changes in the placenta via IL-6. Brain, Behavior and Immunity 25, 604–615.

Huerta, P.T., Kowal, C., DeGiorgio, L.A., Volpe, B.T., Diamond, B., 2006. Immunity and behavior: Antibodies alter emotion.

Proceedings of the National Academy of Sciences of the United States of America 103, 678–683.

Jyonouchi, H., Geng, L., Ruby, A., Zimmerman-Bier, B., 2005. Dysregulated innate immune responses in young children with autism spectrum disorders: Their relationship to gastrointestinal symptoms and dietary intervention. Neuropsychobiology 51, 77–85.

Jyonouchi, H., Geng, L., Streck, D.L., Toruner, G.A., 2011. Children with autism spectrum disorders (ASD) who exhibit chronic gastrointestinal (GI) symptoms and marked fluctuation of behavioral symptoms exhibit distinct innate immune abnormalities and transcriptional profiles of peripheral blood (PB) monocytes. Journal of Neuroimmunology 238, 73–80.

Jyonouchi, H., Sun, S., Itokazu, N., 2002. Innate immunity associated with inflammatory responses and cytokine production against common dietary proteins in patients with autism spectrum disorder. Neuropsychobiology 46, 76–84.

Kowal, C., DeGiorgio, L.A., Nakaoka, T., Hetherington, H., Huerta, P.T., Diamond, B., et al., 2004. Cognition and immunity; antibody impairs memory. Immunity 21, 179–188.

Kuang, F., Wang, B.R., Zhang, P., Fei, L.L., Jia, Y., Duan, X.L., et al., 2004. Extravasation of blood-borne immunoglobulin G through blood-brain barrier during adrenaline-induced transient hypertension in the rat. International Journal of Neuroscience 114, 575–591.

Kugler, S., Bocker, K., Heusipp, G., Greune, L., Kim, K.S., Schmidt, M.A., 2007. Pertussis toxin transiently affects barrier integrity, organelle organization and transmigration of monocytes in a human brain microvascular endothelial cell barrier model. Cell Microbiology 9, 619–632.

Lord, C., Risi, S., Lambrecht, L., Cook Jr., E.H., Leventhal, B.L., DiLavore, P.C., et al., 2000. The autism diagnostic observation schedule-generic: A standard measure of social and communication deficits associated with the spectrum of autism. Journal of Autism and Developmental Disorders 30, 205–223.

Maccioni, R.B., Seeds, N.W., 1986. Transglutaminase and neuronal differentiation. Molecular and Cellular Biochemistry 69, 161–168.

Maenner, M.J., Arneson, C.L., Levy, S.E., Kirby, R.S., Nicholas, J.S., Durkin, M.S., October 20, 2011. Brief Report: Association between behavioral features and gastrointestinal problems among children with autism spectrum disorder. Journal of Autism and Developmental Disorders. [E-Pub. ahead of print].

Mahoney, S.A., Perry, M., Seddon, A., Bohlen, P., Haynes, L., 1996. Transglutaminase forms midkine homodimers in cerebellar neurons and modulates the neurite-outgrowth response. Biochemical and Biophysical Research Communications 224, 147–152.

Martin, L.A., Ashwood, P., Braunschweig, D., Cabanlit, M., Van de Water, J., , D.G.Amaral, 2008. Stereotypies and hyperactivity in rhesus monkeys exposed to IgG from mothers of children with autism. Brain, Behavior and Immunity 22, 806–816.

Martinez, O.P., Longman-Jacobsen, N., Davies, R., Chung, E.K., Yang, Y., Gaudieri, S., et al., 2001. Genetics of human complement component C4 and evolution the central MHC. Frontiers in Bioscience 6, D904–D913.

McAllister, A.K., Van de Water, J., 2009. Breaking boundaries in neural-immune interactions. Neuron 64, 9–12.

Molloy, C.A., Morrow, A.L., Meinzen-Derr, J., Schleifer, K., Dienger, K., Manning-Courtney, P., et al., 2006. Elevated cytokine levels in children with autism spectrum disorder. Journal of Neuroimmunology 172, 198–205.

Mostafa, G.A., AL-ayadhi, L.Y., 2011. Increased serum levels of anti-ganglioside M1 auto-antibodies in autistic children: Relation to the disease severity. Journal of Neuroinflammation 8, 39.

Mostafa, G.A., AL-ayadhi, L.Y., 2011. A lack of association between hyperserotonemia and the increased frequency of serum anti-myelin basic protein auto-antibodies in autistic children. Journal of Neuroinflammation 8, 71.

Mostafa, G.A., Shehab, A.A., 2010. The link of C4B null allele to autism and to a family history of autoimmunity in Egyptian autistic children. Journal of Neuroinflammation 223, 115–119.

Mostafa, G.A., Al Shehab, A., Fouad, N.R., 2010. Frequency of CD4+CD25high regulatory T cells in the peripheral blood of Egyptian children with autism. Journal of Child Neurology 25, 328–335.

Murphy, K., 2011. Janeway's Immunobiology, eighth ed. Garland Science, New York.

Needleman, L.A., Liu, X.B., El-Sabeawy, F., Jones, E.G., McAllister, A.K., 2010. MHC class I molecules are present both pre- and postsynaptically in the visual cortex during postnatal development and in adulthood. Proceedings of the National Academy of Sciences of the United States of America 107, 16999–17004.

Odell, D., Maciulis, A., Cutler, A., Warren, L., McMahon, W.M., Coon, H., et al., 2005. Confirmation of the association of the C4B null allelle in autism. Human Immunology 66, 140–145.

Okada, K., Hashimoto, K., Iwata, Y., Nakamura, K., Tsujii, M., Tsuchiya, K.J., et al., 2007. Decreased serum levels of transforming growth factor-β1 in patients with autism. Progress in Neuro-psychopharmacology & Biological Psychiatry 31, 187–190.

Okunishi, K., Dohi, M., Nakagome, K., Tanaka, R., Mizuno, S., Matsumoto, K., et al., 2005. A novel role of hepatocyte growth factor as an immune regulator through suppressing dendritic cell function. Journal of Immunology 175, 4745–4753.

Onore, C., Careaga, M., Ashwood, P., 2011. The role of immune dysfunction in the pathophysiology of autism. Brain, Behavior and Immunity. [E-Pub. ahead of print].

Rosenspire, A., Yoo, W., Menard, S., Torres, A.R., 2011. Autism spectrum disorders are associated with an elevated autoantibody response to tissue transglutaminase-2. Autism Research 4, 242–249.

Rossi, C.C., Van de Water, J., Rogers, S.J., Amaral, D.G., 2011. Detection of plasma autoantibodies to brain tissue in young children with and without autism spectrum disorders. Brain, Behavior and Immunity. [E-Pub. ahead of print].

Ruan, Q., Johnson, G.V., 2007. Transglutaminase 2 in neurodegenerative disorders. Frontiers in Bioscience 12, 891–904.

Samano, E.S., Ribeiro Lde, M., Gorescu, R.G., Rocha, K.C., Grumach, A.S., 2004. Involvement of C4 allotypes in the pathogenesis of human diseases. Revista do Hospital das Clínicas Faculdade de Medicina, São Paulo 59, 138–144.

Schleinitz, N., Vely, F., Harle, J.R., Vivier, E., 2010. Natural killer cells in human autoimmune diseases. Immunology 131, 451–458.

Singer, H.S., Morris, C.M., Gause, C.D., Gillin, P.K., Crawford, S., Zimmerman, A.W., 2008. Antibodies against fetal brain in sera of mothers with autistic children. Journal of Neuroimmunology 194, 165–172.

Singer, H.S., Morris, C., Gause, C., Pollard, M., Zimmerman, A.W., Pletnikov, M., 2009. Prenatal exposure to antibodies from mothers of children with autism produces neurobehavioral alterations: A pregnant dam mouse model. Journal of Neuroimmunology 211, 39–48.

Singh, V.K., 1996. Plasma increase of interleukin-12 and interferon-gamma. Pathological significance in autism. Journal of Neuroimmunology 66, 143–145.

Singh, V.K., Singh, E.A., Warren, R.P., 1997. Hyperserotoninemia and serotonin receptor antibodies in children with autism but not mental retardation. Biological Psychiatry 41, 753–755.

Singh, V.K., Warren, R., Averett, R., Ghaziuddin, M., 1997. Circulating autoantibodies to neuronal and glial filament proteins in autism. Pediatric Neurology 17, 88–90.

Singh, V.K., Warren, R.P., Odell, J.D., Warren, W.L., Cole, P., 1993. Antibodies to myelin basic protein in children with autistic behavior. Brain, Behavior and Immunity 7, 97–103.

Stranges, P.B., Watson, J., Cooper, C.J., Choisy-Rossi, C.M., Stonebraker, A.C., Beighton, R.A., et al., 2007. Elimination of antigen-presenting cells and autoreactive T cells by Fas contributes to prevention of autoimmunity. Immunity 26, 629–641.

Stubbs, E.G., Crawford, M.L., 1977. Depressed lymphocyte responsiveness in autistic children. Journal of Autism and Childhood Schizophrenia 7, 49–55.

Suzuki, K., Matsuzaki, H., Iwata, K., Kameno, Y., Shimmura, C., Kawai, S., et al., 2011. Plasma cytokine profiles in subjects with high-functioning autism spectrum disorders. PLoS One 6, e20470.

Sweeten, T.L., Bowyer, S.L., Posey, D.J., Halberstadt, G.M., McDougle, C.J., 2003. Increased prevalence of familial autoimmunity in probands with pervasive developmental disorders. Pediatrics 112, e420.

Sweeten, T.L., Odell, D.W., Odell, J.D., Torres, A.R., 2008. C4B null alleles are not associated with genetic polymorphisms in the adjacent gene CYP21A2 in autism. BMC Medical Genetics 9, 1.

Sweeten, T.L., Posey, D.J., McDougle, C.J., 2003. High blood monocyte counts and neopterin levels in children with autistic disorder. American Journal of Psychiatry 160, 1691–1693.

Tang, A.W., Alfirevic, Z., Quenby, S., 2011. Natural killer cells and pregnancy outcomes in women with recurrent miscarriage and infertility: A systematic review. Human Reproduction 26, 1971–1980.

Torrente, F., Ashwood, P., Day, R., Machado, N., Furlano, R.I., Anthony, A., et al., 2002. Small intestinal enteropathy with epithelial IgG and complement deposition in children with regressive autism. Molecular Psychiatry 7, 375–382. 334.

Vargas, D.L., Nascimbene, C., Krishnan, C., Zimmerman, A.W., Pardo, C.A., 2005. Neuroglial activation and neuroinflammation in the brain of patients with autism. Annals of Neurology 57, 67–81.

Vojdani, A., Campbell, A.W., Anyanwu, E., Kashanian, A., Bock, K., Vojdani, E., 2002. Antibodies to neuron-specific antigens in children with autism: Possible cross-reaction with encephalitogenic proteins from milk, Chlamydia pneumoniae and Streptococcus group A. Journal of Neuroimmunology 129, 168–177.

Vojdani, A., Mumper, E., Granpeesheh, D., Mielke, L., Traver, D., Bock, K., et al., 2008. Low natural killer cell cytotoxic activity in autism: The role of glutathione, IL-2 and IL-15. Journal of Neuroimmunology 205, 148–154.

Warren, R.P., Burger, R.A., Odell, D., Torres, A.R., Warren, W.L., 1994. Decreased plasma concentrations of the C4B complement protein in autism. Archives of Pediatrics & Adolescent Medicine 148, 180–183.

Warren, R.P., Foster, A., Margaretten, N.C., 1987. Reduced natural killer cell activity in autism. Journal of the American Academy of Child & Adolescent Psychiatry 26, 333–335.

Warren, R.P., Singh, V.K., Cole, P., Odell, J.D., Pingree, C.B., Warren, W.L., et al., 1991. Increased frequency of the null allele at the complement C4b locus in autism. Clinical & Experimental Immunology 83, 438–440.

Warren, R.P., Yonk, J., Burger, R.W., Odell, D., Warren, W.L., 1995. DR-positive T cells in autism: Association with decreased plasma levels of the complement C4B protein. Neuropsychobiology 31, 53–57.

Wasilewska, J., Jarocka-Cyrta, E., Kaczmarski, M., 2009. Gastrointestinal abnormalities in children with autism. Polski Merkuriusz Lekarski 27, 40–43.

Wills, S., Cabanlit, M., Bennett, J., Ashwood, P., Amaral, D., Van de Water, J., et al., 2007. Autoantibodies in autism spectrum disorders (ASD). Annals of the New York Academy of Sciences 1107, 79–91.

Wills, S., Cabanlit, M., Bennett, J., Ashwood, P., Amaral, D.G., Van de Water, J., 2009. Detection of autoantibodies to neural cells of the cerebellum in the plasma of subjects with autism spectrum disorders. Brain, Behavior and Immunity 23, 64–74.

Wills, S., Rossi, C.C., Bennett, J., Cerdeno, V.M., Ashwood, P., Amaral, D.G., et al., 2011. Further characterization of autoantibodies to GABAergic neurons in the central nervous system produced by a subset of children with autism. Molecular Autism 2, 5–54.

Yonk, L.J., Warren, R.P., Burger, R.A., Cole, P., Odell, J.D., Warren, W.L., et al., 1990. CD4+ helper T cell depression in autism. Immunological Letters 25, 341–345.

Zhao, X., Leotta, A., Kustanovich, V., Lajonchere, C., Geschwind, D.H., Law, K., et al., 2007. A unified genetic theory for sporadic and inherited autism. Proceedings of the National Academy of Sciences of the United States of America 104, 12831–12836.

Zimmerman, A.W., Connors, S.L., Matteson, K.J., Lee, L.C., Singer, H.S., Castaneda, J.A., et al., 2007. Maternal antibrain antibodies in autism. Brain, Behavior and Immunity 21, 351–357.

Zitman, F.M., Todorov, B., Furukawa, K., Willison, H.J., Plomp, J.J., 2010. Total ganglioside ablation at mouse motor nerve terminals alters neurotransmitter release level. Synapse 64, 335–338.

BRAIN IMAGING AND NEUROPATHOLOGY OF AUTISM SPECTRUM DISORDERS

Patrick R. Hof

In recent years, the fields of neuropathology and brain imaging of autism spectrum disorders (ASD) have started to reveal the consequences of disease progression in anatomically defined brain regions and their impact on the function of specific systems. Given the overlap between postmortem histopathology and imaging studies of patients, this section integrates recent evidence from both fields. The section provides an account of recent developments in our understanding of brain dysfunction in autism and emphasizes that the symptoms observed in patients result, in many cases, from subtle changes at the level of regionally constrained neuronal populations occurring on the background of a more global, diffuse pathology.

The first three chapters cover structural and functional magnetic resonance imaging (MRI) findings in ASD (Stigler and McDougle), the application of diffusion MRI to the study of ASD together with presentation of emerging technologies such as high angular resolution diffusion imaging (Roberts, Berman, and Verma), and the pathology of attention in autism using a systems approach to assess deficits in several functions of attention, representing a potential biomarker of ASD (Fan).

The remainder of the section is devoted to neuropathology. Several chapters discuss specific aspects of the neuropathology of ASD, each concentrating on specific systems or structures. Cerebellar pathology is reviewed in detail (Bauman and Kemper), followed by a description of structural and cellular changes in the amygdala (Morgan, Nordahl, and Schumann). Three chapters of this section are concerned with cortical neuropathology, with a review of discrete neuronal pathology occurring at the level of specific regions or even layers of the cerebral cortex, and affecting identifiable neuronal subpopulations. The number of pyramidal cells overall, and localized changes to their morphology and structure in regions like the insula, inferior frontal, and fusiform cortex, are discussed in the context of functional MRI findings, offering a cellular correlate to the *in vivo* observations (Uppal and Hof). Disruption in the architecture of the cerebral cortex in interesting, anatomically relevant elements known as minicolumns is presented in the context of global dysfunction of cortical systems, morphogenesis, and epigenetics (Casanova). Finally, the potential imbalance in excitatory and inhibitory cortical function is discussed in light of recent data on neurotransmitter systems and new mechanistic hypotheses (Blatt).

The final chapter in this section (Wegiel, Schanen, Cook, Brown, Kuchna, Nowicki, Wegiel, Imaki, Ma, London, and Wisniewski) presents new information on the occurrence of neuropathological findings in the brains of patients with ASD and chromosome 15q11–q13 duplication. These cases represent a unique opportunity to assess the degree of pathologic abnormalities as well as a number of comorbidities (such as lesions usually seen in Alzheimer's disease) in a situation in which autism is caused by an identifiable genetic defect.

All of the chapters in Section 3 summarize data that take advantage of the most modern and rigorous approaches in quantitative brain anatomy. The combined knowledge generated by neuropathological and brain imaging studies of ASD is essential to assess key phenotypes, isolate possible biomarkers, and help the development of reliable animal models – discussed in the last section of this book.

3.1

Structural and Functional MRI Studies of Autism Spectrum Disorders

Kimberly A. Stigler*, *Christopher J. McDougle*†

*Department of Psychiatry, Indiana University School of Medicine, Indianapolis, IN, USA †Department of Psychiatry, Harvard Medical School, Boston, MA, USA

INTRODUCTION

Autism spectrum disorders (ASD) are neuropsychiatric conditions characterized by impairments in social skills and communication, as well as repetitive interests and activities. The ASD include autistic disorder (autism), Asperger's disorder, and pervasive developmental disorder not otherwise specified (PDD-NOS). Among the ASD, autism was the first to be characterized, with the publication of a landmark case series by Leo Kanner in 1943. His original report described 11 patients who exhibited symptoms of autistic aloneness, echolalia, pronoun reversal, and need for sameness; an account that closely parallels the current criteria for autism as outlined in the Diagnostic and Statistical Manual of Mental Disorders (fourth edition, Text Revision; DSM-IV-TR) (American Psychiatric Association, 2000).

Kanner (1943) also documented the presence of enlarged head size in 5 of the 11 patients in his case series; an intriguing finding that later led researchers

The Neuroscience of Autism Spectrum Disorders.
http://dx.doi.org/10.1016/B978-0-12-391924-3.00017-X

to investigate head circumference and estimate neuronal numbers in autism. Preliminary studies that included both children and adults were difficult to interpret because head circumference provides a relatively accurate indication of brain size in early childhood, but not in adolescence or adulthood (Aylward et al., 2002; Bailey et al., 1993; Bartholomeusz et al., 2002; Fombonne, 2000; Lainhart et al., 1997). In light of this, researchers focused on infants who later developed autism, finding average or slightly below average head circumference at birth (Courchesne et al., 2003; Dawson et al., 2007; Dementieva et al., 2005; Hazlett et al., 2005; Lainhart et al., 1997). This was followed by accelerated brain growth at or before 1 year of age, with 15% to 20% exhibiting macrocephaly (head size greater than two standard deviations above the mean) by 4 to 5 years of age.

Technological advances have permitted researchers to further investigate these findings via the application of neuroimaging techniques. Computerized tomography (CT) was initially used to search for neuroanatomical abnormalities; however, poor spatial resolution and use of ionizing radiation ultimately restricted its utility in this population (Campbell et al., 1982; Damasio et al., 1980; Rosenbloom et al., 1984). Given these concerns, investigators turned toward a novel imaging approach, magnetic resonance imaging (MRI), to probe brain structure and function in individuals with ASD. Magnetic resonance imaging was found to have many potential advantages, including a high degree of spatial resolution and contrast sensitivity, as well as an absence of ionizing radiation. Research advances led to further improvement of structural MRI (sMRI). In addition, diffusion tensor imaging (DTI), an MRI technique that assesses white matter microstructure, and functional MRI (fMRI), a technique that measures changes in blood oxygenation, were developed (for review, see Huettel et al., 2009). The introduction of these novel neuroimaging approaches using MRI would soon herald a new era of investigation into the neurobiology of ASD. This chapter will review sMRI and fMRI studies in ASD, with an emphasis on well-designed controlled research.

STRUCTURAL MAGNETIC RESONANCE IMAGING

Total Brain Volume

Initial observations of early abnormal brain enlargement, as well as studies of head circumference, suggested a dynamic process of age-dependent brain growth abnormalities in autism. Studies of young children with autism have consistently found increased total brain volume (TBV), with some research suggesting a 5% to 10% enlargement (Carper et al., 2002;

Courchesne et al., 2001; Hazlett et al., 2005; Sparks et al., 2002; Stanfield et al., 2008). An early sMRI study investigated TBV in boys with autism, scanning half at 2 to 4 years, and the other half at 5 to 16 years of age (Courchesne et al., 2001). Neonatal head circumference records suggested that TBV was normal at birth in the autism group. However, sMRI revealed that by 2 to 4 years of age, 90% of the autism group had larger mean TBVs vs. younger controls, with 37% considered macrocephalic. In contrast, the older autism group did not have greater mean TBVs than older controls. A meta-analysis of head circumference, postmortem, and sMRI studies found that children with autism had reduced or normal brain size at birth, exhibited rapid brain overgrowth during early childhood, and then experienced a plateau in brain growth such that brain size was within the normal range by adolescence and adulthood (Figure 3.1.1) (Redcay and Courchesne, 2005). A longitudinal study of brain growth in early childhood (1.5 to 5 years) found significant enlargement of cerebral gray and white matter, suggesting that early brain growth begins before 2 years of age (Schumann et al., 2010). Another longitudinal study found cerebral cortical enlargement at both 2 and 4 to 5 years of age, but rate of cerebral growth was similar to that observed in controls (Hazlett et al., 2011). Whereas some studies have recorded persistent brain enlargement in adolescents and adults with autism (Freitag et al., 2009; Hazlett et al., 2006), other longitudinal research has found

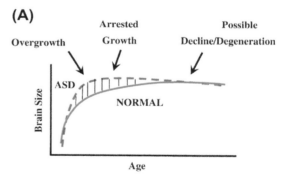

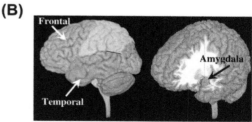

FIGURE 3.1.1 Three phases of growth pathology in autism. (A) Model of early brain overgrowth in autism that is followed by arrest of growth. Red dashed line represents ASD, while blue line represents age-matched typically developing individuals. In some regions and individuals, the arrest of growth may be followed by degeneration. (B) Sites of regional overgrowth in ASD include frontal and temporal cortices, and amygdala. *Source: from Courchesne et al. (2010).*

abnormally slowed white matter development and overgrowth of deep gray matter structures during adolescence in autism (Hua et al., 2011).

Gray and White Matter

Research into early brain enlargement in autism revealed that brain volume did not change in a uniform fashion. In addition, gray and white matter abnormalities were found throughout the brain, illustrating the distributed nature of brain involvement in ASD (Carper et al., 2002; Muller, 2008). Increased frontal lobe volume is one of the most reliable findings (Brun et al., 2009; Hazlett et al., 2006; Palmen et al., 2005), including reports of increased dorsolateral prefrontal cortex (DLPFC) (Mitchell et al., 2009), and DLPFC and medial prefrontal cortex (MPFC) (Carper and Courchesne, 2005; Herbert et al., 2004). However, other studies have found no difference or decreased orbitofrontal cortex (OFC) volume in ASD (Girgis et al., 2007; Hardan et al., 2006b).

Further investigation of gray matter volume revealed differences in multiple brain regions (Figure 3.1.2) (Kates et al., 2004; Palmen et al., 2005). Volumetric differences in gray matter have been predominately found in the frontal cortex (e.g., middle, superior, and inferior frontal gyri, medial OFC) (Bonilha et al., 2008; Hadjikhani et al., 2006; Hardan et al., 2009a; Hyde et al., 2010; McAlonan et al., 2005; Waiter et al., 2004),

but have also been reported in other brain areas, e.g., superior temporal sulcus (STS), fusiform gyrus (FG), insula, inferior parietal lobule (Boddaert et al., 2004; Bonilha et al., 2008; Hadjikhani et al., 2006; Kosaka et al., 2010; McAlonan et al., 2005; Rojas et al., 2006; Waiter et al., 2004). Volumetric differences in white matter have also been observed in several areas (e.g., cerebellum, corpus callosum), with abnormalities primarily recorded in the outer radiate compartments (Amaral et al., 2008; Carper and Courchesne, 2005; Casanova et al., 2011; Herbert et al., 2004; Stanfield et al., 2008). An sMRI study of 13 boys with autism vs. 28 controls (14 with typical development, 14 with developmental language disorder) found increased volume in the outer zone of radiate white matter in all lobes, but mainly in the frontal lobe (Herbert et al., 2004). However, the inner zone of white matter (e.g., corpus callosum, internal capsule) showed no volumetric differences, indicating an excess of intrahemispheric, and a deficit of interhemispheric, corticocortical connections in autism.

Investigations into other characteristics of the cortex have been conducted in ASD. Abnormalities of cortical thickness have begun to suggest age-related differences. Increased cortical thickness was found in children with autism vs. typically developing controls, primarily in the temporal and parietal lobes (Hardan et al., 2006c). In contrast, studies of adolescents and adults with ASD

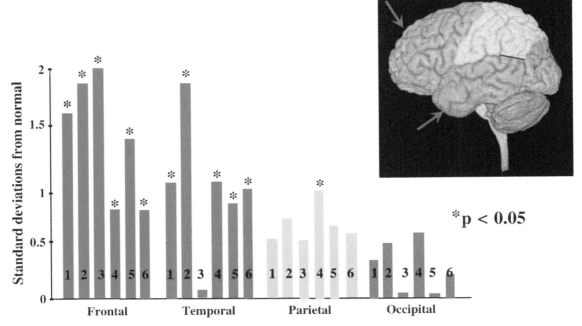

FIGURE 3.1.2 Gray matter overgrowth in ASD. The bars represent abnormalities in different cerebral regions (standard deviations from normal average (in children and adolescents with ASD. Note the general gradient of abnormality. References: 1, Carper et al., 2002, 3.4 years; 2, Bloss and Courchesne, 2007, 3.8 years; 3, Kates et al., 2004, 7.6 years; 4, Palmen et al., 2005, 11.1 years; 5, Hazlett et al., 2006, 19.1 years; 6, Schumann et al., 2010, 2–4 years. *(adapted from Courchesne et al., 2010).*

suggest cortical thinning may take place in the temporal and parietal lobes (Hadjikhani et al., 2006; Wallace et al., 2010), with the study by Hadjikhani and colleagues also finding cortical thinning in frontal regions. Research of cortical shape has also found abnormalities in frontal, parietal, and temporal regions [e.g., STS, inferior frontal gyrus (IFG), sylvian fissure, intraparietal sulcus, right parietal lobe] (Kates et al., 2009; Levitt et al., 2003; Nordahl et al., 2007). Studies of cortical folding found differences in the frontal lobe of boys with autism vs. Asperger's disorder, with the greatest increase recorded in the left inferior frontal region (i.e., Broca's area) (Jou et al., 2010). It is also worth noting that in many instances, structural abnormalities visualized by sMRI (and fMRI) in patients with autism have found correlates in quantitative neuropathological analyses of neuronal and glial cell numbers in a number of brain regions, as reviewed in more detail in other chapters in this section.

Cerebellum

In addition to its involvement in motor coordination, the cerebellum has been found to play a role in modulating language, emotion, and executive function (Hodge et al., 2010). Studies of the cerebellar vermis have shown inconsistent results. Early research recorded decreased volume of cerebellar vermal lobules VI and VII in autism vs. controls (Courchesne et al., 1988). Subsequent studies were unable to replicate these findings (Garber and Ritvo, 1992; Hashimoto et al., 1992; Holttum et al., 1992; Kleiman et al., 1992; Piven et al., 1992). Given these disparate results, a larger study of these vermal regions was conducted, finding 86% exhibited hypoplasia and 14% had hyperplasia (Courchesne et al., 1994). Additional investigations supported the initial finding of decreased volume of vermal lobules VI and VII (Akshoomoff et al., 2004; Kaufmann et al., 2003; Stanfield et al., 2008). Studies of total cerebellum have been more consistent than those of vermis, demonstrating increased volumes in children with ASD (Hardan et al., 2001b; Herbert et al., 2003; Palmen et al., 2005; Sparks et al., 2002).

Amygdala

Volumetric research of the amygdala, a region that has an integral role in emotional and social behavior, has been inconsistent, with age emerging as an important factor (Adolphs, 2008). Increased amygdala volume has been reported in children with autism less than 10 years of age vs. typically developing controls (Schumann et al., 2004; 2009), with some research finding an association between amygdala enlargement and social and communication deficits (Kim et al., 2010; Munson et al., 2006; Schumann et al., 2009; Sparks et al., 2002).

In adolescents and adults, investigators have recorded similar (Haznedar et al., 2000) or smaller amygdala volumes compared to healthy controls (Aylward et al.,

1999; Nacewicz et al., 2006; Pierce et al., 2001). In one study, decreased amygdala volume was positively correlated with time spent fixating on the eye region of faces (Nacewicz et al., 2006). The age-related trajectory of amygdala growth may be related to the pattern of early brain overgrowth observed in autism (Courchesne et al., 2007).

Hippocampus

The hippocampus plays a key role in the integration of information and in associative memory. Volumetric studies have reported inconsistent findings ranging from no difference (Bigler et al., 2003; Haznedar et al., 2000; Howard et al., 2000; Piven et al., 1998; Saitoh et al., 1995) to increased or decreased hippocampal volume in autism vs. healthy controls (Aylward et al., 1999; Nicolson et al., 2006; Schumann et al., 2004; Sparks et al., 2002). These disparate findings may be due to differences in imaging methods and subject heterogeneity.

Insula

The anterior insula is believed to integrate multiple neurocognitive systems related to affective, empathic, and interoceptive processes (Kosaka et al., 2010; Menon and Uddin, 2010; Uddin and Menon, 2009). Compared to healthy controls, adults with ASD were found to exhibit decreased gray matter volume in the right insula and IFG (Kosaka et al., 2010).

Fusiform Gyrus

The fusiform face area (FFA) of the FG is involved in aspects of face processing, including face identification (Haxby et al., 2002). Research using adolescents and adults with ASD has reported unchanged, increased, or decreased FG volumes (Pierce et al., 2001; Toal et al., 2010; Waiter et al., 2004). A study of boys with autism found asymmetries of the FG versus typically developing controls (Herbert et al., 2002).

Superior Temporal Gyrus

The superior temporal gyrus (STG) is implicated in the processing of eye movements, as well as in the visual analysis of social information conveyed by gaze and body movement (Allison et al., 2000; Hoffman and Haxby, 2000; Pelphrey et al., 2005; Puce et al., 1998). In comparison to typically developing controls, youths with autism have been shown to exhibit decreased gray matter volume, as well as anterior and superior displacements of the STG (Boddaert et al., 2004; Levitt et al., 2003).

Planum Temporale

The left planum temporale (PT), often referred to as Wernicke's area, is involved in auditory processing and receptive language (Nakada et al., 2001). As such, it has been associated with lexical processing (Bookheimer, 2002). The left PT has been reported to be larger in children and adolescents with autism vs. typically developing controls (Herbert et al., 2002). In contrast, other controlled research of children and adults with autism found decreased left PT volume (Rojas et al., 2002; 2005). In another study, ASD subjects were divided into younger (7 to 11 years) and older (12 to 19 years) groups, with the older group demonstrating increased left PT volume and stronger leftward asymmetry vs. typically developing controls (Knaus et al., 2009).

Inferior Frontal Gyrus

The left IFG, commonly known as Broca's area, is implicated in sentence comprehension, integration of syntactic and semantic processing regions, and working memory (Bookheimer, 2002). Research on adults with autism reported decreased volume of the IFG (Abell et al., 1999). Children with ASD and language impairment were found to exhibit rightward asymmetry of the IFG (De Fosse et al., 2004; Herbert et al., 2002).

Cingulate Cortex

The anterior cingulate cortex (ACC) is associated with the integration of cognition, emotion, and behavioral expression, while the posterior cingulate cortex (PCC) appears to be involved in visuospatial and memory function. Research has found smaller ACC volume in adults with ASD vs. healthy controls (Haznedar et al., 1997; 2000; McAlonan et al., 2002).

Caudate Nucleus

The caudate nucleus, a part of the basal ganglia that subserve executive function, is believed to play a role in stereotyped and repetitive behaviors (Turner et al., 2006). Research on children and adults with autism found increased caudate nucleus volume, and a positive correlation between caudate volume and repetitive behavior (Brambilla et al., 2003; Hollander et al., 2005; Rojas et al., 2006). Other sMRI research in children and adults with autism has documented an increase in caudate nucleus volume, but found a negative association between caudate nucleus volume and repetitive behavior (Sears et al., 1999). Another study reported that caudate nucleus volume increased with development in children and adults with ASD vs. healthy controls (Langen et al., 2007; 2009). Caudate nucleus volume was negatively correlated with repetitive behavior in the autism group.

Thalamus

The thalamus is implicated in language and emotional processing, as well as aspects of executive function (Katz and Shatz, 1996). Research involving subjects with a wide age range found no volumetric abnormalities of the thalamus (Hardan et al., 2006a; 2008; Haznedar et al., 2006; Tsatsanis et al., 2003). A study of children with autism and typically developing controls demonstrated a positive correlation between thalamic volume and TBV in both groups (Hardan et al., 2008).

Brainstem

The brainstem is implicated in sensory modulation (Ornitz, 1983). Some initial controlled research reported decreased brainstem volume in autism (Gaffney et al., 1988; Hashimoto et al., 1995), while other studies found no volumetric differences (Elia et al., 2000; Hardan et al., 2001a; Herbert et al., 2003; Kleiman et al., 1992; Piven et al., 1992). A study of children with autism vs. typically developing controls reported decreased brainstem gray matter volume in the autism group (Jou et al., 2009). Of interest, brainstem gray matter volume was positively correlated with oral sensory sensitivity in this study.

Corpus Callosum

The corpus callosum is a white matter tract that connects the cerebral hemispheres, facilitating interhemispheric connectivity. Many studies of subjects with autism vs. healthy controls have documented decreased corpus callosum volume (Chung et al., 2004; Egaas et al., 1995; Freitag et al., 2009; Hardan et al., 2000; 2009b; Keary et al., 2009; Manes et al., 1999; Piven et al., 1997; Saitoh et al., 1995; Vidal et al., 2006), although some have not found abnormalities (Elia et al., 2000; Gaffney and Tsai, 1987; Herbert et al., 2004; Tepest et al., 2010). A meta-analysis identified the anterior regions of the corpus callosum as having the largest volumetric deficits in persons with autism (Frazier and Hardan, 2009).

Diffusion Tensor Imaging

The majority of research utilizing DTI, a measure of white matter integrity, has documented decreased fractional anisotropy (coherent fiber tract directionality) in children and adults with ASD in several regions, including ventromedial prefrontal cortex (VMPFC), OFC, ACC, external capsule, internal capsule, corpus callosum, temporal stem, ventral temporal lobe, STG, and superior and middle cerebellar peduncles, among others (Alexander et al., 2007; Barnea-Goraly et al., 2004; Bloemen et al., 2010; Brito et al., 2009; Catani et al., 2008; Cheung et al., 2009; Keller et al., 2007; Lange et al., 2010; Lee et al., 2007; Lo et al., 2011; Pardini et al., 2009; Pugliese et al., 2009; Thakkar et al., 2008).

Summary

Early observations of enlarged head circumference in autism were verified by sMRI research demonstrating increased TBV and an atypical trajectory of brain development. Volumetric differences have been identified in both gray and white matter, but these findings have been inconsistent. Investigators have suggested that these discrepancies may be due to differences in study design, varying methodologies, or subject heterogeneity (Amaral et al., 2008; Craig et al., 2007; Kwon et al., 2004; McAlonan et al., 2008; Stanfield et al., 2008). The use of DTI has begun to delineate white matter abnormalities at a microstructural level in ASD.

FUNCTIONAL MAGNETIC RESONANCE IMAGING

Task-Based Studies of Core Symptoms

Social Cognition

Functional MRI research has increasingly informed the neurobiology of core social impairment in ASD. Face perception, one of the first social impairments to emerge in ASD, is a central component of social cognition (Dawson et al., 2005). Investigations of face perception have demonstrated that typically developing individuals rely on the eye region and use a holistic approach during face processing, while persons with ASD focus more on the mouth region and use a feature-based approach (Klin et al., 2002; Pelphrey et al., 2002; Weeks and Hobson, 1987).

Neutral Face Tasks

Social cognition was investigated in ASD via the use of emotionally neutral face tasks during fMRI, finding either no activation or lower activation in the FFA (Hubl et al., 2003; Pierce et al., 2001; Schultz et al., 2000). In addition, increased activation was found in object-related brain regions in the ASD group. Another study demonstrated decreased activation in the FFA, occipital face area, and STG in adults with autism vs. healthy controls (Humphreys et al., 2008). However, researchers found increased FFA activation in response to a neutral face task when subjects were cued to the eye region by a central fixation cross, suggesting an association between FFA activation and degree of gaze fixation in ASD (Hadjikhani et al., 2004).

Investigators studied abnormal functional connectivity in ASD during a neutral face processing task, finding that greater social impairment was associated with decreased FFA–amygdala connectivity and increased amygdala–right IFG connectivity (Figure 3.1.3) (Kleinhans et al., 2008). These findings suggest that abnormalities within the limbic system may contribute to social deficits in ASD. A subsequent fMRI study investigated whether abnormal habituation to neutral face stimuli characterized amygdala dysfunction in

ASD (Kleinhans et al., 2009). Decreased amygdala habituation was associated with increased social impairment in the ASD group.

Familiar Face Tasks

A fMRI study found significant FFA activation in response to familiar and strange faces in both subjects with autism and healthy controls (Pierce et al., 2004). The inclusion of familiar faces may have enhanced attention and motivation during the task in the autism group. In another study, subjects with autism exhibited normal FFA activation in response to familiar faces, and deficits in FFA activation in response to strangers' faces, suggesting decreased attention during the stranger condition (Pierce and Redcay, 2008).

Emotional Face Tasks

Functional MRI research using emotional face tasks have demonstrated decreased FFA activation (Piggot et al., 2004; Wang et al., 2004), and decreased FFA and amygdala activation (Corbett et al., 2009) in children with ASDs. A dynamic and static emotional face task was used in a study of adolescents and adults with autism. Compared to healthy controls, subjects with autism exhibited reduced activity in the FFA and amygdala in response to the dynamic task (Pelphrey et al., 2007). Another study using an emotional face task found that FFA and amygdala activation were positively correlated with time spent fixating on the eyes (Dalton et al., 2005). Increased right amygdala activation was recorded when attention bias to emotional faces was equivalent between adult subjects with autism and healthy controls (Monk et al., 2010).

Eye Gaze

Controlled fMRI research in adults with autism has demonstrated that brain regions implicated in gaze processing, such as the STG, are not sensitive to intentions conveyed by gaze shifts (Pelphrey et al., 2005). This finding suggests that differences in the response of brain regions underlying gaze processing in autism may contribute to the eye gaze impairments observed in the disorder.

Theory of Mind and the Mirror Neuron System

Early mirror neuron system (MNS) dysfunction is believed to underlie the deficits in theory of mind observed in ASD (Dapretto et al., 2006). The MNS is implicated in action observation and imitation, as well as in the understanding of emotion. Neurophysiological and neuroimaging research has identified the MNS in the pars opercularis of the IFG and the posterior parietal cortex (Buxbaum et al., 2005; Cattaneo and Rizzolatti, 2009; Iacoboni et al., 1999; Johnson-Frey et al., 2003; Rizzolatti and Craighero, 2004).

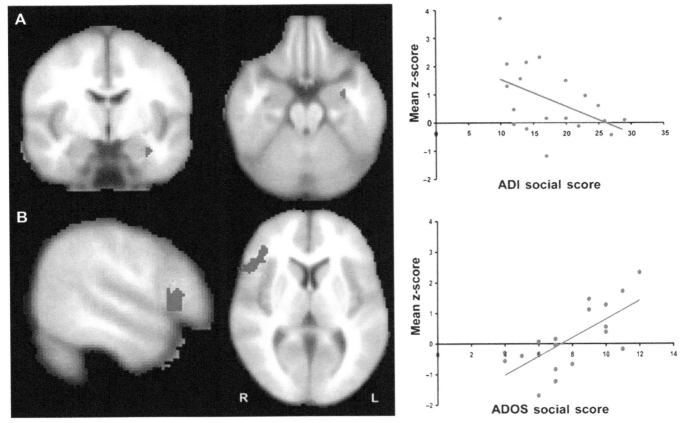

FIGURE 3.1.3   Relationship between functional connectivity and clinical severity in the ASD group. (A) An inverse correlation between fusiform face area–left amygdala connectivity and the Autism Diagnostic Interview-Revised (ADI-R) social score was found. A scatterplot depicting the relationship between face-specific connectivity and social severity on the ADI-R is shown to the right of the functional activation map. The mean z-score value for the amygdala was based on the average z-score of the cluster showing a significant relationship between connectivity and ADI-R social score. (B) A direct relationship between autism diagnostic observation schedule (ADOS) social score and activation in the right inferior frontal gyrus was found in the ASD group. The individuals with ASD with the most severe level of current functioning as measured by the ADOS showed increased connectivity to the right inferior frontal gyrus during face processing. The scatterplot depicts the relationship between the face-specific functional connectivity activation and the ADOS. The mean z-score values for the right inferior frontal gyrus were based on the average z-score of the cluster showing a significant relationship between connectivity and the ADOS social score. *Source: from Kleinhans et al. (2008).*

Investigators conducted a controlled fMRI study of MNS activation during the imitation and observation of emotional facial expressions in children with ASD, finding no MNS activity in the pars opercularis of the IFG in the autism group vs. controls (Dapretto et al., 2006). In addition, MNS activation was found to be inversely correlated with social impairment. Abnormalities in patterns of brain activation, including decreased activation of the MNS, were associated with imitation in adolescents with ASD vs. controls (Williams et al., 2006). These findings may have important implications for imitative development in ASD, which may negatively affect the development of theory of mind in this population. A controlled study of adults with autism reported increased IFG activation during the observation of hand movements compared to a rest condition, suggesting the MNS abnormalities may be associated with social impairment in this disorder (Martineau et al.,

2010). In contrast, normal fMRI responses were found in the MNS during the observation and execution of hand movements in adults with autism vs. healthy controls (Dinstein et al., 2010).

Summary

Functional MRI studies of social cognition have consistently demonstrated abnormalities in FFA activation during face processing in ASD, with findings ranging from decreased to increased activation in this region. Discrepancies regarding the direction of FFA activation may be related to differences in visual attention, motivation, or gaze patterns (Klin and Klin, 2008; Scherf et al., 2010). Research also suggests that early MNS dysfunction may be the basis of theory of mind deficits in ASD.

Language and Communication

Individuals with ASD display a wide range of language and communication impairments. As such, researchers have begun to investigate the underlying neurobiology of these deficits using fMRI approaches. The neural correlates of language development were studied in young children with autism (2 to 3 years old) and typically developing controls during natural sleep, finding a trend for abnormally right-lateralized temporal responses to language in the autism group (Redcay and Courchesne, 2008). A subsequent larger-scale fMRI study of young children (12 to 48 months old) at risk for autism vs. typically developing controls measured brain activity during the presentation of a bedtime story during natural sleep (Eyler et al., 2012). The at-risk subjects who were later diagnosed with autism demonstrated decreased left hemisphere response to speech sounds, and an abnormally right-lateralized temporal cortex response to language, that appeared to worsen with age.

Controlled fMRI research of children and adults with autism has reported decreased left IFG and increased left PT activation during various language tasks (e.g., sentence comprehension, single-word lexical semantic processing, pragmatic language comprehension) (Figure 3.1.4) (Gaffrey et al., 2007; Harris et al., 2006; Just et al., 2004; Mason et al., 2008; Tesink et al., 2009; Wang et al., 2006). Another controlled study that examined semantic processing documented increased activation in the IFG that was less left-lateralized in adolescents with ASD (Knaus et al., 2008).

Studies of children and adults with ASD have demonstrated a dependence on visualization for language processing. Although visualization is not necessary for processing low-imagery sentences, adults with autism vs. healthy controls were found to activate parietal and occipital brain regions associated with imagery during both high- and low-imagery sentence processing tasks (Kana et al., 2006). An fMRI study reported greater activation in the bilateral extrastriate visual cortex in adults with ASD compared to healthy controls, supporting a role for visual imagery during semantic processing (Gaffrey et al., 2007). Children with autism vs. typically developing controls activated occipitoparietal and ventral temporal areas during a pictorial reasoning paradigm, suggesting a dependence on visual mediation in this diagnostic group (Sahyoun et al., 2010).

Summary

Functional MRI research of language and communication suggests that young children with autism may be on a deviant neurodevelopmental trajectory

Control Subjects

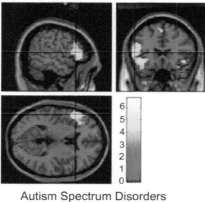

Autism Spectrum Disorders

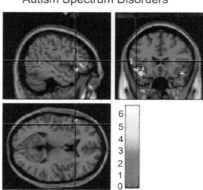

FIGURE 3.1.4 Functional MRI activation patterns for semantic > perceptual word processing tasks in ASD subjects and typically developing controls. Activation local maxima in Broca's area shown at crosshairs corresponds to functional activation in control subjects during semantic contrasted to perceptual word tasks, while ASD subjects had aberrant activation in this region. *Source: adapted from Harris et al. (2006).*

characterized by right hemispheric recruitment for language. A pattern of decreased left IFG and increased left PT activation has been demonstrated in ASD, suggesting an increased propensity to process the meaning of individual words rather than integrate them into a coherent conceptual structure. Finally, research has shown that individuals with ASD demonstrate a reliance on visualization for language processing.

Executive Function and Repetitive Symptoms

Research suggests that the repetitive symptoms commonly observed in ASD may be related to deficits in executive function that impede behavioral control (Lopez et al., 2005). Executive function includes several cognitive domains such as inhibition, working memory, set shifting, and planning, among others (Dichter and Belger, 2007; Russo et al., 2007).

A controlled study found that adults with autism exhibited decreased ACC activation during response inhibition tasks, as well as decreased functional connectivity between the inhibition network (ACC, middle cingulate gyrus, insula) and the right middle and inferior frontal and right parietal regions (Kana et al., 2007). Another study found that relative to healthy controls, adults with ASD showed increased rostral ACC activation to correct and erroneous antisaccades (Thakkar et al., 2008). The abnormally increased rostral ACC activation on correct trials was associated with higher ratings of rigid, repetitive behavior.

Working memory was investigated in a study of adults with autism vs. healthy controls using an n-back working memory task (Koshino et al., 2005). Task accuracy was similar between groups. However, the control group used verbal strategies, while the autism group used a visually oriented processing style. Another study of adults with autism and healthy controls used an oculomotor delayed response task to investigate spatial working memory (Luna et al., 2002). Relative to controls, the autism group showed decreased task-related activation in the DLPFC and PCC. Adolescents with ASD vs. typically developing controls exhibited decreased activation in the ACC, DLPFC, medial and lateral premotor cortex, and caudate during a spatial working memory task, suggesting that frontostriatal networks are dysfunctional in ASD (Silk et al., 2006).

A fMRI study used the Tower of London task to investigate planning in adults with autism and healthy controls (Just et al., 2007). Decreased connectivity between frontal and parietal areas was found in the autism group, indicating that executive function deficits may stem from decreased integration of information across brain regions in this disorder.

Summary

Functional MRI research of executive function suggests that impaired response inhibition may be associated with repetitive symptoms in ASD. Although studies in ASD subjects and controls show similar task accuracy, abnormalities in brain activation and connectivity are often observed in ASD subjects during certain executive function tasks. This finding illustrates that individuals with ASD may use different cognitive strategies to complete these tasks.

Resting State Connectivity and the Default-Mode Network

Resting state studies assess the functional connectivity of a brain region when a subject is not performing any coordinated, purposeful task (Huettel et al., 2009). During the resting state, mental events continue to arise and activate a set of brain regions known as the default-mode network (DMN). Activation of the DMN decreases during active, engaging tasks, and increases during rest and reflection, as well as during tasks involving future prospection and theory of mind (Broyd et al., 2009; Huettel et al., 2009).

Resting state connectivity studies of individuals with ASD have identified abnormalities in the DMN. A continuous resting state study of adolescents and adults with ASD and healthy controls assessed connectivity between three seed regions of the DMN involved in social and emotional processing (MPFC, PCC/precuneus, left angular gyrus) and all brain voxels (Kennedy and Courchesne, 2008a). The ASD group exhibited decreased functional connectivity of the MPFC and left angular gyrus. A subsequent controlled investigation of adolescents and adults with ASD examined abnormalities of the DMN during social and introspective tasks, and at rest (Kennedy and Courchesne, 2008b). Decreased functional activity in the ventral MPFC/ACC was recorded across the task and rest conditions in the ASD group.

A resting state study assessed striatal functional connectivity in children with ASDs and typically developing controls using three caudate nucleus and three putamen seeds for each hemisphere (Di Martino et al., 2011). The ASD group demonstrated a pattern of increased ectopic striatal functional connectivity, with abnormalities involving early developing areas including the insula and brainstem. Intrinsic functional connectivity of the insula was examined using four seeds placed in anterior and posterior regions of the insula in adolescents and young adults with ASD vs. healthy controls (Ebisch et al., 2010). Decreased connectivity was recorded between anterior and posterior insula and brain regions implicated in emotional and sensory processing.

A controlled study of adults with ASD evaluated intrinsic functional connectivity within the DMN, placing a single seed in the PCC (Monk et al., 2009). Decreased connectivity was recorded between PCC and superior frontal gyrus in the ASD group, a finding that was associated with worse social functioning (Figure 3.1.5). Moreover, increased connectivity between PCC and both right temporal lobe and right parahippocampal gyrus was found in the ASD group. Increased severity of repetitive behavior was correlated with stronger connectivity between the PCC and right parahippocampal gyrus. A controlled study of adults with ASD examined the functional connectivity of default mode sub-networks using brief resting fMRI scans (Assaf et al., 2010). Subjects with ASD showed decreased connectivity between the precuneus and MPFC/ACC

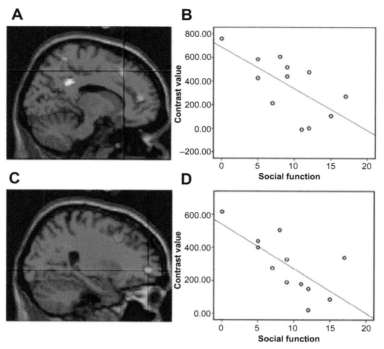

FIGURE 3.1.5   Within the ASD group, social functioning based on the Autism Diagnostic Interview-Revised (ADI-R) measure of total reciprocal social interaction (current), was negatively correlated with functional connectivity with two areas of the superior frontal gyrus, t(10) = 3.02, p = 0.006, *xyz* coordinates 14 26 48 (A) and t(10) = 3.37, p = 0.004, *xyz* coordinates 26 54 −2 (C). A higher score on the ADI-R measure indicates worse social function. For (A) and (C), the threshold was set at p = 0.05 with a minimum cluster size of 50 voxels. To illustrate this association, contrast values were extracted from a 4 mm sphere around the peak activation and plotted with the ADI-R measure of social function, Pearson r = −0.66, p = 0.019 for *xyz* coordinates 14 26 48 (B) and Pearson r = −0.707, p = 0.008 for *xyz* coordinates 26 54 −2 (D). Although other areas correlated with social function, analyses focused on areas of the default network where group differences were found. *Source: from Monk et al. (2009).*

that was negatively correlated with severity of social and communication impairment.

Summary

Research of the DMN, a network implicated in higher-order social cognitive processes such as theory of mind, has demonstrated abnormalities in functional connectivity in ASD. In addition, atypical functional connectivity within the DMN has been associated with severity of core symptoms of ASD, highlighting its potential usefulness as a biomarker in this diagnostic group.

CONCLUSIONS

Structural MRI and fMRI research has meaningfully informed the neurobiology of ASD. Early findings of an above-average head circumference in autism led to sMRI studies that demonstrated increased TBV and an atypical trajectory of neurodevelopment in affected individuals. Structural MRI studies have consistently identified abnormalities in cortical gray and white matter volume in individuals with ASD. White matter

abnormalities have been further elucidated at a microstructural level with DTI. The neural circuitry of ASD has been examined with fMRI using task-based and resting state approaches, finding abnormalities in cortical activation and connectivity. In addition, resting state studies have revealed atypical patterns of functional connectivity in the DMN. Although MRI studies have greatly contributed to our understanding of the neurobiology of ASD, many factors such as small sample sizes, heterogeneous subject characteristics, and varying methodologies potentially limit the reliability and validity of these findings. Future neuroimaging studies that integrate multimodal approaches and address current limitations will serve to advance the field.

ACKNOWLEDGMENTS

This work was supported in part by a Career Development Award (K23 MH082119) from the National Institute of Mental Health and a Daniel X. and Mary Freedman Foundation in Academic Psychiatry Fellowship Award (Dr Stigler); and in partnership with the Nancy Lurie Marks Family Foundation.

References

Abell, F., Krams, M., Ashburner, J., Passingham, R., Friston, K., Frackowiak, R., et al., 1999. The neuroanatomy of autism: A voxel-based whole brain analysis of structural scans. Neuroreport 10, 1647–1651.

Adolphs, R., 2008. Fear, faces, and the human amygdala. Current Opinion in Neurobiology 18, 166–172.

Akshoomoff, N., Lord, C., Lincoln, A.J., Courchesne, R.Y., Carper, R.A., Townsend, J., et al., 2004. Outcome classification of preschool children with autism spectrum disorders using MRI brain measures. Journal of the American Academy of Child and Adolescent Psychiatry 43, 349–357.

Alexander, A.L., Lee, J.E., Lazar, M., Boudos, R., DuBray, M.B., Oakes, T.R., et al., 2007. Diffusion tensor imaging of the corpus callosum in autism. Neuroimage 34, 61–73.

Allison, T., Puce, A., McCarthy, G., 2000. Social perception from visual cues: Role of the STS region. Trends in Cognitive Sciences 4, 267–278.

Amaral, D.G., Schumann, C.M., Nordahl, C.W., 2008. Neuroanatomy of autism. Trends in Neurosciences 31, 137–145.

American Psychiatric Association (APA), 2000. Diagnostic and Statistical Manual of Mental Disorders, fourth ed. Text-Revision, American Psychiatric Association, Washington, DC.

Assaf, M., Jagannathan, K., Calhoun, V.D., Miller, L., Stevens, M.C., Sahl, R., et al., 2010. Abnormal functional connectivity of default mode sub-networks in autism spectrum disorder patients. Neuroimage 53, 247–256.

Aylward, E.H., Minshew, N.J., Field, K., Sparks, B.F., Singh, N., 2002. Effects of age on brain volume and head circumference in autism. Neurology 59, 175–183.

Aylward, E.H., Minshew, N.J., Goldstein, G., Honeycutt, N.A., Augustine, A.M., Yates, K.O., et al., 1999. MRI volumes of amygdala and hippocampus in non-mentally retarded autistic adolescents and adults. Neurology 53, 2145–2150.

Bailey, A., Luthert, P., Bolton, P., Le Couteur, A., Rutter, M., Harding, B., 1993. Autism and megalencephaly. The Lancet 341, 1225–1226.

Barnea-Goraly, N., Kwon, H., Menon, V., Eliez, S., Lotspeich, L., Reiss, A.L., 2004. White matter structure in autism: Preliminary evidence from diffusion tensor imaging. Biological Psychiatry 55, 323–326.

Bartholomeusz, H.H., Courchesne, E., Karns, C.M., 2002. Relationship between head circumference and brain volume in healthy normal toddlers, children, and adults. Neuropediatrics 33, 239–241.

Bigler, E.D., Tate, D.F., Neeley, E.S., Wolfson, L.J., Miller, M.J., Rice, S.A., et al., 2003. Temporal lobe, autism, and macrocephaly. American Journal of Neuroradiology 24, 2066–2076.

Bloemen, O.J., Deeley, Q., Sundram, F., Daly, E.M., Barker, G.J., Jones, D.K., et al., 2010. White matter integrity in Asperger syndrome: A preliminary diffusion tensor magnetic resonance imaging study in adults. Autism Research 3, 203–213.

Bloss, C.S., Courchesne, E., 2007. MRI neuroanatomy in young girls with autism: A preliminary study. Journal of the American Academy of Child and Adolescent Psychiatry 46, 515–523.

Boddaert, N., Chabane, N., Gervais, H., Good, C.D., Bourgeois, M., Plumet, M.H., et al., 2004. Superior temporal sulcus anatomical abnormalities in childhood autism: A voxel-based morphometry MRI study. Neuroimage 23, 364–369.

Bonilha, L., Cendes, F., Rorden, C., Eckert, M., Dalgalarrondo, P., Li, L.M., et al., 2008. Gray and white matter imbalance – typical structural abnormality underlying classic autism? Brain Development 30, 396–401.

Bookheimer, S., 2002. Functional MRI of language: New approaches to understanding the cortical organization of semantic processing. Annual Review of Neuroscience 25, 151–188.

Brambilla, P., Hardan, A., di Nemi, S.U., Perez, J., Soares, J.C., Barale, F., 2003. Brain anatomy and development in autism: Review of structural MRI studies. Brain Research Bulletin 61, 557–569.

Brito, A.R., Vasconcelos, M.M., Domingues, R.C., Hygino da Cruz, L.C., Rodrigues Lde, S., Gasparetto, E.L., et al., 2009. Diffusion tensor imaging findings in school-aged autistic children. Journal of NeuroImaging 19, 337–343.

Broyd, S.J., Demanuele, C., Debener, S., Helps, S.K., James, C.J., Sonuga-Barke, E.J., 2009. Default-mode brain dysfunction in mental disorders: A systematic review. Neuroscience and Biobehavioral Reviews 33, 279–296.

Brun, C.C., Nicolson, R., Lepore, N., Chou, Y.Y., Vidal, C.N., DeVito, T.J., et al., 2009. Mapping brain abnormalities in boys with autism. Human Brain Mapping 30, 3887–3900.

Buxbaum, L.J., Kyle, K.M., Menon, R., 2005. On beyond mirror neurons: Internal representations subserving imitation and recognition of skilled object-related actions in humans. Cognitive Brain Research 25, 226–239.

Campbell, M., Rosenbloom, S., Perry, R., George, A.E., Kricheff II, , Anderson, L., et al., 1982. Computerized axial tomography in young autistic children. American Journal of Psychiatry 139, 510–512.

Carper, R.A., Courchesne, E., 2005. Localized enlargement of the frontal cortex in early autism. Biological Psychiatry 57, 126–133.

Carper, R.A., Moses, P., Tigue, Z.D., Courchesne, E., 2002. Cerebral lobes in autism: Early hyperplasia and abnormal age effects. Neuroimage 16, 1038–1051.

Casanova, M.F., El-Baz, A., Elnakib, A., Switala, A.E., Williams, E.L., Williams, D.L., et al., 2011. Quantitative analysis of the shape of the corpus callosum in patients with autism and comparison individuals. Autism 15, 223–238.

Catani, M., Jones, D.K., Daly, E., Embiricos, N., Deeley, Q., Pugliese, L., et al., 2008. Altered cerebellar feedback projections in Asperger syndrome. Neuroimage 41, 1184–1191.

Cattaneo, L., Rizzolatti, G., 2009. The mirror neuron system. Archives of Neurology 66, 557–560.

Cheung, C., Chua, S.E., Cheung, V., Khong, P.L., Tai, K.S., Wong, T.K., et al., 2009. White matter fractional anisotrophy differences and correlates of diagnostic symptoms in autism. Journal of Child Psychology and Psychiatry 50, 1102–1112.

Chung, M.K., Dalton, K.M., Alexander, A.L., Davidson, R.J., 2004. Less white matter concentration in autism: 2D voxel-based morphometry. Neuroimage 23, 242–251.

Corbett, B.A., Carmean, V., Ravizza, S., Wendelken, C., Henry, M.L., Carter, C., et al., 2009. A functional and structural study of emotion and face processing in children with autism. Psychiatry Research 173, 196–205.

Courchesne, E., Campbell, K., Solso, S., 2011. Brain growth across the life span in autism: Age-specific changes in anatomical pathology. Brain Resource 1380, 138–145.

Courchesne, E., Carper, R., Akshoomoff, N., 2003. Evidence of brain overgrowth in the first year of life in autism. Journal of the American Medical Association 290, 337–344.

Courchesne, E., Karns, C.M., Davis, H.R., Ziccardi, R., Carper, R.A., Tigue, Z.D., et al., 2001. Unusual brain growth patterns in early life in patients with autistic disorder: An MRI study. Neurology 57, 245–254.

Courchesne, E., Pierce, K., Schumann, C.M., Redcay, E., Buckwalter, J.A., Kennedy, D.P., et al., 2007. Mapping early brain development in autism. Neuron 56, 399–413.

Courchesne, E., Saitoh, O., Yeung-Courchesne, R., Press, G.A., Lincoln, A.J., Haas, R.H., et al., 1994. Abnormality of cerebellar vermian lobules VI and VII in patients with infantile autism: Identification of hypoplastic and hyperplastic subgroups with MR imaging. American Journal of Roentgenology 162, 123–130.

Courchesne, E., Yeung-Courchesne, R., Press, G.A., Hesselink, J.R., Jernigan, T.L., 1988. Hypoplasia of cerebellar vermal lobules VI and VII in autism. New England Journal of Medicine 318, 1349–1354.

Craig, M.C., Zaman, S.H., Daly, E.M., Cutter, W.J., Robertson, D.M., Hallahan, B., et al., 2007. Women with autistic-spectrum disorder: Magnetic resonance imaging study of brain anatomy. British Journal of Psychiatry 191, 224–228.

Dalton, K.M., Nacewicz, B.M., Johnstone, T., Schaefer, H.S., Gernsbacher, M.A., Goldsmith, H.H., et al., 2005. Gaze fixation and the neural circuitry of face processing in autism. Nature Neuroscience 8, 519–526.

Damasio, H., Maurer, R.G., Damasio, A.R., Chui, H.C., 1980. Computerized tomographic scan findings in patients with autistic behavior. Archives of Neurology 37, 504–510.

Dapretto, M., Davies, M.S., Pfeifer, J.H., Scott, A.A., Sigman, M., Bookheimer, S.Y., et al., 2006. Understanding emotions in others: Mirror neuron dysfunction in children with autism spectrum disorders. Nature Neuroscience 9, 28–30.

Dawson, G., Munson, J., Webb, S.J., Nalty, T., Abbott, R., Toth, K., 2007. Rate of head growth decelerates and symptoms worsen in the second year of life in autism. Biological Psychiatry 61, 458–464.

Dawson, G., Webb, S.J., McPartland, J., 2005. Understanding the nature of face processing impairment in autism: Insights from behavioral and electrophysiological studies. Developmental Neuropsychology 27, 403–424.

De Fosse, L., Hodge, S.M., Makris, N., Kennedy, D.N., Caviness, V.S., McGrath, L., et al., 2004. Language-association cortex asymmetry in autism and specific language impairment. Annals of Neurology 56, 757–766.

Dementieva, Y.A., Vance, D.D., Donnelly, S.L., Elston, L.A., Wolpert, C.M., Ravan, S.A., et al., 2005. Accelerated head growth in early development of individuals with autism. Pediatric Neurology 32, 102–108.

Dichter, G.S., Belger, A., 2007. Social stimuli interfere with cognitive control in autism. Neuroimage 35, 1219–1230.

Di Martino, A., Kelly, C., Grzadzinski, R., Zuo, X.-N., Mennes, M., Mairena, M.A., et al., 2011. Aberrant striatal functional connectivity in children with autism. Biological Psychiatry 69, 847–856.

Dinstein, I., Thomas, C., Humphreys, K., Minshew, N., Behrmann, M., Heeger, D.J., 2010. Normal movement selectivity in autism. Neuron 66, 461–469.

Ebisch, S.J., Gallese, V., Willems, R.M., Mantini, D., Groen, W.B., Romani, G.L., et al., 2010. Altered intrinsic functional connectivity of anterior and posterior insula regions in high-functioning participants with autism spectrum disorder. Human Brain Mapping 32, 1013–1028.

Egaas, B., Courchesne, E., Saitoh, O., 1995. Reduced size of corpus callosum in autism. Archives of Neurology 52, 794–801.

Elia, M., Ferri, R., Musumeci, S.A., Panerai, S., Bottitta, M., Scuderi, C., 2000. Clinical correlates of brain morphometric features of subjects with low-functioning autistic disorder. Journal of Child Neurology 15, 504–508.

Eyler, L.T., Pierce, K., Courchesne, E., 2012. A failure of left temporal cortex to specialize for language is an early emerging and fundamental property of autism. Brain 135, 949–960.

Fombonne, E., 2000. Is a large head circumference a sign of autism? Journal of Autism and Developmental Disorders 30, 365.

Frazier, T.W., Hardan, A.Y., 2009. A meta-analysis of the corpus callosum in autism. Biological Psychiatry 66, 935–941.

Freitag, C.M., Luders, E., Hulst, H.E., Narr, K.L., Thompson, P.M., Toga, A.W., et al., 2009. Total brain volume and corpus callosum size in medication-naive adolescents and young adults with autism spectrum disorder. Biological Psychiatry 66, 316–319.

Gaffney, G.R., Kuperman, S., Tsai, L.Y., Minchin, S., 1988. Morphological evidence for brainstem involvement in infantile autism. Biological Psychiatry 24, 578–586.

Gaffrey, M.S., Kleinhans, N.M., Haist, F., Akshoomoff, N., Campbell, A., Courchesne, E., et al., 2007. Atypical [corrected] participation of visual cortex during word processing in autism: An fMRI study of semantic decision. Neuropsychologia 45, 1672–1684.

Gaffney, G.R., Tsai, L.Y., 1987. Magnetic resonance imaging of high level autism. Journal of Autism and Developmental Disorders 17, 433–438.

Garber, H.J., Ritvo, E.R., 1992. Magnetic resonance imaging of the posterior fossa in autistic adults. American Journal of Psychiatry 149, 245–247.

Girgis, R.R., Minshew, N.J., Melhem, N.M., Nutche, J.J., Keshavan, M.S., Hardan, A.Y., 2007. Volumetric alterations of the orbitofrontal cortex in autism. Progress in Neuro-psychopharmacology and Biological Psychiatry 31, 41–45.

Hadjikhani, N., Joseph, R.M., Snyder, J., Chabris, C.F., Clark, J., Steele, S., et al., 2004. Activation of the fusiform gyrus when individuals with autism spectrum disorder view faces. Neuroimage 22, 1141–1150.

Hadjikhani, N., Joseph, R.M., Snyder, J., Tager-Flusberg, H., 2006. Anatomical differences in the mirror neuron system and social cognition network in autism. Cerebral Cortex 16, 1276–1282.

Hardan, A.Y., Girgis, R.R., Adams, J., Gilbert, A.R., Keshavan, M.S., Minshew, N.J., 2006. Abnormal brain size effect on the thalamus in autism. Psychiatry Research 147, 145–151.

Hardan, A.Y., Girgis, R.R., Lacerda, A.L., Yorbik, O., Kilpatrick, M., Keshavan, M.S., et al., 2006. Magnetic resonance imaging study of the orbitofrontal cortex in autism. Journal of Child Neurology 21, 866–871.

Hardan, A.Y., Libove, R.A., Keshavan, M.S., Melhem, N.M., Minshew, N.J., 2009. A preliminary longitudinal magnetic resonance imaging study of brain volume and cortical thickness in autism. Biological Psychiatry 66, 320–326.

Hardan, A.Y., Minshew, N.J., Harenski, K., Keshavan, M.S., 2001. Posterior fossa magnetic resonance imaging in autism. Journal of the American Academy of Child and Adolescent Psychiatry 40, 666–672.

Hardan, A.Y., Minshew, N.J., Keshavan, M.S., 2000. Corpus callosum size in autism. Neurology 55, 1033–1036.

Hardan, A.Y., Minshew, N.J., Mallikarjuhn, M., Keshavan, M.S., 2001. Brain volume in autism. Journal of Child Neurology 16, 421–424.

Hardan, A.Y., Minshew, N.J., Melhem, N.M., Srihari, S., Jo, B., Bansal, R., et al., 2008. An MRI and proton spectroscopy study of the thalamus in children with autism. Psychiatry Research 163, 97–105.

Hardan, A.Y., Muddasani, S., Vemulapalli, M., Keshavan, M.S., Minshew, N.J., 2006. An MRI study of increased cortical thickness in autism. American Journal of Psychiatry 163, 1290–1292.

Hardan, A.Y., Pabalan, M., Gupta, N., Bansal, R., Melhem, N.M., Fedorov, S., et al., 2009. Corpus callosum volume in children with autism. Psychiatry Research 174, 57–61.

Harris, G.J., Chabris, C.F., Clark, J., Urban, T., Aharon, I., Steele, S., et al., 2006. Brain activation during semantic processing in autism spectrum disorders via functional magnetic resonance imaging. Brain and Cognition 61, 54–68.

Hashimoto, T., Murakawa, K., Miyazaki, M., Tayama, M., Kuroda, Y., 1992. Magnetic resonance imaging of the brain structures in the posterior fossa in retarded autistic children. Acta Paediatrica 81, 1030–1034.

Hashimoto, T., Tayama, M., Murakawa, K., Yoshimoto, T., Miyazaki, M., Harada, M., et al., 1995. Development of the brainstem and cerebellum in autistic patients. Journal of Autism and Developmental Disorders 25, 1–18.

Haxby, J.V., Hoffman, E.A., Gobbini, M.I., 2002. Human neural systems for face recognition and social communication. Biological Psychiatry 51, 59–67.

Hazlett, H.C., Poe, M.D., Gerig, G., Smith, R.G., Piven, J., 2006. Cortical gray and white brain tissue volume in adolescents and adults with autism. Biological Psychiatry 59, 1–6.

Hazlett, H.C., Poe, M., Gerig, G., Smith, R.G., Provenzale, J., Ross, A., et al., 2005. Magnetic resonance imaging and head circumference study of brain size in autism: Birth through age 2 years. Archives of General Psychiatry 62, 1366–1376.

Hazlett, H.C., Poe, M.D., Gerig, G., Styner, M., Chappell, C., Smith, R.G., et al., 2011. Early brain overgrowth in autism associated with an increase in cortical surface area before age 2 years. Archives of General Psychiatry 68, 467–476.

Haznedar, M.M., Buchsbaum, M.S., Hazlett, E.A., LiCalzi, E.M., Cartwright, C., Hollander, E., 2006. Volumetric analysis and three-dimensional glucose metabolic mapping of the striatum and thalamus in patients with autism spectrum disorders. American Journal of Psychiatry 163, 1252–1263.

Haznedar, M.M., Buchsbaum, M.S., Metzger, M., Solimando, A., Spiegel-Cohen, J., Hollander, E., 1997. Anterior cingulate gyrus volume and glucose metabolism in autistic disorder. American Journal of Psychiatry 154, 1047–1050.

Haznedar, M.M., Buchsbaum, M.S., Wei, T.C., Hof, P.R., Cartwright, C., Bienstock, C.A., et al., 2000. Limbic circuitry in patients with autism spectrum disorders studied with positron emission tomography and magnetic resonance imaging. American Journal of Psychiatry 157, 1994–2001.

Herbert, M.R., Harris, G.J., Adrien, K.T., Ziegler, D.A., Makris, N., Kennedy, D.N., et al., 2002. Abnormal asymmetry in language association cortex in autism. Annals of Neurology 52, 588–596.

Herbert, M.R., Ziegler, D.A., Deutsch, C.K., O'Brien, L.M., Lange, N., Bakardjiev, A., et al., 2003. Dissociations of cerebral cortex, subcortical and cerebral white matter volumes in autistic boys. Brain 126, 1182–1192.

Herbert, M.R., Ziegler, D.A., Makris, N., Filipek, P.A., Kemper, T.L., Normandin, J.J., et al., 2004. Localization of white matter volume increase in autism and developmental language disorder. Annals of Neurology 55, 530–540.

Hodge, S.M., Makris, N., Kennedy, D.N., Caviness, V.S., Howard, J., McGrath, L., et al., 2010. Cerebellum, language, and cognition in autism and specific language impairment. Journal of Autism and Developmental Disorders 40, 300–316.

Hoffman, E.A., Haxby, J.V., 2000. Distinct representations of eye gaze and identity in the distributed human neural system for face perception. Nature Neuroscience 3, 80–84.

Hollander, E., Anagnostou, E., Chaplin, W., Esposito, K., Haznedar, M.M., Licalzi, E., et al., 2005. Striatal volume on magnetic resonance imaging and repetitive behaviors in autism. Biological Psychiatry 58, 226–232.

Holttum, J.R., Minshew, N.J., Sanders, R.S., Phillips, N.E., 1992. Magnetic resonance imaging of the posterior fossa in autism. Biological Psychiatry 32, 1091–1101.

Howard, M.A., Cowell, P.E., Boucher, J., Broks, P., Mayes, A., Farrant, A., et al., 2000. Convergent neuroanatomical and behavioural evidence of an amygdala hypothesis of autism. Neuroreport 11, 2931–2935.

Hua, X., Thompson, P.M., Leow, A.D., Madsen, S.K., Caplan, R., Alger, J.R., et al., 2011. Brain growth rate abnormalities visualized in adolescents with autism. Human Brain Mapping.

Hubl, D., Bolte, S., Feineis-Matthews, S., Lanfermann, H., Federspiel, A., Strik, W., et al., 2003. Functional imbalance of visual pathways indicates alternative face processing strategies in autism. Neurology 61, 1232–1237.

Huettel, S.A., Song, A.W., McCarthy, G. (Eds.), 2009. Functional Magnetic Resonance Imaging, second ed. Sinauer Associates, Sunderland, MA.

Humphreys, K., Hasson, U., Avidan, G., Minshew, N., Behrmann, M., 2008. Cortical patterns of category-selective activation for faces, places and objects in adults with autism. Autism Research 1, 52–63.

Hyde, K.L., Samson, F., Evans, A.C., Mottron, L., 2010. Neuroanatomical differences in brain areas implicated in perceptual and other core features of autism revealed by cortical thickness analysis and voxel-based morphometry. Human Brain Mapping 31, 556–566.

Iacoboni, M., Woods, R.P., Brass, M., Bekkering, H., Mazziotta, J.C., Rizzolatti, G., 1999. Cortical mechanisms of human imitation. Science 286, 2526–2528.

Johnson-Frey, S.H., Maloof, F.R., Newman-Norlund, R., Farrer, C., Inati, S., Grafton, S.T., 2003. Actions or hand-object interactions? Human inferior frontal cortex and action observation. Neuron 39, 1053–1058.

Jou, R.J., Minshew, N.J., Keshavan, M.S., Hardan, A.Y., 2010. Cortical gyrification in autistic and asperger disorders: A preliminary magnetic resonance imaging study. Journal of Child Neurology 25, 1462–1467.

Jou, R.J., Minshew, N.J., Melhem, N.M., Keshavan, M.S., Hardan, A.Y., 2009. Brainstem volumetric alterations in children with autism. Psychological Medicine 39, 1347–1354.

Just, M.A., Cherkassky, V.L., Keller, T.A., Kana, R.K., Minshew, N.J., 2007. Functional and anatomical cortical underconnectivity in autism: Evidence from an FMRI study of an executive function task and corpus callosum morphometry. Cerebral Cortex 17, 951–961.

Just, M.A., Cherkassky, V.L., Keller, T.A., Minshew, N.J., 2004. Cortical activation and synchronization during sentence comprehension in high-functioning autism: Evidence of underconnectivity. Brain 127, 1811–1821.

Kana, R.K., Keller, T.A., Cherkassky, V.L., Minshew, N.J., Just, M.A., 2006. Sentence comprehension in autism: Thinking in pictures with decreased functional connectivity. Brain 129, 2484–2493.

Kana, R.K., Keller, T.A., Minshew, N.J., Just, M.A., 2007. Inhibitory control in high-functioning autism: Decreased activation and underconnectivity in inhibition networks. Biological Psychiatry 62, 198–206.

Kanner, L., 1943. Autistic disturbances of affective contact. The Nervous Child 2, 217–250.

Kates, W.R., Burnette, C.P., Eliez, S., Strunge, L.A., Kaplan, D., Landa, R., et al., 2004. Neuroanatomic variation in monozygotic twin pairs discordant for the narrow phenotype for autism. American Journal of Psychiatry 161, 539–546.

Kates, W.R., Ikuta, I., Burnette, C.P., 2009. Gyrification patterns in monozygotic twin pairs varying in discordance for autism. Autism Research 2, 267–278.

Katz, L.C., Shatz, C.J., 1996. Synaptic activity and the construction of cortical circuits. Science 274, 1133–1138.

Kaufmann, W.E., Cooper, K.L., Mostofsky, S.H., Capone, G.T., Kates, W.R., Newschaffer, C.J., et al., 2003. Specificity of cerebellar vermian abnormalities in autism: A quantitative magnetic resonance imaging study. Journal of Child Neurology 18, 463–470.

Keary, C.J., Minshew, N.J., Bansal, R., Goradia, D., Fedorov, S., Keshavan, M.S., et al., 2009. Corpus callosum volume and neurocognition in autism. Journal of Autism and Developmental Disorders 39, 834–841.

Keller, T.A., Kana, R.K., Just, M.A., 2007. A developmental study of the structural integrity of white matter in autism. Neuroreport 18, 23–27.

Kennedy, D.P., Courchesne, E., 2008. The intrinsic functional organization of the brain is altered in autism. Neuroimage 39, 1877–1885.

Kennedy, D.P., Courchesne, E., 2008. Functional abnormalities of the default network during self- and other-reflection in autism. Social Cognitive Affect Neuroscience 3, 177–190.

Kim, J.E., Lyoo, I.K., Estes, A.M., Renshaw, P.F., Shaw, D.W., Friedman, S.D., et al., 2010. Laterobasal amygdalar enlargement in 6- to 7-year-old children with autism spectrum disorder. Archives of General Psychiatry 67, 1187–1197.

Kleiman, M.D., Neff, S., Rosman, N.P., 1992. The brain in infantile autism: Are posterior fossa structures abnormal? Neurology 42, 753–760.

Kleinhans, N.M., Johnson, L.C., Richards, T., Mahurin, R., Greenson, J., Dawson, G., et al., 2009. Reduced neural habituation in the amygdala and social impairments in autism spectrum disorders. American Journal of Psychiatry 166, 467–475.

Kleinhans, N.M., Richards, T., Sterling, L., Stegbauer, K.C., Mahurin, R., Johnson, L.C., et al., 2008. Abnormal functional connectivity in autism spectrum disorders during face processing. Brain 131, 1000–1012.

Klin, A., Jones, W., Schultz, R., Volkmar, F., Cohen, D., 2002. Visual fixation patterns during viewing of naturalistic social situations as predictors of social competence in individuals with autism. Archives of General Psychiatry 59, 809–816.

Klin, A., Klin, A., 2008. Three things to remember if you are a functional magnetic resonance imaging researcher of face processing in autism spectrum disorders. Biological Psychiatry 64, 549–551.

Knaus, T.A., Silver, A.M., Dominick, K.C., Schuring, M.D., Shaffer, N., Lindgren, K.A., et al., 2009. Age-related changes in the anatomy of language regions in autism spectrum disorder. Brain Imaging Behavior 3, 51–63.

Knaus, T.A., Silver, A.M., Lindgren, K.A., Hadjikhani, N., Tager-Flusberg, H., 2008. FMRI activation during a language task in adolescents with ASD. Journal of International Neuropsychology Society 14, 967–979.

Kosaka, H., Omori, M., Munesue, T., Ishitobi, M., Matsumura, Y., Takahashi, T., et al., 2010. Smaller insula and inferior frontal volumes in young adults with pervasive developmental disorders. Neuroimage 50, 1357–1363.

Koshino, H., Carpenter, P.A., Minshew, N.J., Cherkassky, V.L., Keller, T.A., Just, M.A., 2005. Functional connectivity in an fMRI working memory task in high-functioning autism. Neuroimage 24, 810–821.

Kwon, H., Ow, A.W., Pedatella, K.E., Lotspeich, L.J., Reiss, A.L., 2004. Voxel-based morphometry elucidates structural neuroanatomy of high-functioning autism and asperger syndrome. Developmental Medicine and Child Neurology 46, 760–764.

Lainhart, J.E., Piven, J., Wzorek, M., Landa, R., Santangelo, S.L., Coon, H., et al., 1997. Macrocephaly in children and adults with autism. Journal of the American Academy of Child and Adolescent Psychiatry 36, 282–290.

Lange, N., Dubray, M.B., Lee, J.E., Froimowitz, M.P., Froehlich, A., Adluru, N., et al., 2010. Atypical diffusion tensor hemispheric asymmetry in autism. Autism Research 3, 350–358.

Langen, M., Durston, S., Staal, W.G., Palmen, S.J., van Engeland, H., 2007. Caudate nucleus is enlarged in high-functioning medication-naive subjects with autism. Biological Psychiatry 62, 262–266.

Langen, M., Schnack, H.G., Nederveen, H., Bos, D., Lahuis, B.E., de Jonge, M.V., et al., 2009. Changes in the developmental trajectories of striatum in autism. Biological Psychiatry 66, 327–333.

Lee, J.E., Bigler, E.D., Alexander, A.L., Lazar, M., DuBray, M.B., Chung, M.K., et al., 2007. Diffusion tensor imaging of white matter in the superior temporal gyrus and temporal stem in autism. Neuroscience Letters 424, 127–132.

Levitt, J.G., Blanton, R.E., Smalley, S., Thompson, P.M., Guthrie, D., McCracken, J.T., et al., 2003. Cortical sulcal maps in autism. Cerebral Cortex 13, 728–735.

Lo, Y.C., Soong, W.T., Gau, S.S., Wu, Y.Y., Lai, M.C., Yeh, F.C., et al., 2011. The loss of asymmetry and reduced interhemispheric connectivity in adolescents with autism: A study using diffusion spectrum imaging tractography. Psychiatry Research 192, 60–66.

Lopez, B.R., Lincoln, A.J., Ozonoff, S., Lai, Z., 2005. Examining the relationship between executive functions and restricted, repetitive symptoms of Autistic Disorder. Journal of Autism and Developmental Disorders 35, 445–460.

Luna, B., Minshew, N.J., Garver, K.E., Lazar, N.A., Thulborn, K.R., Eddy, W.F., et al., 2002. Neocortical system abnormalities in autism: An fMRI study of spatial working memory. Neurology 59, 834–840.

Manes, F., Piven, J., Vrancic, D., Nanclares, V., Plebst, C., Starkstein, S.E., 1999. An MRI study of the corpus callosum and cerebellum in mentally retarded autistic individuals. The Journal of Neuropsychiatry and Clinical Neuroscience 11, 470–474.

Martineau, J., Andersson, F., Barthelemy, C., Cottier, J.P., Destrieux, C., 2010. Atypical activation of the mirror neuron system during perception of hand motion in autism. Brain Research 1320, 168–175.

Mason, R.A., Williams, D.L., Kana, R.K., Minshew, N., Just, M.A., 2008. Theory of Mind disruption and recruitment of the right hemisphere during narrative comprehension in autism. Neuropsychologia 46, 269–280.

McAlonan, G.M., Cheung, V., Cheung, C., Suckling, J., Lam, G.Y., Tai, K.S., et al., 2005. Mapping the brain in autism: A voxel-based MRI study of volumetric differences and intercorrelations in autism. Brain 128, 268–276.

McAlonan, G.M., Daly, E., Kumari, V., Critchley, H.D., van Amelsvoort, T., Suckling, J., et al., 2002. Brain anatomy and sensorimotor gating in Asperger's syndrome. Brain 125, 1594–1606.

McAlonan, G.M., Suckling, J., Wong, N., Cheung, V., Lienenkaemper, N., Cheung, C., Chua, S.E., 2008. Distinct patterns of grey matter abnormality in high-functioning autism and Asperger's syndrome. Journal of Child Psychology and Psychiatry 49, 1287–1295.

Menon, V., Uddin, L.Q., 2010. Saliency, switching, attention and control: A network model of insula function. Brain Structure and Function 214, 655–667.

Mitchell, S.R., Reiss, A.L., Tatusko, D.H., Ikuta, I., Kazmerski, D.B., Botti, J.A., et al., 2009. Neuroanatomic alterations and social and communication deficits in monozygotic twins discordant for autism disorder. American Journal of Psychiatry 166, 917–925.

Monk, C.S., Peltier, S.J., Wiggins, J.L., Weng, S.J., Carrasco, M., Risi, S., et al., 2009. Abnormalities of intrinsic functional connectivity in autism spectrum disorders. Neuroimage 47, 764–772.

Monk, C.S., Weng, S.J., Wiggins, J.L., Kurapati, N., Louro, H.M., Carrasco, M., et al., 2010. Neural circuitry of emotional face processing in autism spectrum disorders. Journal of Psychiatry and Neuroscience 35, 105–114.

Muller, R.A., 2008. From loci to networks and back again: Anomalies in the study of autism. Annals of the New York Academy of Sciences 1145, 300–315.

Munson, J., Dawson, G., Abbott, R., Faja, S., Webb, S.J., Friedman, S.D., et al., 2006. Amygdalar volume and behavioral development in autism. Archives of General Psychiatry 63, 686–693.

Nacewicz, B.M., Dalton, K.M., Johnstone, T., Long, M.T., McAuliff, E.M., Oakes, T.R., et al., 2006. Amygdala volume and nonverbal social impairment in adolescent and adult males with autism. Archives of General Psychiatry 63, 1417–1428.

Nakada, T., Fujii, Y., Yoneoka, Y., Kwee, I.L., 2001. Planum temporale: Where spoken and written language meet. European Neurology 46, 121–125.

Nicolson, R., DeVito, T.J., Vidal, C.N., Sui, Y., Hayashi, K.M., Drost, D.J., et al., 2006. Detection and mapping of hippocampal abnormalities in autism. Psychiatry Research 148, 11–21.

Nordahl, C.W., Dierker, D., Mostafavi, I., Schumann, C.M., Rivera, S.M., Amaral, D.G., et al., 2007. Cortical folding abnormalities in autism revealed by surface-based morphometry. Journal of Neuroscience 27, 11,725–11,735.

Ornitz, E.M., 1983. The functional neuroanatomy of infantile autism. International Journal of Neuroscience 19, 85–124.

Palmen, S.J., Hulshoff Pol, H.E., Kemner, C., Schnack, H.G., Durston, S., Lahuis, B.E., et al., 2005. Increased gray-matter volume in medication-naive high-functioning children with autism spectrum disorder. Psychological Medicine 35, 561–570.

Pardini, M., Garaci, F.G., Bonzano, L., Roccatagliata, L., Palmieri, M.G., Pompili, E., et al., 2009. White matter reduced streamline coherence in young men with autism and mental retardation. European Journal of Neurology 16, 1185–1190.

Pelphrey, K.A., Morris, J.P., McCarthy, G., 2005. Neural basis of eye gaze processing deficits in autism. Brain 128, 1038–1048.

Pelphrey, K.A., Morris, J.P., McCarthy, G., Labar, K.S., 2007. Perception of dynamic changes in facial affect and identity in autism. Social Cognitive and Affective Neuroscience 2, 140–149.

Pelphrey, K.A., Sasson, N.J., Reznick, J.S., Paul, G., Goldman, B.D., Piven, J., 2002. Visual scanning of faces in autism. Journal of Autism and Developmental Disorders 32, 249–261.

Pierce, K., Haist, F., Sedaghat, F., Courchesne, E., 2004. The brain response to personally familiar faces in autism: Findings of fusiform activity and beyond. Brain 127, 2703–2716.

Pierce, K., Muller, R.A., Ambrose, J., Allen, G., Courchesne, E., 2001. Face processing occurs outside the fusiform 'face area' in autism: Evidence from functional MRI. Brain 124, 2059–2073.

Pierce, K., Redcay, E., 2008. Fusiform function in children with an autism spectrum disorder is a matter of "who". Biological Psychiatry 64, 552–560.

Piggot, J., Kwon, H., Mobbs, D., Blasey, C., Lotspeich, L., Menon, V., et al., 2004. Emotional attribution in high-functioning individuals with autistic spectrum disorder: A functional imaging study. Journal of the American Academy of Child and Adolescent Psychiatry 43, 473–480.

Piven, J., Bailey, J., Ranson, B.J., Arndt, S., 1997. An MRI study of the corpus callosum in autism. American Journal of Psychiatry 154, 1051–1056.

Piven, J., Bailey, J., Ranson, B.J., Arndt, S., 1998. No difference in hippocampus volume detected on magnetic resonance imaging in autistic individuals. Journal of Autism and Developmental Disorders 28, 105–110.

Piven, J., Nehme, E., Simon, J., Barta, P., Pearlson, G., Folstein, S.E., 1992. Magnetic resonance imaging in autism: Measurement of the cerebellum, pons, and fourth ventricle. Biological Psychiatry 31, 491–504.

Puce, A., Allison, T., Bentin, S., Gore, J.C., McCarthy, G., 1998. Temporal cortex activation in humans viewing eye and mouth movements. Journal of Neuroscience 18, 2188–2199.

Pugliese, L., Catani, M., Ameis, S., Dell'Acqua, F., Thiebaut de Schotten, M., Murphy, C., et al., 2009. The anatomy of extended limbic pathways in asperger syndrome: A preliminary diffusion tensor imaging tractography study. Neuroimage 47, 427–434.

Redcay, E., Courchesne, E., 2005. When is the brain enlarged in autism? a meta-analysis of all brain size reports. Biological Psychiatry 58, 1–9.

Redcay, E., Courchesne, E., 2008. Deviant functional magnetic resonance imaging patterns of brain activity to speech in 2–3-year-old children with autism spectrum disorder. Biological Psychiatry 64, 589–598.

Rizzolatti, G., Craighero, L., 2004. The mirror-neuron system. Annual Review of Neuroscience 27, 169–192.

Rojas, D.C., Bawn, S.D., Benkers, T.L., Reite, M.L., Rogers, S.J., 2002. Smaller left hemisphere planum temporale in adults with autistic disorder. Neuroscience Letters 328, 237–240.

Rojas, D.C., Camou, S.L., Reite, M.L., Rogers, S.J., 2005. Planum temporale volume in children and adolescents with autism. Journal of Autism and Developmental Disorders 35, 479–486.

Rojas, D.C., Peterson, E., Winterrowd, E., Reite, M.L., Rogers, S.J., Tregellas, J.R., 2006. Regional gray matter volumetric changes in autism associated with social and repetitive behavior symptoms. BMC Psychiatry 6, 56.

Rosenbloom, S., Campbell, M., George, A.E., Kricheff, I.I., Taleporos, E., Anderson, L., et al., 1984. High resolution CT scanning in infantile autism: A quantitative approach. Journal of the American Academy of Child and Adolescent Psychiatry 23, 72–77.

Russo, N., Flanagan, T., Iarocci, G., Berringer, D., Zelazo, P.D., Burack, J.A., 2007. Deconstructing executive deficits among persons with autism: Implications for cognitive neuroscience. Brain and Cognition 65, 77–86.

Sahyoun, C.P., Belliveau, J.W., Soulieres, I., Schwartz, S., Mody, M., 2010. Neuroimaging of the functional and structural networks underlying visuospatial vs. linguistic reasoning in high-functioning autism. Neuropsychologia 48, 86–95.

Saitoh, O., Courchesne, E., Egaas, B., Lincoln, A.J., Schreibman, L., 1995. Cross-sectional area of the posterior hippocampus in autistic patients with cerebellar and corpus callosum abnormalities. Neurology 45, 317–324.

Scherf, K.S., Luna, B., Minshew, N., Behrmann, M., 2010. Location, location, location: Alterations in the functional topography of face- but not object- or place-related cortex in adolescents with autism. Frontiers in Human. Neuroscience 4, 26.

Schultz, R.T., Gauthier, I., Klin, A., Fulbright, R.K., Anderson, A.W., Volkmar, F., et al., 2000. Abnormal ventral temporal cortical activity during face discrimination among individuals with autism and Asperger syndrome. Archives of General Psychiatry 57, 331–340.

Schumann, C.M., Barnes, C.C., Lord, C., Courchesne, E., 2009. Amygdala enlargement in toddlers with autism related to severity of social and communication impairments. Biological Psychiatry 66, 942–949.

Schumann, C.M., Bloss, C.S., Barnes, C.C., Wideman, G.M., Carper, R.A., Akshoomoff, N., et al., 2010. Longitudinal magnetic resonance imaging study of cortical development through early childhood in autism. Journal of Neuroscience 30, 4419–4427.

Schumann, C.M., Hamstra, J., Goodlin-Jones, B.L., Lotspeich, L.J., Kwon, H., Buonocore, M.H., et al., 2004. The amygdala is enlarged in children but not adolescents with autism; the hippocampus is enlarged at all ages. Journal of Neuroscience 24, 6392–6401.

Sears, L.L., Vest, C., Mohamed, S., Bailey, J., Ranson, B.J., Piven, J., 1999. An MRI study of the basal ganglia in autism. Progress in Neuropsychopharmacology and Biological Psychiatry 23, 613–624.

Silk, T.J., Rinehart, N., Bradshaw, J.L., Tonge, B., Egan, G., O'Boyle, M.W., et al., 2006. Visuospatial processing and the function of prefrontal-parietal networks in autism spectrum disorders: A functional MRI study. American Journal of Psychiatry 163, 1440–1443.

Sparks, B.F., Friedman, S.D., Shaw, D.W., Aylward, E.H., Echelard, D., Artru, A.A., et al., 2002. Brain structural abnormalities in young children with autism spectrum disorder. Neurology 59, 184–192.

Stanfield, A.C., McIntosh, A.M., Spencer, M.D., Philip, R., Gaur, S., Lawrie, S.M., 2008. Towards a neuroanatomy of autism: A systematic review and meta-analysis of structural magnetic resonance imaging studies. European Psychiatry 23, 289–299.

Tepest, R., Jacobi, E., Gawronski, A., Krug, B., Moller-Hartmann, W., Lehnhardt, F.G., et al., 2010. Corpus callosum size in adults with high-functioning autism and the relevance of gender. Psychiatry Research 183, 38–43.

Tesink, C.M., Buitelaar, J.K., Petersson, K.M., van der Gaag, R.J., Kan, C.C., Tendolkar, I., et al., 2009. Neural correlates of pragmatic language comprehension in autism spectrum disorders. Brain 132, 1941–1952.

Thakkar, K.N., Polli, F.E., Joseph, R.M., Tuch, D.S., Hadjikhani, N., Barton, J.J., et al., 2008. Response monitoring, repetitive behaviour and anterior cingulate abnormalities in autism spectrum disorders (ASD). Brain 131, 2464–2478.

Toal, F., Daly, E.M., Page, L., Deeley, Q., Hallahan, B., Bloemen, O., et al., 2010. Clinical and anatomical heterogeneity in autistic spectrum disorder: A structural MRI study. Psychological Medicine 40, 1171–1181.

Tsatsanis, K.D., Rourke, B.P., Klin, A., Volkmar, F.R., Cicchetti, D., Schultz, R.T., 2003. Reduced thalamic volume in high-functioning individuals with autism. Biological Psychiatry 53, 121–129.

Turner, K.C., Frost, L., Linsenbardt, D., McIlroy, J.R., Muller, R.A., 2006. Atypically diffuse functional connectivity between caudate nuclei and cerebral cortex in autism. Behavioral and Brain Functions 2, 34.

Uddin, L.Q., Menon, V., 2009. The anterior insula in autism: Underconnected and under-examined. Neurosci and Biobehavioral Reviews 33, 1198–1203.

Vidal, C.N., Nicolson, R., DeVito, T.J., Hayashi, K.M., Geaga, J.A., Drost, D.J., et al., 2006. Mapping corpus callosum deficits in autism: An index of aberrant cortical connectivity. Biological Psychiatry 60, 218–225.

Waiter, G.D., Williams, J.H., Murray, A.D., Gilchrist, A., Perrett, D.I., Whiten, A., 2004. A voxel-based investigation of brain structure in male adolescents with autistic spectrum disorder. Neuroimage 22, 619–625.

Wallace, G.L., Dankner, N., Kenworthy, L., Giedd, J.N., Martin, A., 2010. Age-related temporal and parietal cortical thinning in autism spectrum disorders. Brain 133, 3745–3754.

Wang, A.T., Dapretto, M., Hariri, A.R., Sigman, M., Bookheimer, S.Y., 2004. Neural correlates of facial affect processing in children and adolescents with autism spectrum disorder. Journal of the American Academy of Child and Adolescent Psychiatry 43, 481–490.

Wang, A.T., Lee, S.S., Sigman, M., Dapretto, M., 2006. Neural basis of irony comprehension in children with autism: The role of prosody and context. Brain 129, 932–943.

Weeks, S.J., Hobson, R.P., 1987. The salience of facial expression for autistic children. Journal of Child Psychology and Psychiatry 28, 137–151.

Williams, J.H., Waiter, G.D., Gilchrist, A., Perrett, D.I., Murray, A.D., Whiten, A., 2006. Neural mechanisms of imitation and 'mirror neuron' functioning in autistic spectrum disorder. Neuropsychologia 44, 610–621.

3.2

DTI and Tractography in the Autistic Brain

Timothy P.L. Roberts[*,†], *Jeffrey I. Berman*[*,†], *Ragini Verma*[‡]

[*]Department of Radiology [†]Children's Hospital of Philadelphia, Philadelphia, PA, USA
[‡]University of Pennsylvania, Philadelphia, PA, USA

INTRODUCTION

Many techniques exist to investigate the anatomy and physiology of the brain. These methods range from single unit neuron recordings to psychological testing. Each technique has inherent limitations, but together these complementary methods enhance our understanding of brain structure and function. Magnetic resonance imaging (MRI) is a safe, non-invasive method of studying the brain and can be performed on patients, controls, and pediatric populations. Diffusion MR is an MRI technique that uses the random movement of water to characterize the microstructure of brain tissue. This chapter reviews current and emerging diffusion MR techniques and how they are beginning to be used to study the brains of individuals with autism spectrum disorders (ASD). A technical review of the diffusion tensor imaging (DTI) methodology will be followed by a review of the application of DTI to ASD, the development of quantitative metrics of diffusion and pattern classifiers, and finally, emerging advances in diffusion imaging, most notably high-angular-resolution diffusion Imaging (HARDI).

DIFFUSION AS A RANDOM PROCESS

Brownian motion or diffusion refers to the random movement of water (Brown, 1828). This movement is not the result of bulk flow and is driven by the thermal energy of the water molecules. Water diffuses all the time, and this movement does not require active transport or a concentration gradient. Water diffusion occurs *in vivo*, *ex vivo*, and in non-biological materials which contain water. The probable distance which a water molecule moves during a certain time interval can be described by a normal Gaussian distribution. The average distance traveled, r, in a defined time, t, (in one spatial dimension) can be described by:

$$r = \sqrt{2Dt} \qquad (3.2.1)$$

The self-diffusion coefficient, D, has units of square length divided by time and is related to properties of the water molecule and its environment (Einstein, 1905). The diffusion coefficient accurately describes the random movement of unrestricted water molecules. In a system with no structures blocking or hindering water

The Neuroscience of Autism Spectrum Disorders.
http://dx.doi.org/10.1016/B978-0-12-391924-3.00018-1

FIGURE 3.2.1 The goal of diffusion MR is to use the random movement of water to probe tissue microstructure. On the left, brain tissue anatomy and the water diffusion within an axonal bundle are depicted. The right depicts the diffusion MR measurement of the pattern of diffusion and its modeling with the diffusion tensor ellipsoid.

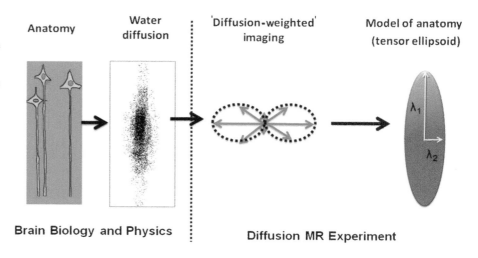

movement, diffusion is equally likely in all directions and the mean distance traveled is equal for all directions. In such an *isotropic* system of diffusion, the diffusion coefficient is the same for each direction. In fact, the self-diffusion coefficient depends only on the molecular weight of the molecule (for water, MW = 18), solvent viscosity, and the absolute temperature. Environments other than pure water, such as brain tissue, however, may affect the random movement of water in such a way that diffusion is best considered as 'apparent diffusion,' and is subject to modulation by additional, biologically interesting, factors. The goal of diffusion MR is to use the measured pattern of diffusion to infer the organization and microstructure of brain tissue (Figure 3.2.1).

DIFFUSION IN THE BRAIN

The brain exhibits a high degree of organization among its billions of neurons. The white matter is arranged into bundles of axons of related function and similar cortical connections ('neurons that fire together, wire together,' attributed to Hebb). Diffusion MR relies upon the high degree of organization found within these white matter pathways. The voxels comprising an MR image are of finite size (typically 2 x 2 x 2 mm). If the billions of axons in the brain were randomly arranged, water diffusion would be isotropic when integrated over the volume of a voxel. However, since white matter pathways typically comprise coherently oriented axons, diffusion-weighted imaging (and the diffusion tensor imaging formalism) can be used to determine the orientation and microstructural properties of axonal bundles.

Water movement in brain tissue is restricted by myelin, membranes, proteins, neurofilaments, microtubules, organelles, and anything else interacting with water (Basser and Pierpaoli, 1996; Beaulieu, 2002; Beaulieu and Allen, 1994; Song et al., 2003). These barriers

cause the measured apparent water diffusivity in brain tissue to be lower than the diffusivity of unrestricted water. If the macromolecules are coherently arranged, such as in an axonal bundle, water will have a preferred direction of diffusion (Figure 3.2.1). Anisotropic diffusion occurs in an environment where the diffusion coefficient of water is directionally dependent. For example, within a bundle of axons, the myelin and axonal membranes act as a barrier and reduce the mean distance that water will diffuse perpendicular to the axons. Parallel to the axons, diffusion is less hindered and the apparent diffusion coefficient *in that direction* is higher.

It is important to note that the measured apparent anisotropy is related to the time period over which diffusion is allowed to occur. If diffusion is observed for a very short amount of time, few water molecules will have moved far enough to 'bump into' an obstacle such as an axonal membrane. In this case, the diffusion will appear to be more isotropic. If the diffusion is allowed to occur for a much longer time period, the majority of water molecules will have reached a barrier and the anisotropic pattern will emerge. For typical diffusion-weighted imaging sequences employed to study diffusion in the living human brain, such observation times are in the range of 10 to 60 ms, corresponding to diffusion path lengths of the order of a few μm (10^{-6} m), and on the scale of cell dimensions.

HOW MR CAN MEASURE DIFFUSION

Diffusion MR observes Brownian motion by tagging populations of water molecules and observing their movements (Tanner and Stejskal, 1968). The diffusion MR experiment is analogous to a simple diffusion experiment where a drop of dye is placed in a bowl of water. Using the equations for diffusion, the observed change in the dye's concentration can be used to calculate the diffusion coefficient of the liquid. MR diffusion techniques are sensitive to the magnitude of the diffusion coefficient and work in much the same way. Instead of visible dye, a known concentration gradient of spin-labeled water molecules is established with the MR scanner and then changes in concentration are measured over time. The MR signal in a diffusion-weighted image is related to the diffusion coefficient as follows:

$$\frac{S}{S_0} = e^{-bD} \qquad (3.2.2)$$

In this relationship, S refers to the intensity of the MR signal when the diffusion gradient is applied. As the diffusion coefficient increases, the value of S decreases. The term S_0 refers to the baseline MR signal level without diffusion weighting. The ratio of S to S_0 is related to the b-value and the (apparent) diffusion coefficient, D, of the water. The b-value is related to the level of diffusion weighting applied. The b-value must be sufficiently high to observe anisotropic diffusion. A typical clinical diffusion tensor scan uses a b-value of approximately 1,000 s/mm^2. Since each scan encodes diffusion in a single specific direction, multiple diffusion-weighted scans are required to represent the directional differences in diffusion (note at least six directions are required to be encoded for simple DTI; more are required for advanced modeling).

THE DIFFUSION TENSOR MODEL OF MICROSTRUCTURE

The brain exhibits complex and varied patterns of anisotropic diffusion reflecting the underlying microstructure. Diffusion MR can probe diffusivity in many directions to measure the associated apparent diffusion coefficients, thereby assessing directional preference for diffusion. It is desirable to precipitate the multiple diffusion-weighted images in scalar metrics that are rotationally invariant and describe the underlying tissue structure. The diffusion tensor is a model which requires a minimum of six probed diffusion directions to describe the three dimensional (3D) pattern of diffusion within a voxel. Diffusion tensor imaging (DTI) refers to the MR acquisition of diffusion-weighted images and subsequent calculation of the diffusion tensor and associated scalar metrics.

The tensor itself is a 3 by 3 matrix that can graphically be represented by a diffusion ellipsoid (Figure 3.2.2). The diffusion ellipsoid is a shape that describes the directional diffusion coefficients of water molecules in each direction at a particular time. For isotropic diffusion, the diffusion ellipsoid is a sphere. Anisotropic diffusion is modeled with an elongated ellipsoid. The longest axis describes diffusivity in the direction with greatest mean water displacement. The diffusion tensor model assumes this orientation is parallel to an axonal bundle. The length of the longest axis is termed the primary eigenvalue of the diffusion tensor and its direction the principal eigenvector. The second and third eigenvalues are the minor eigenvalues describing diffusion perpendicular to the primary eigenvector.

A number of diffusion parameters describing the microstructure of a particular voxel can be defined with the three eigenvalues (Figure 3.2.3). These metrics are only dependent on the geometric shape of the diffusion ellipse and not on the orientation of the ellipse or the MR scanner coordinate system. The directionally averaged diffusion coefficient, (D_{av}), is the mean of the three eigenvalues and describes the spatially averaged diffusivity of water in a voxel. D_{av} is sometimes referred to as the apparent diffusion coefficient (ADC) or mean diffusivity (MD).

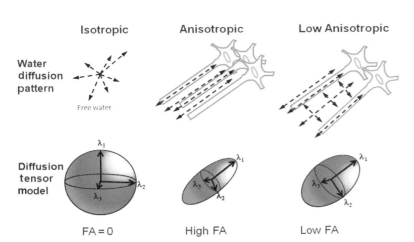

FIGURE 3.2.2 The different modes of diffusion possible within the brain are depicted. Isotropic diffusion occurs where there are no barriers to the movement of water. The diffusion ellipsoid for isotropic diffusion is spherical because diffusion is equally likely in all directions. Within bundles of white matter, diffusion is least restricted along the axons. The corresponding diffusion ellipsoid is elongated. If the arrangement of axons is altered, the pattern of diffusion will also change. FA = fractional anisotropy; λ = eigenvalue.

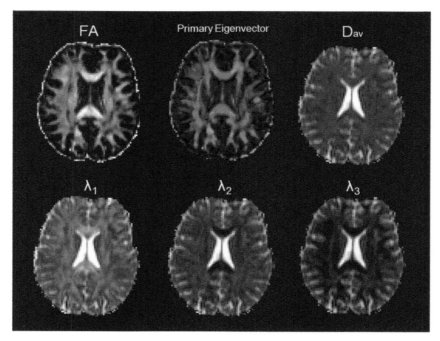

FIGURE 3.2.3   Diffusion metric maps derived from the tensor are shown. On the top row are fractional anisotropy (FA), color-coded primary eigenvector, and the directionally averaged apparent diffusion coefficient. The primary eigenvector is color-coded with blue inferior-superior, red left-right, and green anterior-posterior. On the bottom row are the individual eigenvalues displayed with the same window and level. Notice that the primary eigenvalue map contains the largest values while the third eigenvalue is the smallest.

$$D_{av} = \frac{\lambda_1 + \lambda_2 + \lambda_3}{3} \qquad (3.2.3)$$

The fractional anisotropy (FA) metric describes the degree of directionality of diffusivity within a voxel. If the three eigenvalues are equal, the FA will be zero. The fractional anisotropy approaches its maximum value if the primary eigenvalue is much larger than the minor eigenvalues.

$$FA = \frac{\sqrt{(\lambda_1 - \lambda_2)^2 + (\lambda_2 - \lambda_3)^2 + (\lambda_3 - \lambda_1)^2}}{\sqrt{2}\sqrt{\lambda_1 + \lambda_2 + \lambda_3}} \qquad (3.2.4)$$

So the FA can be seen to vary in the range 0 to 1, with 0 representing isotropic diffusion and 1 representing purely directional diffusion. In practice, most white matter of the brain is characterized by an FA in the range 0.4 to 0.8. The direction of preferred diffusion is not coded in the eigenvalues, but rather in the principal eigenvector of the DTI tensor model (corresponding to the direction of the long axis of the ellipsoid).

DIFFUSION AND SCALAR MEASURES IN ASD

As described above, quantification of water diffusion in the brain can be characterized by scalar metrics (such as MD and FA) that relate to the microstructure of white matter. As such, these measures can be used to characterize normal developmental processes as well as to identify anomalies associated with pathologies and especially neuropsychiatric disorders, such as ASD.

Atypical brain growth has been implicated in ASD by both neuropathologic and imaging studies. Interestingly, while the observations are made generally throughout much of the brain, the temporal and frontal lobes, and especially the white matter fraction of these, appear to be most strongly different in ASD compared to age-matched controls (Herbert, 2005). Given the social and communication impairment evident in ASD, structural changes to these regions may not be surprising. Further, given hypotheses of abnormal connectivity in ASD, involvement of white matter structures may also be intuitive. Interestingly, abnormal development of posterior frontal white matter was also shown to be associated with motor impairments. Furthermore, the more peripheral 'U' fibers for the frontal lobes are also thought to be involved. All these findings suggest that a white matter maturation anomaly may be a hallmark of ASD.

There have been a considerable number of recent publications implicating abnormal diffusion tensor properties in the white matter of children with ASD (Jou et al., 2011; Kleinhans et al., 2008; Langen et al., 2011; Mostofsky et al., 2007; Shukla et al., 2010; 2011a, b; Weinstein et al., 2011). Alexander et al. (2007), in one of the earlier studies, found increased MD and decreased FA in autistic patients along a smaller than normal corpus callosum, more pronounced in a group with lower performance IQ measures. Kumar et al. have found increased length of right arcuate fasciculus in ASD patients, associated with lower FA and higher MD. Lee et al. (2007), demonstrated increase in MD in bilateral white matter of the superior temporal gyrus and right temporal stem in patients with high-functioning autism (HFA) when compared to age-matched typically developing controls (TDC). The authors also found overall reduction in FA and increased radial diffusivity (the average of the second and third eigenvalues, λ_2 and λ_3), and attributed the findings along these pathways, critically involved in language and social cognition, to microstructural disorganization. Even though increases in radial diffusivity have been attributed to abnormalities of myelin, the authors believed that changes in axonal density, organization, and gliosis could equally lead to an increase in radial diffusivity. Sundaram et al. (2008) also found increases in MD with associated reduction in FA in short association fibers in the frontal lobes of ASD patients when compared to TDC; MD was also increased in the long fibers of the frontal lobes in ASD. Likewise, despite descriptions of increased white matter in autism, examining the number of fiber trajectories (or streamlines), no significant difference was found between ASD and typical development (TD), perhaps reflecting a lower density of packing (or an abnormal organization). Fletcher et al. (2010) showed elevated MD in the arcuate fasciculus in a pilot study (N = 10) using an automated fiber selection algorithm. Nagae et al. (2012) recently demonstrated elevated mean diffusivity in the left hemisphere superior longitudinal fasciculus in a large group of children with ASD, and demonstrated an association between degree of diffusivity elevation and impairment of language function (as assessed by the Clinical Evaluation for Language Fundamentals, fourth edition (CELF-4) evaluation). This type of study clearly points towards a neurobiological basis of impaired behavioral performance in ASD.

While the exact biological underpinning of the diffusion observation must at this time remain speculative, one possible etiology that would lead to elevated MD would be an incomplete or insufficient pruning of white matter branches (part of the normal developmental process) preventing axons from bundling tightly and allowing water to diffuse more readily. This might be expected to elevate the radial diffusivity more than the axial (λ_1) and thus lead to decreases in FA, as the eigenvalues become more similar. In general, inspection of the individual eigenvalues (and not just the summary statistics MD and FA) offers more specific insight into the biological basis. Taken together, the studies demonstrate a consistency of observation of white matter anomalies, mostly characterized by elevated MD and decreased FA compared to age-matched non-ASD control subjects. Multiple fiber bundles have been implicated, including

the corpus callosum as well as white matter of the frontal and temporal lobes. Nagae et al. (2012) report much less evidence of abnormality in the corticospinal tracts, perhaps reflecting the lesser contribution of motor impairments to the autism phenotype (compared, for example, to the communication and social functions subserved by white matter of the frontal and temporal lobes, both of which are more frequently reported as abnormal in ASD). Table 3.2.1 summarizes the recent published studies of DTI in ASD, including only those manuscripts with a sample size > 20.

POPULATION STATISTICS AND PATTERN CLASSIFIERS BASED ON DTI

Methods for population-based statistics using DTI have been developed with the aim of elucidating group differences as well as probing certain regions of the brain based on one or more hypotheses. Traditionally, population studies use methods like voxel-based morphometry (VBM) (Ashburner and Friston, 2000) that study the whole brain in the absence of a hypothesis, or investigate spatial-hypothesis-driven region of interest (ROI)-based studies (Alexander et al., 2007). In ASD, as described above, VBM studies using DTI have reported lower white matter integrity mainly in the corpus callosum, internal and external capsule, temporal white matter, superior and inferior longitudinal fasciculus (Alexander et al., 2007; Barnea-Goraly et al., 2004; Keller et al., 2007; Lee et al., 2007; Verhoeven et al., 2010). ROI-based studies have hypothesized abnormalities in the arcuate fasciculus (Fletcher et al., 2010), superior temporal gyrus, and temporal stem (Lee et al., 2007) in ASD. Despite their popularity, VBM methods only identify local group differences and do not lend themselves to the statistical identification of spatially distributed patterns of voxel differences (where the changes in individual voxels or voxel clusters may be sub-threshold and escape identification). ROI-based analyses performed on certain preselected ROIs require *a priori* knowledge of the affected regions, specific to pathology. These methods, therefore, have a restricted exploratory power, based on the separate ROIs used, whose combined change during the course of pathologic progression may be difficult to assess.

This has led to the development of methods that can learn subtle brain pattern differences and provide a quantifiable score that serves as a pathophysiological marker reflecting the extent of pathology, and is expected to augment diagnostic decisions. Furthermore, by identifying key anatomic substrates (features) that provide such group separation, classifiers provide potential neurobiological insight into the basis of the disorder. High dimensional pattern classification

TABLE 3.2.1   A Brief Review of those Studies of DTI in ASD with a Sample Size (in the ASD group) of 20 or Greater

Study author, year	Sample size in ASD group	Structures identified as anomalous	Change in MD, FA, other scalars	Notes
Keller et al., 2006	34	CC	Decreased FA	
Alexander et al., 2007	43	CC	Increased MD, decreased FA	Association with IQ
Lee et al., 2007	43	WM of superior temporal lobe, temporal stem	Increased MD, decreased FA — Radial diffusivity	
Sundaram et al., 2008	50	Short fibers of frontal lobe	Increased MD, decreased FA	Younger children
Kumar et al., 2010	32	Right arcuate fasciculus, right uncinate fasciculus	Increased MD, decreased FA, increased length	Young children, Association with behavior
Pugliese et al., 2009	24	Inferior fronto-occipital fasciculus	Decreased FA	Adults
Cheng et al., 2010	25	PLIC frontal and temporal WM	Decreased FA, increased FA	
Lange et al., 2010	30 + 12	WM of superior temporal lobe, temporal stem	Tskew asymmetry, decreased FA	
Weinstein et al., 2011	22	CC, left SLF	Increased FA, decreased MD	
Shukla et al., 2010	26	Whole brain, CC	Decreased FA, increased MD	These three papers describe analysis methods applied to the same sample
Shukla et al., 2011a	26		Decreased FA	
Shukla et al., 2011b	26		Decreased FA, increased MD	
Ingalhalikar et al., 2011	45	IC, EC, left SLF	Decreased FA	
Nagae et al., 2012	35	Left SLF	Increased MD	Association with language function, mild increase in MD of CST

A number of pilot studies with n < 20 exist, but typically show discrepant findings, probably reflecting the heterogeneity in ASD and the need for larger samples to draw definitive conclusions. As can be seen, even with n > 20, not all findings are consistent. CC = corpus callosum; CST = corticospinal tracts; EC = exterior capsule; IC = internal capsule; SLF = superior longitudinal fasciculus; WM = white matter.

methods (linear discriminant analysis, k-NN classifiers, support vector machines (SVMs)) have been adopted in the neuroimaging community to identify patterns of pathology that differentiate between patients and controls. There are a few classification studies in ASD, which differ based on the features used for classification and the method used to train the classifiers. Figure 3.2.4 shows the steps involved in creating classifiers: feature extraction, in which features are computed from the training samples; feature selection, in which a ranking is assigned to the features based on how discriminative they are; and then classifier training. Finally, the generalizability of a classifier to a new dataset is established via different cross-validation approaches, such as leave-one-out and n-fold cross-validation. Lange et al. 2010 used quadratic classifiers with hypothesis-based specific regions of the brain to create autism-specific classifiers using DTI-based features computed in two regions in the brain. Similarly, Adluru

et al. (2009) trained SVM classifiers on chosen fiber tract shape features.

Although such methods give reasonable classification accuracy, they are hypothesized to certain brain regions, making it difficult to understand brain region interactions. In addition, the components cannot provide a physiological insight into the regions that contribute to the group separability. Ingalhalikar et al., (2011) created ASD classifiers using SVMs based on DTI features of anisotropy and diffusivity computed from atlas-based ROIs. These classifiers capture multivariate relationships among various anatomical regions for more effective characterization of group differences, as well as for quantifying the degree of pathological abnormality associated with each subject, via an abnormality score. Figure 3.2.5 shows a plot of these scores and their ability to differentiate between ASD and TD. This score can then be used to complement clinical scores, thereby aiding in

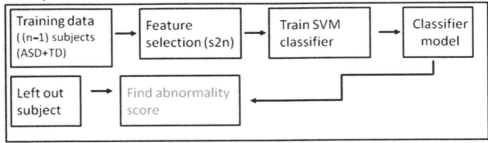

Preprocessing

LOO process (each subject is left out recursively)

FIGURE 3.2.4   The pattern classification pipeline (top) showing the important steps in training classifiers, namely extracting features, selecting and ranking the features, and then using these features computed from the training samples to create classifiers. The bottom part of the figure shows a standard cross-validation pipeline in which leave-one-out cross-validation is used to study the generalizability of a classifier to a new sample.

diagnostic decisions and potentially enhancing disease characterization. The regions ranked by the classifier (Figure 3.2.5, right) provide a neurobiological insight into the pathology of ASD, and the ranking of features can be used for hypothesis generation for studies based on the regions implicated.

DTI TRACTOGRAPHY

One can also exploit the directional information of diffusion anisotropy to allow delineation of axonal fiber tracts in the brain. In each brain voxel, the dominant direction of axonal bundles can be assumed to be

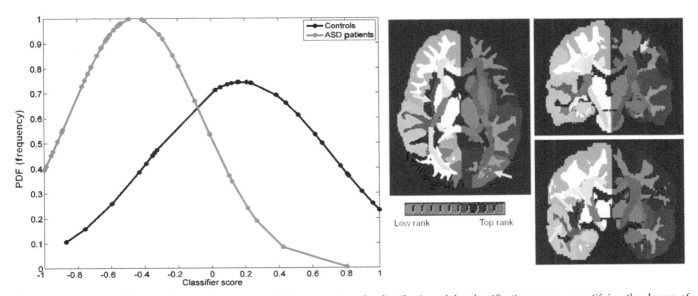

FIGURE 3.2.5   (Left) Probability density function (PDF) representing the distribution of the classification scores, quantifying the degree of pathology of a subject. The separation in the PDF peaks indicates the high separation between two groups. (Right) Regions ranked based on their contribution to the classification.

FIGURE 3.2.6   Diffusion MR fiber-tracking method based upon Fiber Assignment by Continuous Tracking (FACT). The first step is to define a starting region (dotted orange voxels). Starting points (blue dots) are distributed within the starting region of interest. The fiber trajectories (green arrows) follow the primary eigenvectors of the diffusion ellipsoids (grey ellipses). When a fiber track enters a new voxel, the course of the trajectory is altered to match the new voxel's eigenvector. Constraints on FA levels and curvature may also be applied to prevent erroneous fiber tracks.

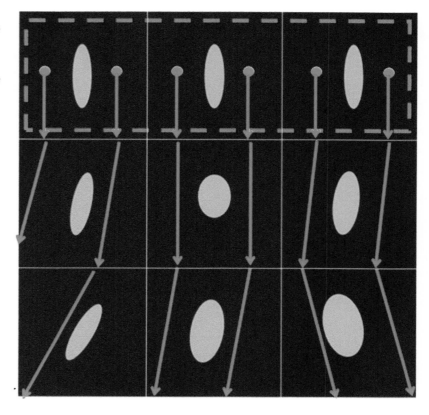

parallel to the primary eigenvector (the direction of the long axis of the diffusion ellipsoid). DTI tractography follows the primary eigenvector from voxel to voxel through the brain and can depict in 3D a specific white matter tract (Basser et al., 2000; Conturo et al., 1999; Mori et al., 1999; Mori and van Zijl, 2002; Parker et al., 2003). Numerous tractography algorithms have been published, but all make the fundamental assumption that water diffusion is correlated with axon orientation. These fiber-tracking algorithms can be divided into deterministic methods and probabilistic methods. Deterministic methods assume the diffusion tensor is an accurate representation of the underlying fiber structure and do not consider estimates of uncertainty in fiber orientation (Figure 3.2.6). Probabilistic methods include an estimate of uncertainty in the tensor and propagate trajectories in multiple possible directions (Behrens et al., 2003).

The first step in tractography is to acquire a DTI dataset and calculate the diffusion tensors and diffusion maps including FA, D_{av}, and color-coded FA maps (Figure 3.2.3). Fiber tracts can be generated for every voxel within the white matter to show a complete and complex set of axonal connections (Figure 3.2.7, left). However, it is desirable to delineate a specific white matter tract by selecting a subset of the fiber tracts. To accomplish this, a starting region of interest is placed within the white matter tract of interest. This step may be aided with subject-specific cortical mapping techniques such as functional MRI (fMRI), magnetoencephaography, or electrocorticography (Engel et al., 2005; Ganslandt et al., 2004; Guye et al., 2003; Krishnan et al., 2004; Nagarajan et al., 2008; Schiffbauer et al., 2002; Schulder et al., 1998). Alternatively, the starting region may be manually placed with the help of anatomical atlases and the direction color-coded FA map (see Figure 3.2.3). Only the fiber trajectories that pass through this ROI are preserved. Additional ROIs may be used to further filter the set of trajectories constituting a specific white matter tract using logical operands AND, OR, and NOT. Rules on the geometry and course of the fiber tracts may be applied, including a threshold on FA and a maximum anatomically plausible turning angle. The result of this process is a depiction in 3D of a group of spatially contiguous fiber tracts representing the position of a white matter tract (Figure 3.2.7, right).

The clinical and scientific utility of DTI fiber tracking is found in the localization and quantitative assessment of specific neuronal pathways. DTI fiber tracking allows individual neuronal pathways to be quantified across regions of the brain where manual segmentation would not be possible. The 3D region encompassing a delineated white matter tract may be used to measure FA, diffusivity, eigenvalues, or any other metric that can be computed

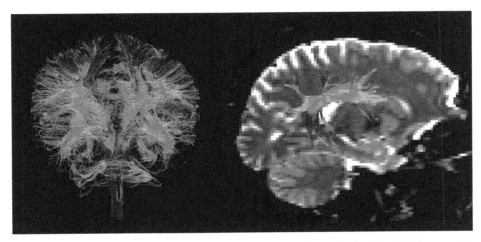

FIGURE 3.2.7   3D tractography in the brain. On the left, full brain DTI tractography is depicted in 3D. Tractography was performed using a deterministic fiber-tracking algorithm. The streamlines are colored according their orientation in the same convention as direction color-coded FA maps (blue: inferior-superior, red: left-right, green: anterior-posterior). The right panel shows the subset of fiber tracks representing the superior longitudinal fasciculus (SLF).

from the diffusion volume. Tractography allows an entire tract to be quantitatively assessed while ROI analysis is restricted to portions of the tract well defined by landmarks (Partridge et al., 2005). Further, tract-level, properties, such as approximations of 'fiber density' or tract length and shape, can also be extracted and used to characterize the white matter. In addition to measures which describe the microstructure within the tract of interest, tractography can also be used to assess patterns of connectivity between the cortices of the brain.

ADVANCED TRACT METRICS AND FULL BRAIN NETWORKS

The theory that ASD is not only a disorder of brain development but also of brain connectivity is receiving increased attention. The *in vivo* mapping of brain connectivity, either structurally or functionally, is now routinely included in research studies investigating neurological development (Hagmann et al., 2010), as well as those looking at specific diseases such as attention deficit/hyperactivity disorder (Konrad and Eickhoff, 2010) and schizophrenia (Yu et al., 2011). These approaches model the brain as a vastly interconnected network of brain regions. Each region or node is treated as an independent functional unit, while the amount of functional or structural connectivity between regions is represented by the strength of the connections between nodes. The most prominent structural connectivity analysis methodologies rely on computing a single set of fiber streamlines used to represent the axonal fiber bundles of the brain. This set of fibers is determined by seeding the tracking algorithm either from all white matter (WM) voxels (Hagmann et al., 2007; 2008) or from all brain voxels (Calamante et al., 2010) and is

then used to either compute a track density image (TDI) or determine connectivity weights between GM regions as the number of streamlines whose endpoints lie in those regions, sometimes normalized by the length of the tracks. The use of every voxel, either white or grey matter, as a seed, may cause an oversampling of large, central fiber bundles that traverse many voxels. In the process, shorter U-fibers or association fibers are undersampled, which might be problematic for studies of pathologies such as autism that may require the investigation of short-as well as long-range connectivity.

Several approaches have been proposed that combine anisotropy measures with fiber-tracking methods to produce a connection weight between nodes (Iturria-Medina et al., 2007; 2008; Robinson et al., 2010). However the inclusion of anisotropy into the connectivity weight, while drawing a parallel to the work on fractional anisotropy, reduces the interpretability of this measure, particularly as an anatomical/structural description. Other work (Gong et al., 2009a, b) computes the connection probability between two nodes in such a way as to yield a non-symmetric connectivity measure due to the inherent dependence on the seed region, which might be difficult to attribute a physiological meaning to. Figure 3.2.8 shows example of a fiber density image, along with a connectivity matrix. Having created connectivity matrices, graph theory and network analysis methods are used to investigate pathology-based group differences in connectivity. In addition to studying the whole connection matrix, graph theoretical measures are derived from them (Rubinov and Sporns, 2010), representative of the underlying graphs, but perhaps challenging to interpret with respect to pathology. To date, there are no diffusion-based network studies in ASD. However, Figure 3.2.9 shows the preliminary application of

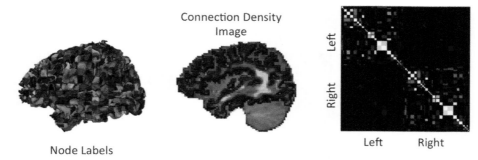

FIGURE 3.2.8 Different measures computed using the tractography between nodes that the brain is parcellated into (left); (middle) fiber density map; (right) connectivity matrix representing connection strengths between nodes.

network analysis methods to a population of ASD versus typically developing children. The left figure shows the dominance of short-range connections (intra-lobar mainly) in the ASD population and the figure on the right shows the dominant long-range connectivity in the typically developing controls.

HIGH-ANGULAR-RESOLUTION DIFFUSION IMAGING (HARDI)

Although DTI is now routinely used in diagnostic radiology and to study compromised WM in autism, it is unable to model complex white matter, such as regions of fiber crossings and branchings, or fibers like the acoustic radiation that turn sharply or overlap with other features. Simply put, the diffusion tensor model assumes for every voxel a single preferred orientation of diffusion – in the presence of even two crossing fibers, the ambiguity in directional preference (e.g., left–right *and* anterior–posterior) is paradoxically represented as diminished anisotropy. Both quantitation and fiber tracking will fail. There is a significant fraction of

complex WM voxels in the brain that contain multiple fiber bundles oriented in different directions where information garnered from the diffusion tensor model is not entirely reliable (Behrens et al., 2007). This has led to the development of DW-MRI acquisition, called HARDI (high-angular-resolution diffusion imaging), that can be fitted with higher-order models (HOMs), to address the modeling of tissue in complex WM regions. In HARDI acquisition protocols, a large number of gradient directions (45 or more) are acquired at a high b-value ($>$ 1,000 s/mm^2), to which different kinds of HOMs could be fitted. HOMs are expected to provide a much richer understanding of pathology-based connectivity changes in these complex regions, as well as a quantification of the degree of abnormality of white matter. Furthermore, this should allow white matter throughout the brain to be included in analyses (not just simply oriented structures). As the field of connectivity develops, this enhanced 'inclusivity' is paramount.

Q-space imaging (QSI) is the most general methodology for investigating diffusion signal using HOMs, but it requires data samples from a wide range of discrete gradient strengths and directions, making

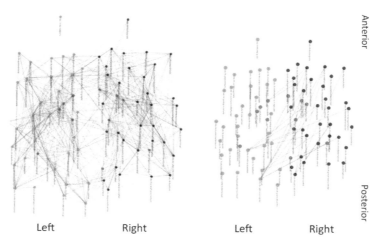

FIGURE 3.2.9 Connectivity networks on 95 nodes computed for an ASD population. (Left) Connections with strengths that are significantly higher in ASD than TD. (Right) Connections with strengths that are higher inTD than ASD. These show that short-range connections dominate in the ASD population over TD.

QSI acquisition time-consuming and currently infeasible for clinical studies. This has led to the widespread popularity of single gradient strength (single *b*-value) acquisition schemes, commonly referred to as *q*-ball imaging (QBI). A number of QBI-based HOMs have been introduced to model complex WM regions containing multiple crossing fiber populations (Descoteaux et al., 2006; 2007; Frank, 2002; Hess et al., 2006; Jian and Vemuri, 2007; Özarslan and Mareci, 2003; Özarslan et al., 2005; Tournier et al., 2004; 2007; 2008; Tuch, 2004; Tuch et al., 2003). Some models of particular interest are:

1. The *Apparent Diffusion Coefficient Profile* (ADC) is commonly represented as an *n*th order fully symmetric Cartesian tensor (Özarslan and Mareci, 2003), which reduces to the well-known diffusion tensor in second order.

2. The *Orientation Distribution Function* (ODF) approximates the radial projection of diffusion signal, using the spherical Funk-Radon transform. Alternative transforms have been proposed, such as the *Diffusion Orientation Transform* (DOT) (Özarslan et al., 2006) with a similar intent of describing the angular components of the underlying diffusion signal.

3. *Gaussian Mixture Models* describe the DW signal as a mixture of Gaussian diffusion processes, either with a discrete number of components (multi-tensor models; Peled et al., 2006) or with a continuous Von Mises–Fisher mixture models (Kumar et al., 2009).

4. In the *Fiber Orientation Distribution* (FOD) model (Tournier et al., 2004; 2007; 2008), the DW-MRI signal is modeled as the spherical convolution of the fiber orientation distribution function and a fiber impulse response function. The FOD has been shown to be robust with a low *b*-value (< 1500 s/mm^2) and a relatively few gradient directions (Tournier et al., 2007).

As the ADC, FOD, and ODF are all functions defined on the unit sphere, it is convenient to represent them by their expansion in the real spherical harmonic basis (RSH). Most of the research in HOMs has concentrated on acquiring high-gradient data as well as in fitting more and more sophisticated models and there is a growing need for developing methods for statistical analyses of HARDI data (Figure 3.2.10).

In summary, the field of diffusion imaging is evolving rapidly and its application to the study of ASD is recent, but rapidly increasing. Offering quantitative insights into local microstructure, as well as providing evidence for structural connectivity (and compromises thereof) between brain regions, its role is self-evident. In combination with functional measures (such as electrophysiological recording of response latency – see, e.g., Roberts et al., 2009), or in combination with measures of functional connectivity (derived from resting-state MRI or magnetoencephalography or electroencephalography (MEG/EEG)), multimodal approaches incorporating diffusion sensitive imaging might offer converging evidence of atypical neurobiology underlying

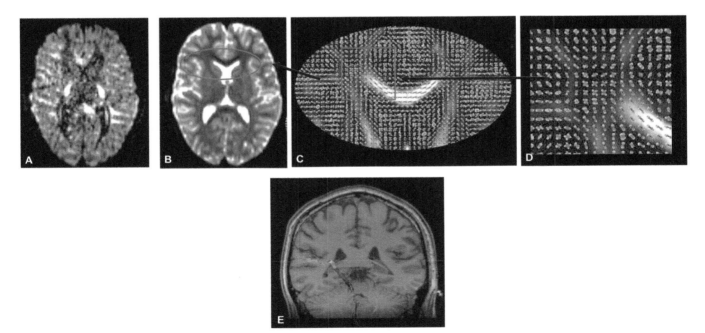

FIGURE 3.2.10   (A, B) Representative slices from the DW and b = 0 images of the HARDI data acquired; (C, D) data fitted with a HOM; (E) acoustic radiation tracked on data fitted with HOM.

behavioral and clinical presentation. Evolution of advanced diffusion techniques, such as HARDI, as well as adoption of network analysis methodologies, offers greater promise of utility, both in terms of neurobiological insight as well as pattern classifier approaches to identify subtypes, stratifying the heterogeneous ASD population into clusters of more homogeneous nature.

GLOSSARY

Autism spectrum disorders – ASD
Clinical Evaluation for Language Fundamentals – fourth edition – CELF 4
Corticospinal tracts – CST
Corpus callosum – CC
Diffusion tensor imaging – DTI
Fractional anisotropy – FA
Mean diffusivity – MD, also known as apparent diffusion coefficient (ADC) or D_{av}
Superior longitudinal fasciculus – SLF
Typically developing children and adolescents – TD/TDC
Support vector machine – SVM
Voxel-based morphometry – VBM
White matter – WM

References

Adluru, N., Hinrichs, C., Chung, M.K., Lee, J.-E., Singh, V., Bigler, E.D., et al., 2009. Classification in DTI using shapes of white matter tracts. Proceedings of IEEE Engineering in Medicine and Biology Conference, 2719–2722.

Alexander, A.L., Lee, J.E., Lazar, M., et al., 2007. Diffusion tensor imaging of the corpus callosum in autism. Neuroimage 34, 61–73.

Ashburner, J., Friston, K.J., 2000. Voxel-based morphometry – the methods. Neuroimage 11, 805–821.

Barnea-Goraly, N., Kwon, H., Menon, V., et al., 2004. White matter structure in autism: Preliminary evidence from diffusion tensor imaging. Biological Psychiatry 55, 323–326.

Basser, P.J., Pajevic, S., Pierpaoli, C., Duda, J., Aldroubi, A., 2000. In vivo fiber tractography using DT-MRI data. Magnetic Resonance in Medicine 44, 625–632.

Basser, P.J., Pierpaoli, C., 1996. Microstructural and physiological features of tissues elucidated by quantitative-diffusion-tensor MRI. Journal of Magnetic Resonance Series B 111, 209–219.

Beaulieu, C., 2002. The basis of anisotropic water diffusion in the nervous system – a technical review. NMR in Biomedicine 15, 435–455.

Beaulieu, C., Allen, P.S., 1994. Determinants of anisotropic water diffusion in nerves. Magnetic Resonance in Medicine 31, 394–400.

Behrens, T.E., Berg, H.J., Jbabdi, S., et al., 2007. Probabilistic diffusion tractography with multiple fibre orientations: What can we gain? Neuroimage 34, 144–155.

Behrens, T.E., Woolrich, M.W., Jenkinson, M., et al., 2003. Characterization and propagation of uncertainty in diffusion-weighted MR imaging. Magnetic Resonance in Medicine 50, 1077–1088.

Brown, R., 1828. A brief account of microscopical investigatons on the particles contained in the pollen of plants. Philosophical Magazine 4, 161–173.

Calamante, F., Tournier, J.D., et al., 2010. Track-density imaging (TDI): Super-resolution white matter imaging using whole-brain track-density mapping. Neuroimage 53, 1233–1243.

Conturo, T.E., Lori, N.F., Cull, T.S., Akbudak, E., Snyder, A.Z., Shimony, J.S., et al., 1999. Tracking neuronal fiber pathways in the living human brain. Proceedings of the National Academy of Sciences of the USA 96, 10,422–10,427.

Descoteaux, M., Angelino, E., Fitzgibbons, S., et al., 2006. Apparent diffusion coefficients from high angular resolution diffusion imaging: Estimation and applications. Magnetic Resonance in Medicine 56, 395–410.

Descoteaux, M., Angelino, E., Fitzgibbons, S., et al., 2007. Regularized, fast, and robust analytical Q-ball imaging. Magnetic Resonance in Medicine 58, 497–510.

Einstein, A., 1905. On the motion of small particles suspended in liquids at rest required by the molecular-kinetic theory of heat. Annalen der Physik 17, 549–560.

Engel, A.K., Moll, C.K., Fried, I., Ojemann, G.A., 2005. Invasive recordings from the human brain: Clinical insights and beyond. Nature Reviews Neuroscience 6, 35–47.

Fletcher, P.T., Whitaker, R.T., Tao, R., et al., 2010. Microstructural connectivity of the arcuate fasciculus in adolescents with high-functioning autism. Neuroimage 51, 1117–1125.

Frank, L.R., 2002. Characterization of anisotropy in high angular resolution diffusion-weighted MRI. Magnetic Resonance in Medicine 47, 1083–1099.

Ganslandt, O., Buchfelder, M., Hastreiter, P., Grummich, R., Fahlbusch, R., Nimsky, C., 2004. Magnetic source imaging supports clinical decision making in glioma patients. Clinical Neurology and Neurosurgery 107, 20–26.

Gong, G., He, Y., Concha, L., et al., 2009a. Mapping anatomical connectivity patterns of human cerebral cortex using in vivo diffusion tensor imaging tractography. Cerebral Cortex 19, 524–536.

Gong, G., Rosa-Neto, P., Carbonell, F., et al., 2009b. Age- and gender-related differences in the cortical anatomical network. The Journal of Neuroscience 29, 15,684–15,693.

Guye, M., Parker, G.J., Symms, M., Boulby, P., Wheeler-Kingshott, C.A., Salek-Haddadi, A., et al., 2003. Combined functional MRI and tractography to demonstrate the connectivity of the human primary motor cortex in vivo. Neuroimage 19, 1349–1360.

Hagmann, P., Cammoun, L., et al., 2008. Mapping the structural core of human cerebral cortex. PLoS Biology 6, e159.

Hagmann, P., Kurant, M., Gigandet, X., et al., 2007. Mapping human whole-brain structural networks with diffusion MRI. PLoS ONE 2, e597.

Hagmann, P., Sporns, O., Madan, N., et al., 2010. White matter maturation reshapes structural connectivity in the late developing human brain. Proceedings of the National Academy of Sciences of the USA 107, 19,067–19,072.

Herbert, M.R., 2005. Large brains in autism: The challenge of pervasive abnormality. Neuroscientist 11, 417–440.

Hess, C.P., Mukherjee, P., Han, E.T., et al., 2006. Q-ball reconstruction of multimodal fiber orientations using the spherical harmonic basis. Magnetic Resonance in Medicine 56, 104–117.

Ingalhalikar, M., Parker, D., et al., 2011. Diffusion based abnormality markers of pathology: Toward learned diagnostic prediction of ASD. Neuroimage.

Iturria-Medina, Y., Canales-Rodríguez, E.J., et al., 2007. Characterizing brain anatomical connections using diffusion weighted MRI and graph theory. Neuroimage 36, 645–660.

Iturria-Medina, Y., Sotero, R.C., Canales-Rodriguez, E.J., et al., 2008. Studying the human brain anatomical network via diffusion-weighted MRI and graph theory. NeuroImage 40, 1064–1076.

Jian, B., Vemuri, B.C., 2007. A unified computational framework for deconvolution to reconstruct multiple fibers from diffusion weighted MRI. IEEE Transactions on Medical Imaging 26, 1464–1471.

Jou, R.J., Mateljevic, N., Kaiser, M.D., Sugrue, D.R., Volkmar, F.R., Pelphrey, K.A., 2011. Structural neural phenotype of autism: Preliminary evidence from a diffusion tensor imaging study using tract-based spatial statistics. American Journal of Neuroradiology.

Keller, T.A., Kana, R.K., Just, M.A., et al., 2007. A developmental study of the structural integrity of white matter in autism. Neuroreport 18, 23–27.

Kleinhans, N.M., Muller, R.A., Cohen, D.N., Courchesne, E., 2008. Atypical functional lateralization of language in autism spectrum disorders. Brain Research 1221, 115–125.

Konrad, K., Eickhoff, S.B., 2010. Is the ADHD brain wired differently? A review on structural and functional connectivity in attention deficit hyperactivity disorder. Human Brain Mapping 31, 904–916.

Krishnan, R., Raabe, A., Hattingen, E., Szelenyi, A., Yahya, H., Hermann, E., et al., 2004. Functional magnetic resonance imaging-integrated neuronavigation: Correlation between lesion-to-motor cortex distance and outcome. Neurosurgery 55, 904–914. 914–915.

Kumar, A., Sundaram, S.K., Sivaswamy, L., et al., 2010. Alterations in frontal lobe tracts and corpus callosum in young children with autism spectrum disorder. Cerebral Cortex 20, 2103–2113.

Kumar, R., Vemuri, B.C., Wang, F., et al., 2009. Multi-fiber reconstruction from DW-MRI using a continuous mixture of hyper-spherical von Mises-Fisher distributions. Information Processing in Medical Imaging.

Lange, N., Dubray, M.B., Lee, J.E., et al., 2010. Atypical diffusion tensor hemispheric asymmetry in autism. Autism Research 3, 350–358.

Langen, M., Leemans, A., Johnston, P., et al., 2011. Fronto-striatal circuitry and inhibitory control in autism: Findings from diffusion tensor imaging tractography. Cortex.

Lee, J.E., Bigler, E.D., Alexander, A.L., et al., 2007. Diffusion tensor imaging of white matter in the superior temporal gyrus and temporal stem in autism. Neuroscience Letters 424, 127–132.

Mori, S., Crain, B.J., Chacko, V.P., van Zijl, P.C., 1999. Three-dimensional tracking of axonal projections in the brain by magnetic resonance imaging. Annals of Neurology 45, 265–269.

Mori, S., van Zijl, P.C., 2002. Fiber tracking: Principles and strategies – a technical review. NMR in Biomedicine 15, 468–480.

Mostofsky, S.H., Burgess, M.P., Gidley Larson, J.C., 2007. Increased motor cortex white matter volume predicts motor impairment in autism. Brain 130, 2117–2122.

Nagae, L.M., Zarnow, D.M., Blaskey, L., et al. Elevated mean diffusivity In the left hemisphere superior longitudinal fasciculus in autism spectrum disorders increases with more profound language impairment. American Journal of Neuroradiology, In press.

Nagarajan, S., Kirsch, H., Lin, P., Findlay, A., Honma, S., Berger, M.S., 2008. Preoperative localization of hand motor cortex by adaptive spatial filtering of magnetoencephalography data. Journal of Neurosurgery 109, 228–237.

Özarslan, E., Mareci, T.H., 2003. Generalized diffusion tensor imaging and analytical relationships between diffusion tensor imaging and high angular resolution diffusion imaging. Magnetic Resonance in Medicine 50, 955–965.

Özarslan, E., Shepherd, T.M., Vemuri, B.C., et al., 2006. Resolution of complex tissue microarchitecture using the diffusion orientation transform (DOT). Neuroimage 31, 1086–1103.

Özarslan, E., Vemuri, B.C., Mareci, T.H., et al., 2005. Generalized scalar measures for diffusion MRI using trace, variance, and entropy. Magnetic Resonance in Medicine 53, 866–876.

Parker, G.J., Haroon, H.A., Wheeler-Kingshott, C.A., 2003. A framework for a streamline-based probabilistic index of connectivity (PICo) using a structural interpretation of MRI diffusion measurements. Journal of Magnetic Resonance Imaging 18, 242–254.

Partridge, S.C., Mukherjee, P., Berman, J.I., Henry, R.G., Miller, S.P., Lu, Y., et al., 2005. Tractography-based quantitation of diffusion tensor imaging parameters in white matter tracts of preterm newborns. Journal of Magnetic Resonance Imaging 22, 467–474.

Peled, S., Friman, O., Jolesz, F., et al., 2006. Geometrically constrained two-tensor model for crossing tracts in DWI. Magnetic Resonance Imaging 24, 1263–1270.

Roberts, T.P., Khan, S.Y., Blaskey, L., et al., 2009. Developmental correlation of diffusion anisotropy with auditory evoked response. Neuroreport 20, 1586–1591.

Robinson, E.C., Hammers, A., et al., 2010. Identifying population differences in whole-brain structural networks: A machine learning approach. NeuroImage 50, 910–919.

Rubinov, M., Sporns, O., 2010. Complex network measures of brain connectivity: Uses and interpretations. NeuroImage 52, 1059–1069.

Schiffbauer, H., Berger, M.S., Ferrari, P., Freudenstein, D., Rowley, H.A., Roberts, T.P., 2002. Preoperative magnetic source imaging for brain tumor surgery: A quantitative comparison with intraoperative sensory and motor mapping. Journal of Neurosurgery 97, 1333–1342.

Schulder, M., Maldjian, J.A., Liu, W.C., Holodny, A.I., Kalnin, A.T., Mun, I.K., et al., 1998. Functional image-guided surgery of intracranial tumors located in or near the sensorimotor cortex. Journal of Neurosurgery 89, 412–418.

Shukla, D.K., Keehn, B., Lincoln, A.J., Muller, R.A., 2010. White matter compromise of callosal and subcortical fiber tracts in children with autism spectrum disorder: A diffusion tensor imaging study. Journal of the American Academy of Child & Adolescent Psychiatry 49, 1269–1278.

Shukla, D.K., Keehn, B., Muller, R.A., 2011. Tract-specific analyses of diffusion tensor imaging show widespread white matter compromise in autism spectrum disorder. Journal of Child Psychology and Psychiatry 52, 286–295.

Shukla, D.K., Keehn, B., Smylie, D.M., Muller, R.A., 2011. Microstructural abnormalities of short-distance white matter tracts in autism spectrum disorder. Neuropsychologia 49, 1378–1382.

Song, S.K., Sun, S.W., Ju, W.K., Lin, S.J., Cross, A.H., Neufeld, A.H., 2003. Diffusion tensor imaging detects and differentiates axon and myelin degeneration in mouse optic nerve after retinal ischemia. NeuroImage 20, 1714–1722.

Sundaram, S.K., Kumar, A., Makki, M.I., Behen, M.E., Chugani, H.T., Chugani, D.C., 2008. Diffusion tensor imaging of frontal lobe in autism spectrum disorder. Cerebral Cortex 18, 2659–2665.

Tanner, J.E., Stejskal, E.O., 1968. Restricted self-diffusion of protons in colloidal systems by the pulsed-gradient, spin-echo method. The Journal of Chemical Physics 49, 1768–1777.

Tournier, J.D., Calamante, F., Connelly, A., et al., 2007. Robust determination of the fibre orientation distribution in diffusion MRI: Non-negativity constrained super-resolved spherical deconvolution. NeuroImage 35, 1459–1472.

Tournier, J.D., Calamante, F., Gadian, D.G., et al., 2004. Direct estimation of the fiber orientation density function from diffusion-weighted MRI data using spherical deconvolution. Neuroimage 23, 1176–1185.

Tournier, J.D., Yeh, C.H., Calamante, F., et al., 2008. Resolving crossing fibres using constrained spherical deconvolution: Validation using diffusion-weighted imaging phantom data. NeuroImage 42, 617–625.

Tuch, D.S., 2004. Q-ball imaging. Magnetic Resonance in Medicine 52, 1358–1372.

Tuch, D.S., Reese, T.G., Wiegell, M.R., et al., 2003. Diffusion MRI of complex neural architecture. Neuron 40, 885–895.

Verhoeven, J.S., De Cock, P., Lagae, L., et al., 2010. Neuroimaging of autism. Neuroradiology 52, 3–14.

Weinstein, M., Ben-Sira, L., Levy, Y., et al., 2011. Abnormal white matter integrity in young children with autism. Human Brain Mapping 32, 534–543.

Yu, Q., Sui, J., Rachakonda, S., et al., 2011. Altered topological properties of functional network connectivity in schizophrenia during resting state: A small-world brain network study. PLoS ONE 6, e25423.

Attentional Network Deficits in Autism Spectrum Disorders

Jin Fan

Department of Psychology, Queens College, The City University of New York, Flushing; Departments of Psychiatry and Neuroscience, and Seaver Autism Center for Research and Treatment, Mount Sinai School of Medicine, New York, NY, USA

OUTLINE

INTRODUCTION

Attention refers to the activity of a set of brain networks that can influence the priority of the computations of other brain networks for access to consciousness. Typical functions of attention involve obtaining and maintaining a state of vigilance or alertness, selection of sensory information, and monitoring and resolving conflict between possible responses. Attention is involved in all cognitive functions as the gateway to voluntary control of thoughts, feelings, and actions, and is critical to the establishment of higher-level cognitive functions. Autism spectrum disorders (ASD) are characterized by deficits of social interaction and communication as well as repetitive behaviors and restricted interest in the environment. While studies have shown significant cognitive abnormalities in autism (e.g., theory of mind), the relative primacy in the development of these deficits remains unclear.

Although attentional difficulties (e.g., deficits of joint/shifting attention) are common in children and adults with ASD, such deficits have not been considered to be a core symptom of ASD. The purpose of this chapter is to provide a neurocognitive framework for the attention deficits observed in autism. The reader will notice that as attention is divided into its component subsystems, the link between specific attention deficits (along with corresponding changes in neurocircuitry) and pathological features of ASD in cognitive and social development will become clear. The evidence presented in this chapter will build the argument that attentional deficits in autism may be part of its primary pathology and show relationships to the core symptom domains. In this review, I will examine behavioral and neuroimaging data that suggest that such deficits play a much more important role in the pathophysiology of autism than previously thought.

ATTENTION AS AN ORGAN SYSTEM

To facilitate understanding of the neural bases of attention, it can be treated as an organ system with its

The Neuroscience of Autism Spectrum Disorders.
http://dx.doi.org/10.1016/B978-0-12-391924-3.00019-3

281

own anatomy and circuitry. A system is defined as a group of differentiated structures made up of various cellular components and adapted to the performance of some specific function. As such, the attentional system has been defined in specific functional and anatomical terms (Posner and Badgaiyan, 1998; Posner and Fan, 2008; Posner and Petersen, 1990).

Attentional functions

Attention comprises three separate functional components: alerting, orienting, and executive control. The *alerting function* is further divided into tonic and phasic alertness. Tonic (or intrinsic) alertness reflects general wakefulness and arousal, whereas phasic alertness refers to changes in response readiness to a target, often following an external warning stimulus. The *orienting function* involves the selection of specific information from numerous sensory inputs. Orienting can be reflexive (exogenous), as when a sudden target event directs attention to its location, or it can be more voluntary (endogenous), as when a person searches the visual field looking for a target. Orienting that involves head and/or eye movements toward the target is called overt orienting, whereas orienting that does not involve head and/or eye movement is referred to as covert orienting. Orienting involves rapid or slow shifting of attention among objects within a modality or among various sensory modalities, and has three elementary operations: disengaging attention from its current focus, moving attention to the new target, and engaging attention on the new target (Posner et al., 1984). The *executive control function* of attention involves the engagement of more complex mental operations during monitoring and resolving conflict between computations or responses, such as in a color Stroop task (MacLeod, 1991) (e.g., the word RED is written in blue color and your task is to name the ink color of the word), in which the competition between the two processes of color naming (blue) and word meaning (red) has to be solved before one can make a response.

Attentional networks

Each of these three attentional functions is mediated by anatomically distinct neural networks and neurotransmitters (Figure 3.3.1 and Table 3.3.1). Alerting has been associated with thalamic, frontal, and parietal regions and is influenced by the cortical distribution of the brain's noradrenergic (NAergic) system, which arises from the locus coeruleus in the midbrain (Coull et al., 1996; Marrocco et al., 1994). Blocking the NAergic system blocks the normal effect of warning signals (Marrocco et al., 1994). The NAergic system has also been implicated in maintaining an alert state (Witte and Marrocco, 1997).

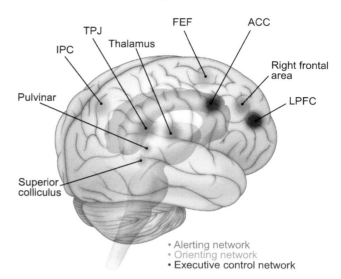

FIGURE 3.3.1 Functional anatomy of the attentional networks. Right frontal and parietal areas, while TPJ is active for tonic and phasic alerting. The pulvinar, superior colliculus, IPC, and FEF are active for orienting. The ACC and LPFC are important regions for executive control. ACC: anterior cingulate cortex; IPC: intraparietal cortex; FEF: frontal eye fields; LPFC: lateral prefrontal cortex; TPJ: temporal parietal junction.

The orienting system for visual events has been associated with brain areas such as the superior parietal lobule, temporal parietal junction (TPJ) and the frontal eye fields (FEF) (Corbetta et al., 2000; Corbetta and Shulman, 2002; Posner, 1980; Posner and Cohen, 1984; Posner et al., 1982). It has been shown that bilaterally, the intraparietal cortex (IPC) and the FEF are involved in orienting, whereas the right TPJ and inferior frontal gyrus are involved in reorienting (Corbetta et al., 2000; Corbetta and Shulman, 2002). Our functional magnetic resonance imaging (fMRI) study showed that the TPJ is involved in alerting rather than orienting (Fan et al., 2005). This finding has subsequently been confirmed by other groups (Thiel and Fink, 2007). Cholinergic systems arising in the basal forebrain play an important role in modulating orienting. Injections of muscarinic antagonist scopolamine into the lateral intraparietal area in nonhuman primates have been shown to increase reaction time and decrease performance accuracy in a covert orienting task (Davidson and Marrocco, 2000), suggesting that this network is related to acetylcholine (ACh). The site of this effect is not in the basal forebrain, but in the parietal lobe. Damage to the parietal lobe is associated with deficits in disengagement of attention (Posner et al., 1984). Damage to the superior colliculus and other midbrain structures is associated with a deficit in movement of attention (Posner and Petersen, 1990). Lesions to the pulvinar nucleus of the thalamus are associated with deficits in engagement of visual attention (Rafal and Posner, 1987).

TABLE 3.3.1   Attentions and Possible Brain Regions and Neurotransmitters Involved

Attentional functions	Subcomponents	Brain regions involved	Neurotransmitters
Alerting	Tonic alerting Phasic alerting	Thalamic, frontal, parietal regions, locus ceruleus, cerebellum and brainstem, temporal parietal junction	Noradrenaline
Orienting	Disengaging Moving Engaging	Superior parietal lobule, frontal eye field, superior colliculus, midbrain structures, pulvinar nucleus of thalamus	Acetylcholine
Executive control		Anterior cingulate cortex, lateral prefrontal cortex	Dopamine

Finally, the executive control of attention involves the anterior cingulate cortex (ACC) and the lateral prefrontal cortex (LPFC) (Matsumoto and Tanaka, 2004) and is modulated by dopamine (Benes, 2000; Lidow et al., 1991). Other regions, such as the anterior insular cortex, also play a role in executive control (Craig, 2009). A number of neuroimaging studies have shown activation of the dorsal ACC in tasks requiring subjects to respond to one dimension of a stimulus rather than a strong conflicting dimension (Botvinick et al., 2001; Bush et al., 2000; Fan et al., 2003; MacDonald et al., 2000).

IMPAIRMENTS OF ATTENTIONAL FUNCTIONS AND THEIR NEURAL SUBSTRATES IN AUTISM

There is accumulating data to support the presence of attention impairments in ASD. In a comprehensive review, Allen and Courchesne (2001) suggested that impairments of attention are among the most consistently reported cognitive deficits in autism. The following section describes deficits of attentional functions and networks in ASD, based on the view of functional separation and specification of attention, providing a framework for a more comprehensive interpretation and better understanding of the attentional impairments observed in affected individuals.

Alerting

Some studies have shown that children with autism possess a normal ability to sustain attention (Pascualvaca et al., 1998), and that their difficulties in sustaining attention may not be a primary impairment but may be due to a developmental delay and to motivational contingencies of a task (Garretson et al., 1990). However, there is evidence that altered arousal mechanisms in ASD, such as a chronically high state of arousal (Hutt et al., 1964) and aberrant response to novelty, may underlie some of the observed behavioral abnormalities such as attention to social and nonsocial stimuli (Dawson and Lewy, 1989). The evidence supporting

the argument of normal ability to sustain attention comes from studies that employed the commonly used Continuous Performance Test (CPT) (Rosvold et al., 1956) to measure sustained attention or vigilance, which failed to show any performance deficits in patients with autism (Buchsbaum et al., 1992; Garretson et al., 1990; Pascualvaca et al., 1998; Siegel et al., 1992; 1995). Although the results from the CPT appeared to show no evidence of deficits related to alerting (Casey et al., 1993; Pascualvaca et al., 1998), the two types of alerting functions, tonic and phasic alertness, were not considered separately. When past data is reanalyzed examining phasic and tonic alerting separately, autistic children benefited less than controls from the presence of a cue (i.e., deficit of phasic alerting), and autistic savants had slower response than controls in the no-cue condition (i.e., deficit of tonic alerting).

Morphometric studies have also shown evidence of anatomical abnormalities in the parietal lobe in ASD (Courchesne et al., 1993), though not in other regions typically associated with the alerting network (see Table 3.3.1). However, numerous studies of individuals with autism provide evidence of anatomical abnormalities in the cerebellum (Courchesne et al., 1994; Hashimoto et al., 1995; Murakami et al., 1989), and brainstem (Courchesne et al., 1994; Hashimoto et al., 1995; Murakami et al., 1989). The cerebellum has been hypothesized to play a role in anticipatory operation, an idea consistent with the concept of phasic alerting (Allen and Courchesne, 2001), while nuclei in the brainstem are known to be related to tonic attention (e.g., locus coeruleus) (Witte and Marrocco, 1997).

The cerebellum may play an important role in anticipating upcoming sensory events and in optimizing neural systems (e.g., brainstem, thalamus, and cerebral cortex) that mediate arousal and are involved in processing such events (Courchesne et al., 1994). In ASD, the abnormally low density of Purkinje cells in the cerebellar cortex may lead to disinhibition of the cerebellar deep nuclei and consequent overexcitement of the thalamus and cerebral cortex. The cerebellum may also influence higher cognitive function, as it has widespread connections with numerous non-motor areas, including the reticular activation system, brainstem, thalamus, and parietal cortex (Itoh and Mizuno, 1979; Kitano et al., 1976; Moruzzi and Magoun, 1949; Nieuwenhuys et al., 1988; Sasaki et al., 1972; Schmahmann and Pandya, 1989; Snider, 1950; Vilensky and van Hoesen, 1981). The cerebellum has also been shown to have modulatory effects on sensory responsiveness (Crispino and Bullock, 1984). Taken together, these findings suggest abnormalities in the alerting function of attention and that these functional abnormalities may be related to structural abnormalities that have frequently been reported in autism.

Orienting

It is a well-documented phenomenon that individuals with ASD do not orient to human faces normally. Although some studies have shown an orienting deficit related to social cues (e.g., Dawson et al., 1998), others provide evidence of an orienting deficit in autistic patients that is not due to social information (Landry and Bryson, 2004; Renner et al., 2006; Teder-Salejarvi et al., 2005). Spatial orienting of attention has been studied extensively in autism using the spatial attention paradigm (Posner et al., 1984) (e.g., Casey et al., 1993; Townsend et al., 1996a, b). In a study by Casey and colleagues (1993), patients with ASD showing savant skills provided evidence for abnormalities of both disengaging and moving of attention. Wainwright-Sharp and Bryson (1993) demonstrated deficits in disengaging and moving attention and difficulty processing briefly presented cue information within the visual modality. Townsend and colleagues (1996a) separated individuals with ASD into groups with (P+) or without (P−) parietal lobe abnormalities as defined by reduced posterior parietal cortex volume. The P+ group showed significantly slower reaction times when detecting a target in an unexpected location relative to in an expected location, emphasizing the important role of the parietal lobes in the functional deficits of orienting in autism.

An orienting deficit is also evident in tasks that require rapid shifting of attention between modalities (Courchesne et al., 1994), between object features (Courchesne et al., 1994; Rinehart et al., 2001), and between spatial locations (Belmonte, 2000; Harris et al., 1999; Townsend et al., 1996a,b; Wainwright and Bryson, 1996; Wainwright-Sharp and Bryson, 1993), and in responding to auditory or visual context stimulation when intensively focused on processing a single piece of information (Lovaas et al., 1971; 1979; Townsend and Courchesne, 1994). In addition, orienting deficits also appeared when adjusting and updating the scope and focus of attention (Burack et al., 1997), in engaging visual attention in the presence of distractors (Burack, 1994), in disengaging attention from a spatial focus (Wainwright and Bryson, 1996),

and in dividing attention between auditory and visual channels (Casey et al., 1993). In other words, when there are multiple parallel inputs from different sensory systems or within one sensory modality, the ability to process the information of the unattended input is significantly reduced in patients with ASD.

It has been observed that both patients with autism and patients with cerebellar damage have impairments in shifting attention between sensory modalities. Some have proposed that such deficits may be a contributor to the development of ASD. Deficits in the ability to disengage and move attention have been reported in autism in relation to abnormal development of the cerebellum (Akshoomoff et al., 2002). Abnormalities of the parietal lobes (Courchesne et al., 1993) have been related to a deficit of the orienting function (Townsend and Courchesne, 1994). In general, evidence suggests that parietal lobe abnormalities are associated with difficulties in disengaging attention from current focus and that cerebellar abnormalities affect the rapid and accurate moving of attention to a new focus in ASD.

Executive control

The over-focused or selective attention found in patients with ASD (Lovaas et al., 1979; Lovaas and Schreibman, 1971) may reflect abnormal function of executive attention. A dysfunction of executive control in autism persists throughout development (Luna et al., 2007), and may be attributed to abnormalities of frontal lobes in patients with ASD (Aylward et al., 2002; Carper and Courchesne, 2000; Courchesne et al., 2001; Koshino et al., 2008; Sparks et al., 2002). Early studies have shown poor performance in patients with autism on executive tasks requiring a shift of mental sets (Kanner, 1943; Lovaas et al., 1971; 1979). In a study by Casey and colleagues (1993), although individuals with ASD with savant skills and normal controls showed no significant difference on single visual and single auditory CPT, those with savantism showed a significant deficit on dual visual and dual auditory CPT, indicating a limited capacity in executive control of attention for task switching. In the non-computerized version of the Wisconsin Card Sorting Test (WCST) (Pascualvaca et al., 1998), individuals with ASD show higher error rates and fewer categories, suggesting deficits of executive control (i.e., mental flexibility).

One study showed that the most consistent deficit in patients with ASD was in their performance of complex verbal tasks requiring cognitive switching and initiation of efficient lexical retrieval strategies, whereas cognitive inhibition was intact (Kleinhans et al., 2005). It was demonstrated that decreased accuracy of response shifting in patients with autism was associated with relatively reduced activation in frontal, striatal, and parietal regions, and that repetitive behavior was negatively correlated with cingulate functional activation (Shafritz et al., 2008). In a recent magnetic resonance spectroscopy study of the attentional networks in ASD, lower glutamate plus glutamine concentration in the right ACC was found (Bernardi et al., 2011), which could potentially underlie deficits in executive control in ASD.

Although a behavioral deficit in cognitive control in general has been demonstrated (Solomon et al., 2008), it has been shown that social stimuli can further interfere with cognitive control and activation of structures subserving this function, including the ACC (Dichter and Belger, 2007). In terms of neuropathology, Kemper and Bauman (1993) have demonstrated that the ACC consistently exhibits abnormalities in postmortem studies of patients with autism. Frith and colleagues (2001) have found ASD to be associated with deficits in midline frontal areas related to theory of mind, and Chiu and colleagues (2008) have demonstrated abnormal patterns of cingulate activity during performance of an interpersonal exchange game, suggesting that cingulate deficits could underlie the social deficits associated with ASD.

The phenomena of 'stimulus overselectivity' (some, usually more relevant, aspects of a stimulus are selected to the exclusion of other aspects of the stimulus) and 'underselectivity' suggest that there are deficits in the monitoring function of the executive control network. Lovaas and colleagues (Lovaas and Schreibman, 1971) showed that children with normal development responded equally to a complex stimulus consisting of visual, auditory, and tactile elements, whereas children with autism responded primarily to only one element. Burack (1994) showed that the performance of patients with autism on a forced-choice reaction time task was impaired in the presence of distractors, with no benefit from the presence of a smaller window to focus attention. Since individuals typically benefit from a smaller window to focus attention in the presence of distractors, these findings suggest an impairment best explained by an abnormal interaction between orienting and executive control functions. The impaired ability to filter extraneous information in ASD (related to deficits in executive control of attention) has also been suggested as a primary source of over-arousal (Burack, 1994; Dawson and Lewy, 1989). Overselectivity and underselectivity correlate with the presence or absence of parietal lobe abnormality in autism (Allen and Courchesne, 2001; Townsend and Courchesne, 1994).

THE ATTENTION MODEL OF AUTISM

An attention model of autism was proposed over 30 years ago (e.g., Gold and Gold, 1975). As discussed, there is evidence to support an atypical pattern of attention in ASD (Goldstein et al., 2001). It has been argued that attention may partly underlie the abnormal patterns of subjective experience reported by patients with autism (Murray et al., 2005). Further, abnormal functional activation related to impaired attention in ASD 'may be the developmental basis of higher order cognitive styles, such as weak central coherence' (Belmonte and Yurgelun-Todd, 2003). In this context, the deficits in social and cognitive development in autism may be conceptualized as having an attentional component. For example, amygdala activity, related to emotion processing, is dynamically modulated by the thalamocortical pathways (Das et al., 2005) related to the alerting and orienting functions. Additionally, orienting and executive control functions of attention are of fundamental importance during the normal exchange of information (e.g., joint attention between infants and mothers), which happens frequently, rapidly, often unpredictably, or with conflict between mental processes or responses.

Courchesne and colleagues (1994) have shown that early damage in one system alters neural organization in other interconnected systems. They hypothesized that the Purkinje neuron loss seen in ASD would result in deficits in timely and accurate direction of attention and the expression of intention. Deficits in direction of attention would then lead to deficits in infant–mother joint social and affective interactions and eventually to more complex verbal and nonverbal communication deficits (Courchesne et al., 1994). In addition to social communication difficulties, deficits in orienting may be associated with executive control, as appears to be the case in schizophrenia (Early et al., 1989a, b; Posner et al., 1988). An orienting deficit could arise based in part on abnormal function of frontal areas that are part of the executive control network. The links between executive control and self-regulation have been established by studies using connectivity analysis (Crottaz-Herbette and Menon, 2006; Etkin et al., 2006) and suggest that deficits in the executive control network could have widespread consequences for cognition and emotion.

Given the widespread impairment of every aspect of attention described above, one question that remains is how an attentional theory of ASD would account for the uneven developmental profile often observed, as well as the specific impairment in social communication that is characteristic of ASD. While mother–child interaction affected in ASD can be explained by deficits in direction of attention, it is not obvious why deficits in direction of attention appear to be more severe for social than nonsocial stimuli (e.g., Dawson et al., 1998; 2004; Maestro et al., 2002), or why young children with autism preferentially orient to nonsocial over social stimuli (e.g., Klin et al., 2009; Kuhl et al., 2005). As we defined attention as functioning to impact the order of the computations of other brain networks for access to consciousness, perhaps the attentional profile in ASD is more related to deficits interacting with the networks related to social functioning, such as social communication, which may differentiate autism from other disorders such as attention deficit/hyperactivity disorder. Potential interactions with other neural networks (e.g., social communication network) require further investigation.

Finally, despite the accumulation of studies supporting an attentional theory for autism, such studies so far have only focused on single components of attention without treating attention as an organ system that has its own functions and networks, as I and my colleagues have proposed (Posner Fan, 2008). The interactions among these attentional functions and networks, and between these attentional networks and other domain-specific networks for social function and communication, would provide a useful heuristic to understand the underlying mechanisms of attentional deficits in ASD and their implications.

CONCLUSION

Data suggest that attentional deficits are a consistent finding in ASD. Viewing such data in the context of an attentional network system (i.e., alerting, orienting, and executive functions), may help identify abnormalities of neurocircuitry in autism that result in attentional dysfunction. The attentional network framework may also allow us to hypothesize about the role of attentional difficulties in the primary pathophysiology of ASD.

ACKNOWLEDGMENTS

This work was supported by a NIH grant R21MH08 3164 to J.F. The author would like to thank Drs Evdokia Anagnostou, Nicholas T. Van Dam, David Grodberg, Xiaosi Gu, Patrick R. Hof, and Michael I. Posner for making insightful comments and for helping in editing.

References

Akshoomoff, N., Pierce, K., Courchesne, E., 2002. The neurobiological basis of autism from a developmental perspective. Development and Psychopathology 14, 613–634.

Allen, G., Courchesne, E., 2001. Attention function and dysfunction in autism. Frontiers in Bioscience 6, D105–D119.

Aylward, E.H., Minshew, N.J., Field, K., Sparks, B.F., Singh, N., 2002. Effects of age on brain volume and head circumference in autism. Neurology 59, 175–183.

Belmonte, M.K., 2000. Abnormal attention in autism shown by steady-state visual evoked potentials. Autism 4, 269–285.

Belmonte, M.K., Yurgelun-Todd, D.A., 2003. Functional anatomy of impaired selective attention and compensatory processing in autism. Cognitive Brain Research 17, 651–664.

Benes, F.M., 2000. Emerging principles of altered neural circuitry in schizophrenia. Brain Research Reviews 31, 251–269.

Bernardi, S., Anagnostou, E., Shen, J., Kolevzon, A., Buxbaum, J.D., Hollander, E., et al., 2011. In vivo (1)H-magnetic resonance spectroscopy study of the attentional networks in autism. Brain Research 1380, 198–205.

Botvinick, M.M., Braver, T.S., Barch, D.M., Carter, C.S., Cohen, J.D., 2001. Conflict monitoring and cognitive control. Psychological Review 108, 624–652.

Buchsbaum, M.S., Siegel, B.V., Wu, J.C., Hazlett, E., Sicotte, N., Haier, R., et al., 1992. Brief report: Attention performance in autism and regional brain metabolic rate assessed by positron emission tomography. Journal of Autism and Developmental Disorders 22, 115–125.

Burack, J.A., 1994. Selective attention deficits in persons with autism: Preliminary evidence of an inefficient attentional lens. Journal of Abnormal Psychology 103, 535–543.

Burack, J.A., Enns, J.T., Stauder, J.E.A., Mottron, L., Randolph, B., 1997. Attention and autism: Behavioral and electrophysiological evidence. In: Cohen, D.J., Volkmar, F.R. (Eds.), Handbook of Autism and Pervasive Developmental Disorders, second ed. John Wiley and Sons, New York, pp. 226–247.

Bush, G., Luu, P., Posner, M.I., 2000. Cognitive and emotional influences in anterior cingulate cortex. Trends in Cognitive Sciences 4, 215–222.

Carper, R.A., Courchesne, E., 2000. Inverse correlation between frontal lobe and cerebellum sizes in children with autism. Brain 123, 836–844.

Casey, B.J., Gordon, C.T., Mannheim, G.B., Rumsey, J.M., 1993. Dysfunctional attention in autistic savants. Journal of Clinical and Experimental Neuropsychology 15, 933–946.

Chiu, P.H., Kayali, M.A., Kishida, K.T., Tomlin, D., Klinger, L.G., Klinger, M.R., et al., 2008. Self responses along cingulate cortex reveal quantitative neural phenotype for high-functioning autism. Neuron 57, 463–473.

Corbetta, M., Kincade, J.M., Ollinger, J.M., McAvoy, M.P., Shulman, G.L., 2000. Voluntary orienting is dissociated from target detection in human posterior parietal cortex. Nature Neuroscience 3, 292–297.

Corbetta, M., Shulman, G.L., 2002. Control of goal-directed and stimulus-driven attention in the brain. Nature Reviews Neuroscience 3, 201–215.

Coull, J.T., Sahakian, B.J., Hodges, J.R., 1996. The alpha(2) antagonist idazoxan remediates certain attentional and executive dysfunction in patients with dementia of frontal type. Psychopharmacology (Berl) 123, 239–249.

Courchesne, E., Chisum, H., Townsend, J., 1994a. Neural activity-dependent brain changes in development: Implications for psychopathology. Development and Psychopathology 6, 697–722.

Courchesne, E., Karns, C.M., Davis, H.R., Ziccardi, R., Carper, R.A., Tigue, Z.D., et al., 2001. Unusual brain growth patterns in early life in patients with autistic disorder: An MRI study. Neurology 57, 245–254.

Courchesne, E., Press, G.A., Yeung-Courchesne, R., 1993. Parietal lobe abnormalities detected with MR in patients with infantile autism. American Journal of Roentgenology 160, 387–393.

Courchesne, E., Townsend, J., Akshoomoff, N.A., Saitoh, O., Yeung-Courchesne, R., Lincoln, A.J., et al., 1994b. Impairment in shifting attention in autistic and cerebellar patients. Behavioral Neuroscience 108, 848–865.

Courchesne, E., Townsend, J., Akshoomoff, N.A., et al., 1994c. A new finding: Impairment in shifting attention in autistic and cerebellar patients. In: Broman, S.H., Grafman, J. (Eds.), Atypical Cognitive Deficits in Developmental Disorders. Lawrance Erlbaum, Hillsdale, NJ, pp. 101–137.

Courchesne, E., Townsend, J., Saitoh, O., 1994d. The brain in infantile autism: Posterior fossa structures are abnormal. Neurology 44, 214–223.

Craig, A.D., 2009. How do you feel - now? The anterior insula and human awareness. Nature Reviews Neuroscience 10, 59–70.

Crispino, L., Bullock, T.H., 1984. Cerebellum mediates modality-specific modulation of sensory responses of midbrain and forebrain in rat. Proceedings of the National Academy of Sciences of the United States of America 81, 2917–2920.

Crottaz-Herbette, S., Menon, V., 2006. Where and when the anterior cingulate cortex modulates attentional response: Combined fMRI and ERP evidence. Journal of Cognitive Neuroscience 18, 766–780.

Das, P., Kemp, A.H., Liddell, B.J., Brown, K.J., Olivieri, G., Peduto, A., et al., 2005. Pathways for fear perception: Modulation of amygdala activity by thalamo-cortical systems. Neuroimage 26, 141–148.

Davidson, M.C., Marrocco, R.T., 2000. Local infusion of scopolamine into intraparietal cortex slows covert orienting in rhesus monkeys. Journal of Neurophysiology 83, 1536–1549.

Dawson, G., Lewy, A., 1989. Arousal, attention, and the socioemotional impairments of individuals with autism. In: Dawson, G. (Ed.), Autism: Nature, diagnosis, and treatment. Guilford Press, New York, pp. 49–74.

Dawson, G., Meltzoff, A.N., Osterling, J., Rinaldi, J., Brown, E., 1998. Children with autism fail to orient to naturally occurring social stimuli. Journal of Autism and Developmental Disorders 28, 479–485.

Dawson, G., Toth, K., Abbott, R., Osterling, J., Munson, J., Estes, A., et al., 2004. Early social attention impairments in autism: Social orienting, joint attention, and attention to distress. Developmental Psychology 40, 271–283.

Dichter, G.S., Belger, A., 2007. Social stimuli interfere with cognitive control in autism. Neuroimage 35, 1219–1230.

Early, T.S., Posner, M.I., Reiman, E.M., Raichle, M.E., 1989. Hyperactivity of the left striato-pallidal projection. Part I: Lower level theory. Psychiatric Developments 7, 85–108.

Early, T.S., Posner, M.I., Reiman, E.M., Raichle, M.E., 1989. Left striato-pallidal hyperactivity in schizophrenia. Part II: Phenomenology and thought disorder. Psychiatric Developments 7, 109–121.

Etkin, A., Egner, T., Peraza, D.M., Kandel, E.R., Hirsch, J., 2006. Resolving emotional conflict: A role for the rostral anterior cingulate cortex in modulating activity in the amygdala. Neuron 51, 871–882.

Fan, J., Flombaum, J.I., McCandliss, B.D., Thomas, K.M., Posner, M.I., 2003. Cognitive and brain consequences of conflict. Neuroimage 18, 42–57.

Fan, J., McCandliss, B.D., Fossella, J., Flombaum, J.I., Posner, M.I., 2005. The activation of attentional networks. Neuroimage 26, 471–479.

Frith, U., 2001. Mind blindness and the brain in autism. Neuron 32, 969–979.

Garretson, H.B., Fein, D., Waterhouse, L., 1990. Sustained attention in children with autism. Journal of Autism and Developmental Disorders 20, 101–114.

Gold, M.S., Gold, J.R., 1975. Autism and attention: Theoretical considerations and a pilot study using set reaction time. Child Psychiatry and Human Development 6, 68–80.

Goldstein, G., Johnson, C.R., Minshew, N.J., 2001. Attentional processes in autism. Journal of Autism and Developmental Disorders 31, 433–440.

Harris, N.S., Courchesne, E., Townsend, J., Carper, R.A., Lord, C., 1999. Neuroanatomic contributions to slowed orienting of attention in children with autism. Cognitive Brain Research 8, 61–71.

Hashimoto, T., Tayama, M., Murakawa, K., Yoshimoto, T., Miyazaki, M., Harada, M., et al., 1995. Development of the brainstem and cerebellum in autistic patients. Journal of Autism and Developmental Disorders 25, 1–18.

Hutt, C., Hutt, S.J., Lee, D., Ounsted, C., 1964. Arousal and childhood autism. Nature 204, 908–909.

Itoh, K., Mizuno, N., 1979. A cerebello-pulvinar projection in the cat as visualized by the use of anterograde transport of horseradish peroxidase. Brain Research 171, 131–134.

Kanner, L., 1943. Autistic disturbances of affective contact. The Nervous Child 2, 217–250.

Kemper, T.L., Bauman, M.L., 1993. The contribution of neuropathologic studies to the understanding of autism. Neurologic Clinics 11, 175–187.

Kitano, K., Ishida, Y., Ishikawa, T., Murayama, S., 1976. Responses of extralemniscal thalamic neurones to stimulation of the fastigial nucleus and influences of the cerebral cortex in the cat. Brain Research 106, 172–175.

Kleinhans, N., Akshoomoff, N., Delis, D.C., 2005. Executive functions in autism and Asperger's disorder: Flexibility, fluency, and inhibition. Developmental Neuropsychology 27, 379–401.

Klin, A., Lin, D.J., Gorrindo, P., Ramsay, G., Jones, W., 2009. Two-year-olds with autism orient to non-social contingencies rather than biological motion. Nature 459, 257–261.

Koshino, H., Kana, R.K., Keller, T.A., Cherkassky, V.L., Minshew, N.J., Just, M.A., 2008. fMRI investigation of working memory for faces in autism: Visual coding and underconnectivity with frontal areas. Cerebral Cortex 18, 289–300.

Kuhl, P.K., Coffey-Corina, S., Padden, D., Dawson, G., 2005. Links between social and linguistic processing of speech in preschool children with autism: Behavioral and electrophysiological measures. Developmental Science 8, F1–F12.

Landry, R., Bryson, S.E., 2004. Impaired disengagement of attention in young children with autism. Journal of Child Psychology and Psychiatry 45, 1115–1122.

Lidow, M.S., Goldman-Rakic, P.S., Gallager, D.W., Rakic, P., 1991. Distribution of dopaminergic receptors in the primate cerebral cortex: Quantitative autoradiographic analysis using [3H] raclopride, [3H]spiperone and [3H]SCH23390. Neuroscience 40, 657–671.

Lovaas, O.I., Koegel, R.L., Schreibman, L., 1979. Stimulus overselectivity in autism: A review of research. Psychological Bulletin 86, 1236–1254.

Lovaas, O.I., Schreibman, L., 1971. Stimulus overselectivity of autistic children in a two stimulus situation. Behavior Research Therapy 9, 305–310.

Lovaas, O.I., Schreibman, L., Koegel, R., Rehm, R., 1971. Selective responding by autistic children to multiple sensory input. Journal of Abnormal Psychology 77, 211–222.

Luna, B., Doll, S.K., Hegedus, S.J., Minshew, N.J., Sweeney, J.A., 2007. Maturation of executive function in autism. Biological Psychiatry 61, 474–481.

MacDonald, A.W., Cohen, J.D., Stenger, V.A., Carter, C.S., 2000. Dissociating the role of the dorsolateral prefrontal and anterior cingulate cortex in cognitive control. Science 288, 1835–1838.

MacLeod, C.M., 1991. Half a century of research on the Stroop effect: An integrative review. Psychological Bulletin 109, 163–203.

Maestro, S., Muratori, F., Cavallaro, M.C., Pei, F., Stern, D., Golse, B., et al., 2002. Attentional skills during the first 6 months of age in autism spectrum disorder. Journal of the American Academy of Child & Adolescent Psychiatry 41, 1239–1245.

Marrocco, R.T., Witte, E.A., Davidson, M.C., 1994. Arousal systems. Current Opinion in Neurobiology 4, 166–170.

Matsumoto, K., Tanaka, K., 2004. Conflict and cognitive control. Science 303, 969–970.

Moruzzi, G., Magoun, H.W., 1949. Brain stem reticular formation and activation of the EEG. Electroencephalography and Clinical Neurophysiology 1, 455–473.

Murakami, J.W., Courchesne, E., Press, G.A., Yeung-Courchesne, R., Hesselink, J.R., 1989. Reduced cerebellar hemisphere size and its relationship to vermal hypoplasia in autism. Archives of Neurology 46, 689–694.

Murray, D., Lesser, M., Lawson, W., 2005. Attention, monotropism and the diagnostic criteria for autism. Autism 9, 139–156.

Nieuwenhuys, R., Voogd, J., van Huijzen, C., 1988. The Human Central Nervous System: A Synopsis and Atlas, third ed. Springer-Verlag, Berlin; New York.

Pascualvaca, D.M., Fantie, B.D., Papageorgiou, M., Mirsky, A.F., 1998. Attentional capacities in children with autism: Is there a general deficit in shifting focus? Journal of Autism and Developmental Disorders 28, 467–478.

Posner, M.I., 1980. Orienting of attention. Quarterly Journal of Experimental Psychology 32, 3–25.

Posner, M.I., Badgaiyan, R.D., 1998. Attention and neural networks. In: Parks, R.W., Levine, D.S., Long, D.L. (Eds.), Fundamentals of Neural Network Modeling: Neuropsychology and Cognitive Neuroscience. Massachusetts Institute of Technology, Massachusetts, pp. 61–76.

Posner, M.I., Cohen, Y., 1984. Components of visual orienting. In: Bouma, H., Bowhuis, D.G. (Eds.), Attention and Performance X. Lawrence Erlbaum Associates, Hillsdale, NJ, pp. 531–556.

Posner, M.I., Cohen, Y., Rafal, R.D., 1982. Neural systems control of spatial orienting. Philosophical Transactions of the Royal Society of London. Series B, Biological Sciences 298, 187–198.

Posner, M.I., Early, T.S., Reiman, E., Pardo, P.J., Dhawan, M., 1988. Asymmetries in hemispheric control of attention in schizophrenia. Archives of General Psychiatry 45, 814–821.

Posner, M.I., Fan, J., 2008. Attention as an organ system. In: Pomerantz, J.R. (Ed.), Topics in Integrative Neuroscience: From Cells to Cognition. Cambridge University Press, Cambridge, pp. 31–61.

Posner, M.I., Petersen, S.E., 1990. The attention system of the human brain. Annual Review of Neuroscience 13, 25–42.

Posner, M.I., Walker, J.A., Friedrich, F.J., Rafal, R.D., 1984. Effects of parietal injury on covert orienting of attention. Journal of Neuroscience 4, 1863–1874.

Rafal, R.D., Posner, M.I., 1987. Deficits in human visual spatial attention following thalamic lesions. Proceedings of the National Academy of Sciences of the United States of America 84, 7349–7353.

Renner, P., Grofer Klinger, L., Klinger, M.R., 2006. Exogenous and endogenous attention orienting in autism spectrum disorders. Child Neuropsychology 12, 361–382.

Rinehart, N.J., Bradshaw, J.L., Moss, S.A., Brereton, A.V., Tonge, B.J., 2001. A deficit in shifting attention present in high-functioning autism but not Asperger's disorder. Autism 5, 67–80.

Rosvold, H.E., Mirsky, A.F., Sarason, I., Bransome, E.D., Beck, L.H., 1956. A continuous performance test of brain damage. Journal of Consulting Psychology 20, 343–350.

Sasaki, K., Matsuda, Y., Kawaguchi, S., Mizuno, N., 1972. On the cerebello-thalamo-cerebral pathway for the parietal cortex. Experimental Brain Research 16, 89–103.

Schmahmann, J.D., Pandya, D.N., 1989. Anatomical investigation of projections to the basis pontis from posterior parietal association cortices in rhesus monkey. Journal of Comparative Neurology 289, 53–73.

Shafritz, K.M., Dichter, G.S., Baranek, G.T., Belger, A., 2008. The neural circuitry mediating shifts in behavioral response and cognitive set in autism. Biological Psychiatry 63, 974–980.

Siegel Jr., B.V., Asarnow, R., Tanguay, P., Call, J.D., Abel, L., Ho, A., et al., 1992. Regional cerebral glucose metabolism and attention in adults with a history of childhood autism. Journal of Neuropsychiatry and Clinical Neuroscience 4, 406–414.

Siegel Jr., B.V., Nuechterlein, K.H., Abel, L., Wu, J.C., Buchsbaum, M.S., 1995. Glucose metabolic correlates of continuous performance test performance in adults with a history of infantile autism, schizophrenics, and controls. Schizophrenia Research 17, 85–94.

Snider, R.S., 1950. Recent contributions to the anatomy and physiology of the cerebellum. Archives of Neurology and Psychiatry 64, 196–219.

Solomon, M., Ozonoff, S.J., Cummings, N., Carter, C.S., 2008. Cognitive control in autism spectrum disorders. International Journal of Developmental Neuroscience 26, 239–247.

Sparks, B.F., Friedman, S.D., Shaw, D.W., Aylward, E.H., Echelard, D., Artru, A.A., et al., 2002. Brain structural abnormalities in young children with autism spectrum disorder. Neurology 59, 184–192.

Teder-Salejarvi, W.A., Pierce, K.L., Courchesne, E., Hillyard, S.A., 2005. Auditory spatial localization and attention deficits in autistic adults. Cognitive Brain Research 23, 221–234.

Thiel, C.M., Fink, G.R., 2007. Visual and auditory alertness: Modality-specific and supramodal neural mechanisms and their modulation by nicotine. Journal of Neurophysiology 97, 2758–2768.

Townsend, J., Courchesne, E., 1994. Parietal damage and narrow spotlight spatial attention. Journal of Cognitive Neuroscience 6, 220–232.

Townsend, J., Courchesne, E., Covington, J., Westerfield, M., Harris, N.S., Lyden, P., et al., 1999. Spatial attention deficits in patients with acquired or developmental cerebellar abnormality. Journal of Neuroscience 19, 5632–5643.

Townsend, J., Courchesne, E., Egaas, B., 1996a. Slowed orienting of covert visual-spatial attention in autism: Specific deficits associated with cerebellar and parietal abnormality. Development and Psychopathology 8, 563–584.

Townsend, J., Harris, N.S., Courchesne, E., 1996b. Visual attention abnormalities in autism: Delayed orienting to location. Journal of the International Neuropsychological Society 2, 541–550.

Vilensky, J.A., van Hoesen, G.W., 1981. Corticopontine projections from the cingulate cortex in the rhesus monkey. Brain Research 205, 391–395.

Wainwright, J.A., Bryson, S.E., 1996. Visual-spatial orienting in autism. Journal of Autism and Developmental Disorders 26, 423–438.

Wainwright-Sharp, J.A., Bryson, S.E., 1993. Visual orienting deficits in high-functioning people with autism. Journal of Autism and Developmental Disorders 23, 1–13.

Witte, E.A., Marrocco, R.T., 1997. Alteration of brain noradrenergic activity in rhesus monkeys affects the alerting component of covert orienting. Psychopharmacology 132, 315–323.

The Cerebellum in Autism Spectrum Disorders

Margaret L. Bauman*, †, Thomas L. Kemper†

*Harvard Medical School, Boston, MA, USA †Departments of Anatomy and Neurobiology, Boston University School of Medicine, Boston, MA, USA

INTRODUCTION

Autism is a behaviorally defined disorder first described by Leo Kanner in 1943. By definition, symptoms first become apparent before three years of age and include the core clinical features of impaired social interaction, delayed and disordered language/communication and isolated areas of interest. Many individuals also show poor eye contact, abnormalities of sensory processing, low muscle tone, poor fine and gross motor skills, an insistence on sameness, and repetitive and stereotypic behaviors. Although it was initially believed that 75% of persons affected with autism were cognitively impaired, it has become evident that many autistic persons are of at least average intelligence. Autism is now recognized to be a complex and heterogeneous disorder, clinically, etiologically and neurobiologically. As a result, the syndrome is now referred to as the autism spectrum disorders (ASD). At the present time, the cause of ASD remains poorly defined but both genetic and environmental factors have been implicated.

In 1985, Bauman and Kemper reported on the neuroanatomy of the brain obtained from a 29-year-old patient with ASD, studied in comparison with that of an age and sex-matched control, using the technique of whole brain serial section. Abnormalities were described primarily involving the limbic lobe and the cerebellum. Since that time, it has become evident that the cerebellum and areas related to it are the most consistently described abnormal regions in the autistic brain.

This chapter will provide an overview of what is known regarding the gross and microscopic anatomy of the cerebellum and the possible clinical implications of these findings.

GROSS ANATOMIC STRUCTURE

Initial efforts to image the brain in ASD began with the pneumoencephalographic study of Hauser et al. in 1975, in which enlargement of the left temporal horn in 15 of 18 autistic children was described. With the subsequent advent of computerized tomographic scanning (CT) technology, further studies were reported, primarily involving asymmetries of the cerebral hemispheres and ventricular size (Hier et al., 1979; Campbell et al., 1982; Rosenbloom et al., 1984; Jacobson et al., 1988). It was not until the magnetic resonance imaging (MRI) study of Courchesne et al. (1988) that observations of the radiographic morphology of the autistic brain began to focus on the structures of the cerebellum. In this study, hypoplasia of vermal lobules VI and VII was described in autistic subjects relative to controls, and it was suggested that these findings might relate to deficits in attention, sensory modulation, motor and behavioral initiation; clinical features that frequently characterize these patients.

Since the publication of this report, a large number of additional MRI studies of the cerebellum have been completed with variable results. Much of the inconsistent findings between studies have been attributable to differing methods of MRI scanning, with dissimilar slice thicknesses, slice orientation and position. Adding to the variations in methodology between imaging investigations is the selection of subjects and control groups with differing levels of inclusion and exclusion criteria, further compounding the challenge of comparing results between studies.

Additional morphometric MRI studies in autistic children, adolescents and adults have reported evidence of increased cerebellar volume, which when observed, appears to be proportional to overall cerebral volumes, rather than being specific to the cerebellum *per se*. Other studies have implicated a more diffuse involvement of the vermis including the anterior vermis (lobules I–V) and lobules VIII–X. Given the differences in findings between studies, there has been the suggestion that there may be a bimodal distribution of vermal differences, with the majority of ASD individuals showing hypoplasia and a subset demonstrating vermal hyperplasia (Courchesne et al., 1994).

In 2009, Scott et al. published the results of a volumetric analysis of the structure of the whole cerebellum and its components in 62 ASD male subjects, ages 7.5 to 18.5 years of age in comparison with age-matched controls. When compared with typically developing children, there was no reduction in the size of the mid-sagittal area of the vermis or subgroups of the lobules in any of the ASD diagnostic groups. However, the total vermal volume was reduced in the subgroup of high functioning autistic subjects, primarily in the more laterally situated portions of the vermis. Neither IQ nor age predicted the size of the vermis. No differences in the volume of the individual vermal lobules or cerebellar hemispheres were found. Thus, changes in vermal size as delineated on magnetic resonance imaging studies does not appear to be a consistent finding in ASD. The authors note that the presence of vermal hypoplasia has been reported in a number of neurodevelopmental and neurogenetic disorders with and without autistic features, suggesting that this form of neuropathology is not specific to ASD nor a sensitive signature for it, but a common feature of atypical development (Ciesielski et al., 1997).

With advances in technology, specific assessments of white and grey matter involvement and connectivity in the cerebellum have increased. Using functional magnetic resonance imaging (fMRI), Mostofsky et al. (2009) studied neural activation and connectivity during sequential appositional finger tapping. They investigated 13 children of 8–12 years of age with high-functioning ASD (HFA) in comparison with 13 age- and sex-matched controls in order to study the underpinnings of complex motor behavior. Children with HFA demonstrated diffusely decreased connectivity across the motor execution network relative to controls. In addition, the controls showed greater activation in the anterior cerebellum while the HFA group showed greater activation in the supplementary motor area. The authors suggested that the decreased cerebellar activation in the HFA group might reflect a difficulty in shifting motor execution from cortical regions associated with effortful control to regions associated with habitual execution. Further, diffusely decreased connectivity may reflect poor coordination within the circuitry necessary for automating patterned motor behavior. The investigators hypothesized that these findings might explain some of the impairments in motor development seen in ASD as well as abnormal and delayed acquisition of gestures important for communication and socialization.

The technology utilized in diffusion tensor imaging (DTI) is only just beginning to be used to study the brain in ASD. One such study examined cerebellar outflow and inflow pathways in 27 autistic children and 16 typically developing controls (Sivaswamy et al., 2010). The results of this study suggested underconnectivity between the cerebellum and neocortex in the autistic subjects. As technology improves in the future, it is likely that more DTI studies of the autistic brain will be implemented, which will provide more specific data regarding neuronal connectivity in specific brain regions.

MICROSCOPIC OBSERVATIONS IN THE CEREBELLUM AND RELATED OLIVE

Although many regions have been found to be abnormal in the postmortem autistic brain, one of the most consistently described abnormal structures has been the cerebellum and regions related to it. In 1985, Bauman and Kemper described their observations in the postmortem brain of a 29-year-old autistic man, processed in whole brain serial section, and studied in comparison to that of an identically prepared brain from a 25-year-old sex-matched control. Both brains were studied by means of a comparison microscope, multiple sections being studied side by side in the same field of view. The most significant findings were confined to the limbic system and cerebellar circuits. Decreased numbers of Purkinje cells were found primarily in the posterolateral neocerebellar cortex and adjacent archicerebellar cortex of the cerebellar hemispheres. Subsequently, Ritvo et al. (1986) quantitatively studied the microscopic anatomy of the cerebellar hemispheres and vermis from four autistic brains and controls. Decreased numbers of Purkinje cells were reported throughout the cerebellum.

Following these initial studies, eight additional brains from well-documented autistic subjects were systematically studied using the technique of gapless serial section (Bauman and Kemper, 1995). These cases included six children, two girls and two boys ages 5–12, and two young adult males ages 22 and 28. All were studied in comparison with age- and sex-matched controls. All eight brains showed a marked reduction in the number of Purkinje cells and a variable decrease in granule cells throughout the cerebellar hemispheres, with the most significant findings being observed in the neocerebellar cortex and adjacent archicerebellar cortex as previously reported (Arin et al., 1991). Despite reports of hypo- and hyperplasia of the vermis in the autistic brain from magnetic resonance imaging (Courchesne et al., 1994), no statistically significant differences were noted in the size or number of Purkinje cells in any area of the autistic vermis compared to the controls (Bauman and Kemper, 1996). Thus, reduced numbers of Purkinje cells have been largely noted in the posterior inferior hemispheric regions of the cerebellum in the brains of both autistic children and adults, with and without seizures or medication usage and these findings appear to be unrelated to cognitive function.

More recently, Whitney et al., (2008) has suggested that reduced numbers of Purkinje cells in the autistic brain may not be present in all cases. In this study, three of the six brains analyzed showed Purkinje cell numbers that closely approximated those of the controls. In addition, the density of Purkinje cells did not correlate with clinical severity of autistic symptoms. This apparent histological heterogeneity is further supported by the observations of reduced Purkinje cell size in some autistic brains (Fatemi et al., 2002).

Although much research has been directed toward Purkinje cell findings in the autistic cerebellum, relatively little attention has been directed toward the deep cerebellar nuclei which were also noted to be abnormal in the early histoanatomical studies.(Bauman and Kemper, 1994). In these initial studies, the neuronal cells of the fastigial, globose, and emboliform nuclei located in the roof of the cerebellum appeared to differ depending on the age of the patient. In the older (adult) cases, ages 22–29 years, the neurons were observed to be small and pale and significantly reduced in number. In

contrast, these same neurons, as well as those in the dentate nucleus, were found to be enlarged and present in adequate numbers in all of the younger autistic brains (5–13 years old) when compared with age- and sex-matched controls (Bauman and Kemper, 1994).

A similar pattern of neuronal differences was also noted in the principal inferior olivary nucleus in the brainstem. As observed in the deep cerebellar nuclei, neuronal cell size appeared to differ with age but not cell number which remained comparable to controls. The olivary neurons in the two adult autistic brains were small and pale, while those in the six child brains were enlarged in size but otherwise normal in appearance. However, unlike the neurons of the deep cerebellar nuclei, some of the olivary neurons tended to cluster along the periphery of the olivary convolutions, a pattern reported in several disorders of prenatal origin associated with mental retardation (Sumi, 1980; DeBassio et al., 1985), and was an observation that appeared to be unrelated to age or sex.

Given the known close relationship of the olivary climbing fiber axons to the Purkinje cell dendrites (Holmes and Stewart, 1908), the preservation of the olivary neurons despite a significant reduction in Purkinje cell number in most of the autistic brains studied strongly suggests that the cerebellar abnormalities are of prenatal origin. In the fetal monkey, studies have shown that the olivary climbing fiber axons synapse with the Purkinje cell dendrites in a transitory zone beneath the Purkinje cell layer called the lamina dissecans, these connections then forming a single unit (Rakic, 1971). In the human fetus, this zone is no longer present after 28–30 weeks gestation (Rakic and Sidman, 1970). Therefore, given the tight connection between the Purkinje cells and olivary climbing fiber axons, once this bond is made, loss or damage to the cerebellar Purkinje cells after 28–30 weeks gestation would result in an obligatory retrograde cell loss of olivary neurons (Holmes and Stewart, 1908; Norman, 1940; Greenfield, 1954). Since, in the autistic brain, the number of olivary neurons appears to be preserved, it is likely that whatever led to the reduction of Purkinje cell numbers in these patients, has to have occurred prior to the establishment of this tight bond, and therefore, prior to 28–30 weeks of gestation.

More recently, Whitney et al. (2009) , using immunocytochemical staining and stereological techniques, evaluated the numbers of GABAergic basket cells and stellate cells in the cerebellar molecular layer in the posterior cerebellar lobe of six autistic and four control brains; cells that are of critical importance for Purkinje cell functioning. No statistically significant differences were detected between autistic and control cases with regard to basket and stellate cell numbers, or in the number of basket cells and stellate cells per Purkinje cell. The investigators concluded that the preservation of the basket and stellate cells, in the presence of reduced number of Purkinje cells, suggested that, at least in some cases, Purkinje cells were generated, migrated to their proper location in the Purkinje cell layer and subsequently died, thus suggesting a later developmental loss of Purkinje cells than previously hypothesized. While these two suggested explanations for reduced Purkinje cell number in the autistic brain may appear to be at variance with each other, it may be that there is more than one neurobiological mechanism that results in reduced numbers of Purkinje cells in ASD and that the differing observations in these and other studies may reflect the heterogeneity of the disorder.

THE ROLE OF THE CEREBELLUM IN ASD – CLINICAL IMPLICATIONS

Although the clinical features of ASD do not typically become evident until sometime during the second year of life, it is generally accepted by experts in the field that ASD is a neurodevelopmental disorder that begins before birth, and that both genetic and environmental factors may play a role in its etiology. There is also a growing appreciation that the disorder is heterogeneous clinically, neurobiologically and etiologically. Further, there appears to be increasing evidence that the underlying biological mechanisms involved in ASD may involve an ongoing process that evolves over time. It has been observed, for example that overall brain weight in young children with ASD is statistically heavier than that of age and sex-matched controls, while the brain weight of autistic adults tends to be less than that of controls (Bauman and Kemper, 1997). More recently, imaging studies have provided evidence for increased brain volume in approximately 20% of ASD children, most prominently between the ages of 2 and 4.5 years of age, a growth parameter that appears to plateau by adolescence (Courchesne et al., 2001; Lainhart et al., 1997). At the microscopic level, neuronal cells in some brain regions, including the deep cerebellar nuclei of the cerebellum and the inferior olivary nucleus of the brainstem have been found to be enlarged in the brains of autistic children aged 5–13 years, but small and pale in the brains of autistic adults over the age of 22 years. These findings, combined with a recent report of reduced cortical thickness with age, measured in cranial magnetic resonance imaging studies (Hardan et al., 2009), support the hypothesis that the underlying neuropathological mechanisms involved in ASD may involve one or more postnatal processes that are ongoing. Clinically and pathologically, in most cases this process does not appear to be a degenerative one, but may reflect the brain's attempt to compensate for its atypical circuitry over time. Assuming that this hypothesis is correct, the effect of changes in the brain with age may have a significant impact on the clinical features of the disorder over time.

Functionally, it is known that the cerebellum connects with many cortical and subcortical areas of the cerebral hemispheres and acts as a modulator for many of the cognitive, language, motor, sensory, emotional and behavioral functions associated with these regions (Schmahmann, 1997). Studies in both animals and humans are beginning to more clearly elucidate significant pathways between the cerebellum and forebrain regions, and to build upon and extend previous research findings. For example, it has been well established that the cerebellum is involved in the acquisition of some types of motor learning and the regulation of motor coordination (Bloedel, 1992). In 2004, Schmahmann et al. delineated the presence of connectivity between the cerebellum and the parietal association cortices through the pons in the brainstem in a series of animal studies, thus providing a circuitry that could be compromised and that could potentially result in motor dysfunction and dyspraxia in ASD. More recently, Mostofsky et al. (2009), using functional magnetic resonance imaging (fMRI) in a series of high functioning autistic (HFA) children and typically developing controls, ages 8–13 years, demonstrated the presence of a diffusely decreased connectivity across the motor execution network in the HFA children relative to the controls during a sequential, appositional finger tapping task. The authors suggested that decreased cerebellar activation in the HFA group might reflect a difficulty in shifting motor execution from those cortical regions associated with effortful control to regions associated with habitual execution. The authors further hypothesized that diffusely decreased connectivity might also reflect poor coordination within the circuitry needed to automate patterned motor behavior and speculated that these findings could explain the presence of abnormal and delayed acquisition of gestures important for communication and socialization in ASD.

Several additional studies have supported the concept of underconnectivity between the cerebellum and forebrain structures. In 2007, Takarae et al. studied saccadic and eye pursuit movement paradigms in a group of HFA and TD children using fMRI. The HFA group showed decreased activation in the cortical eye fields and cerebellar hemispheres during eye movement tasks. In a more recent study, Sivaswamy et al. (2010) conducted an analysis of cerebellar outflow and inflow pathways in 27 autistic children and 16 typically developing children using digital tensor imaging techniques (DTI). The investigators noted an increase in the mean diffusivity of the bilateral superior cerebellar peduncles as well as an asymmetrical patterns in the fractional anisotropy of the middle and inferior cerebellar peduncles in the HFA group when compared with the typically developing children. These findings further support the presence of underconnectivity between the cerebellum and the neocortex in ASD.

In addition to its role in motor function and control, the cerebellum is involved in a range of other developmental and neurological functions. As early as the 1970s, studies in animals had delineated the existence of a direct pathway between the fastigial nucleus of the cerebellum and the amygdala and septal nuclei, as well as a reciprocal circuitry between the fastigial nucleus and the hippocampus, suggesting that the cerebellum may be important for the regulation of emotion and higher cortical thought processes (Heath and Harper, 1974; Heath et al. 1978). Animal and human studies have also implicated the cerebellum in functional psychiatric disorders (Heath et al., 1979) and in the regulation of affective behavior (Berman et al., 1974), as well as in the elaboration of the classical conditioned reflex response (McCormick and Thompson, 1984).

In the 1980s and early 1990s, a number of studies were published suggesting that the cerebellum might be involved in mental imagery and anticipatory planning (Leiner et al., 1987) as well as some aspects of language processing (Petersen et al., 1989). In a positron emission tomographic study, Petersen et al. (1998) examined skilled and unskilled motor and language performance, and noted that the right cerebellum was significantly more active on a naïve verb generation task, while the left cerebellum became active during an unskilled fine motor task, suggesting that the cerebellum is part of the scaffolding circuitry used to cope with novel task demands.

Interest in the mechanisms related to attention in ASD have resulted in a number of studies involving the role of the cerebellum in the control of attention, particularly the voluntary shift of attention between sensory modalities such as auditory and visual modalities (Courchesne et al. 1992; Akshoomoff and Courchesne, 1992). A recent paper by Hodge et al. (2010) reported on the results of structural MRI studies in children, 6–13 years old, with autism and language impairment, children with specific language impairment (SLI) without ASD, and typically developing controls. Abnormalities were found in the neurodevelopment of the fronto-cortico-cerebellar circuits which are important for motor control and the processing of language, cognition, working memory and attention in the autism and language impairment and SLI groups.

It has been suggested that the cerebellum may play a role in cognitive planning, a function that is independent of memory and that is most evident in novel situations (Grafman et al., 1982). Studies in the monkey have shown that the dorsolateral prefrontal cortex, a region believed to be involved in spatial working memory, is the target of output from the dentate nucleus of the cerebellum (Middleton and Strick, 1994). This relationship suggests that the cerebellum may be involved in the timing and planning of future behavior.

FUTURE DIRECTIONS

Although much progress has been made in our understanding of the neurobiology of the brain in ASD, and in particular the role of the cerebellum in this disorder, research has been impacted by the limited availability of quality post-mortem brain samples, small sample sizes, variable detailed symptomatic descriptions of patients during life, and the apparent heterogeneity of the disorder itself. Further, as it is believed by most experts in the field that ASD begins before birth, it is likely that many if not most of the research findings to date represent the result of a pathological cascade that has had its start very early in life. Despite these impediments, however, research is beginning to unlock some of the pieces of this complex puzzle. In the cerebellum, much attention has been paid to the Purkinje cells, overall cerebellar size and the vermis. Relatively little attention has be devoted to the deep cerebellar nuclei which have also been found to be abnormal and which appear to change in size and number with age. The significance of these observations is currently unknown but merits further investigation.

Space does not allow for a discussion of the growing number of studies elucidating the profiles of neurotransmitter and neuropeptide systems as well as receptor binding and synaptic integrity, all involved in cerebellar function and connectivity, nor the growing interest in the significance and role of inflammation and immune factors. Investigations such as these, combined with increasingly refined imaging technology, should provide a more detailed analysis of cerebellar function and circuitry in general and in disorders such as ASD in the future.

CONCLUSION

Research related to the understanding of the underlying neurobiology of ASD has advanced substantially over the past 25 years, yet many questions remain unanswered. It has become clear that ASD is a heterogeneous disorder clinically, etiologically and biologically, thus creating challenges to identifying meaningful commonalities among those affected that could explain underlying causative mechanisms. Studies of post-mortem brains have been confounded by limited detailed clinical data about each patient during life, often making clinico-pathological correlates difficult. It is hoped that with advances in technology, coupled with more refined genetic, neurochemical, immunological and neuroana-tomic profiling of ASD and its broader phenotype, a better understanding of the pathogenesis of the disorder may emerge, ultimately leading to earlier diag-nosis and effective interventions and treatments. There is growing evidence of the importance of the cerebellum in the modulation of emotion, behavior, learning and language. It is likely that the structural and neurochem-ical abnormalities of the cerebellum and regions related to it seen in the autistic brain contribute to at least some of the atypical behaviors and disordered information processing associated with the disorder. However, the precise functional significance of cerebellar abnormali-ties in the autistic brain, the clues that they may be able to provide regarding the etiology and timing of onset and their relationship to the clinical features of the disorder remain to be determined.

ACKNOWLEDGMENTS

We would like to acknowledge the support of the Nancy Lurie Marks Family Foundation, NINDS (NS38975-(05) and Autism Speaks for their support of our research and to thank the many families whose generous donations of postmortem brain tissue has made much of this research possible.

References

Akshoomoff, N.A., Courchesne, E., 1992. A new role for the cere-bellum in cognitive operations. Behavioral Neuroscience 106, 731–738.

Arin, D.M., Bauman, M.L., Kemper, T.L., 1991. The distribution of purkinje cell loss in the cerebellum in autism. Neurology 41, (Suppl.), 307.

Bauman, M.L., Kemper, T.L., 1985. Histoanatomic observations of the brain in early infantile autism. Neurology 35, 866–874.

Bauman, M.L., Kemper, T.L., 1994. Neuroanatomic observations of the brain in autism. In: Bauman, M.L., Kemper, T.L. (Eds.), The Neurobiology of Autism. Johns Hopkins University Press, Balti-more, pp. 119–145.

Bauman, M.L., Kemper, T.L., 1995. Neuroanatomical observations of the brain in autism. In: Panksepp, J. (Ed.), Advances in Biological Psychiatry. JAI Press, New York, pp. 1–26.

Bauman, M.L., Kemper, T.L., 1996. Observations on the purkinje cells in the cerebellar vermis in autism. Journal of Neuropathology and Experimental Neurology 55, 613.

Bauman, M.L., Kemper, T.L., 1997. Is autism a progressive process? Neurology 48 (Suppl.), 285.

Berman, A.J., Berman, D., Prescott, J.W., 1974. The effect of cerebellar lesions on emotional behavior in the rhesus monkey. In: Cooper, I.S., Riklan, M., Snyder, R.S. (Eds.), The Cerebellum, Epilepsy and Behavior. Plenum, New York, pp. 277–284.

Bloedel, J.R., 1992. Functional heterogeneity with structural homoge-neity: How does the cerebellum operate? The Behavioral and Brain Sciences 15, 666–678.

Campbell, M.S., Rosenbloom, S., Perry, R., George, A.E., Krichett, I.L., Anderson, L., et al., 1982. Computerized axial tomography in young autistic children. American Journal of Psychiatry 139, 510–512.

Ciesielski, K.T., Harris, R.J., Hart, B.L., Pabst, H.F., 1997. Cerebellar hypoplasia and frontal lobe cognitive deficits in disorders of early childhood. Neuropsychologia 35, 643–655.

Courchesne, E., Akshoomoff, N.A., Townsend, J., 1992. Recent advances in autism. In: Naruse, H., Ornitz, E.M. (Eds.), Neurobi-ology of Infantile Autism. Elsevier, Amsterdam, pp. 11–128.

Courchesne, E., Karns, C.M., Davids, H.R., et al., 2001. Unusual brain growth patterns in early life in patients with autistic disorder. Neurology 57, 245–254.

Courchesne, E., Saitoh, O., Yeung-Courchesne, R., Press, G.A., Lincoln, A.J., Haas, R.H., et al., 1994. Abnormalities of cerebellar lobules VI and VII in patients with infantile autism: Identification of hypoplasia and hyperplasia subgroups by MRI imaging. American Journal of Roentgenology 162, 123–130.

Courchesne, E., Yeung-Courchesne, R., Press, G.A., Hesselink, J.R., Jernigan, T.L., 1988. Hypoplasia of cerebellar lobules VI and VII in autism. New England Journal of Medicine 318, 1349–1354.

DeBassio, W.A., Kemper, T.L., Knoefel, J.E., 1985. Coffin-siris syndrome: neuropathological findings. Archives of Neurology 42, 350–353.

Fatemi, S.H., Halt, A.R., Realmuto, G., Earle, J., Kist, D.A., Thuras, P., et al., 2002. Purkinje cell size is reduced in cerebellum of patients with autism. Cellular and Molecular Neurobiology 22, 171–175.

Grafman, J., Litvan, I., Massaquoi, S., Stewart, M., Sivigu, A., Hallet, M., 1992. Cognitive planning in patients with cerebellar atrophy. Neurology 42, 1493–1496.

Greenfield, J.G., 1954. The spinocerebellar degenerations. Thomas, Springfield, IL.

Hardan, A.Y., Libove, R.A., Keshavan, M.S., Melhem, N.M., Minshew, N.J., 2009. A preliminary longitudinal magnetic reso-nance imaging study of brain volume and cortical thickness in autism. Biological Psychiatry 66, 313–315.

Hauser, S.I., Delong, G.R., Rosman, N.P., 1975. Pneumoencephalo-graphic findings in the infantile autism syndrome: a correlation with temporal lobe disease. Brain 98, 667–688.

Heath, R.G., Harper, J.W., 1974. Ascending projections of the cerebellar fastigial nucleus to the hippocampus, amygdala and other temporal lobe sites. evoked potential and other histologic studies in monkeys and cats. Experimental Neurology 45, 268–287.

Heath, R.G., Dempsey, C.W., Fontana, C.J., Myers, W.A., 1978. Cere-bellar stimulation: effects on septal region, hippocampus and amygdala of cats and rats. Biological Psychiatry 113, 501–529.

Heath, R.G., Franklin, D.E., Shraberg, D., 1979. Gross pathology of the cerebellum in patients diagnosed and treated as functional psychiatric disorders. The Journal of Nervous and Mental Disease 167, 585–592.

Hier, D.B., LeMay, M., Rosenberger, P.B., 1979. Autism and unfavor-able left-right asymmetries of the brain. Journal of Autism and Developmental Disorders 9, 153–159.

Hodge, S.M., Makris, N., Kennedy, D.N., Caviness, V.S., Howard, J., McGrath, L., et al., 2010. Cerebellum, language and cognition in autism and specific language impairment. Journal of Autism and Developmental Disorders 40, 300–316.

Holmes, G., Stewart, T.G., 1908. On the connection of the inferior olives with the cerebellum in man. Brain 31, 125–137.

Jacobson, R., Lecouteur, A., Howlin, P., Rutter, M., 1988. Selective subcortical abnormalities in autism. Psychological Medicine 18, 39–48.

Kanner, L., 1943. Autistic disturbance of affective contact. The Nervous Child 2, 217–250.

Lainhart, J.E., Piven, J., Wzorek, M., et al., 1997. Macrocephaly in children and adults with autism. Journal of the American Academy of Child & Adolescent Psychiatry 36, 282.

Leiner, H.C., Leiner, A.L., Dow, R.S., 1987. Cerebrocerebellar learning loops in apes and humans. Italian Journal of Neurological Sciences 8, 425–436.

McCormick, D.A., Thompson, R.F., 1984. Cerebellum: essential involvement in the classically conditioned eyelid response. Science 223, 296–299.

Middleton, F.A., Strick, P.I., 1994. Anatomical evidence for cerebellar and basal ganglia involvement in higher cognitive function. Science 266, 458–461.

Mostofsky, S.H., Powell, S.K., Simmonds, D.J., Goldberg, M.C., Caffo, B., Pekar, J.J., 2009. Decreased connectivity and cerebellar activity in autism during motor task performance. Brain 132, 2413–2425.

Norman, R.M., 1940. Cerebellar atrophy associated with état marbré of the basal ganglia. Journal of Neurology and Psychiatry 3, 311–318.

Petersen, S.E., Fos, P.T., Posner, M.I., Mintum, M.A., Raichle, M.E., 1989. Positron emission tomographic studies in the processing of single words. Journal of Cognitive Neuroscience I, 153–170.

Petersen, S.E., van Mier, H., Fiez, J.A., Raichle, M.E., 1998. The effects of practice on the functional anatomy of task performance. Proceedings of the National Academy of Sciences of the United States of America 95, 853–860.

Rakic, P., 1971. Neuron-glia relationship during granule cell migration in developing cerebellar cortex: A Golgi and electron microscopic study in macacus rhesus. Journal of Comparative Neurology 141, 282–312.

Rakic, P., Sidman, R.L., 1970. Histogenesis of the cortical layers in human cerebellum, particularly the lamina dissecans. Journal of Comparative Neurology 139, 473–500.

Ritvo, E.R., Freeman, B.J., Scheibel, A.B., Duong, T., Robinson, H., Guthrie, d., et al., 1986. Lower purkinje cell counts in the cerebella of four autistic subjects: Initial findings of the UCLA-NSAC autopsy research report. American Journal of Psychiatry 146, 862–866.

Rosenbloom, S., Campbell, M., George, A.E., 1984. High resolution CT scanning in infantile autism: a quantitative approach. Journal of the American Academy of Child & Adolescent Psychiatry 23, 72–77.

Schmahmann, J., 1997. The cerebellum and cognition. In: International Review of Neurobiology, vol. 41. Academic Press, San Diego.

Scott, J.A., Schumann, C.M., Goodwin-Jones, B.L., Amaral, D.G., 2009. A comprehensive volumetric analysis of the cerebellum in children and adolescents with autism spectrum disorders. Autism Research 2, 246–257.

Sivaswamy, L., Kumar, A., Rajan, D., Behen, M., Muzik, O., Chugani, D., et al., 2010. A diffusion tensor imaging study of the cerebellar pathways in children with autism spectrum disorder. Journal of Child Neurology 10, 1223–1231.

Sumi, S.M., 1980. Brain malformation in the trisomy 18 syndrome. Brain 93, 821–830.

Takarae, Y., Minshew, N.J., Luna, B., Sweeney, J.A., 2007. Atypical involvement of frontostriatal systems during sensorimotor control in autism. Psychiatry Research 156, 117–127.

Whitney, E.R., Kemper, T.L., Rosene, D.L., Bauman, M.L., Blatt, G.J., 2008. Cerebellar purkinje cells are reduced in a subpopulation of autistic brains: a stereological experiment using calbindin-D28k. Cerebellum 7, 406–416.

Whitney, E.R., Kemper, T.L., Rosene, D.L., Bauman, M.L., Blatt, G.J., 2009. Density of cerebellar basket and stellate cells in autism: evidence for a late developmental loss of purkinje cells. Journal of Neuroscience Research 87, 2245–2254.

3.5

The Amygdala in Autism Spectrum Disorders

John T. Morgan, Christine Wu Nordahl, Cynthia M. Schumann

MIND Institute, Department of Psychiatry and Behavioral Sciences, UC Davis, CA, USA

OUTLINE

INTRODUCTION

The amygdala is a medial temporal lobe structure that occupies barely 0.3% of the volume of the human brain (~ 2 cm^3) (Figure 3.5.1). Despite its size, it has been associated with more neurodevelopmental and psychiatric disorders than perhaps any other brain region. This may be because the amygdala is an integral part of a system that is focused on detecting and responding to danger in the environment. It does this by processing cortical sensory input, linking that sensory information with prior knowledge, and orchestrating a subsequent response. If this system becomes dysfunctional, it may give rise to inappropriate social behavior or anxiety, symptoms that are commonly observed in autism spectrum disorders (ASD).

Although the primary function of the amygdala is to monitor the environment for danger, this basic function is at the heart of our social cognition. For example, to determine if another person is going to bring us harm, or if they are indicating danger somewhere in the environment, we look to their eyes for information on emotional state or the direction of their eye gaze. We maintain a balanced state of vigilance in scanning the environment in order to produce an appropriate response in each situation. However, if this system is hypoactive, we may not detect pertinent social cues, and therefore not evoke the appropriate social response. Alternatively, with a hyperactive system, excessive anxiety may arise during normally non-threatening social situations, leading us to avoid interaction.

The Neuroscience of Autism Spectrum Disorders.
http://dx.doi.org/10.1016/B978-0-12-391924-3.00021-1

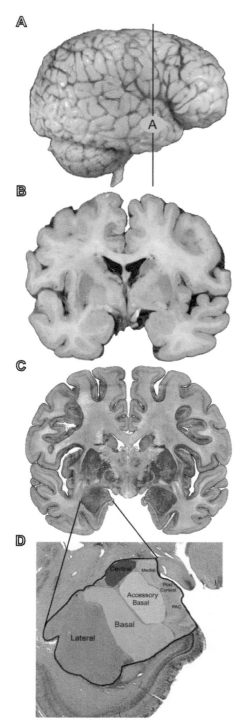

FIGURE 3.5.1   (A) Lateral view of human brain displaying location of amygdala (A, blue circle) within the medial temporal lobe. Vertical line indicates location of the coronal section in panel B. (B) Coronal section at mid-rostrocaudal level of the amygdala. (C) Coronal section at mid-rostrocaudal level of the amygdala stained by Nissl method. Whole amygdala is outlined in red. (D) Coronal Nissl section of mid-rostrocaudal amygdala with major nuclei outlined and colored: lateral, basal, accessory basal, central, and remaining nuclei: medial, posterior cortical, periamygdaloid complex. A = amygdala, PAC = periamygdaloid complex.

Leo Kanner (1943) first described the symptoms of ASD in a group of children who demonstrated atypical social, communicative, and repetitive behaviors. Interestingly, an excerpt from his original description is reminiscent of behaviors we now consider to be modulated by the amygdala.

> Everything that is brought to the child from the outside, everything that changes his external or even internal environment, **represents a dreaded intrusion**…
>
> Behavior is governed by an **anxiously** obsessive desire for the maintenance of sameness….
>
> Their faces give the impression of serious-mindedness and, in the presence of others, an **anxious tenseness**, probably because of the uneasy anticipation of possible interference. When alone with objects, there is often a placid smile… sometimes accompanied by happy though monotonous humming and singing.
> **Leo Kanner (1943)** *Autistic Disturbances of Affective Contact*

In fact, there is more evidence that the amygdala is pathological, both structurally and functionally, in ASD than any other brain region. In this chapter, we will review this evidence. To evaluate how the amygdala could become pathological in ASD, we will first begin with a brief overview of its typical structural and functional development. In Box 3.5.1, we consider the similarities and differences between the behavioral impairments of people with amygdala lesions and those with ASD. We then review functional magnetic resonance imaging (fMRI) research on amygdala activity in ASD. This field provides some evidence for aberrant amygdala function in ASD, particularly during face processing, although more work is needed to isolate the precise nature of these abnormalities. Structural MRI studies provide the strongest evidence for abnormal amygdala development in ASD at present. We discuss findings that reveal that the amygdala may be undergoing an abnormal developmental trajectory which includes early enlargement. However, emerging evidence from MRI studies also reveals that there is considerable heterogeneity in ASD, and subgroups or sub-phenotypes will likely emerge as larger populations are evaluated longitudinally across age groups. Lastly, we review evidence from postmortem brain tissue studies that seek to explain at the cellular and molecular level why the amygdala may be structurally and functionally abnormal in ASD. There are, unfortunately, only a few findings in this area as researchers work to find adequate high-quality brain tissue to study. However, initial studies indicate that there may be fundamental alterations in some major cell populations in the amygdala. We conclude with a summary of current knowledge about the amygdala in ASD and the future of brain research on this structure. It will be critical to develop a comprehensive interdisciplinary program of research on amygdala abnormalities in order to understand the causes of ASD and develop appropriate, targeted therapies.

BOX 3.5.1

ASD VERSUS AMYGDALA LESIONS

People with amygdala lesions do not have ASD (Paul et al., 2010). However, both people with ASD and those with amygdala lesions display similar impairments in social behavior (see Adolphs, 2010 for review). These include directing visual attention to emotionally salient stimuli, eye gaze, interpreting others' emotions, and theory of mind. Beyond these obvious similarities in their impairments, there remain several critical differences between the groups (Birmingham et al., 2011; Paul et al., 2010). The study of their similarities and differences has the potential to provide essential clues to the role of the amygdala in ASD. These studies may help to pinpoint where the impairments in ASD are occurring: in the amygdala itself, or upstream or downstream in another component of the social brain network.

The most well known patient with a bilateral amygdala lesion is SM; Ralph Adolphs and his colleagues have extensively reported on her abilities and impairments. SM spends less time looking at the eye region of the face than typical individuals do. Thus, she has less opportunity to gather information on a person's emotional state. When she does fixate on the eyes, she has difficulty making full use of that information. These impairments are also observed in people who have ASD. Typical individuals scan the face in a classic triangle pattern, between the eyes and mouth, and spend more time looking at the eyes. As shown in the adjacent figure, SM and people with ASD often look at the mouth or nose, or skip the face all together (Adolphs et al., 2005; Klin et al., 2002; Pelphrey et al., 2002). Both groups also show similar impairments in judging the trustworthiness and approachability of another person in social situations (Adolphs, 2001; Adolphs et al., 1998).

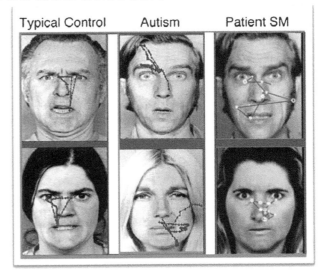

However, the reason these impairments occur may differ between the groups. We cannot automatically assume that dysfunction is attributed solely to the amygdala. Birmingham, Cerf, and Adolphs recently reported that both SM and subjects with ASD spend less time looking at the face, and in particular the eyes, while viewing complex social scenes that contain faces (Birmingham et al., 2011). However, SM was able to increase her gaze to the eyes when the scene required more social attention, while people with ASD did not. Adolphs and colleagues suggest that the amygdala is critical for specifying the relative importance of social features for allocating attention. Based on their findings, they believe that the amygdala is abnormal in ASD, but that the abnormalities in social attention itself lie in upstream regions, such as the prefrontal cortex.

THE TYPICALLY DEVELOPING AMYGDALA

Before examining the ways in which the amygdala is abnormal in ASD, it is helpful to have an understanding of the organization and function of the amygdala in typical development. The cellular structure of the amygdala appears to be well established at the time of birth. Early in prenatal development, the amygdala is derived from the ganglionic eminence (Kordower et al., 1992; O'Rahilly and Muller, 2006). The cells that are to become amygdala neurons migrate along radial glia around the fifth month of gestation (Ulfig et al., 1998). The amygdala consists of 13 well-defined nuclei (Amaral et al., 1992; Freese and Amaral, 2009). The more superficial nuclei of the amygdala, such as the medial and central nuclei, become identifiable and begin to undergo synaptogenesis during the fifth month of gestation. However, the deeper nuclei, such as the lateral and basal nuclei, do not show evidence of synaptogenesis until around the seventh month (Humphrey, 1968; Ulfig et al., 2003). Neuronal migration forming the amygdala is essentially complete by the end of the eighth month of gestation (Setzer and Ulfig, 1999; Ulfig et al., 1998; 2003).

At birth, the cytoarchitecture of the primate amygdala already closely resembles that seen in the adult. Neurotransmitter systems, such as serotonin and opiate receptors, show a distribution similar to that seen in adults (Bauman and Amaral, 2005). The pathways of amygdalo-cortical connectivity are also relatively well developed, although processes such as myelination continue through early childhood (Emery and Amaral, 2000). Despite the rapid development of the basic cellular organization of the amygdala, structural MRI studies indicate that the human amygdala continues to undergo substantial growth throughout childhood and well into adolescence. The dramatic increases in amygdala volume observed over this time period are in striking contrast to what is seen throughout much of the rest of the neocortex, which actually contracts in size during this period. Several independent cross-sectional MRI studies have found that the amygdala increases in size by ~ 40% from 5 years of age to adulthood in typically developing males (Giedd, 1997; Giedd et al., 1996; Ostby et al., 2009; Schumann et al., 2004). There appear to be sex differences in this remarkable growth trajectory, with female children and adolescents showing somewhat earlier enlargement than males (Giedd, 1997; Giedd et al., 1996). The underlying neurobiology that produces the extended developmental trajectory of amygdala growth is currently under investigation.

The mature amygdala maintains a dense network of connections with many other regions of the brain, particularly the 'social brain' (Figure 3.5.2). Information typically enters the amygdala via the lateral, and to some extent basal, nuclei from both higher-order sensory and association cortices. Prominent among these regions are 'social brain' components such as the fusiform face area, superior temporal gyrus, medial prefrontal cortex, anterior cingulate cortex, and orbitofrontal cortex (reviews: Amaral et al., 2008; Adolphs, 2009; Freese and Amaral, 2009). The fusiform face area is predominantly implicated in the recognition of faces. The superior temporal gyrus is critical for language perception and comprehension, and also plays a role in face processing. The anterior cingulate cortex appears to be responsible for detecting and correcting errors, including social errors. The medial prefrontal cortex and orbitofrontal cortex are involved in emotion regulation and calculation of reward.

From the lateral and basal nucleus, information is either returned via reciprocal connections to cortical regions, or flows medially to the central and medial nuclei for output to subcortical and brainstem regions. Via these regions, the amygdala modulates the autonomic nervous system, which is involved in preparing the body for what is sometimes referred to as the 'fight or flight' response. As might be expected given this role, the amygdala is closely linked to anxiety disorders. In the next section, we discuss the roles of the amygdala in both social behaviors and anxiety in more detail.

TYPICAL FUNCTION OF THE AMYGDALA

Deciding whether to run from a bear, or even trust a person we meet for the first time, is critical to our survival. The optimal reaction may be very simple, such as 'run as fast as you can.' In other interactions, we may need to draw from previous knowledge to determine the best course of action. Researchers such as Joseph LeDoux have proposed that there may be two pathways for making such evaluations (Phelps and LeDoux, 2005). The first is rapid, proceeding from the visual pathway to coordinate other brain regions to take appropriate action. The second pathway is slower; cortical regions are recruited to provide additional input to the amygdala which then orchestrates other brain regions to carry out a suitable response (Adolphs, 2010). Information is also fed back through the amygdala, in concert with memory regions such as the hippocampal formation, to add an emotional tag to the event as it is sent to long-term storage. There is extensive evidence from the rodent literature that the amygdala is responsible for learned or conditioned fear (LeDoux, 2007). If an event has strong negative emotional content, the amygdala can contribute to anxiety over that memory and, under certain circumstances, even post-traumatic stress disorder (PTSD) (Roozendaal et al., 2009).

The amygdala is a complex structure that interacts with systems that mediate functions ranging from

FIGURE 3.5.2 Anatomical locations of several major components of the 'social brain'. Arrows indicate major inputs to and outputs from the amygdala. A) A three-dimensional view of the lateral surface view of the brain, showing the amygdala's connections with fusiform face area, orbitofrontal cortex, and superior temporal sulcus. B) A three-dimensional view of the medial surface of the left hemisphere. This view shows the amygdala's connections with anterior cingulate cortex and medial prefrontal cortex. Abbreviations: ACC: anterior cingulate cortex, AMY: amygdala, FFA: fusiform face area, MPFC: medial prefrontal cortex, OFC: orbitofrontal cortex, STS: superior temporal sulcus.

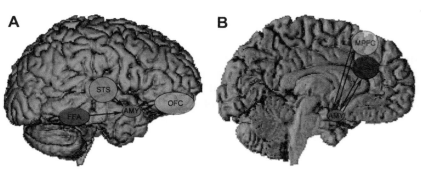

olfaction in rodents to judging trustworthiness in humans (Adolphs, 2010; Kennedy et al., 2009). Evidence from functional imaging studies, alongside studies of people with amygdala lesions, has led Ralph Adolphs to propose the concept of a 'social brain' network, in which the amygdala modulates cortical and subcortical regions during evaluation of the biological significance of affective visual stimuli (reviews: Adolphs, 2009; 2010). The amygdala is not solely responsible for social behavior, but is part of an intricate circuit of structures that each contributes to the process of social cognition and interaction. Patients with amygdala lesions, such as SM, display impairments in identifying the emotion of facial expressions, particularly those depicting fear (Adolphs et al., 1994). Amygdala lesion patients also show deficits in theory of mind, that is, understanding the emotional states of others and attributing beliefs to them (Shaw et al., 2004). Several more subtle impairments have been recently described, such as difficulty in identifying personal space (Kennedy et al., 2009).

One would expect that the amygdala is called upon extensively early in social development, as young children must learn to identify potential dangers by monitoring the responses of their caregivers. As in adults, children and adolescents recruit the amygdala to interpret the emotion in facial expressions, albeit with a different pattern of activity (Baird et al., 1999; Killgore et al., 2001; Thomas et al., 2001). Interestingly, Thomas and colleagues (2001) found that in children, the amygdala is more active in response to neutral facial expressions than to those depicting fear. This suggests that the amygdala plays a dynamic role in learning to interpret emotions when the stimuli may be ambiguous in early development. However, the question of whether this role is diminished later in development once those associations have been formed is still under investigation (Hamann and Adolphs, 1999; Shaw et al., 2004).

As discussed elsewhere in this book (see Chapter 4.2), primate lesion studies have been used to investigate the role of the amygdala in social behavior at various time periods in development. A series of studies from Bauman et al. (Amaral et al., 2003; Bauman et al., 2004a, b) indicate that the amygdala is not essential for the early development of the fundamental components of social cognition. However, it may have a significant modulatory role on social behavior, especially in potentially threatening situations. Amygdala-lesioned primates demonstrate abnormal fear responses to both social and nonsocial stimuli (both heightened fear of conspecifics and absence of fear to normally aversive objects) (Bauman et al., 2004b; Prather et al., 2001). The ability to rapidly and accurately evaluate social signals for signs of impending danger is an essential social skill that must be acquired early in development. If this ability is dependent upon a properly functioning amygdala, then it is reasonable to speculate that amygdala pathology may have a profound influence on aspects of social behavior.

Recent studies have begun to explore the comparability of patients with amygdala lesions, such as SM, to individuals with ASD. Clearly patients with amygdala lesions do not have ASD (Birmingham et al., 2011), and hence the amygdala is not solely responsible for the core impairments of ASD. In Box 3.5.1, we suggest that a comparison between the two populations can provide clues as to how the amygdala may be functioning pathologically in ASD. In the following section we discuss the functional abnormalities that have been observed in the amygdala in ASD.

AMYGDALA FUNCTIONAL ABNORMALITIES IN AUTISM SPECTRUM DISORDERS

Abnormalities in amygdala function have long been suspected in ASD due to the region's involvement in social and emotional processes. The first fMRI study to investigate this possibility examined how the amygdala in people with ASD responded while viewing the eye region of the face (Baron-Cohen et al., 1999). Subjects with ASD were asked to identify what a person might be thinking or feeling, based solely on a rectangle containing emotionally expressive eyes. The amygdala was hypoactive in individuals with ASD relative to typically developing controls during this task. Amygdala hypoactivity in ASD subjects has since been reported during an array of social tasks, including basic facial processing, discrimination of emotions, and attribution of intent (Corbett et al., 2009; Grelotti et al., 2005; Hadjikhani et al., 2007; Kleinhans et al., 2011; Malisza et al., 2011; Pelphrey et al., 2007; Piggot et al., 2004; Pinkham et al., 2008; Wang et al., 2006).

However, there is some evidence that this hypoactivation may reflect the fact that individuals with ASD do not look at the eyes the same way as typical individuals do (Figure 3.5.3) (Klin et al., 2002; Pelphrey et al., 2002; Spezio et al., 2007). Instead, they are likely to spend more time looking at the mouth or other areas of the face. In addition, amygdala activation levels in ASD are strongly correlated with the amount of time spent looking at the eye region (Figure 3.5.3) (Dalton et al., 2005; 2007). Therefore, when eye gaze is controlled for, amygdala activation can be normal or even hyperactive, although this is not always the case (Dalton et al., 2005; Monk et al., 2010; Perlman et al., 2011; Weng et al., 2011). Interestingly, individuals with ASD who show the least fixation on the eyes also have a smaller amygdala, are the most socially impaired in childhood, and are

FIGURE 3.5.3   Abnormalities of facial scanning in autism and fMRI images of amygdala activation. (A) A path of facial scanning in a typically developing individual. The majority of the time is spent moving back and forth between the eyes. (B) A path of facial scanning in an individual with autism. Several other regions of the face, such as the mouth, are examined instead of the eyes. (C) fMRI activation of the left amygdala in coronal (top) and sagittal (bottom) planes of section. (D) fMRI activation of the right amygdala in coronal (top) and sagittal (bottom) planes of section. *Source: (A and B) from Pelphrey et al. (2002); (C and D) from Dalton et al. (2005).*

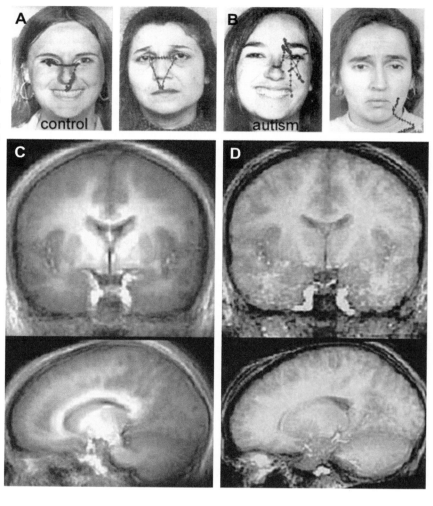

slower to distinguish emotional from neutral expressions (Figure 3.5.3) (Nacewicz et al., 2006).

There are a few theories to explain why people with ASD do not look at the eye region of the face as often as typically developing individuals do. One is a lack of attention to, or motivation for, the presented task. Subjects with ASD show amygdala activation equivalent to controls while viewing faces they are motivated to look at, such as their mother's face (Pierce et al., 2001; 2004). However, when viewing unfamiliar adult women, a lower motivation condition, they show a deficit in activation. Another possible explanation for abnormal eye gaze in ASD is anxiety, which is often increased in patients with ASD and strongly linked to amygdala dysfunction (Davis, 1992; Gillott et al., 2001; Kim and Whalen, 2009; White et al., 2009). Greater self-reported social anxiety is correlated with increased right amygdala activation in ASD (Kleinhans et al., 2010). Subjects with ASD also display amygdala hyperactivation when anticipating the presentation of a face (Dichter

et al., 2012). This excess activation is correlated with the severity of social symptoms.

Regardless of the cause, it is clear that facial scanning is abnormal in ASD, and that it affects the measured levels of amygdala activation. However, differences in facial scanning do not fully account for abnormalities in amygdala activation. When subjects are presented with fearful physical gestures, a task that does not involve any facial information, hypoactivity is still observed (Grezes et al., 2009). The difficulty of the presented task may also be a factor (Hadjikhani et al., 2004; Wang et al., 2004). Another is the length of the stimulus presentation. When subjects with ASD are presented with faces for a long period of time, their amygdala shows a slower habituation, or return to the original activity level, than in controls (Kleinhans et al., 2009). Therefore, studies with longer stimulus presentation times may be examining differences in the habituation of the amygdala to a stimulus rather than its peak activity in response to the initial stimulus presentation.

The amygdala's functional connections to other components of the 'social brain' are also a topic of investigation. The primary method used is functional connectivity MRI, which measures the correlations in activity levels between brain regions during a task. The amygdala appears to have reduced connectivity to neighboring brain regions such as temporal lobe, fusiform face area, and secondary visual areas (Kleinhans et al., 2008; Monk et al., 2010). At the same time, it may be overconnected to more distant, higher-order cognitive areas such as ventromedial prefrontal cortex and dorsolateral prefrontal cortex (Monk et al., 2010; Rudie et al., 2011). In addition to affecting brain function in the moment, these alterations may have long-term effects. Amygdala damage causes significant changes over time in the morphology of many cortical regions to which it is connected (Boes et al., 2011). This suggests that alterations may take place across the cortex in ASD due to changes in connectivity with the amygdala, or vice versa.

In summary, the amygdala demonstrates substantial functional abnormalities in response to many different social stimuli in ASD. However, the precise nature of these differences is currently a matter of debate. Several potential confounds have been identified that may help explain some of the discrepant findings in this field. It will be critical for future studies of this region to carefully examine and control for these experimental variables. As discussed in the next section, it will also be important in future study design to take account of the growing knowledge regarding the heterogeneity and age-related structural changes the amygdala undergoes in different phenotypes of ASD.

STRUCTURAL ABNORMALITIES IN THE AMYGDALA IN AUTISM SPECTRUM DISORDERS

Over the past two decades, structural MRI studies have provided the most consistent evidence that the amygdala is developmentally abnormal in ASD. Collectively, these cross-sectional studies suggest that the amygdala follows an abnormal course of development, with precocious growth early in childhood. The most consistent findings in amygdala development are in studies of very young children. Thus far, all published studies of amygdala volume in young children ranging from 2 to 5 years of age with ASD report abnormal enlargement relative to typically developing controls (Mosconi et al., 2009; Nordahl et al., 2012; Schumann et al., 2009; Sparks et al., 2002). This enlargement appears to persist into middle childhood (Schumann et al., 2004). However, studies of adolescents and adults with ASD are more inconsistent. Whereas some studies report amygdala enlargement (Groen et al., 2010; Howard et al., 2000), others find no difference at all (Haznedar et al., 2000; Palmen et al., 2005; Schumann et al., 2004), and still others find smaller amygdala volumes (Aylward et al., 1999; Nacewicz et al., 2006; Pierce et al., 2001). Some of these inconsistencies are likely due to factors such as sample characterization, age range, and method for delineating amygdala volume (manual vs. automated segmentation). As shown in Figure 3.5.4, these studies collectively suggest an abnormal trajectory of amygdala development that includes increased amygdala volume in childhood,

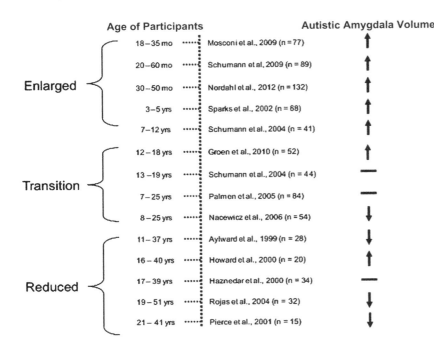

FIGURE 3.5.4 Summary of structural MRI studies that have evaluated amygdala volume in individuals with autism relative to typically developing controls. Collectively, these studies show that volumetric differences depend heavily on the age range being studied. Abnormal enlargement is present during early childhood, but sometime during adolescence, volumetric differences normalize and some studies even report decreased amygdala volume in adulthood.

followed by either no difference or smaller amygdala volume in adulthood. However, the amygdala is continuing to grow in typically developing males through adolescence (Giedd, 1997; Giedd et al., 1996; Ostby et al., 2009; Schumann et al., 2004), and therefore understanding the typical growth trajectory is equally important in determining how and when amygdala growth in children with ASD deviates from that of typical development.

While cross-sectional studies of amygdala volume have been informative, the field still lacks longitudinal studies of amygdala growth. There have only been two published longitudinal studies of amygdala development, and both focus on young children (Mosconi et al., 2009; Nordahl et al., 2012). Most recently, we evaluated amygdala volume over a one-year interval in 3–4-year-old children with ASD (Figure 3.5.5) (Nordahl et al., 2012). We found that the amygdala was already enlarged by age 3, but the rate of amygdala growth was still increasing. Interestingly, we also found a considerable amount of heterogeneity within the growth rates of the amygdalae in children with ASD. Although the group average across the entire ASD sample revealed an increased rate of growth, when we examined individual differences, a more nuanced picture emerged (Figure 3.5.5). While 40% of children with ASD demonstrated rapid amygdala growth of over 18% increase in one year (ASD-Amygdala Rapid), another 40% demonstrated normal amygdala growth, similar in rate to their typically developing peers (ASD-Typical). Yet another 20% actually displayed slower than normal amygdala growth over this time frame, but slightly accelerated total brain growth (ASD-Amygdala Slow). These findings suggest that there are likely multiple trajectories of abnormal amygdala growth within the autism spectrum. The findings are promising, in that identification of different neural phenotypes in children with ASD may eventually be used to guide the selection of treatments for the disorder.

Many questions remain regarding the trajectory of amygdala growth from early childhood through adulthood. For example, when does enlargement of the amygdala begin? How long does precocious growth last? What is the maximal magnitude of abnormal amygdala enlargement and when during development does it peak? And importantly, how heterogeneous is amygdala pathology in ASD, and are there clinical features that correlate with different trajectories of amygdala development? Additional longitudinal studies that span a wider period of development will be critical for answering these questions.

The behavioral and clinical correlates of amygdala enlargement in ASD remain unclear. An association between amygdala enlargement and anxiety has been reported (Juranek et al., 2006). Although anxiety is not a core feature of ASD, it is a common comorbidity, and amygdala enlargement has been associated with anxiety disorders (for review see Shin et al., 2009). Additional studies evaluating associations between amygdala volume and anxiety in ASD are needed. Regarding the core features of ASD, two studies have reported correlations between amygdala volume and social and communications scores on the ADI-R in young children (Munson et al., 2006; Schumann et al., 2009). Munson et al. found that enlarged right amygdala volume at age 3–4 years was predictive of poorer social and communication abilities at age 6. However, in a study of 10–24 year olds, Nacewicz et al. report a negative correlation between amygdala volume and Autism Diagnostic Interview-Revised (ADI-R) social and communication scores in 10–24 year olds with ASD (Nacewicz et al., 2006). They also report that smaller amygdala volume is related to decreased eye fixation and deficits in processing facial emotions. Similarly, Mosconi et al. (2009) evaluated amygdala volume and joint attention in 2–5 year olds with ASD and report that smaller amygdala volumes are related to deficits in joint attention ability. These seemingly inconsistent results have been attributed to an altered developmental trajectory of the amygdala and a potential 'allostatic load' (Matys et al., 2004; Mosconi et al., 2009; Nacewicz et al., 2006; Schumann and Amaral, 2009), wherein early pathological enlargement of the amygdala gives way to eventual atrophy due to hyperactivity of the amygdala early on. Brain tissue studies that report reduced neuron numbers in adults with ASD (Schumann and Amaral, 2006) provide some support for this hypothesis. However, as discussed in the next section, another possibility is that reduced cell numbers in the amygdala may be present all along, and early amygdala overgrowth is due to some other factor besides the number of neurons, such as glial cell number or the extent of neuronal dendritic arborization (Schumann and Amaral, 2009).

Beyond volumetric abnormalities, MRI studies have also shed light on potential biochemical changes within the amygdala in ASD. There is some evidence from MR spectroscopy studies for reduced levels of N-acetyl-aspartate, a marker of neuronal integrity, in the area of the amygdala (Endo et al., 2007; Gabis et al., 2008; Otsuka et al., 1999; Page et al., 2006). However, there is some inconsistency in the findings, likely due to differences in sample characteristics, but also in large part to methodological differences (Kleinhans et al., 2009). In particular, the region of interest defined for spectroscopy studies often includes at least part of the hippocampus. Thus, the specificity of biochemical changes to the amygdala cannot be established with certainty. In a recent study, Nacewicz et al. (2012) identify possible methodological problems related to

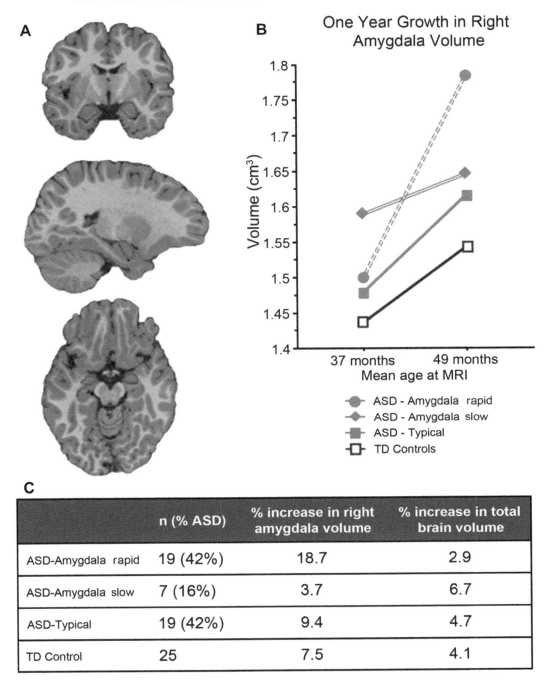

	n (% ASD)	% increase in right amygdala volume	% increase in total brain volume
ASD-Amygdala rapid	19 (42%)	18.7	2.9
ASD-Amygdala slow	7 (16%)	3.7	6.7
ASD-Typical	19 (42%)	9.4	4.7
TD Control	25	7.5	4.1

FIGURE 3.5.5 (A) Example of manual delineation of the amygdala. (B) Averaged amygdala volumes at 37 months and 49 months of age. Several ASD subgroups were apparent. Amygdala volume increased the most dramatically in the ASD-Amygdala Rapid subgroup, while the ASD-Amygdala Slow group exhibited a slower amygdala growth rate. The ASD-Typical group showed a growth rate similar to typically developing (TD) controls. (C) Raw data on percentage increases for amygdala and total brain volume in the amygdala subgroups relative to typically developing controls.

spectroscopy, including age-related variability due to auditory canal and mastoid development and anatomical localization of the amygdala. The authors suggest a protocol to carefully restrict measurement to the amygdala that could help future studies utilizing this methodology to better understand biochemical alterations in the amygdala.

Diffusion tensor imaging (DTI) is an imaging technique that is used to evaluate microstructural differences in white matter. Fractional anisotropy (FA) is a common measurement used in DTI studies and ranges from 0, isotropic movement of water molecules (e.g., cerebrospinal fluid), to 1, anisotropic movement of water molecules (e.g., fiber bundles). Abnormalities in FA have been reported in the amygdala in several small studies using whole-brain analyses (Barnea-Goraly et al., 2004; Jou et al., 2011; Noriuchi et al., 2010). However, much remains to be explored, and probabilistic tractography holds promise in being able to evaluate structural connectivity of the amygdala with other brain regions implicated in ASD, such as orbitofrontal cortex and fusiform gyrus.

The regional specificity of abnormalities within the amygdala is just beginning to be evaluated using structural MRI. As mentioned above, the amygdala is a collection of nuclei, and there is evidence from postmortem studies that suggests that the lateral nucleus may be differentially affected (Schumann and Amaral, 2006). Subregions within the amygdala are not readily discernable on a standard T1-weighted MRI. However, methodologies are emerging that may be used to differentiate subregions of the amygdala. Kim and Whalen (2009) utilized a novel surface-based analysis of the amygdala to look for regional shape differences, reporting that the laterobasal subregion of the amygdala is selectively enlarged in 6 year olds with ASD. Another proposed method for evaluating subregions of the amygdala is to use diffusion-weighted tractography to segment the amygdala into four major nuclei groups (lateral, basal and accessory basal, medial and cortical, and central) based on projection zone (Saygin et al., 2011). Although this method has not yet been applied to ASD, it does hold promise for determining which subregions of the amygdala are most affected.

Another future direction of research should be understanding sex differences in amygdala pathology in ASD. In typical development, the amygdala matures at different rates in females and males (Giedd et al., 1996). However, sexual dimorphism of the amygdala has not been evaluated in ASD. Unfortunately, because ASD occurs at a rate of 4:1 in males to females, most structural imaging studies utilize samples that are heavily weighted towards males. Often, this means that the sample sizes of females with ASD are not large enough to analyze independently. Schumann et al. (2009), with a sample size of nine females with ASD, report that amygdala enlargement is more robust in females than males. This finding is intriguing, but needs to be explored with much larger sample sizes longitudinally in females with ASD.

In summary, structural MRI studies have provided strong evidence that the amygdala follows an abnormal course of development in ASD. The amygdala is already abnormally enlarged by age 2–3 years, and continues this accelerated development into early childhood. Amygdala enlargement in ASD persists into middle childhood, but the amygdala appears have a normal or even reduced volume in adolescence and adulthood. One possible model is that the amygdala grows too large too early in children with ASD, but then its growth levels off during adolescence. In contrast, in typical development, the amygdala continues to grow through late childhood into adolescence, eventually catching up to or even surpassing the volume of the amygdala in ASD. Beyond adolescence, there is some evidence that the amygdala may be smaller in adults with ASD. Whether this reflects continued amygdala growth in typical adolescents, or an actual degenerative reduction in the amygdala of autistic adolescents and adults, is a current topic of investigation. Longitudinal studies that span early childhood through adulthood are needed. While structural MRI studies provide a macroscopic view of the amygdala in ASD, postmortem studies are the key to understanding the underlying cellular basis of abnormal amygdala volumes. In the next section, we review what is known from the postmortem work that has been carried out thus far on the amygdala in ASD.

CELLULAR ABNORMALITIES IN THE AMYGDALA IN AUTISM SPECTRUM DISORDERS

Unusual cellular profiles were reported in the amygdala of postmortem ASD cases in some of the earliest neuropathological studies of the disorder (Bauman and Kemper, 1985; 1994). The first report investigated a 29-year-old male with ASD, seizure disorder, and mental retardation, compared to an age-matched typical control (Bauman and Kemper, 1985). Examining the cellular features of the two cases side by side, the authors observed increased cell-packing density in the cortical, medial, and central nuclei of the amygdala, and reduced neuron size in the subject with ASD. Few abnormalities were noted in the other nuclei, including lateral and basal nuclei.

A larger follow-up study was conducted in five additional cases with ASD, four males and one female of 9–28 years of age (Kemper and Bauman, 1993). This study suggested that cellular density increases were present in several amygdala nuclei in most cases, particularly the cortical, medial, and central nuclei (Kemper and Bauman, 1993). The lateral nucleus appeared unaffected, and the basal nucleus was moderately affected. A reduction in neuron size was also reported, a possible indication of immature morphology (Kemper and Bauman, 1993). However, three of the five cases examined in this study also had a seizure disorder. Studies of

and emotional stimuli, especially during face processing. Future work in this field must be directed towards understanding the impact of several experimental variables on the observed level of activation. Structural imaging studies have identified an abnormal growth trajectory in the amygdala in ASD that includes early overgrowth. However, recent work suggests that there is significant heterogeneity in this abnormality, as well as in other structural features. There is also the possibility of abnormal amygdala connectivity to other brain regions. These findings must be further extended to produce a comprehensive developmental profile of structural abnormalities in the amygdala in ASD. Underlying these macrostructural changes are what appear to be substantial alterations in the cellular composition of the amygdala, including a lower neuron number and the presence of microglial abnormalities in adolescent and adult cases. However, whether these alterations arise during development, or are instead a product of extended aberrant functioning, is a critical question. To arrive at a complete understanding of amygdala dysfunction in ASD, it will be necessary to integrate functional, structural, and cellular approaches, careful examination of clinical phenotypes, and genetic and gene expression techniques. As the amygdala becomes better understood, it has the potential to point the way towards novel behavioral and medical therapies for several features of the disorder. This may include not only frequent comorbid symptoms such as anxiety, but also core social impairments.

References

Adolphs, R., 2001. The neurobiology of social cognition. Current Opinion in Neurobiology 11, 231–239.

Adolphs, R., 2009. The social brain: Neural basis of social knowledge. Annual Review of Psychology 60, 693–716.

Adolphs, R., 2010. What does the amygdala contribute to social cognition? Annals of the New York Academy of Sciences 1191, 42–61.

Adolphs, R., Gosselin, F., Buchanan, T.W., Tranel, D., Schyns, P., Damasio, A.R., 2005. A mechanism for impaired fear recognition after amygdala damage. Nature 433, 68–72.

Adolphs, R., Tranel, D., Damasio, A.R., 1998. The human amygdala in social judgment. Nature 393, 470–474.

Adolphs, R., Tranel, D., Damasio, H., Damasio, A., 1994. Impaired recognition of emotion in facial expressions following bilateral damage to the human amygdala. Nature 372, 669–672.

Amaral, D.G., Bauman, M.D., Capitanio, J.P., Lavenex, P., Mason, W.A., Mauldin-Jourdain, M.L., et al., 2003. The amygdala: Is it an essential component of the neural network for social cognition? Neuropsychologia 41, 517–522.

Amaral, D.G., Price, J.L., Pitkanen, A., Carmichael, S.T., 1992. Anatomical organization of the primate amygdaloid complex. In: The Amygdala: Neurobiological Aspects of Emotion, Memory and Mental Dysfunction. John Wiley and Sons, Hoboken, NJ, pp. 1–66.

Amaral, D.G., Schumann, C.M., Nordahl, C.W., 2008. Neuroanatomy of autism. Trends in Neurosciences 31, 137–145.

Aylward, E., Minshew, N., Goldstein, G., Honeycutt, N., Augustine, A., Yates, K., et al., 1999. MRI volumes of amygdala and hippocampus in non-mentally retarded autistic adolescents and adults. Neurology 53, 2145–2150.

Azmitia, E.C., Singh, J.S., Hou, X.P., Wegiel, J., 2011. Dystrophic serotonin axons in postmortem brains from young autism patients. Anatomical Record 294, 1653–1662.

Azmitia, E.C., Singh, J.S., Whitaker-Azmitia, P.M., 2011. Increased serotonin axons (immunoreactive to 5-HT transporter) in postmortem brains from young autism donors. Neuropharmacology 60, 1347–1354.

Baird, A.A., Gruber, S.A., Fein, D.A., Maas, L.C., Steingard, R.J., Renshaw, P.F., et al., 1999. Functional magnetic resonance imaging of facial affect recognition in children and adolescents. Journal of the American Academy of Child & Adolescent Psychiatry 38, 195–199.

Barnea-Goraly, N., Kwon, H., Menon, V., Eliez, S., Lotspeich, L., Reiss, A.L., 2004. White matter structure in autism: Preliminary evidence from diffusion tensor imaging. Biological Psychiatry 55, 323–326.

Baron-Cohen, S., Ring, H., Wheelwright, S., Bullmore, E.T., Brammer, M.J., Simmons, A., et al., 1999. Social intelligence in the normal and autistic brain: An fMRI study. European Journal of Neuroscience 11, 1891–1898.

Bauman, M.D., Amaral, D.G., 2005. The distribution of serotonergic fibers in the macaque monkey amygdala: An immunohistochemical study using antisera to 5-hydroxytryptamine. Neuroscience 136, 193–203.

Bauman, M., Kemper, T.L., 1985. Histoanatomic observations of the brain in early infantile autism. Neurology 35, 866–875.

Bauman, M.L., Kemper, T.L., 1994. Neuroanatomic observations of the brain in autism. In: Bauman, M.L., Kemper, T.L. (Eds.), The Neurobiology of Autism. Johns Hopkins University Press, Baltimore, MD, pp. 119–145.

Bauman, M.D., Lavenex, P., Mason, W.A., Capitanio, J.P., Amaral, D.G., 2004. The development of mother-infant interactions after neonatal amygdala lesions in rhesus monkeys. Journal of Neuroscience 24, 711–721.

Bauman, M.D., Lavenex, P., Mason, W.A., Capitanio, J.P., Amaral, D.G., 2004. The development of social behavior following neonatal amygdala lesions in rhesus monkeys. Journal of Cognitive Neuroscience 16, 1388–1411.

Bessis, A., Bechade, C., Bernard, D., Roumier, A., 2007. Microglial control of neuronal death and synaptic properties. Glia 55, 233–238.

Birmingham, E., Cerf, M., Adolphs, R., 2011. Comparing social attention in autism and amygdala lesions: Effects of stimulus and task condition. Social Neuroscience 6, 420–435.

Boes, A.D., Mehta, S., Rudrauf, D., Van Der Plas, E., Grabowski, T., Adolphs, R., et al., 2011. Changes in cortical morphology resulting from long-term amygdala damage. Social Cognitive and Affective Neuroscience 7, 588–595.

Corbett, B.A., Carmean, V., Ravizza, S., Wendelken, C., Henry, M.L., Carter, C., et al., 2009. A functional and structural study of emotion and face processing in children with autism. Psychiatry Research 173, 196–205.

Dalton, K.M., Nacewicz, B.M., et al., 2007. Gaze-fixation, brain activation, and amygdala volume in unaffected siblings of individuals with autism. Biological Psychiatry 61, 512–520.

Dalton, K.M., Nacewicz, B.M., Johnstone, T., Schaefer, H.S., Gernsbacher, M.A., Goldsmith, H.H., et al., 2005. Gaze fixation and the neural circuitry of face processing in autism. Nature Neuroscience 8, 519–526.

Davis, M., 1992. The role of the amygdala in fear and anxiety. Annual Review of Neuroscience 15, 353–375.

Dichter, G.S., Richey, J.A., Rittenberg, A.M., Sabatino, A., Bodfish, J.W., 2012. Reward circuitry function in autism during face anticipation and outcomes. Journal of Autism and Developmental Disorders 42, 147–160.

Emery, N.J., Amaral, D.G., 2000. The role of the amygdala in primate social cognition. In: Lane, R.D., Nadel, L. (Eds.), Cognitive Neuroscience of Emotion. Oxford University Press, Oxford.

Endo, T., Shioiri, T., Kitamura, H., Kimura, T., Endo, S., Masuzawa, N., et al., 2007. Altered chemical metabolites in the amygdala-hippocampus region contribute to autistic symptoms of autism spectrum disorders. Biological Psychiatry 62, 1030–1037.

Freese, J., Amaral, D.G., 2009. Neuroanatomy of the Primate Amygdala. In: Whalen, P.J., Phelps, E.A. (Eds.), The Human Amygdala. Guilford Press, New York.

Gabis, L., Wei, H., Azizian, A., DeVincent, C., Tudorica, A., Kesner-Baruch, Y., et al., 2008. 1H-magnetic resonance spectroscopy markers of cognitive and language ability in clinical subtypes of autism spectrum disorders. Journal of Child Neurology 23, 766–774.

Giedd, J.N., 1997. Normal development. Neuroimaging 6, 265–282.

Giedd, J.N., Snell, J.W., Lange, N., et al., 1996. Quantitative magnetic resonance imaging of human brain development: Ages 4–18. Cerebral Cortex 6, 551–560.

Gillott, A., Furniss, F., Walter, A., 2001. Anxiety in high-functioning children with autism. Autism 5, 277–286.

Grelotti, D.J., Klin, A.J., Gauthier, I., Skudlarski, P., Cohen, D.J., Gore, J.C., et al., 2005. fMRI activation of the fusiform gyrus and amygdala to cartoon characters but not to faces in a boy with autism. Neuropsychologia 43, 373–385.

Grezes, J., Wicker, B., Berthoz, S., de Gelder, B., 2009. A failure to grasp the affective meaning of actions in autism spectrum disorder subjects. Neuropsychologia 47, 1816–1825.

Groen, W., Teluij, M., Buitelaar, J., Tendolkar, I., 2010. Amygdala and hippocampus enlargement during adolescence in autism. Journal of the American Academy of Child & Adolescent Psychiatry 49, 552–560.

Hadjikhani, N., Chabris, C., Joseph, R., Clark, J., McGrath, L., Aharon, I., et al., 2004. Early visual cortex organization in autism: An fMRI study. Neuroreport 15, 267–270.

Hadjikhani, N., Joseph, R.M., Snyder, J., Tager-Flusberg, H., 2007. Abnormal activation of the social brain during face perception in autism. Human Brain Mapping 28, 441–449.

Hamann, S.B., Adolphs, R., 1999. Normal recognition of emotional similarity between facial expressions following bilateral amygdala damage. Neuropsychologia 37, 1135–1141.

Haznedar, M.M., Buchsbaum, M.S., Wei, T.-C., Hof, P.R., Cartwright, C., Bienstock, C.A., et al., 2000. Limbic circuitry in patients with autism spectrum disorders studied with positron emission tomography and magnetic resonace imaging. American Journal of Psychiatry 157, 1994–2001.

Howard, M.A., Cowell, P.E., Boucher, J., Broks, P., Mayes, A., Farrant, A., et al., 2000. Convergent neuroanatomical and behavioural evidence of an amygdala hypothesis of autism. Neuroreport 11, 2931–2935.

Humphrey, T., 1968. The development of the human amygdala during early embryonic life. Journal of Comparative Neurology 132, 135–165.

Jou, R.J., Jackowski, A.P., Papademetris, X., Rajeevan, N., Staib, L.H., Volkmar, F.R., 2011. Diffusion tensor imaging in autism spectrum disorders: Preliminary evidence of abnormal neural connectivity. Australian and New Zealand Journal of Psychiatry 45, 153–162.

Juranek, J., Filipek, P.A., Berenji, G.R., Modahl, C., Osann, K., Spence, M.A., 2006. Association between amygdala volume and anxiety level: Magnetic resonance imaging (MRI) study in autistic children. Journal of Child Neurology 21, 1051–1058.

Kanner, L., 1943. Autistic disturbances of affective contact. The Nervous Child 2, 217–250.

Kemper, T.L., Bauman, M.L., 1993. The contribution of neuropathologic studies to the understanding of autism. Neurologic Clinics 11, 175–187.

Kennedy, D.P., Glascher, J., Tyszka, J.M., Adolphs, R., 2009. Personal space regulation by the human amygdala. Nature Neuroscience 12, 1226–1227.

Killgore, W.D., Oki, M., Yurgelun-Todd, D.A., 2001. Sex-specific developmental changes in amygdala responses to affective faces. Neuroreport 12, 427–433.

Kim, M.J., Whalen, P.J., 2009. The structural integrity of an amygdala-prefrontal pathway predicts trait anxiety. Journal of Neuroscience 29, 11,614–11,618.

Kleinhans, N.M., Johnson, L.C., Richards, T., Mahurin, R., Greenson, J., Dawson, G., et al., 2009. Reduced neural habituation in the amygdala and social impairments in autism spectrum disorders. American Journal of Psychiatry 166, 467–475.

Kleinhans, N.M., Richards, T., Johnson, L.C., Weaver, K.E., Greenson, J., Dawson, G., et al., 2011. fMRI evidence of neural abnormalities in the subcortical face processing system in ASD. NeuroImage 54, 697–704.

Kleinhans, N.M., Richards, T., Sterling, L., Stegbauer, K.C., Mahurin, R., Johnson, L.C., et al., 2008. Abnormal functional connectivity in autism spectrum disorders during face processing. Brain 131, 1000–1012.

Kleinhans, N.M., Richards, T., Weaver, K., Johnson, L.C., Greenson, J., Dawson, G., et al., 2010. Association between amygdala response to emotional faces and social anxiety in autism spectrum disorders. Neuropsychologia 48, 3665–3670.

Klin, A., Jones, W., Schultz, R., Volkmar, F., Cohen, D., 2002. Visual fixation patterns during viewing of naturalistic social situations as predictors of social competence in individuals with autism. Archives of Neurology and Psychiatry 59, 809–816.

Kordower, J.H., Piecinski, P., Rakic, P., 1992. Neurogenesis of the amygdaloid nuclear complex in the rhesus monkey. Brain Research and Development 68, 9–15.

LeDoux, J., 2007. The amygdala. Current Biology 17, 868–874.

Malisza, K.L., Clancy, C., Shiloff, D., Holden, J., Jones, C., Paulson, K., et al., 2011. Functional magnetic resonance imaging of facial information processing in children with autistic disorder, attention deficit hyperactivity disorder and typically developing controls. International Journal of Adolescent Medicine and Health 23, 269–277.

Matys, T., Pawlak, R., Matys, E., Pavlides, C., McEwen, B.S., Strickland, S., 2004. Tissue plasminogen activator promotes the effects of corticotropin-releasing factor on the amygdala and anxiety-like behavior. Proceedings of the National Academy of Sciences of the United States of America 101, 16,345–16,350.

Monk, C.S., Weng, S.J., Wiggins, J.L., Kurapati, N., Louro, H.M., Carrasco, M., et al., 2010. Neural circuitry of emotional face processing in autism spectrum disorders. Journal of Psychiatry and Neuroscience 35, 105–114.

Morgan, J.T., Chana, G., Pardo, C.A., Achim, C., Semendeferi, K., Buckwalter, J., et al., 2010. Microglial activation and increased microglial density observed in the dorsolateral prefrontal cortex in autism. Biological Psychiatry 68, 368–376.

Mosconi, M.W., Cody-Hazlett, H., Poe, M.D., Gerig, G., Gimpel-Smith, R., Piven, J., 2009. Longitudinal study of amygdala volume and joint attention in 2- to 4-year-old children with autism. Archives of Neurology and Psychiatry 66, 509–516.

Munson, J., Dawson, G., Abbott, R., Faja, S., Webb, S.J., Friedman, S.D., et al., 2006. Amygdalar volume and behavioral development in autism. Archives of Neurology and Psychiatry 63, 686–693.

Nacewicz, B.M., Dalton, K.M., Johnstone, T., Long, M.T., McAuliff, E.M., Oakes, T.R., et al., 2006. Amygdala volume and nonverbal social impairment in adolescent and adult males with autism. Archives of Neurology and Psychiatry 63, 1417–1428.

Nacewicz, B.M., Angelos, L., Dalton, K.M., Fischer, R., Anderle, M.J., Alexander, A.L., et al., 2012. Reliable non-invasive measurement of human neurochemistry using proton spectroscopy with an anatomically defined amygdala-specific voxel. NeuroImage 59, 2548–2559.

Nordahl, C.W., Scholz, R., Yang, X., Buonocore, M.H., Simon, T., Rogers, S., et al., 2012. Increased rate of amygdala growth in children aged 2 to 4 years with autism spectrum disorders: A longitudinal study. Archives of General Psychiartry 69, 53–61.

Noriuchi, M., Kikuchi, Y., Yoshiura, T., Kira, R., Shigeto, H., Hara, T., et al., 2010. Altered white matter fractional anisotropy and social impairment in children with autism spectrum disorder. Brain Research 1362, 141–149.

O'Rahilly, R., Muller, F., 2006. The Embryonic Human Brain: An Atlas Of Developmental Stages. John Wiley & Sons, Hoboken, NJ.

Ostby, Y., Tamnes, C.K., Fjell, A.M., Westlye, L.T., Due-Tonnessen, P., Walhovd, K.B., 2009. Heterogeneity in subcortical brain development: A structural magnetic resonance imaging study of brain maturation from 8 to 30 years. Journal of Neuroscience 29, 11,772–11,782.

Otsuka, H., Harada, M., Mori, K., Hisaoka, S., Nishitani, H., 1999. Brain metabolites in the hippocampus-amygdala region and cerebellum in autism: An 1H-MR spectroscopy study. Neuroradiology 41, 517–519.

Page, L.A., Daly, E., Schmitz, N., Simmons, A., Toal, F., Deeley, Q., et al., 2006. In vivo 1H-magnetic resonance spectroscopy study of amygdala-hippocampal and parietal regions in autism. American Journal of Psychiatry 163, 2189–2192.

Palmen, S.J., Hulshoff Pol, H.E., Kemner, C., Schnack, H.G., Durston, S., Lahuis, B.E., et al., 2005. Increased gray-matter volume in medication-naive high-functioning children with autism spectrum disorder. Psychological Medicine 35, 561–570.

Paul, L.K., Corsello, C., Tranel, D., Adolphs, R., 2010. Does bilateral damage to the human amygdala produce autistic symptoms? Journal of Neurodevelopmental Disorders 2, 165–173.

Pelphrey, K.A., Morris, J.P., McCarthy, G., Labar, K.S., 2007. Perception of dynamic changes in facial affect and identity in autism. Social Cognitive and Affective Neuroscience 2, 140–149.

Pelphrey, K.A., Sasson, N.J., Reznick, J.S., Paul, G., Goldman, B.D., Piven, J., 2002. Visual scanning of faces in autism. Journal of Autism and Developmental Disorders 32, 249–261.

Perlman, S.B., Hudac, C.M., Pegors, T., Minshew, N.J., Pelphrey, K.A., 2011. Experimental manipulation of face-evoked activity in the fusiform gyrus of individuals with autism. Social Neuroscience 6, 22–30.

Phelps, E.A., LeDoux, J.E., 2005. Contributions of the amygdala to emotion processing: From animal models to human behavior. Neuron 48, 175–187.

Pierce, K., Haist, F., Sedaghat, F., Courchesne, E., 2004. The brain response to personally familiar faces in autism: Findings of fusiform activity and beyond. Brain 127, 2703–2716.

Pierce, K., Müller, R.-A., Ambrose, J., Allen, G., Courchesne, E., 2001. Face processing occurs outside the fusiform 'face area' in autism: Evidence from fMRI. Brain 124, 2059–2073.

Piggot, J., Kwon, H., Mobbs, D., Blasey, C., Lotspeich, L., Menon, V., et al., 2004. Emotional attribution in high-functioning individuals with autistic spectrum disorder: A functional imaging study. Journal of the American Academy of Child & Adolescent Psychiatry 43, 473–480.

Pinkham, A.E., Hopfinger, J.B., Pelphrey, K.A., Piven, J., Penn, D.L., 2008. Neural bases for impaired social cognition in schizophrenia and autism spectrum disorders. Schizophrenia Research 99, 164–175.

Pitkänen, A., Tuunanen, J., Kalviainen, R., Partanen, K., Salmenpera, T., 1998. Amygdala damage in experimental and human temporal lobe epilepsy. Epilepsy Research 32, 233–253.

Prather, M.D., Lavenex, P., Mauldin-Jourdain, M.L., Mason, W.A., et al., 2001. Increased social fear and decreased fear of objects in monkeys with neonatal amygdala lesions. Neuroscience 106, 653–658.

Rojas, D.C., Smith, J.A., Benkers, T.L., Camou, S.L., Reite, M.L., Rogers, S.J., 2004. Hippocampus and amygdala volumes in parents of children with autistic disorder. American Journal of Psychiatry 161, 2038–2044.

Roozendaal, B., McEwen, B.S., Chattarji, S., 2009. Stress, memory and the amygdala. Nature Reviews Neuroscience 10, 423–433.

Rudie, J.D., Shehzad, Z., Hernandez, L.M., Colich, N.L., Bookheimer, S.Y., Iacoboni, M., et al., 2011. Reduced functional integration and segregation of distributed neural systems underlying social and emotional information processing in autism spectrum disorders. Cerebral Cortex 22, 1025–1037.

Saygin, Z.M., Osher, D.E., Augustinack, J., Fischl, B., Gabrieli, J.D., 2011. Connectivity-based segmentation of human amygdala nuclei using probabilistic tractography. Neuroimage 56, 1353–1361.

Schumann, C.M., Amaral, D.G., 2005. Stereological estimation of the number of neurons in the human amygdaloid complex. Journal of Comparative Neurology 491, 320–329.

Schumann, C.M., Amaral, D.G., 2006. Stereological analysis of amygdala neuron number in autism. Journal of Neuroscience 26, 7674–7679.

Schumann, C.M., Amaral, D.G., 2009. The human amygdala in autism. In: Whalen, P.J., Phelps, E.A. (Eds.), The Human Amygdala. Guilford Press, New York.

Schumann, C.M., Barnes, C.C., Lord, C., Courchesne, E., 2009. Amygdala enlargement in toddlers with autism related to severity of social and communication impairments. Biological Psychiatry 66, 942–949.

Schumann, C.M., Hamstra, J., Goodlin-Jones, B.L., Lotspeich, L.J., Kwon, H., Buonocore, M.H., et al., 2004. The amygdala is enlarged in children but not adolescents with autism; the hippocampus is enlarged at all ages. Journal of Neuroscience 24, 6392–6401.

Setzer, M., Ulfig, N., 1999. Differential expression of calbindin and calretinin in the human fetal amygdala. Microscopy Research and Technique 46, 1–17.

Shaw, P., Lawrence, E.J., Radbourne, C., Bramham, J., Polkey, C.E., David, A.S., 2004. The impact of early and late damage to the human amygdala on 'theory of mind' reasoning. Brain 127, 1535–1548.

Shin, L.M., Rauch, S.L., Pitman, R.K., Whalen, P.J., 2009. The Human Amygdala in Anxiety Disorders. In: Whalen, P.J., Phelps, E.A. (Eds.), The Human Amygdala. Guilford Press, New York.

Sparks, B.F., Friedman, S.D., Shaw, D.W., Aylward, E., Echelard, D., Artru, A.A., et al., 2002. Brain sructural abnormalities in young children with autism spectrum disorder. Neurology 59, 184–192.

Spezio, M.L., Adolphs, R., Hurley, R.S., Piven, J., 2007. Analysis of face gaze in autism using "Bubbles". Neuropsychologia 45, 144–151.

Stevens, B., Allen, N.J., Vazquez, L.E., Howell, G.R., Christopherson, K.S., Nouri, N., et al., 2007. The classical complement cascade mediates CNS synapse elimination. Cell 131, 1164–1178.

Thomas, K.M., Drevets, W.C., Whalen, P.J., Eccard, C.H., Dahl, R.E., Ryan, N.D., et al., 2001. Amygdala response to facial expressions in children and adults. Biological Psychiatry 49, 309–316.

Ulfig, N., Setzer, M., Bohl, J., 1998. Transient architectonic features in the basolateral amygdala of the human fetal brain. Acta Anatomica 163, 99–112.

Ulfig, N., Setzer, M., Bohl, J., 2003. Ontogeny of the human amygdala. Annals of the New York Academy of Sciences 985, 22–33.

Vargas, D.L., Nascimbene, C., Krishnan, C., Zimmerman, A.W., Pardo, C.A., 2005. Neuroglial activation and neuroinflammation in the brain of patients with autism. Annals of Neurology 57, 67–81.

Wang, A.T., Dapretto, M., Hariri, A.R., Sigman, M., Bookheimer, S.Y., 2004. Neural correlates of facial affect processing in children and adolescents with autism spectrum disorder. Journal of the American Academy of Child and Adolescent Psychiatry 43, 481–490.

Wang, A.T., Lee, S.S., Sigman, M., Dapretto, M., 2006. Neural basis of irony comprehension in children with autism: The role of prosody and context. Brain 129, 932–943.

Weng, S.J., Carrasco, M., Swartz, J.R., Wiggins, J.L., Kurapati, N., Liberzon, I., et al., 2011. Neural activation to emotional faces in adolescents with autism spectrum disorders. Journal of Child Psychology and Psychiatry 52, 296–305.

White, S.W., Oswald, D., Ollendick, T., Scahill, L., 2009. Anxiety in children and adolescents with autism spectrum disorders. Clinical Psychology Review 29, 216–229.

Zikopoulos, B., Barbas, H., 2010. Changes in prefrontal axons may disrupt the network in autism. Journal of Neuroscience 30, 14,595–14,609.

3.6

Discrete Cortical Neuropathology in Autism Spectrum Disorders

Neha Uppal*,†, Patrick R. Hof†

*Seaver Autism Center for Research and Treatment, †Fishberg Department of Neuroscience, and Friedman Brain Institute, Mount Sinai School of Medicine, New York, NY, USA

WHOLE-BRAIN CHANGES

The study of autism spectrum disorders (ASD) is challenging due its heterogeneous causes and its common phenotype. One way forward is to determine whether there are commonalities amongst patients with ASD from the point of view of changes in brain structure, and in relation to the clinical manifestation of the disease. In the past decade, functional magnetic resonance imaging (fMRI) has proved to be a successful technique for exploring whole-brain changes in ASD. Studies using fMRI techniques have shown clearly that the brain develops differently in ASD (see the section Fusiform Gyrus). Of particular interest to the neuropathology of ASD are the age-specific changes in brain growth that highlight the developmental nature of the disorder (Courchesne et al., 2011a). The brains of very young children with ASD display an overgrowth that is apparent by 2 years of age. After this period, their brain growth rate is similar to controls, signifying that this abnormal brain enlargement begins after birth and before the age of 2 (Courchesne et al., 2003; Hazlett et al., 2011). There is a region-specificity to this enlargement, with the largest growth occurring in the frontal and temporal cortices and no change in the occipital lobe (Carper et al., 2002). This is followed by a subsequently slower increase in brain size later on in childhood, during which patients with ASD and controls have similar brain volumes (Courchesne et al., 2011a). By adulthood, brain size begins to decrease at a slightly faster pace than typically aging brains, and therefore with time, the size of the brain in patients with ASD drops marginally below typical size. Many of the neuronal abnormalities observed in distinct areas in ASD correspond to the changes seen at the whole-brain level. These region-specific differences have been reported in cortical, subcortical, and cerebellar areas as highlighted throughout the section Inferior Frontal Cortex; this subsection will feature the studies that have expanded our knowledge on the cortical changes found in ASD (Figure 3.6.1), starting with the prefrontal cortex.

The Neuroscience of Autism Spectrum Disorders.
http://dx.doi.org/10.1016/B978-0-12-391924-3.00022-3

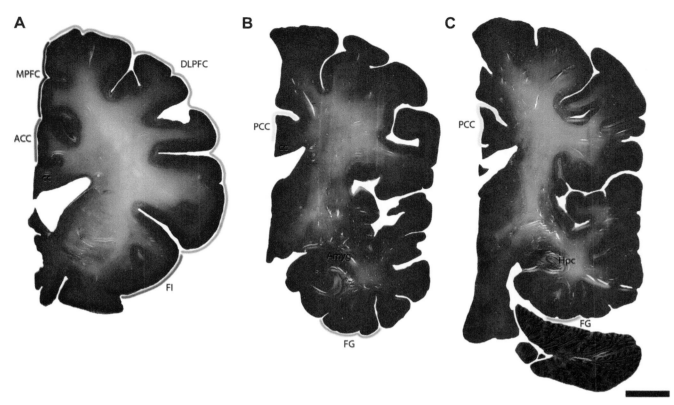

FIGURE 3.6.1　Nissl-stained hemispheres showing cortical areas implicated in ASD, in a rostro-caudal order from A to C. (A) The anterior cingulate cortex (ACC; red), medial prefrontal cortex (MPFC; dark blue), dorsolateral prefrontal cortex (DLPFC; green), and frontoinsular cortex (FI; pink); (B) posterior cingulate cortex (PCC; light blue), fusiform gyrus (FG; orange), and amygdala (Amyg); (C) posterior cingulate cortex (PCC; light blue), fusiform gyrus (FG; orange), and hippocampus (Hpc). Corpus callosum = cc; scale bar = 1 cm.

PREFRONTAL CORTEX

The prefrontal cortex (PFC) is known for its role in cognitive control, as it coordinates activity from individual brain areas to achieve internal goals (Fuster, 2001; Miller and Cohen, 2001). The PFC has consistently been shown to have abnormal overgrowth in young children with ASD from about the age of 2 to 5 years (Carper and Courchesne, 2005; Carper et al., 2002; Hazlett et al., 2011; Schumann et al., 2010), leading Courchesne and colleagues to explore whether cellular defects are the cause of the observed increase in brain size (Courchesne et al., 2011b). These authors assessed neuron and glial number in the dorsolateral and medial PFC in seven males with ASD, aged 2 to 16, compared to six comparably aged controls. Their stereological results showed a striking 79% increase in neuron number in the dorsolateral PFC and a 29% increase in the medial PFC, with an overall increase of 67% in the PFC of male children with ASD (Figure 3.6.2). This increase only occurred in neuronal cells, as the difference in glial number was insignificant between groups. In addition, the brain size of patients with ASD deviated from normal age-based values (Redcay and Courchesne, 2005) by 17.6%, which

was an increase not found in controls. The increase in brain size and neuron number suggests that the overgrowth detected in many patients with ASD is likely due to an increase in neuron number, substantiated by the fact that neuron volume was not altered in ASD. Interestingly, the authors noted that while control neuron numbers were predicted by brain weight, the increase in neuron number found in patients with ASD should have led to a 29.4% enlargement in brain size.

Given the role of the PFC in higher cognitive functioning, one might expect a differential change within the group of patients with ASD depending on the extent of intellectual disability. The authors explored this possibility as well, as there were both low- and high-functioning patients with ASD in this study, but found there was no clear effect of intellect on neuronal number. This provides an interesting possibility that the neuropathology among patients with ASD may be very similar, although their phenotypes may vary across the spectrum.

Future studies assessing differences in these parameters extending to the orbital PFC will provide insight into possible disruptions in social behavior, as this area is known to have a role in processing social information (see, for example, Kringelbach and Rolls, 2004). Recently,

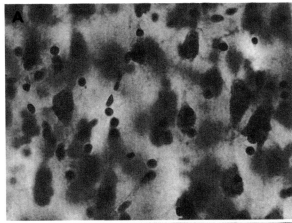

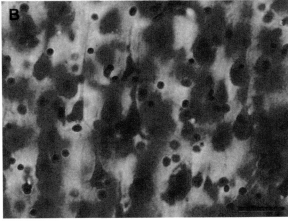

FIGURE 3.6.2 Neuropathological increase in neuron number in layer III of the dorsolateral prefrontal cortex. Note the increase in neurons the patient with ASD (B; 5 years old) compared to the control subject (A; 4 years old). Scale bar = 30 μm.

the size of the orbital PFC was shown to be correlated with the size of a person's social network (Powell et al., 2012), suggesting that patients with ASD would have a smaller region than typically developing controls. In fact, children with ASD (8–12-years-old males) had a reduced right lateral orbital PFC size compared to controls, and more specifically in gray matter volume (Girgis et al., 2007), although this difference was not reported previously (Carper and Courchesne, 2005). It would be beneficial to analyze potential alterations in neuron number in this region. It would also be beneficial to corroborate the results in the dorsolateral and medial PFC by analyzing separate layers as well as individual Brodmann areas in these regions to determine if there are differential results based on functionality.

INFERIOR FRONTAL CORTEX

The posterior inferior frontal cortex, defined by Brodmann as areas 44 and 45, has a well-established role in language production and syntactic processing, as well as empathy in the left hemisphere (Broca, 1861; Liakakis et al., 2011; Tyler et al., 2011), and in fine motor control, response inhibition, and metaphoric meanings of sentences in the right hemisphere (Bookheimer, 2002; Hampshire et al., 2010). Because of its involvement in language processing, this region is of particular interest in ASD, as social communication is affected. Areas 44 and 45 are also thought to be part of the mirror neuron system – a network of areas activated when mimicking action and social-related movements (e.g., Gallese et al., 1996; Heiser et al., 2003; Keuken et al., 2011; Rizzolatti and Arbib, 1998; Rizzolatti et al., 1996). This system has been shown to be dysfunctional in ASD (Le Bel et al., 2009; Williams, 2008; Williams et al., 2001) and is hypothesized to underlie the core deficits in social skills and theory of mind (Baron-Cohen et al., 1985; Senju, 2011), though the presence of an impairment has been challenged by many groups (Dinstein et al., 2010; Hamilton, 2009; Theoret et al., 2005). In addition, imaging studies have reported abnormalities in activation in this region in ASD (De Fosse et al., 2004; Just et al., 2004; Kana et al., 2006; Koshino et al., 2005).

Identifying the neuropathology of areas 44 and 45 began in 1985 with a preliminary study on a 21-year-old female with ASD (Coleman et al., 1985). The results showed no difference in the density of pyramidal neurons, other neurons, or glia in area 44, though the individual variability was very high, with only one patient and two controls. Hof and colleagues continued the exploration of this area using stereological quantification, determining whether there are changes in pyramidal neuron number and size as well as layer volume, in 4- to 66-year-old patients with ASD compared to 4- to 52-year-old controls (Jacot-Descombes et al., 2012). Although no change was found in neuron number or layer volume, the authors found significant decreases in neuron size in layers III, V, and VI in patients with ASD (Figure 3.6.3). While this result is contrary to those found in the PFC by the Courchesne group (Courchesne et al., 2011b), it does support findings of reduced neuron number in the fusiform gyrus (FG) and amygdala, as well as an established hypothesis of globally reduced connectivity in ASD (Courchesne and Pierce, 2005; van Kooten et al., 2008). As the size of the neuron soma is reduced, so are its dendrites, which may result in a reduction in inputs and/or outputs to this area. In support of this hypothesis, functional connectivity is reduced between areas 44 and 45 and temporal language areas (Dinstein et al., 2011; Just et al., 2004) as well as between this region and the primary visual cortex (Villalobos et al., 2005). In addition, low-functioning patients with ASD have reduced activation of the left inferior frontal gyrus during speech stimulation when compared to controls (Lai et al., 2012).

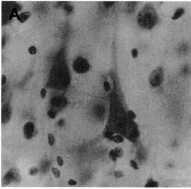

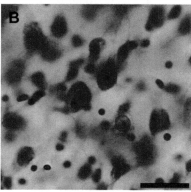

FIGURE 3.6.3   Reduced neuronal size in layer III pyramidal neurons in area 44 in a patient with ASD (B; 5 years old) compared to a control subject (A; 4 years old). Scale bar = 30 μm.

Alterations in connectivity of areas 44 and 45 may disrupt language processing, imitation, and joint attention circuits, leading to the language delay that is characteristic of ASD.

FUSIFORM GYRUS

The fusiform gyrus (FG) is thought to underlie our ability to process faces and is therefore crucial for interacting appropriately in social situations. Several groups have hypothesized that the social impairments seen in ASD may be partially explained by a dysfunction of the FG manifested through differential activation patterns during face-related tasks. Though not conclusive (see for example, Hadjikhani et al., 2004b), most fMRI studies report a hypoactivation of the FG in ASD (Bolte et al., 2006; Kanwisher et al., 1999; Kleinhans et al., 2008; Pierce et al., 2001; 2004; Piggot et al., 2004). Schmitz and colleagues sought to understand the cellular basis of these deficits in face processing from a neuropathological standpoint, assessing differences in neuron density, total neuron number, and mean perikaryal volume (van Kooten et al., 2008). The authors analyzed seven patients with ASD and ten controls

using stereological methods, with ages ranging from 4 to 23 years in the ASD group, and 4 to 65 years for controls. The authors determined that patients with ASD had significantly lower neuron densities in layer III, significantly lower total neuron numbers in layers III, V, and VI, and significantly smaller mean perikaryal volumes in layers V and VI of the FG (Figure 3.6.4). The authors also assessed the primary visual area and the cortical gray matter and found no differences between patients with ASD and controls, confirming that the observed changes are FG-specific.

These results support functional neuroimaging data showing hypoactivation of the FG in ASD (Schultz et al., 2003). The decrease in neuron density, total neuron number, and somal size in these areas suggests that there may be a similarly reduced connectivity between the FG and its cortical input and output areas. More specifically, cortical inputs to the FG are mainly from the inferior occipital gyrus and superior temporal gyrus, involved in the visual analysis and moving aspects of faces (such as eye gaze and mouth movement), respectively (Haxby et al., 2000; Puce et al., 1998). Cortical efferents are sent to the inferior frontal gyrus and orbitofrontal gyrus, where the semantics of facial expression and 'reward' value of faces are evaluated (Ishai, 2007; Ishai et al., 2002). Subcortically, the FG projects to the amygdala, thought to underlie our understanding of the emotional significance of stimuli (Fairhall and Ishai, 2007).

While the reduction in activity as well as number and size of neurons implies a potential impairment in connectivity, the origin of this impairment is not yet known. To date, no alterations have been found in the primary visual area, and therefore cannot be attributed to a reduction in activity in the FG (Hadjikhani et al., 2004a; van Kooten et al., 2008). However, as the authors highlight in their paper, there is reduced activity in the inferior occipital gyrus and superior temporal gyrus in ASD, suggesting that their input may be altered and in turn affect the activity of the FG. One would expect that the neuronal differences in the FG would have a similar effect on efferent areas, namely the amygdala, inferior frontal gyrus, and orbitofrontal cortex. In line with this hypothesis, Schumann and colleagues have found an overall decrease in neurons in the amygdala, which receives input from layer V of the FG (Schumann and Amaral, 2006); more specifically, the number of neurons was significantly reduced in the lateral nucleus, which is the amygdala's principal input area (see Section Inferior Frontal Gyrus for more details). As previously discussed, the inferior frontal gyrus has a similarly reduced neuron size in layers III, V, and VI (Jacot-Descombes et al., 2012).

A more recent study re-examining the FG did not find numerical or cytoarchitectural differences between

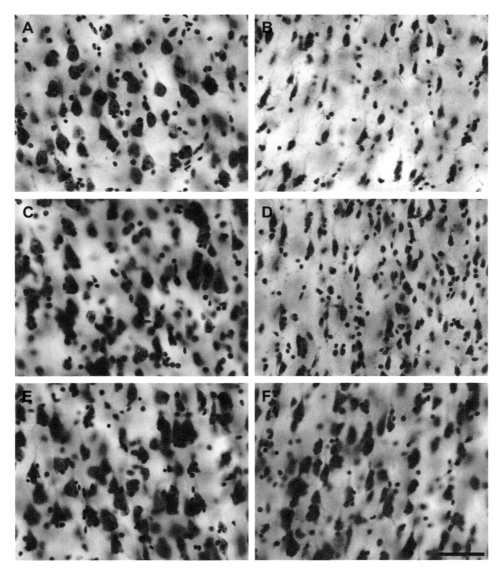

FIGURE 3.6.4 Neuropathological changes in layers III, V, and VI of the fusiform gyrus in a control subject (left hand column; 23 years old) compared to a patient with ASD (right hand column; 21 years old). Note the lower neuron density in layer III (B), the marked decrease in total neuron density and perikaryal size in layer V (D), and the reduced perikaryal size (F) in the patient with ASD compared to the control subject (A, C, and E, respectively). Scale bar = 30 μm.

patients with ASD and controls (Oblak et al., 2011), possibly owing to the study design that grouped layers instead of analyzing them separately. In addition, a difference in the age range of the examined cases should be taken into account, given that Schmitz and collaborators studied a group that included young children and young adult patients, whereas the study carried out by Blatt and colleagues focused on adolescence to late 30s (age range 14–37 years). To further understand the implication of FG neuropathology in ASD, a developmental approach is warranted and future studies would benefit from exploring narrower age ranges and comparing findings from different age groups.

FRONTOINSULAR CORTEX

The presence of consistently impaired social skills in ASD has prompted an intense exploration of cortical areas thought to be implicated in emotional regulation and awareness of oneself and others (Minshew and Keller, 2010). The frontoinsular cortex (FI) is thought to process conscious awareness of bodily sensations involved in emotional perception through its role in polymodal sensory and visceral integration (Craig, 2002; 2003; 2009; Critchley et al., 2004). In addition, this area is home to the specialized von Economo neurons (VENs; see Box 3.6.1), thought to be involved in processing of social information. To explore whether VENs in

---

BOX 3.6.1

VON ECONOMO NEURONS

Von Economo neurons (VENs) are a specialized neuron present in humans and other large-brained mammals, including great apes, cetaceans, and elephants (Allman et al., 2010; Butti and Hof, 2010; Butti et al., 2009; Hakeem et al., 2009; Hof and Van der Gucht, 2007; Nimchinsky et al., 1999). They are large, vertical bipolar neurons found in layer V of the FI and ACC (Nimchinsky et al., 1995; 1999; von Economo, 1926; Watson et al., 2006) and, in fewer numbers, in area 9 of the PFC (Fajardo et al., 2008) of humans (for review, see Butti et al., 2012; Cauda et al., 2012). Their cortical distribution and the bipolar shape of their dendritic tree have been linked to a possible role in the integration of bodily feelings (processed in the FI) and goal-directed cognitive assessments (processed in the ACC and PFC) in our ability to quickly assess and react in complex social situations (Allman et al., 2005; 2010). VENs are selectively and significantly reduced in patients with the behavioral variant of frontotemporal dementia (Kim et al., 2012; Seeley, 2010; Seeley et al., 2006; 2007a), and in patients with agenesis of the corpus callosum (Kaufman et al., 2008), and have a reduced density in patients with early-onset schizophrenia (Brüne et al., 2010). These are disorders in which social conduct is markedly affected, supporting VENs' hypothesized role in social cognition. The presence of similar social deficits in patients with ASD gave rise to the speculation that abnormalities in VENs might also be found in this disorder (Santos et al., 2011; Simms et al., 2009).

---

the FI were specifically altered in ASD, Courchesne and colleagues quantified VENs in four males with ASD (3, 15, 34, and 41 years old) and five age-matched controls (2, 16, 21, 44, and 75 years old), hypothesizing that patients with ASD would have a reduction in VEN number (Kennedy et al., 2007). The authors did not find a significant difference between groups, but did suggest a slight increase in VEN number in a subgroup of patients with ASD; the lack of difference may have been due to the large age range in this study.

Recently, the possible presence of changes in VEN numbers and their relationship with the diagnosis of ASD was re-evaluated (Santos et al., 2011). Using a stereological approach, VENs and pyramidal neurons were quantified in layer V of the FI of four children with ASD and three comparably aged controls, ranging from age 4 to 14. The authors found a robust difference between the two groups: a 53% increase in the ratio of VENs to pyramidal neurons in children with ASD. This finding is consistent with results from the children in this age range analyzed by the Courchesne group, with a 58% increase in VEN number in the 3-year-old patient with ASD compared to the 2-year-old control (Kennedy et al., 2007). These increases suggest possible neuronal overgrowth in young patients with ASD as well as potential alterations in migration, cortical lamination, and apoptosis. Qualitatively, abnormalities in VEN morphology and cortical lamination were also

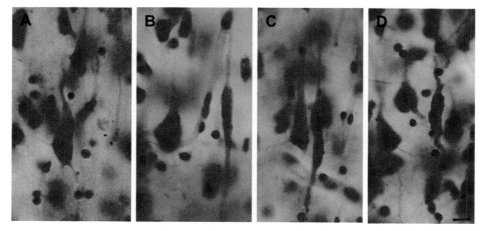

FIGURE 3.6.5   Typical and abnormal morphology of von Economo neurons (VENs). (A) Typical pyramidal cell in a control subject; (B, C) typical VEN alongside a pyramidal cell; (D) abnormal morphology of VENs found in patients with ASD: note the corkscrew dendrites, swollen soma, and surrounding oligodendrocytes. Scale bar = 10 μm.

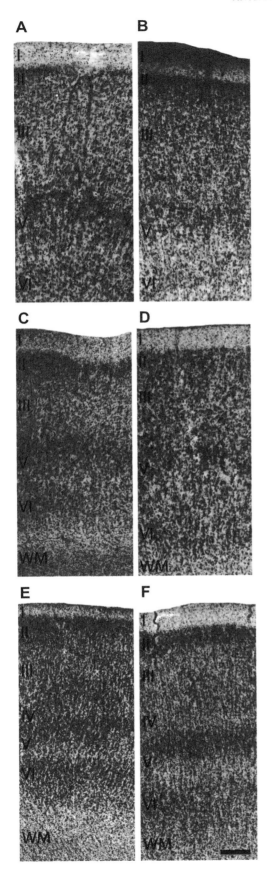

observed, which may underlie a disrupted processing of information (Figure 3.6.5, 3.6.6A–B). As the FI is implicated in our ability to understand our emotions and integrate them into our cognitive processing (Craig, 2009), the phenotype of ASD would be a likely result of irregularities in functioning in this area. In light of the proposed role of VENs in fast intuitive assessments, emotional processing, and social cognition, together with their localization in the anterior insula, a speculative interpretation of the higher total numbers of VENs and ratios of VENs to pyramidal neurons in FI could link these quantitative findings with a heightened interoception clinically described in young patients with ASD (Haag et al., 2005).

ANTERIOR CINGULATE CORTEX

The anterior cingulate cortex (ACC), which works in concert with the FI in processing emotions and their integration in decision-making, can be grossly subdivided into anterior and posterior parts (Allman et al., 2001; Devinsky et al., 1995; Taylor, 2009). The ACC has been implicated in ASD through its known role in value attribution and reward (Schmitz et al., 2008) and has consistent alterations in activation patterns that have been demonstrated in imaging studies of patients with ASD (Barnea-Goraly et al., 2004; Haznedar et al., 2000; Welchew et al., 2005). In parallel, Kemper and Bauman noted that in patients with ASD, the ACC was unusually coarse with poor lamination in five out of six cases (Kemper and Bauman, 1993). The first study to examine the ACC quantitatively using stereology analyzed the size and density of neurons in the three subregions of the ACC (areas 24a, b, c; Vogt et al., 1995) as well as VEN density, size, and distribution in nine males with ASD spanning adolescence and adulthood (15–54 years old; Simms et al., 2009). Significantly higher pyramidal neuron densities in superficial layers I, II, and III were reported in the left hemisphere in area 24a, whereas a reduction in pyramidal neuron size was found in all layers of area 24b and a significant reduction in neuronal density was reported in layers V and VI in area 24c. The results in area 24b are consistent with previously reported reductions in pyramidal neuron density in the FG and amygdala, and the reduced neuron size has also been reported in the FG and IFG (Jacot-Descombes et al., 2012; Schumann and Amaral, 2006;

FIGURE 3.6.6 Cortical layers I–VI of patients with ASD and control subjects in three areas implicated in ASD. Lamination is less distinct in patients with ASD in the frontoinsular cortex (B), anterior cingulate cortex (D), and posterior cingulate cortex (F) compared to controls (A, C, and E, respectively). Scale bar = 200 μm.

van Kooten et al., 2008). The authors suggested that these alterations in pyramidal neuron size and density may represent areas in which neuronal development or circuitry has been affected.

In line with the heterogeneity of the disorder itself, when analyzing VEN density, the authors found distinct subgroups in patients with ASD compared to controls. Three patients with ASD, aged 26, 27, and 32 years, all presented with abnormal cytoarchitecture (Figure 3.6.6C–D) and significantly higher VEN density when compared to controls in areas 24a and 24b. Of the remaining six patients (15, 19, 20, 26, 32, and 54 years old) two had cytoarchitecture irregularities and all had significantly lower density of VENs than controls in subareas 24a, b, and c. Although no correlation with age was found in this study, a larger sample size would provide an interesting perspective for possible differences related to the ages of the patients given the previously discussed results of Hof and colleagues in the FI (Santos et al., 2011). Similar to the effect of increased numbers and an atypical cortical lamination in the FI, a disruption in information processing of the ACC may result in a reduction in the ability to modulate social interaction. A larger number of subjects and a broader age range will be crucial in future studies to allow the exploration of possible subtypes of patients with ASD, which may provide a basis for the discrepancies in VEN numbers described in the ACC. Although difficult to perform, the unveiling of neuropathological distinctions between subgroups, subsequently explored by neuroimaging studies, could provide insight on correlations between activation patterns and behavioral or symptomatic manifestations that would be potentially useful in clinical settings.

POSTERIOR CINGULATE CORTEX

Although not yet widely studied from a neuropathological standpoint, the posterior cingulate cortex (PCC) has been increasingly identified as potentially dysfunctional in ASD (Oblak et al., 2011). The PCC is involved in the processing of the salience of events and faces and is activated by emotionally significant stimuli in neuroimaging studies (Maddock and Buonocore, 1997; Maddock et al., 2001; 2003). Oblak and colleagues (2011) investigated this area at the cellular level in patients with ASD (eight 19–54-year-old males), compared to typically developing controls (seven 20–63-year-old males). Even though no overall significant differences were found in neuron and interneuron densities between groups, individual cases displayed changes in neuron density, size, and distribution, as well as poor lamination, warranting further studies in larger cohorts (Figure 3.6.6D–E).

HIPPOCAMPUS

Neuropathological explorations of limbic system areas have expanded to include the hippocampal formation, involved in learning, memory, and emotion perception. Imaging studies have reported an enlargement in very young children with ASD (3–4 years old, Sparks et al., 2002) as well as in young males with low- and high-functioning ASD (7–18 years old, Schumann et al., 2004), and adolescents with ASD (12–18 years old, Groen et al., 2010). Volume measurements for adolescents and adults have been more inconsistent, with reports of reductions in males with high-functioning ASD (15–40 years old, Howard et al., 2000; 11–37 years old, Aylward et al., 1999), and no difference in hippocampal volume in adolescents and adults (patients with ASD and Asperger's syndrome, 16–39 years old, Haznedar et al., 2000; 12–29 years old, Piven et al., 1998). Preliminary qualitative neuropathology has shown a decrease in neuronal size, an increase in cell packing density, and the presence of limited dendritic arborization in patients with ASD, putatively indicative of disrupted neuronal maturation (Bailey et al., 1998; Kemper and Bauman, 1993; Raymond et al., 1996).

Blatt and colleagues quantitatively analyzed a less-researched cell population in the anterior hippocampus: GABAergic interneurons (producing GABA, γ-aminobutyric acid) (Lawrence et al., 2010). These inhibitory cells are of particular interest because of the emergent hypothesis that ASD is an imbalance in excitation and inhibition, and more specifically that there is a reduced inhibition in ASD (for example, Rubenstein and Merzenich, 2003). Using stereological techniques, the authors found an increased density of specific subtypes of GABAergic interneurons in all five males with ASD compared to age- and gender-matched controls (13–54 years old, Lawrence et al., 2010). In ASD, the dentate gyrus showed a significant increase in density of calbindin-immunoreactive interneurons, whereas CA1 had a higher density of parvalbumin- and calretinin-immunoreactive interneurons, and CA3 had a similar increase in parvalbumin-immunoreactive interneurons. In light of a possible role of these calcium-binding proteins in the modulation of calcium signaling and their location in the hippocampal circuitry, the authors speculated that these abnormalities represent the basis for some of the behavioral abnormalities observed in ASD. More specifically, the changes in inhibitory neuron density support the hypothesis of an imbalance in excitation and inhibition as an underlying factor in social abnormalities in ASD (see Section 3.7).

Other groups exploring the neuropathological correlates of ASD in the hippocampus observed the presence of abnormal growth and development of neurons linked to cytoarchitectural abnormalities in 4 out of 13 patients with ASD (Wegiel et al., 2010). Two males, aged 23 and 60, showed dysplasia in the entorhinal cortex, while abnormal migration and distortion of layers was observed in the dentate gyrus of 11- and 13-year-old patients (female and male, respectively). In addition, dysplasia in CA1 was observed in the 13-year-old and a 56-year-old male with ASD. At a more microscopic level, patients with ASD displayed swollen axon terminals, also known as spheroids, in the hippocampus (Weidenheim et al., 2001). In the 11-year-old patient, spheroids were present in the entorhinal cortex and all CA regions, most prominently in CA3, while in a 20-year-old male, spheroids were observed in the entorhinal cortex, CA1, and CA3.

A more recent study on males with fragile X syndrome (64 and 77 years old), a disorder which is commonly comorbid with ASD, found focal thickening in CA1 as well as abnormalities in the dentate gyrus in both patients analyzed (Greco et al., 2011). The expansions in CA1 contained an increased amount of pyramidal neurons, and the authors observed a parallel decrease in pyramidal neurons in adjacent areas.

Some investigators have hypothesized that pathology in the hippocampus and extending through the medial temporal lobe may separate low- from high-functioning patients with ASD, although this is controversial (Bachevalier, 1994). These alterations suggest a proportional disruption in dendritic and neuropil development and potential underdevelopment in connectivity of these hippocampal areas. Interestingly, volume changes in the amygdala and hippocampus seem to parallel one another, regardless of the inconsistencies between studies on the magnitude and direction of the change.

CONCLUSION

The evident pathology only in specific areas suggests that there are pathways, particularly ones involved in social cognition, that are affected in ASD, while other brain regions involved in unaffected functions are spared. The pattern of reduced neuronal size and density highlights the strong possibility that circuits involving these areas are somehow disrupted. For example, the face-processing circuit involves the FG, ACC, orbital PFC, amygdala, and the superior temporal gyrus, all of which have been implicated in ASD neuropathologically or through abnormal activation. It has been hypothesized that the reduced activity (and potentially the reduced neuron number and size) in the FG stems from the lack of attention to the eye region, which holds salient social information (Davidson and Dalton, 2003). This implies that the impairment in the FG may begin from areas involved in a social-affective brain

circuit, namely the amygdala, PFC, ACC, insula, and striatum (Davidson and Irwin, 1999). Each of these areas, aside from the striatum, which has yet to be studied at the cellular level (although shown to be disrupted in ASD through imaging studies – Di Martino et al., 2011; Langen et al., 2009), has presented with clear neuropathology in this disorder. The inattention to the eyes may be caused by a lack of importance towards facial stimuli, or an active avoidance of socially salient stimuli due to autonomic hyper-reactivity. The latter hypothesis is supported by the increased number of VENs seen in the FI of children with ASD, which the authors speculate underlies a heightened interoception. Irrespective of its basis, this lack of attention to facial stimuli may cause a reduction in input to the FG and thus cause the decrease in neuron number and size over time. As discussed previously, the neuropathology in the FG may also be related to the smaller soma in pyramidal neurons in the IFG, as this area receives efferents from the FG.

Disruptions in neural connectivity in ASD are not only hypothesized when the brain is engaged in a task but also during rest. The default mode network is active during rest (Buckner et al., 2008; Greicius et al., 2003), and is comprised of two key 'nodes': the ventromedial PFC and PCC (Sridharan et al., 2008) along with their connections. The central executive network, which activates during cognitively demanding tasks and is therefore active when the default mode network is not, consists of the dorsolateral PFC and posterior parietal cortex along with their connecting areas. The areas that activate during the switch between these networks are the ACC and FI (Seeley et al., 2007b; Taylor, 2009). In ASD, the default mode network displays both lack of deactivation during cognitive tasks and weaker connectivity amongst areas in the network (Assaf et al., 2010; Cherkassky et al., 2006; Kennedy and Courchesne, 2008; Kennedy et al., 2006; Monk et al., 2009; Weng et al., 2010), which may imply a reduced baseline activity during rest. The abnormalities in the default mode network have been correlated to the social deficits in this disorder, and though the results have not yet been consistent, future studies with larger samples and more comparable study designs may provide clearer evidence for a role of this network in ASD. A dysfunction in this overall network is compounded by the cellular pathology in many of these areas, outlined above.

Yet another circuit has been hypothesized to be affected in ASD, revolving around the amygdala (Baron-Cohen et al., 2000) and additionally implicating the orbital PFC and superior temporal gyrus in impairments in the 'social brain' (see Section 3.4). A closer analysis of all the implicated brain regions in these pathways will be possible with the addition of more cases to brain banks. Studies focusing on specific age groups, genders, and intellect (separating patients with Asperger's syndrome and high-functioning and low-functioning forms of ASD) would be beneficial for understanding the potential differences that have been outlined both behaviorally and through imaging studies. In addition, with a larger collection of resources, studies focusing not only on neuronal differences but also on potential changes in oligodendrocytes, astrocytes, and microglia numbers will help elucidate a more recent hypothesis of immune abnormalities in ASD (Section 2.7). However, regardless of the size, the advantage of the current brain banks is that many groups are looking at different areas in the same cases, and it will be an invaluable resource to bring together information from all areas sampled in a given case to give a broader picture of patterns of neuronal alterations and how these might relate to a certain phenotype.

ACKNOWLEDGMENTS

The authors thank ASD Speaks (the ASD Celloidin Library Project, PRH), the James S. McDonnell Foundation (PRH), and the Seaver Foundation (NU), Drs J. Wegiel, D. Lightfoot, and J. Pickett, as well as Ms E. Xiu, for their help and support.

References

Allman, J.M., Hakeem, A., Erwin, J.M., Nimchinsky, E., Hof, P., 2001. The anterior cingulate cortex: The evolution of an interface between emotion and cognition. Annals of the New York Academy of Sciences 935, 107–117.

Allman, J.M., Tetreault, N.A., Hakeem, A.Y., Manaye, K.F., Semendeferi, K., Erwin, J.M., et al., 2010. The Von Economo neurons in frontoinsular and anterior cingulate cortex of great apes and humans. Brain Structure & Function 214, 495–517.

Allman, J.M., Watson, K.K., Tetreault, N.A., Hakeem, A.Y., 2005. Intuition and ASD: A possible role for Von Economo neurons. Trends in Cognitive Sciences 9, 367–373.

Assaf, M., Jagannathan, K., Calhoun, V.D., Miller, L., Stevens, M.C., Sahl, R., et al., 2010. Abnormal functional connectivity of default mode sub-networks in ASD spectrum disorder patients. Neuroimage 53, 247–256.

Aylward, E.H., Minshew, N.J., Goldstein, G., Honeycutt, N.A., Augustine, A.M., Yates, K.O., et al., 1999. MRI volumes of amygdala and hippocampus in non-mentally retarded autistic adolescents and adults. Neurology 53, 2145–2150.

Bachevalier, J., 1994. Medial temporal lobe structures and ASD: A review of clinical and experimental findings. Neuropsychologia 32, 627–648.

Bailey, A., Luthert, P., Dean, A., Harding, B., Janota, I., Montgomery, M., et al., 1998. A clinicopathological study of ASD. Brain 121, 889–905.

Barnea-Goraly, N., Kwon, H., Menon, V., Eliez, S., Lotspeich, L., Reiss, A.L., 2004. White matter structure in ASD: Preliminary evidence from diffusion tensor imaging. Biological Psychiatry 55, 323–326.

Baron-Cohen, S., Leslie, A.M., Frith, U., 1985. Does the autistic child have a theory of mind? Cognition 21, 37–46.

Baron-Cohen, S., Ring, H.A., Bullmore, E.T., Wheelwright, S., Ashwin, C., Williams, S.C., 2000. The amygdala theory of ASD. Neuroscience and Biobehavioral Reviews 24, 355–364.

Bolte, S., Hubl, D., Feineis-Matthews, S., Prvulovic, D., Dierks, T., Poustka, F., 2006. Facial affect recognition training in ASD: Can we animate the fusiform gyrus? Behavioral Neuroscience 120, 211–216.

Bookheimer, S., 2002. Functional MRI of language: New approaches to understanding the cortical organization of semantic processing. Annual Review of Neuroscience 25, 151–188.

Broca, P., 1861. Remarques sur le siège de la faculté du langage articulé; suivies d'une observation d'aphémie (perte de la parole). Bulletins et Mémoires de la Société Anatomique de Paris 36, 330–357.

Brüne, M., Schobel, A., Karau, R., Benali, A., Faustmann, P.M., Juckel, G., et al., 2010. Von Economo neuron density in the anterior cingulate cortex is reduced in early onset schizophrenia. Acta Neuropathologica 119, 771–778.

Buckner, R.L., Andrews-Hanna, J.R., Schacter, D.L., 2008. The brain's default network: Anatomy, function, and relevance to disease. Annals of the New York Academy of Sciences 1124, 1–38.

Butti, C., Hof, P.R., 2010. The insular cortex: A comparative perspective. Brain Structure and Function 214, 477–493.

Butti, C., Santos, M., Uppal, N., Hof, P.R., 2012. Von Economo neurons: Clinical and evolutionary perspectives. Cortex.

Butti, C., Sherwood, C.C., Hakeem, A.Y., Allman, J.M., Hof, P.R., 2009. Total number and volume of Von Economo neurons in the cerebral cortex of cetaceans. Journal of Comparative Neurology 515, 243–259.

Carper, R.A., Courchesne, E., 2005. Localized enlargement of the frontal cortex in early ASD. Biological Psychiatry 57, 126–133.

Carper, R.A., Moses, P., Tigue, Z.D., Courchesne, E., 2002. Cerebral lobes in ASD: Early hyperplasia and abnormal age effects. Neuroimage 16, 1038–1051.

Cauda, F., Torta, D.M., Sacco, K., D'Agata, F., Geda, E., Duca, S., et al., 2012. Functional anatomy of cortical areas characterized by Von Economo neurons. Brain Structure & Function doi:10.1007/s00429-012-0382-9.

Cherkassky, V.L., Kana, R.K., Keller, T.A., Just, M.A., 2006. Functional connectivity in a baseline resting-state network in ASD. Neuroreport 17, 1687–1690.

Coleman, P.D., Romano, J., Lapham, L., Simon, W., 1985. Cell counts in cerebral cortex of an autistic patient. Journal of Autism and Developmental Disorders 15, 245–255.

Courchesne, E., Pierce, K., 2005. Why the frontal cortex in ASD might be talking only to itself: Local over-connectivity but long-distance disconnection. Current Opinion in Neurobiology 15, 225–230.

Courchesne, E., Campbell, K., Solso, S., 2011. Brain growth across the life span in ASD: Age-specific changes in anatomical pathology. Brain Research 1380, 138–145.

Courchesne, E., Carper, R., Akshoomoff, N., 2003. Evidence of brain overgrowth in the first year of life in ASD. The Journal of American Medical Association 290, 337–344.

Courchesne, E., Mouton, P.R., Calhoun, M.E., Semendeferi, K., Ahrens-Barbeau, C., Hallet, M.J., et al., 2011. Neuron number and size in prefrontal cortex of children with ASD. Journal of the American Medical Association 306, 2001–2010.

Craig, A.D., 2002. How do you feel? Interoception: The sense of the physiological condition of the body. Nature Reviews Neuroscience 3, 655–666.

Craig, A.D., 2003. Interoception: The sense of the physiological condition of the body. Current Opinion in Neurobiology 13, 500–505.

Craig, A.D., 2009. How do you feel now? The anterior insula and human awareness. Nature Reviews Neuroscience 10, 59–70.

Critchley, H.D., Wiens, S., Rotshtein, P., Ohman, A., Dolan, R.J., 2004. Neural systems supporting interoceptive awareness. Nature Neuroscience 7, 189–195.

Davidson, R.J., Dalton, K., 2003. Dysfunction in the neural circuitry of emotional face processing in individuals with ASD. Psychophysiology 40, s3.

Davidson, R.J., Irwin, W., 1999. The functional neuroanatomy of emotion and affective style. Trends in Cognitive Sciences 3, 11–21.

De Fosse, L., Hodge, S.M., Makris, N., Kennedy, D.N., Caviness, V.S., McGrath, L., et al., 2004. Language-association cortex asymmetry in ASD and specific language impairment. Annals of Neurology 56, 757–766.

Devinsky, O., Morrell, M.J., Vogt, B.A., 1995. Contributions of anterior cingulate cortex to behaviour. Brain 118, 279–306.

Di Martino, A., Kelly, C., Grzadzinski, R., Zuo, X.N., Mennes, M., Mairena, M.A., et al., 2011. Aberrant striatal functional connectivity in children with ASD. Biological Psychiatry 69, 847–856.

Dinstein, I., Pierce, K., Eyler, L., Solso, S., Malach, R., Behrmann, M., et al., 2011. Disrupted neural synchronization in toddlers with ASD. Neuron 70, 1218–1225.

Dinstein, I., Thomas, C., Humphreys, K., Minshew, N., Behrmann, M., Heeger, D.J., 2010. Normal movement selectivity in ASD. Neuron 66, 461–469.

Fairhall, S.L., Ishai, A., 2007. Effective connectivity within the distributed cortical network for face perception. Cerebral Cortex 17, 2400–2406.

Fajardo, C., Escobar, M.I., Buritica, E., Arteaga, G., Umbarila, J., Casanova, M.F., et al., 2008. Von Economo neurons are present in the dorsolateral (dysgranular) prefrontal cortex of humans. Neuroscience Letters 435, 215–218.

Fuster, J.M., 2001. The prefrontal cortex – An update: Time is of the essence. Neuron 30, 319–333.

Gallese, V., Fadiga, L., Fogassi, L., Rizzolatti, G., 1996. Action recognition in the premotor cortex. Brain 119, 593–609.

Girgis, R.R., Minshew, N.J., Melhem, N.M., Nutche, J.J., Keshavan, M.S., Hardan, A.Y., 2007. Volumetric alterations of the orbitofrontal cortex in ASD. Progress in Neuropsychopharmacology & Biological Psychiatry 31, 41–45.

Greco, C.M., Navarro, C.S., Hunsaker, M.R., Maezawa, I., Shuler, J.F., Tassone, F., et al., 2011. Neuropathologic features in the hippocampus and cerebellum of three older men with fragile X syndrome. Molecular Autism 2, 2.

Greicius, M.D., Krasnow, B., Reiss, A.L., Menon, V., 2003. Functional connectivity in the resting brain: A network analysis of the default mode hypothesis. Proceedings of the National Academy of Sciences of the United States of America 100, 253–258.

Groen, W., Teluij, M., Buitelaar, J., Tendolkar, I., 2010. Amygdala and hippocampus enlargement during adolescence in ASD. Journal of the American Academy of Child & Adolescent Psychiatry 49, 552–560.

Haag, G., Tordjman, S., Duprat, A., Urwand, S., Jardin, F., Clement, M.C., et al., 2005. Psychodynamic assessment of changes in children with ASD under psychoanalytic treatment. International Journal of Psychoanalysis 86, 335–352.

Hadjikhani, N., Chabris, C.F., Joseph, R.M., Clark, J., McGrath, L., Aharon, I., et al., 2004. Early visual cortex organization in ASD: An fMRI study. Neuroreport 15, 267–270.

Hadjikhani, N., Joseph, R.M., Snyder, J., Chabris, C.F., Clark, J., Steele, S., et al., 2004. Activation of the fusiform gyrus when individuals with ASD spectrum disorder view faces. Neuroimage 22, 1141–1150.

Hakeem, A.Y., Sherwood, C.C., Bonar, C.J., Butti, C., Hof, P.R., Allman, J.M., 2009. Von Economo neurons in the elephant brain. Anatomical Record 292, 242–248.

Hamilton, A.F., 2009. Goals, intentions and mental states: Challenges for theories of ASD. Journal of Child Psychology and Psychiatry 50, 881–892.

Hampshire, A., Chamberlain, S.R., Monti, M.M., Duncan, J., Owen, A.M., 2010. The role of the right inferior frontal gyrus: Inhibition and attentional control. Neuroimage 50, 1313–1319.

Haxby, J.V., Hoffman, E.A., Gobbini, M.I., 2000. The distributed human neural system for face perception. Trends in Cognitive Sciences 4, 223–233.

Hazlett, H.C., Poe, M.D., Gerig, G., Styner, M., Chappell, C., Smith, R.G., et al., 2011. Early brain overgrowth in ASD associated with an increase in cortical surface area before age 2 years. Archives of General Psychiatry 68, 467–476.

Haznedar, M.M., Buchsbaum, M.S., Wei, T.C., Hof, P.R., Cartwright, C., Bienstock, C.A., et al., 2000. Limbic circuitry in patients with ASD spectrum disorders studied with positron emission tomography and magnetic resonance imaging. American Journal of Psychiatry 157, 1994–2001.

Heiser, M., Iacoboni, M., Maeda, F., Marcus, J., Mazziotta, J.C., 2003. The essential role of Broca's area in imitation. European Journal of Neuroscience 17, 1123–1128.

Hof, P.R., Van der Gucht, E., 2007. Structure of the cerebral cortex of the humpback whale Megaptera novaeangliae (Cetacea, Mysticeti, Balaenopteridae). Anatomical Record 290, 1–31.

Howard, M.A., Cowell, P.E., Boucher, J., Broks, P., Mayes, A., Farrant, A., et al., 2000. Convergent neuroanatomical and behavioural evidence of an amygdala hypothesis of ASD. Neuroreport 11, 2931–2935.

Ishai, A., 2007. Sex, beauty and the orbitofrontal cortex. International Journal of Psychophysiology 63, 181–185.

Ishai, A., Haxby, J.V., Ungerleider, L.G., 2002. Visual imagery of famous faces: Effects of memory and attention revealed by fMRI. Neuroimage 17, 1729–1741.

Jacot-Descombes, S., Uppal, N., Wicinski, B., Santos, M., Schmeidler, J., Giannakopoulos, P., et al., 2012. Decreased pyramidal neuron somal size in Brodmann areas 44 and 45 in patients with autism. Acta Neuropathologica 124, 67–79.

Just, M.A., Cherkassky, V.L., Keller, T.A., Minshew, N.J., 2004. Cortical activation and synchronization during sentence comprehension in high-functioning ASD: Evidence of underconnectivity. Brain 127, 1811–1821.

Kana, R.K., Keller, T.A., Cherkassky, V.L., Minshew, N.J., Just, M.A., 2006. Sentence comprehension in ASD: Thinking in pictures with decreased functional connectivity. Brain 129, 2484–2493.

Kanwisher, N., Stanley, D., Harris, A., 1999. The fusiform face area is selective for faces not animals. Neuroreport 10, 183–187.

Kaufman, J.A., Paul, L.K., Manaye, K.F., Granstedt, A.E., Hof, P.R., Hakeem, A.Y., et al., 2008. Selective reduction of Von Economo neuron number in agenesis of the corpus callosum. Acta Neuropathologica 116, 479–489.

Kemper, T.L., Bauman, M.L., 1993. The contribution of neuropathologic studies to the understanding of ASD. Neurologic Clinics 11, 175–187.

Kennedy, D.P., Courchesne, E., 2008. The intrinsic functional organization of the brain is altered in ASD. Neuroimage 39, 1877–1885.

Kennedy, D.P., Redcay, E., Courchesne, E., 2006. Failing to deactivate: Resting functional abnormalities in ASD. Proceedings of the National Academy of Sciences of the United States of America 103, 8275–8280.

Kennedy, D.P., Semendeferi, K., Courchesne, E., 2007. No reduction of spindle neuron number in frontoinsular cortex in ASD. Brain and Cognition 64, 124–129.

Keuken, M.C., Hardie, A., Dev, S., Paulus, M.P., Jonas, K.J., Den Wildenberg, W.P., et al., 2011. The role of the left inferior frontal gyrus in social perception: An rTMS study. Brain Research 1383, 196–205.

Kim, E.J., Sidhu, M., Macedo, M.N., Huang, E.J., Hof, P.R., Miller, B.J., et al., 2012. Selective frontoinsular von Economo neuron and fork cell loss in early behavioral variant frontotemporal dementia. Cerebral Cortex 22, 251–259.

Kleinhans, N.M., Richards, T., Sterling, L., Stegbauer, K.C., Mahurin, R., Johnson, L.C., et al., 2008. Abnormal functional connectivity in ASD spectrum disorders during face processing. Brain 131, 1000–1012.

Koshino, H., Carpenter, P.A., Minshew, N.J., Cherkassky, V.L., Keller, T.A., Just, M.A., 2005. Functional connectivity in an fMRI working memory task in high-functioning ASD. Neuroimage 24, 810–821.

Kringelbach, M.L., Rolls, E.T., 2004. The functional neuroanatomy of the human orbitofrontal cortex: Evidence from neuroimaging and neuropsychology. Progress in Neurobiology 72, 341–372.

Lai, G., Pantazatos, S.P., Schneider, H., Hirsch, J., 2012. Neural systems for speech and song in ASD. Brain 135, 961–975.

Langen, M., Schnack, H.G., Nederveen, H., Bos, D., Lahuis, B.E., de Jonge, M.V., et al., 2009. Changes in the developmental trajectories of striatum in ASD. European Neuropsychopharmacology 19, S678–S679.

Lawrence, Y.A., Kemper, T.L., Bauman, M.L., Blatt, G.J., 2010. Parvalbumin-, calbindin-, and calretinin-immunoreactive hippocampal interneuron density in ASD. Acta Neurologica Scandinavica 121, 99–108.

Le Bel, R.M., Pineda, J.A., Sharma, A., 2009. Motor-auditory-visual integration: The role of the human mirror neuron system in communication and communication disorders. Journal of Communicational Disorders 42, 299–304.

Liakakis, G., Nickel, J., Seitz, R.J., 2011. Diversity of the inferior frontal gyrus – a meta-analysis of neuroimaging studies. Behavioral Brain Research 225, 341–347.

Maddock, R.J., Buonocore, M.H., 1997. Activation of left posterior cingulate gyrus by the auditory presentation of threat-related words: An fMRI study. Psychiatry Research 75, 1–14.

Maddock, R.J., Garrett, A.S., Buonocore, M.H., 2001. Remembering familiar people: The posterior cingulate cortex and autobiographical memory retrieval. Neuroscience 104, 667–676.

Maddock, R.J., Garrett, A.S., Buonocore, M.H., 2003. Posterior cingulate cortex activation by emotional words: fMRI evidence from a valence decision task. Human Brain Mapping 18, 30–41.

Miller, E.K., Cohen, J.D., 2001. An integrative theory of prefrontal cortex function. Annual Review of Neuroscience 24, 167–202.

Minshew, N.J., Keller, T.A., 2010. The nature of brain dysfunction in ASD: Functional brain imaging studies. Current Opinion in Neurology 23, 124–130.

Monk, C.S., Peltier, S.J., Wiggins, J.L., Weng, S.J., Carrasco, M., Risi, S., et al., 2009. Abnormalities of intrinsic functional connectivity in ASD spectrum disorders. Neuroimage 47, 764–772.

Nimchinsky, E.A., Gilissen, E., Allman, J.M., Perl, D.P., Erwin, J.M., Hof, P.R., 1999. A neuronal morphologic type unique to humans and great apes. Proceedings of the National Academy of Sciences of the United States of America 96, 5268–5273.

Nimchinsky, E.A., Vogt, B.A., Morrison, J.H., Hof, P.R., 1995. Spindle neurons of the human anterior cingulate cortex. Journal of Comparative Neurology 355, 27–37.

Oblak, A.L., Rosene, D.L., Kemper, T.L., Bauman, M.L., Blatt, G.J., 2011. Altered posterior cingulate cortical cyctoarchitecture, but normal density of neurons and interneurons in the posterior cingulate cortex and fusiform gyrus in ASD. Autism Research 4, 200–211.

Pierce, K., Haist, F., Sedaghat, F., Courchesne, E., 2004. The brain response to personally familiar faces in ASD: Findings of fusiform activity and beyond. Brain 127, 2703–2716.

Pierce, K., Muller, R.A., Ambrose, J., Allen, G., Courchesne, E., 2001. Face processing occurs outside the fusiform 'face area' in ASD: Evidence from functional MRI. Brain 124, 2059–2073.

Piggot, J., Kwon, H., Mobbs, D., Blasey, C., Lotspeich, L., Menon, V., et al., 2004. Emotional attribution in high-functioning individuals with autistic spectrum disorder: A functional imaging study. Journal of the American Academy of Child & Adolescent Psychiatry 43, 473–480.

Piven, J., Bailey, J., Ranson, B.J., Arndt, S., 1998. No difference in hippocampus volume detected on magnetic resonance imaging in autistic individuals. Journal of Autism and Developmental Disorders 28, 105–110.

Powell, J., Lewis, P.A., Roberts, N., Garcia-Finana, M., Dunbar, R.I., 2012. Orbital prefrontal cortex volume predicts social network size: An imaging study of individual differences in humans. Proceedings of the Royal Society. B, Biological Sciences doi:10.1098/rspb.2011.2574.

Puce, A., Allison, T., Bentin, S., Gore, J.C., McCarthy, G., 1998. Temporal cortex activation in humans viewing eye and mouth movements. Journal of Neuroscience 18, 2188–2199.

Raymond, G.V., Bauman, M.L., Kemper, T.L., 1996. Hippocampus in ASD: A Golgi analysis. Acta Neuropathologica 91, 117–119.

Redcay, E., Courchesne, E., 2005. When is the brain enlarged in ASD? A meta-analysis of all brain size reports. Biological Psychiatry 58, 1–9.

Rizzolatti, G., Arbib, M.A., 1998. Language within our grasp. Trends in Neurosciences 21, 188–194.

Rizzolatti, G., Fadiga, L., Gallese, V., Fogassi, L., 1996. Premotor cortex and the recognition of motor actions. Cognitive Brain Research 3, 131–141.

Rubenstein, J.L., Merzenich, M.M., 2003. Model of ASD: Increased ratio of excitation/inhibition in key neural systems. Genes, Brain and Behavior 2, 255–267.

Santos, M., Uppal, N., Butti, C., Wicinski, B., Schmeidler, J., Giannakopoulos, P., et al., 2011. Von Economo neurons in ASD: A stereologic study of the frontoinsular cortex in children. Brain Research 1380, 206–217.

Schmitz, N., Rubia, K., van Amelsvoort, T., Daly, E., Smith, A., Murphy, D.G., 2008. Neural correlates of reward in ASD. British Journal of Psychiatry 192, 19–24.

Schultz, R.T., Grelotti, D.J., Klin, A., Kleinman, J., Van der Gaag, C., Marois, R., et al., 2003. The role of the fusiform face area in social cognition: Implications for the pathobiology of ASD. Philosophical Transactions of the Royal Society of London. Series B, Biological Sciences 358, 415–427.

Schumann, C.M., Amaral, D.G., 2006. Stereological analysis of amygdala neuron number in ASD. Journal of Neuroscience 26, 7674–7679.

Schumann, C.M., Bloss, C.S., Barnes, C.C., Wideman, G.M., Carper, R.A., Akshoomoff, N., et al., 2010. Longitudinal magnetic resonance imaging study of cortical development through early childhood in ASD. Journal of Neuroscience 30, 4419–4427.

Schumann, C.M., Hamstra, J., Goodlin-Jones, B.L., Lotspeich, L.J., Kwon, H., Buonocore, M.H., et al., 2004. The amygdala is enlarged in children but not adolescents with ASD; the hippocampus is enlarged at all ages. Journal of Neuroscience 24, 6392–6401.

Seeley, W.W., 2010. Anterior insula degeneration in frontotemporal dementia. Brain Structure & Function 214, 465–475.

Seeley, W.W., Allman, J.M., Carlin, D.A., Crawford, R.K., Macedo, M.N., Greicius, M.D., et al., 2007. Divergent social functioning in behavioral variant frontotemporal dementia and Alzheimer disease: Reciprocal networks and neuronal evolution. Alzheimer Disease and Associated Disorders 21, S50–S57.

Seeley, W.W., Carlin, D.A., Allman, J.M., Macedo, M.N., Bush, C., Miller, B.L., et al., 2006. Early frontotemporal dementia targets neurons unique to apes and humans. Annals of Neurology 60, 660–667.

Seeley, W.W., Menon, V., Schatzberg, A.F., Keller, J., Glover, G.H., Kenna, H., et al., 2007. Dissociable intrinsic connectivity networks for salience processing and executive control. Journal of Neuroscience 27, 2349–2356.

Senju, A., 2011. Spontaneous theory of mind and its absence in ASD spectrum disorders. Neuroscientist.

Simms, M.L., Kemper, T.L., Timbie, C.M., Bauman, M.L., Blatt, G.J., 2009. The anterior cingulate cortex in ASD: Heterogeneity of qualitative and quantitative cytoarchitectonic features suggests possible subgroups. Acta Neuropathologica 118, 673–684.

Sparks, B.F., Friedman, S.D., Shaw, D.W., Aylward, E.H., Echelard, D., Artru, A.A., et al., 2002. Brain structural abnormalities in young children with ASD spectrum disorder. Neurology 59, 184–192.

Sridharan, D., Levitin, D.J., Menon, V., 2008. A critical role for the right fronto-insular cortex in switching between central-executive and default-mode networks. Proceedings of the National Academy of Sciences of the United States of America 105, 12,569–12,574.

Taylor, K.S., Semionowicz, D.A., Davis, K.D., 2009. Two systems of resting state connectivity between insula and cingulate cortex. Human Brain Mapping 30, 2731–2745.

Theoret, H., Halligan, E., Kobayashi, M., Fregni, F., Tager-Flusberg, H., Pascual-Leone, A., 2005. Impaired motor facilitation during action observation in individuals with ASD spectrum disorder. Current Biology 15, R84–R85.

Tyler, L.K., Marslen-Wilson, W.D., Randall, B., Wright, P., Devereux, B.J., Zhuang, J., et al., 2011. Left inferior frontal cortex and syntax: Function, structure and behaviour in patients with left hemisphere damage. Brain 134, 415–431.

van Kooten, I.A., Palmen, S.J., von Cappeln, P., Steinbusch, H.W., Korr, H., Heinsen, H., et al., 2008. Neurons in the fusiform gyrus are fewer and smaller in ASD. Brain 131, 987–999.

Villalobos, M.E., Mizuno, A., Dahl, B.C., Kemmotsu, N., Muller, R.A., 2005. Reduced functional connectivity between V1 and inferior frontal cortex associated with visuomotor performance in ASD. Neuroimage 25, 916–925.

Vogt, B.A., Nimchinsky, E.A., Vogt, L.J., Hof, P.R., 1995. Human cingulate cortex: Surface features, flat maps, and cytoarchitecture. Journal of Comparative Neurology 359, 490–506.

von Economo, C., 1926. Eine neue art spezialzellen des lobus cinguli and lobus insulae. Zeitschrift für der Gesamte Neurologie und Psychiatrie 100, 706–712.

Watson, K.K., Jones, T.K., Allman, J.M., 2006. Dendritic architecture of the von Economo neurons. Neuroscience 141, 1107–1112.

Wegiel, J., Kuchna, I., Nowicki, K., Imaki, H., Marchi, E., Ma, S.Y., et al., 2010. The neuropathology of ASD: Defects of neurogenesis and neuronal migration, and dysplastic changes. Acta Neuropathologica 119, 755–770.

Weidenheim, K.M., Goodman, L., Dickson, D.W., Gillberg, C., Rastam, M., Rapin, I., 2001. Etiology and pathophysiology of autistic behavior: Clues from two cases with an unusual variant of neuroaxonal dystrophy. Journal of Child Neurology 16, 809–819.

Welchew, D.E., Ashwin, C., Berkouk, K., Salvador, R., Suckling, J., Baron-Cohen, S., et al., 2005. Functional disconnectivity of the medial temporal lobe in Asperger's syndrome. Biological Psychiatry 57, 991–998.

Weng, S.J., Wiggins, J.L., Peltier, S.J., Carrasco, M., Risi, S., Lord, C., et al., 2010. Alterations of resting state functional connectivity in the default network in adolescents with ASD spectrum disorders. Brain Research 1313, 202–214.

Williams, J.H., 2008. Self-other relations in social development and ASD: Multiple roles for mirror neurons and other brain bases. Autism Research 1, 73–90.

Williams, J.H., Whiten, A., Suddendorf, T., Perrett, D.I., 2001. Imitation, mirror neurons and ASD. Neuroscience and Biobehavioral Reviews 25, 287–295.

3.7

The Minicolumnopathy of Autism Spectrum Disorders

Manuel F. Casanova

Department of Psychiatry, University of Louisville, Louisville, KY, USA

INTRODUCTION

A number of associated medical conditions underscore the neurodevelopmental nature of autism spectrum disorders (ASD). For example, approximately a third of patients with Möbius syndrome (i.e., congenital palsy of the sixth and seventh cranial nerves) have comorbid ASD (Strömland et al., 2002). Physical examination of ASD patients reveals a number of minor malformations attributed to developmental processes. The most common among these malformations is the posterior rotation of the external ears. A report that 5% of thalidomide victims have ASD-like features further supports the developmental nature of ASD, which according to Rodier may be timed around the closure of the neural tube during fetal gestation (Rodier et al., 1996; Rodier, 2002). The fact that thalidomide patients with ASD features have ear abnormalities and normal limbs helps pinpoint the genesis of the disorder as early as 20 to 24 days after conception. This timing coincides with recent reports that the brains of ASD individuals have supernumerary minicolumns or cortical modules. Minicolumns are basic units of cortical processing whose total numbers are normally defined during the first 40 days of development. Exogenous factors may also provide for heterochronic divisions of germinal cells (i.e., outside the first 40 days of gestation) and the formation of abnormal minicolumns.

All subcortical structures are primarily nucleoid in type. The cortex has been the first brain structure during mammalian evolution to develop both a radial and laminar organization. Subcortical lesions result in specific deficits. In contrast, some cortical lesions provide for graded symptoms that can't necessarily be related to individual cellular components. These clinical observations suggest the existence of a hierarchical cortical system where the properties of the whole far exceed the properties of its individual components. At present there is evidence to designate as modules four different but intertwined anatomical structures: 1) minicolumns, 2) multiple minicolumns, 3) macrocolumns, and 4) large scale networks of macrocolumns (Casanova et al., 2003). In this chapter the term minicolumn will be restricted primarily to denote pyramidal cell arrays.

CORTICOGENESIS

In its initial neuroepithelial stage the brain is comprised of ependymal cells attached to both the ventricular and pial surfaces. Closely packed neuroepithelial cells fasten to the pial surface by endfeet that join together *via* tight junctions. The resulting apposition of endfeet provides for the pia glial limiting membrane and its basal lamina. As time goes by astrocytes will become the major source of endfeet to the pia glial limiting membrane and replace the attachment of radial glial fibers (Marin-Padilla, 1995; 2010).

Maturation of the cortex follows a ventro-dorsal gradient that is concomitant to the penetration of primordial corticopetal fibers. These early fibers originate at extracortical sites and travel all the way to the marginal zone of the developing brain. With progressive growth the number of primordial corticopetal fibers increases. Neurons sandwiched among the more superficial fibers acquire a horizontal orientation. These cells, known as Cajal-Retzius neurons, are found in all ammiotes (Tissir et al., 2002).

To a large extent, the cortex can be conceived as a nucleus whose complexity has increased throughout evolution, and most visibly so in mammals, by the addition of neuronal cell layers (Casanova et al., 2009a). Corticogenesis pursues a recursive process of stratification with the lowest (inner) layers being older than the upper (outer) ones (Aboitiz, 1999). This migratory process is mediated, in part, by radial glial fibers being used as scaffold for the movement of neuroblasts and by the attraction caused by extracellular reelin, a specific recognition molecule expressed by Cajal-Retzius cells (see above). Migrating neuroblasts stemming from the germinal neuroepithelium arrive at the developing cortex and split the original primordial plexiform strata into the cortex's first layer (outside) and the subplate zone (interior) (Marin-Padilla, 1998). Both the subplate and first layer represent common anatomical elements to the cortices of amphibians and reptiles.

Neurons reaching the cortex by radial migration lose their attachment to their guiding glial projection. This process in humans is noted at about the 7th week of gestation and is nearly complete by the 15th week of gestation. No additional pyramidal cells are derived after the 17th or 18th week of gestation (Marin-Padilla, 2010). Neurons 'liberated' in this way into the cortical plate will then acquire characteristics of mature pyramidal cells by developing a descending axonal process and an apical dendrite that extends and branches within the first layer. The subplate zone, previously mentioned, will also serve as the residence of pyramidal-like neurons called Martinotti cells. These specialized cells have basal dendrites and an ascending axon that transverse the cortical plate and branch within the first lamina establishing contacts with Cajal-Retzius cells (Myakhar et al., 2011). During corticogenesis, Martinotti neurons are incorporated into the various developing layers of the cortex.

Pyramidal cells will mature in unison with the incorporation into the gray matter of interneurons and an intrinsic microvascular network. All of these systems (i.e., pyramidal cells, interneurons, and vasculature) follow an ascending stratified maturation (Marin-Padilla, 2010). In the case of pyramidal cells maturation will be marked by the formation of basilar dendrites, spines, and functional contacts with ascending corticopetal projections. The demarcation between the subplate and the white matter will become blurred. Cells in the subplate region undergo regressive changes to become deep interstitial neurons. The end result is a core of rectilinearly arranged pyramidal cells with surrounding elements providing a so-called shower curtain of inhibition (Casanova et al., 2010).

CORTICAL MODULARITY

Chords of pyramidal cells spanning the vertical axis of the cerebral cortex were noted by neuroanatomists of the late Nineteenth Century. Von Economo and Koskinas (1925) called these 'radial structures' as they paralleled the so-called radii, that is, myelinated axon bundles observed in the cerebral cortex. More recent investigators have characterized these structures primarily by the use of Nissl staining. Distances between pyramidal cell arrays have been reported as varying between 30 to 80 μm. Peters and colleagues showed a correlation between pyramidal cell arrays and apical dendritic bundles (Peters et al., 1991). Likewise other authors have shown a correspondence of pyramidal cell arrays to double bouquet cells and myelinated bundles. More specifically the axon bundles or 'horsetails' that characterize double bouquet cells have shown a one-to-one alignment with myelinated axon bundles in both monkey visual cortex and human temporal cortex (DeFelipe et al., 1990). It is therefore presumed that the juxtaposition of these features is non-coincidental and contributes to a canonical cortical microcircuit (Casanova et al., 2008).

The minicolumn serves as an elemental unit of information processing and the simplest modular unit of the cortex (Mountcastle, 1998). According to this model, each minicolumn implements stereotypical information processing operations that are executed in parallel throughout the cortex. This operation is modulated by the pattern of connectivity for each brain region (Creutzfeldt, 1977). Evidence in support of this model is derived from experiments with two-photon imaging of calcium fluxes in which the organization of response fields were comprised of columns 1 to 2 cell-wide (Ohki et al., 2005). Similarly, recent studies using labeled retroviruses and multiple cell recording illustrate how the ontogenetic stratified pyramidal cells have a propensity for developing connections between sister cells rather than neighboring non-siblings (Yu et al., 2009). Results of these and other experiments indicate that specific microcircuits preferentially develop within ontogenetic radial clones of excitatory neurons. Variability within this canonical microcircuit is prominent in humans as compared to other species (Casanova et al., 2009b). Most of this variability resides within the peripheral neuropil space; a compartment housing, among other things, various inhibitory elements (Casanova et al., 2009b).

The cerebral cortex is an autopoietic system composed of canonical circuits. The genesis of this system resides in the recursive positioning of cells along a radial glial scaffolding. The end result of this close apposition of cells is a scenario receptive to Hebbian reciprocity. In effect, early cells within ontogenetic minicolumns are connected to each other via gap junctions (Peinado et al., 1993; Peinado, 2001). The end result is a core compartment comprised of pyramidal cells that has not changed much through mammalian evolution. Much of the minicolumnar variability observed across mammalian species resides within its peripheral neuropil space.

THE MINICOLUMNOPATHY OF AUTISM SPECTRUM DISORDER

Our group used an unbiased semiautomated imaging method (Casanova and Switala, 2005) to analyze minicolumnar morphometry of Brodmann areas 9, 21, and 22 in post mortem tissue of ASD subjects (Casanova et al., 2002a) (Figure 3.7.1). Photomicrograph images were decomposed according to a Gaussian gray-scale distribution and thresholded to define cellular kernels (Otsu, 1979). The least squares method was used to fit radial axes through vertical segments of clusters of Nissl-stained elements representing pyramidal neuron soma, i.e., minicolumnar 'cores'. Parameter values for our algorithm were generated for minicolumnar width as determined by mean tangential axis-to-axis distance, width of vertical segments representing core pyramidal neuron columns, relative dispersal of pyramidal neurons around the radial axis, and mean intercellular distance within minicolumns. In our sample of ASD subjects, minicolumnar width was determined to be significantly narrower ($p = 0.034$) with the greatest decrease found in the peripheral neuropil space compartment (Casanova et al., 2002a). Consistent with this finding the number of minicolumns per frame area was proportionately increased and mean within-frame intercellular distance was decreased.

Subsequently, we sought to determine whether proportionate changes in gray matter could be identified in this tissue series as implied by our data (Casanova et al., 2002b). We modified a method developed by Schleicher and colleagues (2005) to assess thresholded

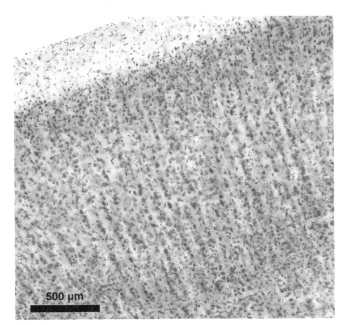

FIGURE 3.7.1 Pyramidal cell arrays are clearly seen in this micrograph of Nissl-stained tissue from Brodmann area 3, right hemisphere, in human postmortem tissue. Arrays actually extend from lamina II all the way to the white matter, but they appear fragmented due to the tissue section, or the focal plane of the of the image, not being parallel to the minicolumnar structure.

images according to a gray level index (GLI) representing the framed proportion of Nissl-stained cell elements (Figure 3.7.2). In our ASD subjects mean distance between core pyramidal neuron columns as represented by cluster segments of GLI maxima was decreased and mean number per image frame was increased indicating greater numbers of narrower minicolumns. GLI segment amplitude was increased consistent with decreased relative cellularity of peripheral neuropil. Mean GLI values for tissue from ASD subjects did not vary significantly in comparison with controls. This finding in addition to the observed increase in density of minicolumns within a cortical sheet of comparable volume suggests that numbers of pyramidal neurons in each minicolumn may be decreased; alternatively, as suggested by increased cortical cell density, average neuron size may be decreased without a concomitant reduction in numbers per minicolumn core.

The genesis for increased cell density in ASD was addressed by a recent study of minicolumnar morphometry from an independent case series of ASD subjects (Casanova et al., 2006). Corroborating our earlier findings, no significant difference in GLI values were found and minicolumnar width as determined by the segmentation and GLI methods was significantly narrower in representative neocortical areas (Brodmann areas 17, 4, and 9, and 3b) of tissue obtained from ASD

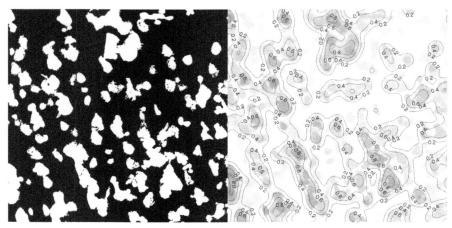

FIGURE 3.7.2   Gray level index (Schleicher et al. 2005) is the fraction of area occupied by Nissl stained neurons, and is essentially a biased estimate of the stereological volume fraction V_V. Left: Stained objects have been identified by thresholding (Otsu, 1979). Right: Smoothing with a kernel approximately 25 μm in width produces estimates of the GLI at every location in the image. The choice of kernel depends upon the features to be analyzed; for minicolumnar structure an asymmetric kernel 110 by 10 μm has been used. *(Casanova et al., 2002b; 2006).*

subjects as compared to controls. In order to assess pyramidal neuron size directly, we applied a Boolean morphometric model (Stoyan et al., 1995) incorporating parameters for kernel size, circumference and intensity. Multivariate analysis yielded significant diagnosis dependence indicating smaller kernel size and increased image frame kernel density. The results suggest that the lack of significant differences in mean GLI values between ASD patients and neurotypicals can be explained by a small reduction in the overall size of neuronal perikarya. Casanova et al. (2006; 2011) indicated that the smaller cell bodies create a bias in terms of brain connectivity favoring shorter projections (e.g., arcuate fibers) at the expense of longer ones (e.g., commissural projections).

Taken together, results of these studies showed an increased neuronal density in the brains of ASD patients explained, in part, by the apposition of narrower minicolumns. The results did not indicate whether increased numbers of minicolumns, increased core column neuronal density, or both were additional contributory factors. To resolve this question, we applied an algorithm to determine the distribution of edge lengths between image frame kernels (Figure 3.7.3) (Casanova et al., 2006). We generated a Gaussian bimodal distribution of interneuronal distances within and between core cell columns. The higher-value mode representing intercolumnar neuron distance was shifted leftward (i.e., lesser values) reflecting decreased peripheral neuropil and reduced minicolumnar width. No significant

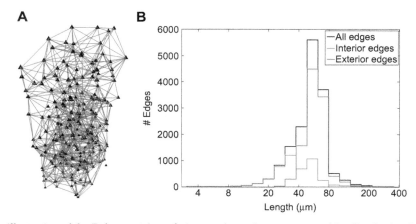

FIGURE 3.7.3   A) As an illustration of the Delaunay triangulation, a schematic was generated by distributing 'neurons' around hexagonally packed 'minicolumn cores' in three dimensions. The Delaunay triangulation of these objects is actually a set of simplices; four neurons are the vertices of a simplex if they lie on a sphere whose interior contains no other neurons. The edges of each simplex have been colored green if both endpoints belong to the same artificial minicolumn (interior edges) and red if they belong to different minicolumns (exterior edges). B) The observed distribution of edge lengths in the Delaunay triangulation can be modeled as a mixture distribution with components corresponding to the lengths of interior, typically shorter, edges, and longer exterior edges.

change was evident in the lower-value mode or its amplitude, consistent with equivalent density and number of minicolumnar core neurons in our sample of ASD subjects. These findings imply that in ASD the number and arrangement of cellular elements and hence basic microcircuit architecture within the minicolumnar pyramidal neuron core are preserved. It also indicates that increased neuronal density in the cerebral cortex of ASD individuals is due to an increased number of minicolumns rather than to an increased number of cells per minicolumn.

The cortical deficits subsumed by a minicolumnopathy were further characterized by comparing minicolumnar widths across layers (Casanova et al., 2010). Brains of seven ASD patients and an equal number of age-matched controls were analyzed by computerized image analysis to determine minicolumnar widths at nine separate neocortical Brodmann areas: 3b, 4, 9, 10, 11, 17, 24, 43, and 44. Each area was assessed at supragranular, granular, and infragranular levels. ASD subjects had smaller minicolumns wherein differences varied according to neocortical areas with the largest difference noted in BA 44. Changes were equally observed across different laminae suggesting involvement of a common anatomical element. As a possible explanation, the authors of the study suggested a possible abnormality among the inhibitory elements present within the peripheral neuropil space of the minicolumn.

Supernumerary minicolumns in ASD are abnormally constructed with significant diminutions in their peripheral neuropil space (Casanova et al. 2002a; 2010). This minicolumnar compartment is defined by the presence of inhibitory elements, which some researchers have opted to call a strong vertical flow of inhibition or, more graphically, a shower curtain of inhibition (Szentagothai and Arbib, 1975; Mountcastle, 1998). It appears possible that certain behavioral traits of ASD (e.g., hypersensitivity) may be rooted in an excitatory/inhibitory imbalance stemming from the abnormal modulation of signals through the cell minicolumn. The author of this chapter has proposed that this imbalance is due to the heterochronic stimulation of germinal cells by an environmental factor in susceptible individuals. In essence, when stimulated at an inopportune time the radial migration of future pyramidal cells is uncoupled from the already existing tangential migration of inhibitory cells (Figure 3.7.4). The heterochronic stimulation of germinal cells offers the most parsimonious explanation to the minicolumnar abnormalities, dysplastic cortical changes, and heterotopias described in the brains of ASD individuals (Bailey et al., 1998; Casanova et al., 2002a; Wegiel et al., 2010).

Our own studies and a summary of the neuropathological literature suggest that the periventricular

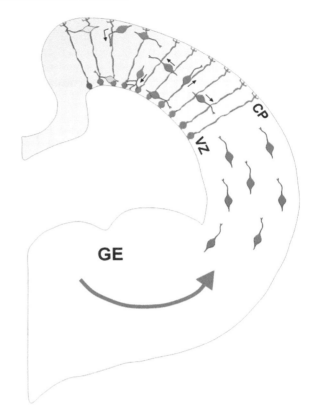

FIGURE 3.7.4 The figure illustrates the radial migration of neuroblasts from the germinal layer of the ventricular zone (VZ) to the cortical plate (CP). These cells will provide for pyramidal (excitatory) cell arrays within the core of minicolumns. A tangential mode of migration is shown as originating, among several places, in the ganglionic eminence (GE). These cells give rise to interneurons (i.e., inhibitory neurons). When properly coupled, both migratory elements provide for a proper excitatory/inhibitory cortical balance. [Graphic from Yokota et al. (2007) used in accordance with a Creative Commons Attribution License.]

germinal cells offer a *loci minoris resistentia* to ASD. Nodular heterotopias of the periventricular zone have been recently reported in the brains of ASD individuals (Wegiel et al., 2010). The malformation is clearly reminiscent of the candle gutterings observed in ventricles of patients with tuberous sclerosis. Features of ASD are present in 25 to 50% of individuals with tuberous sclerosis complex (Wiznitzer, 2004). Brainstem abnormalities described by Bauman and Kemper (2005) can be ascribed to migrational abnormalities stemming from the germinal zone located within the rhombic lip. Viral infections that exhibit neurotropism for periventricular germinal cells (e.g., congenital cytomegalovirus) have been reported to express an ASD phenotype. Imaging of these patients usually exhibits subependymal cysts (Yamashita et al., 2003).

The specificity of GABAergic inhibition in the neocortex is focused around the minicolumn and its core of pyramidal cell arrays (Casanova et al., 2003). Axons of GABAergic neurons target distinct domains of pyramidal neurons (Druga, 2009). The function of these cells is best understood in the context of diads of inhibitory neurons to pyramidal cells: double bouquet-pyramidal cell, basket-pyramidal cell, chandelier-pyramidal cell, and Martinotti-pyramidal cell (Marin-Padilla, 2010). Researchers have explored the possibility that abnormal modulation of interneurons on their minicolumnar substrates can provide for a host of mental disorders (Casanova et al., 2003; Casanova and Tillquist, 2008; Raghanti et al., 2010). It is therefore unsurprising that computer models that alter the excitatory/inhibitory balance have been used to explain representations of core ASD symptoms. More specifically, Gustafsson (1997) proposed that in ASD there is a mismatch between excitation and lateral inhibition. He concluded from his model that there is too much inhibition, whereas Casanova and colleagues (2003) propose the opposite, that there is too little inhibition. A similar idea was proposed by Hussman (2001) who suggested a generalized GABAergic deficit in ASD, a theory known as 'the suppressed GABAergic inhibition hypothesis'. Evidence supporting this way of thinking is derived from pathology relating GABA receptors in several suspected etiologies of ASD (Blatt and Fatemi, 2011). The evidence reviewed in this chapter is therefore supportive of abnormal germinal divisions providing for migratory and cortical dysplastic changes wherein some of the core symptoms are the expression of desynchronized maturation of pyramidal cells (excitatory) and interneurons (inhibitory).

References

Aboitiz, F., 1999. Evolution of isocortical organization. A tentative scenario including roles of reelin, p35/cdk5 and the subplate zone. Cerebral Cortex 9, 655–661.

Bailey, A., Luther, P., Dean, A., Harding, B., Janota, I., Montgomery, M., et al., 1998. A clinicopathological study of autism. Brain 121, 189–905.

Bauman, M.L., Kemper, T.L., 2005. Structural brain anatomy in autism: What is the evidence? In: Bauman, M.L., Kemper, T.L. (Eds.), The Neurobiology of Autism. Johns Hopkins University Press, Baltimore, pp. 121–135.

Blatt, G.J., Fatemi, S.H., 2011. Alterations in GABAergic biomarkers in the autism brain: Research findings and clinical implications. Anatomical Record 294, 1646–1652.

Casanova, M.F., Switala, A.E., 2005. Minicolumnar morphometry: Computerized image analysis. In: Casanova, M.F. (Ed.), Neocortical Modularity and the Cell Minicolumn. Nova Biomedical, New York, pp. 161–179.

Casanova, M.F., Tillquist, C.R., 2008. Encephalization, emergent properties, and psychiatry: A minicolumnar perspective. Neuroscientist 14, 101–118.

Casanova, M.F., Buxhoeveden, D., Gomez, J., 2003. Disruption in the inhibitory architecture of the cell minicolumn: Implications for autism. Neuroscientist 9, 496–507.

Casanova, M.F., Buxhoeveden, D.P., Switala, A.E., Roy, E., 2002. Minicolumnar pathology in autism. Neurology 58, 428–432.

Casanova, M.F., Buxhoeveden, D.P., Switala, A.E., Roy, E., 2002. Neuronal density and architecture (gray level index) in the brains of ASD patients. Journal of Child Neurology 17, 515–521.

Casanova, M.F., El-Baz, A., Switala, A., 2011. Laws of conservation as related to brain growth, aging, and evolution: Symmetry of the minicolumn. Frontiers in Neuroanatomy 5, 66.

Casanova, M.F., El-Baz, A., Vanbogaert, E., Narahari, P., Switala, A., 2010. Minicolumnar core width by lamina comparisons between ASD subjects and controls. Brain Pathology 20, 451–458.

Casanova, M.F., El-Baz, A., Vanbogaert, E., Narahari, P., Trippe, J., 2009. Minicolumnar width: Comparison between supragranular and infragranular layers. Journal of Neuroscience Methods 184, 19–24.

Casanova, M.F., Konkachbaev, A.I., Switala, A.E., Elmaghraby, A.S., 2008. Recursive trace line method for detecting myelinated bundles: A comparison study with pyramidal cell arrays. Journal of Neuroscience Methods 168, 367–372.

Casanova, M.F., Trippe, J., Tillquist, C., Switala, A.E., 2009. Morphometric variability of minicolumns in the striate cortex of Homo sapiens, Macaca mulatta and Pan troglodytes. Journal of Anatomy 214, 226–234.

Casanova, M.F., Van Kooten, I.A.J., Switala, A.E., Van Engeland, H., Heinsen, H., Steinbusch, H.W.M., et al., 2006. Minicolumnar abnormalities in autism. Acta Neuropathologica 112, 287–303.

Creutzfeldt, O.D., 1977. Generality of the functional structure of the neocortex. Naturwissenschaften 64, 507–517.

DeFelipe, J., Hendry, S.H.C., Hashikawa, T., Molinari, M., Jones, E.G., 1990. A microcolumnar structure of monkey cerebral cortex revealed by immunocytochemical studies of double bouquet cell axons. Neuroscience 37, 655–673.

Druga, R., 2009. Neocortical inhibitory system. Folia Biologica 55, 201–217.

Gustafsson, L., 1997. Inadequate cortical feature maps: A neural circuit theory of autism. Biological Psychiatry 42, 1138–1147.

Hussman, J.P., 2001. Suppressed GABAergic inhibition as a common factor in suspected etiologies of autism. Journal of Autism Development and Disorders 31, 247–248.

Marin-Padilla, M., 1995. Prenatal development of fibrous (white matter), protoplasmic (gray matter), and layer I astrocytes in the human cerebral cortex: A Golgi study. Journal of Comparative Neurology 357, 554–572.

Marin-Padilla, M., 1998. Cajal–Retzius cells and the development of the neocortex. Trends in Neurosciences 21, 64–71.

Marin-Padilla, M., 2010. The human brain: Prenatal development and structure. Springer, New York.

Mountcastle, V.B., 1998. Perceptual neuroscience: The cerebral cortex. Harvard University Press, Cambridge, MA.

Myakhar, O., Unichencko, P., Kirischuk, S., 2011. GABAergic projections from the subplate to Cajal-Retzius cells in the neocortex. Neuroreport 22, 525–529.

Ohki, K., Chung, S., Ch'ng, Y.H., Kara, P., Reid, R.C., 2005. Functional imaging with cellular resolution reveals precise micro-architecture in visual cortex. Nature 433, 597–603.

Otsu, N., 1979. A threshold selection method from grey-level histograms. IEEE Transactions on System, Man and Cybernetics 9, 62–66.

Peinado, A., 2001. Immature neocortical neurons exist as extensive syncitial networks linked by dendrodendritic electrical connections. Journal of Neurophysiology 85, 620–629.

Peinado, A., Yuste, R., Katz, L.C., 1993. Gap junctional communication and the development of local circuits in neocortex. Cerebral Cortex 3, 488–498.

Peters, A., Palay, S.L., Webster, H., deF, 1991. The fine structure of the nervous system: Neurons and their supporting cells, third ed. Oxford University Press, New York.

Raghanti, M.A., Spocter, M.A., Butti, C., Hof, P.R., Sherwood, C.C., 2010. A comparative perspective on minicolumns and inhibitory GABAergic interneurons in the neocortex. Frontiers in Neuro-anatomy 4, 3.

Rodier, P.M., 2002. Converging evidence for brain stem injury in autism. Developmental Psychopathology 14, 537–557.

Rodier, P.M., Ingram, J.L., Tisdale, B., Nelson, S., Romano, J., 1996. Embryological origin for autism: Developmental anomalies of the cranial nerve motor nuclei. Journal of Comparative Neurology 370, 247–261.

Schleicher, A., Palomero-Gallagher, N., Morosan, P., Eickhoff, S.B., Kowalski, T., De Vos, K., et al., 2005. Quantitative architectural analysis: A new approach to cortical mapping. Anatomy and Embryology 210, 373–386.

Stoyan, D., Kendall, W.S., Mecke, J., 1995. Stochastic geometry and its applications. Wiley, Chichester.

Strömland, K., Sjögreen, L., Miller, M., Gillberg, C., Wentz, E., Johansson, M., et al., 2002. Möbius sequence: A Swedish multidiscipline study. European Journal of Paediatric Neurology 6, 35–45.

Szentagothai, J., Arbib, M.A., 1975. Conceptual models of neural organization. MIT Press, Cambridge, MA.

Tissir, F., Lambert de Rouvoit, C., Goffinet, A.M., 2002. The role of reelin in the development and evolution of the cerebral cortex. Brazilian Journal of Biological Research 35, 1473–1484.

Von Economo, C., Koskinas, G.N., 1925. Die Cytoarchitektonik der Hirnrinde des erwachsenen Menschen. J. Springer, Wien.

Wegiel, J., Kuchna, I., Nowicki, K., Imaki, H., Wegiel, J., Marchi, E., et al., 2010. The neuropathology of autism: Defects of neurogenesis and neuronal migration, and dysplastic changes. Acta Neuro-pathologica 119, 755–770.

Wiznitzer, M., 2004. Autism and tuberous sclerosis. Journal of Child Neurology 19, 675–679.

Yamashita, Y., Fujimoto, C., Nakajima, E., Isagai, T., Matsuishi, T., 2003. Possible association between congenital cytomegalovirus infection and ASD disorder. Journal of Autism and Developmental Disorders 33, 455–459.

Yokota, Y., Ghashgaei, H.T., Han, C., Watson, H., Campbell, K.J., Anton, E.S., 2007. Radial glial dependent and independent dynamics of interneuronal migration in the developing cerebral cortex. PLoS ONE 2, e794.

Yu, Y.C., Bultje, R.S., Wang, X., Shi, S.H., 2009. Specific synapses develop preferentially among sister excitatory neurons in the neocortex. Nature 458, 501–504.

Inhibitory and Excitatory Systems in Autism Spectrum Disorders

Gene J. Blatt

Department of Anatomy and Neurobiology,
Boston University School of Medicine, Boston MA, USA

OUTLINE

THE EXCITATION: INHIBITION HYPOTHESIS OF AUTISM

Autism spectrum disorders (ASD) include classical autism (autistic disorder) as well as related disorders having less severe manifestations. Autism is a behavioral disorder with deficits in social communication, delayed or severely impaired language, and stereotyped or repetitive behaviors (American Psychiatric Association, 2000). ASD are highly heritable (Folstein and Rosen-Shieldley, 2001; Rutter, 2000; Veenstra-VanderWeele et al., 2003) and there are multiple genes that contribute to the phenotype, making the disorder heterogeneous and complex in nature (see Chapters 2.1–2.4). Approximately 30% of affected individuals have seizures (Gillberg and Billstedt, 2000) and up to 70% have sharp spike activity recorded by electroencephalogram or magnetoencephalography (Lewine et al., 1999; Wheless et al., 2002). Hussman (2001) proposed that inhibitory γ-aminobutyric acid (GABA) is suppressed in the brains of individuals with ASD, suggesting that the excitatory circuitry may be favored. At approximately the same time as Hussman's article appeared, Blatt et al. (2001) published a study using postmortem tissue from adults with ASD demonstrating decreased density of ^{3}[H]-muscimol-labeled GABA-A receptors as well as its associated ^{3}[H]-flunitrazepam-labeled benzodiazepine binding sites in high binding CA and subicular subfields of the hippocampal formation. These results from the same ASD cases were later found by multiple concentration ligand binding to be a deficit in the number of GABA-A receptors and benzodiazepine binding sites [Bmax] and not due to the binding affinity of the ligands [Kd] (Guptill et al., 2007).

The idea that alterations in GABA combined with the higher tonic excitatory activity in the brains of individuals with autism led Rubenstein and Merzenich (2003) to the hypothesis that some forms of autism can be modeled by the idea that there is an increased ratio of excitation/inhibition (E/I) within critical neural systems in the ASD brain. The inherent idea behind the hypothesis is that there is increased 'noise,' due either to a disproportionately high level of excitation or a disproportionately low level of inhibition within the developing neural circuitry in the cerebral cortex. This then results in an unstable cortex that is highly vulnerable to seizure activity (Rubenstein and Merzenich, 2003). In addition, the authors further postulated that the resulting E/I imbalance in the cortex of individuals with ASD may also have delayed synapse maturation, and caused abnormal myelination and/or potential problems within the local circuitry and cellular mechanisms leading to the generation of hyperexcitable states. It is also important to note that the root cause of such imbalance within the synaptic circuitry is still undetermined, and is also complicated by an array of genetic, epigenetic, cellular, and molecular findings. There are also possible environmental influences, that have emerged in parallel with the report that there is an increasing incidence of ASD as high as 11.3 per 1,000 children aged 8 years of age (Centers for Disease Control and Prevention, 2012, based on 2008 survey; see also Chapter 1.1).

Recently, Yizhar et al. (2011) tested the E/I hypothesis in a freely moving animal (mouse) by designing chimeric redshifted opsins and optogenetically elevating the cellular E/I balance in the medial prefrontal cortex while the mice were performing behaviors relevant to learning and social function. Utilizing optrode recordings in anesthetized mice, the authors monitored the expression of step function opsins and modulated excitation, and monitored inhibition in transgenic mice encoded for parvalbumin/opsins where expression of a tagged enhanced yellow fluorescent protein was restricted to GABAergic parvalbumin-expressing neurons. Elevation of the E/I balance in mouse medial prefrontal cortex caused a profound impairment in cellular information processing associated with behavioral impairments, and compensatory elevation of inhibition was found to partially rescue the social deficits caused by E/I elevation (Yizhar et al., 2011).

In a follow-up review on genetic mechanisms known to predispose individuals to ASD, Rubenstein (2010) addressed the issue of how components of genetic pathways can contribute to the E/I imbalance. One way is to determine specific transcriptional pathways that are downstream of transcriptional factors controlling (or modulating) either excitatory or inhibitory neurons. As an example, mouse mutations of Dlx homeodomain transcription factors affect forebrain inhibitory neuronal development, as Dlx genes have widespread expression prenatally in progenitor cells of forebrain GABAergic neurons and postnatally in some types of mature GABAergic cortical interneurons. These mutations can affect development, particularly migration and differentiation of GABAergic interneurons, and mice lacking Dlx1 genes exhibit a selective degeneration of specific cortical

inhibitory neuronal types, resulting in decreased cortical inhibition and epilepsy (see Rubenstein, 2010 for review).

EXPERIMENTAL EVIDENCE OF CHANGES IN THE GABAergic SYSTEM IN AUTISM

Aberrations in the GABA system in ASD were virtually unexplored in the 20th century. In 2001, a treatise appeared suggesting that the GABAergic system potentially played an important role in the disorder (Hussman, 2001). That same year, we published the first account of a specific change in GABA receptors in a pilot study of postmortem tissue sections from the hippocampus, that had initially screened nine different neurotransmitter receptor types from four different systems including GABA, glutamate, 5-HT (5-hydroxytryptamine, or serotonin), and acetylcholine (Blatt et al., 2001). The study reported significantly decreased GABA-A receptor density and benzodiazepine binding site density (i.e., located on most GABA-A receptors) in high-binding hippocampal subfields in the adult autism group compared to age- and postmortem interval (PMI)-matched controls, but normal levels of 5-HT transporters, 5-HT2 receptors, high-affinity choline uptake sites, muscarinic receptors type 1, N-methyl-D-aspartate (NMDA) receptors, and kainate receptors. These results, although from a limited sample size, provided a direction of research to pursue, because prior to that publication, nearly all ASD research had focused on peripheral 5-HT levels due to the observations of increased blood levels of 5-HT (i.e., hyperserotonemia). The initial GABA-A and benzodiazepine results were expanded in a multiple concentration binding study. This found that the decreased density of both markers was due to a decrease in the number of receptors (Bmax) in the CA and subicular subfields, and not due to the binding affinity of the receptors/binding sites of the ligands (Guptill et al., 2007). Fatemi et al. (2002) found significantly lower levels of the two key GABA-synthesizing enzymes, GAD65 and GAD67, in the cerebellum and parietal cortex, suggesting that lower levels of GABA may be present in the ASD brain compared to controls. Yip et al. (2007; 2008; 2009) followed those studies with three *in situ* hybridization investigations to determine which cell types in the cerebellum had decreased levels of GAD isoforms. They reported decreased levels of GAD67 mRNA in the Purkinje cells (Figure 3.8.1), increased levels of GAD67 mRNA in cerebellar interneurons in the molecular layer, and decreased levels of GAD65 mRNA in the dentate nucleus (see Blatt and Fatemi, 2011, for review).

These studies were followed by investigations of various hippocampal and neocortical areas in autism examining ^{3}[H]-muscimol-labeled GABA-A

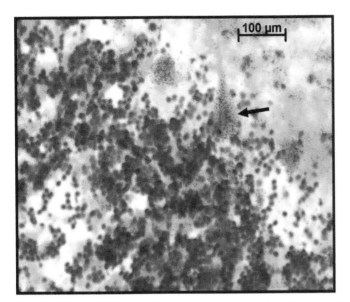

FIGURE 3.8.1 *In situ* hybridization demonstrating labeling of glutamic acid decarboxylase (GAD) 67 mRNA in Purkinje cells of the posterior lateral cerebellar cortex (Crus II region) in a control case (arrow pointing to silver grain accumulations within a Purkinje cell). Results from this study comparing autism cases versus controls demonstrated significant reductions in GAD 67 mRNA in the autism groups (Yip et al., 2007). This suggests that remaining Purkinje cells in the cerebellar hemisphere in autism cases are deficient in a key enzyme critical for the synthesis of GABA.

receptors, [3][H]-CGP54626-labeled GABA-B receptors, and [3][H]-flunitrazepam-labeled benzodiazepine binding site number and binding affinity. In three studies it was found that there were significant reductions in the number of GABA-A receptors and benzodiazepine binding sites, and decreases in the density of GABA-B receptors in the anterior cingulate cortex (Brodmann area 24), posterior cingulate cortex (Brodmann area 23), and the fusiform gyrus (Brodmann area 37), some throughout the superficial and deep layers and others within specific layers (Oblak et al., 2009; 2010; 2011a; see Figures 3.8.2 and 3.8.3 and Table 3.8.1). The cingulate and fusiform cortices are important functionally and related changes in behavioral phenotypes are present in individuals with ASD.

The anterior cingulate cortex plays important roles in social-emotional and social-communicative functions as well as in pain perception; the posterior cingulate cortex is preferentially involved in visuospatial recognition (Olson and Musil, 1992; Olson et al., 1996). It is part of the default network recruited when subjects see the faces or hear the voices of individuals who are emotionally important in their lives (Maddock et al., 2001), and it modulates emotion (Mayberg et al., 1999). The fusiform gyrus is a large region in the inferior temporal cortex that plays important roles in object and face recognition, and recognition of facial expressions is located in the fusiform face area (FFA), which is activated in imaging studies when parts of faces or pictures of facial expressions are presented to the subjects (e.g., Kleinhans et al., 2008; Pelphrey et al., 2007; Perlman et al., 2011; Pierce and Redcay, 2008). All three regions may contribute to ASD-related behaviors.

Reported decreases in GABA receptors suggest an imbalance in the ratio of excitatory/inhibitory drive within these cortical regions. One entity that does not appear to be a contributing factor to the pathologies, at least in the posterior cingulate and fusiform cortices in ASD, is the density of calbindin- and parvalbumin-expressing subpopulations of GABAergic interneurons, since both of these were found to be at normal levels (Oblak et al., 2011b). Levitt (2005) has suggested, however, that disruption of GABAergic interneuron development may underlie ASD. In support of this, GABA interneurons appear to play an important role in Rett syndrome (RTT; Chao et al., 2010), one of the ASD. In RTT, there are mutations in the X-linked *MECP2* gene encoding the methyl-CpG-binding protein 2 (MeCP2) and behaviorally, the syndrome is characterized by developmental regression, motor abnormalities, seizures, and ASD-related behaviors, including stereotyped behaviors (e.g., Chahrour and Zoghbi, 2007; Lam et al., 2000). A study used mice lacking the *MeCP2* gene in a subset of forebrain GABAergic interneurons, and found that these animals displayed features of ASD, including repetitive behaviors. They also had presynaptic reduction in GAD and GABA immunoreactivity, suggesting that MeCP2 is critical for normal GABAergic function (Chao et al., 2010) and that disturbance of GABAergic interneurons in development can upset the E/I balance in neuropsychiatric phenotypes including RTT.

GABA-A receptor downregulation has also been reported in postmortem tissue samples from individuals with ASD, via biochemical analyses. This receptor protein dysregulation showed significantly altered expression of GABRA1, GABRA2, GABRA3, and GABARB3 subunits in parietal cortex (area 40); GABRA1 and GABRB3 subunits in cerebellum; and GABRA1 subunit in superior frontal cortex (area 9) (Fatemi et al., 2009a). Another investigation by the same group examined GABA-B receptor protein expression in the same three cortical areas (Fatemi et al., 2009b). In this study, levels of GABA-B1 and GABA-B2 subunits were also found to be dysregulated. Significant changes in the levels of GABBR1 and GABBR2 were found in the cerebellum, but only GABBR1 subunit expression was altered in area 40 and area 9. Dysregulation of GABA-B receptor subunits may contribute to seizure activity and/or cognitive problems in individuals with autism (Fatemi et al., 2009b). Taken together, experimental results from postmortem tissue studies on the GABAergic system provide strong evidence that

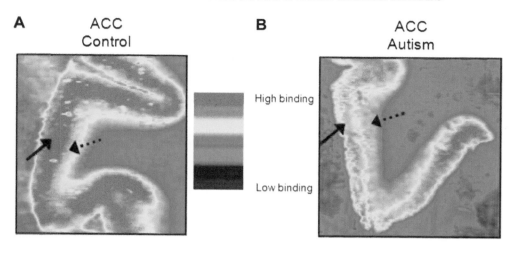

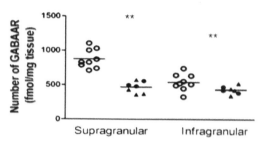

FIGURE 3.8.2   Examples of pseudocolored images of [³H]-muscimol-labeled GABA_A receptors (15 nM concentration selected from a seven concentration binding study) in the anterior cingulate cortex (Brodmann area 24; ACC) in a control (A) and autism (B) case. Solid black arrows demonstrate the location of sampling in the supragranular (superficial) layers (layers I–III); arrows with dashed lines indicate sampling in the infra-granular layers (layers V–VI). In the [³H]-muscimol-binding experiments (C), the number (Bmax) of GABA_A receptors in the supragranular ($p = 0.02$) and infragranular layers ($p = 0.04$) in the autism cases was significantly (**) decreased (student t-test). *Modified from Figure 4 in Oblak et al. (2009).*

inhibitory tone in the cerebellum, limbic cortical areas (hippocampus, anterior and posterior cingulate cortex), and neocortex (parietal area 40, prefrontal area 9) and the fusiform gyrus (area 37) in the temporal lobe is dys-regulated in the ASD brain. These findings suggest that the altered E/I balance may at least include depressed inhibitory influences on neurons and circuits throughout the ASD brain. It is unknown whether these alterations are primary in nature or due to compensatory changes due to glutamatergic dysregulation. A discussion on excitatory systems follows.

EXPERIMENTAL EVIDENCE OF CHANGES IN THE GLUTAMATERGIC SYSTEM IN ASD

The fragile X mental retardation disorder, under the umbrella of ASD, lacks the fragile X mental retardation protein (FMRP) and is the most common form of human mental retardation. The X-linked *FMR1* gene that prevents the expression of FMRP (O'Donnell and Warren, 2002) causes moderate to severe mental retardation and also results in abnormalities, including hyperactivity, anxiety, obsessive-compulsive, and autism-related behaviors (Bakker and Oostra, 2003; Hagerman, 2002; see Bear et al., 2004, and Chapter 4.5 for review). The *Fmr1* knockout mouse (e.g., Bakker and Oostra, 2003) has behavioral abnormalities as well, including increased locomotor activity, increased susceptibility to seizures, and morphological anomalies that include longer dendritic arbors with thin spines (Irwin et al., 2002; Nimchinsky et al., 2001). It was from studies of this mouse model that Huber et al. (2002) suggested that there was a connection between metabotropic glutamate receptor (mGluR) activity and the fragile X phenotype (Bear et al., 2004). A further link to long-term depression (LTD), important for

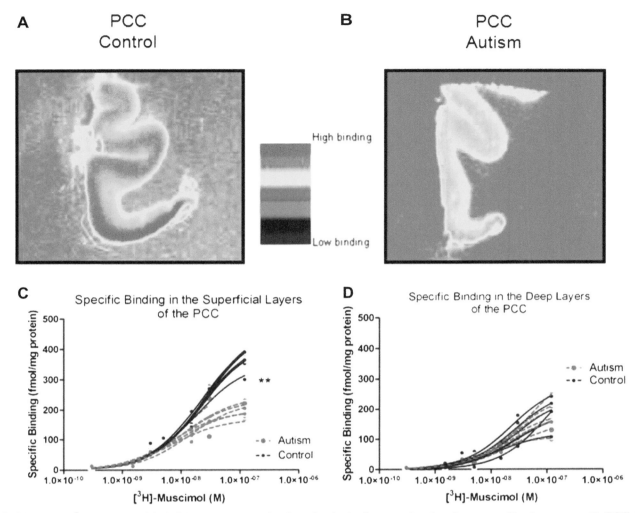

FIGURE 3.8.3 [³H]-muscimol-labeled GABA$_A$ receptor binding density in the posterior cingulate cortex (Brodmann area 23; PCC) from one adult control case (A) and one age- and postmortem-interval-matched case with autism (B). Images were taken from [³H]-sensitive film (concentration 15 nM selected from a seven concentration binding experiment). Note the reduced binding density in the superficial layers (layers I–IV) in the patient with autism (B) compared to the control (A) case. (C and D) Two examples of individual binding curves for the [³H]-muscimol study are illustrated in the superficial (C) and deep (D) layers of the PCC Each line represents an individual case. Smooth curves indicate fit to the hyperbolic binding equation with control in blue and autism in red. Asterisk (**) denotes significant decrease in binding in the superficial layers in the autism group (C) but normal binding levels in the deep (layers V–VI) layers (D). *Modified from Figures 1 and 5 in Oblak et al. (2011a).*

TABLE 3.8.1 Summary of Findings for GABAergic Receptor Subtypes in Superficial and Deep Layers in the Anterior Cingulate (ACC), Posterior Cingulate (PCC) and Fusiform Gyrus (FG) in Adult Autism Cases Compared to Age- and Postmortem-Interval-Matched Controls (Oblak et al., 2009; 2010; 2011a)

	BZD		GABA$_A$		GABA$_B$	
	Superficial layers	**Deep layers**	**Superficial layers**	**Deep layers**	**Superficial layers**	**Deep layers**
ACC	Significant decrease	Significant decrease	Significant decrease	Significant decrease	Significant decrease	Not significant
PCC	Significant decrease	Not significant	Significant decrease	Not significant	Significant decrease	Significant decrease
FG	Significant decrease	Significant decrease	Significant decrease	Not significant	Significant decrease	Significant decrease

activity-guided synapse stabilization/elimination, was made earlier with mGluRs when Oliet et al. (1997) discovered that there were two types of LTD in the hippocampus, one that involved NMDA receptors and the other involving postsynaptic group 1 mGluRs. From this discovery came the development of the animal model, which led Bear et al. (2004) to develop the mGluR theory of fragile X mental retardation.

In brief, the theory argues that overactive signaling by group 1 mGluRs, including mGluR1/5, is the key contributing factor to the psychiatric and neurological symptoms of fragile X syndrome. It was then determined that long-term potentiation (LTP), important for long-term synaptic strength in layer V of the visual neocortex, depends primarily on mGluR5 activation, and that mGluR5-mediated synaptic plasticity is lacking in FMRP knockout mice (Wilson and Cox, 2007). The link between altered synaptic function and mental impairment, however, was still unclear. Nakamoto et al. (2007) cultured hippocampal neurons and used short interfering RNAs (siRNAs) against *Fmr1* to demonstrate that hypersensitive (i.e., action potential driven) AMPA receptor internalization in response to mGluR signaling in dendrites could represent a major molecular defect in fragile X syndrome, which can be corrected by an mGluR5 antagonist (e.g., 2-methyl-6-phenylethynyl-pyridine, MPEP). Such rescue drugs, including allosteric modulators, were also thought to be potentially useful by other investigators (Bear, 2005; Catania et al., 2007; Dölen and Bear, 2008; 2009; Rodriguez and Williams, 2007). *Fmr1* knockout mice are considered ideal for testing the efficacy of therapeutic strategies aimed at treating the cognitive impairments in fragile X (Krueger et al., 2011; see Cleva and Olive, 2011 for review; and Pacey et al., 2011 for subchronic administration of both MPEP and/or the GABA-B receptor orthosteric agonist R-baclofen; Levenga et al., 2011 for discussion of a new mGluR5 antagonist, AFQ056, for treatment of fragile X syndrome; and Jacquemont et al., 2011 for epigenetic modification of the *FMR1* gene in conjunction with the use of AFQ056).

The selective mGluR5 antagonist MPEP has also proved useful in treating repetitive behaviors in a BTBR mouse model that shows robust ASD-related behaviors (Silverman et al., 2010). Recently, Auerbach and Bear (2010) updated the role of group 1 mGluRs in synaptic plasticity. The authors reported their actions on the same set of synapses of both the priming of long-term potentiation and the inducing of long-term depression, responsible for both triggering synaptic modifications and stimulating protein synthesis. Thus, changes in neocortical excitatory synaptic circuitry are likely to play an important role in fragile X syndrome as well as in upsetting the E/I synaptic balance. Postmortem studies in the superior frontal cortex in adult autism cases have recently revealed significantly reduced levels of FMRP protein. Significantly increased levels of mGluR5 receptor protein in children with autism have also been reported (Fatemi and Folsom, 2011). In another postmortem study, increased levels of mGluR5 receptor protein were also found in the vermis in children with ASD (Fatemi et al., 2011). Finally, Piras et al. (unpublished results) have recently demonstrated an increase in mGluR1 mRNA via an *in situ* hybridization study in the lateral cerebellar hemisphere area Crus II. The study used postmortem adult autism cases compared to age- and postmortem-interval-matched controls. mGluR1 is abundant in the cerebellum whereas mGluR5 is robustly expressed in the cerebral cortex.

Carlson (2012) emphasizes that there is evidence that other glutamate-type receptors may be altered in ASD, including NMDA, AMPA, and kainate, although the relationships between these receptors and ASD-associated phenotypes are less well understood. In an early study, Purcell et al. (2001) used postmortem cerebellar tissue from 10 individuals with autism compared to 23 matched controls to identify genes via complementary DNA (cDNA) microarray that were significantly up- or downregulated in autism. Results demonstrated that the mRNA levels of several genes were upregulated in autism, including the excitatory amino acid transporter type 1 (EAAT1) and AMPAR1 glutamate receptors. Ligand-binding studies also revealed significantly decreased AMPA receptor density in the cerebellum in individuals with autism, suggesting that dysregulation of glutamate may be a contributing factor to the pathogenesis of the disorder (Purcell et al., 2001). Interestingly, in a model of serotonin (5-HT) depleted mice, Boylan et al. (2007) reported a significant decrease in cerebral cortical AMPA glutamate receptor binding at postnatal day 15, and suggested that behavioral changes in these animals including sensorimotor, cognitive, and social deficits and, hence, changes in both 5-HT transporters and AMPA receptors, may be due to deficiencies in axonal pruning to critical cortical areas. Shinohe et al. (2006) reported that serum glutamate levels were increased in patients with ASD. This study was performed on a small sample of patients with autism (n = 18) compared with 19 age-matched male controls. It also showed a positive correlation between serum glutamate levels and the Autism Diagnostic Interview-Revised (ADI-R) social scores (Shinohe et al., 2006). This hyperglutamatergic hypothesis, suggesting that an abnormality in transmission, higher seizure risk, and increased inflammatory events plays a role in the pathophysiology of ASD was addressed in a published letter by Fatemi (2007). In that response, Fatemi points to a few prior studies that may support this hypothesis, including his findings of decreased levels of glutamic acid decarboxylase enzymes GAD65 and GAD67, since glutamate production is also part of that synthesis pathway (Fatemi et al., 2002). Decreased GAD67 mRNA in Purkinje cells is also involved in converting glutamate to GABA (Yip et al., 2007). There are also various reports of increased presence of neuroglia in the ASD brain (Vargas et al., 2005), which could take up glutamate from extracellular compartments and participate in the conversion from glutamine to glutamate via the activity of glutaminase (McKenna, 2007). Ongoing experiments in our laboratory are investigating number and affinity of these additional types of glutamate receptors in both the cerebellum and cerebral cortical areas in ASD. Further evidence for ionotropic glutamate receptor dysfunction in ASD is discussed in Chapter 4.7, including genetic evidence from *Shank3*-deficient mice.

NEUROIMAGING STUDIES OF THE GABAergic AND GLUTAMATERGIC SYSTEMS IN ASD

Advances in imaging technology now allow a number of transmitter and metabolite levels in the brain to be determined while the individual is in the scanner. The advent of magnetic resonance spectroscopy (MRS) has added a new, non-invasive dimension to studies of the brain, and interpretation of state-specific cortical and subcortical areas can be analyzed in real time. Harada et al. (2011) evaluated the GABAergic and glutamatergic systems in the frontal lobe and lenticular nucleus of 12 patients with ASD and 10 controls, using a three-tesla MRS. These authors reported lower GABA levels in the frontal lobes of the autism patient group, and a significantly lower ratio of GABA/NAA (*N*-acetyl-aspartate – a derivative of aspartate, an excitatory transmitter found in neurons, which, like glutamate, gives off a strong signal in imaging) but not in the lenticular nucleus. A similar significant reduction in the frontal lobe was demonstrated in the same autism group for the GABA/glutamate ratio compared to normal controls (Harada et al., 2011). These results translate to increased E/I balance in the frontal lobes that would predict increased excitatory activity. New MRS techniques include the administration of radiolabeled tracers; allowing measurements of low molecular weight compounds within a specific volume of brain tissue (see Dager et al., 2008).

Chugani (2012) has summarized GABA-A receptor binding studies using imaging techniques over the last decade. A small percentage of ASD patients have been identified with abnormalities in chromosome 15q11–13, a region that codes for three GABA-A receptor subunit genes (*GABRA5*, *GABRB3*, and *GABRG3*) (Buxbaum et al., 2002; Menold et al., 2001; Silva et al., 2002). In brief,

there were a number of imaging studies in patients with neurological disorders other than autism that exhibit some aspects of the autism-related phenotype. Deletion of the maternal chromosome that contains this region results in Angelman syndrome. These patients have severe mental retardation, lack of speech, and epilepsy. However, deletion of the paternal chromosome results in Prader–Willi syndrome, which is characterized by mild to moderate mental retardation, hypotonia, and obesity. Holopainen et al. (2001) demonstrated decreased ^{11}[C]-flumazenil binding to GABA-A receptor β3 subunit in frontal and parietal lobes, hippocampus, and cerebellum in patients with Angelman syndrome, while Lucignani et al. (2004) found reduced binding of the same radioisotope in the cingulate, frontal, and temporal cortices in Prader–Willi syndrome patients (see Chugani, 2012, for review).

In contrast again to decreased GABA and GABA-A receptor subtype levels, Page and colleagues (2006) found significantly elevated glutamate/glutamine (Glx) peak levels in the amygdala and hippocampus, but not in the parietal cortex, in an early MRS study of 25 adults with autism compared to 21 normal controls. Another study, however, found decreased Glx peaks in the cingulate in high-functioning adults with autism (e.g., Bernardi et al., 2011, in an MRS study; see also Chugani, 2012). New advances in MRS technology should be able to better separate the peaks of glutamate and glutamine as well as more accurately sample GABA levels to gain more insights into how the E/I ratio is changed in specific brain areas in children and adults with ASD.

EXPERIMENTAL EVIDENCE OF CHANGES IN THE SEROTONERGIC SYSTEM IN AUTISM AND ITS IMPORTANCE FOR PHARMACOTHERAPEUTIC TREATMENT

Serotonin (5-HT) acts as a neurotransmitter but also plays important roles as a trophic and differentiation factor in neural development (see Whitaker-Azmitia, 2001, for review). In both nonhuman primates and normal humans, 5-HT is thought to participate in the modulation of social behavior (Knutson et al., 1998; Stein et al., 2002, for review) and in aggression and hostility (Coccaro and Kavoussi, 1997). There is substantial evidence that some individuals with autism have differences in their 5-HT metabolism. Many individuals with ASD and their relatives have elevated levels of whole-blood or platelet serotonin levels (i.e., hyperserotonemia) (Abramson et al., 1989; Anderson et al., 1987; Cook et al., 1993; 1994; Cook and Leventhal, 1996; Lam et al., 2006; Leboyer et al, 1999; Leventhal et al., 1990; Piven et al., 1991; Schain and Freedman, 1961; Singh et al., 1997). Additional studies have revealed genetic variation in the 5-HT transporter (5-HTT) in some individuals with autism (e.g., Wassink et al., 2007). Recent findings from our laboratory provide strong evidence of alterations in brain 5-HT systems of individuals with ASD, with reductions in density of binding to ^{3}[H]-8-OH-DPAT-labeled 5-HT1A receptors and ^{125}[I]-DOI-labeled 5-HT2A receptors in both the anterior and posterior cingulate cortex and in the fusiform gyrus (which play important roles in social-emotional and social-communicative behaviors, and facial-emotional and facial recognition), but no or little change in binding to 5-HTT (unpublished results). This suggests that more specific pharmacotherapies targeted toward affected 5-HT receptor subtypes rather than 5-HTT may lead to improved therapeutic outcomes.

There is a paucity of information on the central 5-HT system in ASD cases, making it extremely difficult to direct useful pharmacotherapies toward affected receptor target sites. In one of the only morphological studies conducted on the 5-HT system in ASD, Azmitia et al. (2011) used postmortem tissue from individual cases of autism aged 2 to 29 years compared to age-matched controls. These investigators utilized an antibody directed toward 5-HTT and analysis of the 5-HT fibers, and they revealed that the number of axons in all ages was increased in forebrain pathways and their terminal regions of temporal lobe cortex. The authors concluded that selective serotonin reuptake inhibitors (SSRIs) directed specifically toward 5-HTT should be used with caution when treating children with ASD. This striking result could also suggest that there may be dysregulation of 5-HT at the synapse and/or a possible downregulation of postsynaptic receptors in brain areas in individuals with autism. The most likely candidate 5-HT receptors are the 5-HT1A autoreceptor (presynaptic) and/or postsynaptic receptor, and the largely postsynaptic 5-HT2A, the latter being the most abundant serotonergic receptor in the brain (see Nichols and Nichols, 2008, for review). The lack of identified targets for drug treatment has led to mixed results, with potentially harmful effects in individuals with ASD.

Although most individuals with ASD receive some type of pharmacotherapy, much of it off-label (Oswald and Sonenklar, 2007, and see Chapters 1.6 and 1.7), the efficacy of the available pharmacological treatments with respect to the core symptoms of ASD is limited (Gibbs, 2010; Chapters 1.6 and 1.7). Based largely on analogy to their effectiveness in treating obsessive compulsive disorder, SSRIs, which inhibit the uptake of 5-HT by the serotonin transporter (5-HTU; 5-HTT; SERT) at the presynaptic terminal, are widely prescribed for treatment of repetitive behaviors in children and adolescents with ASD and constitute the greatest global market share of medications for autism (King et al., 2009). In the most comprehensive clinical

trial to date, 149 patients with ASD, 5–17 years of age, from six academic centers, were administered citalopram hydrobromide (which targets the serotonin uptake site or transporter) or placebo for 12 weeks. Not only did the experimental group fail to show significant improvement, but the citalopram treatment group exhibited an elevated incidence of adverse events including increased energy level and impulsiveness, decreased concentration, hyperactivity, stereotypy, and insomnia (King et al., 2009). These findings are in general agreement with a meta-analysis of clinical trials for SSRIs conducted recently by Williams et al. (2010), which concluded that there is no evidence of effect of SSRIs in children with ASD and emerging evidence of harm.

In addition, there is limited evidence of the effectiveness of SSRIs in adults with ASD but due to the smaller sizes of these studies, the results are less clear and need to be repeated in larger cohorts (Williams et al., 2010). Interestingly, the issue of high 5-HT blood levels in pregnant mothers, including due mothers' intake of SSRIs to treat depression, has been hypothesized as a possible contributing factor toward the increased prevalence of ASD (Hadjikhani, 2010). This may be a result of increased 5-HT crossing the blood–brain barrier, which is not fully formed until about 2 years of age, causing a loss of serotonergic terminals (see Whitaker-Azmitia, 2005). Further, Winter et al. (2008) found significantly decreased levels of 5-HT but not of dopamine in the cerebellum at postnatal day 14 in prenatally (E16) virally exposed mice, indicating that disruption of the 5-HT system following prenatal viral infection can model 5-HT changes in neurodevelopmental disorders such as schizophrenia and autism.

NEUROIMAGING STUDIES OF THE SEROTONERGIC SYSTEM IN ASD

In a positron emission tomography (PET) imaging study, it was reported that there is abnormal 5-HT synthesis in brain regions in ASD (Chandana et al., 2005; Chugani et al., 1997; 1999). Male children with autism have reduced 5-HT synthesis in their frontal and thalamic regions and increased synthesis in the cerebellum (Chugani et al., 1997; 1999). The emerging idea that specific 5-HT receptor types are negatively affected in ASD has renewed focus on the discovery of novel biomarkers in autism, but these studies are limited to high-functioning individuals. In a 2010 study, PET imaging was used on high-functioning young adults with autism (n = 20, aged 18–26 years), to determine the occurrence of changes in 5-HTT (Nakamura et al., 2010). These authors found reduced 5-HTT binding in the anterior and posterior cingulate cortices, that was associated with impairment of social cognition in individuals with high-functioning autism. Reduced 5-HTT binding in the thalamus also correlated with repetitive and/or obsessive behaviors and interests. In contrast, the same study found increased dopamine transporter binding in the orbital frontal cortex in the same study group, indicating a significant inverse relationship between 5-HTT and the binding of the dopamine transporter (Nakamura et al., 2010). In a single photon emission computed tomography (SPECT) study in very high functioning children and adolescents with autism (Leiter method IQ = 70–109), in a very limited study sample Makkonen et al. (2008) found normal 5-HTT (SERT) binding levels in midbrain and temporal lobe areas but reduced binding in the medial frontal lobe (more evident in the adolescents).

In an *in vivo* SPECT study in adults with Asperger's syndrome, Murphy et al. (2006) used the ligand 5-^{123}[I]-R91150 that is selective for 5-HT2A receptors, and found a significant reduction in receptor binding and findings related to abnormal social communication. A PET study by Goldberg et al. (2009) reported that the parents of children with ASD have significantly reduced 5-HT2 receptor binding compared to controls, and that their platelet 5-HT levels were negatively correlated with cortical 5-HT2 binding potential. Moresco et al. (2002) found that 5-HT2A receptors modulate personality traits and Veenstra-VanderWeele (2002) has identified the 5-HT2A gene as a functional candidate gene in autism. In contrast with the increased 5-HTT levels in platelets discussed earlier, significant decreases in platelet 5-HT2A receptor binding were reported in ASD patients (Cook et al., 1993; McBride et al., 1989).

ADDITIONAL COMMENTS AND CONCLUSIONS

There is now emerging experimental evidence that there are abnormalities in a number of neurotransmitter systems in autism, with perhaps the strongest evidence to date focusing on specific aspects of the GABAergic, glutamatergic, and serotonergic systems. Dysregulation of key synthesizing enzymes, and specific types of transporters and receptors in cerebellum, hippocampal, and/or neocortical areas can all contribute to upsetting the E/I balance at the synaptic level, and can influence circuits that participate in autism-related behaviors. The complex nature and heterogeneity of the disorder, coupled with the varying prenatal and postnatal developmental expression of each biomarker, make identifying its many etiologies a daunting task. Nevertheless, molecular geneticists are making progress in identifying the vast array of candidate genes for autism, and are now grouping them into subsets based on

development neural structures/processes and function. For example, Hussman et al. (2011) recently categorized groups of genes identified from genome-wide association studies (GWAS) by applying a linear filter with computer simulations to reveal autism datasets. A large subset of genes were identified that are involved in neurite outgrowth and guidance of axons and dendrites, as well as groups of genes with roles in synaptic function, including those that play roles in E/I balance. Among the many genes identified in the E/I grouping were *GABBR2*, the gene that encodes the GABA-B2 subunit; *GRIK2* and *GRIK4* that encode kainate (glutamate) receptor subtypes; and *GRM3*, important for verbal memory and encoding the metabotropic glutamate receptor 3 (Hussman et al., 2011).

It is clear that we have only just begun to uncover which specific markers are affected in autism, and it will undoubtedly emerge that different combinations of genes, including some that target transporter/receptor proteins, are involved in the ASD subsets affecting particular pathway(s) and, in turn, behaviors. Ultimately, such identified markers will be critical in developing novel pharmacotherapies. Currently, the use of SSRIs has been questioned for treating individuals with autism. Both postmortem and imaging studies are revealing that specific serotonergic receptor subtypes, such as 5-HT2A receptors, appear more affected in different brain regions than the 5-HT transporter, despite findings that there are candidate genes identified as well as robust findings of elevated 5-HT levels in the periphery. Technological advances in imaging, such as magnetic resonance spectroscopy (MRS), have been used to detect separate GABA, glutamine, and glutamate peak levels in specific brain areas, and this is one example of how new, higher resolution data will enable important strides to be made toward understanding the mechanism(s) and pathway(s) that contribute to the multifaceted etiologies of this disorder.

References

Abramson, R.K., Wright, H.H., Carpenter, R., Brennan, W., Lumpuy, O., Cole, E., et al., 1989. Elevated blood serotonin in autistic probands and their first-degree relatives. Journal of Autism and Developmental Disorders 19, 397–407.

American Psychiatric Association (APA), 2000. Diagnostic and statistical manual of mental disorders, fourth ed. Text. Rev. 1994. APA, Washington, DC.

Anderson, G.M., Freedman, D.X., Cohen, D.J., Volkmar, F.R., Hoder, E.L., McPhedran, P., et al., 1987. Whole blood serotonin in autistic and normal subjects. Journal of Child Psychology and Psychiatry 28, 885–900.

Auerbach, B.D., Bear, M.F., 2010. Loss of the fragile X mental retardation protein decouples metabotropic glutamate receptor dependent priming of long-term potentiation from protein synthesis. Journal of Neurophysiology 104, 1047–1051.

Azmitia, E.C., Singh, J.S., Whitaker-Azmitia, P.M., 2011. Increased serotonin axons (immunoreative to 5-HT transporter) in post-mortem brains from young autism donors. Neuropharmacology 60, 1347–1354.

Bakker, C.E., Oostra, B.A., 2003. Understanding fragile X syndrome: Insights from animal models. Cytogenetic and Genome Research 100, 111–123.

Bear, M.F., 2005. Therapeutic implications of the mGluR theory of fragile X mental retardation. Genes, Brain and Behavior 4, 393–398.

Bear, M.F., Huber, K.M., Warren, S.T., 2004. The mGluR theory of fragile X mental retardation. Trends in Neurosciences 27, 370–377.

Bernardi, S., Anagnostou, E., Shen, J., Kolevzon, A., Buxbaum, J.D., Hollander, E., et al., 2011. In vivo ^{1}h-magnetic resonance spectroscopy study of the attentional networks in autism. Brain Research 1380, 198–205.

Blatt, G.J., Fatemi, S.H., 2011. Alterations in GABAergic biomarkers in the autism brain: Research findings and clinical implications. Anatomical Record 294, 1646–1652.

Blatt, G.J., Fitzgerald, C.M., Guptill, J.T., Booker, A.B., Kemper, T.L., Bauman, M.L., 2001. Density and distribution of hippocampal neurotransmitter receptors in autism: An autoradiographic study. Journal of Autism and Developmental Disorders 31, 537–543.

Boylan, C.B., Blue, M.E., Hohmann, C.F., 2007. Modeling early cortical serotonergic deficits in autism. Behavioral Brain Research 176, 94–108.

Buxbaum, J.D., Silverman, J.M., Smith, C.J., Greenberg, D.A., Kilifarski, M., Reichet, J., et al., 2002. Association between a GABRB3 polymorphism and autism. Molecular Psychiatry 7, 311–316.

Carlson, G.C., 2012. Glutamate receptor dysfunction and drug targets across models of autism spectrum disorders. Pharmacology, Biochemistry, and Behavior 100, 850–854.

Catania, M.V., D'Antoni, S., Bonaccorso, C.M., Aronica, E., Bear, M.F., Nicoletti, F., 2007. Group I metabotropic glutamate receptors: A role in neurodevelopmental disorders? Molecular Neurobiology 35, 298–307.

Centers for Disease Control and Prevention (CDC), 2012. Prevalence of autism spectrum disorders – Autism and developmental disabilities monitoring network, 14 sites, United States, 2008. MMWR Surveillance Summary 61, 1–19.

Chahrour, M., Zoghbi, H.Y., 2007. The story of Rett syndrome: From clinic to neurobiology. Neuron 56, 422–437.

Chandana, S.R., Behen, M.E., Juhász, C., Muzik, O., Rothermel, R.D., Mangner, T.J., et al., 2005. Significance of abnormalities in developmental trajectory and asymmetry of cortical serotonin synthesis in autism. International Journal of Developmental Neuroscience 23, 171–182.

Chao, H.T., Chen, H., Samaco, R.C., Xue, M., Chahrour, M., Yoo, J., et al., 2010. Dysfunction in GABA signalling mediates autism-like stereotypies and Rett syndrome phenotypes. Nature 468, 263–269.

Chugani, D.C., 2012. Neuroimaging and neurochemistry of autism. Pediatric Clinics of North America 59, 63–73.

Chugani, D.C., Muzik, O., Behen, M., Rothermel, R., Janisse, J.J., Lee, J., et al., 1999. Developmental changes in brain serotonin synthesis capacity in autistic and nonautistic children. Annals of Neurology 45, 287–295.

Chugani, D.C., Muzik, O., Rothermel, R., Behen, M., Chakraborty, P., Mangner, T., et al., 1997. Altered serotonin synthesis in the dentatothalamocortical pathway in autistic boys. Annals of Neurology 42, 666–669.

Cleva, R.M., Olive, M.F., 2011. Positive allosteric modulators of type 5 metabotropic glutamate receptors (mGluR5) and their therapeutic potential for the treatment of CNS disorders. Molecules 16, 2097–2106.

Coccaro, E.F., Kavoussi, R.J., 1997. Fluoxetine and impulsive aggressive behavior in personality-disordered subjects. Archives of General Psychiatry 54, 1081–1088.

Cook, E., Leventhal, B., 1996. The Serotonin system in autism. Current Opinion in Pediatrics 8, 348–354.

Cook Jr., E.H., Arora, R.C., Anderson, G.M., Berry-Kravis, E.M., Yan, S.Y., Yeoh, H.C., et al., 1993. Platelet serotonin studies in hyperserotonemic relatives of children with autistic disorder. Life Science 52, 2005–2015.

Cook Jr., E.H., Charak, D.A., Arida, J., Spohn, J.A., Roizen, N.J., Leventhal, B.L., 1994. Depressive and obsessive-compulsive symptoms in hyperserotonemic parents of children with autistic disorder. Psychiatry Research 52, 25–33.

Dager, S.R., Corrigan, N.M., Richards, T.L., Posse, S., 2008. Research applications of magnetic resonance spectroscopy to investigate psychiatric disorders. Topics in Magnetic Resonance Imaging 19, 81–96.

Dölen, G., Bear, M.F., 2008. Role for metabotropic glutamate receptor 5 (mGluR5) in the pathogenesis of fragile X syndrome. Journal of Physiology 586, 1503–1508.

Dölen, G., Bear, M.F., 2009. Fragile X syndrome and autism: From disease model to therapeutic targets. Journal of Neurodevelopmental Disorders 1, 133–140.

Fatemi, S.H., 2007. The hyperglutamatergic hypothesis of autism. Progress in Neuropsychopharmacology & Biological Psychiatry 30, 1472–1477.

Fatemi, S.H., Folsom, T.D., 2011. Dysregulation of fragile X mental retardation protein and metabotropic glutamate receptor 5 in superior frontal cortex of individuals with autism: A postmortem brain study. Molecular Autism 2, 1–11.

Fatemi, S.H., Folsom, T.D., Kneeland, R.E., Liesch, S.B., 2011. Metabotropic glutamate receptor 5 upregulation in children with autism is associated with underexpression of both fragile X mental retardation protein and GABAA receptor beta 3 in adults with autism. Anatomical Record 294, 1635–1645.

Fatemi, S.H., Folsom, T.D., Reutiman, T.J., Thuras, P.D., 2009. Expression of GABA(B) receptors is altered in brains of subjects with autism. Cerebellum 8, 64–69.

Fatemi, S.H., Halt, A.R., Stary, J.M., Kanodia, R., Schulz, S.C., Realmuto, G.R., 2002. Glutamic acid decarboxylase 65 and 67 kDa proteins are reduced in autistic parietal and cerebellar cortices. Biological Psychiatry 52, 805–810.

Fatemi, S.H., Reutiman, T.J., Folsom, T.D., Thuras, P.D., 2009. GABA(A) receptor downregulation in brains of subjects with autism. Journal of Autism and Developmental Disorders 39, 223–230.

Folstein, S.E., Rosen-Sheidley, B., 2001. Genetics of autism: Complex aetiology for a heterogeneous disorder. Nature Reviews Genetics 2, 943–955.

Gibbs, T.T., 2010. Pharmacological treatment of Autism. In: Blatt, G.J. (Ed.), The Neurochemical Basis of Autism. Springer, New York, pp. 245–267.

Gillberg, C., Billstedt, E., 2000. Autism and Asperger syndrome: Coexistence with other clinical disorders. Acta Psychiatrica Scandinavica 102, 321–330.

Goldberg, J., Anderson, G.M., Zwaigenbaum, L., Hall, G.B., Nahmias, C., Thompson, A., et al., 2009. Cortical serotonin type-2 receptor density in parents of children with autism spectrum disorders. Journal of Autism Developmental Disorders 39, 97–104.

Guptill,., J.T., Booker, A.B., Gibbs, T.T., Kemper, T.L., Bauman, M.L., Blatt, G.J., 2007. [^{3}H]-flunitrazepam-labeled benzodiazepine binding sites in the hippocampal formation in autism: A multiple concentration autoradiographic study. Journal of Autism and Developmental Disorders 37, 911–920.

Hadjikhani, N., 2010. Serotonin, pregnancy and increased autism prevalence: Is there a link? Medical Hypotheses 74, 880–883.

Hagerman, R.J., 2002. The physical and behavioral phenotype. In: Hagerman, R.J., Hagerman, P. (Eds.), Fragile X Syndrome: Diagnosis, Treatment, and Research. Johns Hopkins University Press, Baltimore, MD, pp. 3–109.

Harada, M., Taki, M.M., Nose, A., Kubo, H., Mori, K., Nishitani, H., et al., 2011. Non-invasive evaluation of the GABAergic/glutamatergic system in autistic patients observed by MEGA-editing proton MR spectroscopy using a clinical 3 tesla instrument. Journal of Autism and Developmental Disorders 41, 447–454.

Holopainen, I.E., Metsähonkala, E.L., Kokkonen, H., Parkkola, R.K., Manner, T.E., Någren, K., et al., 2001. Decreased binding of [^{11}C] flumazenil in Angelman syndrome patients with GABA(A) receptor beta 3 subunit deletions. Annals of Neurology 49, 110–113.

Huber, K.M., Gallagher, S.M., Warren, S.T., Bear, M.F., 2002. Altered synaptic plasticity in a mouse model of fragile X mental retardation. Proceedings of the National Academy of Sciences of the United States of America 99, 7746–7750.

Hussman, J.P., 2001. Suppressed GABAergic inhibition as a common factor in suspected etiologies of autism. Journal of Autism and Developmental Disorders 2, 247–248.

Hussman, J.P., Chung, R.H., Griswold, A.J., Jaworski, J.M., Salyakina, D., Ma, D., et al., 2011. A noise-reduction GWAS analysis implicates altered regulation of neurite outgrowth and guidance in autism. Molecular Autism 2, 1–16.

Irwin, S.A., Idupulapati, M., Gilbert, M.E., Harris, J.B., Chakravarthi, A.B., Rogers, E.J., et al., 2002. Dendritic spine and dendritic field characteristics of layer V pyramidal neurons in the visual cortex of fragile-X knockout mice. American Journal of Medical Genetics 111, 140–146.

Jacquemont, S., Curie, A., des Portes, V., Torrioli, M.G., Berry-Kravis, E., Hagerman, R.J., et al., 2011. Epigenetic modification of the FMR1 gene in fragile X syndrome is associated with differential response to the mGluR5 antagonist AFQ056. Science Translational Medicine 3, 1–9.

King, B.H., Hollander, E., Sikich, L., McCracken, J.T., Scahill, L., Bregman, J.D., et al., 2009. Lack of efficacy of citalopram in children with autism spectrum disorders and high levels of repetitive behavior: Citalopram ineffective in children with autism. Archives of General Psychiatry 66, 583–590.

Kleinhans, N.M., Richards, T., Sterling, L., Stegbauer, K.C., Mahurin, R., Johnson, L.C., et al., 2008. Abnormal functional connectivity in autism spectrum disorders during face processing. Brain 131, 1000–1012.

Knutson, B., Wolkowitz, O.M., Cole, S.W., Chan, T., Moore, E.A., Johnson, R.C., et al., 1998. Selective alteration of personality and social behavior by serotonergic intervention. American Journal of Psychiatry 155, 373–379.

Krueger, D.D., Osterweil, E.K., Chen, S.P., Tye, L.D., Bear, M.F., 2011. Cognitive dysfunction and prefrontal synaptic abnormalities in a mouse model of fragile X syndrome. Proceedings of the National Academy of Sciences of the United States of America 108, 2587–2592.

Lam, K.S., Aman, M.G., Arnold, L.E., 2006. Neurochemical correlates of autistic disorder: A review of the literature. Research in Developmental Disabilities 27, 254–289.

Lam, C.W., Yeung, W.L., Ko, C.H., Poon, P.M., Tong, S.F., Chan, K.Y., et al., 2000. Spectrum of mutations in the MECP2 gene in patients with infantile autism and Rett syndrome. Journal of Medical Genetics 37, 1–4.

Leboyer, M., Philippe, A., Bouvard, M., Guilloud-Bataille, M., Bondoux, D., Tabuteau, F., et al., 1999. Whole blood serotonin and plasma beta-endorphin in autistic probands and their first-degree relatives. Biological Psychiatry 45, 158–163.

Levenga, J., Hayashi, S., de Vrij, F.M., Koekkoek, S.K., van der Linde, H.C., Nieuwenhuizen, I., et al., 2011. AFQ056, a new mGluR5 antagonist for treatment of fragile X syndrome. Neurobiology of Disease 42, 311–317.

Leventhal, B.L., Cook Jr., E.H., Morford, M., Ravitz, A., Freedman, D.X., 1990. Relationships of whole blood serotonin and plasma norepinephrine within families. Journal of Autism and Developmental Disorders 20, 499–511.

Levitt, P., 2005. Disruption of interneuron development. Epilepsia 46, 22–28.

Lewine, J.D., Andrews, R., Chez, M., Patil, A.A., Devinsky, O., Smith, M., et al., 1999. Magnetoencephalographic patterns of epileptiform activity in children with regressive autism spectrum disorders. Pediatrics 104, 405–418.

Lucignani, G., Panzacchi, A., Bosio, L., Moresco, R.M., Ravasi, L., Coppa, I., et al., 2004. GABA A receptor abnormalities in Prader-Willi syndrome assessed with positron emission tomography and [11C] flumazenil. NeuroImage 22, 22–28.

Maddock, R.J., Garrett, A.S., Buonocore, M.H., 2001. Remembering familiar people: The posterior cingulate cortex and autobiographical memory retrieval. Neuroscience 104, 667–676.

Makkonen, I., Riikonen, R., Kokki, H., Airaksinen, M.M., Kuikka, J.T., 2008. Serotonin and dopamine transporter binding in children with autism determined by SPECT. Developmental Medicine and Child Neurology 50, 593–597.

Mayberg, H.S., Liotti, M., Brannan, S.K., McGinnis, S., Mahurin, R.K., Jerabek, P.A., et al., 1999. Reciprocal limbic-cortical function and negative mood: Converging PET findings in depression and normal sadness. American Journal of Psychiatry 156, 675–682.

McBride, P.A., Anderson, G.M., Hertzig, M.E., Sweeney, J.A., Kream, J., Cohen, D.J., et al., 1989. Serotonergic responsivity in male young adults with autistic disorder: Results of a pilot study. Archives of General Psychiatry 46, 213–221.

McKenna, M.C., 2007. The glutamate-glutamine cycle is not stoichiometric: Fates of glutamate in brain. Journal of Neuroscience Research 85, 3347–3358.

Menold, M.M., Shao, Y., Wolpert, C.M., Donnelly, S.L., Raiford, K.L., Martin, E.R., et al., 2001. Association analysis of chromosome 15 GABAA receptor subunit genes in autistic disorder. Journal of Neurogenetics 15, 245–259.

Moresco, F.M., Dieci, M., Vita, A., Messa, C., Gobbo, C., Galli, L., et al., 2002. In vivo serotonin 5HT(2A) receptor binding and personality traits in healthy subjects: A positron emission tomography study. Neuroimage 17, 1470–1478.

Murphy, D.G., Daly, E., Schmitz, N., Toal, F., Murphy, K., Curran, S., et al., 2006. Cortical serotonin 5-HT2A receptor binding and social communication in adults with Asperger's syndrome: An in vivo SPECT study. American Journal of Psychiatry 163, 934–936.

Nakamoto, M., Nalavadi, V., Epstein, M.P., Narayanan, U., Bassell, G.J., Warren, S.T., 2007. Fragile X mental retardation protein deficiency leads to excessive mGluR5-dependent internalization of AMPA receptors. Proceedings of the National Academy of Sciences of the United States of America 104, 15537–15542.

Nakamura, K., Sekine, Y., Ouchi, Y., Tsujii, M., Yoshikawa, E., Futatsubashi, M., et al., 2010. Brain serotonin and dopamine transporter bindings in adults with high-functioning autism. Archives of General Psychiatry 67, 59–68.

Nichols, D.E., Nichols, C.D., 2008. Serotonin receptors. Chemical Reviews 108, 1614–1641.

Nimchinsky, E.A., Oberlander, A.M., Svoboda, K., 2001. Abnormal development of dendritic spines in FMR1 knock-out mice. Journal of Neuroscience 21, 5139–5146.

Oblak, A.L., Gibbs, T.T., Blatt, G.J., 2009. Decreased GABAA receptors and benzodiazepine binding sites in the anterior cingulate cortex in autism. Autism Research 2, 205–219.

Oblak, A.L., Gibbs, T.T., Blatt, G.J., 2010. Decreased GABA(B) receptors in the cingulate cortex and fusiform gyrus in autism. Journal of Neurochemistry 114, 1414–1423.

Oblak, A.L., Gibbs, T.T., Blatt, G.J., 2011. Reduced GABAA receptors and benzodiazepine binding sites in the posterior cingulate cortex and fusiform gyrus in autism. Brain Research 1380, 218–228.

Oblak, A.L., Rosene, D.L., Kemper, T.L., Bauman, M.L., Blatt, G.J., 2011. Altered posterior cingulate cortical cyctoarchitecture, but normal density of neurons and interneurons in the posterior cingulate cortex and fusiform gyrus in autism. Autism Research 4, 200–211.

O'Donnell, W.T., Warren, S.T., 2002. A decade of molecular studies of fragile X syndrome. Annual Reviews of Neuroscience 25, 315–338.

Oliet, S.H., Malenka, R.C., Nicoll, R.A., 1997. Two distinct forms of long-term depression coexist in CA1 hippocampal pyramidal cells. Neuron 18, 969–982.

Olson, C.R., Musil, S.Y., 1992. Posterior cingulated cortex: Sensory and oculomotor properties of single neurons in behaving cat. Cerebral Cortex 2, 485–502.

Olson, C.R., Musil, S.Y., Goldberg, M.E., 1996. Single neurons in posterior singulate cortex of behaving macaque: Eye movement signals. Journal of Neurophysiology 76, 3285–3300.

Oswald, D.P., Sonenklar, N.A., 2007. Medication use among children with autism spectrum disorders. Journal of Child Adolescent Psychopharmacology. 17, 348–355.

Pacey, L.K., Tharmalingam, S., Hampson, D.R., 2011. Subchronic administration and combination metabotropic glutamate and GABAB receptor drug therapy in fragile X syndrome. Journal of Pharmacology and Experimental Therapy 338, 897–905.

Page, L.A., Daly, E., Schmitz, N., Simmons, A., Toal, F., Deeley, Q., et al., 2006. In vivo 1h-magnetic resonance spectroscopy study of amygdale-hippocampal and parietal regions in autism. American Journal of Psychiatry 163, 189–192.

Pelphrey, K.A., Morris, J.P., McCarthy, G., Labar, K.S., 2007. Perception of dynamic changes in facial affect and identity in autism. Social Cognitive and Affective Neuroscience 2, 140–149.

Perlman, S.B., Hudac, C.M., Pegors, T., Minshew, N.J., Pelphrey, K.A., 2011. Experimental manipulation of face-evoked activity in the fusiform gyrus of individuals with autism. Social Neuroscience 6, 22–30.

Pierce, K., Redcay, E., 2008. Fusiform function in children with an autism spectrum disorder is a matter of "who". Biological Psychiatry 64, 552–560.

Piven, J., Tsai, G.C., Nehme, E., Coyle, J.T., Chase, G.A., Folstein, S.E., 1991. Platelet serotonin, a possible marker for familial autism. Journal of Autism and Developmental Disorders 21, 51–59.

Purcell, A.E., Jeon, O.H., Zimmerman, A.W., Blue, M.E., Pevsner, J., 2001. Postmortem brain abnormalities of the glutamate neurotransmitter system in autism. Neurology 57, 1618–1628.

Rodriguez, A.L., Williams, R., 2007. Recent progress in the development of allosteric modulators of mGluR5. Current Opinion in Drug Discovery & Development 10, 715–722.

Rubenstein, J.L., 2010. Three hypotheses for developmental defects that may underlie some forms of autism spectrum disorder. Current Opinion in Neurology 23, 118–123.

Rubenstein, J.L., Merzenich, M.M., 2003. Model of autism: Increased ratio of excitation/inhibition in key neural systems. Brain and Behavior 2, 255–267.

Rutter, M., 2000. Genetic studies of autism: From the 1970s into the millennium. Journal of Abnormal Child Psychology 28, 3–14.

Schain, R.J., Freedman, D.X., 1961. Studies on 5-hydroxyindole metabolism in autistic and other mentally retarded children. Journal of Pediatrics 58, 315–320.

Shinohe, A., Hashimoto, K., Nakamura, K., Tsujii, M., Iwata, Y., Tsuchiya, K.J., et al., 2006. Increased serum levels of glutamate in adult patients with autism. Progress in Neuropsychopharmacology & Biological Psychiatry 30, 1472–1477.

Silva, A.E., Vayego-Lourenco, S.A., Fett-Conte, A.C., Goloni-Bertollo, E.M., Varella-Garcia, M., 2002. Tetrasomy 15q11-q13 identified by fluorescence in situ hybridization in a patient with autistic disorder. Arquivos de Neuro-psiquiatria 60, 290–294.

Silverman, J.L., Tolu, S.S., Barkan, C.L., Crawley, J.N., 2010. Repetitive self-grooming behavior in the BTBR mouse model of autism is blocked by the mGluR5 antagonist MPEP. Neuropsychopharmacology 35, 976–989.

Singh, V.K., Singh, E.A., Warren, R.P., 1997. Hyperserotoninemia and serotonin receptor antibodies in children with autism but not mental retardation. Biological Psychiatry 41, 753–755.

Stein, D.J., Westenberg, H.G., Liebowitz, M.R., 2002. Social anxiety disorder and generalized anxiety disorder: Serotonergic and dopaminergic neurocircuitry. Journal of Clinical Psychiatry 63, 12–19.

Vargas, D.L., Nascimbene, C., Krishnan, C., Zimmerman, A.W., Pardo, C.A., 2005. Neuroglial activation and neuroinflammation in the brain of patients with autism. Annals of Neurology 57, 67–81.

Veenstra-VanderWeele, J., Cook Jr., E., Lombroso, P.J., 2003. Genetics of childhood disorders: XLVI. Autism, part 5: Genetics of autism. Journal of the American Academy of Child & Adolescent Psychiatry 42, 116–118.

Veenstra-VanderWeele, J., Kim, S.J., Lord, C., Courchesne, R., Akshoomoff, N., Leventhal, B.L., et al., 2002. Transmission disequilibrium studies of the serotonin 5-HT2A receptor gene (HTR2A) in autism. American Journal of Medical Genetics 114, 277–283.

Wassink, T.H., Hazlett, H.C., Epping, E.A., Arndt, S., Dager, S.R., Schellenberg, G.D., et al., 2007. Cerebral cortical gray matter overgrowth and functional variation of the serotonin transporter gene in autism. Archives of General Psychiatry 64, 709–717.

Wheless, J.W., Simos, P.G., Butler, I.J., 2002. Language dysfunction in epileptic conditions. Seminars in Pediatric Neurology 9, 218–228.

Whitaker-Azmitia, P.M., 2001. Serotonin and brain development: role in human developmental diseases. Brain Research Bulletin 56, 479–485.

Whitaker-Azmitia, P.M., 2005. Behavioral and cellular consequences of increasing serotonergic activity during brain development: A Role in autism? International Journal of Develpmental Neuroscience 23, 75–83.

Williams, K., Wheeler, D.M., Silove, N., Hazell, P., 2010. Selective serotonin reuptake inhibitors (SSRIs) for autism spectrum disorders (ASD). Cochrane Database Systematic Reviews 4, 1–34.

Wilson, B.M., Cox, C.L., 2007. Absence of metabotropic glutamate receptor-mediated plasticity in the neocortex of fragile X mice. Proceedings of the National Academy of Sciences of the United States of America 104, 2454–2459.

Winter, C., Reutiman, T.J., Folsom, T.D., Sohr, R., Wolf, R.J., Juckel, G., et al., 2008. Dopamine and serotonin levels following prenatal viral infection in mouse – implications for psychiatric disorders such as schizophrenia and autism. European Neuropsychopharmacology 18, 712–716.

Yip, J., Soghomonian, J.J., Blatt, G.J., 2007. Decreased GAD67 mRNA levels in cerebellar Purkinje cells in autism: Pathophysiological implications. Acta Neuropathologia 113, 559–568.

Yip, J., Soghomonian, J.J., Blatt, G.J., 2008. Decreased GAD67 mRNA expression in cerebellar interneurons in autism: Implications for Purkinje cell dysfunction. Journal of Neuroscience Research 86, 525–530.

Yip, J., Soghomonian, J.J., Blatt, G.J., 2009. Decreased GAD65 mRNA levels in select subpopulations of neurons in the cerebellar dentate nuclei in autism: An in situ hybridization study. Autism Research 2, 50–59.

Yizhar, O., Fenno, L.E., Prigge, M., Schneider, F., Davidson, T.J., O'Shea, D.J., et al., 2011. Neocortical excitation/inhibition balance in information processing and social dysfunction. Nature 477, 171–178.

Clinicopathological Stratification of Idiopathic Autism and Autism with 15q11.2–q13 Duplications

Jerzy Wegiel*, N. Carolyn Schanen‡, Edwin H. Cook††, W. Ted Brown†,
Izabela Kuchna*, Krzysztof Nowicki*, Jarek Wegiel*, Humi Imaki*,
Shuang Yong Ma*, Eric London**, Thomas Wisniewski††

*Departments of Developmental Neurobiology, †Human Genetics, **Psychology, New York State Institute for Basic
Research in Developmental Disabilities, Staten Island, NY, USA ‡Nemours Biomedical Research, duPont Hospital for
Children, Wilmington, DE, USA ††Department of Psychiatry, Departments of Neurology, Pathology, and Psychiatry,
NYU Langone Medical Center, New York, NY, USA

OUTLINE

The Neuroscience of Autism Spectrum Disorders.
http://dx.doi.org/10.1016/B978-0-12-391924-3.00025-9

GENETIC FACTORS IN AUTISM

In 1977, Folstein and Rutter (Folstein and Rutter, 1977) demonstrated a striking difference in concordance rates of autism between monozygous and dizygous twins. The studies that followed revealed close to 90% monozygous concordance rates for autism spectrum disorder (ASD) and very low concordance rates for dizygotic twins (Bailey et al., 1995), showing a significant role of genetic factors in autism etiology (Ritvo et al., 1985; Smalley et al., 1988, Steffenburg et al., 1989; Folstein and Piven, 1991; Rutter et al., 1990a, b; Lotspeich and Ciaranello, 1993). Recent studies demonstrate a contribution of both genetic and environmental factors to ASD. Liu et al. (2010) revealed 57.0% and 67.2% concordance rates for monozygotic males and females, respectively, 32.9% concordance rates for same sex dizygotic twins, and 9.7% recurrence risk for siblings, whereas Hallmayer et al. (2011) demonstrated moderate, 37% and 38% genetic heritability for autism and ASD, respectively, and 55% contribution of shared environmental factors to autism and 55% to ASD.

A genetic basis has been revealed for less than 15% of autism cases, whereas no single genetic cause explains more than 2% (Abrahams and Geschwind, 2008; Wang et al., 2009). Chromosomal abnormalities, especially large chromosomal anomalies, such as unbalanced translocations, inversions, rings, and interstitial deletions and duplications, were detected in 1.7% to 4.8% of subjects diagnosed with ASD (Lauritsen et al., 1999; Wassink et al., 2004). They are identified as duplications of 15q [dup(15)], deletions of 18q, Xp, 2q, and such sex chromosome aneuploidies as 47XYY and 45X (Gillberg, 1998; Reddy, 2005). Autism is diagnosed in 69% of subjects with maternal origin duplications 15q11.2–q13 (dup15) (Rineer et al., 1998), in 15% to 28% of individuals with fragile X syndrome (FXS) (Hagerman, 2002), and in 7% of people with Down syndrome (DS) (Kent et al., 1999).

DUPLICATIONS OF CHROMOSOME 15Q11Q13

The imprinted chromosome region 15q11q13 is known for its instability, resulting in the DNA repeats or deletions associated with several syndromes. Prader-Willi syndrome (PWS) is predominantly the result of a paternal deletion of the small nuclear ribonucleoprotein polypeptide N (SNRPN) gene in 15q11q13 (Ozcelik et al., 1992), whereas the Angelman syndrome (AS) is most often the result of maternal deletion of the ubiquitin-protein ligase E3A (UBE3A) gene (Knoll et al., 1993). Subsets of subjects with PWS or AS have been

reported to exhibit autism-like behavior (Arrieta et al., 1994; Demb and Papola, 1995; Dykens and Kasari, 1997; Penner et al., 1993; Steffenburg et al., 1996; Summers et al., 1995). Chromosomal abnormalities of the proximal 15q region belong to the most common genomic aberrations detected in autistic disorder probands (Arrieta et al., 1994; Baker et al., 1994; Bundey et al., 1994; Cook EH et al., 1997; Flejter et al., 1996; Gillberg et al., 1991; Hotopf and Bolton, 1995; Kerbeshian et al., 1990; Martinsson et al., 1996; Schroer et al., 1998; Weidmer-Mikhail et al., 1998; Wolpert et al., 2000a, b). These abnormalities were found in up to 3% of subjects diagnosed with ASD. An especially strong association with autism was revealed in duplications in the range of 8 to 12 Mb derived from the maternal chromosome (Cook EH et al., 1997; Dawson et al., 2002). Interstitial triplications [int trp(15)] are relatively rare but have invariably been associated with a severe phenotype, including intellectual deficit (ID), ASD, and seizures. A few subjects have been diagnosed with duplications of paternal origin; however, they were described as clinically unaffected (Bolton et al., 2001; Cook EH et al., 1997; Mohandas et al., 1999; Schroer et al., 1998) or affected but without ASD (Mao et al., 2000; Mohandas et al., 1999). In only one subject was paternal origin dup(15) associated with ASD (Bolton et al., 2004). Because only maternally inherited aberrations of chromosome 15q11q13 have been reported to be associated with a severe clinical phenotype, one may assume that the copy number of maternal genes within this genomic region contributes to alterations of brain development and the autistic phenotype.

GENE EXPRESSION IN DUP(15)

Postmortem studies of the brain reveal that chromosome 15q11–13 duplications are associated with epigenetic alterations in gene expression that are not predicted from copy number (Hogart et al., 2008). Whole-genome expression profiling of lymphoblast cell lines derived from individuals with autism and isodicentric 15 [idic(15)] revealed 112 transcripts that are significantly dysregulated in samples from subjects with duplications. However, only four of a total of 80 genes located within the duplicated area of chromosome 15 were found to be upregulated, including an 1.5- to 2.0-fold upregulation of ubiquitin protein ligase E3A (UBE3A; 15q11-q13) and a 1.89-fold increase of HERC2. Baron et al. (2006) concluded that the majority of changes are not due to increased gene dosage in a critical chromosome 15 region, but represent potential downstream effects of this duplication, including two downregulated genes, namely, APP encoded by a gene on chromosome 21, and SUMO1 encoded by a gene on chromosome 2.

Several functional categories were identified as being associated with macromolecular catabolic processes, including the ubiquitin-dependent protein catabolism. The increase of UBE3A protein level may indicate dysregulation of ubiquitin-mediated proteasome pathway in cells with dup(15), resulting in enhanced ubiquitination of proteins for non-lysosomal degradation/disposal in response to genotoxic insult. Down regulation of SUMO1, a ubiquitin-like molecule, may indicate other forms of dysregulation of cell catabolic processes leading to decreased cell sensitivity to apoptotic stimuli and tolerance to DNA damage (Baron et al., 2006).

The γ-aminobutyric acid type$_A$ (GABA$_A$) receptor subunit genes (α5, β3, and γ3) are located in the susceptibility segment of duplicated chromosome 15 (Bass et al., 2000; Buxbaum et al., 2002; Cook et al., 1998; Menold et al., 2001). GABA is the main inhibitory neurotransmitter that binds to a complex of GABA$_A$ receptors. Polymorphisms in the GABA$_A$-β3 receptor subunit are associated with ASD (Cook et al., 1998; Martin et al., 2000). Moreover, differential methylations of the GABA$_A$ gene (Bittel et al., 2005; Gabriel et al., 1998; Hogart et al., 2007; Meguro et al., 1997) may result in epigenetic modifications and modifications of clinical phenotypes in dup(15)/autism.

CLINICAL CHARACTERISTICS

Between 1994 and 2008, approximately 160 patients diagnosed with inverted (inv) dup(15) were characterized (Battaglia, 2008; Dennis et al., 2006; Wang et al., 2004; Webb, 1994; Webb et al., 1998; Wolpert et al., 2000a, b), and had a similar male:female ratio (3:1) to that reported in idiopathic autism (Bryson, 1996) and in probands with dup (15q) (Wolpert et al., 2000a).

Clinicopathological correlations in dup(15) cohorts with considerable variations in the breakpoints, copy numbers, additional genetic and epigenetic modifications, and significant clinical differences are limited. In spite of these differences, distinctive clinical features of dup(15) syndrome, including early central hypotonia, developmental delay, intellectual disability, epilepsy, and autistic behavior, can be defined. Battaglia's summary of clinical findings (2008) suggests that:

a) in more than 75% of individuals with dup(15) hypotonia and lax ligaments, developmental delay and intellectual disability, autistic behavior, epilepsy, and minor dysmorphic features, involving mainly the face, are present;

b) from 25% to 50% of subjects are affected by brain abnormalities, growth retardation, and gastrointestinal and uninary tract defects; and

c) in less than 25% of subjects, microcephaly and congenital heart defects are observed.

Wolpert et al. (2000a) documented that multiple maternal copies of the proximal 15q region may lead to one form of autistic disorder involving genes in the 15q11q13 region. Social, communicative, and behavioral function, and many clinical features are similar among individuals with autism associated with dup(15) and those with autism arising from other causes. The authors' review shows a much greater occurrence rate of seizures in dup(15) (69%) than reported in idiopathic autism (33%) (Tuchman and Rapin, 2002; Tuchman et al., 2009), a common delay in achieving motor milestones (77%), and hypotonia (77%) in dup(15) and a much lower occurrence rate of these abnormalities in idiopathic autism. Almost all individuals with inv dup(15) have moderate to profound developmental delay and intellectual disability (Battaglia et al., 1997; Battaglia, 2008; Crolla et al., 1995; Gillberg et al., 1991; Webb, 1994; Webb et al., 1998; Robinson et al., 1993; Wolpert et al., 2000a).

Earlier studies of smaller groups of patients based on non-standardized criteria revealed autism in 33% (Leana-Cox et al., 1994) and 36% (Crolla et al., 1995) of individuals diagnosed with the syndrome. Application of standardized assessment of autistic symptoms to a cohort of 29 children and adults with dup(15) revealed that 69% of these subjects met the criteria for autism diagnosis (Rineer et al., 1998).

NEUROPATHOLOGY OF AUTISM WITH DUP(15) AND OF IDIOPATHIC AUTISM

The current knowledge of brain developmental alterations is based on the results of an examination of the brains of nine individuals diagnosed with dup(15), including seven subjects (78%) diagnosed with autism (Wegiel et al., 2012a,b). These studies demonstrate several striking differences and some similarities between subjects diagnosed with autism associated with dup(15) and idiopathic autism. These patterns indicate that the autistic phenotype might be a product of etiologically, qualitatively, and quantitatively different processes.

INCREASED PREVALENCE OF BRAIN TRANSIENT OVERGROWTH AND MACROCEPHALY IN IDIOPATHIC AUTISM AND MICROCEPHALY IN DUP(15) AUTISM

Macrocephaly, defined as head circumference greater than the 97th percentile of the normal population, has been reported in more than 20% of autistic subjects

(Bailey et al., 1995; Bolton et al., 1994; Fombonne et al., 1999; Lainhart et al., 1997). Increased brain weight was also reported in autistic subjects in postmortem studies (Bailey et al., 1993; Bauman and Kemper, 1985). A short period of increased brain size, starting before the age of 1 year (Lainhart et al., 1997; Redcay and Courchesne, 2005), results in macrocephaly in 37% of autistic children under the age of 4 years (Courchesne et al., 2001) and macrocephaly in 42% of the 19 twins diagnosed with idiopathic autism under the age of 16 years (Bailey et al., 1995). Brain overgrowth is associated with an increased number of neurons (Courchesne et al., 2011). However, approximately 15% of 2- to 16-year-old autistic children are affected by microcephaly (Fombonne et al., 1999), which is frequently associated with a more severe clinical phenotype (Guerin et al., 1996; Hof et al., 1991), including intellectual disability and other disorders (Fombonne et al., 1999).

The characteristics of individuals with dup(15) are few, but published reports show opposite proportions between macrocephalic and microcephalic subjects, unlike in idiopathic autism. In the largest examined cohort (n = 107) with dup(15), macrocephaly was detected in only 2.8%, and microcephaly in six times (16.8%) more subjects (Schroer et al., 1998). The first postmortem study of the brains of nine subjects diagnosed with dup(15), including seven subjects diagnosed with autism (78%) revealed the mean brain weight to be 303 g lower than in the idiopathic autism group (p < 0.001) (Wegiel et al. 2012 a, b). Age-adjusted mean brain weight for dup(15) (n = 9), idiopathic autism (n = 10) and control (n = 7) subjects was 1,171 g, 1474 g, and 1378 g, respectively. The difference between the dup(15) and control group was non-significant but suggestive (p = 0.06; Figure 3.9.1).

Two postmortem studies of idiopathic autism cohorts revealed epilepsy in 6 of 13 subjects (46%; Wegiel et al., 2010) and 3/10 (30%), whereas in the dup(15) group,

epilepsy was diagnosed in seven of nine cases (78%) (Wegiel et al., 2012a). In the dup(15) cohort, sudden and unexplained death in patients with epilepsy (SUDEP) was diagnosed in 6 of 9 subjects (67%), and seizure-related death was determined in one case (10%), resulting in 77% of cases of sudden death (Wegiel et al., 2012a). Sudden death in the idiopathic autism cohort was reported in four of 13 subjects (31%, Wegiel et al., 2010). These data suggest that the microcephaly and very early onset of seizures are risk factors for SUDEP in the subpopulation of dup(15) subjects, and that this risk is at least twice as high in dup(15) than in idiopathic autism.

NEUROPATHOLOGICAL STRATIFICATION OF DEVELOPMENTAL ABNORMALITIES IN DUP(15) AND IDIOPATHIC AUTISM COHORTS

Applications of an extended neuropathological protocol based on examination of approximately 120 serial hemispheric sections per brain resulted in the detection of each developmental abnormality larger than 2–3 mm. Three major types of developmental change were detected, including heterotopias, dysplastic changes, and abnormal neuronal proliferation. They were found in all nine dup(15) and all 10 subjects with idiopathic autism; however, the type, topography, and number of abnormalities show significant differences between these two cohorts (Figure 3.9.2).

HETEROTOPIAS

Defects of migration resulting in heterotopias in the alveus, hilar portion of the CA3, and dentate gyrus (DG) occur very often in the dup(15) group (89%), are rare in individuals with idiopathic autism (10%, p = 0.001), and are not present in control subjects.

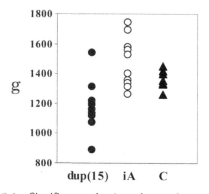

FIGURE 3.9.1 Significant reduction of mean brain weight (g) in the dup(15) autism group (1,171 g) compared to the idiopathic autism (iA) cohort (1,474 g; p < 0.001), and non-significant but suggestive reduction in comparison to the control (C) group (1,378 g; p < 0.06).

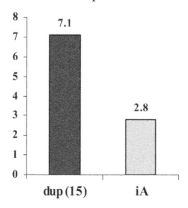

FIGURE 3.9.2 The mean number of developmental alterations detected in postmortem evaluation of serial hemispheric sections was 2.5 times higher in the dup(15) autism group (7.1/case) than in the idiopathic autism (iA) group (2.8/case).

However, the prevalence of the heterotopias in cerebellar white matter is comparable in dup(15) (56%) and idiopathic autism (60%). The heterotopias in cerebral white matter are rare in both cohorts (11% and 10%, respectively). These three patterns illustrate not only striking topographical differences in the distribution of defects of neuronal migration but also significant differences between idiopathic autism and autism associated with dup(15).

DYSPLASIA

Microdysgenesis resulting in focal developmental alterations of cytoarchitecture is also topographically selective and is detected mainly in the DG and CA fields in the hippocampal formation, and in the cerebral and cerebellar cortex. Dysplastic changes in the DG have been identified as hyperconvolution of the DG, duplication of the granular layer, massive protrusions of the granular layer into the molecular layer, focal thickening, thinning and fragmentation of the granular layer. The prevalence of dysplasia in the DG is several times higher (89%) in subjects with dup(15) than in the idiopathic autism group (10%; p < 0.001) (Figure 3.9.3). In the DG, usually only one type of these changes is observed in idiopathic autism, whereas from two to five types are observed in each brain in dup(15) autism. However, dysplastic changes in the CA fields are rare in both cohorts, and the percentage of affected subjects is comparable: 20% in dup(15) autism and 22% in idiopathic autism.

Another feature distinguishing these two cohorts is cerebral cortex dysplasia, which is detected in 50% of

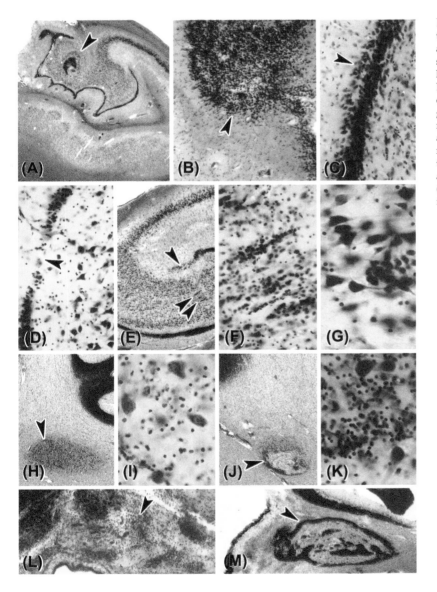

FIGURE 3.9.3 Topography and morphology of 11 types of developmental abnormalities in the brain of a 24-year-old male diagnosed with dup(15), autism, severe seizures, and SUDEP: dentate gyrus (DG) hyperconvolution and DG heterotopia in the CA4 A) DG granule cell layer protrusion (B) arrowhead, duplication (C), focal thinning and discontinuity (D), granule cell layer fragmentation (E); arrowhead; multifocal microdysgenesis within CA4 (E), two arrowheads; larger magnification of different types of microdysgenesis within CA4 (F, G); cerebellar heterotopia with morphology of cerebellar deep nuclei (H, I) and with modified morphology of cerebellar cortex (J, K); and dysplasia in the cerebellar nodulus (L) and flocculus (M).

subjects with dup(15) but is absent in idiopathic autism and in control subjects. The diversity of neocortical dysplastic changes, including multifocal cortical dysplasia with focal hypo- or acellularity, loss of vertical and horizontal organization, focal polymicrogyria and bottom-of-a-sulcus dysplasia, suggests that cortical abnormalities in dup(15) autism are the product of the disruption of several different mechanisms of cortex development.

The subependymal nodular dysplasia detected in the lateral ventricle in the occipital lobe in the brain of 15- and 39-year-old females diagnosed with dup(15) autism, and in 7- and 32-year-old males diagnosed with idiopathic autism are evidence of abnormal neuronal proliferation in some autistic subjects regardless of autism etiology and identify the predilection site for this developmental defect, which is also detectable on MRI scans (Wegiel et al., 2010, 2012a).

CAUSATIVE LINK BETWEEN DEVELOPMENTAL NEUROPATHOLOGICAL CHANGES, EPILEPSY, AND SUDDEN DEATH IN CHILDHOOD

Similar hippocampal developmental abnormalities observed in sudden unexpected and unexplained death in childhood (SUDC) cases (Kinney et al., 2007) are considered an epileptogenic focus that might be triggered by infection, fever, or head trauma and result in seizures and unwitnessed death (Blum et al., 2000; Frysinger and Harper, 1990; Yang et al., 2001). SUDC in two subjects and SUDEP in five cases with dup(15) and autism and several-fold higher prevalence of hippocampal and cortical dysplasia than in idiopathic autism appears to be the clinicopathological criterion for stratification between and within these cohorts. These developmental alterations are not pathognomonic of an 'epileptic brain' (Kinney et al., 2007), but the combination of microcephaly, the 2.5-fold higher prevalence of several types of developmental abnormalities, the 2.3-fold higher prevalence of epilepsy, and the six-times higher prevalence of epilepsy-related death in the dup(15) cohort suggests that unique genetic and molecular modifications and developmental structural defects distinguish these two cohorts of autistic subjects.

THE LINK BETWEEN DYSPLASTIC CHANGES IN THE CEREBELLAR FLOCCULUS AND ATYPICAL GAZE

Cerebellar abnormalities are among the most consistent developmental alterations detected in ASD (Bauman and Kemper, 1996; Courchesne et al., 2001; Kemper and Bauman, 1993; Ritvo et al., 1986; Whitney et al., 2008; 2009). A reduced number of Purkinje cells (PC) has been detected in 72% of the reported ASD cases (Palmen et al. review, 2004), but studies by Whitney et al. suggest that the reduced number of PC is not the effect of a developmental deficit, but is instead the result of early neuronal loss (Whitney et al., 2008; 2009). The prevalence of defective migration of cortical neurons and dentate nucleus neurons in the cerebellar white matter was almost identical in dup(15) autism and idiopathic autism (56% and 60%, respectively). Four types of cerebellar dysplasia, including nodulus, flocculus, and vermis dysplasia, and focal polymicrogyria, were found in dup(15) autism and idiopathic autism. Vermis dysplasia and focal polymicrogyria were rare in both groups.

However, a portion of the flocculus and a small portion of the nodulus, developmentally related to the flocculus ('flocculus-like' region of the ventral paraflocculus; Tan et al., 1995), were affected by dysplastic changes. Flocculus dysplasia is associated with a striking deficit of PC and unipolar brush cells, an almost complete lack of inhibitory basket and stellate cells in the molecular layer, and reduction of the number of granule cells. This abnormal flocculus cytoarchitecture appears to be an indicator of the profound disruption of the olivofloccular circuitry and severe functional alterations. The flocculus participates in the control of eye motion (Leung et al., 2000), and coordination of eye and head movements during active gaze shifts by modulating the vestibulo-ocular reflex (Belton and McCrea, 1999). Dysplastic changes are observed in the nodulus of autistic and control subjects, but the function of the affected region of the nodulus is not clear. The presence of dysplasia in the flocculus of 75% of individuals with dup(15) autism (Wegiel et al., 2012b), in 50% and 67% of idiopathic autism cases (Wegiel et al., 2012a, c), and 20% of control subjects (Wegiel et al., 2012c) and the presence of olivary dysplasia in three of five autistic subjects and ectopic neurons related to the olivary complex in two cases reported by Bailey et al. (1998) indicate that both major structural and functional components of the olivofloccular circuitry are prone to developmental defects, most likely contributing to the atypical gaze of autistic subjects. These findings also suggest that flocculus developmental defects are observed in autistic subjects regardless of etiology. Individuals diagnosed with idiopathic autism and dup(15) autism reveal altered oculomotor functions, including atypical gaze, impairments in smooth pursuit, and deficits in facial perceptions, suggesting defects in the olivofloccular neuronal circuit. These defects are reported early in the development of children with ASD (Mundy et al., 1986; Dawson et al., 1998) and contribute to deficits in using gaze to understand the intentions of other people and their mental states (Baron-Cohen, 1995; Baron-Cohen et al., 1999; 2001; Leekam et al., 1998, 2000).

INCREASED LEVELS OF SECRETED AMYLOID PRECURSOR PROTEIN-α (SAPP-α) AND REDUCED LEVELS OF Aβ40 AND Aβ42 IN THE BLOOD PLASMA

Significantly lower concentrations of both $Aβ_{1-40}$ and $Aβ_{1-42}$, and a reduced ratio of $Aβ_{40/42}$ detected in the blood plasma of 52 autistic children 3 to 16 years of age, compared to 39 age-matched control subjects, were attributed to the loss of Aβ equilibrium between the brain and blood (Al-Ayadhi et al., 2012). Significantly increased levels of sAPP-α in blood plasma in 60% of autistic children (Sokol et al., 2006) indicate enhanced non-amyloidogenic APP processing by α-secretase. Higher levels of sAPP-α in blood plasma were especially prominent in autistic subjects with aggressive behavior (Ray et al., 2011; Sokol et al., 2006). Enhanced non-amyloidogenic cleavage of APP with α-secretase is associated not only with ASD (Bailey et al., 2008; Ray et al., 2011; Sokol et al., 2006; 2011; Wegiel et al., 2012b), but also with FXS (Sokol et al., 2011; Westmark and Malter, 2007; Westmark et al., 2011). Due to the neurotrophic activity of sAPP-α, increased levels of this APP metabolite are considered a co-factor contributing to brain overgrowth in autism and FXS (Sokol et al., 2011). The fragile X mental retardation protein (FMRP) binds to and represses translation of APP mRNA. The absence of FMRP in people diagnosed with FXS results in upregulation of APP, $Aβ_{40}$, and $Aβ_{42}$. Similar upregulation is detected in Fmr1 knock-out ($Fmr1^{KO}$) mice (Westmark and Malter, 2007); however, genetic reduction of AβPP by removal of one App allele in $Fmr1^{KO}$ mice reverses the FXS phenotype and increases blood plasma levels of $Aβ_{1-42}$ to control levels (Westmark et al., 2011).

ENHANCED ACCUMULATION OF N-TERMINAL TRUNCATED Aβ IN NEURONAL CYTOPLASM

Neuronal proteolytic cleavage of APP by β- and γ-secretases (amyloidogenic pathway) results in release of $Aβ_{1-40}$ and $Aβ_{1-42}$, which are able to form fibrillar deposits in the extracellular space (amyloid plaques) and in the wall of brain vessels (amyloid angiopathy). $Aβ_{17-40}$ and $Aβ_{17-42}$ are products of α- and γ-secretases (p3 peptide) in the non-amyloidogenic pathway (Iversen et al. 1995; Selkoe, 2001). Aβ is generated and detected in the endoplasmic reticulum/Golgi apparatus and endosomal-lysosomal pathway (Cook D.G. et al., 1997; Glabe,

2001; Greenfield et al., 1999; Hartmann et al., 1997; Wilson et al., 1999), multivesicular bodies (Takahashi et al., 2002), and mitochondria (Bayer and Wirths, 2010; Caspersen et al., 2005). Aβ peptides differ in oligomerization and fibrillization as well as toxicity. Intraneuronal accumulation has been reported in normal human brain (Wegiel et al., 2007). Enhanced accumulation has been proposed as an early alteration in Alzheimer's disease (AD) and in transgenic mouse models of AD (Bayer and Wirths, 2010; Gouras et al., 2010; Gyure et al., 2001; Mochizuki et al., 2000; Winton et al., 2011).

Intraneuronal Aβ in human brain is mainly N-terminal truncated $Aβ_{17-40}$ and $Aβ_{17-42}$ (Wegiel et al., 2007). Cytoplasmic Aβ in neurons is a reflection of the balance between its rate of synthesis, accumulation in cytoplasmic organelles, and its degradation. The extracellular level of Aβ is a reflection of neuronal production and extracellular oligomerization, fibrilization, deposition, and disposal, including drawing of the excessive amounts through the blood-brain barrier to the blood (Weller et al., 1998). The morphology and amount of intracellular deposits of Aβ are neuron-type-specific, and show a broad spectrum of differences in developing and aging brains and in brains affected by pathology. Increased level of sAPP-α in the blood plasma of autistic subjects is linked to enhanced intraneuronal accumulation of amino-terminally truncated $Aβ_{17-40/42}$ in their neurons (Wegiel et al., 2012b).

STRATIFICATION OF Aβ ACCUMULATION IN NEURONS IN THE DUP(15) AUTISM AND IDIOPATHIC AUTISM

A postmortem study of 12 brain structures and neuronal populations (frontal, temporal, and occipital cortex; amygdala, thalamus, lateral geniculate body, DG; CA1 and CA3 fields and PC) revealed higher Aβ load in neurons in 11 subregions in dup(15) autism than in idiopathic autism ($p < 0.0001$) and in control subjects ($p < 0.0001$). In eight regions, cytoplasmic Aβ load was significantly higher in idiopathic autism than in control subjects ($p < 0.001$).

We found the excessive accumulation of Aβ in two ASD cohorts to be neuron type-specific. Classification of neuronal Aβ immunoreactivity as strong, moderate, and weak revealed two types of alterations. Type 1 is characterized by a significant increase in the percentage of neurons with strong Aβ immunoreactivity, defined as a condensed mass of indistinguishable small and large immunoreactive granules occupying a large portion of neuronal perikarya. Type 1 of Aβ accumulation is typical for the amygdala, thalamus, and lateral geniculate

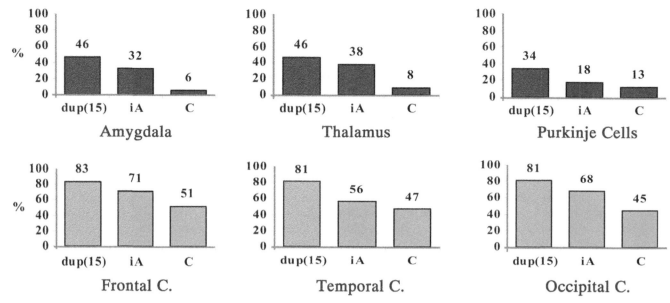

FIGURE 3.9.4   The percentage of neurons with very high intracellular Aβ load is significantly higher in the amygdala, thalamus, and Purkinje cells in dup(15) autism than idiopathic autism and control subjects (p < 0.0001). In the frontal, temporal, and occipital cortex, the total percentage of Aβ-immunoreactive neurons (neurons with strong, moderate, and weak Aβ immunoreactivity) is significantly higher in dup(15) autism than in idiopathic autism and control groups (p < 0.0001).

nucleus (Figure 3.9.4). Stratification of dup(15)autism and idiopathic autism cohorts is reflected in a 7.6-fold increase of the percentage of strongly immunoreactive neurons in the amygdala and thalamus and a 4.5-fold increase in the lateral geniculate nucleus in dup(15) autism in comparison to the control cohort. In idiopathic autism, the increase was 5.3×, 6.3×, and 3.9×, respectively, in comparison to that found in the control subjects. Type 2 of Aβ intraneuronal accumulation is distinguished by a relatively low percentage of neurons with strong Aβ immunoreactivity, but a higher total percentage of Aβ-immunoreactive neurons. This pattern was typical for pyramidal neurons in all three examined

neocortical regions (frontal, temporal, and occipital cortex), and the total percentage of Aβ-immunoreactive neurons was higher in dup(15) than in the autism and control groups (p < 0.001).

$A\beta_{1-40}$ AND $A\beta_{1-42}$ IN DIFFUSE PLAQUES IN AUTISM

Diffuse amorphous nonfibrillar Aβ deposits are classified as preplaques (Mann et al., 1989) or pre-amyloid deposits (Tagliavini et al., 1989). However, diffuse deposits in the human cerebellar cortex and the

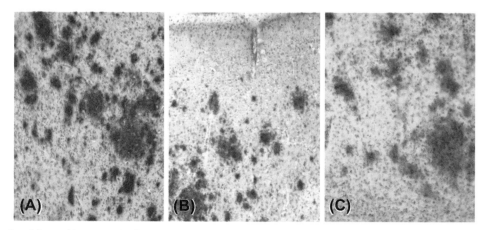

FIGURE 3.9.5   In the oldest subject examined postmortem in the dup(15) group (39-year-old autistic female), and two subjects with autistic disorder of unknown etiology (51 and 52 years old), numerous diffuse $A\beta_{1-40/42}$-immunoreactive plaques were detected in the cortical ribbon (A, B, C), respectively.

parvocellular layer of the presubiculum do not fibrilize, regardless of age or stage of AD (Wisniewski et al., 1998). Diffuse plaques were found in 2 of the 11 subjects diagnosed with ASD (51 and 52 years old) and in 1 of 9 subjects diagnosed with dup(15) and autism (Figure 3.9.5). These subjects were the oldest in both examined groups. Plaques were nonfibrillar, thioflavin S-negative, but in contrast to N-terminal truncated $A\beta_{17-40/42}$ in neurons, they contained full-length $A\beta_{1-40/42}$ (Wegiel et al., 2012b). Diffuse plaques are also observed in young people diagnosed with Down syndrome, but they are $A\beta_{17-40/42}$-immunoreactive (Gowing et al., 1994; Lalowski et al., 1996).

Both in the plaque perimeter and in plaque-free areas, numerous astrocytes and some microglial cells contain amyloid, but only N-terminally truncated $A\beta_{17-40/42}$. Focal enhanced proliferation of astrocytes, accumulation of $A\beta$ in their cytoplasm, and accelerated death also likely results in $A\beta$ deposition, mainly in the perivascular space.

These findings suggest that the pattern of metabolic alterations of APP processing and $A\beta$ accumulation is comparable in the two autistic cohorts, but the severity of metabolic changes is significantly intensified in dup(15) autism in comparison to idiopathic autism. Enhanced APP processing with α- and γ-secretase increases the percentage of $A\beta$-immunoreactive neurons and intracellular amyloid load in dup(15) autism with microcephaly. Increased levels of blood plasma neurotrophic sAPP-α detected in 60% of subjects with idiopathic autism justified the hypothesis that the increased level of the product of α-secretase may help identify a subset of children in which early brain overgrowth is sufficient for development of autism and might be a marker of the mechanism that regulates brain overgrowth (Sokol et al., 2011).

CLOSING REMARKS

Comparative postmortem studies of the brains of individuals diagnosed with dup(15) autism identify a cluster of neuropathological findings differentiating this cohort of autistic subjects with genetically identified autism etiology from a cohort of subjects with idiopathic autism. These studies support the recommendation by Happe et al. (2006) for subclassification of ASD according to different etiologies, clinical presentations, and neuropathologic findings, and most likely in terms of different preventive strategies and different treatments.

Because the complex nature of developmental abnormalities increases the risk of death in childhood and early adulthood in the dup(15) autism cohort, postmortem study appears to reflect both developmental abnormalities associated with this genetic trait, and

a particular combination of factors contributing to early death. The list of factors likely related to the risk of early death and the detected pattern of neuropathological changes includes: (a) maternal origin of dup(15), (b) autism, (c) more severe clinical phenotypes with ID, early-onset and severe or intractable seizures, and increased prevalence of SUDEP, (d) high prevalence of microcephaly, (e) several-fold increase in the number of developmental abnormalities, including defects of migration and multifocal defects of cytoarchitecture, especially numerous in the hippocampal formation, and (f) several-fold increase in the percentage of neurons with increased amyloid load, reflecting enhanced APP processing in non-amyloidogenic pathway with α- and γ-secretase ($A\beta_{17-40/42}$); enhanced proliferation and activation of $A\beta_{17-40/42}$-positive astrocytes, enhanced rate of astrocytes death, and in some cases, an early onset of diffuse plaques containing $A\beta_{1-40/42}$.

ACKNOWLEDGEMENTS

This study was supported in part by funds from the New York State Office for People With Developmental Disabilities, a grant from the US Department of Defense Autism Spectrum Disorders Research Program (AS073234, J.W., T.W.), a grant from Autism Speaks (Princeton, New Jersey, J.W.), and an Autism Center of Excellence (NIH P50 HD055751; EHC). Clinical and molecular investigations of the subjects with chromosome 15 duplications were supported by the Collaborative Programs for Excellence in Autism Research (NIH U19 HD35470; N.C.S.) and Nemours Biomedical Research, duPont Hospital for Children.

References

Abrahams, B.S., Geschwind, D.H., 2008. Advances in autism genetics: on the threshold of a new neurobiology. Nature Reviews Genetics 9, 341–355.

Al-Ayadhi, L.I., Bacha, A.G.B., Kotb, M., El-Ansary, A.K., 2012. A novel study on amyloid β peptide 40, 42 and 40/42 ratio in Saudi autistics. Behavioral and Brain Functions 8, 1–8.

Arrieta, I., Lobato, M.N., Martinez, B., Criado, B., 1994. Parental origin of Robertsonian translocation (15q22q) and Prader-Willi syndrome associated with autism. Psychiatric Genetics 4, 63–65.

Bailey, A.R., Giunta, B.N., Obregon, D., Nikolic, W.V., Tian, J., Sanberg, C.D., et al., 2008. Peripheral biomarkers in autism: secreted amyloid precursor protein-α as a probable key player in early diagnosis. International Journal of Clinics and Experimental Medicine 1, 338–344.

Bailey, A., Le Couteur, A., Gottesman, I., Bolton, P., Simonoff, E., Yuzda, E., et al., 1995. Autism as a strongly genetic disorder: evidence from a British twin study. Psychological Medicine 25, 63–77.

Bailey, A., Luthert, P., Bolton, P., LeCouteur, A., Rutter, M., 1993. Autism and megalencephaly. The Lancet 341, 1225–1226.

Bailey, A., Luthert, P., Dean, A., Harding, B., Janota, I., Montgomery, M., et al., 1998. A clinicopathological study of autism. Brain 121, 889–905.

Baker, P., Piven, J., Schwartz, S., Patil, S., 1994. Brief report: Duplication of chromosome 15q11-13 in two individuals with autistic disorder. Journal of Autism and Developmental Disorders 24, 529–535.

Baron, C.A., Tepper, C.G., Liu, S.Y., Davis, R.R., Wang, N.J., Schanen, N.C., et al., 2006. Genomic and functional profiling of duplicated chromosome 15 cell lines reveal regulatory alterations in UBE3A-associated ubiquitin-proteasome pathway processes. Human Molecular Genetics 15, 853–869.

Baron-Cohen, S., 1995. Mindblindness: An Essay on Autism and Theory of Mind. MIT Press, Cambridge.

Baron-Cohen, S., Campbell, R., Karmiloff-Smith, A., Grant, J., Walker, J., 1999. Are children with autism blind to mentalistic significance of the eyes? British Journal of Developmental Psychology 13, 379–398.

Baron-Cohen, S., Wheelwright, S., Hill, J., 2001. The reading the mind in the eyes test revised version: a study with normal adults, and adults with Asperger syndrome or high-functioning autism. Journal of Child Psychology and Psychiatry 42, 241–252.

Bass, M.P., Menold, M.M., Wolpert, C.M., Donnelly, S.L., Ravan, S.A., Hauser, E.R., et al., 2000. Genetic studies in autistic disorder and chromosome 15. Neurogenetics 2, 219–226.

Battaglia, A., 2008. The inv dup (15) or idic (15) syndrome (tetrasomy 15q). Orphanet Journal of Rare Diseases 3, 30.

Battaglia, A., Gurrieri, F., Bertini, E., Bellacosa, A., Pomponi, M.G., Paravatou-Petsotas, M., et al., 1997. The inv dup(15) syndrome: a clinically recognizable syndrome with altered behavior, mental retardation, and epilepsy. Neurology 48, 1081–1086.

Bauman, M.L., Kemper, T.L., 1985. Histoanatomic observations of the brain in early infantile autism. Neurology 35, 866–867.

Bauman, M.L., Kemper, T.L., 1996. Observations of the Purkinje cells in the cerebellar vermis in autism. Journal of Neuropathology and Experimental Neurology 55, 613.

Bayer, T.A., Wirths, O., 2010. Intracellular accumulation of amyloid-beta–a predictor of synaptic dysfunction and neuron loss in Alzheimer's disease. Frontiers in Aging Neuroscience 2, 8.

Belton, T., McCrea, R.A., 1999. Contribution of the cerebellar flocculus to gaze control during active head movements. Journal of Neurophysiology 81, 3105–3109.

Bittel, D.C., Kibiryeva, N., Talebizadeh, Z., Driscoll, D.J., Butler, M.G., 2005. Microarray analysis of gene/transcript expression in Angelman syndrome: deletion versus UPD. Genomics 85, 85–91.

Blum, A.S., Ives, J.R., Goldberger, A.L., Al-Aweel, I.C., Krishnamurthy, K.B., Drislane, F.W., et al., 2000. Oxygen desaturations triggered by partial seizures: Implications for cardiopulmonary instability in epilepsy. Epilepsia 41, 536–541.

Bolton, P.F., Dennis, N.R., Browne, C.E., Thomas, N.S., Veltman, M.W., Thompson, R.J., et al., 2001. The phenotypic manifestations of interstitial duplications of proximal 15q with special reference to the autistic spectrum disorders. American Journal of Medicinal Genetics 105, 675–685.

Bolton, P., Macdonald, H., Pickles, A., Rios, P., Goode, S., Crowson, M., et al., 1994. A case-control family history study of autism. Journal of Child Psychology and Psychiatry 35, 877–900.

Bolton, P.F., Veltman, M.W., Weisblatt, E., Holmes, J.R., Thomas, N.S., Youings, S.A., et al., 2004. Chromosome 15q11-13 abnormalities and other medical conditions in individuals with autism spectrum disorders. Psychiatric Genetics 14, 131–137.

Bryson, S.E., 1996. Brief report: epidemiology of autism. Journal of Autism and Developmental Disorders 26, 165–167.

Bundey, S., Hardy, C., Vickers, S., Kilpatrick, M.W., Corbett, J.A., 1994. Duplication of the 15q11-13 region in a patient with autism, epilepsy and ataxia. Development Medicine and Child Neurology 36, 736–742.

Buxbaum, J.D., Silverman, J.M., Smith, C.J., Greenberg, D.A., Kilifarski, M., Reichert, J., et al., 2002. Association between a GABRB3 polymorphism and autism. Molecular Psychiatry 7, 311–316.

Caspersen, C., Wang, N., Yao, J., Sosunov, A., Chen, X., Lustbader, J.W., et al., 2005. Mitochondrial Aβ: a potential focal point for neuronal metabolic dysfunction in Alzheimer's disease. FASEB Journal 19, 2040–2041.

Cook, D.G., Forman, M.S., Sung, J.C., Leight, S., Kolson, D.L., Iwatsubo, T., et al., 1997. Alzheimer's Aβ (1–42) is generated in the endoplasmic reticulum/ intermediate compartment of NT2N cells. Nature Medicine 3, 1021–1023.

Cook, E.H., Courchesne, R.Y., Cox, N.J., Lord, C., Gonen, D., Guter, S.J., et al., 1998. Linkage-disequilibrium mapping of autistic disorder, with 15q11-13 markers. American Journal of Human Genetics 62, 1077–1083.

Cook, E.H., Lindgren, V., Leventhal, B.L., Courchesne, R., Lincoln, A., Shulman, C., et al., 1997. Autism or atypical autism in maternally but not paternally derived proximal 15q duplication. American Journal of Human Genetics 60, 928–934.

Courchesne, E., Carper, R., Akshoomoff, N., 2003. Evidence of brain overgrowth in the first year of life in autism. The Journal of American Medical Association 290, 337–344.

Courchesne, E., Karns, C.M., Davis, H.R., Ziccardi, R., Carper, R.A., Tigue, Z.D., et al., 2001. Unusual brain growth patterns in early life in patients with autistic disorder. an MRI study. Neurology 57, 245–254.

Courchesne, E., Mouton, P.R., Calhoun, M.E., Semendeferi, K., Ahrens-Barbeau, C., Hallet, M.J., et al., 2011. Neuron number and size in prefrontal cortex of children with autism. The Journal of American Medical Association 306, 2001–2010.

Crolla, J.A., Harvey, J.F., Sitch, F.L., Dennis, N.R., 1995. Supernumerary marker 15 chromosomes: a clinical, molecular and FISH approach to diagnosis and prognosis. Human Genetics 95, 161–170.

Dawson, G., Meltzoff, A., Osterling, J., Rinaldi, J., 1998. Neuropsychological correlates of early symptoms of autism. Child Development 69, 1276–1285.

Dawson, A.J., Mogk, R., Rothenmund, H., Bridge, P.J., 2002. Paternal origin of a small, class I inv dup (15). American Journal of Medical Genetics 107, 334–336.

Demb, H.B., Papola, P., 1995. PDD and Prader-Willi syndrome. Journal of the American Academy of Child & Adolescent Psychiatry 34, 539–540.

Dennis, N.R., Veltman, M.W., Thompson, R., Craig, E., Bolton, P.F., Thomas, N.S., 2006. Clinical findings in 33 subjects with large supernumerary marker (15) chromosomes and 3 subjects with triplication of 15q11-q13. Amerian Journal of Medical Genetics. Part A 140, 434–441.

Dykens, E.M., Kasari, C., 1997. Maladaptive behavior in children with Prader-Willi syndrome, Down syndrome, and non-specific mental retardation. American Journal of Mental Retardation 102, 228–237.

Flejter, W.L., Bennett-Baker, P.E., Ghaziuddin, M., McDonald, M., Sheldon, S., Gorski, J.L., 1996. Cytogenetic and molecular analysis of inv dup (15) chromosomes observed in two patients with autistic disorder and mental retardation. American Journal of Medical Genetics 61, 182–187.

Folstein, S., Rutter, M., 1977. Infantile autism: a genetic study of 21 twin pairs. Journal of Child Psychology and Psychiatry 18, 297–321.

Folstein, S.E., Piven, J., 1991. Etiology of autism: Genetic influences. Pediatrics 87, 767–773.

Fombonne, E., Rogé, B., Claverie, J., Courty, S., Frémolle, J., 1999. Microcephaly and macrocephaly in autism. Journal of Autism and Developmental Disorders 29, 113–119.

Frysinger, R.C., Harper, R.M., 1990. Cardiac and respiratory correlations with unit discharge in epileptic human temporal lobe. Epilepsia 31, 162–171.

Gabriel, J.M., Higgins, M.J., Gebuhr, T.C., Shows, T.B., Saitoh, S., Nicholls, R.D., 1998. A model system to study genomic imprinting of human genes. Proceedings of the National Academy of Sciences of the United States of America 95, 14857–14862.

Gillberg, C., 1998. Chromosomal disorders and autism. Journal of Autism and Developmental Disorders 28, 415–425.

Gillberg, C., Steffenburg, S., Wahlstrom, J., Gillberg, I.C., Sjostedt, A., Martinson, T., et al., 1991. Autism associated with marker chromosome. Journal of the American Academy of Child & Adolescent Psychiatry 30, 489–494.

Glabe, C., 2001. Intracellular mechanisms of amyloid accumulation and pathogenesis in Alzheimer's disease. Journal of Molecular Neuroscience 17, 137–145.

Gouras, G.K., Tampellini, D., Takahashi, R.H., Capetillo-Zarate, E., 2010. Intraneuronal β-amyloid accumulation and synapse pathology in Alzheimer's disease. Acta Neuropathologica 119, 523–541.

Gowing, E., Roher, A.E., Woods, A.S., Cotter, R.J., Chaney, M., Little, S.P., et al., 1994. Chemical characterization of Aβ17-42 peptide, a component of diffuse amyloid deposits of Alzheimer disease. Journal of Biological Chemistry 269, 10987–10990.

Greenfield, J.P., Tsai, J., Gouras, G.K., Hai, B., Thinakaran, G., Checler, F., et al., 1999. Endoplasmic reticulum and trans-golgi network generate distinct populations of Alzheimer β-amyloid peptides. Proceedings of the National Academy of Sciences of the United States of America 96, 742–747.

Guerin, P., Lyon, G., Barthelemy, C., Sostak, E., Chevrollier, V., Garreau, B., et al., 1996. Neuropathological study of a case of autistic syndrome with severe mental retardation. Developmental Medicine and Child Neurology 38, 203–211.

Gyure, K.A., Durham, R., Stewart, W.F., Smialek, J.E., Troncoso, J.C., 2001. Intraneuronal Aβ-amyloid precedes development of amyloid plaques in Down syndrome. Archives of Pathology & Laboratory Medicine 125, 489–492.

Hagerman, R.J., 2002. The physical and behavioral phenotype. In: Hagerman, R.J., Hagerman, P.J. (Eds.), Fragile X syndrome: Diagnosis, Treatment, and Research, third ed. John Hopkins University Press, Baltimore, pp. 3–109.

Hallmayer, J., Cleveland, S., Torres, A., Phillips, J., Cohen, B., Torigoe, T., et al., 2011. Genetic heritability and shared environmental factors among twin pairs with autism. Archives of General Psychiatry doi:10.1001/archgenpsychiatry.2011.76.

Happe, F., Ronald, A., Plomin, R., 2006. Time to give up on a single explanation for autism. Nature Neuroscience 9, 1218–1220.

Hartmann, T., Bieger, S.C., Brühl, B., Tienari, P.J., Ida, N., Allsop, D., et al., 1997. Distinct sites of intracellular production for Alzheimer's disease Aβ40/42 amyloid peptides. Nature Medicine 3, 1016–1020.

Hof, P.R., Knabe, R., Bovier, P., Bouras, C., 1991. Neuropathological observations in a case of autism presenting with self-injury behavior. Acta Neuropathologica 82, 321–326.

Hogart, A., Leung, K.N., Wang, N.J., Wu, D.J., Driscoll, J., Vellero, R.O., et al., 2008. Chromosome 15q11-13 duplication syndrome brain reveals epigenetic alterations in gene expression not predicted from copy number. Journal of Medical Genetics 46, 86–93.

Hogart, A., Nagarajan, R.P., Patzel, K.A., Yasui, D.H., LaSalle, J.M., 2007. 15q11-13 GABAA receptor genes are normally biallelically expressed in brain yet are subject to epigenetic dysregulation in autism spectrum disorders. Human Molecular Genetics 16, 691–703.

Hotopf, M., Bolton, P., 1995. A case of autism associated with partial tetrasomy 15. Journal of Autism and Developmental Disorders 25, 41–48.

Iversen, L.L., Mortishire-Smith, R.J., Pollack, S.J., Shearman, M.S., 1995. The toxicity in vitro of beta-amyloid protein. Biochemistry Journal 311, 1–16.

Kemper, T.L., Bauman, M.L., 1993. The contribution of neuropathologic studies to the understanding of autism. Neurologic Clinics 11, 175–187.

Kent, L., Evans, J., Paul, M., Sharp, M., 1999. Comorbidity of autistic spectrum disorders in children with Down syndrome. Developmental Medicine and Child Neurology 41, 153–158.

Kerbeshian, J., Burd, L., Randall, T., Martsolf, J., Jalal, S., 1990. Autism, profound mental retardation, and typical bipolar disorder in a 33-year-old female with a deletion of 15q12. Journal of Mental Deficiency Research 34 205–210.

Kinney, H.C., Armstrong, D.L., Chadwick, A.E., Crandall, L.A., Hilbert, C., Belliveau, R.A., et al., 2007. Sudden death in toddlers associated with developmental abnormalities of the hippocampus: a report of five cases. Pediatric and Developmental Pathology 10, 208–223.

Knoll, J.H.M., Wagstaff, J., Lalande, M., 1993. Cytogenetic and molecular studies in the Prader-Willi and Angelman syndromes: an overview. American Journal of Medical Genetics 46, 2–6.

Lainhart, J.E., Piven, J., Wzorek, M., Landa, R., Santangelo, S.L., Coon, H., et al., 1997. Macrocephaly in children and adults with autism. Journal of the American Academy of Child & Adolescent Psychiatry 36, 282–290.

Lalowski, M., Golabek, A., Lemere, C.A., Selkoe, D.J., Wisniewski, H.M., Beavis, R.C., et al., 1996. The "non-amyloidogenic " p3 fragment (amyloid β 17-24) is a major constituent of Down's syndrome cerebellar preamyloid. Journal of Biological Chemistry 271, 33623–33631.

Lauritsen, M., Mors, O., Mortensen, P.B., Ewald, H., 1999. Infantile autism and associated autosomal chromosome abnormalities: a register-based study and a literature survey. Journal of Child Psychology and Psychiatry 40, 335–345.

Leana-Cox, J., Jenkins, L., Palmer, C.G., Plattner, R., Sheppard, L., Flejter, W.L., et al., 1994. Molecular cytogenetic analysis of inv dup(15) chromosomes, using probes specific for the Prader-Willi/Angelman syndrome region: clinical implications. American Journal of Human Genetics 54, 748–756.

Leekam, S.R., Hunnisett, E., Moore, C., 1998. Targets and cues: gaze-following in children with autism. Journal of Child Psychology and Psychiatry 39, 951–962.

Leekam, S.R., Lopez, B., Moore, C., 2000. Attention and joint attention in preschool children with autism. Developmental Psychology 36, 261–273.

Leung, H.C., Suh, M., Kettner, R.E., 2000. Cerebellar flocculus and paraflocculus Purkinje cell activity during circular pursuit in monkey. Journal of Neurophysiology 83, 13–30.

Liu, K., Zerubavel, N., Bearman, P., 2010. Social demographic change in autism. Demography 47, 327–343.

Lotspeich, L.J., Ciaranello, R.D., 1993. The neurobiology and genetics of infantile autism. International Review of Neurobiology 35, 87–129.

Mann, D.M., Brown, A., Prinja, D., Davies, C.A., Landon, M., Masters, C.L., et al., 1989. An analysis of the morphology of senile plaques in Down's syndrome patients of different ages using immunocytochemical and lectin histochemical techniques. Neuropathology and Applied Neurobiology 15, 317–329.

Mao, R., Jalal, S.M., Snow, K., Michels, V.V., Szabo, S.M., Babovic-Vuksanovic, D., 2000. Characteristics of two cases with dup(15)(q11.2-q12): one of maternal and one of paternal origin. Genetics in Medicine. 2, 131–135.

Martin, E.R., Menold, M.M., Wolpert, C.M., Bass, M.P., Donelly, S.L., Ravan, S.A., et al., 2000. Analysis of linkage disequilibrium in γ-aminobutyric acid receptor subunit genes in autistic disorder. American Journal of Medical Genetics 96, 43–48.

Martinsson, T., Johanesson, T., Vujic, M., Sjostedt, A., Steffenburg, S., Gillberg, C., et al., 1996. Maternal origin in inv dup(15) chromosomes in infantile autism. European Child & Adolescent Psychiatry 5, 185–192.

Meguro, M., Mitsuya, K., Sui, H., Shigenami, K., Kugoh, H., Nakao, M., et al., 1997. Evidence for uniparental, paternal expression of the human GABAA receptor subunit genes, using microcell-mediated chromosome transfer. Human Molecular Genetics 6, 2127–2133.

Menold, M.M., Shao, Y., Wolpert, C.M., Donnelly, S.L., Raiford, K.L., Martin, E.R., et al., 2001. Association analysis of chromosome 15 gabaa receptor subunit genes in autistic disorder. Journal of Neurogenetics 15, 245–259.

Mochizuki, A., Tamaoka, A., Shimohata, A., Komatsuzaki, Y., Shoji, S., 2000. Aβ42-positive non-pyramidal neurons around amyloid plaques in Alzheimer's disease. The Lancet 355, 42–43.

Mohandas, T.K., Park, J.P., Spellman, R.A., Filiano, J.J., Mamourian, A.C., Hawk, A.B., et al., 1999. Paternally derived de novo interstitial duplication of proximal 15q in a patient with developmental delay. American Journal of Medical Genetics 82, 294–300.

Mundy, P., Sigman, M., Ungerer, J., Sherman, T., 1986. Defining the social deficits of autism: the contribution of non-verbal communication measures. Journal of Child Psychology and Psychiatry 27, 657–669.

Ozcelik, T., Leff, S., Robinson, W., Donlon, T., Lalande, M., Sanjines, E., et al., 1992. Small nuclear ribonucleoprotein polypeptide N (SNRPN), an expressed gene in the Prader-Willi syndrome critical region. Nature Genetics 2, 265–269.

Palmen, S.J.M.C., van Engeland, H., Hof, P.R., Schmitz, C., 2004. Neuropathological findings in autism. Brain 127, 2572–2583.

Penner, K.A., Johnston, J., Faircloth, B.H., Irish, P., Williams, C.A., 1993. Communication, cognition, and social interaction in the Angelman syndrome. American Journal of Medical Genetics 46, 34–39.

Ray, B., Long, J.M., Sokol, D.K., Lahiri, D.K., 2011. Increased secreted amyloid precursor protein-α (sAPPα) in severe autism: proposal of a specific, anabolic pathway and putative biomarker. PLoS ONE 6, 1–10. e20405.

Redcay, E., Courchesne, E., 2005. When is the brain enlarged in autism? a meta-analysis of all brain size-reports. Biological Psychiatry 58, 1–9.

Reddy, K.S., 2005. Cytogenetic abnormalities and fragile x-syndrome in autism spectrum disorder. BMC Medical Genetics 6, 3.

Rineer, S., Finucane, B., Simon, E.W., 1998. Autistic symptoms among children and young adults with isodicentric chromosome 15. American Journal of Medical Genetics 81, 428–433.

Ritvo, E.R., Freeman, B.J., Mason-Brothers, A., Mo, A., et al., 1985. Concordance for the syndrome of autism in 40 pairs of afflicted twins. American Journal of Psychiatry 142, 74–77.

Ritvo, E.R., Freeman, B.J., Scheibel, A.B., Duong, T., Robinson, H., Guthrie, D., Ritvo, A., 1986. Lower Purkinje cell counts in the cerebella of four autistic subjects: Initial findings of the UCLA-NSAC autopsy research report. American Journal of Psychiatry 143, 862–866.

Robinson, W.P., Wagstaff, J., Bernasconi, F., Baccichetti, C., Artifoni, L., Franzoni, E., Suslak, L., et al., 1993. Uniparental disomy explains the occurrence of the Angelman or Prader-Willi syndrome in patients with an additional small inv dup(15) chromosome. Journal of Medical Genetics 30, 756–760.

Rutter, M., Bolton, P., Harrington, R., Le Couteur, A., Macdonald, H., Simonoff, E., 1990. Genetic factors in child psychiatric disorders: I. a review of research strategies. Journal of Child Psychology and Psychiatry 31, 3–37.

Rutter, M., Macdonald, H., Le Couteur, A., Harrington, R., Bolton, P., Bailey, A., 1990. Genetic factors in child psychiatric disorders: II. empirical findings. Journal of Child Psychology and Psychiatry 31, 39–83.

Schroer, R.J., Phelan, M.C., Michaelis, R.C., Crawford, E.C., Skinner, S.A., Cuccaro, M., et al., 1998. Autism and maternally derived aberrations of chromosome 15q. American Journal of Medical Genetics 76, 327–336.

Selkoe, D.J., 2001. Alzheimer's disease: genes, proteins, and therapy. Physiological Reviews 81, 741–766.

Smalley, S.L., Asarnow, R.F., Spence, M.A., 1988. Autism and genetics. a decade of research. Archives of General Psychiatry 45, 953–961.

Sokol, D.K., Chen, D., Farlow, M.R., Dunn, D.W., Maloney, B., Zimmer, J.A., et al., 2006. High levels of Alzheimer beta- amyloid precursor protein (APP) in children with severely autistic behavior and aggression. Journal of Child Neurology 21, 444–449.

Sokol, D.K., Maloney, B., Long, J.M., Ray, B., Lahiri, D.K., 2011. Autism, Alzheimer disease, and fragile X. APP, FMRP, and mGluR5 are molecular links. Neurology 76, 1344–1352.

Steffenburg, S., Gillberg, C., Hellgren, L., Andersson, L., Gillberg, I.C., Jakobsson, G., et al., 1989. A twin study of autism in Denmark, Finland, Iceland, Norway, and Sweden. Journal of Child Psychology and Psychiatry 30, 405–416.

Steffenburg, S., Gillberg, C.L., Steffenburg, U., Kyllerman, M., 1996. Autism in Angelman syndrome: a population-based study. Pediatric Neurology 14, 131–136.

Summers, J.A., Allison, D.B., Lynch, P.S., Sandler, L., 1995. Behavior problems in Angelman syndrome. Journal of Intellectual Disability Research 39, 97–106.

Tagliavini, F., Giaccone, G., Linoli, G., Frangione, B., Bugiani, O., 1989. Cerebral extracellular preamyloid deposits in Alzheimer's disease, Down syndrome and nondemented elderly individuals. Progress in Clinical and Biological Research 317, 1001–1005.

Takahashi, R.H., Milner, T.A., Li, F., Nam, E.E., Edgar, M.A., Yamaguchi, H., et al., 2002. Intraneuronal Alzheimer Aβ42 accumulates in multivesicular bodies and is associated with synaptic pathology. American Journal of Pathology 161, 1869–1879.

Tan, J., Epema, A.H., Voogd, J., 1995. Zonal organization of the flocculovestibular nucleus projection in the rabbit: A combined axonal tracing and acetylcholinesterase histochemical study. Journal of Comparative Neurology 356, 51–71.

Tuchman, R.F., Rapin, I., 2002. Epilepsy in autism. Lancet Neurology 1, 352–358.

Tuchman, R., Moshe, S.L., Rapin, I., 2009. Convulsing toward the pathophysiology of autism. Brain & Development 31, 95–103.

Wang, N.J., Liu, D., Parokonny, A.S., Schanen, N.C., 2004. High-resolution molecular characterization of 15q11-q13 rearrangements by array comparative genomic hybridization (array CGH) with detection of gene dosage. American Journal of Human Genetics 75, 267–281.

Wang, K., Zhang, H., Ma, D., Bucan, M., Glessner, J.T., Abrahams, B.S., et al., 2009. Common genetic variants on 5p14.1 associate with autism spectrum disorders. Nature 459, 528–533.

Wassink, T.H., Brzustowicz, L.M., Bartlett, C.W., Szatmari, P., 2004. The search for autism disease genes. Mental Retardation and Developmental Disabilities Research Reviews 10, 272–283.

Webb, T., 1994. Inv dup (15) supernumerary marker chromosomes. Journal of Medical Genetics 31, 585–594.

Webb, T., Hardy, C.A., King, M., Watkiss, E., Mitchell, C., Cole, T., 1998. A clinical, cytogenetic and molecular study of ten probands with inv dup (15) marker chromosomes. Clinical Genetics 53, 34–43.

Wegiel, J., Frackowiak, J., Mazur-Kolecka, B., Schanen, N.C., Cook, E.H., Sigman, M., et al., 2012b. Abnormal intracellular accumulation and extracellular Aβ deposition in idiopathic and dup 15q11.2-q13 autism spectrum disorders. PLoS ONE. www.plosone.org 7,5, e35414.

Wegiel, J., Kuchna, I., Nowicki, K., Frackowiak, J., Mazur-Kolecka, B., Imaki, H., et al., 2007. Intraneuronal Aβ immunoreactivity is not a predictor of brain amyloidosis-β or neurofibrillary degeneration. Acta Neuropathologica 113, 389–402.

Wegiel, J., Kuchna, I., Nowicki, K., Imaki, H., Wegiel, J., Ma, S.Y., et al., 2012. Contribution of olivo-floccular circuitry developmental defects to atypical gaze in autism. Journal of Autism and Developmental Disorders, Submitted for publication.

Wegiel, J., Kuchna, I., Nowicki, K., Imaki, H., Wegiel, J., Marchi, E., et al., 2010. The neuropathology of autism: defects of neurogenesis and neuronal migration, and dysplastic changes. Acta Neuropathologica 119, 755–770.

Wegiel, J., Schanen, N.C., Cook, E.H., Sigman, M., Brown, W.T., Kuchna, I., et al., 2012. Differences between the pattern of developmental abnormalities in autism associated with duplications 15q11.2-q13 and idiopathic autism. Journal of Neuropathology and Experimental Neurology 71, 382–397.

Weidmer-Mikhail, E., Sheldon, S., Ghaziuddin, M., 1998. Chromosomes in autism and related pervasive developmental disorders: a cytogenetic study. Journal of Intellectual Disability Research 42, 8–12.

Weller, R.O., Massey, A., Newman, T.A., Hutchings, M., Kuo, Y.M., Roher, A.E., 1998. Cerebral amyloid angiopathy: amyloid beta accumulates in putative interstitial fluid drainage pathways in Alzheimer's disease. American Journal of Pathology 153, 725–733.

Westmark, C.J., Malter, J.S., 2007. FMRP mediates mGluR5-dependent translation of amyloid precursor protein. PLoS Biology 5, e52.

Westmark, C.J., Westmark, P.R., O'Riordan, K.J., Ray, B.C., Hervey, C.M., Salamat, M.S., et al., 2011. Reversal of fragile X phenotypes by manipulation of AβPP/Aβ levels in Fmr1^{KO} mice. PLoS ONE 6, e26549.

Whitney, E.R., Kemper, T.L., Bauman, M.L., Rosene, D.L., Blatt, G.J., 2008. Cerebellar Purkinje cells are reduced in a subpopulation of autistic brains: a stereological experiment using Calbindin-D28k. Cerebellum 7, 406–416.

Whitney, E.R., Kemper, T.L., Rosene, D.L., Bauman, M.L., Blatt, G.J., 2009. Density of cerebellar basket and stellate cells in autism: evidence for a late developmental loss of Purkinje cells. Journal of Neuroscience Research 87, 2245–2254.

Wilson, C.A., Doms, R.W., Lee, V.M.-Y., 1999. Intracellular APP processing and Aβ production in Alzheimer disease. Journal of Neuropathology and Experimental Neurology 58, 787–794.

Winton, M.J., Lee, E.B., Sun, E., Wong, M.M., Leight, S., Zhang, B., et al., 2011. Intraneuronal APP, not free Aβ peptides in 3xTg-AD mice: Implications for tau versus Aβ-mediated Alzheimer neurodegeneration. Journal of Neuroscience 31, 7691–7699.

Wisniewski, H.M., Sadowski, M., Jakubowska-Sadowska, K., Tarnawski, M., Wegiel, J., 1998. Diffuse, lake-like amyloid-ß deposits in the parvopyramidal layer of the presubiculum in Alzheimer disease. Journal of Neuropathology and Experimental Neurology 57, 674–683.

Wolpert, C.M., Menold, M.M., Bass, M.P., Qumsieh, M.B., Donelly, S.L., Ravan, S.A., et al., 2000. Three probands with autistic disorder and isodicentric chromosome 15. American Journal of Medical Genetics 96, 365–372.

Wolpert, C., Pericak-Vance, M.A., Abramson, R.K., Wright, H.H., Cuccaro, M.L., 2000. Autistic symptoms among children and young adults with isodicentric chromosome 15. American Journal of Medical Genetics 96, 128–129.

Yang, T.F., Wong, T.T., Chang, K.P., Kwan, S.Y., Kuo, W.Y., Lee, Y.C., et al., 2001. Power spectrum analysis of heart rate variability in children with epilepsy. Child's Nervous System 17, 602–606.

MODEL SYSTEMS AND PATHWAYS IN AUTISM SPECTRUM DISORDERS
Joseph D. Buxbaum

There is great interest in model systems for autism spectrum disorders (ASD) that can help our understanding of disease mechanisms and pathophysiology, while providing means to aid in drug development. Mouse models remain one of the most widely used animal models for ASD (Wetsel, Moy, and Jiang), while nonhuman primates provide unique opportunities to understand the brain structures involved in high-order cognitive function (Bauman and Amaral). An emerging field is that of inducible pluripotent stem cells (iPSC) from patients, which provide a means of studying human neural cells carrying risk genes and loci in the laboratory setting (Muotri).

The most common known causes of ASD include duplications at 15q11–q13 (Takumi, Fukumoto, and Nomura), as well as mutations of *FMR1* (Brown and Cohen), *MECP2* (Adams and LaSalle), *SHANK* genes (Harony, Gunal, and Buxbaum), and PI3K signaling genes (Kwok, Mellios, and Sur). These genes, loci, and pathways account for as much as 5% of ASD, and it is instructive to survey what is known about them, both in ASD and in model systems. One emerging finding is that the genes and pathways involved are distinct, suggesting that a simple integrated model for ASD is very unlikely. Other genes and pathways that are implicated in ASD are discussed in Section 2, which summarizes the extreme etiological heterogeneity of ASD.

This section concludes with a brief overview of the emerging field of systems biology in ASD (Buxbaum), and shows how such approaches can identify pathways disrupted in a recurrent manner in ASD.

The chapters in Section 4 provide a high-level look at model systems in ASD while underscoring the difficulty in trying to model all ASD genes. The chapters also show the utility of multiple neurobiological approaches when analyzing ASD models, and provide a reminder that there is not likely to be a specific phenotype at any level that is invariably associated with different causes of ASD. This is not that unexpected, as the human genes and loci associated with ASD show variable expressivity as well.

4.1

Mouse Behavioral Models for Autism Spectrum Disorders

William C. Wetsel*, Sheryl S. Moy†, Yong-hui Jiang**

*Departments of Psychiatry and Behavioral Sciences, Cell Biology, and Neurobiology, Duke University Medical Center, Durham, NC, USA †Carolina Institute for Developmental Disabilities and Department of Psychiatry, University of North Carolina at Chapel Hill, Chapel Hill, NC, USA **Departments of Pediatrics and Neurobiology, Duke University Medical Center, Durham, NC, USA

BEHAVIORAL CHARACTERISTICS OF AUTISM SPECTRUM DISORDERS IN HUMANS

Currently, the diagnosis of autism is based primarily on evaluation of behavioral features because there are no reliable biological or imaging markers available (Lord et al., 2000a; Volkmar et al., 2009; see also Section 1). Clinical diagnosis is made according to criteria described in the Diagnostic and Statistical Manual of Mental Disorders (DSM-IV; American Psychiatric Association, 1994) in conjunction with clinical judgment (Table 4.1.1). These criteria include impaired development in social interaction and communication, as well as restricted, repetitive, and stereotyped responses. Some of these features are shared with Asperger syndrome and pervasive developmental disorder not otherwise specified (including atypical autism), or PDD-NOS. Asperger syndrome includes

the same criteria as autism for social interactions and repetitive/stereotyped behaviors; however, there is no clinically significant delay in language (American Psychiatric Association, 1994). A diagnosis of PDD-NOS is rendered when there are severe impairments in the development of reciprocal social interactions or nonverbal or verbal communication, or when stereotyped behavior, activities, or interests are evident (American Psychiatric Association, 1994). These patients should not meet criteria for any other pervasive developmental disorder, schizophrenia, schizotypal personality disorder, or avoidant personality disorder. Autistic disorder, Asperger syndrome, and PDD-NOS are frequently referred to as autism spectrum disorders (ASD).

Many sophisticated diagnostic or screen instruments such ADOS (autism diagnostic observation schedule) and ADI-R (autism diagnostic interview-revised) have been developed over the last decade (Lord et al.,

The Neuroscience of Autism Spectrum Disorders.
http://dx.doi.org/10.1016/B978-0-12-391924-3.00026-0

TABLE 4.1.1   DSM-IV Criteria for Diagnosis of Autism

I. Six or more impairments from categories A, B, and C, with at least two from A and one each from B and C

    A. Qualitative impairment in social interaction by two or more of the following:

        1. Marked impairments in the use of multiple nonverbal responses

        2. Failure to develop relationships with peers at appropriate developmental level

        3. Lack of spontaneous seeking to share interests, enjoyment, or achievements with others

        4. Absence of reciprocal emotional or social interaction

    B. Qualitative impairments in communication by one or more of the following:

        1. Delay or total lack of the development of spoken language

        2. Marked impairment to initiate or sustain a conversation with others in individuals with adequate speech

        3. Idiosyncratic or stereotyped and repetitive use of language

        4. Lack of varied, spontaneous make-believe or social-imitative play appropriate to developmental level

    C. Restricted stereotyped and repetitive behaviors, interests, and activities in at least two of the following:

        1. Encompassing preoccupation with one or more stereotyped and restricted patterns of interest that is abnormal in focus or intensity

        2. Inflexibility to specific nonfunctional rituals or routines

        3. Repetitive and stereotyped motor responses

        4. Persistent preoccupation with parts of objects

II. Delays or abnormal functioning in at least one of the following with onset prior to 3 years of age:

    A. Social interaction

    B. Language as used in social communication

    C. Symbolic or imaginative play

III. The disturbance is not better accounted for by Rett's disorder or childhood disintegrative disorder

---

From: American Psychiatric Association (1994).

2000b; 2001). Because special training or certification is required for clinicians or clinical psychologists to administer these instruments, the use of these tools to assist in the diagnosis of ASD has varied significantly among different centers in United States, and even more in other countries due to the language barriers. These practices have posed some challenges in interpreting and comparing findings from different studies in the field of autism research.

As may be expected, there is considerable clinical heterogeneity in ASD (Lord et al., 2000a). The degree of impairments in core features can vary significantly among individuals with diagnosis of autism (Lord et al., 2001). For example, the impairments in language and communication may range from absence of speech to only mild attenuation – or it may not be affected, as in Asperger syndrome. Co-occurrence of a long list of comorbidities also contributes to the clinical heterogeneity (Bauman, 2010; Micali et al., 2004; Xue et al., 2008). The most common comorbidity in ASD is intellectual disability, which can vary in severity and is observed in about 70% of ASD patients. Other common comorbidities include seizures, sleep disturbances, gastrointestinal abnormalities, attention deficit and hyperactivity, and movement disorders. The pathophysiology of these comorbidities is not well understood, in part because in many cases the etiology of the core behavioral features is still elusive. However, clinical treatment of these comorbidities is important for improving the quality of life of ASD children and their families (Coury et al., 2009).

GENETICS AND PATHOPHYSIOLOGY OF AUTISM SPECTRUM DISORDERS

The high heritability of ASD has been well supported by the high concordance rate (70–90%) in monozygotic twins (Folstein and Rutter, 1977; Ronald and Hoekstra, 2011). However, the inheritance pattern underlying ASD remains elusive (Beaudet, 2007; State and Levitt, 2011; Veenstra-VanderWeele et al., 2004). Although ASD in multiplex families is common, Mendelian inheritance in these families is rare. In some multiplex families, clinical presentations among affected children are quite variable, suggesting that each case may have a different etiology. Over the past decade, strong evidence has emerged supporting the involvement of single genes in the etiology of ASD (Abrahams and Geschwind, 2008; Miles, 2011). These include fragile X, Rett syndrome, and Angelman's syndrome – which are relatively common – and rare metabolic syndromes such as adenylosuccinate lyase deficiency and creatine metabolism disorders (Miles et al., 2010) (Table 4.1.2).

Identification of the molecular basis of other forms of ASD remains a challenge. Several approaches have been taken to identify their genetic basis, including linkage and genome-wide association, copy number variant (CNV), and candidate gene approaches (see Section 2). Traditional linkage and genome-wide association studies have been unsuccessful in identifying genes in the affected individuals. The recent discovery of CNVs within the human genome has led to many large-scale studies (Glessner et al., 2009; Pinto et al., 2010; Sebat et al., 2007; Weiss et al., 2008). These investigations have identified a few highly penetrant gain and loss CNVs that are strongly associated with ASD. Although CNV analysis has become a diagnostic tool in the clinical

TABLE 4.1.2 Genes and Chromosomal Defects Implicated in ASD

Syndromic ASD			Non-syndromic ASD	
Syndrome	*Gene*	*Function*	*Gene*	*Function*
Fragile X	FMR1	RNA binding	NLGN3	Ligand for neurexins
Rett	MeCP2	Methyl-DNA binding	NLGN4	Ligand for neurexins
Angelman	UBE3A	Ubiquitin ligase	SHANK2	Post-synaptic density protein
Timothy	CACNA1C	Ca^{2+} channel	SHANK3	Post-synaptic density protein
Tuberous sclerosis	TSC1/TSC2	Cell cycle	PCDH10	Cell adhesion
Sotos	NSD1	Histone modification	NRXN1	Synaptic receptor
PTEN-macrocephaly	PTEN	Protein phosphatase	CNTN3	Synaptic receptor
Cortical dysplasia[a]	CNTNAP2	Synaptic protein	CNTN4	Synaptic receptor
Phenylketonuria	PAH	Phenylalanine metabolism	NHE9	Na^+/H^+ exchanger
Creatine transporter	GAMT/AGAT/SLC6A8	Creatine metabolism		
Adenylosuccinate lyase deficiency	ADSL	Purine metabolism		
Smith–Lemli–Opitz	DHCR7	Cholesterol metabolism		
Syndrome	*Chromosome*		*Chromosome*	
Phelan–McDermid	22q13.3 deletion		16p11.2 deletion	
Angelman	15q11–q13 maternal deletion		15q11–q13 maternal duplication	
Prader–Willi	15q11–q13 paternal deletion		7q11.3 duplication	
Smith–Magenis	17q11.2 deletion		2q37 deletion	
Potocki–Lupski	17q11.2 duplication		1q21.1 deletion and duplication	
VCFS	22q11.2 deletion		15q13.3 deletion/duplication	

[a] *Also termed focal epilepsy syndrome.*

care of ASD, the overall detection rate is relatively low (5–10%), although it may be higher in individuals with more severe ASD symptoms who have other mild congenital anomalies (Miller et al., 2010; Shen et al., 2010). While most identified CNVs are novel and are found in single families, their clinical significance is unclear.

Besides CNVs, the candidate gene approach has led to the discovery of mutations in several genes in non-syndromic ASD. These genes include NLGN3/4, SHANK2, and SHANK3, and others are listed in Table 4.1.2 (Berkel et al., 2010; Durand et al., 2007; Jamain et al., 2003). The frequency of mutations in these genes is very low, and some have only been found within a single family. Despite their rarity, results from these studies have supported two general conclusions. First, they provide the first evidence that a genetic defect in a single gene or genes may underlie ASD. Second, mutations in these genes support an emerging theme that the molecular pathogenesis of ASD may reside in

dysfunction of synapses (see also chapter 2.1 and other chapters in Section 4). Nonetheless, the molecular bases of the majority of ASD cases remain to be determined (Schaaf et al., 2011). A new generation of sequencing techniques may help to reveal further insights into this problem (State and Levitt, 2011; and see Chapter 2.4). This and other information may allow us in the future to dissect the role of environmental or epigenetic factors implicated in the pathophysiology of ASD.

A number of approaches have been taken to gain insights into the pathophysiology of ASD. Studies using postmortem brain tissues from ASD patients have been used to provide specific clues into the pathophysiology of the condition (Amaral et al., 2008; Bauman and Kemper, 2005; and see Section 3). Importantly, the neuroanatomical basis of the core behavioral features of ASD remains poorly defined. Structural imaging investigations have found numerous alterations in various brain regions that differ from healthy controls (Anagnostou and Taylor, 2011). Functional magnetic resonance imaging studies have revealed hyper- or hypoconnectivity in selected brain regions of ASD patients (Minshew and Keller, 2010). Diffusion tensor imaging approaches have identified alterations in ASD brains (Ameis et al., 2011; Jou et al., 2011; Lange et al., 2010). However, interpretation of these findings is complicated by the small sample sizes in the studies, and by the molecular and clinical heterogeneity of the subjects. Despite inconsistencies, a major theory that has emerged from these studies is that the ASD brain undergoes an early period of overgrowth followed by deceleration (Courchesne et al., 2011a; Dawson et al., 2004). The overgrowth has been found in many different brain regions including both white and gray matter in the cerebral cortex, as well as in the striatum and other non-cortical areas. Despite these observations, little is known about the molecular basis of the overgrowth in brain

(Courchesne and Pierce, 2005). Recent research suggests that it may be due to significantly increased cell densities and sizes within the prefrontal cortex of ASD post-mortem brain (Courchesne et al., 2011b). Since the sample sizes were small, it remains to be determined whether these findings are replicable and whether they can be applied to a broad range of ASD cases.

MODELS OF AUTISM SPECTRUM DISORDERS USING INBRED STRAINS OF MICE

Since the diagnosis of autism is based upon core behavioral symptoms, animal models for the disorder are studied based upon intrinsic behavioral profiles that reflect these features (Table 4.1.3). Many studies

TABLE 4.1.3   Mouse Behavioral Assays to Model Core Symptoms of Autism

Behavioral test	Test description
SOCIAL DEFECTS	
Three-chamber social approach test	This task assesses social motivation and reward. Mice are given a choice between spending time in proximity to an unfamiliar mouse versus a novel object (a measure of sociability), or in proximity to an already-investigated mouse versus a novel mouse (a measure of social novelty preference and social recognition)
Direct interaction and juvenile play	Behavioral profiles during social interaction can provide an index of social reciprocity (a set of back-and-forth responses). Stimulus and partner responses include sniffing, crawling over or under, chasing, grooming or licking, mounting, and fighting
Social conditioned place preference	This choice task provides a measure of the reward value for a given context, without direct presentation of the motivating stimuli during the test. In the conditioning phase, mice learn to associate one set of unique environmental stimuli with social isolation, and another set with a social context (group housing). Mice are then given a choice between the environmental stimuli paired with the social versus non-social contexts
COMMUNICATION DEFICITS	
Social transmission of food preference	Mice can learn to prefer a novel food that has previously been consumed by a 'demonstrator' mouse through the social transfer of olfactory and other information, probably by sniffing food odors on the breath and mouth of the demonstrator
Ultrasonic vocalizations (USVs)	Neonatal mouse pups emit USVs in response to social isolation. Ultrasonic calls are also emitted during juvenile and adult social interaction, and male mice will produce USVs in response to exposure to female mouse urine (a social stimulus)
REPETITIVE BEHAVIOR	
Motor stereotypy	In mice, abnormal perseverative responses can include over-grooming (sometimes to the point of self-injury), 'jack-hammer' jumping, cage-lid back flipping, wall-climbing, locomotor circling, and increased digging in a marble-burying assay[a]
Restricted interests	Reduced interest can be measured by a lack of exploration in a novel environment, restricted pattern of poking in a nose-poke task, lack of preference for novel objects, and failure to dig in a marble-burying assay[a]
Reversal learning	Cognitive flexibility or rigidity can be assessed in the Morris water maze task. Mice learn to find the hidden platform in a fixed location in a circular pool. For reversal learning, the location of the platform is changed and mice are then evaluated for their ability to adapt to the new learning condition. Reversal learning can also be tested in a Barnes maze or T-maze procedure

[a] Note, marble burying is primarily a test for anxiety-like behaviors and it can be used as a screen for antidepressant action. If it is used to examine motor stereotypies and/or restricted interests, then additional tests should be run to exclude anxiety-like responses from the phenotype.

have focused on inbred mouse strains and outbred stock, which provide panels of genetically diverse lines to screen for social deficits, impaired communication, repetitive behavior, and other indices of ASD. For example, researchers have found that social approach and avoidance vary across different inbred and outbred mouse lines (Bolivar et al., 2007; Brodkin et al., 2004; Jacome et al., 2011; Moy et al., 2004; 2007; 2008b; Nadler et al., 2004; Sankoorikal et al., 2006). The use of multi-component phenotyping regimens has shown further that specific constellations of behavioral abnormalities characterize particular strains, in line with the diverse clinical profiles observed in ASD. The evaluation of mouse models across several functional domains can reveal alterations in behavior, such as increased anxiety, hyperactivity, or learning deficits, which all reflect comorbidities in the human disorder, as well as sensory or motor impairments that could confound the evaluation of social interaction or other behaviors.

Studies utilizing inbred mice have identified several strains that have phenotypic profiles reflecting one or more features of autism. Since C57BL/6J mice show high levels of sociability and are widely used as the genetic background for mutant lines, they are often used as a comparison group. One of the inbred strains found to display autism-like behaviors is BALB/c, or the closely related BALB/cByJ mouse. Both substrains have low social approach in a three-chambered choice task (Brodkin, 2007; Brodkin et al., 2004; Fairless et al., 2008; Jacome et al., 2011; Moy et al., 2007; Sankoorikal et al., 2006). BALB/c mice also have deficits in tests of direct social interaction (Jacome et al., 2011; Panksepp et al., 2007) and fail to demonstrate conditioned place preference for an environment associated with a social context (Panksepp et al., 2007; Panksepp and Lahvis, 2007). Social abnormalities reported for male BALB/c mice include deficient ultrasonic vocalizations during direct social interactions in adolescence (Panksepp et al., 2007) and moderate to high levels of aggression (Dow et al., 2011; Guillot and Chapouthier, 1996; Mineur et al., 2003). However, BALB/cJ and BALB/cByJ mice fail to engage in high rates of grooming or other types of motor stereotypies, and they do not show deficits in reversal learning, an index for cognitive rigidity (Jacome et al., 2011; Moy et al., 2007). These latter findings indicate that these BALB substrains do not meet the core symptom criteria for repetitive behavior in autism.

A goal for the use of mouse models is to identify neuroanatomical, biochemical, or genetic correlates to autism-like phenotypes, which could be informative for understanding mechanisms underlying the etiology and symptoms of the disorder. In this regard, BALB/c mice have variable reductions in the volume of the corpus callosum (Wahlsten, 1989; Wahlsten et al., 2003).

Fairless and colleagues (2008) have found that in BALB/cJ mice, the reduction in callosal size is correlated with decreased sociability in a three-chambered social approach test. It is notable that imaging studies in human subjects have provided evidence for deficient connectivity between brain regions in autism (Belmonte et al., 2004; Geschwind and Levitt, 2007; Just et al., 2007; Minshew and Williams, 2007). Thus, hemispheric connectivity may be especially important for responses during complex social encounters that involve rapid information processing across different brain regions.

In contrast to the incomplete penetrance of callosal volume reductions in BALB/c mice, the BTBR T$^+$tf/J inbred strain is devoid of a corpus callosum (Kusek et al., 2007; Wahlsten et al., 2003). This strain also has a behavioral profile that recapitulates many features associated with ASD, including low sociability in a three-chambered choice test, reduced direct social interaction and juvenile play, and deficient social transmission of food preference (Bolivar et al., 2007; Denfensor et al., 2011; McFarlane et al., 2008; Moy et al., 2007; Yang et al., 2007). Additionally, BTBR T$^+$tf/J mice have ultrasonic vocalizations that are different from C57BL/6J mice in a variety of social contexts (Scattoni et al., 2008; 2011; Wohr et al., 2011). The strain also engages in higher levels of self-grooming than C57BL/6J animals (McFarlane et al., 2008; Yang et al., 2007) – although this response could be a consequence of the *tufted* (*tf*) mutation in the BTBR T$^+$tf/J strain, which leads to abnormal hair loss in mice (Lyon, 1956). One study has shown that BTBR T$^+$tf/J mice have a selective impairment in reversal learning in the Morris water maze, suggesting that this strain could be a model of the cognitive rigidity associated with autism (Moy et al., 2007).

The C58/J inbred strain presents a unique behavioral profile, including social deficits and several forms of overt motor stereotypy (Moy et al., 2008b; Ryan et al., 2010). These mice have decreased sociability in the three-chambered choice task and do not exhibit social transmission of food preference. The C58/J mice can be observed to engage in marked repetitive responses both in the home-cage and in novel environments, including cage-lid back flipping, 'jack-hammer' jumping, and upright scrabbling on chamber walls. Altered motor responses can be observed early in the neonatal period, in line with the emergence of autism symptoms in early childhood in humans (Ryan et al., 2010).

One mouse that has been investigated extensively as a model of autism is the fragile X model mouse. Disruption of the *FMR1* (fragile X mental retardation 1) gene leads to fragile X syndrome, the most common heritable cause of intellectual disability in humans (see Chapter 4.5). In addition to cognitive dysfunction, the disorder is characterized by attention deficits, hyperactivity, anxiety, morphological abnormalities, epileptiform seizures, and autism-like behaviors, including impaired social interaction and communication deficits (Hagerman et al., 1986). *Fmr1* knockout mice recapitulate some aspects of this diverse clinical profile, such as hyperactivity, macro-orchidism, and susceptibility to seizures, but have relatively mild or no impairment in some cognitive tasks (Bakker et al., 1994; Kooy et al., 1996; Peier et al., 2000; Thomas et al., 2011; Yan et al., 2004), and can show normal or even enhanced social approach and interaction (Moy et al., 2008a; Spencer et al., 2005; 2008; Thomas et al., 2011). Deficits in social preference can be observed; however, these are dependent upon which particular background strain is used (Moy et al., 2008a; Pietropaolo et al., 2011). These findings suggest that variability of abnormal phenotypes in fragile X mice can be attributed, partially at least, to interactions between *Fmr1* and modifier genes that differ across background strains.

The *FMR1* gene encodes fragile X mental retardation protein (FMRP), an RNA-binding protein that functions as a translational repressor for specific mRNAs. Deficiency of FMRP is associated with aberrant dendritic spine morphology, including elongated, thin, immature spines, and an overall increase in spine density, in both fragile X subjects and in *Fmr1* knockout mice (Comery et al., 1997; Galvez et al., 2003; Grossman et al., 2006; Irwin et al., 2002; Nimchinsky et al., 2001). Because dendritic spines are key locations for excitatory synaptic connections, dendritic abnormalities could play a role in the disruption of synaptic mechanisms implicated in autism and intellectual disability (Abrahams and Geschwind, 2008). Hayashi and colleagues (2007) have investigated inhibition of p21-activated kinase (PAK), which mediates morphogenesis of dendritic spines, as a strategy for genetic rescue in *Fmr1* null mice. PAK inhibition led to a significant reversal of the elongated spines and increased spine density. This inhibition also decreased the hyperlocomotion and stereotypy in these mutants, providing evidence that structural dendritic pathology could underlie behavioral abnormalities relevant to the human syndrome.

The metabotropic glutamate receptor (mGluR) theory of fragile X further implicates FMRP deficiency in excitatory synaptic dysfunction (Bear et al., 2004). The theory proposes that decreased regulation of translation by FMRP leads to exaggerated protein synthesis by group 1 mGluRs, with subsequent alterations in postsynaptic receptor trafficking. A particular focus is the mGluR5 receptor subtype, which mediates protein synthesis required for synaptic plasticity in long-term depression (Luscher and Huber, 2010). *Fmr1* knockout mice with partial disruption of *Grm5*, the gene encoding mGluR5, show several rescued phenotypes, including decreased dendritic spine density, normalized ocular dominance plasticity, reduced susceptibility to audiogenic seizures,

and reversal of alterations in extinction learning (Dolen et al., 2007) (Table 4.1.4). However, some abnormal behaviors are not affected or are only moderately changed (Thomas et al., 2011). In *Fmr1* knockout mice, pharmacological inhibition of mGluR5 signaling with MPEP (2-methyl-6-phenylethynyl-pyridine hydrochloride), a selective mGluR5 antagonist, can attenuate the increased length of dendritic spines; although this effect is age dependent (Su et al., 2011). This compound can decrease hyperactivity in the open field, reduce perseverative digging, enhance motor learning on the rotarod, and suppress seizures (Thomas et al., 2012; Yan et al., 2005). Further, AFQ056, a recently developed mGluR5 antagonist, can reverse impaired sensorimotor gating in *Fmr1* knockout mice (Levenga et al., 2011). Thus, evidence from *Fmr1* mice provides support for inhibition of mGluR5 signaling as a promising strategy for treating humans with fragile X syndrome.

Besides mGluR5 antagonists, investigators have used additional strategies in an attempt to rescue abnormal responses in different mouse models of ASD (Table 4.1.4). The interventions have included environmental, genetic, and pharmacological procedures that have been successful to varying degrees in mice with alterations in *Mecp2*, *Fmr1*, *Ube3a*, *NL1*, *Pten*, and *Oxtr*, as well as the BALB/c and BTBR *T⁺tf/J* inbred strains. A challenge is to determine whether rescue of a given behavioral domain across models occurs through shared or discrete mechanisms.

MODELS OF AUTISM SPECTRUM DISORDERS USING *SHANK3* MICE

Recent studies in human populations have implicated variants of the *SHANK3* gene as risk factors for autism (Awadalla et al., 2010; Durand et al., 2007; Gauthier et al., 2009; Marshall et al., 2008; Moessner et al., 2007; and see Chapter 4.7) In humans, *SHANK3* maps to the critical region of 22q13.3 deletion syndrome, also called Phelan–McDermid syndrome, in which the sizes of the deletions are variable (i.e., 0.1–10 Mb) (Phelan, 2007). Smaller deletions specific to *SHANK3,* or translocations within the *SHANK3* gene, are found in patients with behavioral features indistinguishable from those with large deletions (Anderlid et al., 2002; Bonaglia et al., 2006; Wong et al., 2007). It is noteworthy that SHANK3 protein has an extensive array of mRNA and protein isoforms that result from combinations of six promoters and alternative splicing of coding exons, both in humans and mice (Maunakea et al., 2010; Wang et al., 2011). Full-length SHANK3 has five conserved domains and each domain interacts with different proteins in the postsynaptic density (Gundelfinger et al., 2006; Kreienkamp, 2008). Each protein isoform possesses a distinct

Restricted, stereotyped, or repetitive behaviors	Not tested	No lesions	Home-cage: self-grooming 35% ♂KO[a,b] had lesions by 3–6 months; Morris water maze reversal: plasticity of response ♂WT=♂KO[s]	Social dyadic[k], open field, and novel object in home-cage tests: self-grooming WT<<KO[a]; Social dyadic test[k]: sifting through bedding WT<<KO; Hole-Board: head-pokes WT<<KO; Novel object in home-cage: repeated and restricted contacts WT<<KO; Morris water maze reversal: plasticity of response[s] WT>KO	Marble burying[t]: number of marbles buried WT=HET[a]
Olfaction	Habituation-dishabituation test: ♂WT=♂HET[a,b]	Not tested	Not tested	Olfactory discrimination: WT=KO[a]	Habituation-dishabituation tests[l]: ♂WT=♂HET[a,b]
Anxiety	Not tested	Elevated zero maze: open area ♂WT=♂KO[a,b]	Elevated zero maze: open area ♂WT>♂KO[a,b]; Light-dark box: latency to cross ♂WT<♂KO, time in chambers ♂WT=♂KO	Elevated zero maze: open area WT=KO[a]; Light-dark box: WT=KO	Plus maze, light-dark box, open field, and marble burying: WT=HET[a]
Motor performance	Not tested	Open field: locomotion ♂WT=♂KO[a,b], rearing ♂WT=♂KO	Open field: locomotion ♂WT=♂KO[a,b], rearing ♂WT>♂KO; Rotorod: WT=KO	Open field: locomotion WT>♂KO[a,b], rearing and stereotypy WT=KO; Rotorod: WT>♂KO; Grip strength: WT=KO; TreadScan: WT>KO; Foot-fault: WT<<KO	Open field, Y-maze, plus maze, light-dark box: locomotion WT=HET[a], habituation WT<HET; Rotorod: WT=HET
Cognitive performance	Not tested	Not tested	Morris water maze: acquisition and reversal ♂WT=♂KO[a,b]	Morris water maze: acquisition WT>KO[a], probe WT=KO, reversal and probe WT>KO; Novel object recognition: STM, LTM, RM[u] KO<WT; STFP[u]: LTM and RM KO<WT[t]	Morris water maze (acquisition), Y-maze (spontaneous alternation, spatial memory), contextual and cued fear conditioning and extinction: WT=HET[a]
Seizure	Not tested	Not tested	Occasional ♂KO[a,b,v]	None observed	Not tested
Pain sensitivity	Not tested	Not tested	Not tested	Not tested	Hot plate: WT=HET[a,b]; Foot-shock: WT=HET
Prepulse inhibition (PPI)	Not tested	Not tested	Not tested	Not tested	

(Continued)

TABLE 4.1.5   Behavioral Phenotypes of Shank3 Mutant Mice – cont'd

Variable	Bozdagi et al., 2010	Peça et al., 2011	Wang et al., 2011	Bangash et al., 2011
			Acoustic PPI: null activity, startle response, and PPI WT=KO[a]	Acoustic PPI; startle response to 110 and 120 dB ♂WT>♂HET[a,b], startle latency 110 and 120 dB ♂WT<♂HET, %PPI at 4 dB with 120 dB startle ♂WT>♂HET
MK-801-stimulated locomotion	Not tested	Not tested	Not tested	Open field: ♂WT<♂HET[a,b] only at 0.3 mg/kg
Amphetamine-stimulated locomotion	Not tested	Not tested	Not tested	Open field: ♂WT<♂HET[a,b] only at 2 mg/kg

[a] WT = wild-type, HET = heterozygote, KO = knockout.

[b] ♂ = male, ♀ = female.

[c] Cohorts 1 and 2 were tested sequentially in the zero maze, light-dark box, open field, rotorod, neurophysiological screen, Morris water maze, and prepulse inhibition. Cohort 3 was tested in sociability, hole board, foot-fault, TredScan, novel object recognition, social transmission of food preference, ultrasonic vocalization, novel object in the home cage, and dyadic social behavior. Cohort 4 was tested in the olfactory test. Tests were separated by ~1 week.

[d] Cohort 1 testing: social interaction, olfaction, open field, plus- and T-mazes, prepulse inhibition, MK-801 and amphetamine; Cohort 2 testing: ultrasonic vocalizations, light-dark box, rotorod, marble burying, Morris water maze, fear conditioning, and pain sensitivity. All tests were separated by ≥ 24 hr.

[e] The only test time given was for grooming at 1900–2100 hr; mice were housed individually for this test.

[f] The only test time given was for the Morris water maze at 0800–0100.

[g] Reciprocal male-female social interaction.

[h] Target mice (Stranger 1 or Stranger 2) were 5–6-week-old males, genotype was not given.

[i] WT and KO mice were group-housed and tested in the open field with age-matched WT mice socially naïve to the target mice. Reciprocal social interaction did not distinguish responses of stimulus from target mice.

[j] Target mice (Stranger 1 or Stranger 2) were weight- and sex-matched naïve C3H/HeJ mice.

[k] Weight- and sex-matched naïve C3H/HeJ group-housed partner, 14 day-isolated tester WT or KO mouse.

[l] Stimulus mouse was 28–35-day-old Swiss-Webster, 129, or C57BL/6 male.

[m] Stimulus mouse (male C57BL/6J) in cup.

[n] Stimulus mouse (male C57BL/6J) was 2–3 months of age and housed individually for 4 days for resident-intruder; housing status not stated for test in neutral arena but presumed to be the same as for the resident-intruder test.

[o] Social approach in three-chamber test, novel stimulus mice were C57BL/6 males or hormonally stimulated females.

[p] Estrus female introduced into home-cage of male WT or HET mouse; WT and HET mice group-housed prior to test.

[q] C3H/HeJ female (restrained in cage) was introduced into the WT or KO home-cage for USV test.

[r] Estrus female introduced into home-cage of male WT or HET mouse; WT and HET mice were housed individually 5 days before testing.

[s] Plasticity of response was assessed in the Morris water maze by 'reversal' – changing the location of the hidden platform.

[t] Although marble burying is used as a test of motor stereotypies and restricted interests, it is more often used as a test for anxiety. Since the Shank3Δ21 mice were not anxious, these results suggest this strain of mice do not display motor stereotypies or restricted interests.

[u] STM = short-term memory, LTM = long-term memory, RM = remote memory, STFP = social transmission of food preference.

[v] No spontaneous seizures, but observe occasional handling-induced seizures.

features were quite different among the various *Shank3* studies, it is unclear whether these procedural or other factors contributed to the different phenotypes. This problem is further compounded by the fact that *Shank3* mice with different genetic backgrounds, genotypes and sexes, and residual Shank3 proteins were studied. Hence, it will be important to use protocols that are more uniform, if not identical, to more fully understand the role of the different *Shank3* mutations in the expression of ASD-like phenotypes. More generally, a major challenge in the future with animal models will be to determine whether the various inbred, outbred, and mutant animal models of ASD share common mechanisms of dysfunction and whether these mechanisms can be targeted for therapy in humans.

References

Abrahams, B.S., Geschwind, D.H., 2008. Advances in autism genetics: On the threshold of a new neurobiology. Nature Reviews Genetics 9, 341–355.

Amaral, D.G., Schumann, C.M., Nordahl, C.W., 2008. Neuroanatomy of autism. Trends in Neurosciences 31, 137–145.

Ameis, S.H., Fan, J., Rockel, C., Voineskos, A.N., Lobaugh, N.J., Soorya, L., et al., 2011. Impaired structural connectivity of socio-emotional circuits in autism spectrum disorders: A diffusion tensor imaging study. PLoS ONE 6, e28044.

American Psychiatric Association, Diagnostic and Statistical Manual of Mental Disorders, fourth ed. (DSM-IV), 1994. American Psychiatric Association, Washington, pp. 66–78.

Anagnostou, E., Taylor, M.J., 2011. Review of neuroimaging in autism spectrum disorders: What have we learned and where we go from here. Molecular Autism 2, 4.

Anderlid, B.M., Schoumans, J., Anneren, G., Tapia-Paez, I., Dumanski, J., Blennow, E., et al., 2002. FISH-mapping of a 100-kb terminal 22q13 deletion. Human Genetics 110, 439–443.

Awadalla, P., Gauthier, J., Myers, R.A., Casals, F., Hamdan, F.F., Griffing, A.R., et al., 2010. Direct measure of the *de novo* mutation rate in autism and schizophrenia cohorts. American Journal of Human Genetics 87, 316–324.

Bakker, C.E., Verheij, C., Willemsen, R., van der Helm, R., Oerlemans, F., Vermey, M., et al., 1994. *Fmr1* knockout mice: A model to study fragile X mental retardation. The Dutch-Belgian fragile X Consortium. Cell 78, 23–33.

Bangash, M.A., Park, J.M., Melnikova, T., Wang, D., Jeon, S.K., Lee, D., et al., 2011. Enhanced polyubiquination of Shank3 and NMDA receptor in mouse model of autism. Cell 145, 758–772.

Bauman, M.L., 2010. Medical comorbidities in autism: Challenges to diagnosis and treatment. Neurotherapeutics 7, 320–327.

Bauman, M.L., Kemper, T.L., 2005. Neuroanatomic observations of the brain in autism: A review and future directions. International Journal of Developmental Neuroscience 23, 183–187.

Bear, M.F., Huber, K.M., Warren, S.T., 2004. The mGluR theory of fragile X mental retardation. Trends in Neurosciences 27, 370–377.

Beaudet, A.L., 2007. Autism: Highly heritable but not inherited. Nature Medicine 13, 534–536.

Belmonte, M.K., Allen, G., Beckel-Mitchener, A., Boulanger, L.M., Carper, R.A., Webb, S.J., 2004. Autism and abnormal development of brain connectivity. Journal of Neuroscience 24, 9228–9231.

Berkel, S., Marshall, C.R., Weiss, B., Howe, J., Roeth, R., Moog, U., et al., 2010. Mutations in the SHANK2 synaptic scaffolding gene in autism spectrum disorder and mental retardation. Nature Genetics 42, 489–491.

Bilousova, T.V., Dansie, L., Ngo, M., Aye, J., Charles, J.R., Ethell, D.W., et al., 2009. Minocycline promotes dendritic spine maturation and improves behavioral performance in the fragile X mouse model. Journal of Medical Genetics 46, 94–102.

Blundell, J., Blaiss, C.A., Etherton, M.R., Espinosa, F., Tabuchi, K., Walz, C., et al., 2010. Neuroligin-1 deletion results in impaired spatial memory and increased repetitive behavior. Journal of Neuroscience 30, 2115–2129.

Bolivar, V.J., Walters, S.R., Phoenix, J.L., 2007. Assessing autism-like behavior in mice: Variations in social interactions among inbred strains. Behavioral Brain Research 176, 21–26.

Bonaglia, M.C., Giorda, R., Mani, E., Aceti, G., Anderlid, B.M., Baroncini, A., et al., 2006. Identification of a recurrent breakpoint within the SHANK3 gene in the 22q13.3 deletion syndrome. Journal of Medical Genetics 43, 822–828.

Bozdagi, O., Sakurai, T., Papapetrou, D., Wang, X., Dickstein, D.L., Takahashi, N., et al., 2010. Haplo-insufficiency of the autism-associated *Shank3* gene leads to deficits in synaptic function, social interaction, and social communication. Molecular Autism 1, 15.

Brodkin, E.S., 2007. BALB/c mice: Low sociability and other phenotypes that may be relevant to autism. Behavioral Brain Research 176, 53–65.

Brodkin, E.S., Hagemann, A., Nemetski, S.M., Silver, L.M., 2004. Social approach-avoidance behavior of inbred mouse strains towards DBA/2 mice. Brain Research 1002, 151–157.

Chadman, K.K., 2011. Fluoxetine but not risperidone increases sociability in the BTBR mouse model of autism. Pharmacology Biochemistry and Behavior 97, 586–594.

Comery, T.A., Harris, J.B., Willems, P.J., Oostra, B.A., Irwin, S.A., Weiler, I.J., et al., 1997. Abnormal dendritic spines in fragile X knockout mice: Maturation and pruning deficits. Proceedings of the National Academy of Sciences of the United States of America 94, 5401–5404.

Courchesne, E., Pierce, K., 2005. Brain overgrowth in autism during a critical time in development: Implications for frontal pyramidal neuron and interneuron development and connectivity. International Journal of Developmental Neuroscience 23, 153–170.

Courchesne, E., Campbell, K., Solso, S., 2011. Brain growth across the life span in autism: Age-specific changes in anatomical pathology. Brain Research 1380, 138–145.

Courchesne, E., Mouton, P.R., Calhoun, M.E., Semendeferi, K., Ahrens–Barbeau, C., Hallet, M.J., et al., 2011. Neuron number and size in prefrontal cortex of children with autism. Journal of the American Medical Association 306, 2001–2010.

Coury, D., Jones, N.E., Klatka, K., Winklosky, B., Perrin, J.M., 2009. Healthcare for children with autism: The autism treatment network. Current Opinion in Pediatrics 21, 828–832.

Daily, J.L., Nash, K., Jinwal, U., Golde, T., Rogers, J., Peters, M.M., et al., 2011. Adeno-associated virus-mediated rescue of the cognitive defects in a mouse model for Angelman syndrome. PLoS ONE 6 e27221.

Dawson, G., Webb, S.J., Carver, L., Panagiotides, H., McPartland, J., 2004. Young children with autism show atypical brain responses to fearful versus neutral facial expressions of emotion. Developmental Science 7, 340–359.

Defensor, E.B., Pearson, B.L., Pobbe, R.L., Bolivar, V.J., Blanchard, D.C., Blanchard, R.J., 2011. A novel social proximity test suggests patterns of social avoidance and gaze aversion-like behavior in BTBR T+ tf/J mice. Behavioral Brain Research 217, 302–308.

de Vrij, F.M., Levenga, J., van der Linde, H.C., Koekkoek, S.K., De Zeeuw, C.I., Nelson, D.L., et al., 2008. Rescue of behavioral phenotype and neuronal protrusion morphology in *Fmr1* KO mice. Neurobiology of Disease 31, 127–132.

Dolen, G., Osterweil, E., Rao, B.S., Smith, G.B., Auerbach, B.D., Chattarji, S., et al., 2007. Correction of fragile X syndrome in mice. Neuron 56, 955–962.

Dow, H.C., Kreibich, A.S., Kaercher, K.A., Sankoorikal, G.M., Pauley, E.D., Lohoff, F.W., et al., 2011. Genetic dissection of inter-male aggressive behavior in BALB/cJ and A/J mice. Genes, Brain and Behavior 10, 57–68.

Durand, C.M., Betancur, C., Boeckers, T.M., Bockmann, J., Chaste, P., Fauchereau, F., et al., 2007. Mutations in the gene encoding the synaptic scaffolding protein SHANK3 are associated with autism spectrum disorders. Nature Genetics 39, 25–27.

Fairless, A.H., Dow, H.C., Toledo, M.M., Malkus, K.A., Edelmann, M., Li, H., et al., 2008. Low sociability is associated with reduced size of the corpus callosum in the BALB/cJ inbred mouse strain. Brain Research 1230, 211–217.

Folstein, S., Rutter, M., 1977. Infantile autism: A genetic study of 21 twin pairs. Journal of Child Psychology and Psychiatry 18, 297–321.

Galvez, R., Gopal, A.R., Greenough, W.T., 2003. Somatosensory cortical barrel dendritic abnormalities in a mouse model of the fragile X mental retardation syndrome. Brain Research 971, 83–89.

Gauthier, J., Champagne, N., Lafreniere, R.G., Xiong, L., Spiegelman, D., Brustein, E., et al., 2010. De novo mutations in the gene encoding the synaptic scaffolding protein SHANK3 in patients ascertained for schizophrenia. Proceedings of the National Academy of Sciences of the United States of America 107, 7863–7868.

Gauthier, J., Spiegelman, D., Piton, A., Lafreniere, R.G., Laurent, S., St-Onge, J., et al., 2009. Novel de novo SHANK3 mutation in autistic patients. American Journal of Medical Genetics. Part B, Neuropsychiatric Genetics 150B, 421–424.

Geschwind, D.H., Levitt, P., 2007. Autism spectrum disorders: Developmental disconnection syndromes. Current Opinion in Neurobiology 17, 103–111.

Giacometti, E., Luikenhuis, S., Beard, C., Jaenisch, R., 2007. Partial rescue of MeCP2 deficiency by postnatal activation of MeCP2. Proceedings of the National Academy of Sciences of the United States of America 104, 1931–1936.

Glessner, J.T., Wang, K., Cai, G., Korvatska, O., Kim, C.E., Wood, S., et al., 2009. Autism genome-wide copy number variation reveals ubiquitin and neuronal genes. Nature 459, 569–573.

Gould, G.G., Hensler, J.G., Burke, T.F., Benno, R.H., Onaivi, E.S., Daws, L.C., 2011. Density and function of central serotonin (5-HT) transporters, 5-HT1A and 5-HT2A receptors, and effects of their targeting on BTBR T^+ tf/J mouse social behavior. Journal of Neurochemistry 116, 291–303.

Grauer, S.M., Pulito, V.L., Navarra, R.L., Kelly, M.P., Kelley, C., Graf, R., et al., 2009. Phosphodiesterase 10A inhibitor activity in preclinical models of the positive, cognitive, and negative symptoms of schizophrenia. Journal of Pharmacology and Experimental Therapeutics 331, 574–590.

Gross, C., Berry-Kravis, E.M., Bassell, G.J., 2012. Therapeutic strategies in fragile X syndrome: Dysregulated mGluR signaling and beyond. Neuropsychopharmacology Reviews 37, 178–195.

Grossman, A.W., Elisseou, N.M., McKinney, B.C., Greenough, W.T., 2006. Hippocampal pyramidal cells in adult Fmr1 knockout mice exhibit an immature-appearing profile of dendritic spines. Brain Research 1084, 158–164.

Guillot, P.V., Chapouthier, G., 1996. Intermale aggression and dark/light preference in ten inbred mouse strains. Behavioral Brain Research 77, 211–213.

Guo, W., Murthy, A.C., Zhang, L., Johnson, E.B., Schaller, E.G., Allan, A.M., et al., 2011. Inhibition of GSK3β improves hippocampus-dependent learning and rescues neurogenesis in a mouse model of fragile X syndrome. Human Molecular Genetics 21, 681–691.

Gundelfinger, E.D., Boeckers, T.M., Baron, M.K., Bowie, J.U., 2006. A role for zinc in postsynaptic density asSAMbly and plasticity? Trends in Biochemical Sciences 31, 366–373.

Guy, J., Gan, J., Selfridge, J., Cobb, S., Bird, A., 2007. Reversal of neurological defects in a mouse model of Rett syndrome. Science 315, 1143–1147.

Hagerman, R.J., Jackson, 3rd A.W., Levitas, A., Rimland, B., Braden, M., 1986. An analysis of autism in fifty males with the fragile X syndrome. American Journal Medical Genetics 23, 359–374.

Hayashi, M.L., Rao, B.S., Seo, J.S., Choi, H.S., Dolan, B.M., Choi, S.Y., et al., 2007. Inhibition of p21-activated kinase rescues symptoms of fragile X syndrome in mice. Proceedings of the National Academy of Sciences of the United States of America 104, 11,489–11,494.

Irwin, S.A., Idupulapati, M., Gilbert, M.E., Harris, J.B., Chakravarti, A.B., Rogers, E.J., et al., 2002. Dendritic spine and dendritic field characteristics of layer V pyramidal neurons in the visual cortex of fragile-X knockout mice. American Journal Medical Genetics 111, 140–146.

Jacome, L.F., Burket, J.A., Herndon, A.L., Cannon, W.R., Deutsch, S.I., 2011a. D-serine improves dimensions of the sociability deficit of the genetically-inbred Balb/c mouse strain. Brain Research Bulletin 84, 12–16.

Jacome, L.F., Burket, J.A., Herndon, A.L., Deutsch, S.I., 2011b. Genetically inbred Balb/c mice differ from outbred Swiss-Webster mice on discrete measures of sociability: Relevance to a genetic mouse model of autism spectrum disorders. Autism Research 4, 393–400.

Jamain, S., Quach, H., Betancur, C., Rastam, M., Colineaux, C., Gillberg, I.C., et al., 2003. Mutations of the X-linked genes encoding neuroligins NLGN3 and NLGN4 are associated with autism. Nature Genetics 34, 27–29.

Jou, R.J., Mateljevic, N., Kaiser, M.D., Sugrue, D.R., Volkmar, F.R., Pelphrey, K.A., 2011. Structural neural phenotype of autism: Preliminary evidence from a diffusion tensor imaging study using tract-based spatial statistics. American Journal of Neuroradiology 32, 1607–1613.

Just, M.A., Cherkassky, V.L., Keller, T.A., Kana, R.K., Minshew, N.J., 2007. Functional and anatomical cortical underconnectivity in autism: Evidence from an FMRI study of an executive function task and corpus callosum morphometry. Cerebral Cortex 17, 951–961.

Kondo, M., Gray, L.J., Pelka, G.J., Christodoulou, J., Tam, P.P., Hannan, A.J., 2008. Environmental enrichment ameliorates a motor coordination deficit in a mouse model of Rett syndrome – Mecp2 gene dosage effects and BDNF expression. European Journal of Neuroscience 27, 3342–3350.

Kooy, R.F., D'Hooge, R., Reyniers, E., Bakker, C.E., Nagels, G., De Boulle, K., et al., 1996. Transgenic mouse model for the fragile X syndrome. American Journal of Medical Genetics 64, 241–245.

Kreienkamp, H.J., 2008. Scaffolding proteins at the postsynaptic density: Shank as the architectural framework. Handbook of Experimental Pharmacology 186, 365–380.

Kusek, G.K., Wahlsten, D., Herron, B.J., Bolivar, V.J., Flaherty, L., 2007. Localization of two new X-linked quantitative trait loci controlling corpus callosum size in the mouse. Genes, Brain and Behavior 6, 359–363.

Lange, N., Dubray, M.B., Lee, J.E., Froimowitz, M.P., Froehlich, A., Adluru, N., et al., 2010. Atypical diffusion tensor hemispheric asymmetry in autism. Autism Research 3, 350–358.

Lee, C.T., Ingersoll, D.W., 1983. Pheromonal influences on aggressive behavior. In: Svare, B. (Ed.), Hormones and Aggressive Behavior. Plenum Press, New York, pp. 373–404.

Levenga, J., Hayashi, S., de Vrij, F.M., Koekkoek, S.K., van der Linde, H.C., Nieuwenhuizen, I., et al., 2011. AFQ056, a new mGluR5 antagonist for treatment of fragile X syndrome. Neurobiology of Disease 42, 311–317.

Liu, Z.H., Chuang, D.M., Smith, C.B., 2010. Lithium ameliorates phenotypic deficits in a mouse model of fragile X syndrome. International Journal of Neuropsychopharmacology 14, 618–630.

Lord, C., Cook, E.H., Leventhal, B.L., Amaral, D.G., 2000. Autism spectrum disorders. Neuron 28, 355–363.

Lord, C., Leventhal, B.L., Cook Jr., E.H., 2001. Quantifying the phenotype in autism spectrum disorders. American Journal of Medical Genetics 105, 36–38.

Lord, C., Risi, S., Lambrecht, L., Cook Jr., E.H., Leventhal, B.L., DiLavore, P.C., et al., 2000. The autism diagnostic observation schedule-generic: A standard measure of social and communication deficits associated with the spectrum of autism. Journal of Autism and Developmental Disorders 30, 205–223.

Luikenhuis, S., Giacometti, E., Beard, C.F., Jaenisch, R., 2004. Expression of MeCP2 in postmitotic neurons rescues Rett syndrome in mice. Proceedings of the National Academy of Sciences of the United States of America 101, 6033–6038.

Luscher, C., Huber, K.M., 2007. Group 1 mGluR-dependent synaptic long-term depression: Mechanisms and implications for circuitry and disease. Neuron 65, 445–459.

Lyon, M., 1956. Hereditary hair loss in the tufted mutant of the house mouse. Journal of Heredity 47, 101–103.

Marshall, C.R., Noor, A., Vincent, J.B., Lionel, A.C., Feuk, L., Skaug, J., et al., 2008. Structural variation of chromosomes in autism spectrum disorder. American Journal of Human Genetics 82, 477–488.

Maunakea, A.K., Nagarajan, R.P., Bilenky, M., Ballinger, T.J., D'Souza, C., Fouse, S.D., et al., 2010. Conserved role of intragenic DNA methylation in regulating alternative promoters. Nature 466, 253–257.

McFarlane, H.G., Kusek, G.K., Yang, M., Phoenix, J.L., Bolivar, V.J., Crawley, J.N., 2008. Autism-like behavioral phe notypes in BTBR T+ tf/J mice. Genes, Brain and Behavior 7, 152–163.

Micali, N., Chakrabarti, S., Fombonne, E., 2004. The broad autism phenotype: Findings from an epidemiological survey. Autism 8, 21–37.

Miles, J.H., 2011. Autism spectrum disorders – a genetics review. Genetics in Medicine 13, 278–294.

Miles, J.H., McCathren, R.B., Stichter, J., Shinawi, M., 2010. Autism Spectrum Disorders. In: Pagon, R.A., Bird, T.D., Dolan, C.R., Stephens, K. (Eds.), Gene Reviews. Internet University of Washington, Seattle.

Miller, D.T., Adam, M.P., Aradhya, S., Biesecker, L.G., Brothman, A.R., Carter, N.P., et al., 2010. Consensus statement: Chromosomal microarray is a First-tier clinical diagnostic test for individuals with developmental disabilities or congenital anomalies. American Journal of Human Genetics 86, 749–764.

Mines, M.A., Yuskaitis, C.J., King, M.K., Beurel, E., Jope, R.S., 2010. GSK3 influences social preference and anxiety-related behaviors during social interaction in a mouse model of fragile X syndrome and autism. PLoS ONE 5, e9706.

Mineur, Y.S., Prasol, D.J., Belzung, C., Crusio, W.E., 2003. Agonistic behavior and unpredictable chronic mild stress in mice. Behavior Genetics 33, 513–519.

Minshew, N.J., Keller, T.A., 2010. The nature of brain dysfunction in autism: Functional brain imaging studies. Current Opinion in Neurology 23, 124–130.

Minshew, N.J., Williams, D.L., 2007. The new neurobiology of autism: Cortex, connectivity, and neuronal organization. Archives of Neurology 64, 945–950.

Moessner, R., Marshall, C.R., Sutcliffe, J.S., Skaug, J., Pinto, D., Vincent, J., et al., 2007. Contribution of SHANK3 mutations to autism spectrum disorder. American Journal of Human Genetics 81, 1289–1297.

Moy, S.S., Nadler, J.J., Perez, A., Barbaro, R.P., Johns, J.M., Magnuson, T.R., et al., 2004. Sociability and preference for social novelty in five inbred strains: An approach to assess autistic-like behavior in mice. Genes, Brain and Behavior 3, 287–302.

Moy, S.S., Nadler, J.J., Young, N.B., Nonneman, R.J., Grossman, A.W., Murphy, D.L., et al., 2008. Social approach in genetically engineered mouse lines relevant to autism. Genes, Brain and Behavior 8, 129–142.

Moy, S.S., Nadler, J.J., Young, N.B., Nonneman, R.J., Segall, S.K., Andrade, G.M., et al., 2008. Social approach and repetitive behavior in eleven inbred mouse strains. Behavioral Brain Research 191, 118–129.

Moy, S.S., Nadler, J.J., Young, N.B., Perez, A., Holloway, L.P., Barbaro, R.P., et al., 2007. Mouse behavioral tasks relevant to autism: Phenotypes of 10 inbred strains. Behavioral Brain Research 176, 4–20.

Nadler, J.J., Moy, S.S., Dold, G., Trang, D., Simmons, N., Perez, A., et al., 2004. Automated apparatus for rapid quantitation of autism-like social deficits in mice. Genes, Brain and Behavior 3, 303–314.

Nag, N., Berger-Sweeney, J.E., 2007. Postnatal dietary choline supplementation alters behavior in a mouse model of Rett syndrome. Neurobiology of Disease 26, 473–480.

Nag, N., Moriuchi, J.M., Peitzman, C.G., Ward, B.C., Kolodny, N.H., Berger–Sweeney, J.E., 2009. Environmental enrichment alters locomotor behavior and ventricular volume in $Mecp2^{1lox}$ mice. Behavioural Brain Research 196, 44–48.

Nimchinsky, E.A., Oberlander, A.M., Svoboda, K., 2001. Abnormal development of dendritic spines in FMR1 knock-out mice. Journal of Neuroscience 21, 5139–5146.

Olmos-Serrano, J.L., Corbin, J.G., Burns, M.P., 2011. The $GABA_A$ receptor agonist THIP ameliorates specific behavioral deficits in the mouse model of fragile X syndrome. Developmental Neuroscience 33, 395–403.

Pacey, L.K., Doss, L., Cifelli, C., van der Kooy, D., Heximer, S.P., Hampson, D.R., 2011. Genetic deletion of regulator of G-protein signaling 4 (RGS4) rescues a subset of fragile X related phenotypes in the FMR1 knockout mouse. Molecular and Cellular Neuroscience 46, 563–572.

Panksepp, J.B., Lahvis, G.P., 2007. Social reward among juvenile mice. Genes, Brain and Behavior 6, 661–671.

Panksepp, J.B., Jochman, K.A., Kim, J.U., Koy, J.J., Wilson, E.D., Chen, Q., et al., 2007. Affiliative behavior, ultrasonic communication and social reward are influenced by genetic variation in adolescent mice. PLoS ONE 2, e351.

Paylor, R., Yuva–Paylor, L.A., Nelson, D.L., Spencer, C.M., 2008. Reversal of sensorimotor gating abnormalities in Fmr1 knockout mice carrying a human FMR1 transgene. Behavioral Neuroscience 122, 1371–1377.

Peça, J., Feliciano, C., Ting, J.T., Wang, W., Wells, M.F., Venkatraman, T.N., et al., 2011. Shank3 mutant mice display autistic-like behaviors and striatal dysfunction. Nature 472, 437–442.

Peier, A.M., McIlwain, K.L., Kenneson, A., Warren, S.T., Paylor, R., Nelson, D.L., 2000. (Over)correction of FMR1 deficiency with YAC transgenics: Behavioral and physical features. Human Molecular Genetics 9, 1145–1159.

Phelan, K., 2007. 22q13.3 Deletion Syndrome. In: Pagon, R.A., Bird, T.C., Dolan, C.R., Stephens, K. (Eds.), Gene Reviews. Internet University of Washington, Seattle, WA.

Pietropaolo, S., Guilleminot, A., Martin, B., D'Amato, F.R., Crusio, W.E., 2011. Genetic-background modulation of core and variable autistic-like symptoms in Fmr1 knock-out mice. PLoS ONE 6, e17073.

Pinto, D., Pagnamenta, A.T., Klei, L., Anney, R., Merico, D., Regan, R., et al., 2010. Functional impact of global rare copy number variation in autism spectrum disorders. Nature 466, 368–372.

Restivo, L., Ferrari, F., Passino, E., Sgobio, C., Bock, J., Oostra, B.A., et al., 2005. Enriched environment promotes behavioral and morphological recovery in a mouse model for the fragile X syndrome. Proceedings of the National Academy of Sciences of the United States of America 102, 11,557–11,562.

Ronald, A., Hoekstra, R.A., 2011. Autism spectrum disorders and autistic traits: A decade of new twin studies. American Journal of Medical Genetics. Part B, Neuropsychiatric Genetics 156B, 255–274.

Ryan, B.C., Young, N.B., Crawley, J.N., Bodfish, J.W., Moy, S.S., 2010. Social deficits, stereotypy and early emergence of repetitive behavior in the C58/J inbred mouse strain. Behavioral Brain Research 208, 178–188.

Sala, M., Braida, D., Lentini, D., Busnelli, M., Bulgheroni, E., Capurro, V., et al., 2011. Pharmacologic rescue of impaired cognitive flexibility, social deficits, increased aggression, and seizure susceptibility in oxytocin receptor null mice: a neurobehavioral model of autism. Biological Psychiatry 69, 875–882.

Sankoorikal, G.M., Kaercher, K.A., Boon, C.J., Lee, J.K., Brodkin, E.S., 2006. A mouse model system for genetic analysis of sociability: C57BL/6J versus BALB/cJ inbred mouse strains. Biological Psychiatry 59, 415–423.

Scattoni, M.L., Gandhy, S.U., Ricceri, L., Crawley, J.N., 2008. Unusual repertoire of vocalizations in the BTBR T+tf/J mouse model of autism. PLoS ONE 3, e3067.

Scattoni, M.L., Ricceri, L., Crawley, J.N., 2011. Unusual repertoire of vocalizations in adult BTBR T+tf/J mice during three types of social encounters. Genes, Brain and Behavior 10, 44–56.

Schaaf, C.P., Sabo, A., Sakai, Y., Crosby, J., Muzny, D., Hawes, A., et al., 2011. Oligogenic heterozygosity in individuals with high-functioning autism spectrum disorder. Human Molecular Genetics 20, 3366–3375.

Sebat, J., Lakshmi, B., Malhotra, D., Troge, J., Lese-Martin, C., Walsh, T., et al., 2007. Strong association of de novo copy number mutations with autism. Science 316, 445–449.

Shen, Y., Dies, K.A., Holm, I.A., Bridgemohan, C., Sobeih, M.M., Caronna, E.B., et al., 2010. Clinical genetic testing for patients with autism spectrum disorders. Pediatrics 125, e727–e735.

Silverman, J.L., Tolu, S.S., Barkan, C.L., Crawley, J.N., 2010. Repetitive self-grooming behavior in the BTBR mouse model of autism is blocked by the mGluR5 antagonist MPEP. Neuropsychopharmacology 35, 976–989.

Spencer, C.M., Alekseyenko, O., Serysheva, E., Yuva-Paylor, L.A., Paylor, R., 2005. Altered anxiety-related and social behaviors in the Fmr1 knockout mouse model of fragile X syndrome. Genes, Brain and Behavior 4, 420–430.

Spencer, C.M., Graham, D.F., Yuva-Paylor, L.A., Nelson, D.L., Paylor, R., 2008. Social behavior in Fmr1 knockout mice carrying a human FMR1 transgene. Behavioral Neuroscience 122, 710–715.

State, M.W., Levitt, P., 2011. The conundrums of understanding genetic risks for autism spectrum disorders. Nature Neuroscience 14, 1499–1506.

Su, T., Fan, H.X., Jiang, T., Sun, W.W., Den, W.Y., Gao, M.M., et al., 2011. Early continuous inhibition of group 1 mGlu signaling partially rescues dendritic spine abnormalities in the Fmr1 knockout mouse model for fragile X syndrome. Psychopharmacology 215, 291–300.

Thomas, A.M., Bui, N., Graham, D., Perkins, J.R., Yuva-Paylor, L.A., Paylor, R., 2011. Genetic reduction of group 1 metabotropic glutamate receptors alters select behaviors in a mouse model for fragile X syndrome. Behavioral Brain Research 223, 310–321.

Thomas, A.M., Bui, N., Perkins, J.R., Yuva-Paylor, L.A., Paylor, R., 2012. Group I metabotropic glutamate receptor antagonists alter select behaviors in a mouse model for fragile X syndrome. Psychopharmacology 219, 47–58.

van Woerden, G.M., Harris, K.D., Hojjati, M.R., Gustin, R.M., Qiu, S., de Avila Freire, R., et al., 2007. Rescue of neurological deficits in a mouse model for Angelman syndrome by reduction of αCaMKII inhibitory phosphorylation. Nature Neuroscience 10, 280–282.

Veenstra-Vanderweele, J., Christian, S.L., Cook Jr., E.H., 2004. Autism as a paradigmatic complex genetic disorder. Annual Review of Genomics and Human Genetics 5, 379–405.

Veeraragavan, S., Bui, N., Perkins, J.R., Yuva-Paylor, L.A., Carpenter, R.L., Paylor, R., 2011. Modulation of behavioral phenotypes by a muscarinic M1 antagonist in a mouse model of fragile X syndrome. Psychopharmacology 217, 143–151.

Veeraragavan, S., Graham, D., Bui, N., Yuva-Paylor, L.A., Wess, J., Paylor, R., 2012. Genetic reduction of muscarinic M4 receptor modulates analgesic response and acoustic startle response in a mouse model of fragile X syndrome (FXS). Behavioural Brain Research 228, 1–8.

Volkmar, F.R., State, M., Klin, A., 2009. Autism and autism spectrum disorders: Diagnostic issues for the coming decade. Journal of Child Psychology and Psychiatry 50, 108–115.

Wahlsten, D., 1989. Genetic and developmental defects of the mouse corpus callosum. Experientia 45, 828–838.

Wahlsten, D., Metten, P., Crabbe, J.C., 2003. Survey of 21 inbred mouse strains in two laboratories reveals that BTBR T/+tf/tf has severely reduced hippocampal commissure and absent corpus callosum. Brain Research 971, 47–54.

Wang, X., McCoy, P.A., Rodriguiz, R.M., Pan, Y., Je, H.S., Roberts, A.C., et al., 2011. Synapse dysfunction and abnormal behaviors in mice lacking major isoforms of Shank3. Human Molecular Genetics 20, 3093–3108.

Weiss, L.A., Shen, Y., Korn, J.M., Arking, D.E., Miller, D.T., Fossdal, R., et al., 2008. Association between microdeletion and microduplication at 16p11.2 and autism. New England Journal of Medicine 358, 667–675.

Westmark, C.J., Westmark, P.R., O'Riordan, K.J., Ray, B.C., Hervey, C.M., Salamat, M.S., et al., 2011. Reversal of fragile X phenotypes by manipulation of AβPP/Aβ levels in Fmr1^{KO} mice. PLoS ONE 6, e26549.

Wohr, M., Roullet, F.I., Crawley, J.N., 2011. Reduced scent marking and ultrasonic vocalizations in the BTBR T+tf/J mouse model of autism. Genes, Brain and Behavior 10, 35–43.

Wong, A.C., Ning, Y., Flint, J., Clark, K., Dumanski, J.P., Ledbetter, D.H., et al., 1997. Molecular characterization of a 130-kb terminal microdeletion at 22q in a child with mild mental retardation. American Journal of Human Genetics 60, 113–120.

Xue, M., Brimacombe, M., Chaaban, J., Zimmerman-Bier, B., Wagner, G.C., 2008. Autism spectrum disorders: Concurrent clinical disorders. Journal of Child Neurology 23, 6–13.

Yan, Q.J., Asafo-Adjei, P.K., Arnold, H.M., Brown, R.E., Bauchwitz, R.P., 2004. A phenotypic and molecular characterization of the fmr1-tm1Cgr fragile X mouse. Genes, Brain and Behavior 3, 337–359.

Yan, Q.J., Rammal, M., Tranfaglia, M., Bauchwitz, R.P., 2005. Suppression of two major fragile X syndrome mouse model phenotypes by the mGluR5 antagonist MPEP. Neuropharmacology 49, 1053–1066.

Yang, M., Perry, K., Weber, M.D., Katz, A.M., Crawley, J.N., 2011. Social peers rescue autism-relevant sociability deficits in adolescent mice. Autism Research 4, 17–27.

Yang, M., Zhodzishsky, V., Crawley, J.N., 2007. Social deficits in BTBR T+ tf/J mice are unchanged by cross-fostering with C57BL/6J mothers. International Journal of Developmental Neuroscience 25, 515–521.

Yuskaitis, C.J., Mines, M.A., King, M.K., Sweatt, J.D., Miller, C.A., Jope, R.S., 2010. Lithium ameliorates altered glycogen synthase kinase-3 and behavior in a mouse model of fragile X syndrome. Biochemical Pharmacology 79, 632–646.

Zhou, J., Blundell, J., Ogawa, S., Kwon, C.H., Zhang, W., Sinton, C., et al., 2009. Pharmacological inhibition of mTORC1 suppresses anatomical, cellular, and behavioral abnormalities in neural-specific Pten knock-out mice. Journal of Neuroscience 29, 1773–1783.

4.2

Nonhuman Primate Models for Autism Spectrum Disorders

Melissa D. Bauman, David G. Amaral

Department of Psychiatry and Behavioral Sciences, Center for Neuroscience, California National Primate
Research Center, MIND Institute, University of California at Davis, CA, USA

VALIDITY MEASURES

The strength of an animal model depends on its resemblance to the human disorder that it is intended to model. Three criteria are commonly used to evaluate animal models:

1. Construct validity – the extent to which the model reproduces the etiology and/or pathophysiology of the disorder;
2. Face validity – the degree to which the model resembles symptoms of the disorder;
3. Predictive validity – the extent to which treatment of the animal model provides insight into therapeutic options for the human condition (McKinney, 1984; Crawley, 2004).

Construct validity refers to the degree of similarity between the experimental manipulation used to create the animal model and the proposed underlying cause(s) of the human disease. We would suggest that in order for an animal model to provide a valuable contribution to autism research, it must stem from hypotheses that are directly related to the human disorder. Although this has proven particularly challenging for animal models of autism since a large part of the underlying factors of autism spectrum disorders (ASD) remain unknown, we anticipate that construct validity of ASD models will continuously improve as putative causes of the disorders are discovered. Recent research with ASD patient populations has begun to unravel the complex array of genetic, immunological, environmental, and neurobiological risk factors for autism (Abrahams and Geschwind, 2008; Amaral et al., 2008; Ashwood et al., 2006; Hertz-Picciotto et al., 2008; Pessah et al., 2008). Appropriate animal models can play an essential role in experimentally evaluating these findings and establishing causal links between putative risk factors and autism.

Face validity is the extent to which these changes resemble the phenotype of the human disorder. Sophisticated animal models may produce changes in gene expression, brain anatomy and chemistry, and ultimately

The Neuroscience of Autism Spectrum Disorders.
http://dx.doi.org/10.1016/B978-0-12-391924-3.00027-2

behavior. However, because autism is a behaviorally defined disorder, our current evaluation of face validity is based almost exclusively on behavioral outcomes of the animal model. It is important to emphasize that the goal of animal model research is not necessarily to create 'autistic animals,' but to model one or more behavioral *features* of human autism in another species. Clearly, some symptoms of autism, such as language impairments and theory-of-mind deficits, cannot be modeled in any nonhuman animal. We can, however, use animal models to evaluate species-specific behaviors related to the core symptoms of autism, including deficits in social interactions, aspects of social communication, and stereotyped, repetitive behaviors. An ideal animal model with high face validity would produce behavioral changes in the three diagnostic domains of autism. However, this may not be an attainable standard. Behavioral changes in any one of the three core autism domains (social, communication, repetitive behaviors) may yield a model with face validity. Moreover, as animal models of autism become more sophisticated, the use of other outcome measures, such as eye tracking and functional neuroimaging, may build stronger bridges between human patients and animal models.

Predictive validity refers to treatment trials in an animal model that provide insight into therapeutic options for the human condition. Although we are just beginning to develop valid animal models of autism, the information gained through these models will ultimately move the field towards the goal of developing preventative strategies as well as novel therapies to reduce the incidence of autism. The nonhuman primate has the merit of being the most similar of common animal models to humans in terms of anatomy, physiology, and behavior. It has the capacity to play an essential role in evaluating novel preventative approaches and pharmacological interventions.

ADVANTAGES AND LIMITATIONS OF NONHUMAN PRIMATE MODELS

Mouse models have certain advantages over nonhuman primate models. For example, mice are relatively inexpensive and, because of their shorter gestation and larger litters, a greater number of experiments can be completed in a shorter time. Moreover, mouse models can be used for a variety of experimental approaches, including genetic manipulations, which are not feasible in nonhuman primate models. Mouse models, however, are faced with the challenges of relating the rodent brain to the human brain and rodent behavior to human behavior. Portions of the human 'social brain,' such as the prefrontal cortex and fusiform

gyrus, which have been implicated in autism, are poorly developed or may not exist at all in the mouse brain. Given that autism is a disorder defined by changes in complex human behaviors, likely mediated by regions of the social brain, developing a mouse model with strong face validity poses a considerable challenge. It is possible that a uniquely human disorder such as autism may ultimately require the use of animal species that are more closely related to humans, such as nonhuman primates. This may be particularly germane to attempts at developing novel pharmacological interventions.

In this chapter, we focus our descriptions on research utilizing the rhesus macaque (*Macaca mulatta*), often considered to be the species of choice for biomedical research. Compared with rodents, which are separated from humans by more than 70 million years of evolution (Gibbs et al., 2004; Kumar and Hedges, 1998), macaque monkeys diverged from human evolution closer to 25 million years ago and thus exhibit greater similarity to human physiology, neurobiology, behavior, and susceptibility to diseases. One testimony to the relatedness of the macaque and human is the fact that the macaque genome demonstrates a 90–93% sequence homology with the human genome (Kay et al., 1997). In addition to the genetic similarities between macaques and humans, there are compelling similarities between brain and behavior, which make rhesus macaques the model of choice for studying complex human brain disorders (Capitanio and Emborg, 2008). Nonhuman primates have, for example, advanced our understanding of Parkinson's disease by providing insight into the neural circuitry underlying this disorder (Bergman et al., 1990; Burns et al., 1983). These advances, in turn, led to the development of new therapies for humans, such as targeted surgical ablation and deep brain stimulation (Bergman et al., 1990). Nonhuman primate models of Alzheimer's disease have also provided insight into the neural underpinnings of this disease (Wenk, 1993) and provided a model system for evaluating novel therapeutic interventions (Lemere et al., 2004; 2006; Nagahara et al., 2009; Tuszynski et al., 1996; Tuszynski and Blesch, 2004). Future nonhuman primate models may incorporate genetic susceptibility of central nervous system disorders, as demonstrated by a recent primate transgenic model of Huntington's disease (Yang et al., 2008). Although we are in the very early stages of developing valid animal models of autism, it is likely that nonhuman primate models will play an important role in identifying the neural underpinnings of autism and facilitating the development of future treatment and prevention strategies.

The rich social repertoire of the rhesus monkey makes it an ideal experimental model to evaluate potential etiologies and develop novel therapeutic

BOX 4.2.1

The macaque monkey brain is only one tenth the size of the human brain. Nonetheless, the structure of the macaque monkey brain is remarkably similar to that of the human brain (Figure 4.2.1). While it is beyond the scope of this chapter to provide a detailed review of the comparative neuroanatomy of the rodent, macaque monkey, and human brains, one or two examples will suffice to make the point that the macaque monkey brain is more similar to that of the human than is the rodent brain. Perhaps the frontal lobe is the best region to explore these differences. The human frontal lobe has demonstrated the greatest phylogenetic advancement of any cortical area. There is substantial evidence, in fact, that it is the demands of living in a social environment (Byrne and Whiten, 1988; Jolly, 1966) that has spurred on the evolutionary development of the human frontal lobes, particularly of the

increased complexity of connections of these regions (Semendeferi et al., 2002). Put simply, there are cytoarchitectural divisions of the frontal lobe that are identifiable in the human brain and in the macaque monkey brain but are not identifiable in the rodent brain (Preuss, 1995). As Preuss has argued, based on cytoarchitectonic, connectional, and neurotransmitter distribution grounds, it is unlikely that rats have cortical homologues of the human dorsolateral prefrontal cortex that is also a prominent component of the monkey brain. As, instead, the frontal lobe appears to be one of the brain regions most commonly implicated in the neuropathology of autism (Carper and Courchesne, 2005), it raises the concern of whether any rodent model of autism could truly have face validity for related aspects of autism.

interventions for ASD. Rhesus macaques display sophisticated social behavior that resembles many features of human social behavior. Much like humans, macaques spend their lives in complex societies where survival depends on their ability to quickly and accurately interpret and respond to a variety of social signals. Many generations of macaque female relatives live together and form long-lasting social networks or matrilines (Altmann, 1967; Wrangham, 1980). These matrilines are organized into dominance hierarchies where prediction of social rank is closely linked to the dominance status of kin (i.e., high-ranking mothers produce high-ranking offspring) (Bernstein and Mason, 1963; Drickamer, 1972; Missakian, 1972; Sade, 1967). This complex system of social organization requires an equally sophisticated social communication system that includes facial expressions, vocalizations, and body postures. Infant macaques must rapidly learn to interpret and produce social signals in order to successfully interact with members of their social group. A well-characterized trajectory of social development in many ways parallels that of human infants, but at a maturational rate approximately four times faster (i.e., a 1-month-old monkey is roughly developmentally comparable to a 4-month-old human).

MODELING FEATURES OF AUTISM IN NONHUMAN PRIMATES

The overarching goal of animal models of ASD is to contribute to the development of novel preventative measures or treatment strategies for ASD. A first step

in this process is to demonstrate that a putative cause or risk factor does indeed alter brain development or function and lead to the characteristics of autism. Thus, the nonhuman primate model can be employed to gather evidence in support of a particular etiology. Beyond this, however, an animal model may be able to provide information on the underlying mechanisms leading to autistic symptomatology. For example, it is now well established that a sizable proportion of children with autism have precocious growth of their brains, particularly of the frontal lobe. The best evidence for this has come from magnetic resonance imaging studies. However, it is not clear what the neurobiological substrate of this rapid brain growth is. Is it the production of a greater number of neurons or glial cells? Is the enlargement perhaps due to an early inflammatory process? Given the paucity of postmortem tissue available for study from very young children with autism, it is unlikely that study of the human brain will resolve this issue in the foreseeable future. But, if an animal model could be created that has reliable precocious brain growth due to a clinically relevant putative autism cause, then the cellular mechanisms leading to the brain growth could be thoroughly evaluated in the model system.

Distinctions can be drawn between models that are designed to identify underlying neurobiological mechanisms, those designed to elicit behavioral symptoms, and those designed to provide evidence for a specific etiological theory. In the following sections, we have selected nonhuman primate studies from each of these approaches to highlight current and future directions related to the neuroscience of autism.

Neural Systems Models: Neonatal Amygdala Lesions

Neuroscientists, who take a neural systems approach to understanding the brain, attempt to group interconnected brain regions that appear to be involved in a particular behavioral function. This approach has been useful in identifying regions of the brain that are involved in sensory processing, as well as complex cognitive processes such as learning and memory. For example, it is well accepted that structures in the medial temporal lobe are essential for forming declarative memories (Squire et al., 2004). A combination of both neuroanatomical studies and lesion research in nonhuman primates has specifically identified the hippocampal formation along with the perirhinal and parahippocampal cortices as key structures mediating episodic memory (Suzuki and Amaral, 2004). Damage to these brain regions in the adult nonhuman primate markedly and permanently affects the ability to accomplish certain forms of memory testing. A central question for the field of social neuroscience is to determine if the social brain is organized in a similar fashion. If it is, one would expect that the elimination of candidate social brain regions would dramatically alter normal social behavior.

Unfortunately, we know surprisingly little about the brain regions that are essential for species-typical social development. More than 15 years ago, Brothers proposed that the social brain was composed of several brain regions, including the amygdala, anterior cingulate cortex, orbitofrontal cortex, and temporal cortex (shown in Figure 4.2.1) (Brothers, 1990). The exact role that these structures play in social processing, or even if these structures are essential for social behavior, remains unclear to this day. Animal model lesion research provides a means of evaluating whether a neural structure is essential for specific aspects of social behavior. A general approach that we have taken in our nonhuman primate studies is to explore the dependency of component processes of social behavior on putative brain regions. This is done experimentally by making selective lesions of the regions of interest and then carrying out detailed behavioral observations in order to define how the behavioral repertoire of the subjects has been altered. While primate models of autism based on brain lesions do not demonstrate construct, face, or predictive validity, lesion studies do contribute to our understanding of which brain regions are essential for social behavior, and are therefore relevant to our discussion of animal models of autism.

In the early 1990s, much attention was focused on the potential role of amygdala pathology in autism. This 'amygdala theory of autism' was based on several findings:

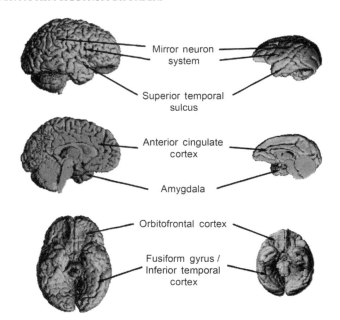

FIGURE 4.2.1 Putative structures of the human (left) and macaque (right) social brain include the mirror neuron system, cortex surrounding superior temporal sulcus, anterior cingulate cortex, amygdala, orbitofrontal cortex and fusiform gryus/inferior temporal cortex.

1. Reports of abnormal cell density in the amygdala of autistic brains (Bauman, 1991: Bauman et al., 1997);
2. Atypical patterns of amygdala activation in human subjects with autism (Baron-Cohen et al., 2000; 1999);
3. A putative animal model of autism resulting from neonatal amygdala damage in rhesus monkeys (Bachevalier, 1994; 1996).

The nonhuman primate model of autism developed by Bachevalier and colleagues was based primarily on a study of six peer-reared monkeys that received aspiration lesions of the amygdala within the first postnatal month (Bachevalier, 1994). When placed in social dyads at 2 months of age, the neonatal amygdala-lesioned infants showed less overall activity, exploration, and social behavior initiation than age-matched controls. At 6 months of age, activity levels were relatively normal, but social interactions were reduced in the amygdalectomized infants compared to the controls. The authors also reported that more extensive lesions of the medial temporal lobe, including the amygdala, hippocampus, and ventromedial temporal cortex, produced a more profound effect on social interactions, including lack of social skills, flat affect, and increased stereotypical behaviors. Given that impaired social communication and a lack of social interest are hallmark features of autism, the authors proposed that lesions of the medial temporal lobe, specifically the amygdala, might provide an animal model of autism (Bachevalier, 1994; 2000).

The studies by Bachevalier and colleagues were some of the first attempts to use the nonhuman primate to model features of autism. One important detail that was not considered in these previous studies was the animals' rearing condition. Rearing nonhuman primates without access to both mothers and peers, even without any other insult to the brain, has a deleterious effect on their social development (Capitanio, 1986). Therefore, the behavioral deficits observed in those studies could have been due to the brain lesion, the rearing environment, or a combination of the two factors. To address this question, we conducted a series of experiments to evaluate the effects of neurotoxic amygdala damage in maternally and socially reared rhesus monkeys (Bauman et al., 2004a, b; Prather et al., 2001). We found that macaque monkeys that are reared by their mothers in a social environment and receive selective amygdala lesions at 2 weeks of age do not demonstrate profound impairments in social development within the first year of life. The amygdala-lesioned monkeys were able to produce and respond to a variety of species-typical social signals and did not differ from control monkeys in the amount and quality of their social interactions (Bauman et al., 2004a, b). The amygdala-lesioned monkeys did, however, show abnormal fear responses to both social and nonsocial stimuli (e.g., heightened fear of conspecifics and absence of fear to normally aversive objects) (Bauman et al., 2004a; Bliss-Moreau et al., 2010; 2011a; Prather et al., 2001). Thus, neonatal lesions of the macaque amygdala resulted in a sparing of species-typical social behavior, while profoundly impacting fear-processing abilities during the window of time that would be relevant to the onset of ASD symptoms.

Our interpretation of the results from the studies described above indicates that the amygdala is not essential for the production of social behavior in adult macaque monkeys or for the early development of fundamental components of social behavior. The current research does, however, suggest that the amygdala plays an essential role in modulating social behavior, especially in potentially threatening contexts. Observations of these animals are ongoing, and we have observed additional changes in their behavior over time. For example, the neonatal amygdala-lesioned subjects were lower ranking in their social groups compared to hippocampus-lesioned or control subjects (Bauman et al., 2006). Interestingly, both the neonatal amygdala- and hippocampus-lesioned subjects develop repetitive behaviors in the second year of life (Bauman et al., 2008). The emergence of stereotypies after a period of relatively normal development bears some resemblance to developmental disorders, such as autism, where abnormal behaviors may become apparent or worsen following a seemingly typical developmental trajectory. In adulthood, the neonatal amygdala-lesioned subjects demonstrate a blunted affective response (reduced facial expression and vocalizations) to both social and nonsocial videos (Bliss-Moreau et al., 2011b). Despite the overall reduction in affective responding, amygdala-lesioned animals did respond most robustly to socially engaging stimuli and least robustly to nonsocial stimuli. These findings indicate that neonatal amygdala damage may ultimately lead to a blunting of affective responding in adulthood, while leaving intact the ability to assess the intensity of social stimuli and respond appropriately.

The absence of pronounced social deficits or repetitive behaviors early in development indicates that neonatal amygdala lesions do not result in an animal model of autism with high face validity. In order to produce a model with high face validity, we would have expected to see pronounced changes in social behavior and communication by the time the monkeys reached 12 months of age (roughly equivalent to a 4-year-old human). Moreover, the construct validity of an amygdala lesion model is questionable. Although there is compelling evidence for structural and functional amygdala abnormalities in individuals with autism (Dalton et al., 2005; Nordahl et al., 2012; Schumann and Amaral, 2005; Schumann et al., 2004), complete amygdala lesions in an animal model clearly do not replicate this neuropathology. Likewise, human subjects who do suffer from bilateral amygdala damage display subtle deficits in social processing, but are clearly not autistic (Adolphs et al., 1994; 1995; 1998; 2005; Adolphs and Tranel, 2003). The low construct and face validity of the neonatal amygdala lesion model would argue against this approach as a valid animal model of autism.

Fortunately, as technology advances, so does our ability to utilize nonhuman primate models to determine the brain regions that are essential for social development and, by extrapolation, may be involved in autism spectrum disorders. Recent advances in the use of non-invasive neuroimaging techniques (e.g., micro-PET (micro positron emission tomography) or fMRI (functional magnetic resonance imaging)), new molecular approaches to temporarily deactivating specific neural regions or specific neural types, and multi-method approaches (e.g., combining transient deactivation with functional neuroimaging) will make tremendous headway in our understanding of the neural basis of social behavior. This research will undoubtedly have important implications not only for understanding the neural basis of typical social behavior, but also for understanding the impairments of social processing that are relevant to ASD.

Behavioral Outcome Models: Isolate Rearing Models

Beginning in the 1960s, Harlow and colleagues initiated a series of experiments to evaluate the effects of raising monkeys in partial or complete social isolation. While these controversial studies were not originally intended as animal models of autism, we have chosen to include these studies in our discussion of nonhuman primate models of autism because of the high face validity associated with this model. Nonhuman primates reared in isolation from conspecifics develop abnormal behaviors such as self-clasping, huddling, self-orality, and rocking with stereotypic movements (Griffin and Harlow, 1966; Harlow and Zimmermann, 1959; Harlow et al., 1965). Even more striking, nonhuman primates reared in complete isolation for the first six months of life fail to develop species-typical social behaviors (Harlow et al., 1965; Harlow and Harlow, 1965) as evidenced by their failure to initiate or reciprocate play and grooming behaviors (Harlow, 1965; Harlow and Harlow, 1962; Harlow et al., 1964) and by their inability to respond to a variety of species-specific social signals (Mason, 1960). Deficits in social and communication development, combined with the presence of self-directed repetitive behaviors, in many ways parallel symptoms of human autism. This is not to suggest that restricted rearing practices are a cause of autism. Parents and therapists of children with autism put forth heroic efforts to create an environment that will help a young child with autism acquire social and communication skills. It is possible, however, that extreme social deprivation conditions such as found in substandard orphanages, may parallel the experimental manipulations of nonhuman primate isolate-rearing models, and ultimately result in behaviors that resemble autism. From a theoretical perspective, it is possible that these adverse rearing conditions affect the same brain regions that are also affected, albeit through different causes, and lead to the social impairments of autism. A 1999 study by Rutter and colleagues reported that 6% of 111 children adopted from Romanian orphanages showed autistic-like patterns of behavior between 4 and 6 years of age (Rutter et al., 1999). Rutter's findings suggest that early deprivation of social stimuli in human children may alter brain development and result in behavioral symptoms that resemble autism.

Both the isolate-reared nonhuman primate studies and the reports of children raised in substandard orphanages indicate that there are critical periods of development when social interaction is required to develop species-typical social behavior. If social interaction is withheld during these critical periods, the resulting behavior resembles autistic symptomatology. Clearly, social interaction is not intentionally withheld from children who go on to develop autism. However, it is possible that autism is caused by a failure to develop the neural circuitry required for infants to attend to and engage in social interaction during these critical periods. Thus, a disruption in the neural circuitry required to

engage in early social interactions may mimic the effects of early social deprivation. Schultz has proposed that early abnormalities in visual attention mediated by the amygdala results in an inability to identify salient signals, which in turn alters overall development of social perception and knowledge of others (Schultz, 2005). Dawson and colleagues have suggested that a primary deficit in social motivation mediated by dopaminergic reward systems underlies the early inattention to social signals that is characteristic of autism (Dawson et al., 2005a, b). Either a disruption in processing capabilities or a deficit in social reward systems could conceivably lead to an inability to attend to social information early in development.

In addition to high face validity, the nonhuman primate isolate-rearing studies demonstrated predictive validity by providing valuable insight into the potential for therapeutic interventions. Studies of the isolate-reared monkeys revealed that recovery of social behavior was possible under specific circumstances. While young isolate-reared monkeys exposed to age-matched peers showed only limited recovery of social responses, if 6-month-old isolates were exposed to much younger monkeys, they achieved almost complete recovery of social behavior (Harlow and Suomi, 1971). The authors suggested that the younger monkeys proved to be therapeutically valuable because they posed no threat to the isolate-reared subjects, thus allowing the isolate-reared monkeys to 'learn' species-typical social behaviors as the younger monkeys passed through their own stages of socialization. These studies suggest that the neural systems affected by isolate rearing retain neural plasticity to respond to specific therapeutic interventions. This is consistent with the intensive behavioral interventions used for children with ASD, which are most effective when delivered early in development (Dawson et al., 2010; Vismara and Rogers, 2010; Wallace and Rogers, 2010).

The parallels between primate deprivation studies and autistic symptoms raises the possibility that this model could have been used to identify neural regions that are essential for normal social development and guide efforts to determine the neuropathology underlying human autism. Alas, this was apparently a missed opportunity. Despite the numerous nonhuman primate isolate rearing studies carried out in the 1960s and 1970s, relatively little information is available regarding the neural systems that were altered. Only a small number of studies have assessed the neuropathology associated with nonhuman primate isolate rearing models, focusing on measures of dendritic arborization in motor and somatosensory cortex (Bryan and Riesen, 1989; Struble and Riesen, 1978), or Purkinje cell size and morphology in isolate-reared monkeys compared to controls (Floeter and Greenough, 1979). Other groups have evaluated changes in dopamine receptor function following apomorphine challenge in adult monkeys that had been reared in social isolation for the first nine months of life (Lewis et al., 1990). In adulthood, the isolate monkeys demonstrated significantly increased rates of blinking and whole-body stereotypies compared to socially reared controls in response to apomorphine challenge. These results suggest that early isolate rearing leads to long-term changes in dopamine receptor sensitivity. A follow-up immunohistochemical study from this same cohort revealed altered neurochemistry in the striatum (i.e., reduced substance P, leucine-enkephalin, calbindin, and tyrosine hydroxylase immunoreactivity), though similar changes were not found in the amygdala (Martin et al., 1991).

Ethical concerns now rightfully preclude the implementation of the isolate rearing protocols carried out in the 1950s and 1960s. Yet, naturally occurring experiments may provide a fertile laboratory for investigating the neurobiology of social behavior. At all major primate colonies, it is common to find cohorts of animals that are socially isolated. The neurobiology of these endogenously hyposocial monkeys has not been investigated, and it would be of interest to determine whether there are characteristic neural alterations associated with these animals. Moreover, it would be intriguing to evaluate whether genetic mutations that are associated with risk of autism are also observed in these animals. If so, it may prove to be the case that they would provide an attractive model for testing potential therapeutics for autism spectrum disorders.

Etiology Models: Prenatal Risk Factors

A previous limitation to the development of additional primate models of autism was the dearth of convincing evidence on specific etiologies of autism. In recent years, the prenatal environment, and particularly the fetal/maternal immune environment, has been highlighted as playing a potential role in the etiology of some forms of ASD (Hallmayer et al., 2011). Our research group is utilizing a nonhuman primate model to evaluate one prenatal risk factor implicated in ASD – maternal auto-antibodies that target fetal brain tissue (described below). Other prenatal challenges, such as maternal infection during pregnancy, have also been associated with an increased risk of neurodevelopmental disorders, including ASD (Atladottir et al., 2010; Meyer et al., 2011; Patterson, 2011). Coe and colleagues have developed sophisticated nonhuman primate models to evaluate brain and behavioral changes related to prenatal infection exposure (Short et al., 2010; Willette et al., 2011). While these studies were not specifically designed as animal models of autism, their findings demonstrate the power of pairing sophisticated behavioral assessments with structural MRI to systematically evaluate the effects of a prenatal insult on both brain and behavior development.

MATERNAL AUTO-ANTIBODY MODEL

Converging evidence indicates that immune dysfunction may play an important role in a subset of autism cases (van Gent et al., 1997). Some patients with autism demonstrate abnormalities and/or deficits of immune system function, including inappropriate immune response to pathogen challenge (Ashwood et al., 2004), recurrent infections (Stern et al., 2005), peripheral immune abnormalities (Ashwood et al., 2003; Croonenberghs et al., 2002; Singh, 1996), and neuroinflammatory responses in the central nervous system (CNS) (Vargas et al., 2005). In addition to general immune system dysfunction, recent evidence suggests that certain forms of autism are associated with autoimmune conditions (Ashwood and Van de Water, 2004). Autoimmunity occurs when the immune system inappropriately identifies and reacts to 'self' components. Several studies have also reported that autoimmune disorders are more common in family members of individuals with autism compared to typically developing controls (Comi et al., 1999; Richler et al., 2006; Sweeten et al., 2003). Moreover, antibodies directed against CNS proteins have been found in the sera of children with autism (Cook et al., 1993; Kozlovskaia et al., 2000; Plioplys et al., 1994; Singh and Rivas, 2004; Singh et al., 1993; 1997; Todd and Ciaranello, 1985).

In addition to the presence of auto-antibodies in individuals with autism, recent evidence raises the possibility that maternal auto-antibodies to fetal brain tissue may play a role in a subset of autism cases (Vincent et al., 2003). Maternal immune factors that cross the placenta during pregnancy have the potential to profoundly impact fetal neurodevelopment. During gestation, immunoglobulin G (IgG) isotype antibodies from the mother are transported across the placenta in order to equip the immunologically naïve fetus with protection (Garty et al., 1994). However, in addition to immunoprotective antibodies, auto-antibodies that react to fetal 'self'-proteins can also cross the placenta, resulting in a number of neonatal autoimmune diseases such as certain forms of arthrogryposis multiplex congenital (Brueton et al., 2000; Vincent et al., 1995). Reports of maternal IgG antibodies reactive to brain proteins in mothers of children with autism suggest a potentially similar role for these auto-antibodies in ASD (Dalton et al., 2003; Singer et al., 2008; Vincent et al., 2003).

While there are multiple patterns of reactivity to brain proteins associated with these maternal auto-antibodies, substantial progress has been made in characterizing which reactivity patterns are specific to ASD. Van de Water and colleagues have identified fetal-brain-specific auto-antibodies in approximately 10% of mothers of children with autism (Braunschweig et al., 2008; 2011). Retrospective analysis of banked blood samples indicates that some women who went on to deliver children diagnosed with ASD had anti-brain antibodies circulating during their pregnancy (Croen et al., 2008). Moreover, maternal auto-antibodies persist in the woman's circulation for up to 18 years, and therefore have the potential to impact fetal development in subsequent pregnancies (Zimmerman et al., 2007). Thus, it is plausible that the presence of specific anti-fetal-brain antibodies in the circulation of mothers during pregnancy may disrupt finely orchestrated events underlying neurodevelopment. Maternal IgG can be detected in the fetal circulation as early as 13 weeks gestation (Simister, 2003) – a time that coincides with both neurogenesis and neuronal migration. The blood–brain barrier in the fetus is incompletely formed, thereby allowing pathogenic maternal antibodies to potentially gain access to the developing brain at critical time-points through gestation (Heininger, 2006). Maternal IgG transport across the placenta increases throughout mid to late pregnancy (Malek et al., 1994; 1996; Martin et al., 2008), thus overlapping with neuronal differentiation, synaptogenesis, dendritic and axonal arborization, myelination, and apoptosis. Slight alterations in any of these processes stemming from *in utero* exposure to anti-brain auto-antibodies could disrupt the trajectory of brain development and ultimately lead to one form of ASD.

Although evidence for pathogenic maternal antibodies is very provocative, it is not feasible to establish a causal relationship in human subjects. Animal models are needed to evaluate the effects of prenatal exposure to potentially pathogenic antibodies. A preliminary rodent model of developmental disorders reported behavioral abnormalities in mice prenatally exposed to serum from a woman whose children have autism and other developmental disorders (Dalton et al., 2003). Similarly, Martin et al. (2008) published a study on the effects of exposing gestating rhesus monkeys to IgG-class antibodies obtained from human mothers of children with autism. Beginning at one month following weaning (at about 7 months of age), the monkey offspring were observed for behavioral differences, either while alone or while paired with a familiar conspecific from their social rearing group. Significantly higher frequencies of whole-body stereotypies were observed in the maternal-autism IgG-treated monkeys compared to the control IgG-treated and control untreated monkeys. A similar pattern of whole-body stereotypies was also observed during interactions with unfamiliar

conspecifics. One month following the pairings with familiar peers, monkeys were removed from their social groups and placed with one of four unfamiliar monkeys in large testing enclosures. Once again, there was a higher frequency of whole-body stereotypies in the maternal-autism IgG-treated monkeys compared to control IgG-treated and control untreated monkeys. In addition to these three behavioral settings, the autism IgG-exposed monkeys produced an increased number of midline crossings (an indication of hyperactivity) in the mother preference task that is administered over the first four days following weaning. In this task, infants are provided access to their mothers or to another familiar adult female. The species-typical response is to identify the location of the mother and then to remain in proximity for the remainder of the trial. The autism IgG-treated animals, however, demonstrated significantly more cross-cage pacing and did not settle in proximity with their mothers. Finally, all animals in this study were fitted with actimeters that measured activity throughout three weeks of testing. No differences in activity were detected when the animals remained in their social groups. However, when the animals were housed individually, the autism IgG-treated group demonstrated significantly higher levels of activity than the control group.

These preliminary data indicated that prenatal exposure to IgG-class antibodies from mothers of children with autism potentially alters the behavioral development of rhesus monkeys. Profound stereotypies were observed in several behavioral settings across seven months of testing. In addition to these striking results, this study provided evidence for the feasibility of examining the effects of potentially pathological maternal antibodies in nonhuman primate models. While these results are provocative, it is premature to consider them indicative of an animal model of autism. Replication is clearly needed. It is also clear that repetitive stereotypies represent only one facet of autistic symptomatology. We have thus far not observed deficits in social behavior and communication in the maternal-IgG-exposure model. It is also noteworthy that repetitive behaviors are not specific to autism. Indeed, motor stereotypies are a common feature of many developmental disorders, including Rett syndrome and mental retardation (Berkson, 1983; Berkson et al., 1995; Bodfish et al., 2000; Wales et al., 2004). In spite of these limitations, we find the results obtained from the initial study promising for several reasons: The proposed model comes directly from families of children with autism and therefore demonstrates high construct validity. The immunological challenge utilized was derived from mothers who have produced multiple children with autism, thus identifying a putative human cause of autism. At the very least, this immunological model has created an animal that demonstrates one of the core features of autism, thus demonstrating moderate face validity.

We are currently conducting a large-scale study attempting to replicate the behavioral results of this preliminary study. In our current study, we have added longitudinal MRI to quantify brain growth in the antibody-exposed animals. Despite an increasing emphasis on structural MRI analysis of the autistic brain, there is currently no pattern of brain changes that is diagnostic of the disorder as a whole (Amaral et al., 2008). Because multiple etiologies and neural phenotypes of ASD are likely to exist, clinical samples invariably include a heterogeneous mix of different subtypes of ASD (Alexander et al. 2007; Nordahl et al., 2011). The situation is quite different for animal models of autism, where we are imposing a known treatment during a defined period of gestation. If exposure to the maternal auto-antibodies has an impact on brain development, we would expect to detect these changes using longitudinal MRI. Another advantage of animal models is the ability to integrate behavioral evaluations, volumetric analyses of brain development, and ultimately postmortem neuropathological assessments in the same individual. Human MRI data alone cannot be used to determine the cellular mechanisms that underlie the neuropathology of autism, and progress in postmortem analysis of brain tissue is hindered by the scarcity of ASD brain tissue. If validated, the nonhuman primate maternal antibody model will allow, for the first time, a histological evaluation of the neural changes associated with a specific risk factor for ASD. We foresee important clinical implications if the maternal antibody model is validated. For example, screening for brain-directed antibodies may provide an indication of risk factors for women who intend to become pregnant. This information may be particularly important to women who have had previous children with autism, since the probability of having a child with autism who has an autistic sibling is much higher. More importantly, the detection of brain-directed auto-antibodies holds the prospect of implementing therapeutic interventions that may decrease the probability of a pregnancy leading to a child with autism.

CONCLUSIONS

Animal models have played an essential role in identifying genetic and environmental factors that contribute to human disorders. They are often essential for understanding the cellular and molecular mechanisms underlying human disease. It is likely that animal models will continue to play an important role in evaluating the biological underpinnings of autism and facilitating the development of prevention and treatment strategies. The validity of animal models is based on:

1. Construct validity (degree of similarity between the experimental manipulation and the underlying cause of the human disease);
2. Face validity (the extent to which the resulting model resembles the phenotype of the human disorder);
3. Predictive validity (treatment discoveries in an animal model which may provide insight into therapeutic options for the human condition).

Nonhuman primates, compared to rodents, more closely resemble humans in both sophistication of their social behavior and their neural organization, thus making them an ideal group to model features of autism. A current limitation to the development of additional primate models is the dearth of convincing evidence on specific etiologies of autism that can be modulated in primate models. Assuming this information will be forthcoming in the near future, it will also be essential to develop behavioral probes for nonhuman primates that are sensitive to the core features of autism. With these developments, the nonhuman primate can provide a valuable test bed for evaluating preventative measures and innovative treatments.

ACKNOWLEDGMENTS

Original research described in this chapter was supported by grants from the National Institute of Mental Health (R37 MH57502 and MH80218) and by the base grant (RR00169) of the California National Primate Research Center (CNPRC).

References

Abbott, N.J., et al., 2010. Structure and function of the blood-brain barrier. Neurobiology of Disease 37, 13–25.

Abrahams, B.S., Geschwind, D.H., 2008. Advances in autism genetics: On the threshold of a new neurobiology. Nature Reviews Genetics 9, 341–355.

Adolphs, R., Tranel, D., 2003. Amygdala damage impairs emotion recognition from scenes only when they contain facial expressions. Neuropsychologia 41, 1281–1289.

Adolphs, R., et al., 1994. Impaired recognition of emotion in facial expressions following bilateral damage to the human amygdala. Nature 372, 669–672.

Adolphs, R., et al., 1995. Fear and the human amygdala. Journal of Neuroscience 15, 5879–5891.

Adolphs, R., Tranel, D., Damasio, A.R., 1998. The human amygdala in social judgment. Nature 393, 470–474.

Adolphs, R., et al., 2005. A mechanism for impaired fear recognition after amygdala damage. Nature 433, 68–72.

Alexander, A.L., et al., 2007. Diffusion tensor imaging of the corpus callosum in autism. NeuroImage 34, 61–73.

Altmann, S., 1967. The structure of primate social communication. In: Altmann, S. (Ed.), Social Communication Among Primates. University of Chicago Press, Chicago, IL.

Amaral, D.G., Schumann, C.M., Nordahl, C.W., 2008. Neuroanatomy of autism. Trends in Neurosciences 31, 137–145.

Ashwood, P., Van de Water, J., 2004. Is autism an autoimmune disease? Autoimmunity Reviews 3, 557–562.

Ashwood, P., et al., 2003. Intestinal lymphocyte populations in children with regressive autism: Evidence for extensive mucosal immunopathology. Journal of Clinical Immunology 23, 504–517.

Ashwood, P., et al., 2004. Spontaneous mucosal lymphocyte cytokine profiles in children with autism and gastrointestinal symptoms: Mucosal immune activation and reduced counter regulatory interleukin-10. Journal of Clinical Immunology 24, 664–673.

Ashwood, P., Wills, S., Van de Water, J., 2006. The immune response in autism: A new frontier for autism research. Journal of Leukocyte Biology 80, 1–15.

Atladottir, H.O., et al., 2010. Maternal infection requiring hospitalization during pregnancy and autism spectrum disorders. Journal of Autism and Developmental Disorders 40, 1423–1430.

Bachevalier, J., 1994. Medial temporal lobe structures and autism – a review of clinical and experimental findings. Neuropsychologia 32, 627–648.

Bachevalier, J., 1996. Brief report – medial temporal lobe and autism – a putative animal model in primates. Journal of Autism and Developmental Disorders 26, 217–220.

Bachevalier, J., 2000. The amygdala, social cognition, and autism. In: Aggleton, J.P. (Ed.), The Amygdala: A Functional Analysis. Oxford University Press, New York, pp. 509–543.

Ballabh, P., Braun, A., Nedergaard, M., 2004. The blood-brain barrier: An Overview – structure, regulation, and clinical implications. Neurobiology of Disease 16, 1–13.

Baron-Cohen, S., et al., 1999. Social intelligence in the normal and autistic brain: An fMRI study. European Journal of Neuroscience 11, 1891–1898.

Baron-Cohen, S., et al., 2000. The amygdala theory of autism. Neuroscience and Biobehavioral Reviews 24, 355–364.

Bauman, M.L., 1991. Microscopic neuroanatomic abnormalities in autism. Pediatrics 87, 791–796.

Bauman, M.L., Filipek, P.A., Kemper, T.L., 1997. Early infantile autism. International Review of Neurobiology 41, 367–386.

Bauman, M.D., et al., 2004. The development of social behavior following neonatal amygdala lesions in rhesus monkeys. Journal of Cognitive Neuroscience 16, 1388–1411.

Bauman, M.D., et al., 2004. The development of mother-infant interactions after neonatal amygdala lesions in rhesus monkeys. Journal of Neuroscience 24, 711–721.

Bauman, M.D., et al., 2006. The expression of social dominance following neonatal lesions of the amygdala or hippocampus in rhesus monkeys (Macaca mulatta). Behavioral Neuroscience 120, 749–760.

Bauman, M.D., et al., 2008. Emergence of stereotypies in juvenile monkeys (Macaca mulatta) with neonatal amygdala or hippocampus lesions. Behavioral Neuroscience 122, 1005–1015.

Bergman, H., Wichmann, T., DeLong, M.R., 1990. Reversal of experimental Parkinsonism by lesions of the subthalamic nucleus. Science 249, 1436–1438.

Berkson, G., 1983. Repetitive stereotyped behaviors. American Journal of Mental Deficiency 88, 239–246.

Berkson, G., Gutermuth, L., Baranek, G., 1995. Relative prevalence and relations among stereotyped and similar behaviors. American Journal of Mental Retardation 100, 137–145.

Bernstein, I.S., Mason, W.A., 1963. Group formation by rhesus monkeys. Animal Behavior 11, 28–31.

Bliss-Moreau, E., et al., 2010. Neonatal amygdala or hippocampus lesions influence responsiveness to objects. Developmental Psychobiology 52, 487–503.

Bliss-Moreau, E., et al., 2011. Neonatal amygdala lesions alter responsiveness to objects in juvenile macaques. Neuroscience 178, 123–132.

Bliss-Moreau, E., Bauman, M.D., Amaral, D.G., 2011. Neonatal amygdala lesions result in globally blunted affect in adult rhesus macaques. Behavioral Neuroscience 125, 848–858.

Bodfish, J.W., et al., 2000. Varieties of repetitive behavior in autism: Comparisons to mental retardation. Journal of Autism and Developmental Disorders 30, 237–243.

Braunschweig, D., et al., 2008. Autism: Maternally derived antibodies specific for fetal brain proteins. Neurotoxicology 29, 226–231.

Braunschweig, D., et al., 2011. Behavioral correlates of maternal antibody status among children with autism. Journal of Autism and Developmental Disorders.

Brothers, L., 1990. The social brain: A project for integrating primate behavior and neurophysiology in a new domain. Concepts in Neuroscience 1, 27–51.

Brueton, L.A., et al., 2000. Asymptomatic maternal myasthenia as a cause of the Pena-Shokeir phenotype. American Journal of Medical Genetics 92, 1–6.

Bryan, G.K., Riesen, A.H., 1989. Deprived somatosensory-motor experience in stumptailed monkey neocortex: Dendritic spine density and dendritic branching of layer IIIB pyramidal cells. Journal of Comparative Neurology 286, 208–217.

Burns, R.S., et al., 1983. A primate model of Parkinsonism: Selective destruction of dopaminergic neurons in the pars compacta of the substantia nigra by N-methyl-4-phenyl-1,2,3,6-tetrahydropyridine. Proceedings of the National Academy of Sciences of the United States of America 80, 4546–4550.

Byrne, R., Whiten, A., 1988. Machiavellian Intelligence: Social Expertise and the Evolution of Intellect in Monkeys Apes and Humans. Oxford.

Capitanio, J., 1986. Behavioral pathology. In: Mitchell, G., Erwin, J. (Eds.), Comparative Primate Biology: Behavior, Conservation, and Ecology. Alan R. Liss, New York, pp. 411–454.

Capitanio, J.P., Emborg, M.E., 2008. Contributions of non-human primates to neuroscience research. The Lancet 371, 1126–1135.

Carper, R.A., Courchesne, E., 2005. Localized enlargement of the frontal cortex in early autism. Biological Psychiatry 57, 126–133.

Comi, A.M., et al., 1999. Familial clustering of autoimmune disorders and evaluation of medical risk factors in autism. Journal of Child Neurology 14, 388–394.

Cook E.H., Jr., et al., 1993. Receptor inhibition by immunoglobulins: Specific inhibition by autistic children, their relatives, and control subjects. Journal of Autism and Developmental Disorders 23, 67–78.

Crawley, J.N., 2004. Designing mouse behavioral tasks relevant to autistic-like behaviors. Mental Retardation and Developmental Disabilities Research Reviews 10, 248–258.

Croen, L.A., et al., 2008. Maternal mid-pregnancy auto-antibodies to fetal brain protein: The early markers for autism study. Biological Psychiatry 64, 583–588.

Croonenberghs, J., et al., 2002. Activation of the inflammatory response system in autism. Neuropsychobiology 45, 1–6.

Dalton, K.M., et al., 2005. Gaze fixation and the neural circuitry of face processing in autism. Nature Neuroscience 8, 519–526.

Dalton, K.M., et al., 2007. Gaze-fixation, brain activation, and amygdala volume in unaffected siblings of individuals with autism. Biological Psychiatry 61, 512–520.

Dalton, P., et al., 2003. Maternal neuronal antibodies associated with autism and a language disorder. Annals of Neurology 53, 533–537.

Dawson, G., et al., 2005. Neurocognitive and electrophysiological evidence of altered face processing in parents of children with autism: Implications for a model of abnormal development of social brain circuitry in autism. Developmental Psychopathology 17, 679–697.

Dawson, G., Webb, S.J., McPartland, J., 2005. Understanding the nature of face processing impairment in autism: Insights from behavioral and electrophysiological studies. Developmental Neuropsychology 27, 403–424.

Dawson, G., et al., 2010. Randomized, controlled trial of an intervention for toddlers with autism: The early start Denver model. Pediatrics 125, e17–e23.

Drickamer, L.C., 1975. Quantitative observation of behavior in free-ranging Macaca mulatta: Methodology and aggression. Behavior 55, 209–236.

Floeter, M.K., Greenough, W.T., 1979. Cerebellar plasticity: Modification of Purkinje cell structure by differential rearing in monkeys. Science 206, 227–229.

Garty, B.Z., et al., 1994. Placental transfer of immunoglobulin G subclasses. Clinical and Diagnostic Laboratory Immunology 1, 667–669.

Gibbs, R.A., et al., 2004. Genome sequence of the Brown Norway rat yields insights into mammalian evolution. Nature 428, 493–521.

Gibbs, R.A., et al., 2007. Evolutionary and biomedical insights from the rhesus macaque genome. Science 316, 222–234.

Griffin, G.A., Harlow, H.F., 1966. Effects of three months of total social deprivation on social adjustment and learning in the rhesus monkey. Child Development 37, 533–547.

Hallmayer, J., et al., 2011. Genetic heritability and shared environmental factors among twin pairs with autism. Archives of General Psychiatry 68, 1095–1102.

Harlow, H.F., 1965. Total social isolation: Effects on macaque monkey behavior. Science 148, 666.

Harlow, H.F., Harlow, M., 1962. Social deprivation in monkeys. Scientific American 207, 136–146.

Harlow, H.F., Harlow, M.K., 1965. The effect of rearing conditions on behavior. International Journal of Psychiatry 1, 43–51.

Harlow, H.F., Suomi, S.J., 1971. Social recovery by isolation-reared monkeys. Proceedings of the National Academy of Sciences of the United States of America 68, 1534–1538.

Harlow, H.F., Zimmermann, R.R., 1959. Affectional responses in the infant monkey; orphaned baby monkeys develop a strong and persistent attachment to inanimate surrogate mothers. Science 130, 421–432.

Harlow, H.F., Dodsworth, R.O., Harlow, M.K., 1965. Total social isolation in monkeys. Proceedings of the National Academy of Sciences of the United States of America 54, 90–97.

Harlow, H.F., Rowland, G.L., Griffin, G.A., 1964. The effect of total social deprivation on the development of monkey behavior. Psychiatric Research Reports 19, 116–135.

Heininger, U., Desgrandchamps, D., Schaad, U.B., 2006. Seroprevalence of Varicella-Zoster virus IgG antibodies in Swiss children during the first 16 months of age. Vaccine 24, 3258–3260.

Hertz-Picciotto, I., et al., 2008. Prenatal exposures to persistent and non-persistent organic compounds and effects on immune system development. Basic & Clinical Pharmacology & Toxicology 102, 146–154.

Jolly, A., 1966. Lemur social behavior and primate intelligence. Science 153, 501–506.

Kay, R.F., Ross, C., Williams, B.A., 1997. Anthropoid origins. Science 275, 797–804.

Kozlovskaia, G.V., et al., 2000. [Nerve growth factor auto-antibodies in children with various forms of mental dysontogenesis and in schizophrenia high risk group]. Zhurnal Nevrologii i Psikhiatrii Imeni S.S. Korsakova 100, 50–52.

Kumar, S., Hedges, S.B., 1998. A molecular timescale for vertebrate evolution. Nature 392, 917–920.

Lemere, C.A., et al., 2004. Alzheimer's disease abeta vaccine reduces central nervous system abeta levels in a non-human primate, the Caribbean vervet. American Journal of Pathology 165, 283–297.

Lemere, C.A., et al., 2006. Amyloid-beta immunotherapy for the prevention and treatment of Alzheimer disease: Lessons from mice, monkeys, and humans. Rejuvenation Research 9, 77–84.

Lewis, M.H., et al., 1990. Long-term effects of early social isolation in Macaca mulatta: Changes in dopamine receptor function following apomorphine challenge. Brain Research 513, 67–73.

Malek, A., Sager, R., Schneider, H., 1994. Maternal-fetal transport of immunoglobulin G and its subclasses during the third trimester of human pregnancy. American Journal of Reproductive Immunology 32, 8–14.

Malek, A., et al., 1996. Evolution of maternofetal transport of immunoglobulins during human pregnancy. American Journal of Reproductive Immunology 36, 248–255.

Malek, A., Sager, R., Schneider, H., 1998. Transport of proteins across the human placenta. American Journal of Reproductive Immunology 40, 347–351.

Martin, L.A., et al., 2008. Stereotypies and hyperactivity in rhesus monkeys exposed to IgG from mothers of children with autism. Brain Behavior Immunity 22, 806–816.

Martin, L.J., et al., 1991. Social deprivation of infant rhesus monkeys alters the chemoarchitecture of the brain: I. Subcortical regions. Journal of Neuroscience 11, 3344–3358.

Mason, W.A., 1960. The effects of social restriction on the behavior of rhesus monkeys: I. Free social behavior. Journal of Comparative and Physiological Psychology 53, 582–589.

McKinney, W.T., 1984. Animal models of depression: An overview. Psychiatric Developmental 2, 77–96.

Meyer, U., Feldon, J., Dammann, O., 2011. Schizophrenia and autism: Both shared and disorder-specific pathogenesis via perinatal inflammation? Pediatric Research 69, 26R–33R.

Missakian, E.A., 1972. Genealogical and cross-genealogical dominance relations in a group of free ranging rhesus monkeys (Macaca mulatta) on Cayo Santiago. Primates 13, 169–180.

Nagahara, A.H., et al., 2009. Neuroprotective effects of brain-derived neurotrophic factor in rodent and primate models of Alzheimer's disease. Nature Medicine 15, 331–337.

Nordahl, C.W., et al., 2011. Brain enlargement is associated with regression in preschool–age boys with autism spectrum disorders. Proceedings of the National Academy of Sciences of the United States of America.

Nordahl, C.W., et al., 2012. Increased rate of amygdala growth in children aged 2 to 4 years with autism spectrum disorders: A longitudinal study. Archives of General Psychiatry 69, 53–61.

Patterson, P.H., 2011. Maternal infection and immune involvement in autism. Trends in Molecular Medicine 17, 389–394.

Pessah, I.N., et al., 2008. Immunologic and neurodevelopmental susceptibilities of autism. Neurotoxicology 29, 532–545.

Plioplys, A.V., et al., 1994. Lymphocyte function in autism and Rett syndrome. Neuropsychobiology 29, 12–16.

Prather, M.D., et al., 2001. Increased social fear and decreased fear of objects in monkeys with neonatal amygdala lesions. Neuroscience 106, 653–658.

Preuss, T., 1995. Do rats have a prefrontal cortex? The Rose-Woolsey-Akert reconsidered. Journal of Cognitive Neuroscience, 1–24.

Richler, J., et al., 2006. Is there a 'regressive phenotype' of autism spectrum disorder associated with the measles-mumps-rubella vaccine? A CPEA Study. Journal of Autism and Developmental Disorders.

Rutter, M., et al., 1999. Quasi-autistic patterns following severe early global privation. English and Romanian Adoptees (ERA) Study Team. Journal of Child Psychology and Psychiatry 40, 537–549.

Sade, D.S., 1967. Determinants of dominance in a group of free-ranging rhesus monkeys. In: Altmann, S.A. (Ed.). Social Communication Among Primates. University of Chicago Press, Chicago, IL, pp. 99–114.

Schultz, R.T., 2005. Developmental deficits in social perception in autism: The role of the amygdala and fusiform face area. International Journal of Developmental Neuroscience 23, 125–141.

Schumann, C.M., Amaral, D.G., 2005. Stereological estimation of the number of neurons in the human amygdaloid complex. Journal of Comparative Neurology 491, 320–329.

Schumann, C.M., et al., 2004. The amygdala is enlarged in children but not adolescents with autism; the hippocampus is enlarged at all ages. Journal of Neuroscience 24, 6392–6401.

Semendeferi, K., et al., 2002. Humans and great apes share a large frontal cortex. Nature Neuroscience 5, 272–276.

Short, S.J., et al., 2010. Maternal influenza infection during pregnancy impacts postnatal brain development in the rhesus monkey. Biological Psychiatry 67, 965–973.

Simister, N.E., 2003. Placental transport of immunoglobulin G. Vaccine 21, 3365–3369.

Singer, H.S., et al., 2008. Antibodies against fetal brain in sera of mothers with autistic children. Journal of Neuroimmunology 194, 165–172.

Singh, V.K., 1996. Plasma increase of interleukin-12 and interferon-gamma: Pathological significance in autism. Journal of Neuroimmunology 66, 143–145.

Singh, V.K., Rivas, W.H., 2004. Prevalence of serum antibodies to caudate nucleus in autistic children. Neuroscience Letters 355, 53–56.

Singh, V.K., et al., 1993. Antibodies to myelin basic protein in children with autistic behavior. Brain, Behavior, and Immunity 7, 97–103.

Singh, V.K., et al., 1997. Circulating auto-antibodies to neuronal and glial filament proteins in autism. Pediatric Neurology 17, 88–90.

Squire, L.R., Stark, C.E., Clark, R.E., 2004. The medial temporal lobe. Annual Review of Neuroscience 27, 279–306.

Stern, L., et al., 2005. Immune function in autistic children. Annals of Allergy, Asthma, & Immunology 95, 558–565.

Struble, R.G., Riesen, A.H., 1978. Changes in cortical dendritic branching subsequent to partial social isolation in stumptailed monkeys. Developmental Psychobiology 11, 479–486.

Suzuki, W.A., Amaral, D.G., 2004. Functional neuroanatomy of the medial temporal lobe memory system. Cortex 40, 220–222.

Sweeten, T.L., et al., 2003. Increased prevalence of familial autoimmunity in probands with pervasive developmental disorders. Pediatrics 112, e420.

Todd, R.D., Ciaranello, R.D., 1985. Demonstration of inter- and intra-species differences in serotonin binding sites by antibodies from an autistic child. Proceedings of the National Academy of Sciences of the United States of America 82, 612–616.

Tuszynski, M.H., Blesch, A., 2004. Nerve growth factor: From animal models of cholinergic neuronal degeneration to gene therapy in Alzheimer's disease. Progress in Brain Research 146, 441–449.

Tuszynski, M.H., et al., 1996. Gene therapy in the adult primate brain: Intraparenchymal grafts of cells genetically modified to produce nerve growth factor prevent cholinergic neuronal degeneration. Gene Therapy 3, 305–314.

van Gent, T., Heijnen, C.J., Treffers, P.D., 1997. Autism and the immune system. Journal of Child Psychology and Psychiatry 38, 337–349.

Vargas, D.L., et al., 2005. Neuroglial activation and neuroinflammation in the brain of patients with autism. Annals of Neurology 57, 67–81.

Vincent, A., et al., 1995. Arthrogryposis multiplex congenita with maternal auto-antibodies specific for a fetal antigen. The Lancet 346, 24–25.

Vincent, A., et al., 2003. Antibodies to neuronal targets in neurological and psychiatric diseases. Annals of the New York Academy of Sciences 992, 48–55.

Vismara, L.A., Rogers, S.J., 2010. Behavioral treatments in autism spectrum disorder: What do we know? Annual Review of Clinical Psychology 6, 447–468.

Wales, L., Charman, T., Mount, R.H., 2004. An analogue assessment of repetitive hand behaviors in girls and young women with Rett syndrome. Journal of Intellectual Disability Research 48, 672–678.

Wallace, K.S., Rogers, S.J., 2010. Intervening in infancy: Implications for autism spectrum disorders. Journal of Child Psychology and Psychiatry 51, 1300–1320.

Wenk, G.L., 1993. A primate model of Alzheimer's disease. Behavioral Brain Research 57, 117–122.

Willette, A.A., et al., 2011. Brain enlargement and increased behavioral and cytokine reactivity in infant monkeys following acute prenatal endotoxemia. Behavioral Brain Research 219, 108–115.

Wrangham, R.W., 1980. An ecological model of female-bonded primate groups. Behavior 75, 262–300.

Yang, S.H., et al., 2008. Towards a transgenic model of Huntington's disease in a non-human primate. Nature 453, 921–924.

Zimmerman, A.W., et al., 2007. Maternal antibrain antibodies in autism. Brain, Behavior, and Immunity 21, 351–357.

4.3

Inducible Pluripotent Stem Cells In Autism Spectrum Disorders

Alysson Renato Muotri

University of California San Diego, School of Medicine, Department of Pediatrics/Rady Children's Hospital San Diego, Department of Cellular and Molecular Medicine, Stem Cell Program, La Jolla, CA, USA

A NOVEL AND COMPLEMENTARY MODEL FOR STUDYING AUTISM SPECTRUM DISORDERS

Science has improved human life and the understanding of human disease by taking advantage of models to mimic several conditions in the laboratory. Models are simplified representations or reflections of the reality. Thus, all models are useful in certain situations. Models are inaccurate by their nature, and all models have specific intrinsic limitations, but the best models allow the complexity of a system to approach the complexity of a human disease.

Autism spectrum disorders (ASD) are complex neuropsychiatric conditions, involving multiple genetic targets across several neural circuits in the brain. The lack of usable neuronal samples from postmortem brains and the inability to isolate populations of neurons from living subjects has blocked progress toward studying the underlying cellular and molecular mechanisms of ASD. Studies of cadaver tissue are problematic

in developmental disorders as disease onset usually precedes death by decades. Frozen tissue sections are of limited use for studying cellular physiology and neural networks. Most of the time, the tissue is not well preserved and even information about gene expression or anatomy can be lost due to inappropriate handling. Additionally, the long-term medication history of patients could affect the observed phenotype in the tissue. Peripheral tissues, such as blood or skin, have being extremely helpful to the understanding of ASD genetics, but have limited suitability for follow-up with relevant biological questions. The case of computational methods is similar, thus far restricted to data collected from peripheral tissue. Brain imaging allows the study of circuits, but only at a very low resolution, under the influence of the environment, and has also limited experimental power.

Finally, animal models often do not recapitulate more than a few aspects of complex human disease, if at all, and this has been particularly problematic in the case of ASD. The lack of ASD-like behaviors in several knockout

The Neuroscience of Autism Spectrum Disorders.
http://dx.doi.org/10.1016/B978-0-12-391924-3.00028-4

mouse models, based upon knowledge of genes related to ASD, reflects the inherent differences between the two species' genetic backgrounds and neural circuits. In fact, while there are multiple genetic mutations that disrupt social behavior in mice, the vast majority do not appear to have direct relevance to ASD. Conversely, many ASD mutations have no effect in mice or lead to phenotypes that do not mimic the human disease (Silverman et al., 2010). These observations illustrate the challenge associated with complex neuropsychiatric modeling in animals and future translation into human therapies (Dragunow, 2008). Thus, the ASD field lacks an appropriate human model, and would greatly benefit from unlimited supplies of neurons so experiments can be performed in controlled situations.

Pluripotent human embryonic stem cells (hESCs) have been successfully isolated from early-stage human embryos (blastocysts). They can self-renew, and differentiate into various cell types, offering an unlimited source of cell types for research (Thomson et al., 1998). However, for ethical and moral reasons, it is not possible to demonstrate that hESCs can actually contribute to different cell types and tissues in a real person. Perhaps the more rigorous demonstration that hESCs can actually become functional human neurons, fully integrated into the neuronal network, is through the successful transplantation of hESCs in the ventricles of embryonic mouse brains (Muotri et al., 2005b). These 'chimeric brains' carried human cells that were differentiated into functional neural lineages and generated mature, active human neurons that successfully integrated into the adult mouse forebrain. A small fraction of the transplanted cells integrated individually or in small clusters into the host tissue with similar morphometric dimensions as adjacent host cells, including shape, size, and orientation, and adjusted to the pre-existing cellular architecture. Transplanted cells colocalized, localized with markers specific for neuronal subtypes. Evidence of synaptic inputs was apparent in the presence of arborized dendrites with spines, suggesting that glutamate-containing terminals contacted these dendrites. Ultrastructural analysis also confirmed that human cells received synaptic input and exhibited mature features, such as pools of presynaptic vesicles adjacent to a postsynaptic density. Moreover, transplanted cells showed neuronal properties similar to neurons under comparable electrophysiological recording conditions. Such observations, plus several other pieces of in vitro evidence, made a convincing argument that human pluripotent stem cells could actually form functional neurons, and thus function as a model for early stages of brain development.

However, to develop cellular models of human disease, it is necessary to generate new cell lines with genomes that are predisposed to diseases. By taking advantage of pre-implantation genetic diagnosis, it was possible to generate hESCs that carried mutations in specific genes known to cause human diseases. This was conducted with cystic fibrosis, Huntington's disease, Marphan syndrome, fragile X, and other monogenetic diseases (Bradley et al., 2011; Mateizel et al., 2006; Pickering et al., 2005; Verlinsky et al., 2005). Forward genetics was also used to generate hESC disease models by homologous recombination. Perhaps the first example was generated by the Benvenisty group, which used gene targeting to knockout the HPRT1 gene, responsible for Lesch–Nyhan syndrome (Urbach et al., 2004). Unfortunately, apart from the ethical and political concerns related to hESC-line derivation, this strategy is also limited by the availability of human blastocysts and by the number of genes one can manipulate in hESCs – notoriously resilient for gene targeting (Giudice and Trounson, 2008). Complex disorders, where multiple genes are affected, or 'sporadic' diseases such as ASD, schizophrenia, or amyotrophic lateral sclerosis (ALS), where the genetic alteration is not previously known, cannot be modeled using forward genetics in hESCs.

Reprogramming technology provides a possible solution to this problem, as it allows the genomes of human individuals afflicted with ASD to be captured in a pluripotent stem cell line. Recently, reprogramming of somatic cells to a pluripotent state by over-expression of specific genes has been accomplished using mouse fibroblasts (Takahashi and Yamanaka, 2006). To reprogram somatic cells, Takahashi and Yamanaka tried 24 genes that were previously demonstrated to be expressed in ESCs, to test their ability to induce somatic cells into ESC-like cells. Surprisingly, they found that only four retroviral-mediated transcription factors – the octamer-binding protein 4 (OCT4, also known as POU5F1), SOX2, Krüppel-like factor 4 (KLF4) and MYC – were sufficient to jump-start the expression of endogenous pluripotency genes in somatic cells. Despite the fact that the biology of reprogramming is not yet completely understood, it is clear that the repression of gene expression by the binding of transcription factors and epigenetic marks in the chromatin observed in donor somatic cells can be reversed by reprogramming factors to developmentally regress the cells to an earlier state (Ho et al., 2011). These reprogrammed cells were able to form embryoid bodies in vitro and teratomas in vivo, and contributed to several tissues in chimeric embryos when injected into mouse blastocysts. The report of human reprogrammed cells using the same set of transcriptional factors was published soon after (Takahashi et al., 2007; Yu et al., 2007). These cells, named induced pluripotent stem cells (iPSCs), can be derived from cells isolated from peripheral tissues of normal individuals or people affected by several conditions.

iPSCs and hESCs are very similar, but significant differences can be detected when they are carefully compared (Marchetto et al., 2009). Gene expression differences between iPSCs and hESCs can be caused by incomplete silencing of genes expressed in donor cells and failure to fully induce pluripotent genes in reprogrammed cells, likely reflecting incomplete resetting of somatic expression (Chin et al., 2009). Epigenetic markers also seem to differ between the two types of pluripotent cells. Hotspots of aberrant epigenomic reprogramming were reported to be found in methylated regions proximal to centromeres and telomeres in iPSCs (Lister et al., 2011). It is also important to mention that, besides epigenetic modifications, genetic alterations can also occur during the reprogramming process. Sometimes iPSC lines display abnormal karyotype (Mayshar et al., 2010) and large copy number variations (CNVs) (Laurent et al., 2011). Interestingly, some of these CNV alterations tend to disappear after several passages of the cells, probably due to selection in culture. Nonetheless, it is important to note that extensive genetic and epigenetic assessments should become a standard procedure to identify the truly reprogrammed cells from those that are only partially reprogrammed or unstable and to ensure the quality of iPSCs used for experiments.

Isogenic pluripotent cells are attractive not only for their potential therapeutic use with lower risk of immune rejection, but also for their potential use in gaining further understanding of complex diseases with heritable and sporadic conditions (Marchetto et al., 2010b; Muotri, 2009). Such cells could be differentiated to human neurons to evaluate whether the captured genome alters a cellular phenotype in a manner similar to that predicted by mechanistic models of ASD (Figure 4.3.1). An iPSC model may also address human-specific effects and avoid some of the well-known limitations of animal models – such as the absence of a human genetic background. Although iPSCs have been generated for several neurological diseases (Marchetto et al., 2011), the demonstration of disease-specific pathogenesis

and phenotypic rescue in relevant cell types is a current challenge in the field, with only a handful of proof-of-principle examples available to date, including spinal muscular atrophy (Ebert et al., 2009), Down syndrome (Baek et al., 2009), Rett syndrome (Marchetto et al., 2010a), schizophrenia (Brennand et al., 2011), and others (Grskovic et al., 2011; Robinton and Daley, 2012; Saporta et al., 2011).

LIMITATIONS OF iPSCs FOR DISEASE MODELING

As with other models of ASD, the iPSC system also has important limitations. The mechanisms behind cellular reprogramming are currently unknown. Understanding the current pitfalls of this technology is crucial to making correct interpretations and plausible extrapolations to the human brain. As mentioned before, some regions of the genome may not be completely reprogrammed. The implications of epigenetically resilient regions of the genome to disease modeling were demonstrated by comparing hESCs and iPSCs as models for fragile X (Urbach et al., 2010). Fragile X is a common form of mental retardation characterized by a lack of expression of *FMR1*, a gene that is normally expressed in hESCs but prompted to silence during differentiation. Interestingly, the mutant FMR locus in iPSCs derived from fragile X patients is not epigenetically reset during the reprogramming process, an important difference between the hESC and iPSC models.

Cells in culture represent an artifact; they are not in the exact same environment as they would be *in vivo*. They are missing important signaling pathways, interaction with other cells, and the holistic environment of different tissues in a living organism. Moreover, our culture conditions for maintenance, propagation, and differentiation of iPSCs are not optimized, but were achieved based on previous data from mice. Thus, it is possible that important signaling information is missing or over-stimulated in the culture system, masking

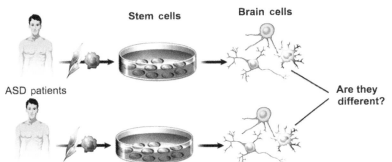

FIGURE 4.3.1 Modeling ASD with induced pluripotent stem cells. Peripheral cells, isolated from skin or dental pulp, can be reprogrammed to a pluripotent state and propagated in large amounts. These cells can be coaxed to differentiate into brain cells, including distinct neuronal subtypes for further phenotypic evaluation. If differences are observed between a cohort of ASD and control neurons, these alterations can be used as readouts in drug-screening platforms.

potential cellular phenotypes. Additional limits to the neural conversion of iPSCs are the lower efficiency and higher variability of neural differentiation in iPSCs compared to ESC lines (Hu et al., 2010), and existence of intra-individual variation within different clones from the same individual.

Another challenge in the 'disease-in-a-dish' field is the derivation of relevant neuronal subtypes. In theory, pluripotent stem cells can be differentiated into all neuronal types of the human brain (Muotri and Gage, 2006). Practically, there are only a few protocols to induce the iPSC differentiation into specific subtypes of neurons. Even there, the differentiation usually contains a heterogeneous population of cell types, such as astrocytes, oligodendrocytes, or even non-neuronal cell types, and the relevant neuronal subtypes need to be sorted out or visualized using specific reporter genes. The use of the synapsin promoter driving EGFP has been instrumental to visualize and sort neurons from the mixed population (Marchetto et al., 2010a). However, the synapsin promoter is not specific to any neuronal subtypes, and characterization of promoter-specific markers will be necessary to isolate these cells in the future. The different types of neurons can then be characterized by their morphology, gene expression, and electrical activity to demonstrate their specificity, maturity, and connectivity.

While for some neurological diseases it is clear what type of neurons are mostly affected, this is not the case for ASD. One way forward would be to use the iPSC system as a toolbox to help determine the impact of ASD risk in different neuronal types. It is the only model that allows progressive time-course analyses of the different neuronal types. It will be possible to investigate the precise neuronal types that are affected in ASD and elucidate the cellular and molecular defects that contribute to disease initiation and progression. As the protocols become more robust, one could systematically differentiate neurons from distinct brain regions to look for phenotypes. This strategy would provide insights on timing and neuronal-specific information about early stages of the disease process.

However, having the relevant neuronal type in culture does not guarantee that disease neurons will behave differently to controls. It is possible that non-cell autonomous effects, such as different cell types, three-dimensional scaffolding, or maturation timing may also contribute to neuronal phenotypes. In that sense, it is expected that neurodevelopmental phenotypes will be easier to spot than phenotypes in late-onset diseases. The latter may need some external stimuli, such as presence of stressors, to reveal the differences in patient-derived neurons.

Another important limitation is the use of appropriate controls. Intuitively, for well-characterized monogenetic diseases, the ideal controls are the ones that differ from the patient only by the genetic defect. Efforts in this direction can be achieved by manipulation of the iPSCs to introduce genetic mutations in control cell lines or to restore the mutation from a patient cell line (Liu et al., 2011; Soldner et al., 2011). Another strategy for generating 'isogenic' cell lines is to take advantage of X-inactivation in female cell lines. Due to the fast X-inactivation process during reprogramming, it is possible to generate iPSC cell clones carrying the mutant or the wild-type version of an X-linked affected gene. This strategy was used to model Rett syndrome, which affects female patients with mutations in the X-linked MECP2 gene (Cheung et al., 2012; Marchetto et al., 2010a). However, it is important to consider that even isogenic clones in culture will accumulate mutations in their genome over time, and thus there will never be an ideal control line. Although the implications of these alterations may be small, we should not underestimate the selection process going on in a dish. For non-monogenetic diseases, or when the mutations are not known, such as sporadic ASD, the challenge is even bigger. Variations between cell lines and even between iPSC clones from the same individual can influence the phenotypic readout. In such cases, a large cohort of well-characterized control cell lines is invaluable. Real phenotypes could be identified when the variation between controls and patients is significantly higher than the intrinsic variation inside each group. Unfortunately, the generation and characterization of individual iPSC clones is currently very expensive and time-consuming, restricting the number of cell lines that an individual can handle. A possible useful strategy for these types of diseases is the coordination of consortium initiatives, where multiple laboratories would contribute to the pool of different cell types and development of phenotypic assays. Consortium initiatives could also be useful for creating banks of genetically well-characterized controls that could be used to research the closest controls to pathological cases.

A final challenge for the iPSC model is the validation of phenotypes observed in human neurons to show that this model can recapitulate the disease in a dish. Comparison with postmortem brain tissues is perhaps the most obvious step towards validation, however, the lack of consistency does not mean that the phenotype is not valid. Important neuronal alterations during development may not be present in adult tissues due to brain compensation, for instance. Validation in animals is an attractive alternative and may reveal important conserved neural pathways between the two species. But again, a negative correlation with mouse models does not imply the phenotypes are not important for humans. Moreover, in the case of sporadic ASD, where animal models offer limited information about the human brain and there is not a large amount of data describing phenotypic variations in neuroanatomical circuits and molecular pathways, validation can be problematic.

MODELING MONOGENETIC AND SINGLE LOCUS ASD USING iPSCs

The use of monogenetic forms of ASD was wisely chosen as proof-of-principle that neurons derived from these patients can recapitulate important aspects of the disease *in vitro*. Studies of single gene mutations accelerated the discovery of causal mechanisms related to neuronal phenotypes. Monogenic disorder modeling gives the opportunity to perform gain- and loss-of-function experiments to confirm that the phenotypes observed are disease-specific as opposed to a general non-specific effect. These models can bring new insights to other forms of ASD. Moreover, by capturing the genetic heterogeneity of ASD in a pluripotent state, the iPSC model has the potential to determine whether patients carrying distinct mutations in disparate genes share common cellular and molecular neuronal phenotypes.

To date, two syndromic ASD were modeled using the iPSC strategy. We recently demonstrated the utility of iPSCs to investigate the functional consequences of mutations in the gene encoding the methyl CpG-binding protein-2 (MeCP2) on neurons from patients with Rett syndrome (RTT), a syndromic form of ASD (Marchetto et al., 2010a). Neurons derived from RTT-iPSCs carrying four different *MECP2* mutations showed several alterations compared to five healthy non-affected individuals, such as decreased soma size, altered dendritic spine density, and reduced excitatory synapses (Figure 4.3.2). Importantly, these phenotypes were validated using wild-type MeCP2 complementary DNA (cDNA) and specific short hairpin RNAs (shRNAs)

against *MECP2* in gain- and loss-of-function experiments. Some of these cellular defects were immediately validated by independent groups, revealing the robustness and reproducibility of the system (Ananiev et al., 2011; Cheung et al., 2012; Kim et al., 2011). We were able to rescue the defects in the number of glutamatergic synapses using two candidate drugs, insulin growth factor 1 (IGF1) and gentamicin. IGF1 is considered to be a candidate for pharmacological treatment of RTT and potentially other central nervous system disorders in ongoing clinical trials (Tropea et al., 2009). Gentamicin, a read-through drug, was also used to rescue neurons carrying a nonsense *MECP2* mutation, by elevating the amount of MeCP2 protein. These observations bring valued information for RTT and, potentially, other ASD patients, since they suggest that pre-symptomatic defects may represent novel biomarkers to be exploited as diagnostic tools. The data also suggest that early intervention may be beneficial.

Moreover, we took advantage of the RTT-iPSCs to demonstrate that neural progenitor cells carrying *MECP2* mutations have increased susceptibility for L1 retrotransposition. Long interspersed nuclear elements-1 (LINE-1 or L1s) are abundant retrotransposons that comprise approximately 20% of mammalian genomes (Gibbs et al., 2004; Lander et al., 2001; Waterston et al., 2002) and are highly active in the nervous system (Coufal et al., 2009; Muotri et al., 2005a). Our data demonstrate that L1 retrotransposition can be controlled in a tissue-specific manner and that disease-related genetic mutations can influence the frequency of neuronal L1 retrotransposition (Muotri et al., 2010). The work revealed an unexpected and novel phenomenon, adding a new layer of complexity to the understanding of genomic plasticity, which may have direct implications for ASD.

Timothy syndrome (TS) is caused by a point mutation in the *CACNA1C* gene, encoding the alpha1 subunit of Ca$_v$1.2 protein (Splawski et al., 2004). There are only a few dozen people in the world with TS. Patients

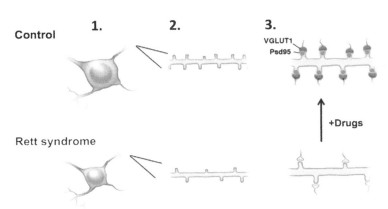

FIGURE 4.3.2   Examples of neuronal differences observed in Rett syndrome (RTT) neurons compared to controls. Neurons derived from RTT-iPSCs showed reduced soma size, low density of dendritic spines, and defects in glutamatergic synapses. Some of these defects were shown to be rescued with candidate drugs, as a proof-of-principle that human RTT neurons can be reverted and behave like neurons derived from non-affected control individuals. The red (VGLUT1) and the green (Psd95) puncta represent markers for glutamatergic connections.

suffering from this condition often display cardiac arrhythmia, hypoglycemia, and global developmental delay. Some individuals are also diagnosed with ASD (Splawski et al., 2004; 2006). To investigate this rare syndromic form of ASD, the Dolmetsch group derived iPSCs from two TS patients and four controls and then stimulated these cells to differentiate into precursor cells and neurons. The protocol used favored the differentiation into cortical neurons. TS-derived neurons showed abnormal calcium signaling leading to differences in gene expression. The data also suggest that TS-iPSCs produce fewer callosal projection neurons. Moreover, TS neurons produced more catecholamines when compared to neurons derived from healthy individuals (Pasca et al., 2011). Catecholamines, such as norepinephrene and dopamine, are important for sensory gating and social behavior, suggesting an important role in the pathophysiology of ASD. The excess of catecholamines could be rescued by treating TS neurons with roscovitine, a cyclin-dependent kinase inhibitor that blocks calcium influx across cell membranes. This experiment suggests a potential novel clinical intervention. Interestingly, while many of the differences between control and TS neurons could be recapitulated in a TS mouse model, the excess of catecholamines could not. One interpretation is that species-specific differences in gene regulation may affect the cellular phenotypes associated with TS patients. Alternatively, the differences that could not be recapitulated in mice may have a less important role in the disease. In the end, differences that provide a therapeutic lead can be transferred to clinical trials for future validation.

MODELING IDIOPATHIC ASD USING iPSCs

The examples of RTT and TS show that functional studies using iPSC-derived neuronal cultures of ASD patients can be useful for exploring the contribution of rare variants to ASD etiology. The notion that very rare mutations may point to key etiological pathways and mechanisms has been repeatedly demonstrated in a wide range of common human disorders, such as Alzheimer's disease (Scheuner et al., 1996) and hypertension (Ji et al., 2008).

Similarly, a rapidly increasing number of ASD loci regions in risk genes have recently been identified, and there is now considerable effort focused on moving from gene discovery to an understanding of the biological substrates influenced by these various mutations (Bozdagi et al., 2010; Gilman et al., 2011; Gutierrez et al., 2009; Levy et al., 2011; Sanders et al., 2011). While the allelic architecture of ASD is still being clarified, at present there is already definitive evidence for

a high degree of locus heterogeneity and a contribution by rare and *de novo* variants (El-Fishawy and State, 2010; Geschwind, 2011). However, estimating the penetrance for these low-frequency variants is challenging, particularly as many such mutations defy Mendelian expectations and carry only intermediate risks (Bucan et al., 2009; State and Levitt, 2011; Weiss et al., 2008). The sample sizes necessary to demonstrate these types of effects will be large. Moreover, the use of rodent models to evaluate complex human behaviors presents considerable obstacles (Silverman et al., 2010) and access to patients' brain tissue is typically unavailable, requiring the use of peripheral tissues (i.e., blood) for biological studies, with all the inherent limitations previously discussed. The lack of relevant human-derived cellular models to study ASD forms an important obstacle in the effort to link genetic alterations to molecular mechanisms and complex behavioral and cognitive phenotypes. Thus, the study of iPSCs offers an important alternative strategy to investigate the functional consequences of genetic alterations in human neurons *in vitro*. Creation of large numbers of iPSC lines from patients with idiopathic ASD could be a novel approach to identify common mechanisms and pathways within cases with different genetic backgrounds.

Merging new sequencing techniques with cellular reprogramming may allow us to characterize alterations in the genomes of thousands of ASD patients and to link specific genetic alterations to cellular and molecular phenotypes. At the moment, this would be cost-prohibitive, but it is expected that both iPSC and sequencing costs will drop exponentially in the near future. Nonetheless, methods for generating neurons on a large scale and automated phenotypic analyses will be essential for taking this idea forward. The stratification of subtypes of ASD will allow us to recognize molecular pathways that are altered in each individual.

USING HUMAN NEURONS AS A DRUG-SCREENING PLATFORM FOR NEW TREATMENTS FOR ASD

Contrary to cardiovascular diseases or cancer, in mental disorders it is not possible to compare a set of screened molecules to drugs that have previously demonstrated some benefit in humans. In cancer, for example, it is possible to isolate a biopsy of the tumor, and use it to test several drugs for efficiency and toxicity before applying these to the patient. In contrast, live human neurons are not available for drug-screening thus far. The lack of drugs in brain disease is a reflection of the missing human model. The studies performed in RTT and TS highlighted the potential of iPSC models in toxicology and drug-screening. Even better, the IGF1 overcorrection observed in some RTT neurons (Marchetto et al., 2010a) indicates that the iPSC technology can not only recapitulate some aspects of a genetic disease but also can be used to better design and anticipate results from translational medicine. This cellular model has the potential to lead to the discovery of new compounds to treat different forms of ASD.

Drug-screening platforms require 'screenable' robust phenotypes in target cell types, such as iPSC-derived neurons. The neuronal differentiation strategies reported to date are not capable of providing vast numbers of homogeneous subtypes of neurons in a reliable, reproducible, and cost-effective fashion. While it seems possible to develop scale-up methods for neuronal differentiation in the near future, cellular readouts are already coming from pioneering published work. Cellular morphology, such as soma size or dendritic spine density, can be measured using high-content imaging software. This may be the case for RTT neurons, where morphological aspects of iPSC-derived neurons could be reproduced by independent laboratories. Early biochemical and gene expression readouts could be an alternative. However, late readouts, such as electrophysiological recordings, may not be ideal, due to the time in culture to reach proper neuronal maturation. It is certainly possible to use stressors or other environmental agents to speed up neuronal maturation or enhance the differences between control and patient groups. However, the impact on ASD pathways of these agents is still unknown. An alternative solution may emerge from the direct conversion of neurons from peripheral cells, skipping the pluripotent state (Pang et al., 2011; Vierbuchen et al., 2010). This technology may be faster than neurons generated from iPSCs but is currently inefficient in humans, difficult to scale-up, and has the disadvantage that it does not mimic neuronal development (Vierbuchen and Wernig, 2011). Although it is expected that more robust protocols for human neuronal direct conversion will be reported in the near future, it remains to be seen how and whether the strategy would be suitable for mimicking aspects of neurodevelopmental diseases. It is possible that direct conversion would bypass the developmental period in which ASD phenotype can be observed. In addition, the use of direct conversion to produce suitable numbers of neurons for high-throughput screening is limited by the fact that cells produced using direct conversion do not self-renew. Large amounts of starting material (fibroblasts or other peripheral somatic cells) are therefore required to produce large amounts of neurons. Fibroblasts, for instance, have a finite capacity for replication and cannot be expended indefinitely.

Finally, readouts need to be suitable for the high-throughput instrumentation screening used in drug discovery. More scalable assays will allow the characterization of increased numbers of control and patient neurons. Finally, there are several chemical libraries that could be used in ASD neurons. It makes sense to use small molecules that cross the blood–brain barrier and have good penetration in the brain. Drug repositioning is a fantastic opportunity. Although this strategy may face some intellectual property challenges, repurposed drugs can bypass much of the early cost and time needed to bring a drug to market. Optimistically, the *in vitro* system using human neurons will accelerate the discovery of novel drugs for RTT and other ASD.

CONCLUSION AND PERSPECTIVES

The iPSC strategy is a novel and complementary approach to modeling ASD. This new model has the capacity to unify data generated from brain imaging, animal work, and genetics, generating downstream hypotheses that could be tested in well-controlled experiments with relevant cell types. Future work should take advantage of better-characterized ASD cohorts, with well-defined clinical endophenotypes, pharmacological history, and genetic predisposition. By generating hiPSC neurons from these ASD cohorts, one could test whether the clinical outcome is predictive of the magnitude of cellular phenotype, whether specific mutations correlate to gene expression differences, or whether clinical pharmacological response is predictable by human neuronal drug response. In the future, this strategy will give us diagnostic tools to group individual patients into specific classes of autism, and make predictions regarding whether certain drugs will be beneficial or not. Reproducible and robust ASD neuronal phenotypes can be achieved by intense collaborative consortia involving several independent laboratories, for instance, sharing the same patient cohorts.

ACKNOWLEDGMENTS

The work in the Muotri laboratory is supported by grants from the California Institute for Regenerative Medicine (CIRM) TR2-01814, the Emerald Foundation and the National Institutes of Health through the NIH Director's New Innovator Award Program, 1-DP2-OD006495-01.

References

Ananiev, G., Williams, E.C., Li, H., Chang, Q., 2011. Isogenic pairs of wild type and mutant induced pluripotent stem cell (iPSC) lines from Rett syndrome patients as in vitro disease model. PLoS One 6, e25255.

Baek, K.H., Zaslavsky, A., Lynch, R.C., Britt, C., Okada, Y., Siarey, R.J., et al., 2009. Down's syndrome suppression of tumor growth and the role of the calcineurin inhibitor DSCR1. Nature 459, 1126–1130.

Bozdagi, O., Sakurai, T., Papapetrou, D., Wang, X., Dickstein, D.L., Takahashi, N., et al., 2010. Haploinsufficiency of the autism-associated Shank3 gene leads to deficits in synaptic function, social interaction, and social communication. Molecular Autism 1, 15.

Bradley, C.K., Scott, H.A., Chami, O., Peura, T.T., Dumevska, B., Schmidt, U., et al., 2011. Derivation of Huntington's disease-affected human embryonic stem cell lines. Stem Cells and Development 20, 495–502.

Brennand, K.J., Simone, A., Jou, J., Gelboin-Burkhart, C., Tran, N., Sangar, S., et al., 2011. Modelling schizophrenia using human induced pluripotent stem cells. Nature 473, 221–225.

Bucan, M., Abrahams, B.S., Wang, K., Glessner, J.T., Herman, E.I., Sonnenblick, L.I., et al., 2009. Genome-wide analyses of exonic copy number variants in a family-based study point to novel autism susceptibility genes. PLoS Genetics 5, e1000536.

Cheung, A.Y., Horvath, L.M., Grafodatskaya, D., Pasceri, P., Weksberg, R., Hotta, A., et al., 2012. Isolation of MECP2-null Rett Syndrome patient hiPS cells and isogenic controls through X-chromosome inactivation. Human Molecular Genetics 20, 2103–2115.

Chin, M.H., Mason, M.J., Xie, W., Volinia, S., Singer, M., Peterson, C., et al., 2009. Induced pluripotent stem cells and embryonic stem cells are distinguished by gene expression signatures. Cell Stem Cell 5, 111–123.

Coufal, N.G., Garcia-Perez, J.L., Peng, G.E., Yeo, G.W., Mu, Y., Lovci, M.T., et al., 2009. L1 retrotransposition in human neural progenitor cells. Nature 460, 1127–1131.

Dragunow, M., 2008. The adult human brain in preclinical drug development. Nature Reviews Drug Discovery 7, 659–666.

Ebert, A.D., Yu, J., Rose Jr., F.F., Mattis, V.B., Lorson, C.L., Thomson, J.A., et al., 2009. Induced pluripotent stem cells from a spinal muscular atrophy patient. Nature 457, 277–280.

El-Fishawy, P., State, M.W., 2010. The genetics of autism: Key issues, recent findings, and clinical implications. Psychiatric Clinics of North America 33, 83–105.

Geschwind, D.H., 2011. Genetics of autism spectrum disorders. Trends in Cognitive Sciences 15, 409–416.

Gibbs, R.A., Weinstock, G.M., Metzker, M.L., Muzny, D.M., Sodergren, E.J., Scherer, S., et al., 2004. Genome sequence of the Brown Norway rat yields insights into mammalian evolution. Nature 428, 493–521.

Gilman, S.R., Iossifov, I., Levy, D., Ronemus, M., Wigler, M., Vitkup, D., 2011. Rare de novo variants associated with autism implicate a large functional network of genes involved in formation and function of synapses. Neuron 70, 898–907.

Giudice, A., Trounson, A., 2008. Genetic modification of human embryonic stem cells for derivation of target cells. Cell Stem Cell 2, 422–433.

Grskovic, M., Javaherian, A., Strulovici, B., Daley, G.Q., 2011. Induced pluripotent stem cells – opportunities for disease modelling and drug discovery. Nature Reviews Drug Discovery 10, 915–929.

Gutierrez, R.C., Hung, J., Zhang, Y., Kertesz, A.C., Espina, F.J., Colicos, M.A., 2009. Altered synchrony and connectivity in neuronal networks expressing an autism-related mutation of neuroligin 3. Neuroscience 162, 208–221.

Ho, R., Chronis, C., Plath, K., 2011. Mechanistic insights into reprogramming to induced pluripotency. Journal of Cellular Physiology 226, 868–878.

Hu, B.Y., Weick, J.P., Yu, J., Ma, L.X., Zhang, X.Q., Thomson, J.A., et al., 2010. Neural differentiation of human induced pluripotent stem cells follows developmental principles but with variable potency. Proceedings of the National Academy of Sciences of the United States of America 107, 4335–4340.

Ji, W., Foo, J.N., O'Roak, B.J., Zhao, H., Larson, M.G., Simon, D.B., et al., 2008. Rare independent mutations in renal salt handling genes contribute to blood pressure variation. Nature Genetics 40, 592–599.

Kim, K.Y., Hysolli, E., Park, I.H., 2011. Neuronal maturation defect in induced pluripotent stem cells from patients with Rett syndrome. Proceedings of the National Academy of Sciences of the United States of America 108, 14,169–14,174.

Lander, E.S., Linton, L.M., Birren, B., Nusbaum, C., Zody, M.C., Baldwin, J., et al., 2001. Initial sequencing and analysis of the human genome. Nature 409, 860–921.

Laurent, L.C., Ulitsky, I., Slavin, I., Tran, H., Schork, A., Morey, R., et al., 2011. Dynamic changes in the copy number of pluripotency and cell proliferation genes in human ESCs and iPSCs during reprogramming and time in culture. Cell Stem Cell 8, 106–118.

Levy, D., Ronemus, M., Yamrom, B., Lee, Y.H., Leotta, A., Kendall, J., et al., 2011. Rare de novo and transmitted copy-number variation in autistic spectrum disorders. Neuron 70, 886–897.

Lister, R., Pelizzola, M., Kida, Y.S., Hawkins, R.D., Nery, J.R., Hon, G., et al., 2011. Hotspots of aberrant epigenomic reprogramming in human induced pluripotent stem cells. Nature 471, 68–73.

Liu, G.H., Suzuki, K., Qu, J., Sancho-Martinez, I., Yi, F., Li, M., et al., 2011. Targeted gene correction of laminopathy-associated LMNA mutations in patient-specific iPSCs. Cell Stem Cell 8, 688–694.

Marchetto, M.C., Brennand, K.J., Boyer, L.F., Gage, F.H., 2011. Induced pluripotent stem cells (iPSCs) and neurological disease modeling: Progress and promises. Human Molecular Genetics 20, R109–R115.

Marchetto, M.C., Carromeu, C., Acab, A., Yu, D., Yeo, G.W., Mu, Y., et al., 2010. A model for neural development and treatment of Rett syndrome using human induced pluripotent stem cells. Cell 143, 527–539.

Marchetto, M.C., Winner, B., Gage, F.H., 2010. Pluripotent stem cells in neurodegenerative and neurodevelopmental diseases. Human Molecular Genetics 19, R71–R76.

Marchetto, M.C., Yeo, G.W., Kainohana, O., Marsala, M., Gage, F.H., Muotri, A.R., 2009. Transcriptional signature and memory retention of human-induced pluripotent stem cells. PLoS ONE 4, e7076.

Mateizel, I., De Temmerman, N., Ullmann, U., Cauffman, G., Sermon, K., Van de Velde, H., et al., 2006. Derivation of human embryonic stem cell lines from embryos obtained after IVF and after PGD for monogenic disorders. Human Reproduction 21, 503–511.

Mayshar, Y., Ben-David, U., Lavon, N., Biancotti, J.C., Yakir, B., Clark, A.T., et al., 2010. Identification and classification of chromosomal aberrations in human induced pluripotent stem cells. Cell Stem Cell 7, 521–531.

Muotri, A.R., 2009. Modeling epilepsy with pluripotent human cells. Epilepsy Behavior 14, 81–85.

Muotri, A.R., Chu, V.T., Marchetto, M.C., Deng, W., Moran, J.V., Gage, F.H., 2005. Somatic mosaicism in neuronal precursor cells mediated by L1 retrotransposition. Nature 435, 903–910.

Muotri, A.R., Gage, F.H., 2006. Generation of neuronal variability and complexity. Nature 441, 1087–1093.

Muotri, A.R., Nakashima, K., Toni, N., Sandler, V.M., Gage, F.H., 2005. Development of functional human embryonic stem cell-derived neurons in mouse brain. Proceedings of the National Academy of Sciences of the United States of America 102, 18,644–18,648.

Muotri, A.R., Marchetto, M.C., Coufal, N.G., Oefner, R., Yeo, G., Nakashima, K., Gage, F.H., 2010. L1 retrotransposition in neurons is modulated by MeCP2. Nature 468, 443–446.

Pang, Z.P., Yang, N., Vierbuchen, T., Ostermeier, A., Fuentes, D.R., Yang, T.Q., et al., 2011. Induction of human neuronal cells by defined transcription factors. Nature 476, 220–223.

Pasca, S.P., Portmann, T., Voineagu, I., Yazawa, M., Shcheglovitov, A., Pasca, A.M., et al., 2011. Using iPSC-derived neurons to uncover cellular phenotypes associated with Timothy syndrome. Nature Medicine 17, 1657–1662.

Pickering, S.J., Minger, S.L., Patel, M., Taylor, H., Black, C., Burns, C.J., et al., 2005. Generation of a human embryonic stem cell line encoding the cystic fibrosis mutation deltaF508, using preimplantation genetic diagnosis. Reproductive Biomedicine Online 10, 390–397.

Robinton, D.A., Daley, G.Q., 2012. The promise of induced pluripotent stem cells in research and therapy. Nature 481, 295–305.

Sanders, S.J., Ercan-Sencicek, A.G., Hus, V., Luo, R., Murtha, M.T., Moreno-De-Luca, D., et al., 2011. Multiple recurrent de novo CNVs, including duplications of the 7q11.23 Williams syndrome region, are strongly associated with autism. Neuron 70, 863–885.

Saporta, M.A., Grskovic, M., Dimos, J.T., 2011. Induced pluripotent stem cells in the study of neurological diseases. Stem Cell Research and Therapy 2, 37.

Scheuner, D., Eckman, C., Jensen, M., Song, X., Citron, M., Suzuki, N., et al., 1996. Secreted amyloid beta-protein similar to that in the senile plaques of alzheimer's disease is increased in vivo by the presenilin 1 and 2 and APP mutations linked to familial Alzheimer's disease. Nature Medicine 2, 864–870.

Silverman, J.L., Yang, M., Lord, C., Crawley, J.N., 2010. Behavioral phenotyping assays for mouse models of autism. Nature Reviews Neuroscience 11, 490–502.

Soldner, F., Laganiere, J., Cheng, A.W., Hockemeyer, D., Gao, Q., Alagappan, R., et al., 2011. Generation of isogenic pluripotent stem cells differing exclusively at two early onset Parkinson point mutations. Cell 146, 318–331.

Splawski, I., Timothy, K.W., Sharpe, L.M., Decher, N., Kumar, P., Bloise, R., et al., 2004. Ca(V)1.2 calcium channel dysfunction causes a multisystem disorder including arrhythmia and autism. Cell 119, 19–31.

Splawski, I., Yoo, D.S., Stotz, S.C., Cherry, A., Clapham, D.E., Keating, M.T., 2006. CACNA1H mutations in autism spectrum disorders. Journal of Biological Chemistry 281, 22,085–22,091.

State, M.W., Levitt, P., 2011. The conundrums of understanding genetic risks for autism spectrum disorders. Nature Neuroscience.

Takahashi, K., Yamanaka, S., 2006. Induction of pluripotent stem cells from mouse embryonic and adult fibroblast cultures by defined factors. Cell 126, 663–676.

Takahashi, K., Tanabe, K., Ohnuki, M., Narita, M., Ichisaka, T., Tomoda, K., et al., 2007. Induction of pluripotent stem cells from adult human fibroblasts by defined factors. Cell 131, 861–872.

Thomson, J.A., Itskovitz-Eldor, J., Shapiro, S.S., Waknitz, M.A., Swiergiel, J.J., Marshall, V.S., et al., 1998. Embryonic stem cell lines derived from human blastocysts. Science 282, 1145–1147.

Tropea, D., Giacometti, E., Wilson, N.R., Beard, C., McCurry, C., Fu, D.D., et al., 2009. Partial reversal of Rett syndrome-like symptoms in MeCP2 mutant mice. Proceedings of the National Academy of Sciences of the United States of America 106, 2029–2034.

Urbach, A., Bar-Nur, O., Daley, G.Q., Benvenisty, N., 2010. Differential modeling of fragile X syndrome by human embryonic stem cells and induced pluripotent stem cells. Cell Stem Cell 6, 407–411.

Urbach, A., Schuldiner, M., Benvenisty, N., 2004. Modeling for Lesch-Nyhan disease by gene targeting in human embryonic stem cells. Stem Cells 22, 635–641.

Verlinsky, Y., Strelchenko, N., Kukharenko, V., Rechitsky, S., Verlinsky, O., Galat, V., et al., 2005. Human embryonic stem cell lines with genetic disorders. Reproductive Biomedicine Online 10, 105–110.

Vierbuchen, T., Wernig, M., 2011. Direct lineage conversions: Unnatural but useful? Nature Biotechnology 29, 892–907.

Vierbuchen, T., Ostermeier, A., Pang, Z.P., Kokubu, Y., Sudhof, T.C., Wernig, M., 2010 Direct conversion of fibroblasts to functional neurons by defined factors. Nature.

Waterston, R.H., Lindblad-Toh, K., Birney, E., Rogers, J., Abril, J.F., Agarwal, P., et al., 2002. Initial sequencing and comparative analysis of the mouse genome. Nature 420, 520–562.

Weiss, L.A., Shen, Y., Korn, J.M., Arking, D.E., Miller, D.T., Fossdal, R., et al., 2008. Association between microdeletion and microduplication at 16p11.2 and autism. New England Journal of Medicine 358, 667–675.

Yu, J., Vodyanik, M.A., Smuga-Otto, K., Antosiewicz-Bourget, J., Frane, J.L., Tian, S., et al., 2007. Induced pluripotent stem cell lines derived from human somatic cells. Science 318, 1917–1920.

4.4

A 15q11–q13 Duplication Mouse Model of Autism Spectrum Disorders

Toru Takumi*, †, Keita Fukumoto*, Jun Nomura*

*Graduate School of Biomedical Sciences, Hiroshima University, Minami, Hiroshima, Japan †Japan Science and Technology Agency (JST), CREST, Chiyoda, Tokyo, Japan

AUTISM

Autism is a developmental brain disorder that is part of a spectrum of related conditions termed autism spectrum disorders (ASD), which includes pervasive development disorder – not otherwise specified and Asperger syndrome (Levitt and Campbell, 2009; see Section 1 of this volume). The prevalence of ASD is estimated at more than 1 in every 150 individuals (see Chapter 1.1). The impact of ASD in modern society is becoming greater, especially in developed countries with lower birth rates, where how to manage this problem is a serious social issue. However, the causes of ASD and its underlying pathophysiology remain to be clarified, awaiting further research from diverse fields. Among psychiatric disorders, autism is considered a target disorder to approach from a neurobiological perspective, in part because genetic studies show that the concordance rate of autism for identical twins is over 90%; higher than that for other psychiatric

diseases, including schizophrenia and mood disorders (Abrahams and Geschwind, 2008).

Most instances of ASD have an unidentified cause, however, 10–20% of cases are known to be due to either genetic disorders (such as fragile X syndrome, tuberous sclerosis, Rett syndrome, etc.); genome abnormalities including copy number variations (CNVs), such as at 15q11–q13 and 16q11.2; or rare mutations in genes such as *NLGN3/4*, *NRXN1*, and *SHANK2/3* (Abrahams and Geschwind, 2008; Berkel et al., 2010; Cook and Scherer, 2008; Kumar et al., 2008; Marshall et al., 2008; Pinto et al., 2010; Toro et al., 2010; Vorstman et al., 2006; Weiss et al., 2008; and see Chapters 2.1 and 2.2). Recent genetic screening using cutting-edge technologies has revealed more examples of CNVs in ASD than previously appreciated (Cook and Scherer, 2008). As the technology for CGH (comparative genomic hybridization) arrays and next-generation sequencing continues to progress, and as these technologies become more widely used, both in research and clinically, the number of individuals with identifiable CNVs and affected genes is likely to increase.

HUMAN CHROMOSOME 15q11–q13

Chromosomal abnormalities have been implicated as a cause of autism even before the era of current high-throughput genome technology. Among chromosomal abnormalities, variation at 15q11–q13 is most notable in terms of recurrent findings in a specific chromosome region (Takumi, 2011; Vorstman et al., 2006; and see Chapter 3.4) (Figure 4.4.1). This region is also known to be imprinted (Chamberlain and Lalande, 2010; Nicholls and Knepper, 2001), giving rise to paternally, maternally and biallelically expressed genes.

The paternally expressed genes in 15q11–q13 include *MKRN3, MAGEL2, NDN* (encoding the protein Necdin), *C15orf2, SNRPN-SNURF,* and clusters of small nucleolar RNAs (snoRNAs). *Magel2* is involved in hypothalamic functions and *Magel2*-deficient mice showed abnormal circadian rhythm, body weight, and hormonal secretion, including abnormal secretion of testosterone (Bischof et al., 2007; Kozlov et al., 2007; Mercer and Wevrick, 2009). *NDN* was first identified as a gene related to neural differentiation (Maruyama et al., 1991) and Necdin knockout mice have been generated in multiple laboratories, however, the animals display differing phenotypes (Gerard et al., 1999; Kuwako et al., 2005; Muscatelli et al., 2000; Tsai et al., 1999). Thus, the role of Necdin in Prader–Willi syndrome remains unclear. Snrpn is the small nuclear ribonucleoprotein N and the *SNRPN* promoter is located in a maternally methylated CpG island that lies within an imprinting center (IC).

The non-coding RNA region of 15q11–q13 includes HBII-52 and HBII-85. Knockout mice lacking MBII-85 (the mouse homolog of HBII-85) showed growth retardation, increased anxiety, and hyperphagia (Ding

et al., 2008; Skryabin et al., 2007). Recently HBII-85 was reported to be a definitive etiological factor in Prader–Willi syndrome (Sahoo et al., 2008). Knockout mice lacking MBII-52, the mouse homolog of HBII-52, displayed an increase in RNA editing of the serotonin 2c receptor (5-HT2cR) and less locomotor activity (Doe et al., 2009).

Maternally expressed genes in the region include *UBE3A* and *ATP10A*. Ube3a is an E3 ubiquitin ligase and mutations in this gene can cause Angelman syndrome (Kishino et al., 1997; Matsuura et al., 1997; and see Chapter 2.1). *Ube3a* knockout mice showed impaired motor function, inducible seizures, and learning deficits (Jiang et al., 1998). Ube3a is well characterized in neurons and is involved in synaptic plasticity (Greer et al., 2010; Margolis et al., 2010; Sato and Stryker, 2010; Yashiro et al., 2009). Recent reports also highlight the involvement of Ube3a in ASD (Glessner et al., 2009). *ATP10A* remains under-studied and its imprinting status remains unclear (Kayashima et al., 2003).

There is a cluster of γ-aminobutyric acid A (GABA$_A$) receptor subunits ((*GABRB3, GABRA5, GABRG3*), *OCA2,* and *HERC2* in the region with biallelic expression. The GABA$_A$ receptor is one of the major neurotransmitter receptors and a notable target in this region, since imbalance between excitatory and inhibitory neurons during development is a pathophysiological hypothesis of causation of developmental brain disorders, including ASD. There is also some evidence of association, although the results are inconsistent (Rubenstein and Merzenich, 2003; and see Chapters 2.3 and 3.9). The GABAβ3 subunit has been extensively investigated and its disruption in mice led to epileptic seizures, deficits in learning and memory, and poor motor skills (DeLorey et al., 1998; Homanics et al., 1997). GABAα5 knockout mice displayed enhanced spatial learning, decreased amplitudes of IPSC (inhibitory postsynaptic currents), and enhanced amplitudes of EPSP (excitatory postsynaptic potentials) in a paired-pulse facilitation paradigm (Collinson et al., 2002; Crestani et al., 2002). Herc2

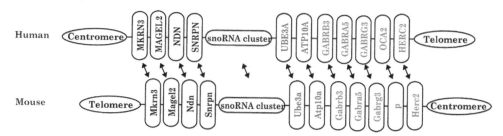

FIGURE 4.4.1　Comparison of genes between the human 15q11–q13 region and the corresponding region of mouse chromosome 7. Blue = paternally expressed gene; red = maternally expressed gene; green = biallelically expressed gene.

contains a COOH-terminal HECT domain and functions as an assembly factor for a complex with E3 ubiquitin ligase (Bekker-Jensen et al., 2010). *Herc2* mutant mice showed defects in growth (Lehman et al., 1998).

In humans, deletion of the paternal 15q11–q13 region causes Prader–Willi syndrome, in which the patient shows hypotonia, obesity, cognitive deficit, and behavioral problems including obsessive-compulsive disorder (Cassidy and Driscoll, 2009; Chamberlain and Lalande, 2010). Deletion of the maternal allele causes Angelman syndrome, which includes motor dysfunction, frequent seizures, learning disabilities, absent speech, and a characteristic happy demeanor (Van Buggenhout and Fryns, 2009). Some cases of Prader–Willi and Angelman syndromes display ASD-like phenotypes.

Duplication of the 15q11–q13 region is considered to be the most frequent cytogenetic abnormality in ASD (Vorstman et al., 2006; and see Chapter 2.1). Autism with 15q duplication syndrome was first reported as partial trisomy of chromosome 15 (Gillberg et al., 1991). After the work of Cook et al. (1997), it has become common to think that maternally duplicated events contribute to ASD while paternally duplicated events do not. However, there are examples of ASD with paternal duplication (Bolton et al., 2004; Mao et al., 2000; Mohandas et al., 1999; Roberts et al., 2002; Veltman et al., 2005). A recent report suggests that ASD cases with maternal duplication are not as common in some studies as in others (Depienne et al., 2009).

MOUSE CHROMOSOME ENGINEERING

Recent embryonic stem (ES) cell technology has provided many mouse models for disease. Notwithstanding the obvious limitations in trying to understand mind or mental functions from mouse models and mouse behavior, many knockout or transgenic mice have been generated and the sum of these analyses has shed light on the molecular pathophysiology of autism (see other chapters in Section 4). Such findings reinforce the importance of establishing animal models of human diseases for gaining an understanding of their pathophysiology.

The generation of mice with a large duplication is technically more challenging than generating conventional knockout mice and requires the chromosome-engineering method developed by Bradley and van der Weyden (2005). This technique is based on the Cre-loxP system (Figure 4.4.2) and, unlike conditional knockout techniques, the target region is extremely large and usually spans Mb-sized regions. Compared to generating deletions by chromosome engineering, creating duplications is more difficult. Two targeting vectors containing the loxP sequence, corresponding to each end of the duplicated region, are required. After double targeting these sites in mouse ES cells, clones in which two loxP sequences are inserted in *trans* orientation are used. In ES cells with a *trans* orientation of the loxP sequence, Cre recombinase can generate an interstitial duplication, although its efficiency is very low even compared with conventional targeting. Although

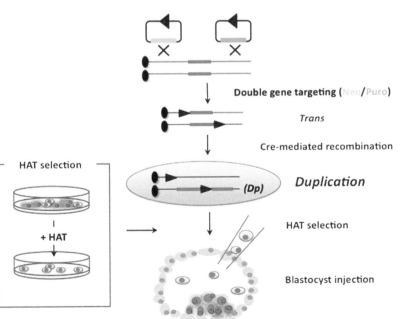

FIGURE 4.4.2 Summary of the chromosome-engineering technique. HAT = hypoxanthine-aminopterin-thymidine.

theoretically possible due to the development of the chromosome-engineering technique, no successful examples of such a long distance interstitial duplication had been performed until very recently, when Nakatani et al. (2009) succeeded in generating a model for human chromosome 15q duplication. The duplication was confirmed, not only in ES cells by Southern blotting, but also in mice by fluorescence *in situ* hybridization (FISH) and CGH-array. Moreover, Southern blot analysis using methylation sensitive and insensitive restriction enzymes and a probe near the IC indicated that allele-specific methylation is conserved in mice with the duplication. As the region is an imprinted one, the authors followed up on two types of duplication, one, in the patDp/+ mice, in which the duplicated region was derived from the paternal allele, and the other (matDp/+ mice), in which the duplication was derived from the maternal allele. The gene expression profiles were consistent with the imprinting status (Figure 4.4.3).

A MOUSE MODEL FOR 15q DUPLICATION

Both patDp/+ and matDp/ mice breed normally and are fertile (Nakatani et al., 2009). The patDp/+ male mice begin to show an increase in body weight after 15 weeks, and the body weight of patDp/+ mice is significantly greater than that of wild-type (WT) mice after 20 weeks. The fact that both decreased (Prader–Willi syndrome) and increased (15q duplication) gene expressions of the PWA region lead to obesity is contradictory but intriguing. The PWA region appears to be involved in some aspects of metabolism, and deviation in levels of key gene products, whether by increase or decrease, may cause abnormalities of metabolism.

		Biallelic	Paternal	Maternal
WT	(PA)–(BmP) — (MA)–(BMp) —	2 fold	1 fold	1 fold
patDp/+	(PA)–(BmP)–(BmP)— (MA)–(BMp) —	3 fold	2 fold	1 fold
matDp/+	(PA)–(BmP) — (MA)–(BMp)–(BMp)—	3 fold	1 fold	2 fold

FIGURE 4.4.3 Predicted expression level of genes in mice with the duplication allele. PA = paternal allele; MA = maternal allele; B = biallelically expressed gene; M = maternally expressed gene; P = paternally expressed gene; WT = wild type.

Histological analyses at both macroscopic and microscopic levels by hematoxylin-eosin or Bodian staining detected no significant difference between mice with the duplication and WT mice (Nakatani et al., 2009). As described above (and in Section 2), recent studies reveal that synaptic cell adhesion molecules and their associated proteins are impacted by rare mutations in autism (Betancur et al., 2009; Bourgeron, 2009; Toro et al., 2010). It will be quite interesting to determine whether spine or synaptic abnormalities are observed in the 15q duplication mice.

ASD-LIKE BEHAVIOR OF 15q DUPLICATION MICE

Behavioral analyses are essential for animal models of autism, because ASD are behavioral abnormalities and diagnosis is made on the basis of the presence of three major phenotypes: impairments in social interaction, impaired social communication, and restricted interests and behavior, or resistance to change. Crawley and others have defined mouse behavioral tests which correspond to human autistic phenotypes (Moy and Nadler, 2008; Silverman et al., 2010).

Systematic behavioral analyses were performed for 15q duplication mice (Nakatani et al., 2009). First, in the three-chamber test – a test of social interaction – wild-type mice spend more time near a novel mouse than near an empty cage, whereas no difference in time spent between the novel mouse and the empty cage is observed in patDp/+ mice. In contrast, when comparing time spent with an inanimate object and an empty cage, both patDp/+ and WT mice spent more time near the novel object than empty cage, indicating that patDp/+ mice were able to recognize novelty. Interestingly, WT mice spent more time around a novel mouse compared to a novel inanimate object, whereas in patDp/+ mice, no difference was seen in the time spent near the novel mouse and near the inanimate object. Beyond these differences, there were no significant differences between matDp/+ and WT mice in the three-chamber test. These results indicate that patDp/+ mice exhibit impaired social interaction.

Second, patDp/+ mice displayed abnormal ultrasonic vocalizations (USVs), elicited when pups are separated from their dams. In WT pups, the number of USVs peaked around postnatal day 5 (P5) and then gradually decreased until P14, when their eyes are open. In contrast, the number of USVs was still high at P7 and even at P14 in patDp/+ mice, suggesting that the developmental course of USVs in patDp/+ mice was delayed compared with WT mice. These results demonstrated that patDp/+ mice may be developmentally abnormal in comparison with WT mice, although the larger number of USVs in patDp/+ pups may reflect higher anxiety and fear in response to isolation stress. No difference in USVs between matDp/+ and WT mice was observed.

Third, the behavioral inflexibility seen in ASD patients was examined with reversal tasks. In the Barnes maze, wild-type, patDp/+ and matDp/+ mice exhibited intact spatial learning and memory. In a reversal test, in which a target, once learned, was moved to a different position, WT and matDp/+ were more likely than patDp/+ mice to learn the new target position, with patDp/+ mice going more often to the original position, indicating that patDp/+ mice displayed resistance to change, or perseveration. patDp/+ mice also showed a similar behavior in the Morris water maze. These results suggest that patDp/+ mice exhibit behavioral inflexibility.

In addition to these phenotypes, patDp/+ mice displayed novelty-induced anxiety and decreased exploratory activity (Tamada et al., 2010). In several tests using food deprivation, such as the novelty suppressed feeding test, radial maze, and Y-maze, patDp/+ mice displayed atypical behavior. Even after food deprivation, patDp/+ mice do not rush to feed and take more time to proceed to feeding than WT mice.

ABNORMAL SEROTONIN IN 15q DUPLICATION MICE

The primary benefit of the model mouse system is that it allows us to study abnormalities at the molecular and cellular levels. Because major behavioral phenotypes appear not in matDp/+ but in patDp/+ mice (Nakatani et al., 2009), maternally imprinted loci could be candidates to be responsible for abnormal behaviors. Among them is MBII-52, mouse brain specific snoRNA 52, found in a large cluster of non-coding RNAs, and an interesting candidate for the following reasons. First, *Mbii-52* is a paternally expressed gene. Second, HBII-52, the human homolog of MBII-52, is reported to be involved in the post-transcriptional modification of the serotonin 2c receptor (5-HT2cR) (Kishore and Stamm, 2006). Third, serotonin (5-HT) is well known to be frequently dysregulated in ASD (Whitaker-Azmitia, 2005). Fourth, 5-HT2cR is a G-protein-coupled receptor that undergoes A to I RNA editing, resulting in an amino acid substitution in the second loop of cytoplasmic domains (Seeburg, 2002), which may affect G-protein coupling efficiency. MBII-52 RNA displayed a roughly two-fold increase in expression in the patDp/+ mouse brain, compared with matDp/+ and WT mice (Nakatani et al., 2009). Pyrosequencing revealed that the RNA editing ratio in potential editing sites of 5-HT2cR in patDp/+ mice was higher than that in matDp/+ or WT mice, suggesting that increased snoRNA in the patDp/+ brains may affect

the RNA editing of 5-HT2cR. Furthermore, a specific agonist for 5-HT2cR induced higher intracellular Ca^{2+} concentration in primary cultures of patDp/+ neurons compared with matDp/+ and WT neurons, indicating that serotonergic signals in patDp/+ neurons are different from matDp/+ and WT neurons. This result suggests that alteration in RNA editing of 5-HT2cR may affect serotonergic signals in neurons, and this alteration may contribute to abnormal behavior in patDp/+ mice.

Neurochemical analyses have revealed abnormal levels of 5-HT and of its metabolites in adult cerebellum and midbrain (see Figure 4.4.4). Interestingly, it was also shown that 5-HT in patDp/+ mice was lower in all brain regions tested during postnatal weeks 1–3 (Tamada et al., 2010). These results suggest that abnormal 5-HT levels during these developmental stages affect the development of neurons and neural circuits, and this may contribute to the abnormal behavior seen in patDp/+ mice.

A MOUSE MODEL OF AUTISM

The model mouse for 15q duplication described here fulfills not only face validity, i.e., showing similar phenotypes to those of human patients, but also construct validity, in that it possesses the same chromosomal abnormality as human patients. Thus, the model can be considered to be an important mouse model for autism (Takumi, 2010). In terms of other recent models with construct and face validity, Tabuchi et al. (2007) reported a knock-in mouse for the *NLGN3* R541C mutation. However, the same knock-in mouse independently generated from Heintz's group displayed no significant or only mild social abnormality (Chadman et al., 2008). Further model mice with rare mutations of other molecules will be expected to recapitulate ASD phenotypes.

At present it is not known which gene or regions within 15q11–q13 are critical for ASD phenotypes. The model mouse for 15q duplication represents one means of addressing this question. A series of bacterial artificial chromosome (BAC), yeast artificial chromosome (YAC), or other engineered mice with longer insertions that cover the duplicated region will provide useful material for further investigation. Alternatively, genetic rescue experiments crossed with a series of knockout or deficient mice will be useful to help identify genes in the interval which contribute to ASD.

EPIGENETICS OF 15q DUPLICATION

It is noteworthy that patDp/+, but not matDp/+, mice display abnormal social behaviors, while maternally duplicated cases in humans are more likely to

FIGURE 4.4.4   Levels of serotonin in patDp/+ and wild-type (WT) mice. Cb = cerebellum; MB = midbrain; OB = olfactory bulb; PFC = prefrontal cortex; MO = medulla oblongata; Ctx = cortex; Hip = hippocampus; Hy = hypothalamus; 5-HT = 5-hydroxytryptamine; 5-HIAA = 5-hydroxyindolacetic acid; DA = dopamine; DOPAC = 3,4-dihydroxyphenylacetic acid; HVA = homovanillic acid.

Adult

	Cb	MB	OB	PFC	Pons & MO
5-HT	—	↓	↓	—	—
5-HIAA	↓	↓	↓	—	—
5-HIAA/5-HT	—	—	—	—	—
DA	—	—	—	—	—
DOPAC	—	—	—	—	—
NE	—	—	—	—	—

Infant stage

	Cb	Ctx	Hip	Hy	MB	Pons & MO
5-HT	↓	↓	↓	↓	↓	↓
5-HIAA	—	↓	↓	—	—	—
5-HIAA/5-HT	↑	—	—	—	—	↑
DA	—	—	—	—	—	↑
DOPAC	↑	—	—	—	↑	↑
HVA	↑	—	—	↓	↑	↑

show severe ASD phenotypes; although paternal cases with autism have been reported (Bolton et al., 2004; Mao et al., 2000; Mohandas et al., 1999; Roberts et al., 2002; Veltman et al., 2005). Recent advances in genetic analysis such as CGH-array and its clinical application are expected to result in an increase in numbers of identified clinical cases (Depienne et al., 2009). Although allele-specific methylation seems to be conserved at least around the IC in mice with a duplication, we cannot exclude the possibility that the imprinting status in other regions is different between human and mouse. Recent systematic analyses of the mouse epigenome revealed that *Ube3a* and a GABA receptor subunit are differentially imprinted in different brain areas (Gregg et al., 2010). In addition, epigenetic changes other than those involving DNA methylation and imprinting in mice may be different from those in humans. Further detailed epigenetic analyses will provide an insight into the mechanisms underlying the effects in patDp/+ mice.

ACKNOWLEDGMENT

The authors acknowledge all members of the Takumi laboratory, especially Jin Nakatani for his persistent efforts that enabled us to provide a useful mouse model. The authors also thank all collaborators including Allan Bradley, Tsuyoshi Miyakawa, and Hisashi Ohta.

References

Abrahams, B.S., Geschwind, D.H., 2008. Advances in autism genetics: On the threshold of a new neurobiology. Nature Reviews Genetics 9, 341–355.

Bekker-Jensen, S., Rendtlew Danielsen, J., Fugger, K., Gromova, I., Nerstedt, A., Lukas, C., et al., 2010. HERC2 coordinates ubiquitin-dependent assembly of DNA repair factors on damaged chromosomes. Nature Cell Biology 12, 80–86.

Berkel, S., Marshall, C.R., Weiss, B., Howe, J., Roeth, R., Moog, U., et al., 2010. Mutations in the *SHANK2* synaptic scaffolding gene in autism spectrum disorder and mental retardation. Nature Genetics 42, 489–491.

Betancur, C., Sakurai, T., Buxbaum, J.D., 2009. The emerging role of synaptic cell-adhesion pathways in the pathogenesis of autism spectrum disorders. Trends in Neurosciences 32, 402–412.

Bischof, J.M., Stewart, C.L., Wevrick, R., 2007. Inactivation of the mouse *Magel2* gene results in growth abnormalities similar to Prader–Willi syndrome. Human Molecular Genetics 16, 2713–2719.

Bolton, P.F., Veltman, M.W., Weisblatt, E., Holmes, J.R., Thomas, N.S., Youings, S.A., et al., 2004. Chromosome 15q11–13 abnormalities and other medical conditions in individuals with autism spectrum disorders. Psychiatric Genetics 14, 131–137.

Bourgeron, T., 2009. A synaptic trek to autism. Current Opinion in Neurobiology 19, 231–234.

Bradley, A., van der Weyden, L., 2005. Mouse: Chromosome engineering for modeling human disease. Annuau Review of Genomics and Human Genetics 7, 247–276.

Cassidy, S.B., Driscoll, D.J., 2009. Prader–Willi syndrome. European Journal of Human Genetics 17, 3–13.

Chadman, K.K., Gong, S., Scattoni, M.L., Boltuck, S.E., Gandhy, S.U., Heintz, N., et al., 2008. Minimal aberrant behavioral phenotypes of neuroligin-3 R451C knock-in mice. Autism Research 1, 147–158.

Chamberlain, S.J., Lalande, M., 2010. Neurodevelopmental disorders involving genomic imprinting at human chromosome 15q11–q13. Neurobiology of Disease 39, 13–20.

Collinson, N., Kuenzi, F.M., Jarolimek, W., Maubach, K.A., Cothliff, R., Sur, C., et al., 2002. Enhanced learning and memory and altered GABAergic synaptic transmission in mice lacking the alpha 5 subunit of the GABAA receptor. Journal of Neuroscience 22, 5572–5580.

Cook Jr., E.H., Lindgren, V., Leventhal, B.L., Courchesne, R., Lincoln, A., Shulman, C., et al., 1997. Autism or atypical autism in maternally but not paternally derived proximal 15q duplication. American Journal of Human Genetics 60, 928–934.

Cook Jr., E.H., Scherer, S.W., 2008. Copy-number variations associated with neuropsychiatric conditions. Nature 455, 919–923.

Crestani, F., Keist, R., Fritschy, J.M., Benke, D., Vogt, K., Prut, L., et al., 2002. Trace fear conditioning involves hippocampal alpha5 GABA(A) receptors. Proceedings of the National Academy of Sciences of the United States of America 99, 8980–8985.

DeLorey, T.M., Handforth, A., Anagnostaras, S.G., Homanics, G.E., Minassian, B.A., Asatourian, A., et al., 1998. Mice lacking the beta3 subunit of the GABAA receptor have the epilepsy phenotype and many of the behavioral characteristics of Angelman syndrome. Journal of Neuroscience 18, 8505–8514.

Depienne, C., Moreno-De-Luca, D., Heron, D., Bouteiller, D., Gennetier, A., Delorme, R., et al., 2009. Screening for genomic rearrangements and methylation abnormalities of the 15q11–q13 region in autism spectrum disorders. Biological Psychiatry 66, 349–359.

Ding, F., Li, H.H., Zhang, S., Solomon, N.M., Camper, S.A., Cohen, P., et al., 2008. SnoRNA Snord116 (Pwcr1/MBII-85) deletion causes growth deficiency and hyperphagia in mice. PLoS ONE 3, e1709.

Doe, C.M., Relkovic, D., Garfield, A.S., Dalley, J.W., Theobald, D.E., Humby, T., et al., 2009. Loss of the imprinted snoRNA mbii-52 leads to increased 5htr2c pre-RNA editing and altered 5HT2CR-mediated behaviour. Human Molecular Genetics 18, 2140–2148.

Gerard, M., Hernandez, L., Wevrick, R., Stewart, C.L., 1999. Disruption of the mouse necdin gene results in early post-natal lethality. Nature Genetics 23, 199–202.

Gillberg, C., Steffenburg, S., Wahlstrom, J., Gillberg, I.C., Sjostedt, A., Martinsson, T., et al., 1991. Autism associated with marker chromosome. Journal of the American Academy of Child and Adolescent Psychiatry 30, 489–494.

Glessner, J.T., Wang, K., Cai, G., Korvatska, O., Kim, C.E., Wood, S., et al., 2009. Autism genome-wide copy number variation reveals ubiquitin and neuronal genes. Nature 459, 569–573.

Greer, P.L., Hanayama, R., Bloodgood, B.L., Mardinly, A.R., Lipton, D.M., Flavell, S.W., et al., 2010. The Angelman syndrome protein Ube3A regulates synapse development by ubiquitinating arc. Cell 140, 704–716.

Gregg, C., Zhang, J., Weissbourd, B., Luo, S., Schroth, G.P., Haig, D., et al., 2010. High-resolution analysis of parent-of-origin allelic expression in the mouse brain. Science 329, 643–648.

Homanics, G.E., DeLorey, T.M., Firestone, L.L., Quinlan, J.J., Handforth, A., Harrison, N.L., et al., 1997. Mice devoid of gamma-aminobutyrate type A receptor beta3 subunit have epilepsy, cleft palate, and hypersensitive behavior. Proceedings of the National Academy of Sciences of the United States of America 94, 4143–4148.

Jiang, Y.H., Armstrong, D., Albrecht, U., Atkins, C.M., Noebels, J.L., Eichele, G., et al., 1998. Mutation of the Angelman ubiquitin ligase in mice causes increased cytoplasmic p53 and deficits of contextual learning and long-term potentiation. Neuron 21, 799–811.

Kayashima, T., Ohta, T., Niikawa, N., Kishino, T., 2003. On the conflicting reports of imprinting status of mouse ATP10a in the adult brain: Strain-background-dependent imprinting? Journal of Human Genetics 48, 492–493 (author reply 494).

Kishino, T., Lalande, M., Wagstaff, J., 1997. UBE3A/E6-AP mutations cause Angelman syndrome. Nature Genetics 15, 70–73.

Kishore, S., Stamm, S., 2006. The snoRNA HBII-52 regulates alternative splicing of the serotonin receptor 2C. Science 311, 230–232.

Kozlov, S.V., Bogenpohl, J.W., Howell, M.P., Wevrick, R., Panda, S., Hogenesch, J.B., et al., 2007. The imprinted gene Magel2 regulates normal circadian output. Nature Genetics 39, 1266–1272.

Kumar, R.A., KaraMohamed, S., Sudi, J., Conrad, D.F., Brune, C., Badner, J.A., et al., 2008. Recurrent 16p11.2 microdeletions in autism. Human Molecular Genetics 17, 628–638.

Kuwako, K., Hosokawa, A., Nishimura, I., Uetsuki, T., Yamada, M., Nada, S., et al., 2005. Disruption of the paternal necdin gene diminishes TrkA signaling for sensory neuron survival. Journal of Neuroscience 25, 7090–7099.

Lehman, A.L., Nakatsu, Y., Ching, A., Bronson, R.T., Oakey, R.J., Keiper-Hrynko, N., et al., 1998. A very large protein with diverse functional motifs is deficient in rjs (runty, jerky, sterile) mice. Proceedings of the National Academy of Sciences of the United States of America 95, 9436–9441.

Levitt, P., Campbell, D.B., 2009. The genetic and neurobiologic compass points toward common signaling dysfunctions in autism spectrum disorders. Journal of Clinical Investigation 119, 747–754.

Mao, R., Jalal, S.M., Snow, K., Michels, V.V., Szabo, S.M., Babovic-Vuksanovic, D., 2000. Characteristics of two cases with dup(15)(q11.2–q12): one of maternal and one of paternal origin. Genetics in Medicine 2, 131–135.

Margolis, S.S., Salogiannis, J., Lipton, D.M., Mandel-Brehm, C., Wills, Z.P., Mardinly, A.R., et al., 2010. EphB-mediated degradation of the RhoA GEF Ephexin5 relieves a developmental brake on excitatory synapse formation. Cell 143, 442–455.

Marshall, C.R., Noor, A., Vincent, J.B., Lionel, A.C., Feuk, L., Skaug, J., et al., 2008. Structural variation of chromosomes in autism spectrum disorder. American Journal of Medical Genetics 82, 477–488.

Maruyama, K., Usami, M., Aizawa, T., Yoshikawa, K., 1991. A novel brain-specific mRNA encoding nuclear protein (necdin) expressed in neurally differentiated embryonal carcinoma cells. Biochemical and Biophysical Research Communications 178, 291–296.

Matsuura, T., Sutcliffe, J.S., Fang, P., Galjaard, R.J., Jiang, Y.H., Benton, C.S., et al., 1997. De novo truncating mutations in E6-AP ubiquitin-protein ligase gene (UBE3A) in Angelman syndrome. Nature Genetics 15, 74–77.

Mercer, R.E., Wevrick, R., 2009. Loss of Magel2, a candidate gene for features of Prader–Willi syndrome, impairs reproductive function in mice. PLoS ONE 4, e4291.

Mohandas, T.K., Park, J.P., Spellman, R.A., Filiano, J.J., Mamourian, A.C., Hawk, A.B., et al., 1999. Paternally derived de novo interstitial duplication of proximal 15q in a patient with developmental delay. American Journal of Medical Genetics 82, 294–300.

Moy, S.S., Nadler, J.J., 2008. Advances in behavioral genetics: Mouse models of autism. Molecular Psychiatry 13, 4–26.

Muscatelli, F., Abrous, D.N., Massacrier, A., Boccaccio, I., Le Moal, M., Cau, P., et al., 2000. Disruption of the mouse Necdin gene results in hypothalamic and behavioral alterations reminiscent of the human Prader–Willi syndrome. Human Molecular Genetics 9, 3101–3110.

Nakatani, J., Tamada, K., Hatanaka, F., Ise, S., Ohta, H., Inoue, K., et al., 2009. Abnormal behavior in a chromosome-engineered mouse model for human 15q11–13 duplication seen in autism. Cell 137, 1235–1246.

Nicholls, R.D., Knepper, J.L., 2001. Genome organization, function, and imprinting in Prader–Willi and Angelman syndromes. Annual Review of Genomics and Human Genetics 2, 153–175.

Pinto, D., Pagnamenta, A.T., Klei, L., Anney, R., Merico, D., Regan, R., et al., 2010. Functional impact of global rare copy number variation in autism spectrum disorders. Nature 466, 368–372.

Roberts, S.E., Dennis, N.R., Browne, C.E., Willatt, L., Woods, G., Cross, I., et al., 2002. Characterisation of interstitial duplications and triplications of chromosome 15q11–q13. Human Genetics 110, 227–234.

Rubenstein, J.L., Merzenich, M.M., 2003. Model of autism: Increased ratio of excitation/inhibition in key neural systems. Genes, Brain and Behavior 2, 255–267.

Sahoo, T., del Gaudio, D., German, J.R., Shinawi, M., Peters, S.U., Person, R.E., et al., 2008. Prader–Willi phenotype caused by paternal deficiency for the HBII-85 C/D box small nucleolar RNA cluster. Nature Genetics 40, 719–721.

Sato, M., Stryker, M.P., 2010. Genomic imprinting of experience-dependent cortical plasticity by the ubiquitin ligase gene Ube3a.

Proceedings of the National Academy of Sciences of the United States of America 107, 5611–5616.

Seeburg, P.H., 2002. A-to-I editing: New and old sites, functions and speculations. Neuron 35, 17–20.

Silverman, J.L., Yang, M., Lord, C., Crawley, J.N., 2010. Behavioural phenotyping assays for mouse models of autism. Nature Reviews Neuroscience 11, 490–502.

Skryabin, B.V., Gubar, L.V., Seeger, B., Pfeiffer, J., Handel, S., Robeck, T., et al., 2007. Deletion of the MBII-85 snoRNA gene cluster in mice results in postnatal growth retardation. PLoS Genetics 3, e235.

Tabuchi, K., Blundell, J., Etherton, M.R., Hammer, R.E., Liu, X., Powell, C.M., et al., 2007. A neuroligin-3 mutation implicated in autism increases inhibitory synaptic transmission in mice. Science 318, 71–76.

Takumi, T., 2010. A humanoid mouse model of autism. Brain Development 32, 753–758.

Takumi, T., 2011. The neurobiology of mouse models syntenic to human chromosome 15q. Journal of Neurodevelopmental Disorders 3, 270–281.

Tamada, K., Tomonaga, S., Hatanaka, F., Nakai, N., Takao, K., Miyakawa, T., et al., 2010. Decreased exploratory activity in a mouse model of 15q duplication syndrome: Implications for disturbance of serotonin signaling. PLoS ONE 5, e15126.

Toro, R., Konyukh, M., Delorme, R., Leblond, C., Chaste, P., Fauchereau, F., et al., 2010. Key role for gene dosage and synaptic homeostasis in autism spectrum disorders. Trends in Genetics 26, 363–372.

Tsai, T.F., Armstrong, D., Beaudet, A.L., 1999. Necdin-deficient mice do not show lethality or the obesity and infertility of Prader–Willi syndrome. Nature Genetics 22, 15–16.

Van Buggenhout, G., Fryns, J.P., 2009. Angelman syndrome (AS, MIM 105830). European Journal of Human Genetics 17, 1367–1373.

Veltman, M.W., Thompson, R.J., Craig, E.E., Dennis, N.R., Roberts, S.E., Moore, V., et al., 2005. A paternally inherited duplication in the Prader–Willi/Angelman syndrome critical region: A case and family study. Journal of Autism and Developmental Disorders 35, 117–127.

Vorstman, J.A., Staal, W.G., van Daalen, E., van Engeland, H., Hochstenbach, P.F., Franke, L., 2006. Identification of novel autism candidate regions through analysis of reported cytogenetic abnormalities associated with autism. Molecular Psychiatry 11, 18–28.

Weiss, L.A., Shen, Y., Korn, J.M., Arking, D.E., Miller, D.T., Fossdal, R., et al., 2008. Association between microdeletion and microduplication at 16p11.2 and autism. New England Journal of Medicine 358, 667–675.

Whitaker-Azmitia, P.M., 2005. Behavioral and cellular consequences of increasing serotonergic activity during brain development: A role in autism? International Journal of Developmental Neuroscience 23, 75–83.

Yashiro, K., Riday, T.T., Condon, K.H., Roberts, A.C., Bernardo, D.R., Prakash, R., et al., 2009. Ube3a is required for experience-dependent maturation of the neocortex. Nature Neuroscience 12, 777–783.

4.5

Fragile X Syndrome and Autism Spectrum Disorders

W. Ted Brown*, Ira L. Cohen[†]

*Department of Human Genetics and [†]New York State, Institute for Basic Research in Developmental Disabilities, Staten Island, NY, USA

BACKGROUND ON FRAGILE X SYNDROME

Fragile X syndrome (FXS) is the most common monogenic form of intellectual disability (ID). The name fragile X comes from the presence of a gap or break near the end of the X chromosome at band q27.3, which appears when cells from an affected individual are cultured in a low folate medium. FXS is usually caused by expansion of an unstable CGG repeat region located within the *FMR1* (Fragile X mental retardation 1) gene, which then becomes inactivated, preventing gene expression. This X-linked form of ID was first recognized as a common and distinct entity around 1980. Current estimates are that approximately 1 in 4,000 males and 1 in 8,000 females in the general population have ID as a result of the syndrome, and that approximately 1 in 300 females and 1 in 700 males are carriers. However, various studies have given somewhat differing estimates and there are likely to be founder effects in some ethnic populations (Coffee et al., 2009; Crawford et al., 2001; Hagerman 2008; Hantash et al., 2011).

Compared to individuals diagnosed with many genetic or chromosomal syndromes, affected fragile X males usually are often typical in physical appearance. This helps to explain why they are frequently undiagnosed and why the syndrome was only recently recognized as a distinct entity. As adults, they usually have enlarged testicular volume, known as macroorchidism. This is typically in the range of 30 to 60 ml, as compared to the normal adult male mean volume of 17 ml. Other recognizable physical features that are variably present include large or prominent ears, highly arched palate, narrow mid-facial diameter, narrow inter-eye distance, long face, large head circumference, prominent forehead, facial asymmetry, prominent thumbs, hyperextensible joints, and mitralvalve prolapse.

The Neuroscience of Autism Spectrum Disorders.
http://dx.doi.org/10.1016/B978-0-12-391924-3.00030-2

Approximately 95% of adult fragile X males have an IQ below 70. Approximately 70% have an IQ in the moderate to severe range, between 20 and 50, while about 10% have an IQ below 20, and 20% have an IQ above 50. There appears to be a decline in measured IQ among young males as they grow from prepubertal to pubertal ages (Bennetto and Pennington, 2002). This appears to be consistent with the findings that young boys with FXS have often been considered to be only mildly impaired or learning disabled, while adults with the syndrome are usually moderately to severely impaired. The reason for this decline in measured IQ may be a relative inability of young affected males to continue to acquire more complex cognitive abilities with maturity. Both IQ and adaptive skills tend to be less severely affected in mosaics (Cohen et al., 1996), see below.

Common neurological features in fragile X males include a static central nervous system encephalopathy without focal lateralizing signs, and impairment of fine motor coordination. Approximately 15% have a history of seizures (Berry-Kravis et al., 2010). These may be transient, but occasionally subjects have persistent seizures that are usually well controlled with anticonvulsant medication. Neuropathological studies have shown immaturity and dysgenesis of dendritic spines (Hinton et al., 1991; Irwin et al., 2001). Volumetric magnetic resonance imaging (MRI) studies have indicated an enlarged caudate nucleus, a decreased amygdala size, and a decreased ratio of posterior to anterior cerebellar vermis and increased volume of fourth and posterior ventricles, similar to findings reported for a subgroup of males with autism spectrum disorders (ASD) (Lightbody and Reiss, 2009).

CLINICAL ASSOCIATION WITH AUTISM/ASD

ASD are disorders of development with both genetic and environmental factors playing a role (see Section 2). They ares phenotypically quite heterogeneous with respect to such factors as presence of regression, presence vs. absence of seizures, syndromic vs. non-syndromic features, degree of intellectual impairment, and severity subtype (autistic disorder, pervasive developmental disability – not otherwise specified (PDD-NOS), Asperger disorder, Rett's disorder, childhood disintegrative disorder – we use the terms autism or ASD here to include all subtypes). First described in 1943 by Kanner, autistic disorder was initially found to be rare, occurring in about 3 to 4 out of every 10,000 persons in the population, but more recent studies have seen a > 10-fold increase in prevalence (Nygren et al., 2011). This is related in part to changes in how

ASD is diagnosed (King and Bearman, 2009), demographics (King and Bearman, 2011; Schieve et al., 2011), increased survival rates of preterm infants (Karmel et al., 2010; Pinto-Martin et al., 2011), and other factors (see Chapter 1.1).

Etiologically, Kanner (1943) speculated that autism was present at birth. Others were certain it was due to deficient mothering. Subsequent discoveries that ASD co-occurs with known syndromes such as phenylketonuria (Friedman, 1969) and, more recently, many other syndromes (see Chapter 2.1) showed that this disorder may have an organic basis, leading to the notion that it is etiologically as well as phenotypically heterogeneous, consisting of separate syndromes (Coleman, 1976), also referred to as the 'autisms' (Coleman and Gilberg, 2012; discussed in detail in Chapter 2.1). Others speculate that the heterogeneity is at a lower level, e.g., with the triad of impairments that define it (in socialization, communication, and imagination) being linked to different genetic and environmental mechanisms (Happe and Ronald, 2008; Robinson et al., 2012). As research continues to identify new mechanisms for ASD, those cases defined as 'idiopathic' represent a smaller and smaller portion of the pie (Shen et al., 2010).

Perhaps most striking aspect of ASD is the sex ratio difference, with males making up about 80% of cases. It is in this light that the association of ASD with FXS stimulated such interest when it was initially described; although it should be noted that ASD can occur in females with FXS (Cohen et al., 1989). In 1982, we and others reported an apparent association between autism and FXS (Brown et al., 1982a, b; Meryash et al., 1982). These reports were quite exciting at the time, as they provided the first hard evidence that a subgroup of persons with ASD, disorders that predominantly affect males, may have a defect in the X chromosome. Subsequent reports at the time replicated these initial observations (Blomquist et al., 1985; Brown et al., 1986; Gillberg, 1983; Levitas et al., 1983; Partington, 1984) using existing diagnostic assessment tools. Newer studies have yielded similar findings using state-of-the-art observational (Autism Diagnostic Observation Schedule-Generic, or ADOS-G) (Lord et al., 1999) and interview (Autism Diagnostic Interview-Revised, or ADI-R) (Le Couteur et al., 1989) assessment tools for autism.

For example, based on ADI-R, ADOS-G, and the American Psychiatric Association's Diagnostic and Statistical Manual IV, text revision (DSM-IV-TR) criteria, approximately 25–30% of males with FXS were found to meet the full criteria for autism, and another 25–30% had a milder autism spectrum disorder or PDD-NOS (Harris et al., 2008). Conversely, the prevalence of FXS in autism varies from 0 to 16% depending on the population tested (see Chapter 2.1). Some of this variance may be related to the fact that ASD is a 'moving target' (Hall et al., 2010) with changes in the DSMs that have taken place over time as well as changes in our assessment tools. FXS is thus widely considered to be the single most common biomedical condition specifically associated with ASD.

DIFFERENCES BETWEEN FXS AUTISM AND NON-FXS AUTISM

As noted, ASD is phenotypically heterogeneous. Unlike FXS, it is a disorder defined on the basis of overt behavior and not on etiology. The association of the two disorders, however, presents a unique opportunity to understand some of the behavioral heterogeneity that one sees in ASD. It is important to reiterate that prior to the identification of the genetic basis of FXS by Lubs (Lubs, 1969) and to its subsequent link to ASD in the early 1980s, many of the people with ASD now known to have FXS would be considered to have idiopathic autism. The discovery of the ASD–FXS link helped to narrow the phenotypic range that we see.

Indeed, many of the characteristics described in FXS first suggested a link to ASD. These included hyperactivity with a short attention span; stereotypic movements and unusual hand mannerisms such as hand-flapping and hand-biting, which often leads to callus formation at the site of biting; speech delay and a relative lack of expressive language ability; and repetitive speech patterns including stereotypical vocalizations, jargon, dysrhythmia, perseveration, echolalia, conditionalized statements, inappropriate tangential comments, and talking to self. Coupled with this, it is often noted that many FXS males are quite social and have an outgoing personality, but they generally have poor eye contact, are hypersensitive to sensory stimuli, and are tactilely defensive, which may interfere with social interactions and development (Hagerman 2002; Tsiouris and Brown, 2004).

This paradox led us to investigate the similarities and differences in males with ASD who do or do not have FXS (Cohen, 1992; 1995; Cohen et al., 1988; 1989; 1991c). These investigations indicated that:

1. Males with FXS and ASD had more adaptive skills impairments than males with FXS alone, with this effect being most evident in those older than 5 years of age. These problems persisted over time (Cohen, 1995).
2. Males with FXS and ASD exhibited more aggressive and verbal repetitive behaviors than males with idiopathic ASD, but were otherwise similar in terms of social communication skills and non-verbal repetitive behaviors (Cohen, 1995).

3. The most significant difference between the idiopathic ASD and FXS ASD groups was in their social avoidance behaviors.

Compared with idiopathic ASD and males with Down syndrome, those with FXS were much more likely to avoid social interaction with their parents and strangers (Cohen et al., 1988). They were also much more likely to specifically avoid eye contact (depending on age and language skills) as opposed to looking at others who were not looking at them (Cohen et al., 1989; 1991c). In general, older and more verbal males with FXS were more likely to specifically avoid eye contact. The children with idiopathic ASD had no such specific aversion to eye contact and appeared more oblivious to social conventions that require eye contact when interacting with others. This latter observation was interesting in light of an early model of ASD (Hutt and Ounsted, 1966) that invoked gaze aversion as pathognomonic of the syndrome. Our data suggested that the model may be correct, but only for the FXS subtype (Cohen et al., 1991c). Several more recent studies have replicated many of these observations (Arron et al., 2011; Bailey et al., 2001; Dissanayake et al., 2009; Lewis et al., 2006) and have also indicated that those affected with both FXS and ASD are at greater risk of other medical complications than those with FXS alone (Garcia-Nonell et al., 2008). On the other hand, it has been argued that cognitive impairment, as assessed by a full-scale IQ, may solely account for the comorbidity between FXS and ASD (Clifford et al., 2007).

The results of our studies on ASD and social avoidance in FXS led to two hypothetical models as to what was the nature of this association. These are shown in Figure 4.5.1 (modified from Figure 3 in Cohen et al., 1991a). Model 1 hypothesizes that, in FXS, the two behavioral phenotypes are independent phenomena, while model 2

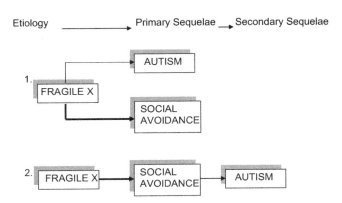

FIGURE 4.5.1 Two possible pathogenetic sequences relating FXS to social avoidance and to autism. The thicker arrow indicates a stronger relation between FXS and social avoidance. *Modified with permission from Cohen et al. (1991a).*

hypothesizes that ASD is secondary to elevated social avoidance in FXS. In this 1991 article and in a subsequent paper (Cohen, 1996), it was speculated that model 2 was more likely to be the correct one. Recently, Kaufmann and his group (Budimirovic et al., 2006) have reported data supporting model 2 as a predictor of ASD diagnosis in FXS, modifying it by taking into account the magnitude of deficits in social skills (the first criterion for an ASD diagnosis in the DSMs).

We suspected that the basis for this social avoidance behavior in FXS was related to a more primary problem with arousal regulation (Cohen, 1996) which, in turn, was related to problems with development of emotion-controlling structures in the brain, such as the amygdala (Cohen, 1996) as well as with neurotransmitters such as -aminobutyric acid (GABA) (Cohen et al., 1991a). It is therefore of interest that autonomic regulation has been found to be altered, such as increased heart rate, in at least two studies of males with FXS (Hall et al., 2009; Heilman et al 2011) and several studies have demonstrated anatomical differences in the amygdala in those with the full and pre-mutation (Gothelf et al., 2008; Hazlett et al., 2009; Hessl et al., 2007; 2011) as well as problems with GABA function (Fatemi et al 2011; Paluszkiewicz et al., 2011).

The behaviors we and others have described in those with both FXS and ASD not only help to allocate some of the heterogeneity seen in ASD but also have implications for treatment, as others have noted (Hall et al., 2010). For example, if eye contact is poor and/or aggression occurs as a result of arousal regulation problems secondary to social demands (a 'fight or flight' reaction) (Cohen, 1996), then a desensitization model may be the first choice to establish rapport and build social skills (perhaps coupled with monitoring of autonomic activity) (Cohen, 1996). Pharmacologically, there may also be a benefit in the use of drugs that suppress autonomic arousal, such as beta blockers (Cohen et al., 1991b), in combination with desensitization and environmental modification.

POTENTIAL GENE MODIFIERS OF THE FXS BEHAVIORAL PHENOTYPE

As noted above, self-injurious behaviors are common in full-mutation FXS, along with stereotyped behaviors and aggression, and there exists a wide range in IQ, as with idiopathic autism. The mechanisms responsible for this wide disparity in phenotype remain to be clearly elucidated. Although FXS is a single-gene disorder, other genes that impact on arousal regulation and central nervous system development may help to explain some of this variation. For example, we have reported

that a common functional polymorphism in the X-linked gene that codes for monoamine oxidase A (MAOA; Xp11.23~11.4) affects the severity of idiopathic ASD in young males (mean age 4.3 years) (Cohen et al., 2003a). Those males with the 'low-activity' allele exhibited more severe stereotypies, lower IQs, and worse social communication skills than those with the 'high-activity' form of the allele. Hessl et al. (2008), however, found no such effect on stereotyped behaviors in older full-mutation FXS males (mean age 15.6 years), but they did note that those with the high-activity allele were more likely to be receiving medications affecting the serotonin system (the primary substrate for MAOA is serotonin).

The differences between the two studies may relate to age, to differences in assessment tools, or to etiology, but another factor that may play a role is the maternal genotype. Using the PDD Behavior Inventory (PDDBI), an informant checklist developed by our group that is age-standardized on an ASD sample and covers both maladaptive and adaptive behaviors (Cohen, 2003; Cohen et al., 2003b; Cohen & Sudhalter, 2005), we found that the behavioral profile of idiopathic ASD differed depending on whether or not the mother was hetero- or homozygous for the high-activity allele. In a sample of 119 males (mean age 6.9 years), those who carried the low-activity allele were all severely affected with high levels of stereotypies and poor social communication skills irrespective of the mother's genotype. However, boys who received the high-activity allele from homozygous mothers presented with severe problems with ritualistic behaviors, arousal regulation, fears, and aggression, while maintaining relatively good language (resembling high-functioning ASD males with comorbid behavior problems). Conversely, boys who received the high-activity allele from heterozygous mothers presented with relatively few behavior problems, along with relatively intact language (resembling mildly affected PDD-NOS cases). It would be interesting to see if such a maternal effect explains some of the Hessl et al. (2008) findings. These authors did find, however, that polymorphism in another gene that affects serotonin, the serotonin transporter, modified the severity of aggressive and stereotyped behaviors, with those homozygous for the L genotype more severely affected.

Some males with FXS have been found to have a Prader–Willi phenotype (PWP), with obesity and hyperphagia. An analysis of 13 such subjects revealed they had a high incidence of delayed puberty, a small penis or testicles, infant hypotonia, and ASD. Further, analysis of the levels of an *FMR1*-interacting protein (CYFIP1) showed that mRNA levels for CYFIP1 were significantly reduced in FXS patients with the PWP as compared to those without the PWP (Nowicki et al., 2007).

FEMALE AND CARRIER PHENOTYPES

Female carriers of a premutation (see gene definitions below) are usually cognitively normal and unaffected. However, remitting recurrent depressive episodes and anxiety disorder have been described among some female carriers (Roberts et al., 2009). Approximately 16% of carrier females experience premature ovarian failure before age 40, compared to about 1% in the general population (Allingham-Hawkins et al., 1999).

Among females who have a full mutation, approximately 50% have a full-scale IQ score below 70. A characteristic profile of cognitive deficits may be present with relatively low Wechsler IQ performance scores, decreased subtest scores on arithmetic, digit span, block design, and object assembly. They may have increased verbal performance scores and do very well academically. Subtle defects in emotional development may exist, based on mild neurocognitive functioning deficits. Shy and socially withdrawn behavior is common. Other, variable, manifestations include socially inappropriate comments, inappropriate affect, poor modulation of verbal tone, tangential speech, and odd communication patterns (Hagerman, 2002). ASD has been reported in females with the full mutation (Bolton et al., 1989; Cohen et al., 1989; Edwards et al., 1988). Clifford et al. (2007) studied 33 males and 31 females with the full mutation, finding 67% of males and 23% of females met relaxed criteria for ASD; while using more restricted ADOS plus ADI-R criteria, 27% of males and 13% of females had ASD.

About 1 in 700 males in the general population inherit the fragile X mutation in a non-expressed or premutation form and are considered to be normal carriers. They are non-penetrant for the mutation and do not express the fragile site. They transmit the premutation only to their daughters, who are also generally non-expressing and carriers of the premutation, but who then can have affected sons. However, ASD has also been reportedly seen in males and females with the premutation (Chonchaiya et al., 2011; Clifford et al., 2007; Farzin et al., 2006; Hagerman et al., 2011).

It has been found that some 20–35% of males with the premutation over the age of 50 develop a multisystem progressive neurological disorder featuring intention tremor and cerebellar ataxia. This new fragile X tremor/ataxia syndrome (FXTAS) is progressive, with a variety of developing symptoms that include short-term memory loss, executive function deficits, cognitive decline, parkinsonism, peripheral neuropathy, lower limb proximal muscle weakness, and autonomic dysfunction. Symmetrical regions of increased T2 signal intensity on MRI in the middle cerebellar peduncles is thought to be a highly sensitive indicator of this syndrome (Jacquemont et al., 2003).

THE MOLECULAR NATURE OF THE FRAGILE X MUTATION

The molecular mutation underlying the fragile X syndrome is usually an expanded string of CGG triplet repeats near the 5' end of the *FMR1* gene, within a transcribed but untranslated promoter region. The CGG repeat region of the gene is variable in length and undergoes tremendous length amplification in affected individuals. Expansion of the CGG repeat in the 5'-untranslated region of *FMR1* results in methylation of the upstream CpG island, lack of gene expression, and the fragile X phenotype. The length of the repeat region is polymorphic in typically developing individuals, with lengths ranging of approximately 5–54 CGGs. The most frequent Caucasian repeat number is 30, followed by 29, 20, 23, and 31. Approximately 5% of normal alleles have 40 repeats or greater (Brown et al., 1996). Interspersed AGGs occur within the normal CGG repeat region that may stabilize the sequence and prevent slippage during DNA replication. Carrier females and transmitting males have an enlargement of the region to a range of approximately 56 to 200 repeats, designated as a premutation. Offspring of carrier females, but not of transmitting males, can have enlargements of the repeat to values ranging from 200 to over 2,000 repeats, referred to as the full mutation. Affected individuals have such a full mutation (Nolin et al., 2003).

A minority of affected individuals have a mosaic pattern, with some proportion of cells showing less than 200 repeats and partially active gene expression. Affected full-mutation males have fathered normal daughters who carry a premutation-sized allele. Analysis of their sperm samples reveals only premutation-sized alleles, suggesting the amplification process occurs post-zygotically (Reyniers et al., 1991). The risk of amplification to the full mutation rises with increasing size of the premutation in the carrier mother (Nolin et al., 2003). As the premutation is transmitted through subsequent generations within families, it demonstrates 'anticipation,' i.e., greater numbers of affected individuals are observed in later generations than in earlier ones.

Molecular diagnostic testing, including prenatal diagnosis, is conducted using two methods. The first method is direct genomic Southern blot analysis, which uses a probe that flanks the CGG repeat region. One such probe, StB12.3, uses a double digestion with two restriction enzymes. Digestion with the first enzyme (EcoRI) produces a 5.2 kb band on a Southern blot. The second, methylation-sensitive, enzyme (EagI) cuts unmethylated DNA at the CpG island, producing a 2.8 kb band, but leaves methylated DNA uncut. Thus, a normal female DNA sample will have both a 2.8 kb band, reflecting the active unmethylated X chromosome, and a 5.2 kb band, reflecting the inactive, methylated, X chromosome. Premutation alleles generally produce bands in the range of 2.9 to 3.2 kb for the active X, such as are present in transmitting males, and 5.3 to 5.7 kb for the inactive X. Normal carrier females generally have two doublets on such DNA analysis. Affected males generally have bands or smears in the 5.8 to 9 kb range.

The second molecular method for detecting the fragile X mutation employs the polymerase chain reaction (PCR). PCR analysis for fragile X mutations is rapid and uses small amounts of starting DNA for analysis. However, because the region has a high CG content, special methods are needed for successful amplification of full mutations (Brown et al., 1993). Some of the larger alleles from both males and affected females may fail to amplify successfully. Hence there is a need to have both methods available for routine diagnostic and prenatal testing purposes. Newer DNA methods are in development to both increase the information provided and reduce the costs of testing (Chen et al., 2010; 2011; Filipovic-Sadic et al., 2010; Godler et al., 2010; Lyon et al., 2010).

While the repeat amplification is far and away the most common cause of the syndrome, a small number of FXS patients have been identified that have either a deletion of the gene region or a point mutation within the gene. This shows that it is the absence of *FMR1* gene expression that causes the syndrome. If one of these rare deletion-type patients is suspected, more detailed molecular investigations are needed for diagnosis (Collins et al., 2010).

Because FXS accounts for approximately 1 to 2% of ID and ASD overall, children with ID or ASD of unexplained etiology should be evaluated for the syndrome. Since reliable prenatal diagnosis by molecular testing is now available, screening of pregnant women for their carrier status is appropriate, particularly in the setting of a family history of ID (Hill et al., 2010).

FMRP

The fragile X gene codes for the fragile X protein (FMRP), which is an RNA-binding protein. Its lack of expression is the underlying cause of the syndrome. *FMR1* is evolutionarily highly conserved and has been identified in diverse organisms, such as the human, chicken, frog, fish, and fruit fly. The human gene spans approximately 38 kb and is composed of 17 exons, which show significant alternative splicing. The longest of the translated protein products contains 614 amino acids. FMRP has been found to contain two different RNA-binding motifs (two KH domains and an RGG box region). It selectively binds to and modulates the expression, primarily by suppression, of a limited set of other mRNAs, estimated to be about 4% of brain mRNAs (Ashley et al., 1993). Absence of FMRP may lead to impaired synaptic plasticity – which could account for the cognitive deficits found in affected individuals.

The *FMR1* gene is widely expressed early in development. With maturation, it is expressed strongly in the brain, gonads, and lymphocytes, but weakly or not at all in the liver, kidney, or lung. Immunocytochemistry with monoclonal antibodies has been shown to be potentially effective for the detection of the full mutation in males, both pre- and postnatally, in whole blood lymphocyte, amniocentesis, and chorionic villus samples (de Vries et al., 1998). Further improvements in the ability to use antibody-based assays for quantization of FMRP are under development (Iwahashi et al., 2009; LaFauci et al., 2010). These should soon allow low-cost newborn screening to identify affected males.

ANIMAL MODELS

An *Fmr1* knockout mouse model has been created, which grossly appears physically normal, fertile, and generally non-disabled (Dutch–Belgian Fragile X Consortium, 1994). However, on detailed testing, the knockout mouse shows enlarged testicular volume, hyperactivity, maze learning deficits, and increased sensitivity to audiogenic epileptic seizures. *Fmr1* knockout mice display a number of abnormal behavioral features of relevance to ASD, including inappropriate social interactions, perseverative behaviors, anxiety, learning and memory alterations, and hyperactivity (Bernardet and Crusio, 2006).

Mammals have two other genes closely related to the fragile X gene, which are autosomal and are termed *FXR1* and *FXR2* (for fragile X mental retardation, autosomal homolog 1 and 2). They encode two proteins, FXR1P and FXR2P, and along with FMRP have been well conserved in mammalian evolution (Kirkpatrick et al., 2001). They share a high amino acid homology with FMRP and have similar functional motifs, including two KH domains and an RGG box. FXR1P and FXR2P are found mainly in the cytoplasm and are able to form complexes with FMRP, and with themselves (Zhang et al., 1995). All three proteins are expressed in neurons and can be found in dendrites. *Fxr1* and *Fxr2* knockout mouse models have been developed (Bontekoe et al., 2002; Mientjes et al., 2004). FXR1P and FXR2P are expressed widely during embryonic development, but display different expression patterns to FMRP in some tissues. FXR1P is highly expressed in muscle and heart, whereas FMRP shows almost no expression in these tissues (Coy et al., 1995). Due to the early postnatal death of *Fxr1* knockout mice, a conditional *Fxr1* knockout model was produced (Mientjes et al., 2004). Unlike FMRP, FXR2P has a nucleolar localization signal and shuttles between the cytoplasm and the nucleolus (Tamanini et al., 2000).

Zebra fish, like mammals, have three FXS-related genes (Tucker et al., 2004). A zebra fish FXS model has been created in which the *fmr1* gene is deleted by genetic knockout (den Broeder et al., 2009). A *Drosophila* model has also been generated (Wan et al., 2000). Unlike mammals, *Drosophila* has a single *Fmr1*-like gene termed *Drosophila FMR1* (*dFmr1*) or *Drosophila Fmr1-related gene* (*dfxr*) (Wan et al., 2000). Both fly and mouse models of FXS display an excess of immature and tortuous dendritic spines, suggesting slowed maturation and abnormal pruning (Dockendorff et al., 2002; Morales et al., 2002). Fly mutants are less active than wild-type flies, interact with each other less often, and have deficient courtship behaviors (Bolduc et al., 2010; Dockendorff et al., 2002); these social deficits may be of relevance to ASD.

THE mGluR THEORY OF FRAGILE X

Abnormalities in the hippocampus of *Fmr1* knockout mice have been found to be related to synaptic plasticity. Glutamate is the major excitatory neurotransmitter and a form of long-lasting, protein synthesis-dependent synaptic plasticity, known as metabotropic glutamate receptor-dependent long-term depression (mGluR-LTD), was found to be enhanced (Huber et al., 2002). Another form of long-term plasticity, in the form of long-term potentiation (LTP) at cortical synapses has also been shown to be impaired in *Fmr1* knockout mice (Li et al., 2002; Zhao et al., 2005). Based on the evidence that FMRP functions primarily as a translational repressor, it has been proposed that it acts as a brake to inhibit the synthesis of more LTD-related proteins in response to the activation of mGluRs. In this model, in the absence of FMRP, the brake is removed and the synthesis of more LTD proteins results in enhanced mGluR-LTD. Evidence supporting the function of FMRP as a translational repressor includes the observation that in the absence of FMRP there is elevated cerebral protein synthesis in the FXS mouse cortex (Qin et al., 2005). One prediction of the 'mGluR theory' is that excessive mGluR5 signaling could contribute to the altered neuronal development in FXS (Bear et al., 2004). Consistent with this prediction, it was demonstrated that a 50% reduction of mGluR5 expression can rescue several phenotypes in *Fmr1* knockout mice, including

behavioral abnormalities, dendritic spine abnormalities in cortical pyramidal neurons, and the elevated basal protein synthesis levels in the hippocampus (Dolen et al., 2007). These results further support the mGluR theory and suggest that mGluRs may be appropriate therapeutic targets for the treatment of FXS.

The most robust behavioral assays to evaluate new treatment strategies in FXS mouse models are those focused on neuronal hyperexcitability – symptoms of this, such as epilepsy and hyperactivity, are also found in subjects with FXS. Increased susceptibility to audiogenic seizures has been reliably observed in *Fmr1* knockout mice and has become a very useful endpoint to evaluate potential therapeutic strategies (Dolen et al., 2007; Musumeci et al., 2000; Yan et al., 2005). Investigations administering receptor antagonists for mGluR5 receptors in mouse FXS models have provided further support for the mGluR theory. For example, MPEP (2-methyl-6-phenylethynyl pyridine hydrochloride) is a potent, highly selective antagonist of mGluR5 receptors in the mouse (Gasparini et al., 1999). When given to *Fmr1* knockout mice, MPEP reversed audiogenic seizures, epileptiform discharges, and abnormal behavioral defects (de Vrij et al., 2008; Yan et al., 2005). When MPEP was given to *dFmr1 Drosophila* mutants, various abnormal phenotypes were reversed, including behavioral defects and brain structural abnormalities (McBride et al., 2005).

NEW DRUG TRIALS IN FXS

This is an exciting time for research in FXS. We are seeing the beginnings of targeted treatment trials of drugs for the syndrome. MPEP is not suitable for humans due to its short half-life and potential toxic effects, but derivative mGluR5 antagonists have been developed by at least three pharmaceutical companies. Jacquemont et al. (2011) reported an early phase II double-blind placebo-controlled trial with the Novartis compound AFQ056 in 30 subjects with FXS. Of the subjects that completed the protocol, 7, with full *FMR1* promoter methylation as assayed by a bisulfate method and with no detectable *FMR1* mRNA, showed improved behavior, as measured with the ABC-C, after AFQ056 treatment as compared with placebo (P < 0.001). The authors detected no response in 18 patients with partial promoter methylation. The reasons why only those with full methylation would show improvements are unclear at this time. A large follow-up trail is now underway (see http://www.ClinicalTrials.gov). Trials are also underway with the Hoffmann-La Roche mGluR5 inhibitor, RO4917523, and the Seaside Therapeutics compound STX107. Results of these exciting studies should be known within a one-year time frame.

GABA is the major inhibitory neurotransmitter in the brain and abnormally low levels of GABA-mediated transmission have been found in *Fmr1* knockout mice (D'Hulst et al., 2006; El Idrissi et al., 2005). Administration of the GABAergic drug (R)-baclofen (arbaclofen) decreases mGluR signaling and was found to reduce seizure susceptibility in *Fmr1* knockout mice (Pacey et al., 2009). A double-blind placebo-controlled crossover trial was performed at 12 sites in the United States using the Seaside Therapeutics drug STX209 (arbaclofen) (Brown et al., 2010). A total of 49 subjects with a full mutation of *FMR1*, and who met the severity criteria on the Aberrant Behavior Checklist – Irritability (ABC-I) subscale, completed the study. Significantly more subjects showed improved behavior and socialization while on the studied drug, indicating a significant potential for the treatment of behavioral symptoms in FXS. Larger, phase III, double-blind trials are now under way with this GABAergic drug to determine the potential benefits in children and adults with FXS. A large trial is also under way to test this drug in children and adolescents with ASD (http://www.ClinicalTrials.gov).

Several other drugs are also in various stages of development and in preliminary trials having shown potential beneficial effects in *Fmr1* knockout animals. These include minocycline, lithium, memantine, ampakines, inhibitors of PI3K/ERK signaling, and inhibitors of p21 kinase (Gross et al., 2011). It is anticipated that many of these targeted treatments, if found beneficial for FXS, may also be useful for at least a subset of individuals with ASD.

References

Allingham-Hawkins, D.J., Babul-Hirji, R., Chitayat, D., Holden, J.J., Yang, K.T., Lee, C., et al., 1999. Fragile X premutation is a significant risk factor for premature ovarian failure: The International Collaborative POF in Fragile X study – preliminary data. American Journal of Medical Genetics 83, 322–325.

Arron, K., Oliver, C., Moss, J., Berg, K., Burbidge, C., 2011. The prevalence and phenomenology of self-injurious and aggressive behavior in genetic syndromes. Journal of Intellectual Disability Research 55, 109–120.

Ashley, C.T., Wilkinson, K.D., Reines, D., Warren, S.T., 1993. FMR1 protein: Conserved RNP family domains and selective RNA binding. Science 262, 563–566.

Bailey, D.B., Jr., Hatton, D.D., Skinner, M., Mesibov, G., 2001. Autistic behavior, FMR1 protein, and developmental trajectories in young males with fragile X syndrome. Journal of Autism and Developmental Disorders 31, 165–174.

Bear, M.F., Huber, K.M., Warren, S.T., 2004. The mGluR theory of fragile X mental retardation. Trends in Neuroscience 27, 370–377.

Bennetto, L., Pennington, B.F., 2002. Neuropsychology. In: Hagerman, R.J., Hagerman, P.J. (Eds.), Fragile X Syndrome: Diagnosis, Treatment and Research, third ed. Johns Hopkins University Press, Baltimore, MD, pp. 206–250.

Bernardet, M., Crusio, W.E., 2006. Fmr1 KO mice as a possible model of autistic features. Scientific World Journal 6, 1164–1176.

Berry-Kravis, E., Raspa, M., Loggin-Hester, L., Bishop, E., Holiday, D., Bailey, D.B., 2010. Seizures in fragile X syndrome: Characteristics and comorbid diagnoses. American Journal of Intellectual and Developmental Disabilities 115, 461–472.

Blomquist, H.K., Bohman, M., Edvinsson, S.O., Gillberg, C., Gustavson, K.H., Holmgren, G., et al., 1985. Frequency of the fragile X syndrome in infantile autism. A Swedish multicenter study. Clinical Genetics 27, 113–117.

Bolduc, F.V., Valente, D., Mitra, P., Tully, T., 2010. An assay for social interaction in *Drosophila* Fragile X mutants. Fly (Austin) 4 (3) [Epub ahead of print].

Bolton, P., Rutter, M., Butler, L., Summers, D., 1989. Females with autism and the fragile X. Journal of Autism and Developmental Disorders 19, 473–476.

Bontekoe, C.J., McIlwain, K.L., Nieuwenhuizen, I.M., Yuva-Paylor, L.A., Nellis, A., Willemsen, R., et al., 2002. Knockout mouse model for Fxr2: A model for mental retardation. Human Molecular Genetics 11, 487–498.

Brown, W.T., 2002. The Molecular Biology of the Fragile X Mutation. In: Hagerman, R.J., Hagerman, P.J. (Eds.), Fragile X Syndrome: Diagnosis, Treatment and Research, third ed. Johns Hopkins University Press, Baltimore, MD, pp. 110–135.

Brown, W.T., Friedman, E., Jenkins, E.C., Brooks, J., Wisniewski, K., Raguthu, S., et al., 1982a. Association of Fragile X syndrome with autism. The Lancet 1, 100.

Brown, W.T., Jenkins, E.C., Cohen, I.L., Fisch, G.S., Wolf-Schein, E.G., Gross, A., et al., 1986. Fragile X and autism: A multicenter survey. American Journal of Medical Genetics 23, 341–352.

Brown, W.T., Jenkins, E.C., Friedman, E., Brooks, J., Wisniewski, K., Raguthu, S., et al., 1982b. Autism is associated with the fragile-X syndrome. Journal of Autism and Developmental Disorders 12, 303–308.

Brown, W.T., Houck, G., Jr., Jeziorowska, A., Levinson, F., Ding, X.-H., Dobkin, C., et al., 1993. Rapid Fragile X carrier screening and prenatal diagnosis by a non-radioactive PCR test. Journal of the American Medical Association 270, 1569–1575.

Brown, W.T., Nolin, S., Houck, G., Ding, X., Glicksman, A., Li, S.-Y., et al., 1996. Prenatal diagnosis and carrier screening by PCR. American Journal of Human Genetics 64, 191–195.

Brown, W.T., Hagerman, R., Rathmell, B., Wang, P., Carpenter, R., Bear, M., et al., 2010. Arbaclofen treatment is associated with global behavioral improvement in fragile X syndrome (FXS): Results of a randomized, controlled phase 2 trial. Presentation 3071 at American Society of Human Genetics 2010 meeting, Baltimore, MD.

Budimirovic, D.B., Bukelis, I., Cox, C., Gray, R.M., Tierney, E., Kaufmann, W.E., 2006. Autism spectrum disorder in Fragile X syndrome: Differential contribution of adaptive socialization and social withdrawal. American Journal of Medical Genetics. Part A 140A, 1814–1826.

Chen, L., Hadd, A., Sah, S., Filipovic-Sadic, S., Krosting, J., Sekinger, E., et al., 2010. An information-rich CGG repeat primed PCR that detects the full range of fragile X expanded alleles and minimizes the need for southern blot analysis. Journal of Molecular Diagnostics 12, 589–600.

Chen, L., Hadd, A.G., Sah, S., Houghton, J.F., Filipovic-Sadic, S., Zhang, W., et al., 2011. High-resolution methylation polymerase chain reaction for fragile X analysis: Evidence for novel FMR1 methylation patterns undetected in Southern blot analyses. Genetics in Medicine 13, 528–538.

Chonchaiya, W., Au, J., Schneider, A., Hessl, D., Harris, S.W., Laird, M., et al., 2011. Increased prevalence of seizures in boys who were probands with the FMR1 premutation and co-morbid autism spectrum disorder. Human Genetics [Epub ahead of print].

Clifford, S., Dissanayake, C., Bui, Q.M., Huggins, R., Taylor, A.K., Loesch, D.Z., 2007. Autism spectrum phenotype in males and females with Fragile X full mutation and premutation. Journal of Autism and Developmental Disorders 37, 738–747.

Coffee, B., Keith, K., Albizua, I., Malone, T., Mowrey, J., Sherman, S.L., et al., 2009. Incidence of Fragile X syndrome by newborn screening for methylated FMR1 DNA. American Journal of Medical Genetics 85, 503–514.

Cohen, I.L., 1992. The behavioral phenotype of Fragile X Syndrome and its association with autism. In: Hagerman, R.J. (Ed.), Third International Fragile X Conference. Spectra Publishing, Denver, CO.

Cohen, I.L., 1995. Behavioral profiles of autistic and non-autistic fragile X males. Developmental Brain Dysfunction 8, 252–269.

Cohen, I.L., 1996. A theoretical analysis of the role of hyperarousal in the behavior and learning of fragile X males. Mental Retardation and Developmental Disabilities Research Reviews 1, 286–291.

Cohen, I.L., 2003. Criterion-related validity of the PDD behavior inventory. Journal of Autism and Developmental Disorders 33, 47–53.

Cohen, I.L., Brown, W.T., Jenkins, E.C., Krawczun, M.S., French, J.H., Raguthu, S., et al., 1989. Fragile X syndrome in females with autism. American Journal of Medical Genetics 34, 302–303.

Cohen, I.L., Fisch, G.S., Sudhalter, V., Wolf-Schein, E.G., Hanson, D., Hagerman, R., et al., 1988. Social gaze, social avoidance, and repetitive behavior in Fragile X males: A controlled study. American Journal of Mental Retardation 92, 436–446.

Cohen, I.L., Liu, X., Schutz, C., White, B.N., Jenkins, E.C., Brown, W.T., et al., 2003a. Association of autism severity with a monoamine oxidase A functional polymorphism. Clinical Genetics 64, 190–197.

Cohen, I.L., Nolin, S.L., Sudhalter, V., Ding, X.H., Dobkin, C.S., Brown, W.T., 1996. Mosaicism for the FMR1 gene influences adaptive skills development in Fragile X-affected males. American Journal of Medical Genetics 64, 365–369.

Cohen, I.L., Schmidt-Lackner, S., Romanczyk, R., Sudhalter, V., 2003b. The PDD Behavior Inventory: A rating scale for assessing response to intervention in children with pervasive developmental disorder. Journal of Autism and Developmental Disorders 33, 31–45.

Cohen, I.L., Sudhalter, V., Pfadt, A., Jenkins, E.C., Brown, W.T., Vietze, P.M., 1991a. Why are autism and the fragile-X syndrome associated? Conceptual and methodological issues. American Journal of Medical Genetics 48, 195–202.

Cohen, I.L., Sudhalter, V., 2005. The PDD Behavior Inventory. Psychological Assessment Resources, Lutz, FL.

Cohen, I.L., Tsiouris, J.A., Pfadt, A., 1991b. Effects of long-acting propranolol on agonistic and stereotyped behaviors in a male with pervasive developmental disorder and Fragile X syndrome: A double-blind, placebo controlled study. Journal of Clinical Psychopharmacology 11, 898–899.

Cohen, I.L., Vietze, P.M., Sudhalter, V., Jenkins, E.C., Brown, W.T., 1991c. Effects of age and communication level on eye contact in Fragile X males and non-Fragile X autistic males. American Journal of Medical Genetics 38, 498–502.

Coleman, M., 1976. The Autistic Syndromes. North-Holland.

Coleman, M., Gilberg, C., 2012. The Autisms. Oxford University Press, New York.

Collins, S.C., Bray, S.M., Suhl, J.A., Cutler, D.J., Coffee, B., Zwick, M.E., et al., 2010. Identification of novel FMR1 variants by massively parallel sequencing in developmentally delayed males. American Journal of Medical Genetics. Part A 52A, 2512–2520.

Coy, J, F., Sedlacek, Z., Bachner, D., Hameister, H., Joos, S., Lichter, P., et al., 1995. Highly conserved 3′UTR and expression pattern of FXR1 points to a divergent gene regulation of FXR1 and FMR1. Human Molecular Genetics 4, 2209–2218.

Crawford, D.C., Acuña, J.M., Sherman, S.L., 2001. Fmr1 and the fragile X syndrome: Human genome epidemiology review. Genetics in Medicine 3, 359–371.

den Broeder, M.J., van der Linde, H., Brouwer, J.R., Oostra, B.A., Willemsen, R., Ketting, R.F., 2009. Generation and characterization of Fmr1 knockout zebrafish. PLoS ONE 4, e7910.

de Vries, B.B., Mohkamsing, S., van den Ouweland, A.M., Halley, D.J., Niermeijer, M.F., Oostra, B.A., et al., 1998. Screening with the FMR1 protein test among mentally retarded males. Human Genetics 103, 520–522.

de Vrij, F.M., Levenga, J., van der Linde, H.C., Koekkoek, S.K., De Zeeuw, C.I., Nelson, D.L., et al., 2008. Rescue of behavioral phenotype and neuronal protrusion morphology in Fmr1 KO mice. Neurobiology of Disease 31, 127–132.

D'Hulst, C., De Geest, N., Reeve, S.P., Van Dam, D., De Deyn, P.P., Hassan, B.A., et al., 2006. Decreased expression of the GABAA receptor in Fragile X syndrome. Brain Research 1121, 238–245.

Dissanayake, C., Bui, Q., Bulhak-Paterson, D., Huggins, R., Loesch, D.Z., 2009. Behavioral and cognitive phenotypes in idiopathic autism versus autism associated with Fragile X syndrome. Journal of Child Psychology and Psychiatry 50, 290–299.

Dockendorff, T.C., Su, H.S., McBride, S.M., Yang, Z., Choi, C.H., Siwicki, K.K., et al., 2002. Drosophila lacking dfmr1 activity show defects in circadian output and fail to maintain courtship interest. Neuron 34, 973–984.

Dolen, G., Osterweil, E., Rao, B.S., Smith, G.B., Auerbach, B.D., Chattarji, S., et al., 2007. Correction of Fragile X syndrome in mice. Neuron 56, 955–962.

Dutch–Belgian Fragile X Consortium, 1994. Fmr1 knockout mice: A model to study fragile X mental retardation. Cell 78, 23–33.

Edwards, D.R., Keppen, L.D., Ranells, J.D., Gollin, S.M., 1988. Autism in association with Fragile X syndrome in females: Implications for diagnosis and treatment in children. Neurotoxicology 9, 359–365.

El, Idrissi, Ding, A., X., H., Scalia, J., Trenkner, E., Brown, W.T., Dobkin, C., 2005. Decreased GABA(A) receptor expression in the seizure-prone Fragile X mouse. Neuroscience Letters 377, 141–146.

Farzin, F., Perry, H., Hessl, D., Loesch, D., Cohen, J., Bacalman, S., et al., 2006. Autism spectrum disorders and attention-deficit/hyperactivity disorder in boys with the Fragile X premutation. Journal of Developmental and Behavioral Pediatrics 27, S137–S144.

Fatemi, S.H., Folsom, T.D., Kneeland, R.E., Liesch, S.B., 2011. Metabotropic glutamate receptor 5 upregulation in children with autism is associated with underexpression of both Fragile X mental retardation protein and GABAA receptor beta 3 in adults with autism. Anatomical Record (Hoboken) 294, 1635–1645.

Filipovic-Sadic, S., Sah, S., Chen, L., Krosting, J., Sekinger, E., Zhang, W., et al., 2010. A novel FMR1 PCR method for the routine detection of low abundance expanded alleles and full mutations in Fragile X syndrome. Clinical Chemistry 56, 399–408.

Friedman, E., 1969. The autistic syndrome and phenylketonuria. Schizophrenia 1, 249–261.

Garcia-Nonell, C., Ratera, E.R., Harris, S., Hessl, D., Ono, M.Y., Tartaglia, N., Marvin, E., et al., 2008. Secondary medical diagnosis in Fragile X syndrome with and without autism spectrum disorder. American Journal of Medical Genetics. Part A 146A, 1911–1916.

Gasparini, F., Lingenhohl, K., Stoehr, N., 1999. 2-Methyl-6-(phenylethynyl)-pyridine (MPEP), a potent, selective and systemically active mGlu5 receptor antagonist. Neuropharmacology 38, 1493–1503.

Gillberg, C., 1983. Identical triplets with infantile autism and the fragile-X syndrome. British Journal of Psychiatry 143, 256–260.

Godler, D.E., Tassone, F., Loesch, D.Z., Taylor, A.K., Gehling, F., Hagerman, R.J., et al., 2010. Methylation of novel markers of Fragile X alleles is inversely correlated with FMRP expression and FMR1 activation ratio. Human Molecular Genetics 191, 618–1632.

Gothelf, D., Furfaro, J.A., Hoeft, F., Eckert, M.A., Hall, S.S., O'Hara, R., et al., 2008. Neuroanatomy of Fragile X syndrome is associated with aberrant behavior and the Fragile X mental retardation protein (FMRP). Annals of Neurology 63, 40–51.

Gross, C., Berry-Kravis, E.M., Bassell, G.J., 2011. Therapeutic strategies in Fragile X syndrome: Dysregulated mGluR signaling and beyond. Neuropsychopharmacology. July, 1–18 [Epub].

Hagerman, P.J., 2008. The Fragile X prevalence paradox. Medical Genetics 45, 498–499.

Hagerman, R.J., 2002. The Physical and Behavioral Phenotype. In: Hagerman, R.J., Hagerman, P.J. (Eds.), Fragile X Syndrome: Diagnosis, Treatment and Research, third ed. Johns Hopkins University Press, Baltimore, pp. 3–109.

Hagerman, R., Au, J., Hagerman, P., 2011. FMR1 premutation and full mutation molecular mechanisms related to autism. Journal of Neurodevelopmental Disorders 3, 211–224.

Hall, S.S., Lightbody, A.A., Hirt, M., Rezvani, A., Reiss, A.L., 2010. Autism in Fragile X syndrome: A category mistake? Journal of the American Academy of Child & Adolescent Psychiatry 49, 921–933.

Hall, S.S., Lightbody, A.A., Huffman, L.C., Lazzeroni, L.C., Reiss, A.L., 2009. Physiological correlates of social avoidance behavior in children and adolescents with Fragile X syndrome. Journal of the American Academy of Child & Adolescent Psychiatry 48, 320–329.

Hantash, F.M., Goos, D.M., Crossley, B., Anderson, B., Zhang, K., Sun, W., et al., 2011. FMR1 premutation carrier frequency in patients undergoing routine population-based carrier screening: Insights into the prevalence of Fragile X syndrome, Fragile X-associated tremor/ataxia syndrome, and Fragile X-associated primary ovarian insufficiency in the United States. Genetics in Medicine 13, 39–45.

Happe, F., Ronald, A., 2008. The 'fractionable autism triad': A review of evidence from behavioral, genetic, cognitive and neural research. Neuropsychological Reviews 18, 287–304.

Harris, S.W., Hessl, D., Goodlin-Jones, B., Ferranti, J., Bacalman, S., Barbato, I., et al., 2008. Autism profiles of males with Fragile X syndrome. American Journal of Mental Retardation 113, 427–438.

Hazlett, H.C., Poe, M.D., Lightbody, A.A., Gerig, G., Macfall, J.R., Ross, A.K., et al., 2009. Teasing apart the heterogeneity of autism: Same behavior, different brains in toddlers with Fragile X syndrome and autism. Journal of Neurodevelopmental Disorders 1, 81–90.

Heilman, K.J., Harden, E.R., Zageris, D.M., Berry-Kravis, E., Porges, S.W., 2011. Autonomic regulation in Fragile X syndrome. Developmental Psychobiology 53, 785–795.

Hessl, D., Rivera, S., Koldewyn, K., Cordeiro, L., Adams, J., Tassone, F., et al., 2007. Amygdala dysfunction in men with the Fragile X premutation. Brain 130, 404–416.

Hessl, D., Tassone, F., Cordeiro, L., Koldewyn, K., McCormick, C., Green, C., et al., 2008. Brief report: Aggression and stereotypic behavior in males with Fragile X syndrome–moderating secondary genes in a 'single gene' disorder. Journal of Autism and Developmental Disorders 38, 184–189.

Hessl, D., Wang, J.M., Schneider, A., Koldewyn, K., Le, L., Iwahashi, C., et al., 2011. Decreased Fragile X mental retardation protein expression underlies amygdala dysfunction in carriers of the Fragile X premutation. Biological Psychiatry 70, 859–865.

Hill, M.K., Archibald, A.D., Cohen, J., Metcalfe, S.A., 2010. A systematic review of population screening for Fragile X syndrome. Genetics in Medicine 12, 396–410.

Hinton, V.J., Brown, W.T., Wisniewski, K., Rudelli, R.D., 1991. Analysis of neocortex in three males with the Fragile X Syndrome. American Journal of Medical Genetics 411, 289–294.

Huber, K.M., Gallagher, S.M., Warren, S.T., Bear, M.F., 2002. Altered synaptic plasticity in a mouse model of Fragile X mental retardation. Proceedings of the National Academy of Sciences of the United States of America 99, 7746–7750.

Hutt, C., Ounsted, C., 1966. The biological significance of gaze aversion with particular reference to the syndrome of infantile autism. Behavioral Sciences 11, 346–356.

Irwin, S.A., Patel, B., Idupulapati, M., Harris, J.B., Crisostomo, R.A., Larsen, B.P., et al., 2001. Abnormal dendritic spine characteristics in the temporal and visual cortices of patients with fragile-X syndrome: A quantitative examination. American Journal of Medical Genetics 98, 161–167.

Iwahashi, C., Tassone, F., Hagerman, R.J., Yasui, D., Parrott, G., Nguyen, D., et al., 2009. A quantitative ELISA assay for the Fragile X mental retardation 1 protein. Journal of Molecular Diagnostics 11, 281–289.

Jacquemont, S., Curie, A., des Portes, V., Torrioli, M.G., Berry-Kravis, E., Hagerman, R.J., et al., 2011. Epigenetic modification of the FMR1 gene in Fragile X syndrome is associated with differential response to the mGluR5 antagonist AFQ056. Science Translational Medicine 3, 64. 64ra1.

Jacquemont, S., Hagerman, R.J., Leehey, M., Grigsby, J., Zhang, L., Brunberg, J.A., et al., 2003. Fragile X premutation tremor/ataxia syndrome: Molecular, clinical, and neuroimaging correlates. American Journal of Medical Genetics 72, 869–878.

Kanner, L., 1943. Autistic disturbances of affective contact. The Nervous Child 2, 217–250.

Karmel, B.Z., Gardner, J.M., Meade, L.S., Cohen, I.L., London, E., Flory, M.J., et al., 2010. Early medical and behavioral characteristics of NICU infants later classified with ASD. Pediatrics 126, 457–467.

King, M., Bearman, P., 2009. Diagnostic change and the increased prevalence of autism. International Journal of Epidemiology 38, 1224–1234.

King, M.D., Bearman, P.S., 2011. Socioeconomic status and the increased prevalence of autism in California. American Sociological Review 76, 320–346.

Kirkpatrick, L.L., McIlwain, K.A., Nelson, D.L., 2001. Comparative genomic sequence analysis of the FXR gene family: FMR1, FXR1, and FXR2. Genomics 78, 169–177.

LaFauci, G., Kascsak, R., Kerr, D., Kascsak, R., Chen, C., Hong, H., et al., 2010. A highly sensitive capture immunoassay for the detection of the fragile X protein (FMRP) using the luminex platform. In: Abstracts of the National Fragile X Foundation Meeting, Detroit, MI.

Le Couteur, C.A., Rutter, M., Lord, C., Rios, P., Robertson, S., Holdgrafer, M., et al., 1989. Autism diagnostic interview: A standardized investigator-based instrument. Journal of Autism and Developmental Disorders 19, 363–387.

Levitas, A., Hagerman, R.J., Braden, M., Rimland, B., McBogg, P., Matus, I., 1983. Autism and the fragile X syndrome. Journal of Developmental and Behavioral Pediatrics 4, 151–158.

Lewis, P., Abbeduto, L., Murphy, M., Richmond, E., Giles, N., Bruno, L., et al., 2006. Cognitive, language and social-cognitive skills of individuals with fragile X syndrome with and without autism. Journal of Intellectual Disability Research 50, 532–545.

Li, J., Pelletier, M.R., Perez Velazquez, J.L., Carlen, P.L., 2002. Reduced cortical synaptic plasticity and GluR1 expression associated with fragile X mental retardation protein deficiency. Molecular and Cellular Neurosciences 19, 138–151.

Lightbody, A.A., Reiss, A.L., 2009. Gene, brain, and behavior relationships in Fragile X syndrome: Evidence from neuroimaging studies. Developmental Disabilities Research Reviews 15, 343–352.

Lord, C., Rutter, M., DiLavore, P.C., Risi, S., 1999. Autism Diagnostic Observation Schedule (ADOS). Western Psychological Services, Los Angeles.

Lubs, H.A., 1969. A marker X chromosome. American Journal of Human Genetics 21, 231–244.

Lyon, E., Laver, T., Yu, P., Jama, M., Young, K., Zoccoli, M., et al., 2010. A simple, high-throughput assay for fragile X expanded alleles using triple repeat primed PCR and capillary electrophoresis. Journal of Molecular Diagnostics 12, 505–511.

McBride, S.M., Choi, C.H., Wang, Y., Liebelt, D., Braunstein, E., Ferreiro, D., et al., 2005. Pharmacological rescue of synaptic plasticity, courtship behavior, and mushroom body defects in a *Drosophila* model of fragile X syndrome. Neuron 45, 753–764.

Meryash, D.L., Szymanski, L.S., Gerald, P.S., 1982. Infantile autism associated with the fragile-X syndrome. Journal of Autism and Developmental Disorders 12, 295–301.

Mientjes, E.J., Willemsen, R., Kirkpatrick, L.L., Nieuwenhuizen, I.M., Hoogeveen-Westerveld, M., Verweij, M., et al., 2004. Fxr1 knockout mice show a striated muscle phenotype: Implications for Fxr1p function in vivo. Human Molecular Genetics 13, 1291–1302.

Morales, J., Hiesinger, P.R., Schroeder, A.J., Kume, K., Verstreken, P., Jackson, F.R., et al., 2002. *Drosophila* fragile X protein, DFXR, regulates neuronal morphology and function in the brain. Neuron 34, 961–972.

Musumeci, S.A., Bosco, P., Calabrese, G., Bakker, C., De Sarro, G.B., Elia, M., et al., 2000. Audiogenic seizures susceptibility in transgenic mice with Fragile X syndrome. Epilepsia 41, 19–23.

Nolin, S., Brown, W.T., Glicksman, A., Houck, G.E., Jr., Gargano, A.D., Sullivan, A., et al., 2003. Expansion of the fragile X CGG repeat in females with premutation or intermediate alleles. American Journal of Medical Genetics 72, 454–464.

Nowicki, S.T., Tassone, F., Ono, M.Y., Ferranti, J., Croquette, M.F., Goodlin-Jones, B., et al., 2007. The Prader-Willi phenotype of Fragile X syndrome. Journal of Developmental and Behavioral Pediatrics 28, 133–138.

Nygren, G., Cederlund, M., Sandberg, E., Gillstedt, F., Arvidsson, T., Carina-Gillberg, I., et al., 2011. The prevalence of autism spectrum disorders in toddlers: A population study of 2-year-old Swedish children. Journal of Autism and Developmental Disorders.

Pacey, L.K., Heximer, S.P., Hampson, D.R., 2009. Increased GABAB receptor-mediated signaling reduces the susceptibility of Fragile X knockout mice to audiogenic seizures. Molecular Pharmacology 76, 18–24.

Paluszkiewicz, S.M., Martin, B.S., Huntsman, M.M., 2011. Fragile X syndrome: The GABAergic system and circuit dysfunction. Developmental Neuroscience.

Partington, M.W., 1984. The fragile X syndrome II: Preliminary data on growth and development in males. American Journal of Medical Genetics 17, 175–194.

Pinto-Martin, J.A., Levy, S.E., Feldman, J.F., Lorenz, J.M., Paneth, N., Whitaker, A.H., 2011. Prevalence of autism spectrum disorder in adolescents born weighing <2000 grams. Pediatrics 128, 883–891.

Qin, M., Kang, J., Burlin, T.V., Jiang, C., Smith, C.B., 2005. Post-adolescent changes in regional cerebral protein synthesis: An in vivo study in the FMR1 null mouse. Journal of Neuroscience 25, 5087–5095.

Reyniers, E., Vits, L., De Boulle, K., Van Roy, B., Van Velzen, D., de Graaff, E., et al., 1991. The full mutation in the FMR-1 gene of male Fragile X patients is absent in their sperm. Nature Genetics 4, 143–146.

Roberts, J.E., Bailey, D.B., Jr., Mankowski, J., Ford, A., Sideris, J., Weisenfeld, L.A., et al., 2009. Mood and anxiety disorders in females with the FMR1 premutation. American Journal of Medical Genetics. Part B, Neuropsychiatric Genetics 150B, 130–139.

Robinson, E.B., Koenen, K.C., McCormick, M.C., Munir, K., Hallett, V., Happé, F., Plomin, R., Ronald, A., 2012. A multivariate twin study of autistic traits in 12-year-olds: Testing the fractionable autism triad hypothesis. Behavioral Genetics 42, 245–255.

Schieve, L.A., Rice, C., Devine, O., Maenner, M.J., Lee, L.C., Fitzgerald, R., et al., 2011. Have secular changes in perinatal risk factors contributed to the recent autism prevalence increase? Development and application of a mathematical assessment model. Annals of Epidemiology 21, 930–945.

Shen, Y., Dies, K.A., Holm, I.A., Bridgemohan, C., Sobeih, M.M., Caronna, E.B., et al., 2010. Clinical genetic testing for patients with autism spectrum disorders. Pediatrics 125, e727–e735.

Tamanini, F., Kirkpatrick, L.L., Schonkeren, J., van Unen, L., Bontekoe, C., Bakker, C., et al., 2000. The fragile X-related proteins FXR1P and FXR2P contain a functional nucleolar-targeting signal equivalent to the HIV-1 regulatory proteins. Human Molecular Genetics 9, 1487–1493.

Tsiouris, J.A., Brown, W.T., 2004. Neuropsychiatric symptoms of Fragile X syndrome: Pathophysiology and pharmacotherapy. CNS Drugs 18, 687–703.

Tucker, B., Richards, R., Lardelli, M., 2004. Expression of three zebrafish orthologs of human FMR1-related genes and their phylogenetic relationships. Developmental Genes and Evolution 214, 567–574.

Wan, L., Dockendorff, T.C., Jongens, T.A., Dreyfuss, G., 2000. Characterization of dFMR1, a *Drosophila melanogaster* homolog of the Fragile X mental retardation protein. Molecular and Cellular Biology 20, 8536–8547.

Yan, Q.J., Rammal, M., Tranfaglia, M., Bauchwitz, R.P., 2005. Suppression of two major Fragile X syndrome mouse model phenotypes by the mGluR5 antagonist MPEP. Neuropharmacology 49, 1053–1066.

Zhang, Y., O'Connor, J.P., Siomi, M.C., Srinivasan, S., Dutra, A., Nussbaum, R.L., et al., 1995. The Fragile X mental retardation syndrome protein interacts with novel homologs FXR1 and FXR2. EMBO Journal 14, 5358–5366.

Zhao, M.G., Toyoda, H., Ko, S.W., Ding, H.K., Wu, L.J., Zhuo, M., 2005. Deficits in trace fear memory and long-term potentiation in a mouse model for fragile X syndrome. Journal of Neuroscience 25, 7385–7392.

MeCP2 and Autism Spectrum Disorders

Sarrita Adams*,†, Janine M. LaSalle†

*Department of Biochemistry, University of Cambridge, Cambridge, UK †Medical Microbiology and Immunology, Genome Center, MIND Institute, University of California, Davis, CA, USA

INTRODUCTION

Rett syndrome (RTT) is a neurodevelopmental disorder mostly caused by mutations in the X-linked gene *MECP2*. RTT primarily affects females, due to mutations typically occurring *de novo* in the paternal germline (Girard et al., 2001; Trappe et al., 2001), and is one of the most common causes of female mental retardation, with an incidence of 1/10,000. RTT is characterized by normal neonatal development followed by rapid regression of developmental milestones at the age of 6–18 months. This regression is marked by microcephaly, loss of purposeful hand movements, loss of acquired speech, hypotonia, epilepsy, and autism (Avivi and Feldman, 1980). Some 95% of individuals with RTT have mutations in *MECP2*, and these mutations vary and include missense, nonsense, and frameshift mutations (Fukuda et al., 2005). *MECP2* is located on chromosome Xq28 and is a member of the methyl-CpG-binding domain (MBD) gene family which also includes *MBD1–4* (Hendrich et al., 1999). Congenital variants of RTT have been defined and are due to mutations in

one of the following genes: cyclin-dependent kinase-like 5, (*CDKL5*) (Nectoux et al., 2006; Sprovieri et al., 2009); forkhead box G1 (*FOXG1*) (Ariani et al., 2008; Mencarelli et al., 2010), and myocyte enhancer factor 2c (*MEF2C*) (Novara et al., 2010; Zweier et al., 2010). The congenital variants of RTT have been observed in males as well as females. Moreover, a distinct variant of RTT is caused by a duplication of *MECP2*. *MECP2* duplication syndrome occurs primarily in males and results in increased expression of MeCP2 protein. Individuals with RTT and *MECP2* duplication syndrome reportedly fulfill the diagnostic criteria for autism spectrum disorders (ASD) (Ramocki et al., 2009), suggesting that *MECP2* and other RTT-associated genes may be common and critical players in the molecular pathogenesis of ASD.

Support for the role of MeCP2 in the etiology of ASD comes from findings that mutations and single nucleotide polymorphisms (SNPs) in *MECP2* have been identified in individuals with ASD who do not fulfill the diagnostic criteria for RTT (Coutinho et al., 2007; Loat et al., 2008; Piton et al., 2011;). Moreover, MeCP2

The Neuroscience of Autism Spectrum Disorders.
http://dx.doi.org/10.1016/B978-0-12-391924-3.00031-4

expression is decreased in a number of different forms of cognitive disability, including autism and attention deficit/hyperactivity disorder (Nagarajan et al., 2006; Samaco et al., 2004). Further, mutations in other members of the MBD gene family have been identified in non-syndromic cases of ASD, including *MBD1*, *MBD2*, and *MBD5* (Li et al., 2005; Cukier et al., 2010). For example, in a sample of 226 autistic patients, 46 alterations were identified in the four MBD genes, including missense mutations and deletions that are predicted to cause functional alterations (Talkowski et al., 2011). These findings suggest that in addition to its role in the pathogenesis of RTT, alterations in the expression of MeCP2 and other methyl-binding proteins play a more general role in the etiology of neurodevelopmental disorders (Gonzales, and LaSalle, 2010; Hammer et al., 2002).

Irregularities in the development and formation of neural circuits are proposed to play a causal role in the ASD phenotype. An overwhelming proportion of autism candidate genes are involved in molecular pathways needed for the accurate development of excitatory and inhibitory cell development and synaptogenesis (Gilman et al., 2011). The correct balance in the ratio of inhibitory to excitatory neurotransmission is necessary for accurate neural circuit formation during postnatal development. As a result, a growing body of evidence suggests that deviations in cortical circuit formation are responsible for the variability in severity of the ASD phenotype (Figure 4.6.1) (Qiu et al., 2011; Yizhar et al., 2011). The multisensory differences observed in ASD involve multiple cortical and subcortical regions (Kwakye et al., 2011). These findings suggest that any factor implicated in ASD must act in a global manner during distinct developmental time frames. MeCP2 fulfills the criteria of being globally expressed throughout embryonic and postnatal brain development (Balmer et al., 2003; Braunschweig et al., 2004; Shahbazian et al., 2002). The observation that RTT patients exhibit autistic features in the early stages of disease, around late infancy, is of relevance and suggests that MeCP2 is required for the refinement of cortical circuitry during postnatal development, a stage that is also likely of critical importance for a broader spectrum of ASD.

STRUCTURE AND FUNCTION OF MeCP2

Structural and functional studies of MeCP2 have revealed it to be a versatile and complex protein with multiple ascribed functions. MeCP2 contains an MBD which binds with higher affinity to methylated than unmethylated CpG dinucleotides (Nan et al., 1993). Missense mutations of *MECP2* in RTT most frequently target the MBD, suggesting its strong clinical relevance (Neul and Zoghbi, 2004). The activity of the MBD is predicted to work in concert with the transcriptional repression domain (TRD) that mediates association with a number of chromatin factors, including the transcriptional repressor Sin3A, histone deacetylase (HDAC) (Nan et al., 1998), transcription factor YY1 (Forlani et al., 2010), and DNA methyltransferase DNMT1 (Kimura and Shiota, 2003). The C-terminal domain (CTD) of MeCP2 has been inferred as necessary for the protein's integrity, mainly based on human cases of RTT in which truncating mutations were observed (Matijevic et al., 2009). The CTD contains a WW-domain-binding region, which allows for binding of MeCP2 to Group II WW domains. A WW domain is a short conserved region containing two tryptophan residues that bind proline-rich peptide motifs. This binding activity is proposed to contribute to Rett syndrome pathogenesis (Buschdorf and Stratling, 2004).

The N-terminal domain (NTD) is the least understood portion of MeCP2 in terms of function, but it is the differential basis of the two alternatively spliced isoforms: MeCP2e1/MeCP2α, which consists of exons 1, 3, and 4 and lacks exon 2 due to alternative splicing, and MeCP2e2/MeCPβ, which consists of exons 1, 2, 3, and 4. As a result of this splicing event the two MeCP2 isoforms differ only in having 9 (MeCP2e2/MeCP2α) or 21 (MeCP2e1/ MeCP2β) amino acids at their NTD (Kriaucionis and Bird, 2004; Mnatzakanian et al., 2004). Mutations in RTT have been found in multiple individuals in exon 1 (Amir et al., 2005; Chunshu et al., 2006; Evans et al., 2005; Poirier et al., 2005), but none have yet been found in exon 2. Furthermore, MeCP2e1/ MeCP2α protein is observed in classic RTT patient lymphocytes with *MECP2* exon 1 mutations (Gianakopoulos et al., 2012), suggesting that the MeCP2e1/ MeCP2α isoform is the most critical to the pathogenesis of RTT. In addition, MeCP2e1/MeCP2α is more highly expressed in the brain, and is translated approximately 10 times more efficiently than MeCP2e2/MeCPβ (Kriaucionis and Bird, 2004). Furthermore, a mouse mutant with only MeCP2e2/MeCP2β deficiency but normal expression of MeCP2e1/MeCP2α exhibited no detectable neurodevelopmental phenotypes (Itoh et al., 2012). While the function of the NTD is primarily unknown, the NTD of MeCP2e2/MeCPβ was found to increase the affinity of the MBD to methylated DNA (Ghosh et al., 2010), suggesting a possible role in modifying MeCP2 binding.

In addition to the roles and activities played by the different domains of the protein, post-translational modifications (PTMs) are a means by which differential MeCP2 activities can be modulated. Phosphorylation of serine residues, particularly those at serine 80 (pS80) and

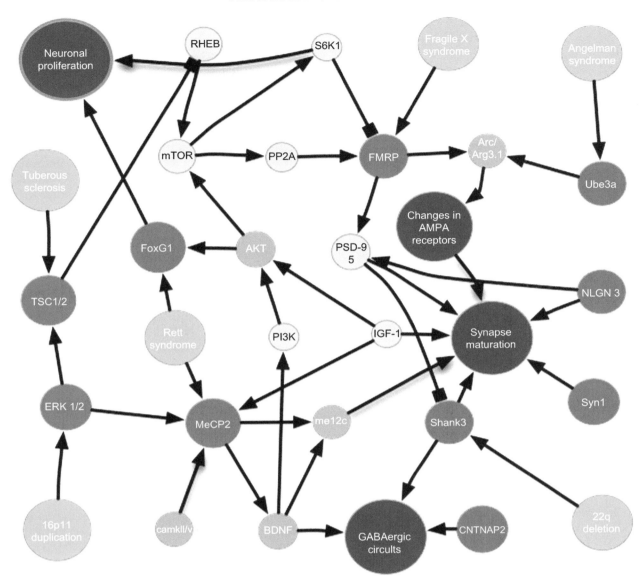

FIGURE 4.6.1 Molecular pathways implicated in Rett Syndrome and ASD overlap during development and adulthood. MeCP2 and ASD candidate genes are important upstream regulators of neuronal maturation and synaptogenesis. Disruption of these molecular pathways causes dysregulation of neuronal circuits. **Blue:** disease; **pink:** ASD candidate gene; **Green:** direct gene targets; **gray:** downstream effect genes. **FMRP** = fragile X mental retardation protein; **MeCP2** = methyl-CpG-binding protein; **TSC1/2** = tuberous sclerosis complex 1/2; **FoxG1** = forkhead box G1; **Ube3a** = ubiquitin protein ligase E3A; **CNTNAP2** = contactin associated like protein 2; **Shank3** = SH3 and multiple ankyrin repeat domains 3; **Erk1/2** = epidermal growth factor receptor; **Syn1** = synapsin 1; **NLGN3** = neuroligin 3; **BDNf** = brain derived neurotrophic factor; **Arc/Arg3.1** = activity-regulated cytoskeleton-associated protein; **PSD-95** = disc, large homolog 4; **Mef2c** = myocyte enhancer factor 2c; **Akt1** = v-akt thymona viral oncogene homolog 1; **CamKII/V** = calcium/calmodulin-dependent protein kinase II/V; **PI3K** = phosphoinositide-3-kinase; **IGF-1** = insulin-like growth factor; **PP2A** = serine/threonine-protein phosphatase 2A; **mTOR** = mechanistic target of rapamycin; **S6K1** = ribosomal protein S6 kinase; **RHEB** = Ras homolog enriched in brain.

serine 421 (pS421) were the best characterized modifications. pS80 is primarily observed in resting neurons (Tao et al., 2009), while pS421 is involved in activity-dependent neuronal response, which is necessary for neuronal maturation and aspects of synaptogenesis (Cohen et al., 2011; Zhou et al., 2006). The calcium/calmodulin kinases CamKII and CamKV, are activity-dependent kinases that have been implicated in S421

phosphorylation of MeCP2. The effect of MeCP2 phosporylation on neuronal maturation is of interest given that aberrant synapse formation has been implicated in ASD, and is evident in transgenic mouse models of both autism and RTT. However, the understanding of the complete spectrum of MeCP2 PTMs and their functional relevance in synapse formation is still in its infancy (Gonzales et al., 2012).

DEVELOPMENTAL MeCP2 EXPRESSION IN THE BRAIN

MECP2 transcripts are expressed in all tissues of the body, but the level of MeCP2 protein is quite variable, with highest levels found in the central nervous system (CNS) (LaSalle et al., 2001). MeCP2 protein levels are also heterogeneous across the CNS and increase during postnatal development, as neurons mature. The abundance of MeCP2 also differs among cell populations within the brain. While glial cells such as astrocytes and microglia have low but detectable MeCP2 (Ballas et al., 2009; LaSalle et al., 2001; Maezawa et al., 2009), mature neurons have high MeCP2 levels. Genome-wide chromatin analyses of MeCP2 in the adult mouse brain have estimated MeCP2 levels to be near those of histone H1, making MeCP2 an extremely abundant nuclear protein in mature neurons (Skene et al., 2010).

The mechanisms that control the dynamics of MeCP2 expression levels are just beginning to be understood. MeCP2 mRNA stability and translation were recently shown to be regulated by microRNAs (miRNAs) that bind to recognition elements in the MeCP2 3′ untranslated regions (UTRs) (Klein et al., 2007). MeCP2 3′UTRs possess multiple polyadenylation sites, which allows for the generation of at least four different transcripts, with different lengths in the 3′UTR. The longest MeCP2 transcript possesses a 3′UTR which is 10.2 kb in length and is highly expressed in the brain, whereas the shorter transcripts (1.8 kb, 5.4 kb, and 7.2 kb) are expressed in visceral organs and muscle (Pelka et al., 2005). In primary cortical neurons the microRNA miR132 negatively regulates the translation of *MECP2* mRNA, and does so through binding to conserved miRNA-recognition elements in the 10.2 kb 3′UTR of *MECP2* (Klein et al., 2007).

Of significance to this finding is the involvement of miRNAs in other X-linked mental retardation syndromes, such as fragile X syndrome. The miRNAs miR132 and miR125b associate with the fragile X mental retardation protein (FMRP). This activity regulates dendritogenesis and synaptic function in cultured hippocampal neurons (Edbauer et al., 2010). Interestingly, two miRNAs encoded on chromosome 21 and upregulated in Down syndrome (DS, trisomy 21) appear to downregulate MeCP2 protein levels (Kuhn et al., 2010), providing support for a potential explanation for reduced MeCP2 levels observed in DS postmortem brains (Samaco et al., 2004). These results suggest that the control of MeCP2 protein levels in the brain could be a common intersecting pathway in different disorders that are characterized by learning disability and autism.

MeCP2 AND ASD MOUSE MODELS

RTT is considered to be a good model for the study of ASD, given that all affected individuals fulfill the diagnostic criteria for ASD. Moreover, there exist strong similarities in the abnormalities in brain morphology and function observed in RTT and ASD. For example, alterations in cortical activity (Dinstein et al., 2011), coupled with changes in white matter density (Carter et al., 2008; Duerden et al., 2012), and neuronal cell size and maturity (Muotri et al., 2010; van Kooten et al., 2008) are common findings in both RTT and ASD brains. The onset of RTT symptoms occurs during early postnatal life, and mouse models of RTT have been used to assess alterations in neuronal activity and function during this developmental time frame. Mouse models of RTT and ASD have been beneficial in identifying neural correlates of ASD. MeCP2-deficient mice share comparable alterations in biophysical, biochemical, and morphological parameters associated with mouse models of ASD. Disruption in learning and memory, coupled with deviations in social behavior, are evident in both RTT and ASD mouse models (Moy et al., 2009). A comparison of mouse models of MeCP2 deficiency with transgenic models of ASD have identified key pathways that are disrupted in ASD, and the impact this has on the ASD phenotype (Table 4.6.1).

Several transgenic mouse models of RTT have been generated, all of which seek to disrupt the function or expression of MeCP2 (Table 4.6.1). The most commonly used model was generated by Cre-LoxP technology to target deletion of exons 3 and 4 (Guy et al., 2001). A different mouse generated around the same time exclusively targeted exon 3 by Cre-LoxP, but exhibited a similar phenotype (Chen et al., 2001). Unlike in humans, where males with RTT causing *MECP2* mutations are rare, *Mecp2*-deficient male mice are viable and exhibit most of the symptoms of RTT, whereas female mice that are heterozygous for the mutation exhibited a milder and more variable phenotype. Since the generation of the $Mecp2^{tm1.1Bird/y}$ and $Mecp2^{tm1.1Jae}$ mice, several other transgenic mouse models of RTT have been developed. These include the $Mecp2^{308/y}$ truncation model (Moretti et al., 2005), the $Mecp2^{tg/y}$ duplication model (Collins et al., 2004), and two MeCP2 phosphorylation mutants (Tao et al., 2009). $Mecp2^{308/y}$ and $Mecp2^{tg/y}$ mice exhibit a similar phenotype to the MeCP2-deficient mouse model, however, their neurological symptoms are less severe and their life span is greatly increased. The MeCP2-phosphorylation mutants display a minor RTT phenotype and demonstrate the subtle effect that MeCP2-dependent phosphorylation has on the aspects of the RTT phenotype. The fact that the full RTT phenotype is not

TABLE 4.6.1

Mouse model	Mutation	Allele type	Human disorder	Brain size	Social behavior	Memory, learning, and motor systems	Repetitive behaviors
Mecp2^tm1.1Bird (62)	Deletion of exons 3 and 4	Knockout	Rett syndrome	Microcephaly	Decreased social interaction	Hypoactivity, ataxia	Hind-limb clasping, tremors
Mecp2^tm1Hzo/J (64, 65)	Deletion of exon 4	C-terminal truncation	Rett syndrome	None	Decreased social interaction	Hypoactivity, ataxia	Hind-limb clasping
Mecp2^Tg (66)	Insertion of full human copy of MECP2	2-fold over-expression	X-linked mental retardation	Unknown	Unknown	Unknown	Hind-limb clasping
Mecp2^S421A,S424A/y (67)	Substitution of alanine at serine 421 and 424	Knock-in	Rett syndrome Removal of phosphorable residues	Increased brain weight	Unknown	Enhanced motor learning (MWM), hyperactivity	None
Mecp2^S80/y (38)	Substitution of alanine at serine 80	Knock-in	Rett syndrome Removal of phosphorable residues	Increased brain weight	Unknown	Hypoactivity	None
Mecp2^Viaat (75)	Deletion of Mecp2 in GABAergic neurons	Conditional deletion	Rett syndrome	None	Decreased social activity	Motor dysfunction, decreased motor learning (MWM)	Overgrooming, hind-limb clasping
Shank3b^-/- (76)	Deletion of exons 13–16	Knockout	22q13.3 deletion	Normal; abnormal striatum	Decreased social activity	Increased anxiety	Overgrooming
Shank3^(+/-)ΔC (103)	C terminus deletion	Gain of function	22q13.3 deletion	Unknown	Unknown	Unknown	Overgrooming
Cntnap2^-/- (72)		Knockout	SNP/CNV	Normal	Decreased social interaction	Decreased spatial learning (MWM)	Overgrooming
Nlgn4^Gt(XST093)Byg (100)	Insertion of gene trap vector	Knockout	SNP/CNV	Small reduction (1.5%)	Decreased social interaction and aggression	Abnormal vocalization	None
Nlgn3^tm1Sud (99)	Ag451→Cys451 mutations	Gain of function	Familial autism	Normal	Decreased social interaction	Enhanced spatial learning (MWM)	None
Fmr1^tm1Cgr (112)	Disruption of exon 5	Knockout	Fragile X syndrome	Normal	Decreased aggression	Decreased spatial learning (MWM), decreased object recognition, hyperactivity	None
Tsc1^tm1.1Djk (114)	Deletion of exons 17 and 18	Knockout	Tuberous sclerosis syndrome	Normal; abnormal cortical morphology	Decreased social interaction	Decreased spatial learning (MWM)	Limb clasping and tremors
Tsc2^tm1Djk (114)	Insertion of gene trap vector	Knockout	Tuberous sclerosis	Normal	Decreased social interaction	Decreased spatial learning, decreased context-dependent fear conditioning	Unknown
Ube3a^Tm1Alb/J (108)	Disruption of 3 kb sequence in exon 2	Knockout	Angelman syndrome	Reduction in size of cerebral cortex and cerebellum	None	Deficits in context-dependent fear conditioning	Hind-limb clasping

observed in MeCP2-phosphorylation mutants may be specifically relevant to ASD, given that alterations in MeCP2-specific PTMs have a greater impact on ASD-related behaviors. For example, there are abnormalities in cognitive and social behaviors in *Mecp2*^{tm3.1Jae} mice (Cohen et al., 2011; Li et al., 2011). This suggests that activity-dependent phosphorylation of MeCP2 is required to mediate these ASD-related behaviors.

Over the past decade, many distinct mouse models of autism have been generated and generally the phenotypes of these models resemble those observed in human individuals with ASD. For example, alterations in sociability, stereotyped behavior, and cognitive performance are observed across these models. Human conditions where autism is comorbid with another multisystem disorder led to the identification of specific genes that are implicated in ASD. For example, mouse models of fragile X syndrome, tuberous sclerosis, Angelman syndrome, and 22q13 microdeletion syndrome are used extensively to study molecular pathways implicated in ASD. By comparing the MeCP2-deficient mouse models with other ASD mouse models, it is possible to gain insight into how molecular, physiological, and behavioral abnormalities converge across mouse models with distinct genotypes. In doing so it may be possible to identify specific pathways that imply susceptibility to ASD, which would be beneficial in the design of future treatment solutions.

Behavioral Phenotypes: Motor, Social, and Cognitive Deficits

Individuals with ASD show a range of irregularities in the acquisition of motor (Matson et al., 2011), social, and cognitive skills (Kuenssberg et al., 2011). These differences range from a total lack of acquired social skills to superior performance in some cognitive tasks, and the disparity in performance is thought to correlate with the severity of neuronal circuitry alterations. In RTT, individuals exhibit a loss of motor skills early on in postnatal development, and the acquisition of stereotyped behavior, such has hand wringing, arm flapping, and rocking (Avivi and Feldman, 1980). Changes in sociability in RTT are also apparent early in infancy, and are demonstrated by the failure to acquire speech, poor eye-contact, and lack of joint attention. The RTT phenotype might be best described as a compound phenotype because as the child progresses through childhood and adolescence, other physiological symptoms are observed that are not related to ASD. Scoliosis, spasticity, and seizures emerge in early juvenile development at around 4 years of age, while parkinsonism-like features are first observed around adolescence (Chahrour and Zoghbi, 2007). These

secondary conditions in RTT may have the effect of diminishing the ASD phenotype. Nevertheless, the emergence of core features of the ASD phenotype in RTT during early development suggests that analysis of MeCP2 function will shed light on molecular pathways involved in ASD.

Stereotyped and obsessive compulsive movements are commonly observed in ASD, and can have a debilitating effect on the individual. A common feature observed in most MeCP2-deficient mouse models is stereotyped hind-paw wringing, and this behavior becomes apparent towards the end of postnatal development at around 6–8 weeks (Moretti et al., 2005; Stearns et al., 2007). Motor stereotypies have been found in other mouse models of ASD. The contactin-associated protein-like 2 knockout mice (*Cntnap2*^{−/−}) exhibit stereotyped behavior in the form of self-grooming (Penagarikano et al., 2011). *CNTNAP2* mutations have been associated with ASD via association, linkage, and gene expression studies (Mikhail et al., 2011; O'Roak et al., 2011). The excessive self-grooming phenotype has been observed in a mouse model of RTT where MeCP2 is deficient specifically in GABAergic neurons (neurons producing GABA, or γ-aminobutyric acid) (Viaat-*Mecp2*^{−/y}). Viaat-*Mecp2*^{−/y} mice exhibited hind-limb clasping and spent 300% more time grooming than wild-type mice (Chao et al., 2010). GABAergic neurotransmission may be a general core regulator of stereotyped behavior. During embryonic development, CNTNAP2 is expressed in the ganglionic eminences which give rise to GABAergic interneurons. Further, *Cntnap2*-deficient mice exhibit a reduced number of GABAergic interneurons in the striatum, a region which is implicated in the generation of habit-forming behaviors. In addition, alterations in electrical properties of striatal glutamatergic neurons also cause repetitive grooming behaviors in *Shank3B*^{−/−} mice (Peça et al., 2011).

Tuberous sclerosis protein (TSC1/2)-deficient mice also exhibit differences in social and motor learning. Specifically, *Tsc2*-deficient mice exhibit mild impairments in rotarod motor learning, as they failed to improve their performance on the task over a two-day training period. However the *Tsc2*-deficient mice did not show any differences in other memory and learning tasks, such as the Morris water maze and contextual fear conditioning (Chevere-Torres et al., 2012). The motor changes may be due to loss of Purkinje cells in the cerebellum, as TSC2 deficiency causes increased apoptosis in this cell population (Reith et al., 2011). Changes in cerebellum morphology and cell survival are a common finding in RTT humans and mouse models. *MECP2* duplication in seven affected human males caused a reduction in white matter, and in three cases the individuals displayed cerebellar degeneration (Reardon et al., 2010). In MeCP2-deficient mice, the cerebellum is decreased in size by approximately 12% (Belichenko et al., 2008). Granule cell death, in response to hypoxia and excitotoxicity, is markedly increased in MeCP2-deficient neuronal cultures, suggesting that the cerebellum in RTT may be sensitive to neuronal insults that could further exacerbate deficits in motor learning and behavior (Abney et al., 1997). Granule cell development is also impaired in neuronal cultures from *Foxg1*-deficient mice, suggesting that both the FOXG1 transcription factor and MeCP2 are important in regulating neuronal survival in the cerebellum. FOXG1 expression is decreased in granule cells undergoing apoptosis, while over-expression protects granule cells from cell death (Dastidar et al., 2011). More recently it has been discovered that FOXG1 and MeCP2 are able to form a molecular complex (Dastidar et al., 2012), which is of importance given that mutations in *FOXG1* are responsible for causing a congenital variant of RTT (Ariani et al., 2008).

Behavioral Phenotypes: Learning and Memory

Although the extent to which learning and memory are impaired in ASD is variable, individuals characterized as having low-functioning autism (LFA) have an identifiable learning disability. Mouse models of ASD have been beneficial in the assessment of different types of learning and memory. The combined usage of a variety of cellular, molecular, and behavioral assessments makes it possible to identify specific cortical circuits that may be disrupted in ASD. The most common findings in ASD mouse models are alterations in neuronal cell maturation and neuronal excitability (Deng et al., 2011; Etherton et al., 2011b). These changes are evident in two brain regions, the hippocampus and the cortex, which are both indispensable for social and cognitive learning and memory.

Despite the expression of MeCP2 throughout the brain, MeCP2-deficient mice show that molecular and electrophysiological alterations are not consistent throughout the CNS. This implies a temporal and spatial regulation of MeCP2 function, meaning that the activity and necessity of MeCP2 differs depending on the brain age and region. For example, long-term potentiation (LTP) in MeCP2-deficient mice is not impaired in layer V cortical pyramidal neurons at 5 weeks old (Dani and Nelson, 2009). However, cortical activity is decreased at both presymptomatic ($<$ 5 weeks) and symptomatic stages in MeCP2-deficient layer V neurons (Dani and Nelson, 2009). Conversely, the $Mecp2^{308/y}$ mutant mouse exhibits a decrease in LTP in synaptic connections of layers II and III in both the motor (M1) and sensory (S1) at 22 weeks old. Similar alterations in neuronal excitability are present in the hippocampus of $Mecp2^{308/y}$ mice; however, these

changes are evident much earlier in postnatal development. For example, long-term depression (LTD) and LTP are impaired in area CA1, which results in increased basal synaptic transmission in this region (Moretti et al., 2006). Support for the alterations in hippocampal neurotransmission has also been identified in $Mecp2^{Bird/y}$ mice. However, decreased inhibitory neurotransmission in the CA3 region of the hippocampus is assumed to cause increased neuronal excitability (Zhang et al., 2008); this is in contrast to increased LTP and LTD observed in $Mecp2^{308/y}$ mice. Enhanced synaptogenesis and altered hippocampal LTP has been observed in phosphorylation mutant $Mecp2^{S421A;S424A/y}$ mice, (Li et al., 2011). This finding suggests that deficits in LTP are due to the inability of MeCP2 to undergo activity-dependent post-translational modifications. The observation that increased hippocampal LTP is evident in mutant $Mecp2^{308/y}$ mice lacking the C-terminal domain provides further support for the role of S421/S424 phosphorylation as being important to learning deficits in RTT and ASD.

Alterations in membrane-bound proteins necessary for maintaining synaptic transmission have also been identified in MeCP2-deficient mouse models. The α-amino-3-hydroxy-5-methyl-4-isoxazole-propionic acid receptor (AMPAR) scaffolding protein, postsynaptic density protein-95 (PSD-95), and the vesicular glutamate transporter (VGlut1) are increased in hippocampal and cortical neuronal cultures derived from $Mecp2^{S421A;S424A/y}$ mice after 21 days *in vitro*. The mechanism by which these postsynaptic proteins are increased may be in part related to MeCP2's role in the regulation of genes involved in cell maturation and synapse formation.

Loss of either of the tuberous sclerosis complex genes, *TSC1* or *TSC2*, in humans causes ASD. The TSC1/2 protein products form a heterodimeric complex that regulates the phosphorylation of the mammalian target of rapamycin (MTOR1), via the AKT pathway. Deletion of *TSC1/TSC2* causes an increase in protein translation, which is brought about by increased activity of MTOR1 and downstream proteins that control translation, cell growth, and metabolism (Zoncu et al., 2011). The mechanisms by which *TSC1/TSC2* mutations cause ASD is not known, however transgenic mouse models of TSC1/2 deficiency have provided an insight into the impact of these mutations on neuronal electrophysiology. Similar to transgenic mouse models of RTT, TSC1/2-deficient mice have alterations in excitatory synaptic currents in the hippocampus. The frequency of mEPSCs is significantly increased in TSC1-deficient CA1 hippocampal slices at P24–31. This increase in mEPSC frequency is mediated by AMPAR and NMDAR activity and is wholly postsynaptic, suggesting that TSC1/2 deficiency causes increased synapse number on postsynaptic neurons (Bateup et al., 2011).

The mads domain gene, *MEF2C*, which plays an important role in the development and function of the nervous system, is a target of MeCP2 regulation, bound by MeCP2 in its promoter region (Chahrour et al., 2008). *MEF2C* is proposed to be an autism candidate gene due to the occurrence of an ASD microdeletion syndrome that removes a 216 kb to 8.8 Mb region on chromosome 5q14.3, containing *MEF2C* (Le Meur et al., 2010). The phenotype of *MEF2C* haploinsufficiency resembles that of RTT, with the main difference being that the onset of postnatal regression occurs within weeks or months after birth (Nowakowska et al., 2010). *Mef2c*-deficient mice are phenotypically similar to *Mecp2*-deficient mice, as both transgenic models exhibit hind-paw clasping and deficits in learning and memory. MeCP2 binding to the promoter of *Mef2c* is increased in the $Mecp2^{Tg/y}$ mouse model (Chahrour et al., 2008) and in $Mecp2^{S421A;S424A/y}$ mice. It is predicted that MeCP2 negatively regulates transcription of *Mef2c* by binding to its promoter, as *Mef2c* decreased transcript levels were found to coordinate with the increased binding of MeCP2 to the *Mef2c* promoter in $Mecp2^{S421A;S424A/y}$ mice (Li et al., 2011). In addition, short interfering RNA (siRNA) knockdown of MeCP2 leads to increased levels of Mef2c (Kuhn et al., 2010). This is of interest given that Mef2c is a transcription factor that functions as a negative regulator of synapse formation. Brain-specific deletion of *Mef2c* results in an increase in the number of excitatory synapses and potentiation of basal synaptic transmission in the hippocampus (Barbosa et al., 2008). Moreover, alterations in hippocampus-dependent learning and memory in *Mef2c*-deficient mice were comparable to those observed in *Mecp2*-deficient mice. Altered context-dependent fear conditioning in adult mice was observed in *Mef2c*-deficient mice, and $Mecp2^{308/y}$ mice, as a decreased fear response to the conditioned stimulus (Barbosa et al., 2008; Moretti et al., 2006). $Mecp2^{S421A;S424A/y}$ mice exhibited the inverse phenotype to the *Mef2c*-deficient and $Mecp2^{308/y}$ mice in the same contextual fearconditioning paradigm.

Mouse Models of Deficiencies in Synaptic Adhesion

Many mouse models of ASD display aberrant expression of glutamatergic and GABAergic synaptic markers, and in some cases mutations in transmembrane proteins have been identified in individuals with ASD. Synaptic adhesion molecules are required for accurate circuit formation and are needed to acquire a functional balance in the ratio of excitatory to inhibitory neurotransmission. Mutations in the postsynaptic scaffolding protein SH3 and multiple ankyrin repeat domains 3 (*SHANK3*) gene have been identified in several cases

of ASD (Durand et al., 2007). Members of the SHANK family of proteins are required to form postsynaptic scaffolding complexes in concert with discs, large (*Drosophila*) homolog-associated protein DLGAP1/3 and PSD-95. However, $Shank3b^{-/-}$ mice did not exhibit any deficits in basal synaptic transmission in the hippocampus, nor did they perform differently to WT (wild-type) mice in hippocampus-dependent learning tasks (Peca et al., 2011).

Different Shank3 mouse models have been developed, and the different mutations expose the complex role of Shank3 in neuronal development and maintenance. In mice haploinsufficient for *Shank3*, in which the exons for the ankyrin repeat domain were deleted and expression of full-length *Shank3* was disrupted, specific deficits in basal glutamatergic synaptic transmission in the hippocampus were identified (Bozdagi et al., 2010). This is in stark contrast to the $Shank3b^{-/-}$ mouse model and suggests that a full knockout of *Shank3* may result in a compensatory gain-of-function activity. In humans, *SHANK3* mutations arise in 22q13 deletion syndrome and result in *SHANK3* haploinsufficiency, therefore the haploinsufficient *Shank3* mouse model better resembles the human phenotype. In a separate mouse model, deletion of exons 4–9 in the *Shank3* open reading frame ($Shank3^{e4-9}$ mice) also caused a similar phenotype to that observed in *Shank3* haploinsufficient mice. Synaptic plasticity was impaired in $Shank3^{e4-9}$ mice and there were clear defects in the AMPAR-dependent phase of LTP, as well as repetitive behaviors, deficiencies in learning and memory, and altered motor skills (Wang et al., 2011). Together, these results suggest that the ankyrin repeat domain of Shank3 encodes susceptibility to the autism phenotype. For example, a human *de novo SHANK3* mutation in the ankyrin domain (Q321R) impairs growth cone formation. This is of importance given that Shank3 is important for early stages of neuronal growth and synapse development through actin polymerization that is necessary for neurite outgrowth (Durand et al., 2012) and the alterations in dendritic spine density observed in many *Shank3* mouse models.

Neuroligin-neurexin complexes are required to form post- and presynaptic terminals, and mutations in both genes have been implicated in ASD, although mouse models have produced disparate results. In humans, the identification of several different mutations in the X-linked genes neuroligin 3 (*NLGN3*) and neuroligin 4 (*NLGN4*) provides strong support for a defect in synaptic connections in ASD (Chih et al., 2004; Yu et al., 2011). A point substitution, R451C, in *NLGN3* has been identified in patients with familial autism (Jamain et al., 2003). NLGN3-R451C knock-in mice were generated and were shown to have increased inhibitory synaptic transmission in the somatosensory cortex, as well as enhanced hippocampus-dependent learning and diminished social behaviors (Tabuchi et al., 2007). In addition, *Nlgn4*-deficient mice also show deficits in social interaction as well as increased aggression (Jamain et al., 2008). However, this phenotype was not observed in the *Nlgn3*-deficient mice (Radyushkin et al., 2009), suggesting that the R451C substitution is a gain-of-function mutation. Similar to *Mecp2*-deficient mice, NLGN3-R451C mice exhibit enhanced hippocampal LTP in area CA1 and altered dendritic branching (Etherton et al., 2011a).

Post-Translational Modifications in RTT and ASD Mouse Models

Changes in activity-dependent gene regulation and subsequent modifications in accurate synapse formation may be a unifying feature of RTT and ASD. Activity-dependent stimulation in gene transcription changes is the core means by which a neuron can adapt and respond to an external stimulus. All aspects of higher cognitive function require a high degree of cortical plasticity that is governed by molecular and electrical changes. As previously stated, upon calcium influx and activation of calcium-dependent kinases, MeCP2 is able to undergo distinct post-translational modifications. However, only recently has it been possible to gain any insight into the impact this has on the pathophysiology of RTT. Although phosphorylation of serine residues on MeCP2 has received the most attention, other PTMs have been observed, including acetylation and ubiquitination (Gonzales et al., unpublished results).

A defect in ubiquitination was observed in the *Shank3*(+/ΔC) mouse model of autism, which mimics a human mutation in *SHANK3* that results in the truncation of the C-terminal domain of the protein (Bozdagi et al., 2010). Similar to the NLGN3-R451C mutation in mice, the *Shank3*(+/ΔC) mutation produces a gain-of-function phenotype resulting in increased polyubiquitination of WT Shank3 protein. The increased polyubiquitination of Shank3 allows for premature targeting of Shank3 to the proteasome and enhanced degradation of WT Shank3. Decreased expression in the NR1 subunit of the NMDAR is evident in *Shank3*(+/ΔC) mice and is also due to increased polyubiquitination (Bangash et al., 2011). The combined effect of a decrease in NR1 and Shank3 is an alteration in hippocampus-dependent LTP and LTD. However, no changes in synaptic plasticity were observed, and hippocampus-dependent learning was intact. These assays were performed at postnatal days 21–28, a relatively short developmental time frame, and so may display temporal and spatial regulation (Bangash et al., 2011). The role of MeCP2 ubiquitination is

currently unknown but, unlike Shank3, it appears that MeCP2 can be ubiquitinated on specific residues, which may alter the stability or functions of the protein (Gonzales et al., unpublished results).

A different cause of ASD, Angelman syndrome, is produced by mutations or deficiencies in the ubiquitin ligase E3 gene (*UBE3A*) on the imprinted chromosomal region 15q11–13 (Lalande et al., 2007). Over-expression of UBE3A at approximately two-fold higher levels in the brain is observed in 15q duplication syndrome individuals with features of autism (Scoles et al., 2011). Among the multiple potential targets of ubiquitination by UBE3A is Arc, a synaptic protein which regulates AMPA receptor (AMPAR) internalization (Greer et al., 2010). Alterations in AMPAR density and activity are apparent in several mouse models of ASD, and are likely the main contributor to alterations in mEPSCs observed in these models. In addition to its role in regulating AMPAR density in neuronal postsynaptic terminals, UBE3A targets the polycomb complex ubiquitin ligase RING1B for degradation, and UBE3A deficiency results in higher levels of RING1B and ubiquitinated histone H2A, which serves to silence developmentally regulated gene expression (Zaaroor-Regev et al., 2010). *Ube3a*-deficient mice have more subtle neurological deficits than other ASD models, but deficits in context-dependent fear conditioning have been observed (Jiang et al., 1998).

Post-translational modifications are also involved in fragile X syndrome (FXS), as phosphorylation of serine 500 of FMRP is necessary for its ability to bind RNA and repress translation (Narayanan et al., 2007). This is important given that loss of FMRP-dependent translational regulation plays a causative role in the generation of the FXS phenotype. Transfection of a S500 phosphomimetic complementary DNA construct of human *FMR1* (S500-*hFMR1*) into the *Drosophila fmr1* (*dfmr1*) null mutant was sufficient to restore brain protein translation levels (Coffee et al., 2012). Moreover, the increased synapse number observed in postmortem cortical samples of human FXS patients and *Fmr1*-deficient mouse models (Bakker et al., 1994; Mineur et al., 2002) was recapitulated in the dfmr1 null mutant at the neuromuscular junction. Transfection of the S500-*hFMR1* construct in *dfmr1* null flies restored synaptic bouton numbers to WT levels and corrected abnormalities in synaptic architecture (Coffee et al., 2012). Phosphorylation of MeCP2 on serine 421 may have a similar global function to FMRP-pS500; however, a serine to alanine substitution at amino acid 421 of MeCP2 in mice had no impact on the protein levels of MeCP2. The *Mecp2*-S421A mutant did exhibit increased complexity of layer V pyramidal neurons. MeCP2-S421 is phosphorylated upon neuronal stimulation and mEPSCs are shifted in layers II and III primary visual cortex of MeCP2-S421A mice, suggesting that an aspect of activity-dependent regulation is disrupted by changes in a post-translational modification of MeCP2 (Cohen et al., 2011). However, phosphorylation of MeCP2 on S421 is insufficient to cause the motor deficits observed in RTT patients and mouse models.

Phosphorylation of S80 appears to respond more specifically to neuronal activity, as calcium influx causes dephosphorylation at S80, which is necessary to regulate MeCP2 chromatin association and MeCP2 binding to specific gene promoters (Tao et al., 2009). A transgenic knock-in model (MeCP2-S80A), in which the serine residue at amino acid 80 is mutated to alanine, reproduces the deficit in locomotor activity observed in RTT patients and mouse models (Guy et al., 2001; Lane et al., 2011). In contrast, MeCP2-S421A;S424 knock-in mice show increased locomotor activity, concomitant with increased neuronal excitability (Tao et al., 2009). The phosphorylation events at S80 and S421;S424 demonstrate that the regulation of MeCP2 by post-translational modifications is complex, and additional investigation of other modifications will be required before there is a full understanding of their relevance to the phenotype of RTT and ASD.

One of the most well defined defects in phosphorylation has been identified in TSC1/2-deficient mice (Kwiatkowski et al., 2002). The TSC1/2 complex is a core translator of protein signal transduction and is able to respond to different physiological events upon the addition and removal of phosphate groups to TSC2. Phosphorylation of TSC2 inhibits mTOR activity, via suppression of the small G protein, RHEB, which restricts cell growth and metabolism (Inoki et al., 2005). This suggests that a failure to regulate these discrete phosphorylation events has a wide and far-reaching effect on neuronal development and function.

The X-linked gene synapsin 1 (SYN1) has been implicated in autism, learning disability, and schizophrenia. The synapsin genes encode neuronal phosphoproteins and are required for the modulation of neurotransmitter release and early synaptogenesis (Bogen et al., 2009). A nonsense mutation at Q555X in SYN1 was identified in a case of familial autism in which individuals had ASD and epilepsy, with the Q555X mutation dramatically reducing phosphorylation by CAMKII and MapK/ERK. It is likely that the changes in phosphorylation impeded neuronal development, similar to Syn1-null mice that exhibit abnormal neurite outgrowth and impaired axon elongation at later stages of development (Fassio et al., 2011). The MapK/ERK pathway has also been implicated in ASD, as ERK1/2 signaling is increased in the frontal cortex of autistic subjects (Piton et al., 2011). Further, deletion of downstream effectors of the MapK/ERK pathway causes defects in brain development and higher cognitive function. This is particularly relevant for ASD as both

22q11 deletion syndrome and 16p11.2 duplication syndrome include the ERK2 and ERK1 gene loci, respectively (Samuels et al., 2009).

The phosphorylation events observed in MeCP2, FMRP, TSC2, and SYN1 share similarities, in that they allow these proteins to modify their activity in response to external stimuli. In turn, neurons can work in cooperation to modify cortical circuitry through altering synapse number and dendritic branching. The failure to accurately integrate external neuronal activity may explain the consistent aberrations in neuronal connectivity in mouse models of ASD. The observation that MeCP2-phosphorylation mutants recapitulate many aspects of the ASD phenotype is of interest because it demonstrates that a core function of MeCP2 is to integrate changes in neuronal activity.

RTT RESCUE IN MOUSE MODELS

Due to the emergence of RTT symptoms in early postnatal development, it has been assumed that re-expression of MeCP2 during this developmental period should be sufficient to reverse the RTT phenotype. The MeCP2 'rescue' approach has been attempted with disparate results depending on the experiment, with most models showing that MeCP2 re-expression delays the onset of RTT symptoms. While these rescue models have provided hope that RTT and related ASD may be reversible after birth, there are still problems to overcome, as MeCP2-rescue mice have a life span that is decreased in comparison to wild-type mice, and subtle features of the RTT phenotype remain present.

A reversible Mecp2-null mouse line was engineered by the insertion of a Lox-stop cassette into intron 2 of Mecp2, which allowed for silencing of the endogenous gene. Subsequently, the silenced gene was conditionally activated by a tamoxifen-inducible Cre-recombinase-mediated cassette excision (Guy et al., 2007). The MeCP2-stop mouse allowed for tamoxifen-induced reactivation of Mecp2 in MeCP2-null mice. Reactivation of MeCP2 during postnatal development in $Mecp2^{-/+}$ heterozygous females rescued changes in LTP, which occurs at symptom onset. However, the same analyses were not performed in $Mecp2^{-/y}$ mice and so it is difficult to infer whether re-expression of MeCP2 in postnatal development is sufficient for rescue. In a separate study, mice expressing a Mecp2e2-specific transgene with a stop cassette were crossed with different Cre-expressing lines to allow for developmentally specific expression of MeCP2 (Giacometti et al., 2007). Despite successful reactivation of MeCP2 at different pre- and postnatal stages, only a partial rescue of the RTT phenotype was achieved with postnatal expression of MeCP2e2. However, early restoration of MeCP2e2 expression, during embryonic development using Cre expression mediated by *Nestin* or *Tau*, significantly increased the life span of the mutant mice. Since *Mecp2e1* is translated 10 times more efficiently than *Mecp2e2*, the experimental difference between expression from the endogenous locus versus only the *Mecp2e2* isoform is a likely reason for the differences in postnatal rescue between these experimental systems. When both isoforms were expressed in different transgenic mouse lines, the *Mecp2e1* high expressing lines were somewhat more efficient than a *Mecp2e2* transgenic mouse in rescuing the *Mecp2*-null phenotype, although both could mediate alleviation of symptoms (Kerr et al., 2012).

Pharmacological approaches to rescuing the RTT phenotype have also shed some light on the molecular pathways that may be implicated in ASD and possible treatment options. Focus on growth factors required for neuronal survival and maturation has received considerable interest since the finding that MeCP2 binds multiple promoters of a member of the neurotrophin family, brain-derived neurotrophic factor (BDNF). *Bdnf* is an activity-dependent gene encoding a growth factor important for neuronal and synapse maturation.

The involvement of BDNF in the pathogenesis of RTT has received a great deal of attention since conditional knockdown of *Bdnf* by 70% in the mouse produces a pathology that closely resembles that found in MeCP2-null mice (Chang et al., 2006). Several studies demonstrate that binding of MeCP2 to the *Bdnf* promoter IV regulates expression in an activity-dependent manner (Chen et al., 2003; Martinowich et al., 2003). Chen and colleagues found that membrane depolarization, which occurs due to neuronal excitation, caused phosphorylation of MeCP2 and induced transcription of *Bdnf* (Chen et al., 2003). These findings provided support for the assumption that in some instances MeCP2 is a negative regulator of gene transcription. However, if MeCP2 is a negative regulator of *Bdnf* expression then *Bdnf* levels would be expected to be higher in RTT samples, due to the lack of negative repression. In reality, reduced levels of *Bdnf* transcript and protein are consistently observed in *Mecp2*-null mice at the beginning of the symptomatic stage (6–8 weeks of age) (Chang et al., 2006; Kline et al., 2010). Furthermore, over expression of a *Bdnf* transgene in *Mecp2*-null mice partially rescued aspects of the RTT phenotype (Chang et al., 2006). Similar *Bdnf* over-expression studies have confirmed that increased *Bdnf* in MeCP2-null mice rescues or delays the onset of other aspects of the RTT phenotype, suggesting that BDNF is deficient in RTT and could be a target for therapy.

A further member of the neurotrophin family, insulin-like growth factor 1 (IGF-1) has been shown to improve aspects of the RTT phenotype in MeCP2-null mice. IGF-1 plays a similar role to BDNF during embryonic and postnatal development and is necessary for cell survival and maturation (O'Kusky et al., 2000). Administration of IGF-1 in MeCP2$^{-/y}$ mice during early postnatal development increased their life expectancy by 50% and improved locomotor defects (Tropea et al., 2009). IGF-1 also increased spontaneous ESPCs in the sensorimotor cortex of MeCP2$^{-/y}$ mice, however it did not restore synaptic activity to WT levels.

As the phenotypes associated with MeCP2 deficiency in neuronal development are indicative of decreased response to activity and subsequent synaptic maturation, neuronal growth factors such as BDNF and IGF-1 may be simply bypassing the MeCP2-dependent pathway by providing a maturational response. If so, understanding the proper regulation and delivery of these neuronal growth factors will be essential to designing improved therapies for RTT and ASD.

FUTURE DIRECTIONS

Induced pluripotent stem cells (iPSCs) have become important in the exploration of the impact MeCP2 mutations have on neuronal development and function. An initial study demonstrated that the neurons generated from RTT-iPSCs displayed similar alterations in electrophysiological properties to those identified in MeCP2-deficient mouse models. Further, there was a reduction in glutamatergic synapse number and cell soma size, implying that properties of neuronal circuit formation are impaired (Muotri et al., 2010 see also Chapter 4.3.); In subsequent studies, the electrophysical properties of RTT-iPSC-derived neurons have been better characterized. These patient-derived neurons fired fewer action potentials, and showed a decrease in the frequency of spontaneous mEPS (Farra et al., 2012). These findings further support the assumption that MeCP2 is required for the development and maintenance of neural network activity.

A drawback of the iPSC-derived neurons is that their neuronal identity has not been fully confirmed. The cerebral cortex possesses a multitude of neuronal cell types that exhibit distinct molecular and electrical characteristics. The neurons derived from iPSCs are unlikely to be truly representative of organically derived neurons, and may only be applicable to a specific type of *in vivo* neurons. Genetic and epigenetic alterations in individual iPSC lines are also common, making it somewhat difficult to ensure the causality of phenotypes ascribed to *MECP2* mutations. However, the rapid progress in iPSC technologies, combined with genomic and epigenomic sequencing technologies, is likely to ensure a better understanding of the impact of human *MECP2* mutations on neuronal phenotypes in the future.

CONCLUSIONS

Taken together, these findings suggest that MeCP2 is similar to other autism candidate genes, in that its function is required throughout the developing and mature brain. Moreover, MeCP2 shares a common feature with ASD candidate genes, such as *FMR1*, *TSC1/2*, *SYN1*, and *NLGN3/4*, in that its activity can be modulated by external events. It is likely that a failure to process neuronal activity accurately has a secondary effect of impeding neuronal circuit formation. Indeed, the prevailing disruption observed in all transgenic mouse models of ASD is altered neuronal electrical potentials. These changes in neurotransmission and efficacy are likely hallmarks of altered neuronal connectivity that is derived at the synapse. These deviations in cortical activity are further exemplified by the presence of abnormalities in social, cognitive, and motor behaviors in MeCP2-deficient mouse models and ASD mouse models.

The finding that transgenic mouse models of RTT and autism exhibit neuronal alterations in synaptic transmission, adhesion, and function in a region-specific manner provides key information into the different brain regions that are implicated in ASD. Analysis of MeCP2 function is especially noteworthy, given that MeCP2 deficiency causes severe autism in which language and social reciprocity are absent and severe stereotypies are present. In summary, the study of MeCP2 deficiency as a means of understanding ASD pathophysiology has important implications for future clinical treatments and interventions. Given that RTT rescue studies have produced some positive results, it will be important to further enhance our understanding of the impact of MeCP2 on neuronal development and maturation.

ACKNOWLEDGMENTS

We thank Rima Woods for critical reading of the manuscript and ongoing funding support from NIH R01 HD041462, R01 ES015171, R01 HD048799, and R01 NS076263 (JL), and The Denman Trust and Talisman Trust (SA).

References

Abney, J., Cutler, B., Fillbach, M., Axelrod, D., Scalettettar, B., 1997. Chromatin dynamics in interphase nuclei and its implications for nuclear structure. Journal of Cell Biology 137, 1459–1468.

Amir, R.E., Fang, P., Yu, Z., Glaze, D.G., Percy, A.K., Zoghbi, H.Y., et al., 2005. Mutations in exon 1 of MECP2 are a rare cause of Rett syndrome. Journal of Medical Genetics 42, e15.

Ariani, F., Hayek, G., Rondinella, D., Artuso, R., Mencarelli, M.A., Spanhol-Rosseto, A., et al., 2008. FOXG1 is responsible for the congenital variant of Rett syndrome. American Journal of Medical Genetics 83, 89–93.

Avivi, L., Feldman, M., 1980. Arrangement of chromosomes in the interphase nucleus. Human Genetics 55, 281–295.

Bakker, C.E., Verheij, C., Willemsen, R., Vanderhelm, R., Oerlemans, F., Vermey, M., et al., 1994. Fmr1 knockout mMice – a model to study fragile-X mental-retardation. Cell 78, 23–33.

Ballas, N., Lioy, D.T., Grunseich, C., Mandel, G., 2009. Non-cell autonomous influence of MeCP2-deficient glia on neuronal dendritic morphology. Nature Neuroscience 12, 311–317.

Balmer, D., Goldstine, J., Rao, Y.M., LaSalle, J.M., 2003. Elevated methyl-CpG-binding protein 2 expression is acquired during postnatal human brain development and is correlated with alternative polyadenylation. Journal of Molecular Medicine 81, 61–68.

Bangash, M.A., Park, J.M., Melnikova, T., Wang, D., Jeon, S.K., Lee, D., et al., 2011. Enhanced polyubiquitination of Shank3 and NMDA receptor in a mouse model of autism. Cell 145, 758–772.

Barbosa, A.C., Kim, M.S., Ertunc, M., Adachi, M., Nelson, E.D., McAnally, J., et al., 2008. MEF2C, a transcription factor that facilitates learning and memory by negative regulation of synapse numbers and function. Proceedings of the National Academy of Sciences of the United States of America 105, 9391–9396.

Bateup, H.S., Takasaki, K.T., Saulnier, J.L., Denefrio, C.L., Sabatini, B.L., 2011. Loss of Tsc1 *in vivo* impairs hippocampal mGluR-LTD and increases excitatory synaptic function. Journal of Neuroscience 31, 8862–8869.

Belichenko, N.P., Belichenko, P.V., Li, H.H., Mobley, W.C., Francke, U., 2008. Comparative study of brain morphology in Mecp2 mutant mouse models of Rett syndrome. Journal of Comparative Neurology 508, 184–195.

Bogen, I.L., Jensen, V., Hvalby, O., Walaas, S.I., 2009. Synapsin-dependent development of glutamatergic synaptic vesicles and presynaptic plasticity in postnatal mouse brain. Neuroscience 158, 231–241.

Bozdagi, O., Sakurai, T., Papapetrou, D., Wang, X., Dickstein, D.L., Takahashi, N., et al., 2010. Haploinsufficiency of the autism-associated shank3 gene leads to deficits in synaptic function, social interaction, and social communication. Molecular Autism 1, 15.

Braunschweig, D., Simcox, T., Samaco, R.C., LaSalle, J.M., 2004. X-chromosome inactivation ratios affect wild-type MeCP2 expression within mosaic Rett syndrome and Mecp2/+ mouse brain. Human Molecular Genetics 13, 1275–1286.

Buschdorf, J.P., Stratling, W.H., 2004. A WW domain binding region in methyl-CpG-binding protein MeCP2: Impact on Rett syndrome. Journal of Molecular Medicine 82, 135–143.

Carter, J.C., Capone, G.T., Kaufmann, W.E., 2008. Neuroanatomic correlates of autism and stereotypy in children with Down syndrome. NeuroReport 19, 653–656.

Chahrour, M., Zoghbi, H.Y., 2007. The story of Rett syndrome: From clinic to neurobiology. Neuron 56, 422–437.

Chahrour, M., Jung, S.Y., Shaw, C., Zhou, X., Wong, S.T., Qin, J., et al., 2008. MeCP2, a key contributor to neurological disease, activates and represses transcription. Science 320, 1224–1229.

Chang, Q., Khare, G., Dani, V., Nelson, S., Jaenisch, R., 2006. The disease progression of mecp2 mutant mice is affected by the level of BDNF expression. Neuron 49, 341–348.

Chao, H.T., Chen, H., Samaco, R.C., Xue, M., Chahrour, M., Yoo, J., et al., 2010. Dysfunction in GABA signaling mediates autism-like stereotypies and Rett syndrome phenotypes. Nature 468, 263–269.

Chao, H.T., Zoghbi, H.Y., Rosenmund, C., 2007. MeCP2 controls excitatory synaptic strength by regulating glutamatergic synapse number. Neuron 56, 58–65.

Chen, R.Z., Akbarian, S., Tudor, M., Jaenisch, R., 2001. Deficiency of methyl-CpG binding protein-2 in CNS neurons results in a Rett-like phenotype in mice. Nature Genetics 27, 327–331.

Chen, W.G., Chang, Q., Lin, Y., Meissner, A., West, A.E., Griffith, E.C., et al., 2003. Derepression of BDNF transcription involves calcium-dependent phosphorylation of MeCP2. Science 302, 885–889.

Chevere-Torres, I., Maki, J.M., Santini, E., Klann, E., 2012. Impaired social interactions and motor learning skills in tuberous sclerosis complex model mice expressing a dominant/negative form of tuberin. Neurobiology of Disease 45, 156–164.

Chih, B., Afridi, S.K., Clark, L., Scheiffele, P., 2004. Disorder-associated mutations lead to functional inactivation of neuroligins. Human Molecular Genetics 13, 1471–1477.

Chunshu, Y., Endoh, K., Soutome, M., Kawamura, R., Kubota, T., 2006. A patient with classic Rett syndrome with a novel mutation in MECP2 exon 1. Clinical Genetics 70, 530–531.

Coffee Jr., R.L., Williamson, A.J., Adkins, C.M., Gray, M.C., Page, T.L., Broadie, K., 2012. In vivo neuronal function of the fragile X mental retardation protein is regulated by phosphorylation. Human Molecular Genetics 21, 900–915.

Cohen, S., Gabel, H.W., Hemberg, M., Hutchinson, A.N., Sadacca, L.A., Ebert, D.H., et al., 2011. Genome-wide activity-dependent MeCP2 phosphorylation regulates nervous system development and function. Neuron 72, 72–85.

Collins, A.L., Levenson, J.M., Vilaythong, A.P., Richman, R., Armstrong, D.L., Noebels, J.L., et al., 2004. Mild overexpression of MeCP2 causes a progressive neurological disorder in mice. Human Molecular Genetics 13, 2679–2689.

Coutinho, A.M., Oliveira, G., Katz, C., Feng, J., Yan, J., Yang, C., et al., 2007. MECP2 coding sequence and 3′UTR variation in 172 unrelated autistic patients. American Journal of Medical Genetics. Part B, Neuropsychiatric Genetics 144B, 475–483.

Cukier, H.N., Rabionet, R., Konidari, I., Rayner-Evans, M.Y., Baltos, M.L., Wright, H.H., et al., 2010. Novel variants identified in methyl-CpG-binding domain genes in autistic individuals. Neurogenetics 11, 291–303.

Dani, V.S., Chang, Q., Maffei, A., Turrigiano, G.G., Jaenisch, R., Nelson, S.B., 2005. Reduced cortical activity due to a shift in the balance between excitation and inhibition in a mouse model of Rett syndrome. Proceedings of the National Academy of Sciences of the United States of America 102, 12,560–12,565.

Dani, V.S., Nelson, S.B., 2009. Intact long-term potentiation but reduced connectivity between neocortical layer 5 pyramidal neurons in a mouse model of Rett syndrome. Journal of Neuroscience 29, 11,263–11,270.

Dastidar, S.G., Bardai, F.H., Ma, C., Price, V., Rawat, V., Verma, P., et al., 2012. Isoform-specific toxicity of Mecp2 in postmitotic neurons: Suppression of neurotoxicity by foxG1. Journal of Neuroscience 32, 2846–2855.

Dastidar, S.G., Landrieu, P.M., D'Mello, S.R., 2011. FoxG1 promotes the survival of postmitotic neurons. Journal of Neuroscience 31, 402–413.

Deng, P.Y., Sojka, D., Klyachko, V.A., 2011. Abnormal presynaptic short-term plasticity and information processing in a mouse model of Fragile X syndrome. Journal of Neuroscience 31, 10,971–10,982.

Dinstein, I., Pierce, K., Eyler, L., Solso, S., Malach, R., Behrmann, M., et al., 2011. Disrupted neural synchronization in toddlers with autism. Neuron 70, 1218–1225.

Duerden, E.G., Mak-Fan, K.M., Taylor, M.J., Roberts, S.W., 2011. Regional differences in grey and white matter in children and adults with autism spectrum disorders: An activation likelihood estimate (ALE) meta-analysis. Autism Research 5, 49–66.

Durand, C.M., Betancur, C., Boeckers, T.M., Bockmann, J., Chaste, P., Fauchereau, F., et al., 2007. Mutations in the gene encoding the synaptic scaffolding protein SHANK3 are associated with autism spectrum disorders. Nature Genetics 39, 25–27.

Durand, C.M., Perroy, J., Loll, F., Perrais, D., Fagni, L., Bourgeron, T., et al., 2012. SHANK3 mutations identified in autism lead to modification of dendritic spine morphology via an actin-dependent mechanism. Molecular Psychiatry 17, 71–84.

Edbauer, D., Neilson, J.R., Foster, K.A., Wang, C.F., Seeburg, D.P., Batterton, M.N., et al., 2010. Regulation of synaptic structure and function by FMRP-associated microRNAs miR-125b and miR-132. Neuron 65, 373–384.

Etherton, M., Foldy, C., Sharma, M., Tabuchi, K., Liu, X., Shamloo, M., et al., 2011. Autism-linked neuroligin-3 R451C mutation differentially alters hippocampal and cortical synaptic function. Proceedings of the National Academy of Sciences of the United States of America 108, 13,764–13,769.

Etherton, M.R., Tabuchi, K., Sharma, M., Ko, J., Südhof, T.C., 2011. An autism-associated point mutation in the neuroligin cytoplasmic tail selectively impairs AMPA receptor-mediated synaptic transmission in hippocampus. EMBO Journal 30, 2908–2919.

Evans, J.C., Archer, H.L., Whatley, S.D., Kerr, A., Clarke, A., Butler, R., 2005. Variation in exon 1 coding region and promoter of MECP2 in Rett syndrome and controls. European Journal of Human Genetics 13, 124–126.

Farra, N., Zhang, W.B., Pasceri, P., Eubanks, J.H., Salter, M.W., Ellis, J., 2012. Rett syndrome induced pluripotent stem cell-derived neurons reveal novel neurophysiological alterations. Molecular Psychiatry Jan 10, doi: 10.1038/mp.2011.180. [Epub ahead of print.].

Fassio, A., Patry, L., Congia, S., Onofri, F., Piton, A., Gauthier, J., et al., 2011. SYN1 loss-of-function mutations in autism and partial epilepsy cause impaired synaptic function. Human Molecular Genetics 20, 2297–2307.

Forlani, G., Giarda, E., Ala, U., Di Cunto, F., Salani, M., Tupler, R., et al., 2010. The MeCP2/YY1 interaction regulates ANT1 expression at 4q35: Novel hints for Rett syndrome pathogenesis. Human Molecular Genetics 19, 3114–3123.

Fukuda, T., Yamashita, Y., Nagamitsu, S., Miyamoto, K., Jin, J.J., Ohmori, I., et al., 2005. Methyl-CpG binding protein 2 gene (MECP2) variations in Japanese patients with Rett syndrome: Pathological mutations and polymorphisms. Brain and Development 27, 211–217.

Ghosh, R.P., Horowitz-Scherer, R.A., Nikitina, T., Shlyakhtenko, L.S., Woodcock, C.L., 2010. MeCP2 binds cooperatively to its substrate and competes with histone H1 for chromatin binding sites. Molecular Cell Biology 30, 4656–4670.

Giacometti, E., Luikenhuis, S., Beard, C., Jaenisch, R., 2007. Partial rescue of MeCP2 deficiency by postnatal activation of MeCP2. Proceedings of the National Academy of Sciences of the United States of America 104, 1931–1936.

Gianakopoulos, P.J., Zhang, Y., Pencea, N., Orlic-Milacic, M., Mittal, K., Windpassinger, C., et al., 2012. Mutations in MECP2 exon 1 in classical Rett patients disrupt MECP2_e1 transcription, but not transcription of MECP2_e2. American Journal of Medical Genetics B, Neuropsychiatry 159B, 210–216.

Gilman, S.R., Iossifov, I., Levy, D., Ronemus, M., Wigler, M., Vitkup, D., 2011. Rare de novo variants associated with autism implicate a large functional network of genes involved in formation and function of synapses. Neuron 70, 898–907.

Girard, M., Couvert, P., Carrie, A., Tardieu, M., Chelly, J., Beldjord, C., et al., 2001. Parental origin of de novo MECP2 mutations in Rett syndrome. European Journal of Human Genetics 9, 231–236.

Gonzales, M.L., LaSalle, J.M. The role of MeCP2 in brain development and neurodevelopmental disorders. Current Opinion in Psychiatry Report 12, 127–134.

Gonzales, M.L., Adams, S., Dunaway, K.W., LaSalle, J.M., 2012. Phosphorylation of distinct sites in MeCP2 modifies cofactor associations and the dynamics of transcriptional regulation. Mol. Cell Biol 32, 2894–2903.

Greer, P.L., Hanayama, R., Bloodgood, B.L., Mardinly, A.R., Lipton, D.M., Flavell, S.W., et al., 2010. The Angelman syndrome protein

Ube3A regulates synapse development by ubiquitinating arc. Cell 140, 704–716.

Guy, J., Gan, J., Selfridge, J., Cobb, S., Bird, A., 2007. Reversal of neurological defects in a mouse model of Rett syndrome. Science 315, 1143–1147.

Guy, J., Hendrich, B., Holmes, M., Martin, J.E., Bird, A., 2001. A mouse Mecp2-null mutation causes neurological symptoms that mimic rett syndrome. Nature Genetics 27, 322–326.

Hammer, S., Dorrani, N., Dragich, J., Kudo, S., Schanen, C., 2002. The phenotypic consequences of MECP2 mutations extend beyond Rett syndrome. Mental Retardation and Developmental Disabilities Research Reviews 8, 94–98.

Hendrich, B., Abbott, C., McQueen, H., Chambers, D., Cross, S., Bird, A., 1999. Genomic structure and chromosomal mapping of the murine and human Mbd1, Mbd2, Mbd3, and Mbd4 genes. Mammalian Genome 10, 906–912.

Inoki, K., Corradetti, M.N., Guan, K.L., 2005. Dysregulation of the TSC-mTOR pathway in human disease. Nature Genetics 37, 19–24.

Itoh, M., Tahimic, C.G., Ide, S., Otsuki, A., Sasaoka, T., Noguchi, S., et al., 2012. Methyl CpG-binding protein isoform MeCP2_e2 is dispensable for Rett syndrome phenotypes but essential for embryo viability and placenta development. Journal of Biological Chemistry.

Jamain, S., Quach, H., Betancur, C., Rastam, M., Colineaux, C., Gillberg, I.C., et al., 2003. Mutations of the X-linked genes encoding neuroligins NLGN3 and NLGN4 are associated with autism. Nature Genetics 34, 27–29.

Jamain, S., Radyushkin, K., Hammerschmidt, K., Granon, S., Boretius, S., Varoqueaux, F., et al., 2008. Reduced social interaction and ultrasonic communication in a mouse model of monogenic heritable autism. Proceedings of the National Academy of Sciences of the United States of America 105, 1710–1715.

Jiang, Y.H., Armstrong, D., Albrecht, U., Atkins, C.M., Noebels, J.L., Eichele, G., et al., 1998. Mutation of the Angelman ubiquitin ligase in mice causes increased cytoplasmic p53 and deficits of contextual learning and long-term potentiation. Neuron 21, 799–811.

Kerr, B., Soto, C.J., Saez, M., Abrams, A., Walz, K., Young, J.I., 2011. Transgenic complementation of MeCP2 deficiency: Phenotypic rescue of Mecp2-null mice by isoform-specific transgenes. Journal of Biological Chemistry 287 13,859–13,867.

Kimura, H., Shiota, K., 2003. Methyl-CpG-binding protein, MeCP2, is a target molecule for maintenance DNA methyltransferase, dnmt1. Journal of Biological Chemistry 278, 4806–4812.

Klein, M.E., Lioy, D.T., Ma, L., Impey, S., Mandel, G., Goodman, R.H., 2007. Homeostatic regulation of MeCP2 expression by a CREB-induced microRNA. Nature Neuroscience 10, 1513–1514.

Kline, D.D., Ogier, M., Kunze, D.L., Katz, D.M., 2010. Exogenous brain-derived neurotrophic factor rescues synaptic dysfunction in Mecp2-null mice. Journal of Neuroscience 30, 5303–5310.

Kriaucionis, S., Bird, A., 2004. The major form of MeCP2 has a novel N-terminus generated by alternative splicing. Nucleic Acids Research 32, 1818–1823.

Kuenssberg, R., McKenzie, K., Jones, J., 2011. The association between the social and communication elements of autism, and repetitive/restrictive behaviors and activities: A review of the literature. Research in Developmental Disabilities 32, 2183–2192.

Kuhn, D.E., Nuovo, G.J., Terry Jr., A.V., Martin, M.M., Malana, G.E., Sansom, S.E., et al., 2010. Chromosome 21-derived microRNAs provide an etiological basis for aberrant protein expression in human Down syndrome brains. Journal of Biological Chemistry 285, 1529–1543.

Kwakye, L.D., Foss-Feig, J.H., Cascio, C.J., Stone, W.L., Wallace, M.T., 2011. Altered auditory and multisensory temporal processing in autism spectrum disorders. Frontiers in Integrative Neuroscience 4, 129.

Kwiatkowski, D.J., Zhang, H., Bandura, J.L., Heiberger, K.M., Glogauer, M., el-Hashemite, N., et al., 2002. A mouse model of TSC1 reveals sex-dependent lethality from liver hemangiomas, and up-regulation of p70S6 kinase activity in Tsc1 null cells. Human Molecular Genetics 11, 525–534.

Lalande, M., Calciano, M.A., 2007. Molecular epigenetics of Angelman syndrome. Cellular and Molecular Life Sciences 64, 947–960.

Lane, J.B., Lee, H.S., Smith, L.W., Cheng, P., Percy, A.K., Glaze, D.G., et al., 2011. Clinical severity and quality of life in children and adolescents with Rett syndrome. Neurology 77, 1812–1818.

LaSalle, J., Goldstine, J., Balmer, D., Greco, C., 2001. Quantitative localization of heterologous methyl-CpG-binding protein 2 (MeCP2) expression phenotypes in normal and Rett syndrome brain by laser scanning cytometry. Human Molecular Genetics 10, 1729–1740.

Le Meur, N., Holder-Espinasse, M., Jaillard, S., Goldenberg, A., Joriot, S., Amati-Bonneau, P., et al., 2010. MEF2C haploinsufficiency caused by either microdeletion of the 5q14.3 region or mutation is responsible for severe mental retardation with stereotypic movements, epilepsy and/or cerebral malformations. Journal of Medical Genetics 47, 22–29.

Li, H., Yamagata, T., Mori, M., Yasuhara, A., Momoi, M.Y., 2005. Mutation analysis of methyl-CpG binding protein family genes in autistic patients. Brain and Development 27, 321–325.

Li, H., Zhong, X., Chau, K.F., Williams, E.C., Chang, Q., 2011. Loss of activity-induced phosphorylation of MeCP2 enhances synaptogenesis, LTP and spatial memory. Nature Neuroscience 14, 1001–1008.

Loat, C.S., Curran, S., Lewis, C.M., Duvall, J., Geschwind, D., Bolton, P., et al., 2008. Methyl-CpG-binding protein 2 polymorphisms and vulnerability to autism. Genes Brain and Behavior 7, 754–760.

Maezawa, I., Swanberg, S., Harvey, D., LaSalle, J.M., Jin, L.W., 2009. Rett syndrome astrocytes are abnormal and spread MeCP2 deficiency through gap junctions. Journal of Neuroscience 29, 5051–5061.

Martinowich, K., Hattori, D., Wu, H., Fouse, S., He, F., Hu, Y., et al., 2003. DNA methylation–related chromatin remodeling in activity-dependent BDNF gene regulation. Science 302, 890–893.

Matijevic, T., Knezevic, J., Slavica, M., Pavelic, J., 2009. Rett syndrome: From the gene to the disease. European Neurology 61, 3–10.

Matson, M.L., Matson, J.L., Beighley, J.S., 2011. Comorbidity of physical and motor problems in children with autism. Research in Developmental Disabilities 32, 2304–2308.

Mikhail, F.M., Lose, E.J., Robin, N.H., Descartes, M.D., Rutledge, K.D., Rutledge, S.L., et al., 2011. Clinically relevant single gene or intragenic deletions encompassing critical neurodevelopmental genes in patients with developmental delay, mental retardation, and/or autism spectrum disorders. American Journal of Medical Genetics. A 155A, 2386–2396.

Mineur, Y.S., Sluyter, F., de Wit, S., Oostra, B.A., Crusio, W.E., 2002. Behavioral and neuroanatomical characterization of the fmr1 knockout mouse. Hippocampus 12, 39–46.

Mnatzakanian, G.N., Lohi, H., Munteanu, I., Alfred, S.E., Yamada, T., MacLeod, P.J., et al., 2004. A previously unidentified MECP2 open reading frame defines a new protein isoform relevant to Rett syndrome. Nature Genetics 36, 339–341.

Moretti, P., Bouwknecht, J.A., Teague, R., Paylor, R., Zoghbi, H.Y., 2005. Abnormalities of social interactions and home-cage behavior in a mouse model of Rett syndrome. Human Molecular Genetics 14, 205–220.

Moretti, P., Levenson, J.M., Battaglia, F., Atkinson, R., Teague, R., Antalffy, B., et al., 2006. Learning and memory and synaptic plasticity are impaired in a mouse model of Rett syndrome. Journal of Neuroscience 26, 319–327.

Moy, S.S., Nadler, J.J., Young, N.B., Nonneman, R.J., Grossman, A.W., Murphy, D.L., et al., 2009. Social approach in genetically engineered mouse lines relevant to autism. Genes Brain and Behavior 8, 129–142.

Muotri, A.R., Marchetto, M.C., Coufal, N.G., Oefner, R., Yeo, G., Nakashima, K., et al., 2010. L1 retrotransposition in neurons is modulated by MeCP2. Nature 468, 443–446.

Nagarajan, R.P., Hogart, A.R., Gwye, Y., Martin, M.R., Lasalle, J.M., 2006. Reduced MeCP2 expression is frequent in autism frontal cortex and correlates with aberrant MECP2 promoter methylation. Epigenetics 1, 172–182.

Nan, X., Meehan, R.R., Bird, A., 1993. Dissection of the methyl-CpG binding domain from the chromosomal protein MeCP2. Nucleic Acids Research 21, 4886–4892.

Nan, X., Ng, H.H., Johnson, C.A., Laherty, C.D., Turner, B.M., Eisenman, R.N., et al., 1998. Transcriptional repression by the methyl-CpG-binding protein MeCP2 involves a histone deacetylase complex. Nature 393, 386–389.

Narayanan, U., Nalavadi, V., Nakamoto, M., Pallas, D.C., Ceman, S., Bassell, G.J., et al., 2007. FMRP phosphorylation reveals an immediate-early signaling pathway triggered by group I mGluR and mediated by PP2A. Journal of Neuroscience 27, 14,349–14,357.

Nectoux, J., Heron, D., Tallot, M., Chelly, J., Bienvenu, T., 2006. Maternal origin of a novel C-terminal truncation mutation in CDKL5 causing a severe atypical form of Rett syndrome. Clinical Genetics 70, 29–33.

Neul, J.L., Zoghbi, H.Y., 2004. Rett syndrome: A prototypical neurodevelopmental disorder. Neuroscientist 10, 118–128.

Novara, F., Beri, S., Giorda, R., Ortibus, E., Nageshappa, S., Darra, F., et al., 2010. Refining the phenotype associated with MEF2C haploinsufficiency. Clinical Genetics 78, 471–477.

Nowakowska, B.A., Obersztyn, E., Szymanska, K., Bekiesinska-Figatowska, M., Xia, Z., Ricks, C.B., et al., 2010. Severe mental retardation, seizures, and hypotonia due to deletions of MEF2C. American Journal of Medical Genetics B, Neuropsychiatric Genetics 153B, 1042–1051.

O'Kusky, J.R., Ye, P., D'Ercole, A.J., 2000. Insulin-like growth factor-I promotes neurogenesis and synaptogenesis in the hippocampal dentate gyrus during postnatal development. Journal of Neuroscience 20, 8435–8442.

O'Roak, B.J., Deriziotis, P., Lee, C., Vives, L., Schwartz, J.J., Girirajan, S., et al., 2011. Exome sequencing in sporadic autism spectrum disorders identifies severe de novo mutations. Nature Genetics 43, 585–589.

Peca, J., Feliciano, C., Ting, J.T., Wang, W., Wells, M.F., Venkatraman, T.N., et al., 2011. Shank3 mutant mice display autistic-like behaviors and striatal dysfunction. Nature 472, 437–442.

Pelka, G.J., Watson, C.M., Christodoulou, J., Tam, P.P., 2005. Distinct expression profiles of Mecp2 transcripts with different lengths of 3'UTR in the brain and visceral organs during mouse development. Genomics 85, 441–452.

Penagarikano, O., Abrahams, B.S., Herman, E.I., Winden, K.D., Gdalyahu, A., Dong, H., et al., 2011. Absence of CNTNAP2 leads to epilepsy, neuronal migration abnormalities, and core autism-related deficits. Cell 147, 235–246.

Piton, A., Gauthier, J., Hamdan, F.F., Lafreniere, R.G., Yang, Y., Henrion, E., et al., 2011. Systematic resequencing of X-chromosome synaptic genes in autism spectrum disorder and schizophrenia. Molecular Psychiatry 16, 867–880.

Poirier, K., Francis, F., Hamel, B., Moraine, C., Fryns, J.P., Ropers, H.H., et al., 2005. Mutations in exon 1 of MECP2B are not a common cause of X-linked mental retardation in males. European Journal of Human Genetics 13, 523–524.

Qiu, S., Anderson, C.T., Levitt, P., Shepherd, G.M., 2011. Circuit-specific intracortical hyperconnectivity in mice with deletion of the autism-associated met receptor tyrosine kinase. Journal of Neuroscience 31, 5855–5864.

Radyushkin, K., Hammerschmidt, K., Boretius, S., Varoqueaux, F., El-Kordi, A., Ronnenberg, A., et al., 2009. Neuroligin-3-deficient mice: Model of a monogenic heritable form of autism with an olfactory deficit. Genes, Brain and Behavior 8, 416–425.

Ramocki, M.B., Peters, S.U., Tavyev, Y.J., Zhang, F., Carvalho, C.M., Schaaf, C.P., et al., 2009. Autism and other neuropsychiatric symptoms are prevalent in individuals with MeCP2 duplication syndrome. Annals of Neurology 66, 771–782.

Reardon, W., Donoghue, V., Murphy, A.M., King, M.D., Mayne, P.D., Horn, N., et al., 2010. Progressive cerebellar degenerative changes in the severe mental retardation syndrome caused by duplication of MECP2 and adjacent loci on xq28. European Journal of Pediatrics 169, 941–949.

Reith, R.M., Way, S., McKenna 3rd, J., Haines, K., Gambello, M.J., 2011. Loss of the tuberous sclerosis complex protein tuberin causes Purkinje cell degeneration. Neurobiology of Disease 43, 113–122.

Samaco, R.C., Nagarajan, R.P., Braunschweig, D., LaSalle, J.M., 2004. Multiple pathways regulate MeCP2 expression in normal brain development and exhibit defects in autism-spectrum disorders. Human Molecular Genetics 13, 629–639.

Samuels, I.S., Saitta, S.C., Landreth, G.E., 2009. MAP'ing CNS development and cognition: An ERKsome process. Neuron 61, 160–167.

Scoles, H.A., Urraca, N., Chadwick, S.W., Reiter, L.T., Lasalle, J.M., 2011. Increased copy number for methylated maternal 15q duplications leads to changes in gene and protein expression in human cortical samples. Molecular Autism 2, 19.

Shahbazian, M.D., Antalffy, B., Armstrong, D.L., Zoghbi, H.Y., 2002. Insight into Rett syndrome: MeCP2 levels display tissue- and cell-specific differences and correlate with neuronal maturation. Human Molecular Genetics 11, 115–124.

Skene, P.J., Illingworth, R.S., Webb, S., Kerr, A.R., James, K.D., Turner, D.J., et al., 2010. Neuronal MeCP2 is expressed at near histone-octamer levels and globally alters the chromatin state. Molecular Cell 37, 457–468.

Sprovieri, T., Conforti, F.L., Fiumara, A., Mazzei, R., Ungaro, C., Citrigno, L., et al., 2009. A novel mutation in the X-linked cyclin-dependent kinase-like 5 (CDKL5) gene associated with a severe Rett phenotype. American Journal of Medical Genetics A 149A, 722–725.

Stearns, N.A., Schaevitz, L.R., Bowling, H., Nag, N., Berger, U.V., Berger-Sweeney, J., 2007. Behavioral and anatomical abnormalities in Mecp2 mutant mice: A model for Rett syndrome. Neuroscience 146, 907–921.

Tabuchi, K., Blundell, J., Etherton, M.R., Hammer, R.E., Liu, X., Powell, C.M., et al., 2007. A neuroligin-3 mutation implicated in autism increases inhibitory synaptic transmission in mice. Science 318, 71–76.

Talkowski, M.E., Mullegama, S.V., Rosenfeld, J.A., van Bon, B.W., Shen, Y., Repnikova, E.A., et al., 2011. Assessment of 2q23.1 microdeletion syndrome implicates MBD5 as a single causal locus of intellectual disability, epilepsy, and autism spectrum disorder. American Journal of Human Genetics 89, 551–563.

Tao, J., Hu, K., Chang, Q., Wu, H., Sherman, N.E., Martinowich, K., et al., 2009. Phosphorylation of MeCP2 at serine 80 regulates its chromatin association and neurological function. Proceedings of the National Academy of Sciences of the United States of America 106, 4882–4887.

Trappe, R., Laccone, F., Cobilanschi, J., Meins, M., Huppke, P., Hanefeld, F., et al., 2001. MECP2 mutations in sporadic cases of Rett syndrome are almost exclusively of paternal origin. American Journal of Human Genetics 68, 1093–1101.

Tropea, D., Giacometti, E., Wilson, N.R., Beard, C., McCurry, C., Fu, D.D., et al., 2009. Partial reversal of Rett syndrome–like symptoms in MeCP2 mutant mice. Proceedings of the National Academy of Sciences of the United States of America 106, 2029–2034.

van Kooten, I.A., Palmen, S.J., von Cappeln, P., Steinbusch, H.W., Korr, H., Heinsen, H., et al., 2008. Neurons in the fusiform gyrus are fewer and smaller in autism. Brain 131, 987–999.

Wang, X., McCoy, P.A., Rodriguiz, R.M., Pan, Y., Je, H.S., Roberts, A.C., et al., 2011. Synaptic dysfunction and abnormal behaviors in mice lacking major isoforms of shank3. Human Molecular Genetics 20, 3093–3108.

Yizhar, O., Fenno, L.E., Prigge, M., Schneider, F., Davidson, T.J., O'Shea, D.J., et al., 2011. Neocortical excitation/inhibition balance in information processing and social dysfunction. Nature 477, 171–178.

Yu, J., He, X., Yao, D., Li, Z., Li, H., Zhao, Z., 2011. A sex-specific association of common variants of neuroligin genes (NLGN3 and NLGN4X) with autism spectrum disorders in a Chinese Han cohort. Behavioral and Brain Functions 7, 13.

Zaaroor-Regev, D., de Bie, P., Scheffner, M., Noy, T., Shemer, R., Heled, M., et al., 2010. Regulation of the polycomb protein ring1B by self-ubiquitination or by E6-AP may have implications to the pathogenesis of Angelman syndrome. Proceedings of the National Academy of Sciences of the United States of America 107, 6788–6793.

Zhang, R., Yamada, J., Hayashi, Y., Wu, Z., Koyama, S., Nakanishi, H., 2008. Inhibition of NMDA-induced outward currents by interleukin-1beta in hippocampal neurons. Biochemical and Biophysical Research Communications 372, 816–820.

Zhou, Z., Hong, E.J., Cohen, S., Zhao, W.N., Ho, H.Y., Schmidt, L., et al., 2006. Brain-specific phosphorylation of MeCP2 regulates activity-dependent bdnf transcription, dendritic growth, and spine maturation. Neuron 52, 255–269.

Zoncu, R., Bar-Peled, L., Efeyan, A., Wang, S., Sancak, Y., Sabatini, D.M., 2011. mTORC1 senses lysosomal amino acids through an inside-out mechanism that requires the vacuolar H(+)-ATPase. Science 334, 678–683.

Zweier, M., Gregor, A., Zweier, C., Engels, H., Sticht, H., Wohlleber, E., et al., 2010. Mutations in MEF2C from the 5q14.3q15 microdeletion syndrome region are a frequent cause of severe mental retardation and diminish MECP2 and CDKL5 expression. Human Mutation 31, 722–733.

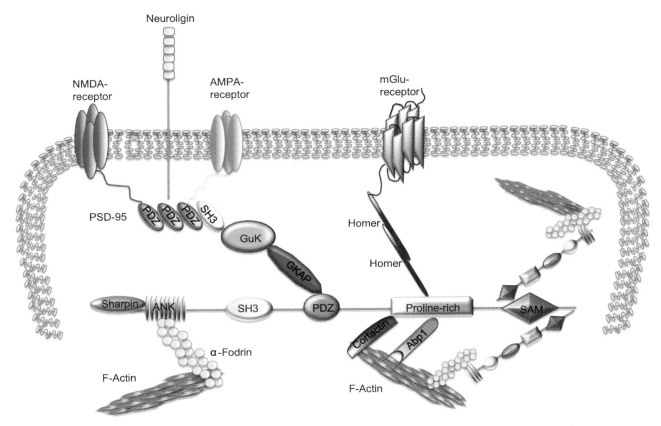

FIGURE 4.7.2 Shank proteins and the postsynaptic compartment. Please see text for further details.

Shank multimerization (Naisbitt et al., 1999). The SAM domains on adjacent molecules associate with each other and form large sheets composed of helical fibers that stack tightly side by side and form a highly ordered array, which is further organized and regulated in the presence of Zn^{2+} ions (Baron et al., 2006). Increasing levels of Zn^{2+} ions in the postsynaptic compartment following neuronal activity were found to affect the amount of Shank proteins at the PSD, and thus were implicated in the proper formation, maturation, and transmission of the synapse (Grabrücker et al., 2011a, b; Gündelfinger et al., 2006).

The PDZ Domain

Self-association of Shank molecules can be also achieved by an interaction between the PDZ (PSD95/discs large/zona-occludens-1) domains. Shank1, 2, and 3 were first identified in a yeast two-hybrid assay using the guanylate-kinase-associated protein (GKAP, also called SAPAP or DAP) as bait (Naisbitt et al., 1999). This study showed that Shank proteins bind the PDZ domain of GKAP, which is a PSD-95-binding protein that forms important components of the PSD.

The PDZ domain is widely found in scaffold proteins and is known to be essential in mediating different processes in the synapse (Feng and Zhang, 2009). In Shank proteins, besides its ability to form dimers (Im et al., 2003), the PDZ domain can also bind several PSD proteins at their C-termini through a characteristic motif (–X–T/S–R/K–L–*, where X is any amino acid, and the asterisk represents a stop codon) (Naisbitt et al., 1999). Among these interacting proteins are other scaffolding proteins, cell adhesion molecules, ion channels, transport proteins, and G-coupled receptors (Feng and Zhang, 2009). The latter group includes the somatostatin receptor type 2 (SSTR2) (Zitzer et al., 1999a, b), the CL1 receptor (Tobaben et al., 2000), and the metabotropic glutamate receptors (mGluRs) (Tu et al., 1999). Furthermore, indirect interaction between Shanks and mGluRs was found to be mediated by the Homer scaffolding proteins (Tu et al., 1999) and to be essential for mGluR5 signaling (Verpelli et al., 2011). In addition, ionotropic glutamate receptors were shown to interact directly with the Shank PDZ domain (Uemura et al., 2004) and to form an indirect interaction mediated by stargazin, which in turn binds to α-amino-3-hydroxyl-5-methyl-4-isoxazole-propionic acid (AMPA) receptors (Chen et al., 2000), and GKAP and PSD-95, which mediate binding to *N*-methyl-D-aspartic acid (NMDA) receptors (Boeckers, 2006; Gündelfinger et al., 2006; Kornau et al., 1995). This tripartite interaction of Shank, GKAP, and PSD-95 was also shown to provide linkage between Shank proteins and neuroligins, which are postsynaptic cell adhesion molecules (CAMs) that interact with the presynaptic CAMs, neurexins, to mediate synapse formation and function (Prange et al., 2004).

The Proline-Rich Domain

The proline-rich region of Shank proteins is composed of proline-rich motifs, each forming different sets of interactions. For example, Shank is known to interact with Homer through the PPXXF motif (Tu et al., 1999). Since a proline-rich motif is also found at the C terminal of the mGluRs, a dimer of Homer can interact simultaneously with both Shank and mGluR molecules, thus forming an indirect link between the two molecules (Tu et al., 1999). In this way, through the interactions of Shank with both the NMDA and mGluR receptors on the one hand, and with mGluRs on the other, Shanks provide functional integration between the metabotropic and the ionotropic glutamate receptor systems. In addition, Homer is known to be essential for the physical link between mGluRs and phospholipase C (PLC), which is further required for the signaling between the mGluR-PLC complex and IP3 receptors (Xiao et al., 1998). Since Shank proteins are known to bind Homer, mGluRs, and PLCβ (Hwang et al., 2005), it has been suggested they play a role in the organization of the mGluR/PLC/IP3/Ca^{2+} signaling pathway (Kreienkamp, 2008).

The interaction between Homer and Shank has been found to play an essential role in enhancing functional maturation of dendritic spines (Hayashi et al., 2009; Sala et al., 2001; 2003; 2005). This process depends on both the interaction between Shank and Homer and a second interaction between Homer and the endoplasmic reticulum (ER) inositol triphosphate receptor (IP3R), which stimulates the recruitment of the ER membranes to the spines.

In addition to its role in mediating Homer interaction, the proline-rich region also mediates the binding of Shank molecules with cytoskeletal components, as it was shown to interact with the SH3 domain of Abp-1 (Haeckel et al., 2008; Qualmann et al., 2004) and IRSp53 (Soltau et al., 2004) actin-binding proteins. Also, both the cortactin and the Abi-1 proteins were found to interact with Shank proteins through the proline-rich region. Cortactin promotes polymerization of the actin cytoskeleton and is an important modulator of long-term synaptic plasticity (Cingolani and Goda, 2008; Du et al., 1998) while Abi-1 regulates the RAC-dependent pathway and thus is involved in actin organization (Leng et al., 2005; Stradal et al., 2001).

The ANK Repeats Domain

The Shank ANK repeats domain (ARD) binds to the spectrin repeat 21 of α-fodrin, providing another link to the cytoskeleton. α-fodrin is a major constituent of the PSD (Carlin et al., 1983) and interacts with actin and calmodulin. This interaction may mediate calmodulin-dependent processes following synaptic stimulation. The ARD can also contribute to the self-association of Shank molecules (Romorini et al., 2004) via their interaction with an SH3 domain of a second Shank molecule. Recently, sharpin was also found to interact through the ARD (Lim et al., 2001). Sharpin is a subunit of the linear ubiquitin chain assembly complex, which is required for activation of nuclear factor kappa-B (NF-κB) signaling (Ikeda et al., 2011). NF-κB, a transcription factor, is known to be activated in synapses in response to excitatory synaptic transmission and may play a role in signaling to the nucleus and in processes such as neuronal survival, learning, and memory (Freudenthal et al., 2004; Meffert et al., 2003). Activation of NF-κB in cultured rat hippocampal neurons modulates AMPA subunits (Furukawa and Mattson, 1998) and loss of NF-κB reduces spine density and the amplitude of synaptic responses in hippocampal cultures (Boersma et al., 2011). Interestingly, in one of the Shank3 mutant mouse models, which will be discussed later in this chapter, targeting the C-terminal and disrupting the Homer-Shank3 complex leads to increased ubiquitination and proteasomal degradation of the remaining wild-type Shank3 (Bangash et al., 2011), which links the mutant Shank3 to the ubiquitin/proteasome pathway.

PSD Targeting and Subcellular Localization

Localization of Shank proteins shows defined patterns of expression and localization during neuronal development. Immunoelectron microscopy has shown that the Shank molecules are located in deeper parts of the PSD than other scaffolding proteins (Valtschanoff and Winberg, 2001). Studies in cultured neurons and in the developing rat brain revealed that in early stages of PSD development, Shank molecules are highly enriched in growth cones of neurons, while later in neuronal development, at the time synaptic contacts are formed, Shank molecules are relocalized to the PSD (Boeckers et al., 1999a; Du et al., 1998; Lim et al., 1999; Naisbitt et al., 1999). For Shank1, the targeting to the PSD depends on its PDZ domain and occurs only after the PSD-95-GKAP complex is recognized (Naisbitt et al., 1999; Sala et al., 2001), whereas Shank2 and Shank3 targeting is dependent on the SAM domain and occurs prior to Shank1 recruitment (Boeckers et al., 2005). This process is tightly coordinated, with Shank2 shown to be the first Shank protein that becomes concentrated at the synapse, followed by Shank3, and finally the clustering of Shank1 leads to maturation of the synaptic contacts (Grabrücker et al., 2011a, b). Activity-induced changes in the distribution of Shanks at hippocampal synapses are also different and Shank1 appears to be a dynamic element within the spine (Tao-Cheng et al., 2010).

Studies on Shank mRNA subcellular distribution revealed that, although the vast majority of the Shank mRNA molecules are localized in the cell bodies of the neurons, there is a dendritic localization of Shank1 transcripts (Bockers et al., 2004; Zitzer et al., 1999b). These transcripts were suggested to be locally translated in the postsynaptic compartment, a process that could be initiated upon synaptic stimulation (Steward and Levy, 1982; Steward and Schuman, 2001), hence implicating the Shank proteins in underlying mechanisms of synaptic plasticity.

PHYSIOLOGICAL FUNCTION OF SHANK PROTEINS

Quantitative analysis has indicated that the number of Shank3 molecules in a single postsynaptic site is 100–450, representing ~ 5% of the total protein molecules and total protein mass (Sugiyama et al., 2005). Therefore, it is not surprising that alteration in Shank expression could profoundly affect synaptic morphology and function. This observation was supported by over-expression experiments in transfected hippocampal neurons, which demonstrated that increased levels of Shank1 and Shank3, independently, led to an increased spine size (Sala et al., 2001). On the other hand, decreased levels of Shank1 have been shown to lead to decreased spine number and size and to reduced PSD thickness (Hung et al., 2008). Most dramatically, introducing Shank3 into aspiny cerebellar neurons *in vitro* led to the generation of spines with functional glutamatergic synapses expressing NMDA, AMPA, and mGlu receptors (Roussignol et al., 2005). In addition, recent studies showed that altering the synaptic levels of Shank2 and Shank3 by changing the extracellular Zn^{2+} concentration influenced PSD size and affected the assembly of the immature synapse (Grabrücker et al., 2011b; Sugiyama et al., 2005).

Taken together, these findings support a role of Shank proteins in the maturation, morphology, and functioning of the synapse. These findings were recently extended by studies from four different groups, each of which has developed and characterized

a Shank-deficient mouse. The results from these studies will be discussed later in this chapter. Notably, much of the *in vivo* work has targeted the Shank3 gene. This choice was made based on the substantial evidence from both genetic and molecular studies that demonstrated the important clinical significance of the Shank3 gene in developmental delay syndromes and autism spectrum disorders (ASD).

CLINICAL RELEVANCE

Chromosome deletion 22q13 deletion syndrome (22q13DS), also known as Phelan–McDermid syndrome, was first described in 1994. Since then, more than 100 cases have been reported in the literature and share common characteristic features including global developmental delay, moderate to profound intellectual disability, decreased muscle tone (hypotonia), and absent or delayed speech (Phelan, 2008), while in 50% or more of the patients, autistic-like behaviors were reported (Cusmano-Ozog et al., 2007; Dhar et al., 2011).

This disorder is caused by microdeletions of terminal segments at the long arm of chromosome 22 (Phelan et al., 2001). Careful analysis of the extent of the deletion in dozens of independent cases revealed that the size of the deleted segment could vary from less than 100 kb to more than 9 Mb. Analysis of the shortest deletion detected by traditional methods indicated the presence of a small 'critical region' which harbors three genes: *ACR*, *RABL2B*, and *SHANK3* (Anderlid et al., 2002). Among these genes, *SHANK3* was found to be the strongest candidate for the neurobehavioral symptoms observed in individuals with 22q13, providing the first line of evidence that a dysfunction in *SHANK3* may be responsible for the neurobehavioral aspects of 22q13DS (Dhar et al., 2011; Luciani et al., 2003; Wilson et al., 2003). This has been reinforced further by the discovery of microdeletions that preserve the other genes in the interval, leaving only *SHANK3* as the causal gene (Bonaglia et al., 2011). A second line of evidence was the demonstration of breakpoints within *SHANK3* in several cases with 22q13DS (Phelan, 2008). The first case was described by Bonaglia et al. (2001), who reported a breakpoint in the *SHANK3* gene due to a *de novo* balanced translocation between chromosomes 12 and 22 (Bonaglia et al., 2001). In 2006, the same group of researchers reported a recurrent breakpoint, in two unrelated patients, within intron 8 of the *SHANK3* gene (Bonaglia et al., 2006). These findings were further supported by discoveries from recent studies that also identified translocations or deletions at the *SHANK3* gene in ASD subjects (Bonaglia et al., 2011; Dhar et al., 2011; Durand et al., 2007; Marshall et al., 2008; Moessner et al., 2007).

Finally, several studies have reported deletions and point mutations in the *SHANK3* gene in patients ascertained with ASD (but having all common phenotypes of 22q13DS including absent or delayed speech and mild to moderate intellectual disability). The *de novo* mutations included insertion or deletion of amino acids that led to the production of a truncated protein through the introduction of a stop codon or by affecting donor or acceptor splicing sites (Durand et al., 2007; Gauthier et al., 2009; Hamdan et al., 2011; Moessner et al., 2007) (Figure 4.7.3). It is also worth mentioning that *de novo* missense and nonsense mutations in *SHANK3* have also been described in atypical schizophrenia, suggesting a molecular genetic link between these two neurodevelopmental disorders (Gauthier et al., 2010). Recently, an *in vitro* study has evaluated the contribution of the two inherited variations (R12C and R300C) and two of the *de novo* mutations (A962G and InsG3680) to the development of dendritic spines and synaptic transmission (Durand et al., 2011). Interestingly, overexpression of *SHANK3* may also result in ASD, as evidenced by a report of Asperger syndrome in an individual with three copies of *SHANK3* locus (Moessner et al., 2007).

As for the other Shank members, *de novo* mutations and deletions in the *SHANK2* gene were recently reported in individuals with ASD and/or intellectual disability (Berkel et al., 2010; Leblond et al., 2012; Pinto et al., 2010). One recent report analyzed copy number variants from 996 individuals with ASD and discovered a deletion removing most exons of *SHANK1* in an individual with ASD (Sato et al., 2011).

ANIMAL MODELS DERIVED FROM SHANK MUTATIONS

Genetically engineered mice that lack members of the Shank family of proteins are important, both to study the function of the proteins and as animal models for ASD. These models are one means of understanding the pathophysiology of ASD, and discovering new treatments.

Shank1-Deficient Mice

A first mouse model to investigate the function of Shank *in vivo* was generated by disruption of the *SHANK1* gene (Hung et al., 2008). Shank1 mutants showed altered PSD protein composition with reduced dendritic spine size, smaller and thinner PSDs, and reduced basal synaptic transmission. GKAP and Homer 1b/c levels in PSD fractions were reduced, but levels of the NMDA and AMPA receptors and mGluR subunits that were tested, as well as levels of PSD-95, were unchanged. Synaptic plasticity was normal in these mice. Behaviorally, they had increased anxiety-related behavior and impaired contextual fear memory. Performance in a spatial learning task was enhanced, but long-term memory retention in this task was impaired in these mice. Subsequent studies support the interpretation that Shank1 knockout mice do not demonstrate ASD-relevant social interaction deficits, but confirm and extend a role for Shank1 in motor functions (Silverman et al., 2011). Interestingly, another recent study of Shank1 knockout pups showed deficits in ultrasonic vocalization production, indicating a specific deficit in communicative behavior in Shank1 knockout mice (Wöhr et al., 2011). In adulthood, Shank1 mutant males deposited fewer scent marks in proximity to female urine than controls (Wöhr et al., 2011).

Shank3-Deficient Mice

Given the importance of Shank3 in synaptic structure and function, as well as the relation between ASD behaviors and mutations in this gene, four independent research teams created mouse models with *Shank3* mutations, in order to further understand the function of Shank3, the pathophysiology of Shank3 deficiency, the phenotypic consequences of the mutations, and to identify therapeutic targets (Bangash et al., 2011; Bozdagi et al., 2010; Peça et al., 2011; Wang et al., 2011) (Figure 4.7.4, Table 4.7.1).

A mouse model with a targeted disruption of *Shank3* exons 4–9 (coding for the ANK domain), disrupting full-length Shank3 (also referred as Shank3a), was the first published mouse model of Shank3 deficiency

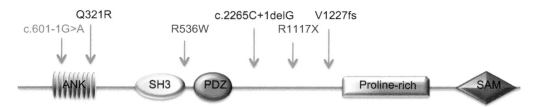

FIGURE 4.7.3 Published pathogenic human mutations in *SHANK3*. *De novo* missense, nonsense, frameshift, and splice site mutations found in ASD (black), intellectual disability (red), and atypical schizophrenia (blue) are shown. The two splice site mutations have been confirmed to introduce aberrant splicing and a premature stop. Additional *de novo* loss-of-function variants have been identified in clinical sequencing studies.

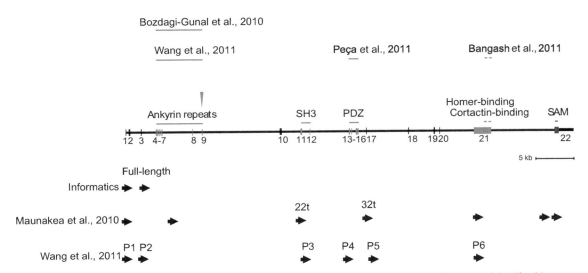

FIGURE 4.7.4 *Shank3* gene structure, mouse models, and alternative gene products. Top: targeted domains of the *Shank3* gene are shown at the ANK, PDZ, and Homer-binding domains. Bottom: start sites for alternate gene products are shown for bioinformatic analysis of full-length Shank3, as well as for two *in vitro* studies. Shank3a corresponds to the full-length protein, Shank3b likely corresponds to products beginning at the SH3 domain, and Shank3c likely corresponds to products beginning just after the PDZ domain.

(Bozdagi et al., 2010). Data from patients show that point mutations in the ANK domain lead to ASD and ID, making this mutation of direct clinical relevance (Hamdan et al., 2011; Moessner et al., 2007) (see Figure 4.7.3). Bozdagi and colleagues examined excitatory glutamatergic synaptic transmission in hippocampal slices from Shank3 heterozygous and wild-type littermates. Heterozygous mice showed deficits in synaptic function and plasticity, specifically in long-term potentiation

(LTP) and reduced basal synaptic transmission, particularly in the AMPA receptor-dependent component. The authors also examined the effect of Shank3 deficiency on spine structure during LTP. Parallel electrophysiological and two photon analyses of spine volume demonstrated persistent expansion of spines in control mice after LTP-inducing stimuli, while only transient spine expansion was observed in *Shank3* heterozygous mice. The group then studied the density of GluR1-immunoreactive

TABLE 4.7.1 Summary of Shank3-Deficient Mouse Models

Measure	Shank3a (e4−9) heterozygotes	Shank3a (e4−9) knockouts	Shank3a (e4−8) knockouts	Shank3b (PDZ) knockouts	Shank3+/ΔC heterozygotes
Electrophysiology	Impaired I/O function and LTP (CA1)	Impaired LTP (CA1)	Modest reduction in I/O function (striatum)	Impaired I/O function and reduced LTP (striatum)	Impaired LTP, NMDA-LTD, increased mGluR-LTD (CA1)
Biochemistry		Reduced Homer1b/c, GKAP, GluR1, and NR2A (CA1)		Reduced Homer 1b/c, GluR2, NR2A, and NR2B (striatum)	Reduced NR1 (CA1)
Morphology	Reduced GluR1 puncta (CA1), impaired spine stability	Increased spine length and decreased spine density (CA1)		Increased dendritic arborization and decreased spine density (striatum)	Normal synaptic morphology
Behavior	Decreased social sniffing and US (male-female), motor deficit; normal MWM and novel object recognition	Impaired US, increased self-grooming and repetitive behavior, motor deficit, impaired MWM and novel object recognition		Reduced social interaction, increased self-grooming, increased anxiety, normal motor function	Reduced social interaction, impaired US, impaired PPI, normal MWM and fear conditioning

I/O = input/output; LTD = long-term depression; MWM = Morris water maze; PPI = paired-impulse inhibition; US = ultrasonic vocalization.

puncta in the CA1 stratum radiatum, and observed a decrease in GluR1-immunoreactive puncta in Shank3 heterozygous mice. Behavioral analysis of these mice documented reduced reciprocal social interactions, as evidenced by less social sniffing and reduced numbers of ultrasonic vocalizations during interactions between male Shank3 heterozygous mice and estrus female mice. Further analyses of behavioral parameters in two additional cohorts representing Shank3 knockout mice, along with their heterozygous and wild-type littermates, also revealed deficits in motor functions (Yang et al., 2011).

In a second study two lines were generated, targeting either the ANK or PDZ domains. The former disrupted full-length Shank3, and the latter disrupted additional shorter forms (Peca et al., 2011). In these mice, each mutant allele had distinct effects on what are identified as three Shank3 isoforms, Shank3a, 3b, and 3c. ANK-domain-targeted knockout mice lacked expression of Shank3a, while other isoforms were unaffected. In the PDZ-targeted knockout mice, both the Shank3a and Shank3b isoforms were absent and the level of Shank3c was reduced.

The authors showed that mice with knockout of the PDZ domain developed potential ASD-like behaviors, evidenced by deficits in social interaction as measured by time spent with a conspecific, as well as increased anxiety and excessive grooming. Mice with targeted disruption of the ANK domain showed little behavioral change compared to controls. Electrophysiological analyses showed altered corticostriatal input-output functions in the mice with a knockout of the PDZ domain, without any change in hippocampal synaptic function. There were also reductions in AMPAR-mEPSC frequency and peak mEPSC amplitude in striatal medium spiny neurons in mice with knockout of the PDZ domain. The striatum of the Shank3b knockout mice showed several morphological features consistent with reduced neuronal signaling. Thus, dendritic arborizations in medium spiny neurons showed increased complexity with increase in total dendritic length and surface area but decrease in spine density, without any change in spine head diameter. Levels of several scaffolding proteins, including SAPAP3, Homer1, PSD93, and glutamate receptor subunits GluR2, NR2A, and NR2B were reduced in PDZ-targeted knockout mice.

An additional mouse model was created by using a strategy similar to the one followed by Bozdagi et al. (2010), targeting the ANK domain and disrupting full-length Shank3 (Shank3a), and the effects of the loss of both copies of *Shank3* were studied (Wang et al., 2011). Behavioral studies showed that Shank3a knockout led to impairments in social approach and affiliation, and communication deficits. These mice do not initiate interaction, while also spending more time grooming. There

were modest learning difficulties as measured in the Morris water maze test, as well as obsessive behaviors and mild motor abnormalities with tests in vertical placement, climbing down a vertical pole, foot-misplacement tasks, and accelerating rotarod, particularly in Shank3a knockout males. Additionally, when presented with a novel object, these mice demonstrated reduced exploratory behavior. Knockout mice also displayed impaired LTP and altered dendritic spine morphology. Biochemical analyses revealed decreased levels of synaptic proteins including GKAP, Homer 1b/c, and subunits of AMPA (GluR1 subunit) and NMDA (NR2A subunit) receptors.

Using a different approach, Bangash et al. (2011) created a Shank3 mouse with deletion of the Homer-interacting region of the Shank3 protein, referred to as Shank3+/ΔC. The model was based on clinical cases that disrupt exon 21, one with a balanced translocation affecting this region and the other with a guanine insertion in exon 21 (Bonaglia et al., 2001; Durand et al., 2007). Interestingly, in this model the heterozygous Shank3 mutation resulted in downregulation of wild-type Shank3 and also the NR1 subunit of NMDA receptor, through increased polyubiquitination; hence this model seems to generate a product that is a dominant negative. The decrease in Shank3 levels resulted in a phenotype that included deficits in social approach and communication; however, these mice did not show any deficits in long-term and short-term spatial memory, context or cue-related fear memory, anxiety or learning of motor skills. Electrophysiological results demonstrated reduced amplitude of NMDAR responses together with reduced NMDAR-dependent LTP and long-term depression (LTD), and enhanced mGluR-dependent LTD, in the heterozygote mice.

Shank2-Deficient Mice

Given that several mutations and small deletions in *SHANK2* have been identified in patients (Berkel et al., 2010), characterization of a rodent model with *Shank2* disruption is important in ASD. Berkel et al. (2012) have analyzed the functional impact caused by two inherited and one *de novo SHANK2* mutation from ASD individuals' (L1008_P1009dup, T1127M, R462X) cells. This group observed a dominant-negative effect when expressing *SHANK2*-R462X for two to three weeks. All mutations led to smaller spines, fewer synapses, and more complex dendritic branches, and one of the mutated forms, R462X, was shown to be mislocalized. Mice over expressing R462X show reduction in miniature postsynaptic AMPA receptor currents in hippocampal-infected neurons compared with neurons over expressing the *SHANK2* wild-type isoform and wild-type neurons. These mice are also less likely to investigate a novel object, and are less capable at navigating a maze (Berkel et al., 2012). Shank2-deficient mice were recently created and characterized by two different groups (Schmeisser et al., 2012; Won et al., 2012). In both mouse models, the targeted deletion resulted in the loss of the Shank2a and Shank2b isoforms and led to reduced social interaction, impairment in social communication, hyperactivity, and repetitive and anxiety-like behaviors. Despite the similarity in behavioral phenotypes, these mouse models exhibited different phenotypes in regard to synaptic transmission. Electrophysiological analysis of the Shank2-deficient mice produced by Schmeisser et al. (2012) revealed reduced basal synaptic transmission, significant reduction in mEPSC frequency, and increased NMDA/AMPA ratio in the CA1 pyramidal cells, when compared to their wild-type littermates. In contrast, analysis of the Shank2-deficient mice produced by Won et al. (2012) revealed that basal transmission in the same brain region was normal, while the LTP and LTD measures were impaired due to NMDA hypofunction, supported by reduced NMDA/AMPA ratio in Shank2-deficient mice, when compared to their wild-type littermates. In agreement with the electrophysiological measures, biochemical analysis of the Shank2-deficint mice by the Schmeisser group revealed an early brain region-specific increase in synaptic levels of NMDAR subunits. This group also reported elevated levels of Shank3 in all analyzed brain regions. No changes were detected in the levels of the glutamate receptor subunits or the Shank3 protein in other Shank2-deficient mice, but a reduction in the phosphorylated fraction of NMDAR-associated signaling components, including CaMKII-/, ERK1/2, and P38, were revealed. Based on these findings, the Won group hypothesized that Shank2 deficiency could lead to reduced NMDAR function. They further supported their hypothesis by demonstrating that enhancement of NMDAR function can reverse the impairment in NMDAR/AMPA ratio and improve the social behavior of the knockout mice.

SHANK AND OTHER MONOGENIC FORMS OF ASD AND GLUTAMATE SIGNALING

The studies above highlight the importance of Shank proteins in glutamatergic signaling and the role of disruptedv glutamatergic signaling in ASD. Several monogenic forms of ASD are the result of disruptions of proteins that are part of the empirically defined AMPA or NMDA receptor complex. In addition to the Shank mutations, in *GRIA3, GRIN2B, HRAS, L1CAM, MAP2K1, NF1, NLGN3, NLGN4, PTPN11, STXBP1, SYN-GAP1,* and *YWHAE,* all of which are found in AMPA or NMDA receptor complexes, can produce an ASD

phenotype. This underscores the importance of alterations in glutamate signaling, and especially ionotropic signaling, where perturbing different components of the pathway can contribute to the same core symptoms characteristic of ASD.

At the same time, there is likely overlap in pathways even for genes not associated with the receptor complexes. For example, a recent protein interactome study revealed high connectivity between Shank and TCS1, suggesting that common molecular pathways underlie ASD phenotypes in distinct syndromes (Sakai et al., 2011). Another recent study identified protein targets for FMRP using a CLIP assay, which identified Shank3 as an FMRP target, supporting glutamate synaptic dysfunction as a key hypothesis for neural mechanisms of ASD (Darnell et al., 2011). Note that in an earlier study (Schütt et al., 2009), concentrations of Shank1 mRNA and protein levels were found to be altered in the neocortex and hippocampus of Fmrp-deficient mice.

CONCLUSIONS

There is strong evidence for a role for Shank proteins and the Shank pathway in ASD. Shank proteins, as key functional components of the excitatory synapse, provide evidence that synaptic dysfunction is part of the etiology of ASD. Pharmacological treatments targeting the primary deficits in ASD do not yet exist. However, recent experimental therapies have been developed, which target underlying pathophysiology using discoveries made through the neurobiological analyses of model systems, including fragile X syndrome, tuberous sclerosis, and Rett syndrome (Bear et al. 2004; Ehninger and Silva 2009; Tropea et al., 2009). Unpublished research (Bozdagi et al.,) shows beneficial effects of IGF-1 treatment in reversing the defects in synaptic function and plasticity in Shank3 heterozygous mice, and this has in turn led to a clinical trial with IGF-1. These various studies provide a basis for optimism around improved therapeutics for ASD, arising out of basic neurobiological studies of genetic models. Considering the role of Shank proteins in ASD and in glutamatergic function, the glutamatergic system could be an important target for treatment in Shank deficiencies and in ASD broadly.

References

Anderlid, B.M., Schoumans, J., Anneren, G., Tapia-Paez, I., Dumanski, J., Blennow, E., et al., 2002. FISH-mapping of a 100-kb terminal 22q13 deletion. Human Genetics 110, 439–443.

Bangash, M.A., Park, J.M., Melnikova, T., Wang, D., Jeon, S.K., Lee, D., et al., 2011. Enhanced polyubiquitination of Shank3 and NMDA receptor in a mouse model of autism. Cell 145, 758–772.

Baron, M.K., Boeckers, T.M., Vaida, B., Faham, S., Gingery, M., Sawaya, M.R., et al., 2006. An architectural framework that may lie at the core of the postsynaptic density. Science 311, 531–535.

Bear, M.F., Huber, K.M., et al., 2004. The mGluR theory of fragile X mental retardation. Trends in Neurosciences 27, 370–377.

Beri, S., Tonna, N., Menozzi, G., Bonaglia, M.C., Sala, C., Giorda, R., 2007. DNA methylation regulates tissue-specific expression of Shank3. Journal of Neurochemistry 101, 1380–1391.

Berkel, S., Marshall, C.R., Weiss, B., Howe, J., Roeth, R., Moog, U., et al., 2010. Mutations in the SHANK2 synaptic scaffolding gene in autism spectrum disorder and mental retardation. Nature Genetics 42, 489–491.

Berkel, S., Tang, W., Treviño, M., Vogt, M., Obenhaus, H.A., Gass, P., et al., 2012. Inherited and *de novo* SHANK2 variants associated with autism spectrum disorder impair neuronal morphogenesis and physiology. Human Molecular Genetics 21, 344–357.

Boeckers, T.M., 2006. The postsynaptic density. Cell and Tissue Research 326, 409–422.

Boeckers, T.M., 2011. Autism Symposium. Society for Neuroscience Meeting.

Boeckers, T.M., Bockmann, J., Kreutz, M.R., Gündelfinger, E.D., 2002. ProSAP/Shank proteins – a family of higher order organizing molecules of the postsynaptic density with an emerging role in human neurological disease. Journal of Neurochemistry 81, 903–910.

Boeckers, T.M., Kreutz, M.R., Winter, C., Zuschratter, W., Smalla, K.H., Sanmarti-Vila, L., et al., 1999. Proline-rich synapse-associated protein-1/cortactin binding protein 1 (ProSAP1/CortBP1) is a PDZ-domain protein highly enriched in the postsynaptic density. Journal of Neuroscience 19, 6506–6518.

Boeckers, T.M., Liedtke, T., Spilker, C., Dresbach, T., Bockmann, J., Kreutz, M.R., et al., 2005. C-terminal synaptic targeting elements for postsynaptic density proteins ProSAP1/Shank2 and ProSAP2/Shank3. Journal of Neurochemistry 92, 519–524.

Bockers, T.M., Segger-Junius, M., Iglauer, P., Bockmann, J., Gündelfinger, E.D., Kreutz, M.R., et al., 2004. Differential expression and dendritic transcript localization of Shank family members: Identification of a dendritic targeting element in the 3′ untranslated region of Shank1 mRNA. Molecular and Cellular Neuroscience 26, 182–190.

Boeckers, T.M., Winter, C., Smalla, K.H., Kreutz, M.R., Bockmann, J., Seidenbecher, C., et al., 1999. Proline-rich synapse-associated proteins ProSAP1 and ProSAP2 interact with synaptic proteins of the SAPAP/GKAP family. Biochemical and Biophysical Research Communications 264, 247–252.

Boersma, M.C., Dresselhaus, E.C., De Biase, L.M., Mihalas, A.B., Bergles, D.E., Meffert, M.K., 2011. A requirement for nuclear factor-kappaB in developmental and plasticity-associated synaptogenesis. Journal of Neuroscience 31, 5414–5425.

Bonaglia, M.C., Giorda, R., Beri, S., De Agostini, C., Novara, F., Fichera, M., et al., 2011. Molecular mechanisms generating and stabilizing terminal 22q13 deletions in 44 subjects with Phelan/McDermid syndrome. PLoS Genetics 7, e1002173.

Bonaglia, M.C., Giorda, R., Borgatti, R., Felisari, G., Gagliardi, C., Selicorni, A., et al., 2001. Disruption of the ProSAP2 gene in a t(12;22)(q24.1;q13.3) is associated with the 22q13.3 deletion syndrome. American Journal of Medical Genetics 69, 261–268.

Bonaglia, M.C., Giorda, R., Mani, E., Aceti, G., Anderlid, B.M., Baroncini, A., et al., 2006. Identification of a recurrent breakpoint within the SHANK3 gene in the 22q13.3 deletion syndrome. Journal of Medical Genetics 43, 822–828.

Bozdagi, O., Sakurai, T., Anderson, T., Patil, S., Buxbaum, J.D., 2011. IGF-1 reverses LTP deficits in a Shank3-deficient mouse. Autism Spectrum, Disorders Cell Symposia.

Bozdagi, O., Sakurai, T., Papapetrou, D., Wang, X., Dickstein, D.L., Takahashi, N., et al., 2010. Haploinsufficiency of the autism-associated Shank3 gene leads to deficits in synaptic function, social interaction, and social communication. Molecular Autism 1, 15.

Carlin, R.K., Bartelt, D.C., Siekevitz, P., 1983. Identification of fodrin as a major calmodulin-binding protein in postsynaptic density preparations. Journal of Cell Biology 96, 443–448.

Chen, L., Chetkovich, D.M., Petralia, R.S., Sweeney, N.T., Kawasaki, Y., Wenthold, R.J., et al., 2000. Stargazin regulates synaptic targeting of AMPA receptors by two distinct mechanisms. Nature 408, 936–943.

Ching, T.T., Maunakea, A.K., Jun, P., Hong, C., Zardo, G., Pinkel, D., et al., 2005. Epigenome analyses using BAC microarrays identify evolutionary conservation of tissue-specific methylation of SHANK3. Nature Genetics 37, 645–651.

Cingolani, L.A., Goda, Y., 2008. Actin in action: The interplay between the actin cytoskeleton and synaptic efficacy. Nature Reviews Neuroscience 9, 344–356.

Cusmano-Ozog, K., Manning, M.A., Hoyme, H.E., 2007. 22q13.3 deletion syndrome: A recognizable malformation syndrome associated with marked speech and language delay. American Journal of Medical Genetics. Part C, Seminars in Medical Genetics 145C, 393–398.

Darnell, J.C., Van Driesche, S.J., Zhang, C., Hung, K.Y., Mele, A., Fraser, C.E., et al., 2011. FMRP stalls ribosomal translocation on mRNAs linked to synaptic function and autism. Cell 146, 247–261.

Dhar, S.U., del Gaudio, D., German, J.R., Peters, S.U., Ou, Z., Bader, P.I., et al., 2011. 22q13.3 deletion syndrome: Clinical and molecular analysis using array CGH. American Journal of Medical Genetics. Part A 152A, 573–581.

Du, Y., Weed, S.A., Xiong, W.C., Marshall, T.D., Parsons, J.T., 1998. Identification of a novel cortactin SH3 domain-binding protein and its localization to growth cones of cultured neurons. Molecular and Cellular Biology 18, 5838–5851.

Durand, C.M., Betancur, C., Boeckers, T.M., Bockmann, J., Chaste, P., Fauchereau, F., et al., 2007. Mutations in the gene encoding the synaptic scaffolding protein SHANK3 are associated with autism spectrum disorders. Nature Genetics 39, 25–27.

Durand, C.M., Perroy, J., Loll, F., Perrais, D., Fagni, L., Bourgeron, T., et al., 2011. SHANK3 mutations identified in autism lead to modification of dendritic spine morphology via an actin-dependent mechanism. Molecular Psychiatry 17, 71–84.

Ehninger, D., Silva, A.J., 2009. Genetics and neuropsychiatric disorders: Treatment during adulthood. Nature Medicine 15, 849–850.

Feng, W., Zhang, M., 2009. Organization and dynamics of PDZ-domain-related supramodules in the postsynaptic density. Nature Reviews Neuroscience 10, 87–99.

Freudenthal, R., Romano, A., Routtenberg, A., 2004. Transcription factor NF-kappaB activation after in vivo perforant path LTP in mouse hippocampus. Hippocampus 14, 677–683.

Furukawa, K., Mattson, M.P., 1998. The transcription factor NF-kappaB mediates increases in calcium currents and decreases in NMDA- and AMPA/kainate-induced currents induced by tumor necrosis factor-alpha in hippocampal neurons. Journal of Neurochemistry 70, 1876–1886.

Gauthier, J., Champagne, N., Lafreniere, R.G., Xiong, L., Spiegelman, D., Brustein, E., et al., 2010. *De novo* mutations in the gene encoding the synaptic scaffolding protein SHANK3 in patients ascertained for schizophrenia. Proceedings of the National Academy of Sciences of the United States of America 107, 7863–7868.

Gauthier, J., Spiegelman, D., Piton, A., Lafreniere, R.G., Laurent, S., St-Onge, J., et al., 2009. Novel *de novo* SHANK3 mutation in autistic patients. American Journal of Medical Genetics. Part B, Neuropsychiatric Genetics 150B, 421–424.

Grabrücker, A.M., Knight, M.J., Proepper, C., Bockmann, J., Joubert, M., Rowan, M., et al., 2011. Concerted action of zinc and ProSAP/Shank in synaptogenesis and synapse maturation. EMBO Journal 30, 569–581.

Grabrücker, A.M., Schmeisser, M.J., Udvardi, P.T., Arons, M., Schoen, M., Woodling, N.S., et al., 2011. Amyloid beta protein-induced zinc sequestration leads to synaptic loss via dysregulation of the ProSAP2/Shank3 scaffold. Molecular Neurodegeneration 6, 65.

Gündelfinger, E.D., Boeckers, T.M., Baron, M.K., Bowie, J.U., 2006. A role for zinc in postsynaptic density asSAMbly and plasticity? Trends in Biochemical Sciences 31, 366–373.

Haeckel, A., Ahuja, R., Gündelfinger, E.D., Qualmann, B., Kessels, M.M., 2008. The actin-binding protein Abp1 controls dendritic spine morphology and is important for spine head and synapse formation. Journal of Neuroscience 28, 10,031–10,044.

Hamdan, F.F., Gauthier, J., Araki, Y., Lin, D.T., Yoshizawa, Y., Higashi, K., et al., 2011. Excess of de novo deleterious mutations in genes associated with glutamatergic systems in nonsyndromic intellectual disability. American Journal of Human Genetics 88, 306–316.

Hayashi, M.K., Tang, C., Verpelli, C., Narayanan, R., Stearns, M.H., Xu, R.M., et al., 2009. The postsynaptic density proteins Homer and Shank form a polymeric network structure. Cell 137, 159–171.

Hung, A.Y., Futai, K., Sala, C., Valtschanoff, J.G., Ryu, J., Woodworth, M.A., et al., 2008. Smaller dendritic spines, weaker synaptic transmission, but enhanced spatial learning in mice lacking Shank1. Journal of Neuroscience 28, 1697–1708.

Hwang, J.I., Kim, H.S., Lee, J.R., Kim, E., Ryu, S.H., Suh, P.G., 2005. The interaction of phospholipase C-β3 with Shank2 regulates mGluR-mediated calcium signal. Journal of Biological Chemistry 280, 12,467–12,473.

Ikeda, F., Deribe, Y.L., Skanland, S.S., Stieglitz, B., Grabbe, C., Franz-Wachtel, M., et al., 2011. SHARPIN forms a linear ubiquitin ligase complex regulating NF-kappaB activity and apoptosis. Nature 471, 637–641.

Im, Y.J., Lee, J.H., Park, S.H., Park, S.J., Rho, S.H., Kang, G.B., et al., 2003. Crystal structure of the Shank PDZ-ligand complex reveals a class I PDZ interaction and a novel PDZ-PDZ dimerization. Journal of Biological Chemistry 278, 48,099–48,104.

Kornau, H.C., Schenker, L.T., Kennedy, M.B., Seeburg, P.H., 1995. Domain interaction between NMDA receptor subunits and the postsynaptic density protein PSD-95. Science 269, 1737–1740.

Kreienkamp, H.J., 2008. Scaffolding proteins at the postsynaptic density: Shank as the architectural framework. Handbook of Experimental Pharmacology, 365–380.

Leblond, C.S., Heinrich, J., Delorme, R., Proepper, C., Betancur, C., Huguet, G., et al., 2012. Genetic and functional analyses of SHANK2 mutations suggest a multiple hit model of autism spectrum disorders. PLoS Genetics 8, e1002521.

Leng, Y., Zhang, J., Badour, K., Arpaia, E., Freeman, S., Cheung, P., et al., 2005. Abelson-interactor-1 promotes WAVE2 membrane translocation and Abelson-mediated tyrosine phosphorylation required for WAVE2 activation. Proceedings of the National Academy of Sciences of the United States of America 102, 1098–1103.

Lim, S., Naisbitt, S., Yoon, J., Hwang, J.I., Suh, P.G., Sheng, M., et al., 1999. Characterization of the Shank family of synaptic proteins: Multiple genes, alternative splicing, and differential expression in brain and development. Journal of Biological Chemistry 274, 29,510–29,518.

Lim, S., Sala, C., Yoon, J., Park, S., Kuroda, S., Sheng, M., et al., 2001. Sharpin, a novel postsynaptic density protein that directly interacts with the shank family of proteins. Molecular and Cellular Neurosciences 17, 385–397.

Luciani, J.J., de Mas, P., Depetris, D., Mignon-Ravix, C., Bottani, A., Prieur, M., et al., 2003. Telomeric 22q13 deletions resulting from rings, simple deletions, and translocations: Cytogenetic, molecular, and clinical analyses of 32 new observations. Journal of Medical Genetics 40, 690–696.

Marshall, C.R., Noor, A., Vincent, J.B., Lionel, A.C., Feuk, L., Skaug, J., et al., 2008. Structural variation of chromosomes in autism spectrum disorder. American Journal of Human Genetics 82, 477–488.

Maunakea, A.K., Nagarajan, R.P., Bilenky, M., Ballinger, T.J., D'Souza, C., Fouse, S.D., et al., 2010. Conserved role of intragenic DNA methylation in regulating alternative promoters. Nature 466, 253–257.

McWilliams, R.R., Gidey, E., Fouassier, L., Weed, S.A., Doctor, R.B., 2004. Characterization of an ankyrin repeat-containing Shank2 isoform (Shank2E) in liver epithelial cells. Biochemistry Journal 380, 181–191.

Meffert, M.K., Chang, J.M., Wiltgen, B.J., Fanselow, M.S., Baltimore, D., 2003. NF-kappa B functions in synaptic signaling and behavior. Nature Neuroscience 6, 1072–1078.

Moessner, R., Marshall, C.R., Sutcliffe, J.S., Skaug, J., Pinto, D., Vincent, J., et al., 2007. Contribution of SHANK3 mutations to autism spectrum disorder. American Journal of Human Genetics 81, 1289–1297.

Naisbitt, S., Kim, E., Tu, J.C., Xiao, B., Sala, C., Valtschanoff, J., et al., 1999. Shank, a novel family of postsynaptic density proteins that binds to the NMDA receptor/PSD-95/GKAP complex and cortactin. Neuron 23, 569–582.

Peça, J., Feliciano, C., Ting, J.T., Wang, W., Wells, M.F., Venkatraman, T.N., et al., 2011. Shank3 mutant mice display autistic-like behaviors and striatal dysfunction. Nature 472, 437–442.

Phelan, M.C., 2008. Deletion 22q13.3 syndrome. Orphanet Journal of Rare Diseases 3, 14.

Phelan, M.C., Rogers, R.C., Saul, R.A., Stapleton, G.A., Sweet, K., McDermid, H., et al., 2001. 22q13 deletion syndrome. American Journal of Medical Genetics 101, 91–99.

Pinto, D., Pagnamenta, A.T., Klei, L., Anney, R., Merico, D., Regan, R., et al., 2010. Functional impact of global rare copy number variation in autism spectrum disorders. Nature 466, 368–372.

Prange, O., Wong, T.P., Gerrow, K., Wang, Y.T., El-Husseini, A., 2004. A balance between excitatory and inhibitory synapses is controlled by PSD-95 and neuroligin. Proceedings of the National Academy of Sciences of the United States of America 101, 13,915–13,920.

Qualmann, B., Boeckers, T.M., Jeromin, M., Gündelfinger, E.D., Kessels, M.M., 2004. Linkage of the actin cytoskeleton to the postsynaptic density via direct interactions of Abp1 with the ProSAP/Shank family. Journal of Neuroscience 24, 2481–2495.

Redecker, P., Gündelfinger, E.D., Boeckers, T.M., 2001. The cortactin-binding postsynaptic density protein proSAP1 in non-neuronal cells. Journal of Histochemistry and Cytochemistry 49, 639–648.

Romorini, S., Piccoli, G., Jiang, M., Grossano, P., Tonna, N., Passafaro, M., et al., 2004. A functional role of postsynaptic density-95-guanylate kinase-associated protein complex in regulating Shank assembly and stability at synapses. Journal of Neuroscience 24, 9391–9404.

Roussignol, G., Ango, F., Romorini, S., Tu, J.C., Sala, C., Worley, P.F., et al., 2005. Shank expression is sufficient to induce functional dendritic spine synapses in aspiny neurons. Journal of Neuroscience 25, 3560–3570.

Sakai, Y., Shaw, C.A., Dawson, B.C., Dugas, D.V., Al-Mohtaseb, Z., Hill, D.E., et al., 2011. Protein interactome reveals converging molecular pathways among autism disorders. Science Translational Medicine 3, 86ra49.

Sala, C., Futai, K., Yamamoto, K., Worley, P.F., Hayashi, Y., Sheng, M., 2003. Inhibition of dendritic spine morphogenesis and synaptic transmission by activity-inducible protein Homer1a. Journal of Neuroscience 23, 6327–6337.

Sala, C., Piech, V., Wilson, N.R., Passafaro, M., Liu, G., Sheng, M., 2001. Regulation of dendritic spine morphology and synaptic function by Shank and Homer. Neuron 31, 115–130.

Sala, C., Roussignol, G., Meldolesi, J., Fagni, L., 2005. Key role of the postsynaptic density scaffold proteins Shank and Homer in the functional architecture of Ca^{2+} homeostasis at dendritic spines in hippocampal neurons. Journal of Neuroscience 25, 4587–4592.

Sato, D., Marshall, C.R., Lionel, A.C., Prasad, A., Pinto, D., Howe, J.L., et al., 2011. Mutations in the SHANK1 synaptic scaffolding gene in autism spectrum disorder and intellectual disability. ICGH Meeting.

Schmeisser, M.J., Ey, E., Wegener, S., Bockmann, J., Stempel, A.V., Kuebler, A., et al., 2012. Autistic-like behaviors and hyperactivity in mice lacking ProSAP1/Shank2. Nature 486, 256–260.

Schütt, J., Falley, K., Richter, D., Kreienkamp, H.J., Kindler, S., 2009. Fragile X mental retardation protein regulates the levels of scaffold proteins and glutamate receptors in postsynaptic densities. Journal of Biological Chemistry 284, 25,479–25,487.

Sheng, M., Kim, E., 2000. The shank family of scaffold proteins. Journal of Cell Science 113, 1851–1856.

Silverman, J.L., Turner, S.M., Barkan, C.L., Tolu, S.S., Saxena, R., Hung, A.Y., et al., 2011. Sociability and motor functions in Shank1 mutant mice. Brain Research 1380, 120–137.

Soltau, M., Berhorster, K., Kindler, S., Buck, F., Richter, D., Kreienkamp, H.J., 2004. Insulin receptor substrate of 53 kDa links postsynaptic shank to PSD-95. Journal of Neurochemistry 90, 659–665.

Steward, O., Levy, W.B., 1982. Preferential localization of poly-ribosomes under the base of dendritic spines in granule cells of the dentate gyrus. Journal of Neuroscience 2, 284–291.

Steward, O., Schuman, E.M., 2001. Protein synthesis at synaptic sites on dendrites. Annual Review of Neuroscience 24, 299–325.

Stradal, T., Courtney, K.D., Rottner, K., Hahne, P., Small, J.V., Pendergast, A.M., 2001. The Abl interactor proteins localize to sites of actin polymerization at the tips of lamellipodia and filopodia. Current Biology 11, 891–895.

Sugiyama, Y., Kawabata, I., Sobue, K., Okabe, S., 2005. Determination of absolute protein numbers in single synapses by a GFP-based calibration technique. Nature Methods 2, 677–684.

Tao-Cheng, J.H., Dosemeci, A., Gallant, P.E., Smith, C., Reese, T., 2010. Activity induced changes in the distribution of Shanks at hippocampal synapses. Neuroscience 168, 11–17.

Tobaben, S., Sudhof, T.C., Stahl, B., 2000. The G protein-coupled receptor CL1 interacts directly with proteins of the shank family. Journal of Biological Chemistry 275, 36,204–36,210.

Tropea, D., Giacometti, E., et al., 2009. Partial reversal of Rett Syndrome-like symptoms in MeCP2 mutant mice. Proceedings of the National Academy of Sciences of the United States of America, 2029–2034.

Tu, J.C., Xiao, B., Naisbitt, S., Yuan, J.P., Petralia, R.S., Brakeman, P., et al., 1999. Coupling of mGluR/Homer and PSD-95 complexes by the Shank family of postsynaptic density proteins. Neuron 23, 583–592.

Uemura, T., Mori, H., Mishina, M., 2004. Direct interaction of GluR-delta2 with Shank scaffold proteins in cerebellar Purkinje cells. Molecular and Cellular Neuroscience 26, 330–341.

Valtschanoff, J.G., Weinberg, R.J., 2001. Laminar organization of the NMDA receptor complex within the postsynaptic density. Journal of Neuroscience 21, 1211–1217.

Verpelli, C., Dvoretskova, E., Vicidomini, C., Rossi, F., Chiappalone, M., Schoen, M., et al., 2011. Importance of Shank3 protein in regulating metabotropic glutamate receptor 5 (mGluR5) expression and signaling at synapses. Journal of Biological Chemistry 286, 34,839–34,850.

Wang, X., McCoy, P.A., Rodriguiz, R.M., Pan, Y., Je, H.S., Roberts, A.C., et al., 2011. Synaptic dysfunction and abnormal behaviors in mice lacking major isoforms of Shank3. Human Molecular Genetics 20, 3093–3108.

Wilson, H.L., Wong, A.C., Shaw, S.R., Tse, W.Y., Stapleton, G.A., Phelan, M.C., et al., 2003. Molecular characterisation of the 22q13 deletion syndrome supports the role of haploinsufficiency of SHANK3/PROSAP2 in the major neurological symptoms. Journal of Medical Genetics 40, 575–584.

Wöhr, M., Roullet, F.I., Hung, A.Y., Sheng, M., Crawley, J.N., 2011. Communication impairments in mice lacking Shank1: Reduced levels of ultrasonic vocalizations and scent marking behavior. PLoS ONE 6, e20631.

Won, H., Lee, H.R., Gee, H.Y., Mah, W., Kim, J.I., Lee, J., et al., 2012. Autistic-like social behavior in Shank2-mutant mice improved by restoring NMDA receptor function. Nature 486, 261–265.

Xiao, B., Tu, J.C., Petralia, R.S., Yuan, J.P., Doan, A., Breder, C.D., et al., 1998. Homer regulates the association of group 1 metabotropic glutamate receptors with multivalent complexes of Homer-related, synaptic proteins. Neuron 21, 707–716.

Yang, M., Bozdagi, O., Scattoni, M., Silverman, J., Buxbaum, J., Crawley, J., 2011. Evaluation of phenotypes relevant to autism and Phelan-McDermid Syndrome in Shank3 mutant mice. Autism Spectrum Disorders, Cell Symposia.

Yao, I., Hata, Y., Hirao, K., Deguchi, M., Ide, N., Takeuchi, M., et al., 1999. Synamon, a novel neuronal protein interacting with synapse-associated protein 90/postsynaptic density-95-associated protein. Journal of Biological Chemistry 274, 27,463–27,466.

Zitzer, H., Hönck, H.H., Bächner, D., Richter, D., Kreienkamp, H.J., 1999. Somatostatin receptor interacting protein defines a novel family of multidomain proteins present in human and rodent brain. Journal of Biological Chemistry 274, 32,997–33,001.

Zitzer, H., Richter, D., Kreienkamp, H.J., 1999b. Agonist-dependent interaction of the rat somatostatin receptor subtype 2 with cortactin-binding protein 1. Journal of Biological Chemistry 274, 18,153–18,156.

PI3K Signaling and miRNA Regulation in Autism Spectrum Disorders

Showming Kwok, Nikolaos Mellios, Mriganka Sur

Simons Center for the Social Brain, Picower Institute for Learning and Memory, Department of Brain and Cognitive Sciences, Massachusetts Institute of Technology, Cambridge, MA, USA

INTRODUCTION

Autism spectrum disorders (ASD) are highly heterogeneous neurodevelopmental disorders characterized by varying degrees of cognitive impairment. The three core behavioral features observed in ASD are impaired social interaction, deficits in communication and language ability, and repetitive and restricted behavior (American Psychiatric Association, 2000). Accompanying these characteristic behaviors are comorbid conditions such as intellectual disability, epilepsy, anxiety, and gastrointestinal conditions (Matson et al., 2011; see also Section 1). The striking diversity of clinical manifestation and polygenic nature of ASD present major hurdles to the understanding of its etiology.

GENETIC INFLUENCES

Although factors such as environment, paternal age, and imprinting are thought to be important in ASD (Cantor et al., 2007; Hogart et al., 2007; Lawler et al., 2004; Persico and Bourgeron, 2006), ASD has a strong genetic component (see Section 2). The genetic contribution is evident in twin studies, which show concordance rates of 60–90% in monozygotic twins and 0–10% in dizygotic twins (Bailey et al., 1995; Folstein and Rutter, 1977; Steffenburg et al., 1989), though a recently reported high concordance rate for dizygotic twins (Hallmayer et al., 2011) points to additional shared environmental factors for ASD (Chapter 2.7). Many genes are involved in ASD, giving rise to its complex etiology (Chapters 2.1–2.4). Currently, there are several dozen genes and loci known to contribute to ASD and accounting for at most 30% of ASD cases, with more loci being discovered (Abrahams and Geschwind, 2008; Sakai et al., 2011; see also Chapters 2.1–2.4).

How can a multitude of genetic variants cause the disease specificity of ASD? Emerging views of the field indicate that:

1. Functions of the susceptible genes must converge onto a few common molecular pathways that subserve the observed ASD phenotypes;
2. The core features of ASD are the most difficult tasks that involve association of multiple areas, and therefore any mild global impairment has the greatest impact on these tasks while sparing the simpler ones; and/or
3. The expression patterns of the affected genes collectively affect specific brain regions that give rise to the normal functions which are disrupted in ASD.

Very few currently identified ASD genes, however, show regionally restricted expression patterns (such as CNTNAP2 enrichment in the anterior regions of the developing cerebral cortex) (Geschwind, 2008; Geschwind and Levitt, 2007; Sakai et al., 2011; Voineagu et al., 2011; Walsh et al., 2008). In the following sections, we will focus on one converging molecular signaling pathway in detail.

MONOGENIC DISORDERS IN ASD

Much of the insight into mechanisms underlying ASD comes from a subset of cases where the phenotype is secondary to a known genetic disorder, though these account for only a small fraction (about 10%) of all ASD patients (Hampson et al., 2012; see also Chapter 2.1). Four such monogenic disorders are fragile X syndrome (FXS), PTEN hamartoma tumor syndrome (PHTS), tuberous sclerosis (TSC), and Rett syndrome (RTT), which are caused by mutations in the *FMR1* (fragile X mental retardation 1), *PTEN* (phosphatase and tensin homolog), *TSC1/TSC2* (tuberous sclerosis protein 1/2), and *MECP2* (methyl-CpG-binding protein 2) genes respectively. FXS and RTT are discussed in detail in Chapters 4.5 and 4.6, but will be summarized here as well.

FXS is an inherited disorder of intellectual disability and is the leading monogenetic cause of ASD (Chapter 4.5). It is caused by an expansion of CGG repeats in the 5′ untranslated region (UTR) of the *FMR1* gene, leading to hypermethylation of the *FMR1* promoter, silencing of FMR1 transcription and, subsequently, deficit of its encoded product, fragile X mental retardation protein (FMRP) (Verkerk et al., 1991). The

metabotropic glutamate receptor (mGluR) theory of FXS suggests that in the absence of FMRP there is exaggerated mGluR-dependent protein synthesis, resulting in increased long-term depression (LTD) at synapses (Bear et al., 2004; Krueger and Bear, 2011). Deficiency of FMRP is also shown to result in excess activity of phosphoinositide 3-kinase (PI3K) and mammalian target of rapamycin (mTOR), a downstream effector of PI3K (Gross et al., 2010; Sharma et al., 2010). These findings provide a mechanistic link between hyperactivity of group 1 mGluR signaling and the abnormal synaptic phenotypes seen in *Fmr1* knockout (KO) mice.

PHTS categorizes a collection of autosomal dominant syndromes, including Cowden syndrome, Lhermitte–Duclos disease, and Proteus and Proteus-like syndromes, characterized by multiple hamartomas, neurological deficits, developmental disorders, and higher risk of cancer (Salmena et al., 2008). *PTEN* mutations are frequently identified in human cancers and have been found in a subset of patients with ASD and extreme macrocephaly (Butler et al., 2005; Herman et al., 2007). *Pten* haploinsufficient mice are macrocephalic and are impaired in social approach behavior (Page et al., 2009). PTEN mutation-mediated PI3K/Akt pathway activation in subsets of mouse cerebral cortical and hippocampal neurons leads to abnormal neuronal features and behavioral changes (Kwon et al., 2006).

TSC is an autosomal dominant genetic disorder caused by heterozygous mutations in the *TSC1* or *TSC2* gene (van Slegtenhorst et al., 1997). Approximately half of TSC patients have intellectual disabilities and other neurological phenotypes such as seizures and ASD behaviors. Additionally, TSC is associated with cerebral cortical tubers in the majority of patients (Joinson et al., 2003; Prather and de Vries, 2004). The *TSC1* gene product, hamartin, binds to tuberin, the product of the *TSC2* gene, and the formation of this heterodimer inactivates small GTP-binding protein Ras homolog enriched in brain (RHEB), which activates mTOR downstream (Ehninger and Silva, 2011; Rosner et al., 2008). Dysregulation of the mTOR pathway as a result of loss of function of the *TSC1* or *TSC2* gene is central to the pathogenesis of TSC.

RTT is a postnatal developmental disorder that affects girls (Chahrour and Zoghbi, 2007; see also Chapter 4.6). Individuals initially appear developmentally normal, followed by the onset of growth deceleration and regression of developed skills. Most girls suffer from stereotypic hand movements, intellectual and learning disability, ASD behaviors, seizure, breathing abnormalities, and loss of motor coordination. More than 95% of RTT cases are caused by mutations in the *MECP2* gene, a global transcriptional regulator that affects the expression of many genes (Amir et al., 1999; Chahrour et al., 2008; Nan et al., 1997). The best-known target of

MeCP2, brain-derived neurotrophic factor (BDNF), is decreased in the $Mecp2^{-/Y}$ mouse model of RTT (Chang et al., 2006; Chen et al., 2003; Martinowich et al., 2003). Over expression of BDNF *in vivo* rescues specific RTT phenotypes in mutant mice (Chang et al., 2006). Systemic administration of a tripeptide form of insulin-like growth factor 1 (IGF-1) restores a range of structural, functional, and behavioral phenotypes in *Mecp2* mutant mice (Tropea et al., 2009), as does administration of recombinant human IGF-1 to the mutant mice (Castro et al., 2011). Consistent with the mouse findings, a recent report found synaptic and calcium signaling defects in neurons developed from RTT patient fibroblasts by using induced pluripotent stem cell (iPSC) technology (Marchetto et al., 2010), and showed that IGF-1 is able to reverse part of the synaptic phenotypes. Both the growth factors BDNF and IGF-1 signal via PI3K/Akt/mTOR and mitogen-activated protein kinase (MAPK) pathways to promote neuronal cell survival and maturation of developing cortical plasticity (Carvalho et al., 2008; Dijkhuizen and Ghosh, 2005; Herman et al., 2007; Joseph D'Ercole and Ye, 2008; Tropea et al., 2006; Yoshii and Constantine-Paton, 2007; Zheng and Quirion, 2004). Direct evidence of the involvement of Akt in RTT comes from a mouse study demonstrating that phosphorylation of rpS6 is reduced in *Mecp2* mutant mice. This hypoactivity of rpS6 is specific to signaling via Akt and not Erk1/2 kinases (Ricciardi et al., 2011).

COMMON MOLECULAR PATHWAY: PI3K/Akt/mTOR PATHWAY

One emerging pathway common to all four syndromic ASD disorders is thus the PI3K/Akt/mTOR pathway (Figure 4.8.1). This pathway has been extensively studied in cancer and diabetes and has been found to be important for an array of cellular functions such as survival, growth, metabolism, cell cycle, and protein synthesis (Guertin and Sabatini, 2007; Manning, 2004; Wullschleger et al., 2006; Zoncu et al., 2011). The PI3K pathway can be activated by multiple extracellular signals whose effects are transduced via receptors on the cell membrane (Figure 4.8.1). Of particular interest, the major categories of surface receptors include receptor tyrosine kinases (RTKs), which are activated by growth factors (e.g., BDNF and IGF-1), and G-protein coupled receptors (GPCRs) such as metabotropic glutamate receptors. The latter are activated by neurotransmitters, including glutamate and dopamine (Hoeffer and Klann, 2010). The ionotropic N-methyl-D-aspartate (NMDA) receptor, which is critical for synaptic plasticity and learning, is also reported to activate this pathway and

its downstream mTOR-dependent translation (Gong et al., 2006).

Upon RTK activation, insulin receptor substrate (IRS) is recruited to RTK and activated via phosphorylation at multiple sites. IRS mediates activation of PI3K at the plasma membrane, which converts phosphatidylinositol-4,5-biphosphate ($PI(4,5)P_2$) to phosphatidylinositol-3,4,5-triphosphate ($PI(3,4,5)P_3$). $PI(3,4,5)P_3$ is a lipid second messenger that activates Akt (also known as PKB) by membrane recruitment and subsequent phosphorylation by phosphoinositide-dependent kinase 1 (PDK1) and mTOR complex 2 (mTORC2) (Guertin and Sabatini, 2007). This activation of Akt is antagonized by PTEN, a lipid phosphatase whose dysfunction is found in ASD, by converting $PI(3,4,5)P_3$ back to $PI(4,5)P_2$ (Di Cristofano and Pandolfi, 2000; Stambolic et al., 1998). Akt is also negatively regulated by tumor suppressor protein phosphatase 2A (PP2A), a ubiquitous serine/threonine protein phosphatase known to dephosphorylate Akt at Thr308 site (Resjo et al., 2002; Switzer et al., 2009; Zhang and Claret, 2012). Of the many downstream molecules inhibited by active Akt, such as the forkhead box O (FOXO) family of transcription factors, glycogen synthase kinase 3 (GSK3), and pro-apoptotic Bcl-2-associated death promoter (BAD) protein, the TSC1/TSC2 heterodimer is the critical link to the regulation of mTOR activity (Manning and Cantley, 2007). Akt phosphorylates and inactivates tuberin/TSC2, a GTPase-activating protein encoded by the *TSC2* gene (Dan et al., 2002; Manning et al., 2002). Tuberin/TSC2 and hamartin/TSC1 are stabilized by forming a heterodimer that protects them from ubiquitination-dependent degradation (Benvenuto et al., 2000). This heterodimer inactivates small G-protein RHEB, which in turn activates mTORC1 downstream (Ehninger and Silva, 2011; Rosner et al., 2008). Therefore, Akt releases the inhibition of TSC1/TSC2 complex on mTORC1.

mTOR kinase nucleates two distinct multiprotein complexes, mTOR complex 1 (mTORC1) and mTOR complex 2 (mTORC2), which control many cellular processes (Guertin and Sabatini, 2007; Zoncu et al., 2011). mTORC1 is rapamycin- and nutrient-sensitive (Kim et al., 2002). It is activated by GTP-loaded RHEB and by Akt via disinhibition of PRAS40, a component in mTORC1 (Haar et al., 2007; Sancak et al., 2007). Downstream effectors of mTORC1 that regulate mRNA translation are S6 kinase 1 (S6K1) and eIF4E-binding protein 1 (4E-BP1) (Wullschleger et al., 2006). S6K1 activation by mTORC1 and PDK1 leads to phosphorylation of 40S ribosomal protein S6, which in turn upregulates translation of target mRNA. Phosphorylation of 4E-BP1 by mTORC1 releases its inhibition on the elongation initiation factor 4E (eIF4E). eIF4E binds to other partners including eIF4B, which is activated by S6K1 and eIF4A (Hoeffer and Klann, 2010). This complex increases protein

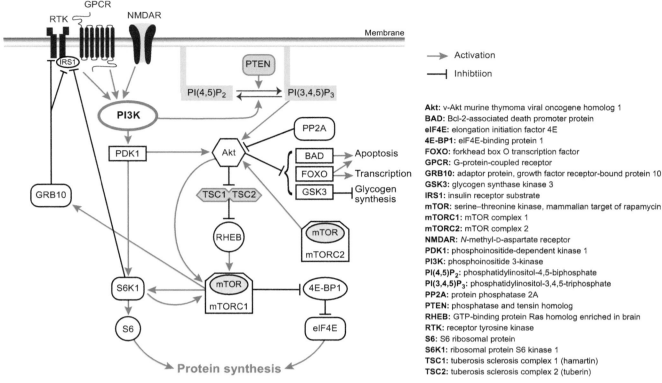

FIGURE 4.8.1 The PI3K signaling pathway. Schematic diagram illustrating the major components of the PI3K signaling pathway, their interactions, and downstream cellular functions. Signaling molecules that are involved in ASD are highlighted in green.

synthesis by affecting translation initiation and elongation. Relative to mTORC1, mTORC2 is less understood. It is a rapamycin-insensitive complex that directly phosphorylates (at Ser473) and activates Akt, amongst other proteins (Zoncu et al., 2011). Recent evidence points to the involvement of TSC1/TSC2 complex in mTORC2 activation (Huang and Manning, 2009). Therefore, mTOR signaling is both upstream (mTORC2) and downstream (mTORC1) of Akt.

In addition to the antagonizing effects of PTEN and PP2A on PI3K signaling, it is worth highlighting the negative feedback loops of PI3K/Akt/mTOR (Figure 4.8.1). Upstream of PI3K, mTORC1-mediated activation of S6K1 phosphorylates (at Ser302) and inhibits IRS1 by preventing its association with the RTK (Harrington et al., 2004; Zick, 2005). Without IRS1 transducing the signal to PI3K, PI3K no longer turns on its downstream effectors. A recent report has also identified an adaptor protein, growth factor receptor-bound protein 10 (GRB10), as the mTORC1 substrate that inhibits and destabilizes IRS1 (Hsu et al., 2011). Together with PTEN and PP2A, these two negative self-regulatory switches maintain the delicate balance of this critical pathway.

In summary, the PI3K/Akt/mTOR pathway is an extensive regulatory network that contains multiple

signal integration nodes whose activities are tightly regulated by extracellular and intracellular signals. Its regulation by small non-coding RNAs will be discussed in the second half of this chapter. We limit the scope of our discussion to protein synthesis, given its critical role in plasticity, memory, and disease (Hoeffer and Klann, 2010). With an understanding of this pathway and its signal integration nature, we now revisit the question of how the diverse genetic variations converge on a number of ASD-specific features by looking at the ultimate site of action: the synapse.

SYNAPTIC DYSFUNCTION IN ASD – EFFECTS OF PI3K/Akt/mTOR SIGNALING

Several lines of evidence point to synapses as the substrates of pathogenesis in ASD (Kelleher and Bear, 2008; Penzes et al., 2011; Persico and Bourgeron, 2006; Walsh et al., 2008; Zoghbi, 2003). Direct evidence comes from the postmortem cortices of ASD subjects, which show increased spine density in various cortical regions (Hutsler and Zhang, 2010). TSC, FXS, and RTT all have defects in spine morphology and/or spine density.

Local protein translation in dendrites is required for synaptic plasticity, and disruption of this process is seen in ASD (Hoeffer and Klann, 2010; Kelleher and Bear, 2008). Both MECP2 and FMRP1 can directly or indirectly (via BDNF) regulate this process. The PI3K/Akt/mTOR pathway is known to control cell size and dendritic growth and arborization through protein synthesis (Jaworski et al., 2005). This local protein translation via PI3K signaling is, at least in part, regulated by glutamate receptor-dependent mechanisms (Gong et al., 2006). Given the critical roles of these glutamate receptors in synaptic plasticity and dendritic protein translation, ASD mutations that affect these receptor functions are instrumental in offering insight into synaptic dysfunction and ASD. A recent study of the protein interactome of ASD revealed high connectivity between the postsynaptic organizer SHANK and TSC1, implying SHANK's potential role in influencing TSC1/TSC2/mTOR signaling (Sakai et al., 2011; see also Chapter 4.7). Together, these examples reinforce the idea that synaptic dysregulation can underlie ASD etiology (although there are additional organelles and systems that can be involved, see Chapter 2.1).

BIOGENESIS AND FUNCTION OF BRAIN-EXPRESSED microRNAs

Although the interplay between protein-coding genes and ASD has been extensively investigated (including the elucidation of their role in regulating the PI3K/Akt/mTOR pathway as discussed above), non-coding RNAs are emerging as potential novel molecular players that could be of relevance for brain function and disease (Qureshi and Mehler, 2011). One specific category of non-coding RNA that has been shown to regulate brain development and maturation, and to be of relevance to neuropsychiatric disorders such as ASD, is that of the evolutionarily conserved small non-coding RNAs known as microRNAs, or miRNAs (Coolen and Bally-Cuif, 2009; Forero et al., 2010). Although miRNAs were initially identified as peculiar molecules that inhibited the expression of worm RNAs by interacting with them in a sequence-specific manner (Lee et al., 1993; Wightman et al., 1993), they were gradually shown to be highly abundant in plants and animals, and to participate in various physiological processes.

Despite their tiny size (approximately 20 nts), miRNAs are initially transcribed either alone or as part of multicistronic miRNA transcripts from intergenic or intronic chromosomal regions in the form of long primary RNA precursor molecules, known as pri-miRNAs (Bartel, 2004; Krol et al., 2010). Pri-miRNAs are cleaved inside the nucleus by the combined action of Drosha and Dgcr8, in order to generate the approximately 70 nts in length hairpin structure miRNA precursors called pre-miRNAs, which in turn are transported

into the cytoplasm and further cleaved by the RNAse III enzyme Dicer (Bartel, 2004; Krol et al., 2010). The cytoplasmic cleavage of pre-miRNAs generates double stranded miRNA duplexes, which, after unwinding, liberate the functionally mature miRNAs. The mature miRNA molecules are then incorporated into the RNA-induced silencing complex (RISC), which scans mRNAs for areas of complementarity to the mature miRNA sequence – particularly the first 2–7 nts of the miRNA, also known as the 'seed sequence' (Bartel, 2004; Krol et al., 2010). Once a proper degree of complementarity is detected between the mRNA target and the miRNA seed sequence, translational inhibition and subsequent mRNA decay can occur, with the exact mechanism of action being still a matter of debate (Pillai et al., 2007).

In the mammalian nervous system, miRNAs are abundantly expressed and have been shown to modulate various aspects of brain development, maturation, and plasticity (Coolen and Bally-Cuif, 2009; Forero et al., 2010), processes that are perturbed in ASD. In most cases, one miRNA can affect only a single brain process during a given developmental time-window. However, there are examples in which the same miRNA exerts different effects during early or late development by regulating multiple target genes, which in some cases are expressed in a cell-specific manner. For example, brain enriched miR-124 can regulate neuronal differentiation by promoting the neuronal identity of mouse neuronal progenitors and neural stem cells (Cheng et al., 2009; Makeyev et al., 2007), block serotonin-induced plasticity in mature neurons in the sea slug *Aplysia* (Rajasethupathy et al., 2009), and at the same time regulate microglial activation in mice (Ponomarev et al., 2011).

ACTIVITY-DEPENDENT microRNAs REGULATE BRAIN PLASTICITY

Activity-dependent gene expression is considered to be necessary for brain function and plasticity. A number of activity-dependent protein-coding genes have been linked to ASD. However, little is known about the role of activity-dependent non-coding RNAs in brain plasticity, or their potential significance in ASD pathophysiology or pathogenesis. To cast some light on this, recent studies have revealed a subset of activity-dependent miRNAs that regulate both structural and functional plasticity, such as miR-132, miR-212, and miR-134 (Gao et al., 2010; Hollander et al., 2010; Mellios et al., 2011; Tognini and Pizzorusso, 2012).

In the case of miR-132 and miR-212, two co-transcribed miRNAs with highly similar sequences, initial studies in rat and mouse neuronal cultures suggested that they respond to neuronal activation through the cyclic AMP (cAMP) response element-binding protein (CREB) signaling pathway and are over-expressed following treatment with BDNF (Remenyi et al., 2010; Vo et al., 2005; Wayman et al., 2008). Furthermore, experiments in rat neuronal cultures and slices suggest that miR-132 promotes dendritic spine maturation, by targeting the spine inhibitor GTPase p250GAP (Impey et al., 2010; Wayman et al., 2008). In addition, miR-132 also stimulates dendritic branching and synaptic integration of newborn neurons in the mouse hippocampus (Luikart et al., 2011; Magill et al., 2010), providing another example in which miRNA function is time- and cell-dependent. On a similar note, miR-212 was found to be over-expressed in rat striatum following cocaine administration, and virus-mediated manipulation of miR-212 expression *in vivo* affected cocaine-induced seeking behavior (Hollander et al., 2010). A similar role for experience-dependent cortical plasticity was uncovered for miR-132, which was shown to be induced by visual experience and to be reduced in mouse visual cortex after visual deprivation (Mellios et al., 2011; Tognini and Pizzorusso, 2012). Interestingly, both over-expression and inhibition of *in vivo* miR-132 function altered dendritic spine maturation and abrogated ocular dominance plasticity (Mellios et al., 2011; Tognini and Pizzorusso, 2012). In the case of miR-132 inhibition, the observed structural deficits were reminiscent of delayed cortical maturation, with the upregulation of miR-132 target p250GAP expression being the proposed mechanism (Mellios et al., 2011). Conversely, over-expression of miR-132 led to increased spine maturation (Tognini and Pizzorusso, 2012), suggesting that balanced levels of this experience-dependent miRNA are required for visual cortex maturation and plasticity. Not surprisingly, the experience-dependent nature of miR-132 has been uncovered in several mouse brain areas other than the visual cortex (Nudelman et al., 2010), thus adding value to the hypothesis that miR-132 could be an important, widespread regulator of experience-dependent plasticity.

Activity-dependent expression of miR-134 has also been demonstrated through the recruitment of transcription factor Mef2 (Fiore et al., 2009). Increased miR-134 levels then inhibit the expression of the translational repressor Pumilio2, and promote neurite morphogenesis in rat hippocampal cultures (Fiore et al., 2009). However, the actions of miR-134 on dendritic maturation are also developmental stage-dependent, since miR-134 can inhibit dendritic spine growth in rat hippocampal neurons through its inhibitory effect on Limk1 (Schratt et al., 2006). On a similar note, miR-134 can also affect the differentiation of mouse cortical progenitors, as well as the migration of immature neurons, by regulating chordin-like 1 (Chrdl-1) and the microtubule-associated protein, doublecortin (Dcx) (Gaughwin

et al., 2011). Furthermore, an interesting link between miR-134 and plasticity and memory was recently uncovered, through the finding that miR-134 is downstream of the mammalian homologue of histone deacetylase Sir2, sirtuin 1 (SIRT1), and inhibits expression of CREB (directly) and BDNF (indirectly) in the mouse hippocampus (Gao et al., 2010). Moreover, the deficits of Sirt1 knockdown on brain plasticity and memory can be rescued following *in vivo* knockdown of miR-134 in the hippocampus (Gao et al., 2010).

POTENTIAL REGULATION OF THE PI3K/Akt/mTOR PATHWAY BY ASD-ALTERED microRNAs

A few studies using brain samples or lymphoblastoid cell cultures derived from subjects diagnosed with ASD have provided the first glimpse of which miRNAs might be dysregulated in autism (Abu-Elneel et al., 2008; Sarachana et al., 2010; Seno et al., 2011; Talebizadeh et al., 2008). Among them is a subset of miRNAs with known links to the PI3K/Akt/mTOR pathway, either directly, such as miR-21, miR-486, and miR-7, or through their interplay with BDNF, such as mir-132/212, and miR-381 (Abu-Elneel et al., 2008; Sarachana et al., 2010; Seno et al., 2011; Talebizadeh et al., 2008). For example, a large number of studies have validated the ASD-related gene *PTEN* as a target of miR-21 (Iliopoulos et al., 2010; Liu et al., 2011), a miRNA that was initially discovered for its oncogenic properties, and is highly expressed in the normal brain. Notably, levels of miR-21 are dysregulated in ASD (Abu-Elneel et al., 2008), as are levels of miR-486 (Seno et al., 2011), another miRNA proven to target *PTEN* expression (Downs et al., 2010). As described above, deficits in PTEN are expected to result in increased activation of Akt, which in turn is known to further upregulate miR-21 levels (Sayed et al., 2010), but also to directly increase miR-21 precursor processing (Aldinger et al., 2011), thus creating a 'toxic' regulatory loop. Furthermore, ASD-altered miRNA miR-7 (Abu-Elneel et al., 2008) is found to target both mTOR and PI3K catalytic subunit delta (PIK3CD), thus negatively regulating PI3K/Akt/mTOR signaling activity (Fang et al., 2012; Kefas et al., 2008). However, further studies are needed to elucidate the exact role of miR-21- and miR-486-mediated regulation of PTEN expression for ASD pathophysiology.

miR-381 and miR-132/212 interact more directly with BDNF, with mouse miR-381 being shown to target BDNF expression (Wu et al., 2011), and rat and mouse miR-132/212 shown to be induced following BDNF treatment (Kawashima et al., 2010; Numakawa et al., 2011; Remenyi et al., 2010). The fact that miR-212 also increases CREB activation and that miR-132 and miR-

212 both target ASD-related gene *Mecp2*, both of which then activate BNDF transcription in rodents (Hollander et al., 2010; Klein et al., 2007), suggests the existence of a complex regulatory loop, with potential implications for ASD. Interestingly, miR-132 changes in ASD samples were reported in three related studies (Abu-Elneel et al., 2008; Sarachana et al., 2010; Talebizadeh et al., 2008); its expression is induced by endotoxins and cytomegalovirus (CMV) (Taganov et al., 2006; Wang et al., 2008), both of which are linked to ASD (Onore et al., 2011; Stubbs et al., 1984). On a similar note, a recent study showed that miR-132 is well positioned to regulate mouse brain–immune system interaction through its effect on acetylcholinesterase (AChE) (Shaked et al., 2009). The intricate interactions between miR-132 and neuroimmune function position miR-132 as an attractive candidate for ASD pathogenesis, especially given the known links between miR-132 and brain plasticity described above, as well as its consistent dysregulation reported in ASD studies.

Although the above studies on miR-132 function and targeting were conducted in rodent models, miR-132 mature miRNA sequence is 100% conserved within mammalian species, a characteristic shared by other brain-expressed miRNAs (Bartel, 2004; Krol et al., 2010). In addition, a high degree of evolutionary conservation has been suggested for the mRNA target sequences of miRNAs (Bartel, 2004; Krol et al., 2010), which allows any mechanistic knowledge obtained in other species to be applied to humans. Therefore, the use of animal models for studying the role of miRNAs in ASD-related brain processes such us neuronal maturation and synaptic plasticity shows great promise for uncovering novel miRNA-mediated mechanisms behind ASD pathogenesis.

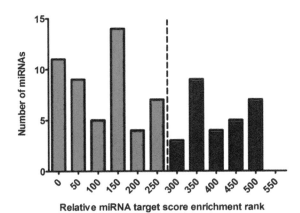

FIGURE 4.8.2 Number of ASD-altered miRNAs plotted against their degree of enrichment for targeting autism related genes. Figure showing the distribution of the ranks of ASD-altered miRNAs based on the number of predicted targets among autism-related genes as calculated by DIANA-mirExTra *in silico* tool. The median miRNA target score enrichment rank is noted with a dotted line, and ranks higher and lower than the median are shown in red and blue, respectively. Lower values denote higher enrichment for ASD gene targets. Notice that ASD-altered miRNAs display enrichment for autism gene targets (the distribution is skewed towards lower values, and deviates substantially from random).

ENRICHMENT OF AUTISM-RELATED GENES AS TARGETS OF ASD DYSREGULATED microRNAs

Aside from the alterations in specific miRNAs linked to certain ASD-related pathways, such as PI3K/Akt/mTOR, one unanswered question remains: are the reported dysregulated miRNAs simply an epiphenomenon of the disease without a major impact on its pathophysiology, or are they capable of modulating a significant number of genes related to ASD? To begin to answer this question, we used *in silico* analysis using the DIANA-mirExTra *in silico* tool (Alexiou et al., 2010) to demonstrate whether ASD-related genes are enriched as predicted targets of the reported ASD-altered miRNAs. The results of this analysis (Figure 4.8.2), which involved ranking miRNAs based on a calculated score that depends on the number of predictive genes reported in SFARI autism gene database (Banerjee-Basu

and Packer, 2010), showed that ASD-altered miRNAs are enriched in target genes linked to the disorder, since they were more likely to be among the top-ranked miRNAs. These findings suggest that the reported changes in miRNA expression in ASD could potentially influence a plethora of autism-related genes, which positions them as promising molecules for understanding the complex ASD pathophysiology. Future studies are needed to further elucidate the role of miRNAs in ASD.

microRNAs CONTROLLING THE PI3K/Akt/mTOR PATHWAY ARE ALTERED IN RETT SYNDROME

The potential role of miRNAs in the regulation of the PI3K/Akt/mTOR pathway can also be extrapolated from studies in RTT. As described above, RTT is one of the most prevalent syndromic forms of ASD and results from disruption of epigenetic modifier *MECP2*. In this case, two miRNAs from the same family, miR-221 and miR-222, have been shown to be reduced in the cerebellum of *Mecp2* KO mice (Wu et al., 2011) and in neural stem cells derived from such mice (Szulwach et al., 2010). These miRNAs are known to target *PTEN* (Garofalo et al., 2009). Their downregulation is, therefore, expected to result in increased PTEN levels and reduced PI3K/Akt/mTOR signaling. Adding to this miRNA-mediated inhibition of PI3K/Akt/mTOR signaling is the simultaneous increase of miR-199a-3p, which inhibits mTOR directly, and Akt activation indirectly by inhibiting MET (Fornari et al., 2010). Lastly, BDNF-targeting miRNAs miR-30a,d, miR-381, and miR-495 are known to be upregulated in *Mecp2* KO brain (Wu et al., 2011) and are expected to result in an indirect reduction in PI3K/Akt/mTOR signaling, by targeting BDNF (Mellios et al., 2008; Wu et al., 2011).

CONCLUSION

Protein-coding genes and non-coding RNAs that influence the PI3K/AKT/mTOR pathway hold much promise for revealing the mechanisms of ASD. In addition, this pathway could be significant for identifying biomarkers for ASD as well as drug targets and potential therapeutics for at least specific subsets of ASD (Bartholomeusz and Gonzalez-Angulo, 2012). The heterogeneity of ASD genotype and phenotype suggests that mechanisms and therapeutics for different subsets of ASD would likely involve multiple signals and approaches. This also highlights the need for personalized medicine, which requires cellular materials derived from ASD patients for revealing mechanisms and for drug screening, for example, through iPSC technology. Given the emerging role of miRNAs in ASD, further work is needed to determine whether the orchestrated action of a subset of ASD-altered miRNAs is adequate to result in a deleterious silencing of components of the PI3K/Akt/mTOR pathway. Last but not least, it would be intriguing to test whether molecules that are known to influence the pathway and be effective in specific subsets of ASD, such as BDNF and IGF-1 in Rett syndrome, can also be effective in other ASD that involve downregulation of PI3K/Akt/mTOR signaling.

References

Abrahams, B.S., Geschwind, D.H., 2008. Advances in autism genetics: On the threshold of a new neurobiology. Nature Review Genetics 9, 341–355.

Abu-Elneel, K., Liu, T., Gazzaniga, F.S., Nishimura, Y., Wall, D.P., Geschwind, D.H., et al., 2008. Heterogeneous dysregulation of microRNAs across the autism spectrum. Neurogenetics 9, 153–161.

Aldinger, K.A., Plummer, J.T., Qiu, S., Levitt, P., 2011. SnapShot: Genetics of autism. Neuron 72, 418–418, e411.

Alexiou, P., Maragkakis, M., Papadopoulos, G.L., Simmosis, V.A., Zhang, L., Hatzigeorgiou, A.G., 2010. The DIANA-mirExTra web server: From gene expression data to microRNA function. PLoS ONE 5, e9171.

American Psychiatric Association, 2000. DSM-IV-TR-2000: Diagnostic and Statistical Manual of Mental Disorders. American Psychiatric Association, Washington, DC.

Amir, R.E., Van den Veyver, I.B., Wan, M., Tran, C.Q., Francke, U., Zoghbi, H.Y., 1999. Rett syndrome is caused by mutations in X-linked MECP2, encoding methyl-CpG-binding protein 2. Nature Genetics 23, 185–188.

Bailey, A., Le Couteur, A., Gottesman, I., Bolton, P., Simonoff, E., Yuzda, E., et al., 1995. Autism as a strongly genetic disorder: Evidence from a British twin study. Psychological Medicine 25, 63–77.

Banerjee-Basu, S., Packer, A., 2010. SFARI Gene: An evolving database for the autism research community. Disease Models & Mechanisms 3, 133–135.

Bartel, D.P., 2004. MicroRNAs: Genomics, biogenesis, mechanism, and function. Cell 116, 281–297.

Bartholomeusz, C., Gonzalez-Angulo, A.M., 2012. Targeting the PI3K signaling pathway in cancer therapy. Expert Opinion on Therapeutic Targets 16, 121–130.

Bear, M.F., Huber, K.M., Warren, S.T., 2004. The mGluR theory of Fragile X mental retardation. Trends in Neurosciences 27, 370–377.

Benvenuto, G., Li, S., Brown, S.J., Braverman, R., Vass, W.C., Cheadle, J.P., et al., 2000. The tuberous sclerosis-1 (TSC1) gene product hamartin suppresses cell growth and augments the expression of the TSC2 product tuberin by inhibiting its ubiquitination. Oncogene 19, 6306–6316.

Butler, M.G., Dasouki, M.J., Zhou, X.P., Talebizadeh, Z., Brown, M., Takahashi, T.N., et al., 2005. Subset of individuals with autism spectrum disorders and extreme macrocephaly associated with germline PTEN tumor suppressor gene mutations. Journal of Medical Genetics 42, 318–321.

Cantor, R.M., Yoon, J.L., Furr, J., Lajonchere, C.M., 2007. Paternal age and autism are associated in a family-based sample. Molecular Psychiatry 12, 419–421.

Carvalho, A.L., Caldeira, M.V., Santos, S.D., Duarte, C.B., 2008. Role of the brain-derived neurotrophic factor at glutamatergic synapses. British Journal of Pharmacology 153, S310–S324.

Castro, J., Kwok, S., Garcia, R., Sur, M., 2011. Effects of Recombinant Human IGF1 Treatment in a Mouse Model of Rett Syndrome. Program No. 59.16/DD25. Neuroscience Meeting Planner. Society for Neuroscience, Washington DC.

Chahrour, M., Jung, S.Y., Shaw, C., Zhou, X., Wong, S.T., Qin, J., et al., 2008. MeCP2, a key contributor to neurological disease, activates and represses transcription. Science 320, 1224–1229.

Chahrour, M., Zoghbi, H.Y., 2007. The story of Rett Syndrome: From clinic to neurobiology. Neuron 56, 422.

Chang, Q., Khare, G., Dani, V., Nelson, S., Jaenisch, R., 2006. The disease progression of Mecp2 mutant mice is affected by the level of BDNF expression. Neuron 49, 341–348.

Chen, W.G., Chang, Q., Lin, Y., Meissner, A., West, A.E., Griffith, E.C., et al., 2003. Derepression of BDNF transcription involves calcium-dependent phosphorylation of MeCP2. Science 302, 885–889.

Cheng, L.C., Pastrana, E., Tavazoie, M., Doetsch, F., 2009. miR-124 regulates adult neurogenesis in the subventricular zone stem cell niche. Nature Neuroscience 12, 399–408.

Coolen, M., Bally-Cuif, L., 2009. MicroRNAs in brain development and physiology. Current Opinion in Neurobiology 19, 461–470.

Dan, H.C., Sun, M., Yang, L., Feldman, R.I., Sui, X.M., Ou, C.C., et al., 2002. Phosphatidylinositol 3-kinase/Akt pathway regulates tuberous sclerosis tumor suppressor complex by phosphorylation of tuberin. Journal of Biological Chemistry 277, 35,364–35,370.

Di Cristofano, A., Pandolfi, P.P., 2000. The multiple roles of PTEN in tumor suppression. Cell 100, 387–390.

Dijkhuizen, P.A., Ghosh, A., 2005. BDNF regulates primary dendrite formation in cortical neurons via the PI3-kinase and MAP kinase signaling pathways. Journal of Neurobiology 62, 278–288.

Downs, J., Bebbington, A.M.I., Jacoby, P., Williams, A.-M., Ghosh, S., Kaufmann, W.E., et al., 2010. Level of purposeful hand function as a marker of clinical severity in Rett syndrome. Developmental Medicine and Child Neurology 52, 817–823.

Ehninger, D., Silva, A.J., 2011. Rapamycin for treating sclerosis and autism spectrum disorders. Trends in Molecular Medicine 17, 78–87.

Fang, Y., Xue, J.-L., Shen, Q., Chen, J., Tian, L., 2012. miR-7 inhibits tumor growth and metastasis by targeting the PI3K/AKT pathway in hepatocellular carcinoma. Hepatology.

Fiore, R., Khudayberdiev, S., Christensen, M., Siegel, G., Flavell, S.W., Kim, T.K., et al., 2009. Mef2-mediated transcription of the miR379-410 cluster regulates activity-dependent dendritogenesis by fine-tuning Pumilio2 protein levels. EMBO Journal 28, 697–710.

Folstein, S., Rutter, M., 1977. Infantile autism: A genetic study of 21 twin pairs. Journal of Child Psychology and Psychiatry 18, 297–321.

Forero, D.A., van der Ven, K., Callaerts, P., Del-Favero, C., Harris, T., Bolton, P.F., 2010. miRNA genes and the brain: Implications for psychiatric disorders. Human Mutation 31, 1195–1204.

Fornari, F., Milazzo, M., Chieco, P., Negrini, M., Calin, G.A., Grazi, G.L., et al., 2010. MiR-199a-3p regulates mTOR and c-Met to influence the doxorubicin sensitivity of human hepatocarcinoma cells. Cancer Research 70, 5184–5193.

Gao, J., Wang, W.Y., Mao, Y.W., Graff, J., Guan, J.S., Pan, L., et al., 2010. A novel pathway regulates memory and plasticity via SIRT1 and miR-134. Nature 466, 1105–1109.

Garofalo, M., Di Leva, G., Romano, G., Nuovo, G., Suh, S.S., Ngankeu, A., et al., 2009. miR-221&222 regulate TRAIL resistance and enhance tumorigenicity through PTEN and TIMP3 downregulation. Cancer Cell 16, 498–509.

Gaughwin, P., Ciesla, M., Yang, H., Lim, B., Brundin, P., 2011. Stage-specific modulation of cortical neuronal development by Mmu-miR-134. Cerebral Cortex 21, 1857–1869.

Geschwind, D.H., 2008. Autism: Many genes, common pathways? Cell 135, 391–395.

Geschwind, D.H., Levitt, P., 2007. Autism spectrum disorders: Developmental disconnection syndromes. Current Opinion in Neurobiology 17, 103–111.

Gong, R., Park, C.S., Abbassi, N.R., Tang, S.-J., 2006. Roles of glutamate receptors and the mammalian target of rapamycin (mTOR) signaling pathway in activity-dependent dendritic protein synthesis in hippocampal neurons. Journal of Biological Chemistry 281, 18,802–18,815.

Gross, C., Nakamoto, M., Yao, X., Chan, C.B., Yim, S.Y., Ye, K., et al., 2010. Excess phosphoinositide 3-kinase subunit synthesis and activity as a novel therapeutic target in Fragile X syndrome. Journal of Neuroscience 30, 10,624–10,638.

Guertin, D.A., Sabatini, D.M., 2007. Defining the role of mTOR in cancer. Cancer Cell 12, 9–22.

Haar, E.V., Lee, S.-I., Bandhakavi, S., Griffin, T.J., Kim, D.-H., 2007. Insulin signaling to mTOR mediated by the Akt/PKB substrate PRAS40. Nature Cell Biology 9, 316–323.

Hallmayer, J., Cleveland, S., Torres, A., Phillips, J., Cohen, B., Torigoe, T., et al., 2011. Genetic heritability and shared environmental factors among twin pairs with autism. Archives of General Psychiatry 68, 1095–1102.

Hampson, D.R., Gholizadeh, S., Pacey, L.K.K., 2012. Pathways to drug development for autism spectrum disorders. Clinical Pharmacology and Therapeutics 91, 189–200.

Harrington, L.S., Findlay, G.M., Gray, A., Tolkacheva, T., Wigfield, S., Rebholz, H., et al., 2004. The TSC1-2 tumor suppressor controls insulin-PI3K signaling via regulation of IRS proteins. Journal of Cell Biology 166, 213–223.

Herman, G.E., Butter, E., Enrile, B., Pastore, M., Prior, T.W., Sommer, A., 2007. Increasing knowledge of PTEN germline mutations: Two additional patients with autism and macrocephaly. American Journal of Medical Genetics Part A 143, 589–593.

Hoeffer, C.A., Klann, E., 2010. mTOR signaling: At the crossroads of plasticity, memory and disease. Trends in Neurosciences 33, 67–75.

Hogart, A., Nagarajan, R.P., Patzel, K.A., Yasui, D.H., Lasalle, J.M., 2007. 15q11-13 GABAA receptor genes are normally biallelically expressed in brain yet are subject to epigenetic dysregulation in autism-spectrum disorders. Human Molecular Genetics 16, 691–703.

Hollander, J.A., Im, H.I., Amelio, A.L., Kocerha, J., Bali, P., Lu, Q., et al., 2010. Striatal microRNA controls cocaine intake through CREB signaling. Nature 466, 197–202.

Hsu, P.P., Kang, S.A., Rameseder, J., Zhang, Y., Ottina, K.A., Lim, D., et al., 2011. The mTOR-regulated phosphoproteome reveals a mechanism of mTORC1-mediated inhibition of growth factor signaling. Science 332, 1317–1322.

Huang, J., Manning, B.D., 2009. A complex interplay between Akt, TSC2 and the two mTOR complexes. Biochemical Society Transactions 37, 217–222.

Hutsler, J.J., Zhang, H., 2010. Increased dendritic spine densities on cortical projection neurons in autism spectrum disorders. Brain Research 1309, 83–94.

Iliopoulos, D., Jaeger, S.A., Hirsch, H.A., Bulyk, M.L., Struhl, K., 2010. STAT3 activation of miR-21 and miR-181b-1 via PTEN and CYLD are part of the epigenetic switch linking inflammation to cancer. Molecular Cell 39, 493–506.

Impey, S., Davare, M., Lasiek, A., Fortin, D., Ando, H., Varlamova, O., et al., 2010. An activity-induced microRNA controls dendritic spine formation by regulating Rac1-PAK signaling. Molecular and Cellular Neuroscience 43, 146–156.

Jaworski, J., Spangler, S., Seeburg, D.P., Hoogenraad, C.C., Sheng, M., 2005. Control of dendritic arborization by the phosphoinositide-3'-kinase-Akt-mammalian target of rapamycin pathway. Journal of Neuroscience 25, 11300–11312.

Joinson, C., O'Callaghan, F.J., Osborne, J.P., Martyn, C., Harris, T., Bolton, P.F., 2003. Learning disability and epilepsy in an epidemiological sample of individuals with tuberous sclerosis complex. Psychological Medicine 33, 335–344.

Joseph D'Ercole, A., Ye, P., 2008. Expanding the mind: Insulin-like growth factor I and brain development. Endocrinology 149, 5958–5962.

Kawashima, H., Numakawa, T., Kumamaru, E., Adachi, N., Mizuno, H., Ninomiya, M., et al., 2010. Glucocorticoid attenuates brain-derived neurotrophic factor-dependent upregulation of glutamate receptors via the suppression of microRNA-132 expression. Neuroscience 165, 1301–1311.

Kefas, B., Godlewski, J., Comeau, L., Li, Y., Abounader, R., Hawkinson, M., et al., 2008. microRNA-7 inhibits the epidermal growth factor receptor and the Akt pathway and is down-regulated in glioblastoma. Cancer Research 68, 3566–3572.

Kelleher, R.J., 3rd, Bear, M.F., 2008. The autistic neuron: Troubled translation? Cell 135, 401–406.

Kim, D.H., Sarbassov, D.D., Ali, S.M., King, J.E., Latek, R.R., Erdjument-Bromage, H., et al., 2002. mTOR interacts with raptor to form a nutrient-sensitive complex that signals to the cell growth machinery. Cell 110, 163–175.

Klein, M.E., Lioy, D.T., Ma, L., Impey, S., Mandel, G., Goodman, R.H., 2007. Homeostatic regulation of MeCP2 expression by a CREB-induced microRNA. Nature Neuroscience 10, 1513–1514.

Krol, J., Loedige, I., Filipowicz, W., 2010. The widespread regulation of microRNA biogenesis, function and decay. Nature Reviews Genetics 11, 597–610.

Krueger, D.D., Bear, M.F., 2011. Toward fulfilling the promise of molecular medicine in Fragile X syndrome. Annual Review of Medicine 62, 411–429.

Kwon, C.-H., et al., 2006. Pten regulates neuronal arborization and social interaction in mice. Neuron 50, 377–388.

Lawler, C.P., Croen, L.A., Grether, J.K., Van de Water, J., 2004. Identifying environmental contributions to autism: Provocative clues and false leads. Mental Retardation and Developmental Disabilities Research Review 10, 292–302.

Lee, R.C., Feinbaum, R.L., Ambros, V., 1993. The *C. elegans* heterochronic gene lin-4 encodes small RNAs with antisense complementarity to lin-14. Cell 75, 843–854.

Liu, L.Z., Li, C., Chen, Q., Jing, Y., Carpenter, R., Jiang, Y., et al., 2011. MiR-21 induced angiogenesis through AKT and ERK activation and HIF-1alpha expression. PLoS ONE 6, e19139.

Luikart, B.W., Bensen, A.L., Washburn, E.K., Perederiy, J.V., Su, K.G., Li, Y., et al., 2011. miR-132 mediates the integration of newborn neurons into the adult dentate gyrus. PLoS ONE 6, e19077.

Magill, S.T., Cambronne, X.A., Luikart, B.W., Lioy, D.T., Leighton, B.H., Westbrook, G.L., et al., 2010. microRNA–132 regulates dendritic growth and arborization of newborn neurons in the adult hippocampus. Proceedings of the National Academy of Sciences of the United States of America 107, 20,382–20,387.

Makeyev, E.V., Zhang, J., Carrasco, M.A., Maniatis, T., 2007. The MicroRNA miR–124 promotes neuronal differentiation by triggering brain-specific alternative pre-mRNA splicing. Molecular Cell 27, 435–448.

Manning, B.D., 2004. Balancing Akt with S6K: Implications for both metabolic diseases and tumorigenesis. Journal of Cell Biology 167, 399–403.

Manning, B.D., Cantley, L.C., 2007. AKT/PKB signaling: Navigating downstream. Cell 129, 1261–1274.

Manning, B.D., Tee, A.R., Logsdon, M.N., Blenis, J., Cantley, L.C., 2002. Identification of the tuberous sclerosis complex-2 tumor suppressor gene product tuberin as a target of the phosphoinositide 3-kinase/akt pathway. Molecular Cell 10, 151–162.

Marchetto, M.C., Carromeu, C., Acab, A., Yu, D., Yeo, G.W., Mu, Y., et al., 2010. A model for neural development and treatment of Rett syndrome using human induced pluripotent stem cells. Cell 143, 527–539.

Martinowich, K., Hattori, D., Wu, H., Fouse, S., He, F., Hu, Y., et al., 2003. DNA methylation-related chromatin remodeling in activity-dependent BDNF gene regulation. Science 302, 890–893.

Matson, M.L., Matson, J.L., Beighley, J.S., 2011. Comorbidity of physical and motor problems in children with autism. Research in Developmental Disabilities 32, 2304–2308.

Mellios, N., Huang, H.S., Grigorenko, A., Rogaev, E., Akbarian, S., 2008. A set of differentially expressed miRNAs, including miR-30a-5p, act as post-transcriptional inhibitors of BDNF in prefrontal cortex. Human Molecular Genetics 17, 3030–3042.

Mellios, N., Sugihara, H., Castro, J., Banerjee, A., Le, C., Kumar, A., et al., 2011. miR-132, an experience-dependent microRNA, is essential for visual cortex plasticity. Nature Neuroscience 14, 1240–1242.

Nan, X., Campoy, F.J., Bird, A., 1997. MeCP2 Is a transcriptional repressor with abundant binding sites in genomic chromatin. Cell 88, 471–481.

Nudelman, A.S., DiRocco, D.P., Lambert, T.J., Garelick, M.G., Le, J., Nathanson, N.M., et al., 2010. Neuronal activity rapidly induces transcription of the CREB-regulated microRNA-132, in vivo. Hippocampus 20, 492–498.

Numakawa, T., Yamamoto, N., Chiba, S., Richards, M., Ooshima, Y., Kishi, S., et al., 2011. Growth factors stimulate expression of neuronal and glial miR-132. Neuroscience Letters 505, 242–247.

Onore, C., Careaga, M., Ashwood, P., 2011. The role of immune dysfunction in the pathophysiology of autism. Brain, Behavior, and Immunity.

Page, D.T., Kuti, O.J., Sur, M., 2009. Computerized assessment of social approach behavior in mouse. Frontiers in Behavioral Neuroscience 3, 48.

Penzes, P., Cahill, M.E., Jones, K.A., VanLeeuwen, J.E., Woolfrey, K.M., 2011. Dendritic spine pathology in neuropsychiatric disorders. Nature Neuroscience 14, 285–293.

Persico, A.M., Bourgeron, T., 2006. Searching for ways out of the autism maze: Genetic, epigenetic and environmental clues. Trends in Neurosciences 29, 349–358.

Pillai, R.S., Bhattacharyya, S.N., Filipowicz, W., 2007. Repression of protein synthesis by miRNAs: How many mechanisms? Trends in Cell Biology 17, 118–126.

Ponomarev, E.D., Veremeyko, T., Barteneva, N., Krichevsky, A.M., Weiner, H.L., 2011. MicroRNA-124 promotes microglia quiescence and suppresses EAE by deactivating macrophages via the C/EBP-alpha-PU.1 pathway. Nature Medicine 17, 64–70.

Prather, P., de Vries, P.J., 2004. Behavioral and cognitive aspects of tuberous sclerosis complex. Journal of Child Neurology 19, 666–674.

Qureshi, I.A., Mehler, M.F., 2011. Non-coding RNA networks underlying cognitive disorders across the lifespan. Trends in Molecular Medicine 17, 337–346.

Rajasethupathy, P., Fiumara, F., Sheridan, R., Betel, D., Puthanveettil, S.V., Russo, J.J., et al., 2009. Characterization of small RNAs in *Aplysia* reveals a role for miR-124 in constraining synaptic plasticity through CREB. Neuron 63, 803–817.

Remenyi, J., Hunter, C.J., Cole, C., Ando, H., Impey, S., Monk, C.E., et al., 2010. Regulation of the miR-212/132 locus by MSK1 and CREB in response to neurotrophins. Biochemical Journal 428, 281–291.

Resjo, S., Goransson, O., Härndahl, L., Zolnierowicz, S., Manganiello, V., Degerman, E., 2002. Protein phosphatase 2A is the main phosphatase involved in the regulation of protein kinase B in rat adipocytes. Cell Signalling 14, 231–238.

Ricciardi, S., Boggio, E.M., Grosso, S., Lonetti, G., Forlani, G., Stefanelli, G., et al., 2011. Reduced AKT/mTOR signaling and protein synthesis dysregulation in a Rett syndrome animal model. Human Molecular Genetics 20, 1182–1196.

Rosner, M., Hanneder, M., Siegel, N., Valli, A., Fuchs, C., Hengstschlager, M., 2008. The mTOR pathway and its role in human genetic diseases. Mutation Research 659, 284–292.

Sakai, Y., Shaw, C.A., Dawson, B.C., Dugas, D.V., Al-Mohtaseb, Z., Hill, D.E., et al., 2011. Protein interactome reveals converging molecular pathways among autism disorders. Science Translational Medicine 3, 86ra49.

Salmena, L., Carracedo, A., Pandolfi, P.P., 2008. Tenets of PTEN tumor suppression. Cell 133, 403–414.

Sancak, Y., Thoreen, C.C., Peterson, T.R., Lindquist, R.A., Kang, S.A., Spooner, E., et al., 2007. PRAS40 is an insulin-regulated inhibitor of the mTORC1 protein kinase. Molecular Cell 25, 903–915.

Sarachana, T., Zhou, R., Chen, G., Manji, H.K., Hu, V.W., 2010. Investigation of post-transcriptional gene regulatory networks associated with autism spectrum disorders by microRNA expression profiling of lymphoblastoid cell lines. Genome Medicine 2, 23.

Sayed, D., He, M., Hong, C., Gao, S., Rane, S., Yang, Z., et al., 2010. MicroRNA-21 is a downstream effector of AKT that mediates its antiapoptotic effects via suppression of Fas ligand. Journal of Biological Chemistry 285, 20281–20290.

Schratt, G.M., Tuebing, F., Nigh, E.A., Kane, C.G., Sabatini, M.E., Kiebler, M., et al., 2006. A brain-specific microRNA regulates dendritic spine development. Nature 439, 283–289.

Seno, M.M., Hu, P., Gwadry, F.G., Pinto, D., Marshall, C.R., Casallo, G., et al., 2011. Gene and miRNA expression profiles in autism spectrum disorders. Brain Research 1380, 85–97.

Shaked, I., Meerson, A., Wolf, Y., Avni, R., Greenberg, D., Gilboa-Geffen, A., et al., 2009. MicroRNA-132 potentiates cholinergic anti-inflammatory signaling by targeting acetylcholinesterase. Immunity 31, 965–973.

Sharma, A., Hoeffer, C.A., Takayasu, Y., Miyawaki, T., McBride, S.M., Klann, E., et al., 2010. Dysregulation of mTOR signaling in Fragile X syndrome. Journal of Neuroscience 30, 694–702.

Stambolic, V., Suzuki, A., de la Pompa, J.L., Brothers, G.M., Mirtsos, C., Sasaki, T., et al., 1998. Negative regulation of PKB/Akt-dependent cell survival by the tumor suppressor PTEN. Cell 95, 29–39.

Steffenburg, S., Gillberg, C., Hellgren, L., Andersson, L., Gillberg, I.C., Jakobsson, G., et al., 1989. A twin study of autism in Denmark, Finland, Iceland, Norway and Sweden. Journal of Child Psychology and Psychiatry 30, 405–416.

Stubbs, E.G., Ash, E., Williams, C.P., 1984. Autism and congenital cytomegalovirus. Journal of Autism and Developmental Disorders 14, 183–189.

Switzer, C.H., Ridnour, L.A., Cheng, R.Y.S., Sparatore, A., Del Soldato, P., Moody, T.W., et al., 2009. Dithiolethione compounds inhibit Akt signaling in human breast and lung cancer cells by increasing PP2A activity. Oncogene 28, 3837–3846.

Szulwach, K.E., Li, X., Smrt, R.D., Li, Y., Luo, Y., Lin, L., et al., 2010. Cross talk between microRNA and epigenetic regulation in adult neurogenesis. Journal of Cell Biology 189, 127–141.

Taganov, K.D., Boldin, M.P., Chang, K.J., Baltimore, D., 2006. NF-kappaB-dependent induction of microRNA miR-146, an inhibitor targeted to signaling proteins of innate immune responses. Proceedings of the National Academy of Sciences of the United States of America 103, 12,481–12,486.

Talebizadeh, Z., Butler, M.G., Theodoro, M.F., 2008. Feasibility and relevance of examining lymphoblastoid cell lines to study role of microRNAs in autism. Autism Research 1, 240–250.

Tognini, P., Pizzorusso, T., 2012. MicroRNA212/132 family: Molecular transducer of neuronal function and plasticity. International Journal of Biochemistry & Cell Biology 44, 6–10.

Tropea, D., Giacometti, E., Wilson, N.R., Beard, C., McCurry, C., Fu, D.D., et al., 2009. Partial reversal of Rett Syndrome-like symptoms in MeCP2 mutant mice. Proceedings of the National Academy of Sciences of the United States of America 106, 2029–2034.

Tropea, D., Kreiman, G., Lyckman, A., Mukherjee, S., Yu, H., Horng, S., et al., 2006. Gene expression changes and molecular pathways mediating activity-dependent plasticity in visual cortex. Nature Neuroscience 9, 660–668.

van Slegtenhorst, M., de Hoogt, R., Hermans, C., Nellist, M., Janssen, B., Verhoef, S., et al., 1997. Identification of the tuberous sclerosis gene TSC1 on chromosome 9q34. Science 277, 805–808.

Verkerk, A.J., Pieretti, M., Sutcliffe, J.S., Fu, Y.H., Kuhl, D.P., Pizzuti, A., et al., 1991. Identification of a gene (FMR-1) containing a CGG repeat coincident with a breakpoint cluster region exhibiting length variation in Fragile X syndrome. Cell 65, 905–914.

Vo, N., et al., 2005. A cAMP-response element binding protein-induced microRNA regulates neuronal morphogenesis. Proceedings of the National Academy of Sciences of the United States of America 102, 16426–16431.

Voineagu, I., Wang, X., Johnston, P., Lowe, J.K., Tian, Y., Horvath, S., et al., 2011. Transcriptomic analysis of autistic brain reveals convergent molecular pathology. Nature 474, 380–384.

Walsh, C.A., Morrow, E.M., Rubenstein, J.L.R., 2008. Autism and Brain Development. Cell 135, 396–400.

Wang, F.Z., Weber, F., Croce, C., Liu, C.G., Liao, X., Pellett, P.E., 2008. Human cytomegalovirus infection alters the expression of cellular microRNA species that affect its replication. Journal of Virology 82, 9065–9074.

Wayman, G.A., Davare, M., Ando, H., Fortin, D., Varlamova, O., Cheng, H.Y., et al., 2008. An activity-regulated microRNA controls dendritic plasticity by down-regulating p250GAP. Proceedings of the National Academy of Sciences of the United States of America 105, 9093–9098.

Wightman, B., Ha, I., Ruvkun, G., 1993. Posttranscriptional regulation of the heterochronic gene lin-14 by lin-4 mediates temporal pattern formation in C. elegans. Cell 75, 855–862.

Wu, X.M., Shao, X.Q., Meng, X.X., Zhang, X.N., Zhu, L., Liu, S.X., et al., 2011. Genome-wide analysis of microRNA and mRNA expression signatures in hydroxycamptothecin-resistant gastric cancer cells. Acta Pharmacologica Sinica 32, 259–269.

Wullschleger, S., Loewith, R., Hall, M.N., 2006. TOR signaling in growth and metabolism. Cell 124, 471–484.

Yoshii, A., Constantine-Paton, M., 2007. BDNF induces transport of PSD-95 to dendrites through PI3K-AKT signaling after NMDA receptor activation. Nature Neuroscience 10, 702.

Zhang, Q., Claret, F.X., 2012. Phosphatases: The new brakes for cancer development? Enzyme Research 2012, 659649.

Zheng, W.-H., Quirion, R., 2004. Comparative signaling pathways of insulin-like growth factor-1 and brain-derived neurotrophic factor in hippocampal neurons and the role of the PI3 kinase pathway in cell survival. Journal of Neurochemistry 89, 844–852.

Zick, Y., 2005. Ser/Thr phosphorylation of IRS proteins: A molecular basis for insulin resistance. Science STKE: Signal Transduction Knowledge Environment 268, pe4.

Zoghbi, H.Y., 2003. Postnatal neurodevelopmental disorders: Meeting at the synapse? Science 302, 826–830.

Zoncu, R., Efeyan, A., Sabatini, D.M., 2011. mTOR: From growth signal integration to cancer, diabetes and ageing. Nature Reviews Molecular Cell Biology 12, 21–35.

Getting from 1,000 Genes to a Triad of Symptoms: The Emerging Role of Systems Biology in Autism Spectrum Disorders

Joseph D. Buxbaum

Seaver Autism Center for Research and Treatment, Departments of Psychiatry, Genetics and Genomics Sciences, and Neuroscience, The Friedman Brain Institute, Mount Sinai School of Medicine, New York

INTRODUCTION

Autism spectrum disorders (ASD) are amongst the most heritable psychiatric disorders known. Many dozens of genes and loci have been identified (see Chapters 2.1–2.4) and there is now good evidence that there are in the order of 500–1,000 ASD loci in the genome (Neale et al., 2012; Sanders et al., 2011). This generates a profound challenge in neuroscience: how to understand the mechanisms that relate an etiologically extremely heterogeneous disorder to its behavioral manifestation which, although associated with some heterogeneity, can still be reduced to core features involving deficits in social communication, deficits in language (minimally the social use of language), and the presence of repetitive behaviors or circumscribed interests.

There are several alternative approaches to this challenge. The first is to focus on a risk gene or locus and dissect the relationship of the risk variants to multiple levels of brain function, with the aim of developing an understanding of how a given risk factor for ASD manifests at these multiple levels. This might be called a bottom up approach. A second approach would be from the top down, focusing on the behaviors and using improved methods to dissect the pathways underlying these behaviors. A third approach, discussed here, would be to use the integrative methods of systems biology to identify pathways (when starting from the bottom up) or systems (when approaching this from a top-down perspective) that are adversely impacted in ASD in a recurrent manner. The systems biological approach has the key advantage of being able to make use of unbiased data to inform pathways and systems, and it can also identify high-value targets for therapeutics (Schadt et al., 2009). This latter point will be critical in multifactorial disorders such as ASD. It will simply not be possible to have a drug development pipeline for all the myriad of genes that contribute to ASD; systems biological approaches can identify driver genes that warrant the large investment in drug development.

In the current chapter we provide a brief summary of examples of recent systems-level analyses of common and rare genetic variation in ASD, and of genes that are differentially expressed in postmortem ASD brain samples. Where informative, we describe some of our own systems biological analyses on high-risk ASD genes and on differentially expressed ASD genes. Finally, we highlight some issues that will need to be resolved before systems biological approaches will be reliably useful in ASD research.

SYSTEMS-LEVEL ANALYSIS OF HIGH-RISK ASD GENES

As noted in Chapters 2.1–2.4, there is good evidence for a large number of genes of intermediate to high effect in ASD. Current estimates are around 500–1,000 ASD genes and loci (Neale et al., 2012; Sanders et al., 2011), of which over 100 have been identified so far (Betancur, 2011; Cooper et al., 2011; see also Chapters 2.1–2.4). Systems-level analyses of genes and loci providing high risk for ASD can help identify pathways that underlie an appreciable proportion of ASD risk and can also identify driver genes for such pathways. To do this, we used a list of 112 ASD genes, that when disrupted are high-risk ASD genes. We used a list from a prior study (Betancur, 2011) that had been further updated by the same author (found in Neale et al., 2012). We asked three questions with these genes. First, do they show increased connectivity, which would provide objective support for the existence of pathways that are enriched for ASD genes? Second, we asked whether these gene lists are associated with specific pathways, including Gene Ontology categories. Finally, in published studies, we asked what mouse and human phenotypes are known to be associated with these genes (Buxbaum et al., 2012; and brief summary below).

It should be evident that with a large number of ASD genes, apparent pathways/connectivity can arise by chance. To assess whether there was excess connectivity amongst ASD genes we made use of DAPPLE (Rossin et al., 2011), which looks for connectivity between genes using a large protein–protein interaction (PPI) network. We analyzed the network relating the high-risk ASD genes with four network statistics and all were significant based on permutation-based P values. The metrics were: the number of direct connections between ASD proteins (expected $= 16.6$; observed $= 41$; $P < 1 \times 10^{-3}$); the average ASD protein direct connectivity (or the direct binding degree) (expected $= 1.44$; observed $= 3.42$; $P < 1 \times 10^{-3}$); the average ASD protein indirect connectivity (or indirect binding degree) (expected $= 38.1$; observed $= 60.8$; $P < 1 \times 10^{-3}$); and the average common interactor binding degree (the average number of ASD proteins

that common interactors bind to) (expected $= 2.50$; observed $= 2.80$; $P = 5 \times 10^{-3}$). The simplest metric (the number of direct connections between ASD proteins) makes it clear that there are definite pathways in the gene set. Moreover, the significant results from the latter three metrics indicate that there are additional gene products that take part in these pathways, and that the gene products also cluster (i.e., the gene products are enriched for both edge and node metrics).

In terms of direct interactions between high-risk ASD genes, DAPPLE identified some of the direct interactions that have been discussed in prior reviews (Figure 4.9.1). The inclusion of indirect interactions identified many clusters of genes around key hub genes (Figure 4.9.2). The ASD genes that were associated with the most significant P values (when assessing the probability that by chance the seed protein would be as connected to other seed proteins as is observed) included 14 with a corrected P value < 0.005 (dark orange in Figure 4.9.2), and an additional 12 with a corrected $P < 0.05$ (light orange in Figure 4.9.2). In the first category were *AFF2*, *CACNA1C*, *CACNA1F*, *FOLR1*, *GNS*, *KRAS*, *L1CAM*, *MAP2K1*, *NF1*, *SHANK3*, *YWHAE*, *CDKL5*, *GRIN2B*, and *SHANK2*, while in the second category were *TSC2*, *BRAF*, *PTPN11*, *NLGN4X*, *SYNGAP1*, *NLGN3*, *OCRL*, *HRAS*, *PTEN*, *VPS1B*, *TSC1*, and *CASK*. These genes are more highly connected to other ASD genes and can be considered hub genes.

The two calcium channel genes and their subnetwork (Figure 4.9.2) might be worthy of more attention, given the evidence for the involvement of *CACNA1C* (as reflected in replicated common variant association studies) in schizophrenia (Ripke et al., 2011) and bipolar disorder (Sklar et al., 2008) and the evidence of a role for the associated single nucleotide polymorphisms (SNPs) in brain function including, for example, working memory (Zhang et al., 2012). There is also emerging evidence of a role for common variation in an additional calcium channel gene (*CACNB2*) in several psychiatric disorders, including ASD (Cross-Disorder Group of the Psychiatric GWAS Consortium, unpublished data).

It is interesting that there is a cluster of significantly connected ASD genes that includes not only *SHANK2* and *SHANK3* (see Chapter 4.7), but also *GNS* and *CDKL5* (Figure 4.9.2). *GNS* is mutated in very rare forms of the recessive Sanfillipo syndrome D, leading to a lysosomal storage disorder. In this group, it is connected to SHANK3 via ABL1. ABL1 binds CDK5L, which also binds MECP2. Mutation of the X-linked gene *CDK5L* causes a Rett syndrome-like disorder (see Chapters 2.1 and 4.6).

The RAS-RAF-MAP2K pathway does not get the same attention in ASD compared to, for example, the other arm of the PI3K signaling pathway, involving Akt, TSC1/TSC2, PTEN, and mTOR (see Chapter 4.8),

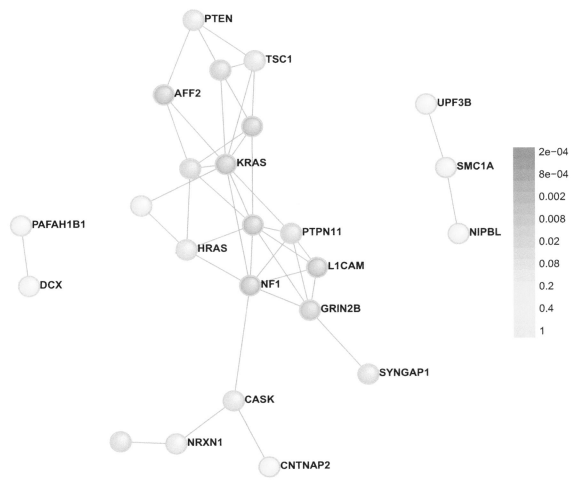

FIGURE 4.9.1 Direct interactions between high-risk ASD genes. High-risk ASD genes were taken from an updated list derived from Betancur, 2011. Direct physical interactions between high-risk ASD genes were determined using DAPPLE, which makes use of a large protein–protein interaction (PPI) network (for all figures, see text for more information). Parameters for DAPPLE were: number of permutations, 1000; and, common interactor binding degree cutoff, 2.

but RAS-RAF-MAP2K clearly includes significantly connected genes and a clear biological pathway with several of the genes already implicated in ASD (Figure 4.9.2, and see Chapter 2.1). It is also interesting that while FMR1 is not a significantly connected protein in this network (which, however, does not include protein–RNA interactions), AFF2/FMR2 is.

We next made use of ToppGene (Chen et al., 2009) to perform an enrichment analysis of high-risk ASD genes in Gene Ontology (GO) categories. Using a cutoff of Bonferroni corrected $P < 1 \times 10^{-5}$, there were significant findings in biological process categories, including those involved in nerve and nervous system development and function (the latter including synaptic transmission) as well as findings in cognition, learning or memory, social behavior, and behavioral interaction between organisms (Table 4.9.1). For cellular component categories, there were significant findings for cell and neuron projection, as well as dendrite, synapse, and axon part (Table 4.9.2).

While these are expected findings in these GO categories, it is important to note how many categories associated with nerve and nervous system development are implicated – highlighting the importance of a neurodevelopmental approach to understanding ASD pathogenesis.

Our analysis of behavioral features observed with disruption of these genes has been reported elsewhere (Buxbaum et al., 2012). Briefly, we observed four classes of neurobiological phenotypes associated with disruption of a large proportion of ASD genes, including:

1. Changes in brain and neuronal morphology;
2. Electrophysiological changes;
3. Neurological changes;
4. Higher-order behavioral changes.

Alterations in brain and neuronal morphology represent quantitative measures that can be more widely adopted in models of ASD to understand cellular and

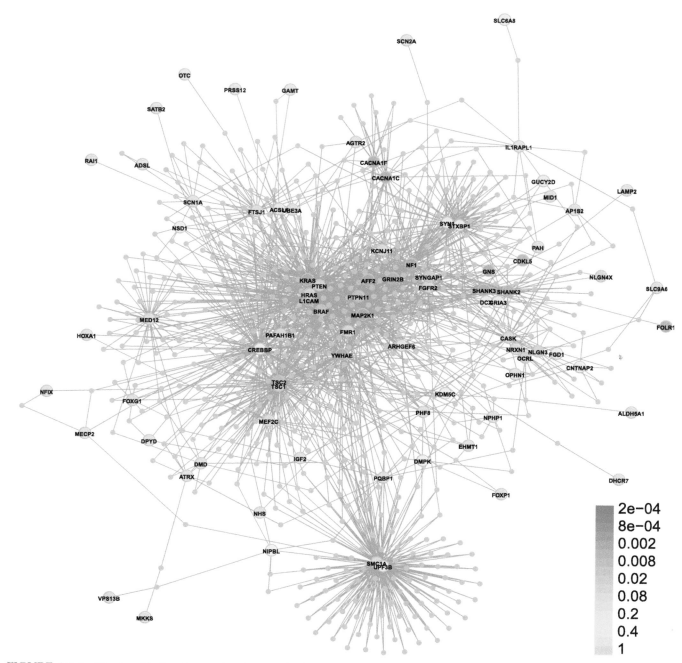

FIGURE 4.9.2 Direct and indirect interactions between high-risk ASD genes. High-risk ASD genes were taken from an updated list derived from Betancur, 2011. Direct and indirect physical interactions between high-risk ASD genes were determined using DAPPLE. Parameters are found in the legend to Figure 4.9.1.

network changes. The electrophysiological changes differed across different genes, indicating that the excitation/inhibition imbalance hypothesis for ASD needs to be considered very carefully. Finally, in analyses of both mouse and human databases, many of the behavioral alterations were neurological changes, encompassing sensory alterations, motor abnormalities, and seizures, as opposed to higher-order behavioral changes in learning and memory and social behavior paradigms.

The conclusions from that study that are particularly germane to the neurosciences are that mutations in high-risk ASD genes result in defined groups of phenotypes. This in turn supports a broad neurobiological approach to phenotyping rodent models for ASD, with a focus on biochemistry and molecular biology, brain and neuronal morphology electrophysiology, and both neurological and additional behavioral analyses.

TABLE 4.9.1   GO Biological Processes Categories Enriched for High-Risk ASD Genes

	ID	Name	P-value	Term in query	Term in genome
1	GO:0007399	Nervous system development	1.79×10^{-18}	47	1570
2	GO:0030030	Cell projection organization	3.72×10^{-14}	31	776
3	GO:0007417	Central nervous system development	1.06×10^{-13}	27	572
4	GO:0003008	System process	8.61×10^{-13}	45	1980
5	GO:0009653	Anatomical structure morphogenesis	1.27×10^{-12}	42	1730
6	GO:0050877	Neurological system process	1.55×10^{-12}	40	1568
7	GO:0007420	Brain development	6.97×10^{-12}	22	405
8	GO:0048666	Neuron development	2.59×10^{-11}	27	715
9	GO:0050890	Cognition	5.78×10^{-11}	15	155
10	GO:0048699	Generation of neurons	9.74×10^{-11}	30	960
11	GO:0007610	Behavior	1.98×10^{-10}	22	477
12	GO:0019226	Transmission of nerve impulse	2.02×10^{-10}	25	651
13	GO:0035637	Multicellular organismal signaling	2.02×10^{-10}	25	651
14	GO:0022008	Neurogenesis	4.26×10^{-10}	30	1016
15	GO:0030182	Neuron differentiation	7.79×10^{-10}	28	894
16	GO:0048468	Cell development	2.33×10^{-9}	32	1244
17	GO:0007154	Cell communication	3.12×10^{-9}	39	1877
18	GO:0031175	Neuron projection development	5.52×10^{-9}	23	625
19	GO:0048513	Organ development	1.77×10^{-8}	41	2184
20	GO:0048869	Cellular developmental process	3.17×10^{-8}	43	2432
21	GO:0048858	Cell projection morphogenesis	4.53×10^{-8}	21	564
22	GO:0032990	Cell part morphogenesis	5.52×10^{-8}	21	570
23	GO:0007268	Synaptic transmission	7.38×10^{-8}	21	579
24	GO:0007611	Learning or memory	1.49×10^{-7}	12	144
25	GO:0035176	Social behavior	1.67×10^{-7}	7	24
26	GO:0030154	Cell differentiation	2.86×10^{-7}	41	2384
27	GO:0007267	Cell−cell signaling	4.37×10^{-7}	26	1005
28	GO:0051705	Behavioral interaction between organisms	6.42×10^{-7}	8	46
29	GO:0000902	Cell morphogenesis	2.25×10^{-6}	21	698
30	GO:0010646	Regulation of cell communication	3.44×10^{-6}	26	1107
31	GO:0007632	Visual behavior	4.66×10^{-6}	7	37
32	GO:0048812	Neuron projection morphogenesis	5.03×10^{-6}	18	523
33	GO:0032989	Cellular component morphogenesis	6.21×10^{-6}	21	739
34	GO:0021987	Cerebral cortex development	6.72×10^{-6}	8	61
35	GO:0071842	Cellular component organization at cellular level	8.21×10^{-6}	39	2438
36	GO:0009790	Embryo development	9.06×10^{-6}	22	831

High-risk ASD genes were taken from an updated list derived from Betancur, 2011. ToppGene was used to create lists of GO terms enriched for high-risk ASD genes. Parameters for ToppGene were: correction, Bonferroni; P-value cutoff, 0.00001; gene limits, 1–2500.

TABLE 4.9.2   GO Cellular Component Categories Enriched for High-Risk ASD Genes

	ID	Name	P-value	Term in query	Term in genome
1	GO:0042995	Cell projection	3.405×10^{-12}	32	1074
2	GO:0044463	Cell projection part	6.298×10^{-10}	21	510
3	GO:0043005	Neuron projection	1.096×10^{-9}	22	586
4	GO:0005624	Membrane fraction	5.032×10^{-9}	28	1071
5	GO:0005626	Insoluble fraction	1.290×10^{-8}	28	1115
6	GO:0000267	Cell fraction	1.456×10^{-8}	32	1466
7	GO:0030425	Dendrite	1.152×10^{-7}	15	308
8	GO:0045202	Synapse	7.582×10^{-7}	17	473

High-risk ASD genes were taken from an updated list derived from Betancur, 2011. ToppGene was used to create lists of GO terms enriched for high-risk ASD genes. Parameters for ToppGene were: correction, Bonferroni; P-value cutoff, 0.00001; gene limits, 1–2500.

SYSTEMS-LEVEL ANALYSIS OF COPY NUMBER VARIANTS IN ASD

Copy number variants (CNV) have been associated with ASD in multiple large-scale studies that included extensive controls (Pinto et al., 2010; Sanders et al., 2011; see also Chapter 2.2). These studies included pathway analyses for gene sets that were enriched in cases over controls. Pinto and colleagues identified enrichment in pathways associated with cell and neuronal development (including proliferation, projection, and motility), GTPase/Ras signaling, and kinase activity and regulation. Sanders and coworkers observed 22 pathways significantly disrupted by CNV in cases, and only 4 pathways disrupted by CNV in unaffected siblings. One cautionary note was that the pathways disrupted in siblings included those involved in transmission of nerve impulses and neurogenesis, reminding us that central nervous system (CNS) genes are large and more likely to be disrupted by chance, and that caution must be exercised before deciding that a given finding is disease-related. In the individuals affected by ASD, the most highly associated gene sets/pathways included those associated with (from most significant down) cell adhesion, muscle contraction, regulation of cytoskeleton rearrangement, blood vessel morphogenesis, and cytoskeleton.

SYSTEMS-LEVEL ANALYSIS OF ASD-ASSOCIATED SINGLE NUCLEOTIDE POLYMORPHISMS

It is fair to say that there are no universally accepted, reliably replicated, common single nucleotide polymorphism (SNP) variants in ASD. However, there is some evidence that such variants exist, although they will require much larger sample sizes for identification and confirmation (Devlin et al., 2011; see also Chapter 2.3). If there are SNP variants associated with ASD, one can begin to ask whether SNPs that show lower P values in genome-wide association studies (GWAS) highlight certain pathways in ASD. These studies are underpowered at this point, but two filters have been used to increase the reliability of the conclusions. In one approach, a two-stage design is used, providing a confirmation dataset (e.g., Anney et al., 2011). One of the strongest findings from this two-stage study was enrichment for GO term GO:0031146 (SCF-dependent proteasomal ubiquitin-dependent protein catabolic process). This category includes only two genes (*FBXO31* and *FBXO6*), members of the F-box family of proteins, which are involved in a variety of pathways, including protein degradation, synapse formation, and circadian rhythm. *FBXO6* has been observed to show altered expression in lymphoblasts from patients with ASD (Nishimura et al., 2007). Other pathways showing replication included GO:0006090 (pyruvate metabolic process), GO:0042156 (zinc-mediated transcriptional activator activity), GO:0032872 (regulation of stress-activated MAPK cascade), and GO:0032874 (positive regulation of stress-activated MAPK cascade).

A second approach to validation is to compare genes implicated by both common variation (typically SNP) associations and by rare variants. A recent example used both replication of SNP findings and overlap with rare variants to show that two neuronal/synaptic modules were found to be significantly enriched for genes affected by both common and rare variants (Ben-David and Shifman, 2012). In this study, the modules were defined from expression data from the Allen Brain Bank. Such weighted gene coexpression network analysis (WGCNA) is becoming a common means of defining pathways and modules in an unbiased manner.

Unfortunately, the reliability of these modules is still less than ideal. For example, these authors showed that, when comparing the modules developed from the Allen Brain with another study (which used gene expression from microarray data from 160 brain samples) 10 out of 19 modules in the authors' study showed no corresponding module in the other dataset, 4 showed one corresponding module, and 5 showed two or three corresponding modules.

SYSTEMS-LEVEL ANALYSIS OF GENE EXPRESSION CHANGES IN ASD BRAIN SAMPLES

There are very few postmortem brain samples from subjects with ASD. Some of those that do exist suffer from concerns around factors such as diagnosis, agonal state, and tissue preservation. However, many important studies have been carried out using the available samples

TABLE 4.9.3 GO Categories Enriched for Genes Showing Reduced Expression in ASD Brain

GO: BIOLOGICAL PROCESS

	ID	Name	P-value	Term in query	Term in genome
1	GO:0007268	Synaptic transmission	5.21×10^{-5}	29	579
2	GO:0006836	Neurotransmitter transport	1.33×10^{-4}	14	147
3	GO:0019226	Transmission of nerve impulse	1.87×10^{-4}	30	651
4	GO:0035637	Multicellular organismal signaling	1.87×10^{-4}	30	651
5	GO:0007269	Neurotransmitter secretion	9.58×10^{-3}	10	104

GO: CELLULAR COMPONENT

	ID	Name	P-value	Term in query	Term in genome
1	GO:0030659	Cytoplasmic vesicle membrane	1.25×10^{-6}	20	263
2	GO:0045202	Synapse	1.28×10^{-6}	27	473
3	GO:0012506	Vesicle membrane	2.85×10^{-6}	20	276
4	GO:0044456	Synapse part	3.63×10^{-6}	22	338
5	GO:0012505	Endomembrane system	2.24×10^{-5}	52	1573
6	GO:0044433	Cytoplasmic vesicle part	2.58×10^{-5}	20	315
7	GO:0043005	Neuron projection	2.95×10^{-5}	28	586
8	GO:0030665	Clathrin-coated vesicle membrane	6.55×10^{-5}	11	95
9	GO:0030662	Coated vesicle membrane	1.59×10^{-4}	12	126
10	GO:0030136	Clathrin-coated vesicle	2.16×10^{-4}	14	180
11	GO:0030672	Synaptic vesicle membrane	2.95×10^{-4}	8	51
12	GO:0030135	Coated vesicle	4.10×10^{-4}	15	218
13	GO:0008021	Synaptic vesicle	2.01×10^{-3}	10	109
14	GO:0016023	Cytoplasmic membrane-bounded vesicle	3.76×10^{-3}	28	751
15	GO:0031090	Organelle membrane	4.98×10^{-3}	56	2088
16	GO:0031410	Cytoplasmic vesicle	5.44×10^{-3}	29	809
17	GO:0031988	Membrane-bounded vesicle	6.35×10^{-3}	28	773
18	GO:0060053	Neurofilament cytoskeleton	7.46×10^{-3}	4	12

Brain expression data were taken from Voineagu et al., 2011, and differentially expressed genes identified. ToppGene was used to create hierarchal lists of GO terms for differentially expressed ASD genes, focusing on those showing reduced expression. Parameters for ToppGene were: correction, Bonferroni; P-value cutoff, 0.01; gene limits, 1–2500.

TABLE 4.9.4   GO Categories Enriched for Genes Showing Increased Expression in ASD Brain

GO: BIOLOGICAL PROCESS

	ID	Name	P-value	Term in query	Term in genome
1	GO:0002376	Immune system process	1.53×10^{-4}	42	1450
2	GO:0043066	Negative regulation of apoptotic process	1.60×10^{-4}	23	517
3	GO:0043069	Negative regulation of programmed cell death	2.04×10^{-4}	23	524
4	GO:0042981	Regulation of apoptotic process	2.25×10^{-4}	36	1147
5	GO:0043067	Regulation of programmed cell death	2.91×10^{-4}	36	1159
6	GO:0060548	Negative regulation of cell death	3.74×10^{-4}	23	542
7	GO:0010941	Regulation of cell death	4.62×10^{-4}	36	1181
8	GO:0010033	Response to organic substance	7.68×10^{-4}	36	1206
9	GO:0002366	Leukocyte activation involved in immune response	9.84×10^{-4}	10	102
10	GO:0002263	Cell activation involved in immune response	9.84×10^{-4}	10	102
11	GO:0006915	Apoptotic process	1.26×10^{-3}	40	1453
12	GO:0001775	Cell activation	1.28×10^{-3}	26	720
13	GO:0008283	Cell proliferation	1.57×10^{-3}	39	1409
14	GO:0012501	Programmed cell death	1.62×10^{-3}	40	1467
15	GO:0007154	Cell communication	1.64×10^{-3}	47	1877
16	GO:0042127	Regulation of cell proliferation	2.03×10^{-3}	32	1041
17	GO:0042221	Response to chemical stimulus	2.44×10^{-3}	53	2273
18	GO:0002286	T cell activation involved in immune response	2.58×10^{-3}	6	29
19	GO:0048523	Negative regulation of cellular process	3.00×10^{-3}	55	2415
20	GO:0009607	Response to biotic stimulus	3.28×10^{-3}	22	568
21	GO:0007243	Intracellular protein kinase cascade	4.71×10^{-3}	25	723
22	GO:0023014	Signal transduction by phosphorylation	4.71×10^{-3}	25	723
23	GO:0045321	Leukocyte activation	5.91×10^{-3}	20	498
24	GO:0035556	Intracellular signal transduction	7.65×10^{-3}	41	1620

GO: CELLULAR COMPONENT

	ID	Name	P-value	Term in query	Term in genome
1	GO:0032587	ruffle membrane	8.42×10^{-3}	5	31

Brain expression data were taken from Voineagu et al., 2011, and differentially expressed genes identified. ToppGene was used to create hierarchal lists of GO terms for differentially expressed ASD genes, focusing on those showing increased expression. Parameters for ToppGene were: correction, Bonferroni; P-value cutoff, 0.01; gene limits, 1–2500.

(see Section 3). One recent study carried out detailed gene expression analyses in three brain regions (Voineagu et al., 2011). This study made use of WGCNA to integrate gene expression changes into pathways and modules. One finding was that there were differences in gene expression between two cortical regions (prefrontal cortex and superior temporal gyrus) observed in controls that were not observed in ASD. This suggests that typical regional differences are attenuated in ASD and that these genes highlight an abnormal developmental profile in ASD.

In a second analysis, the authors looked for modules that were correlated with disease status. The M12 module included genes generally under-expressed in ASD and genes involved in synaptic function, vesicular transport, and neuronal projection. This module included ASD genes such as *CNTNAP2* (Strauss et al., 2006; see also Chapter 2.1) and potential risk loci such as *SLC25A12* (Ramoz et al., 2004; see also Chapter 2.3). It includes a submodule that appears to capture parvalbumin-positive interneurons. The second module (M16), which was upregulated in ASD, included markers for astrocytes and for activated microglia, and for genes involved in immune and inflammatory processes (see Chapter 2.9). Importantly, the M12 module showed enrichment for association signals from GWAS data, but the M16 module did not. This suggests that the changes in gene expression around the neuronal genes in module M12 are more likely causal, while the changes in gene expression around glial, immune, and inflammatory markers are more likely reactive.

To help summarize these findings, we analyzed the data independently, to identify differential expression signatures, differentiating ASD and control samples. We then made use of ToppGene to perform an analysis of differentially expressed genes against Gene Ontology (GO) categories. We made use of all differentially expressed genes identified within the three brain regions profiled in Voineagu et al. (2011) and then combined the gene lists. However, similar findings were observed when just looking at the two cortical brain regions profiled by Voineagu's group. As shown in Table 4.9.3, genes with reduced expression in ASD include those involved in the biological process categories of synapse and synaptic and nerve impulse transmission, neurotransmitter transport and secretion, and signaling. Cellular component categories include many associated with synapse and synaptic vesicle components as well as with one category associated with the neurofilament cytoskeleton.

There was a very different pattern of categories for genes upregulated in ASD brains (Table 4.9.4). Upregulated genes included those involved in immune system processes, cell death, response to stress, xenobiotic stimuli, and cellular metabolism.

In a follow-up analysis, we also asked what phenotypes are associated with such genes in mouse models (Table 4.9.5). To do this we made use of ToppGene to survey the mouse phenotype databases. Mice with alterations in genes that showed reduced expression in ASD showed abnormalities in synaptic transmission, including excitatory transmission and elevated risk of

TABLE 4.9.5 Mouse Phenotypes Associated with Genes that Show Altered Expression in ASD Brain Samples

ID	Name	P-value	Term in query	Term in genome
UPREGULATED GENES				
MP:0003635	Abnormal synaptic Transmission	2.1×10^{-3}	26	466
MP:0002910	Abnormal excitatory postsynaptic currents	2.1×10^{-3}	11	85
MP:0002206	Abnormal CNS synaptic transmission	2.2×10^{-3}	23	397
MP:0003633	Abnormal nervous system physiology	3.6×10^{-3}	48	1384
MP:0002064	Seizures	7.9×10^{-3}	18	284
DOWNREGULATED GENES				
MP:0002451	Abnormal macrophage physiology	3.1×10^{-4}	22	306
MP:0002419	Abnormal innate immunity	6.9×10^{-4}	25	422

Brain expression data were taken from Voineagu et al., 2011, and differentially expressed genes identified. ToppGene was used to survey mouse phenotype databases. Parameters were FDR of 0.01.

seizures. In contrast, mice with alterations in genes that showed increased expression in ASD showed abnormal macrophage physiology, and abnormal innate immunity.

SYSTEMS-LEVEL ANALYSIS OF GENES IMPACTED BY *DE NOVO* SINGLE NUCLEOTIDE VARIATION IN ASD

Several studies have made use of massively parallel sequencing to identify genes with *de novo* single nucleotide variation (SNV) in ASD (see Chapter 2.4). While these 'next-generation' sequencing approaches are only now becoming widespread, systems-level analysis of the first several hundred samples already exists. In one study (Sanders et al., 2012), there was clear enrichment for *de novo* SNVs that impact brain-expressed genes in cases, as compared to unaffected siblings. In another study (Neale et al., 2012), the genes harboring *de novo* SNVs showed a higher degree of connectivity among themselves (using DAPPLE, see above for an explanation) and to prior ASD genes, using the PPI database as a background network.

CONCLUSIONS

Systems biology is just becoming possible in ASD as datasets with high-risk ASD genes, high-risk ASD CNV, SNP associations from GWAS, and gene expression profiles are being developed.

One real limitation of systems biological approaches is the availability of appropriate control and ASD data. For example, WGCNA has been carried out on various control brain samples and in one set of ASD brains. Even amongst the control samples, there have been only modest attempts to test whether the findings in each study agree and, as noted above, when this is examined in two such studies, the agreement is low. The situation is further complicated by questions of sample quality, and many ASD samples are quite compromised. It is easy to run a program on a dataset, but an understanding of all of the clinical and biological issues around the samples needs to precede this. In additions to questions around which brain region was sampled, tissue quality, agonal state, etc., there is the question of risk loci in case samples. For example, the Voineagu study included a sample with a known high-risk CNV. What happens when this sample is left out of the WGCNA?

These issues abound. One favorite approach to assess causality in datasets is to use SNP association data, frequently focusing on SNPs that appear to regulate the expression of adjacent mRNA (expression SNPs, or eSNPs). Here again, there are a number of papers on generating eSNPs from peripheral (e.g., blood) and brain samples. Only infrequent efforts have been made to see if different eSNP datasets agree, and this is something that would not be accepted in any other domain of human genetics. This leads to a situation where even amongst high-profile papers one can find studies in which eSNPs are being applied to brain networks, and neither the eSNPs nor the networks are validated in independent samples. This is a clear sign that the field needs to mature significantly before we can expect reliable results.

In ASD, it is fair to say that systems biological approaches will be absolutely required as a means of understanding how a very diverse set of genes can, when mutated, lead to a well-defined behavioral phenotype. As our understanding of convergent pathways increases, we will begin to understand more about brain development and the molecular basis for brain function and behavior. One important outcome from systems biological analyses is the ability to identify driver genes within pathways and networks. Driver genes can be used for validation of networks (for example by disrupting them in model systems) and also represent high-impact genes for drug development. In this way, systems biological approaches will also inform drug discovery efforts.

References

Anney, R.J., Kenny, E.M., O'Dushlaine, C., Yaspan, B.L., Parkhomenka, E., Buxbaum, J.D., et al., 2011. Gene-ontology enrichment analysis in two independent family-based samples highlights biologically plausible processes for autism spectrum disorders. European Journal of Human Genetics 19, 1082–1089.

Ben-David, E., Shifman, S., 2012. Networks of neuronal genes affected by common and rare variants in autism spectrum disorders. PLoS Genetics 8, e1002556.

Betancur, C., 2011. Etiological heterogeneity in autism spectrum disorders: more than 100 genetic and genomic disorders and still counting. Brain Research 1380, 42–77.

Buxbaum, J.D., Betancur, C., Bozdagi, O., Dorr, N.P., Elder, G.A., Hof, P.R., 2012. Optimizing the phenotyping of rodent ASD models: Enrichment analysis of mouse and human neurobiological phenotypes associated with high-risk autism genes identifies morphological, electrophysiological, neurological, and behavioral features. Molecular Autism 3, 1.

Chen, J., Bardes, E.E., Aronow, B.J., Jegga, A.G., 2009. ToppGene Suite for gene list enrichment analysis and candidate gene prioritization. Nucleic Acids Research 37, W305–W311.

Cooper, G.M., Coe, B.P., Girirajan, S., Rosenfeld, J.A., Vu, T.H., Baker, C., et al., 2011. A copy number variation morbidity map of developmental delay. Nature Genetics 43, 838–846.

Devlin, B., Melhem, N., Roeder, K., 2011. Do common variants play a role in risk for autism? Evidence and theoretical musings. Brain Research 1380, 78–84.

Neale, B.M., Kou, Y., Liu, L., Ma'ayan, A., Samocha, K.E., Sabo, A., et al., 2012. Patterns and rates of exonic *de novo* mutations in autism spectrum disorders. Nature 485, 242–245.

Nishimura, Y., Martin, C.L., Vazquez-Lopez, A., Spence, S.J., Alvarez-Retuerto, A.I., Sigman, M., et al., 2007. Genome-wide expression profiling of lymphoblastoid cell lines distinguishes different forms of autism and reveals shared pathways. Human Molecular Genetics 16, 1682–1698.

Pinto, D., Pagnamenta, A.T., Klei, L., Anney, R., Merico, D., Regan, R., et al., 2010. Functional impact of global rare copy number variation in autism spectrum disorders. Nature 466, 368–372.

Ramoz, N., Reichert, J.G., Smith, C.J., Silverman, J.M., Bespalova, I.N., Davis, K.L., et al., 2004. Linkage and association of the mitochondrial aspartate/glutamate carrier SLC25A12 gene with autism. American Journal of Psychiatry 161, 662–669.

Ripke, S., Sanders, A.R., Kendler, K.S., Levinson, D.F., Sklar, P., Holmans, P.A., et al., 2011. Genome-wide association study identifies five new schizophrenia loci. Nature Genetics 43, 969–976.

Rossin, E.J., Lage, K., Raychaudhuri, S., Xavier, R.J., Tatar, D., Benita, Y., et al., 2011. Proteins encoded in genomic regions associated with immune-mediated disease physically interact and suggest underlying biology. PLoS Genetics 7, e1001273.

Sanders, S.J., Ercan-Sencicek, A.G., Hus, V., Luo, R., Murtha, M.T., Moreno-De-Luca, D., et al., 2011. Multiple recurrent de novo CNVs, including duplications of the 7q11.23 Williams syndrome region, are strongly associated with autism. Neuron 70, 863–885.

Sanders, S.J., Murtha, M.T., Gupta, A.R., Murdoch, J.D., Raubeson, M.J., Willsey, J., et al., 2012. De novo point mutations, revealed by whole-exome sequencing, are strongly associated with autism spectrum disorders. Nature 485, 237–241.

Schadt, E.E., Zhang, B., Zhu, J., 2009. Advances in systems biology are enhancing our understanding of disease and moving us closer to novel disease treatments. Genetica 136, 259–269.

Sklar, P., Smoller, J.W., Fan, J., Ferreira, M.A., Perlis, R.H., Chambert, K., et al., 2008. Whole-genome association study of bipolar disorder. Molecular Psychiatry 13, 558–569.

Strauss, K.A., Puffenberger, E.G., Huentelman, M.J., Gottlieb, S., Dobrin, S.E., Parod, J.M., et al., 2006. Recessive symptomatic focal epilepsy and mutant contactin-associated protein-like 2. New England Journal of Medicine 354, 1370–1377.

Voineagu, I., Wang, X., Johnston, P., Lowe, J.K., Tian, Y., Horvath, S., et al., 2011. Transcriptomic analysis of autistic brain reveals convergent molecular pathology. Nature 474, 380–384.

Zhang, Q., Shen, Q., Xu, Z., Chen, M., Cheng, L., Zhai, J., et al., 2012. The effects of CACNA1C gene polymorphism on spatial working memory in both healthy controls and patients with schizophrenia or bipolar disorder. Neuropsychopharmacology 37, 677–684.

Index

Printed and bound by CPI Group (UK) Ltd, Croydon, CR0 4YY

08/05/2025

01865034-0005